The Royal Marsden Hospital
Manual of Clinical
Nursing Procedures

To Friends, Colleagues ~ Students
at Omayal Achi College
of Nursing with all
Good wishes

from.

Amanda L Lyone
Head of Nursing
Queen Margaret University
College, Edinburgh
19 July 2005

The Royal Marsden Hospital Manual of Clinical Nursing Procedures

Sixth Edition

Edited by

Lisa Dougherty
RN, RM, Onc Cert, MSc
Clinical Nurse Specialist
Intravenous Services
The Royal Marsden Hospital

and

Sara E. Lister
RN, PGDAE, BSc (Hons), MSc
Assistant Chief Nurse/Head of School
The Royal Marsden Hospital School of Cancer Nursing & Rehabilitation
The Royal Marsden Hospital

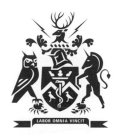

LABOR OMNIA VINCIT

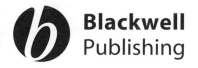

Blackwell
Publishing

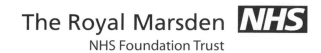

The Royal Marsden **NHS**
NHS Foundation Trust

© 1992, 1996, 2000, 2004 by The Royal Marsden Hospital

Editorial offices:
Blackwell Publishing Ltd, 9600 Garsington Road,
Oxford OX4 2DQ, UK
  Tel: +44 (0)1865 776868
Blackwell Publishing Inc., 350 Main Street,
Malden, MA 02148-5020, USA
  Tel: +1 781 388 8250
Blackwell Publishing Asia Pty Ltd, 550 Swanston Street,
Carlton, Victoria 3053, Australia
  Tel: +61 (0)3 8359 1011

The right of the Author to be identified as the Author of this Work has been asserted in
accordance with the Copyright, Designs and Patents Act 1988.

First edition published by Harper and Row Ltd 1984
Second edition published 1988
Reprinted by HarperCollins 1990
Third edition published by Blackwell Scientific Publications 1992
Fourth edition published by Blackwell Science 1996
Fifth edition published by Blackwell Science 2000
Sixth edition published by Blackwell Publishing Ltd 2004

Library of Congress Cataloging-in-Publication Data

The Royal Marsden Hospital manual of clinical nursing procedures/edited by
Sara Lister and Lisa Dougherty. –6th ed.
    p. cm.
  Includes bibliographical references and index.
  ISBN 1-4051-0161-X (Paperback : alk. paper)
  1. Nursing – Handbooks, manuals, etc. I. Lister, Sara. II. Dougherty, Lisa.
III. Royal Marsden Hospital (London, England)

  RT42.R68 2004
  610.73–dc22   2003023832

ISBN 1-4051-0161-X

A catalogue record for this title is available from the British Library

Set in 9.5/11 pt Minion by Gray Publishing, Tunbridge Wells
Printed and bound in Spain by Mateu Liber, Pinto, Madrid

The publisher's policy is to use permanent paper from mills that operate a sustainable forestry policy,
and which has been manufactured from pulp processed using acid-free and elementary chlorine-free
practices. Furthermore, the publisher ensures that the text paper and cover board used have met
acceptable environmental accreditation standards.

Products and services that are referred to in this book may be either trademarks and/or registered
trademarks of their respective owners. The publisher and authors make no claim to these trademarks.

For further information on Blackwell Publishing, visit our website:
www.blackwellpublishing.com

Every effort has been made in the writing of this book to present accurate and up-to-date information from the best and most reliable
sources. However, the results of caring for individuals depends upon a variety of factors not under the control of the authors or the
publishers of this book. Therefore, neither the authors nor the publishers assume responsibility for, nor make any warranty with
respect to, the outcomes achieved from the procedures described herein.

Contents

Quick reference to the guidelines

Contributors to sixth edition

Edited by

Lisa Dougherty, *RN, RM, Onc Cert, MSc*
Clinical Nurse Specialist – Intravenous Services,
The Royal Marsden Hospital

Sara Lister, *RN, PGDAE, BSc (Hons), MSc*
Assistant Chief Nurse/Head of School, The Royal Marsden
Hospital School of Cancer Nursing & Rehabilitation,
The Royal Marsden Hospital

Contributors

Karen Allen, *RN, ENB 998, BSc (Hons) Cancer Nursing*
Senior Staff Nurse – Smithers Ward   (CHAPTER 33)

Emma Allum, *RN, BN (Hons)*
Formerly Senior Staff Nurse –
Wiltshaw Ward   (CHAPTER 34)

Sarah Aylott, *RN, BSc (Hons) Cancer Nursing*
Formerly Practice Development Facilitator
                                        (CHAPTER 24)

Amanda Baxter, *RN, RMN, Onc Cert, BSc (Hons)*
Clinical Nurse Specialist – Pelvic Care
                        (CHAPTERS 12, 13, 14, 15, 16)

Rachel Bennett, *RN, ENB 998, 934, A11,*
BSc (Hons) Cancer Nursing
Formerly Ward Sister – Wilson Ward   (CHAPTER 25)

David Brighton, *RN, BSc (Hons) Cancer Nursing*
Professional Development
Facilitator (IT)   (CHAPTER 25)

Susannah Button, *RN, Cert Couns, Onc Cert, BSc (Hons)*
Cancer Nursing
Formerly Ward Sister – Ellis Ward   (CHAPTER 6)

Neve Carter, *RN Onc Cert,*
BSc (Hons) Nursing Studies
Senior Staff Nurse – Horder Ward and
Practice Development Facilitator   (CHAPTER 21)

Anne Chandler, *RN, Onc Cert, BSc (Hons) Nursing Studies,*
MSc Pain Management
Clinical Nurse Specialist in Pain Management
                                (CHAPTERS 27, 28, 29)

Belinda Crawford, *RN, BSc (Hons), Postgraduate*
Neurosciences Course (NZ)
Matron – Neurointensive Care,
Atkinson Morley Hospital   (CHAPTERS 26, 40)

Shelley Dolan, *RN, BA (Hons) English,*
MSc Cancer Care, ENB 100, Onc Cert
Nurse Consultant Cancer – Critical Care
                                (CHAPTERS 25, 36)

Lisa Dougherty, *RN, RM, Onc Cert, MSc*
Clinical Nurse Specialist – Intravenous Services
                        (CHAPTERS 10, 11, 38, 44)

Ann Duncan, *RN, Onc Cert,*
ENB 931, 901, 998
Ward Sister – Smithers Ward   (CHAPTER 33)

Stephen Evans, *BSc, MSc, MIPEM, MSRP*
Radiation Protection Adviser,
Physics Department   (CHAPTERS 34, 35)

Emma Foulds, *RN, ENB 264, 998, PGC (Management),*
PATHE, MA
Lecturer Practitioner, The Royal Marsden Hospital School
of Cancer Nursing & Rehabilitation
                                        (CHAPTER 30)

Tracey Gibson, *RN, ENB 100, 998, 237,*
Diploma in Nursing
Senior Staff Nurse – Critical Care Unit   (CHAPTER 7)

Aileen Grant, *RN, Onc Cert*
Staff Nurse – Children's Unit   (CHAPTER 35)

Jagdesh Grewal, *RN, ENB A13, 188, City & Guilds 7307, BA (Hons) Health Studies, PG Dip Nurse Education*
Senior Sister Theatres (CHAPTER 30)

Douglas Guerrero, *RN, DN, ENB 930, 998, Onc Cert, Counselling Cert, BSc (Hons), MSc Clinical Neurosciences*
Clinical Nurse Specialist – Neuro-oncology (CHAPTERS 26, 40)

Shujina Haq, *BSc (Hons), MBBS, DRCOG, DCH, MRCGP*
Specialist Registrar – Occupational
Health (CHAPTER 10)

Sarah Hart, *RN, FETC Oncology, HIV Infection Control Cert, MSc, BSc(Hons) Biological Science (Immunology), MSc Research and Development*
Clinical Nurse Specialist – Infection Control/Radiation
Protection (CHAPTERS 4, 5, 18, 34, 35)

Patricia Hunt, *RN, Palliative Care Cert, MSc Advanced Clinical Practice (Cancer Nursing)*
Clinical Nurse Specialist, Palliative Care/
Lecturer Practitioner, The Royal Marsden Hospital School
of Cancer Nursing & Rehabilitation (CHAPTER 43)

Lorraine Hyde, *RN, Onc Cert, ENB 998, 934, Diploma in Professional Nursing Studies, BSc (Hons) Nursing*
Senior Sister – Day Care Services (CHAPTER 10)

Betti Kirkman, *RM, RN, BSc*
Formerly Clinical Nurse Specialist – Breast
Diagnostic Unit (CHAPTER 6)

Diane Laverty, *RN, Onc Cert, BSc*
Clinical Nurse Specialist – Palliative Care (CHAPTERS 11, 27, 47)

Maria Law, *RN, Onc Cert*
Ward Sister – Kennaway Ward
(CHAPTER 3)

Susan J. Lee, *RN, MBA, MSc*
Formerly Occupational Health Manager
(CHAPTER 23)

Sally Legge, *RN, Onc Cert, MSc*
Clinical Nurse Specialist – GI Cancer
(CHAPTER 3)

Sara Lister, *RN, PGDAE, BSc (Hons), MSc*
Assistant Chief Nurse/Head of School
The Royal Marsden Hospital School of Cancer
Nursing & Rehabilitation (CHAPTERS 1, 9)

Philippa A. Lloyd, *RN, ENB 237, 998, BSc Nursing, BSc Cancer Nursing*
Senior Staff Nurse – Wiltshaw Ward (CHAPTER 15)

Jane Machin, *BA (Hons), DipCCS, Reg MCSLT, DALF*
Specialist Speech and Language Therapist
(CHAPTER 41)

Hazel Mack, *RN, ENB 931, BSc (Hons) Psychology, Post-grad Dip Onc, MSc Cancer Care*
Formerly Acting Ward Sister – Horder Ward
(CHAPTER 21)

Elizabeth MacKenzie, *RN, ENB 100, ENB 237, 998 Teaching and Assessing, BSc (Hons) Human Physiology*
Sister – Critical Care Unit (CHAPTERS 20, 37)

Jean Maguire, *RN, ENB 998, Diploma Palliative Care Nursing, BSc Hons Respiratory Nursing*
Ward Sister/Specialist Sister for Lung
Cancer (CHAPTERS 20, 33)

Chris McNamara, *RN, ENB 237, 937, N23, 998, BSc (Hons) Cancer Nursing, MSc*
Teaching Charge Nurse, The Royal Marsden
Hospital School of Cancer Nursing
& Rehabilitation (CHAPTER 25)

Lisa Mercer, *RD BSc MNutriDiet*
Senior Dietitian (CHAPTER 24)

Wayne Naylor, *RN, ENB 237, Dip Nurs, BSc (Hons) Cancer Nursing*
Clinical Nurse Specialist, Wellington Cancer Centre,
Wellington, New Zealand
Formerly Wound Management Research Nurse,
The Royal Marsden Hospital (CHAPTER 47)

Liz O'Brien, *RN, SEN, FETC, DPSN, BSc (Hons)Nursing, BSc (Hons)Specialist Practice District Nursing*
Clinical Team Leader, District Nursing,
Croydon Primary Care Trust (CHAPTER 8)

Emma Osenton, *RN, BSc (Hons) Cancer Nursing*
Ward Sister – Wiltshaw Ward (CHAPTER 16)

Evelyn Otunbade, *RN, BSc (Hons) Occupational Health and Safety*
Backcare Adviser (CHAPTER 23)

Buddy Joe Paris, *RN, BSc (Hons)*
Staff Nurse – Critical Care Unit (CHAPTER 41)

Gillian Parker, *RN, ENB 237, 980, 100, 998, Onc Health Studies Diploma, BSc*
Senior Staff Nurse – Burdett Coutts Ward (CHAPTER 16)

Rachelle Pearce, *RN, ENB 980, 998, BSc Cancer Nursing*
Formerly Sister – Medical Day Unit (CHAPTER 14)

Emma Pennery, *RN, ENB A11, 931,*
Counselling Cert, MSc
Formerly Senior Clinical Nurse Specialist/Honorary
Clinical Research Fellow   (CHAPTER 6)

Joanne Preece, *BSc (Hons), MIOSH, RSP, MBA*
Formerly Head of Risk Management   (CHAPTER 18)

Ffion M. Read, *RN, Onc Cert*
Senior Staff Nurse – Medical Day Unit   (CHAPTER 44)

Elizabeth Rees, *RN, Onc Cert, BSc (Hons) Cancer Nursing*
Formerly Research Nurse Palliative Care   (CHAPTER 1)

Francis Regan, *RN, BSc (Hons) Cancer Nursing*
Formerly Senior Staff Nurse – Burdett Coutts
Ward   (CHAPTER 13)

Jean Maurice Robert, *RN Dip HE*
Staff Nurse – Critical Care Unit   (CHAPTER 29)

Corinne Rowbotham, *RN*
Senior Staff Nurse – IV Services   (CHAPTER 44)

Patricia Ryan, *RN, BN (Bachelor of Nursing), Onc Cert*
Senior Sister – Haemato-oncology Unit   (CHAPTER 42)

Mave Salter *RN, NDN (Cert), Onc Cert, Cert Ed., Dip*
Couns, BSc (Hons) Nursing, MSc Research and Evaluation
Clinical Nurse Specialist – Community Liaison
                    (CHAPTER 8)

Neelam Sarpal, *RN, ENB 237, 998, 934, N23,*
BSc Cancer Nursing
Teaching Sister, The Royal Marsden Hospital School of
Cancer Nursing & Rehabilitation   (CHAPTERS 9, 11)

Steve Scholtes, *RN, ENB 998, 980, BSc Cancer Nursing*
Charge Nurse – Burdett Coutts
Ward   (CHAPTERS 12, 14)

Kate Scott, *RN, RMN, Onc Cert, Counselling Cert,*
ENB 870, 998, BSc (Hons) Nursing Studies
Clinical Nurse Specialist – Psychological Care
                    (CHAPTER 46)

Clare Shaw, *RD, BSc (Hons), Dip in Dietetics, PhD*
Consultant Dietitian   (CHAPTER 24)

Caroline Soady, *RN, BSc (Hons) Cancer Nursing*
Clinical Nurse Specialist – Head & Neck
                (CHAPTERS 31, 32, 41, 47)

Moira Stephens, *RN, Onc Cert, ENB 934, C&G 7306,*
DPSN, BSc (Hons) Health Studies, MSc Advancing
Professional Health Care Practice
Clinical Nurse Specialist – Haemato-oncology
                (CHAPTERS 19, 22)

Anna-Marie Stevens, *RN, RM, BSc (Hons), Onc Cert*
Clinical Nurse Specialist – Palliative Care
                (CHAPTER 43)

Rebecca Verity, *RN, BSc (Hons) Nursing Studies, MSc*
Advanced Practice (Cancer Nursing)
Formerly Senior Staff Nurse – Bud Flanagan Ward
                (CHAPTER 39)

Chris Viner, *RN, Onc Cert, FETC, MSc in*
Advanced Clinical Practice
Clinical Nurse Specialist – Ambulatory Chemotherapy
                (CHAPTER 44)

Jen Watson *RN, ENB 100*
Sister – Critical Care Unit   (CHAPTER 44)

Caro Watts, *RGN, Dip Onc, Cert Mgt (OU), BSc (Hons),*
MSc
Senior Sister – Private Patients   (CHAPTER 13)

Clare Webb, *BN (Hons), RGN, District Nursing Cert,*
Postgraduate Diploma in Therapeutic Counselling
(Integrative)
Specialist Sister in Psychological Care   (CHAPTER 2)

Barbara Witt, *RN*
Nurse Phlebotomist   (CHAPTER 45)

Miriam Wood, *RN, Onc Cert, BSc (Hons) Cancer Nursing*
Senior Practice Development Facilitator   (CHAPTER 2)

Mary Woods, *RN, Onc Cert, BSc (Hons), MSc Advanced*
Practice Nursing
Clinical Nurse Specialist/
Head of Lymphoedema Services   (CHAPTER 17)

Foreword to sixth edition

The Royal Marsden Hospital Manual of Clinical Nursing Procedures has become a legend. When I look back at the first edition, an internally produced procedure manual just for use at The Royal Marsden, it is quite amazing to think that 'the manual' has become such an important source for nurses everywhere. The fifth edition, in particular, has enjoyed enormous success. This may be because of the nursing profession's growing interest in evidence-based practice and clinical governance, but regardless of the rationale we are confident this work makes a significant contribution to improving the quality of patient care.

There have been a number of major conceptual changes in the development of this new edition. First, we undertook a major evaluation and market research exercise before embarking on the development of the sixth edition. This involved practitioners from the UK and abroad, many of whom had views about the content and structure of the manual. As a result, numerous changes have been made and I would like to take this opportunity to thank everyone who has helped us by contributing comments and suggestions.

Secondly, we believe that this book should not only be a way of The Royal Marsden sharing good practice, but that its publication should also present developmental opportunities for our staff. You will notice that in this edition we have, for the first time, partnered experienced nurse-authors with new authors, mostly staff nurses, to write chapters. This not only provides staff nurses with structured and developmental writing experience, but also means that the content is grounded in the realities of current day-to-day nursing practice from the perspective of staff nurses.

Thirdly, we have had a number of requests from nurse leaders and educators to present the information contained within the sixth edition in different ways, such as on a CD-ROM, in a ring-binder format and on prompt cards for use in skills laboratories. The editors have worked tirelessly to ensure that these different resources will now be available.

The benefits of ensuring that nursing care is, where possible, evidence based and consistent are well documented and I believe that *The Royal Marsden Hospital Manual of Clinical Nursing Procedures* helps us to do this. However, of equal importance is ensuring that the nursing care we provide is individual, therapeutic, culturally sensitive and that it is centred on that special relationship between the nurse, the patient and their loved ones and the partnership that develops between them. It would be almost impossible to write a procedure on creating an environment in which this sort of nursing practice could flourish. Creating a professional practice model, such as this, and an environment in which nurses can think critically, is the responsibility of all nurses.

The sixth edition is the product of an enormous amount of effort by nurses and other staff throughout The Royal Marsden Hospital, especially the editors Lisa Dougherty and Sara Lister. As always, it is with many thanks and great pride, that I am able to support their work.

Dr Dickon Weir-Hughes,
Chief Nurse/Deputy Chief Executive
The Royal Marsden Hospital (London & Surrey)

Foreword to sixth edition

Acknowledgements

In 1984 the first edition of *The Royal Marsden Hospital Manual* was published, thanks to the vision and support of Robert Tiffany, the then Director of Patient Services and Phylip Pritchard, the first editor. Over the next 20 years, the *Manual* has developed going from strength to strength. This process was aided by the innovation and enthusiasm of former editors such as: Jennifer Hunt, Jill David, Valerie Anne Walker, Chris Bailey and Jane Mallett.

This edition introduces many new authors, some of whom are contributing for the first time. There have been changes in the structure of some of the chapters as well as a new layout to increase the readability of the text. Each chapter represents not only nursing in theory, but also nursing in practice. Staff at all levels were encouraged to contribute, and to review and reflect on how the procedures were used in their own areas with the aim to make the practical aspects truly user friendly.

The chapters also rely on the authors' appraisal of the literature, national recommendations such as National Institute for Clinical Excellence (NICE), local guidelines, benchmarking and audit, as well as utilizing the authors' wealth of expertise and experience.

We extend our thanks to all those who wrote, reviewed and contributed to the text and the procedures. We would also like to thank all those who took the time to write to us and highlight sections that may have been unclear or incorrect – we have responded to all suggestions and made changes as appropriate.

Finally our thanks go to Griselda Campbell at Blackwell Publishing for advice and continual support in all aspects of the publishing process.

Lisa Dougherty
Sara Lister
Editors

Introduction

There is an expectation from patients that the nursing care they receive will be based on the best available evidence. Clinical procedures are a fundamental aspect of nursing care so it is essential that they are evidence based. This sixth edition of *The Royal Marsden Hospital Manual of Clinical Nursing Procedures* includes the clinical procedures, and the latest evidence underpinning the fundamental nursing care of any sick adult, whatever their diagnosis.

The findings from a survey of readers, particularly student nurses, informed the writing of this edition. There were a number of requests for additional chapters relating to a broad variety of aspects of nursing practice. We considered all of these and have included those that relate to the clinical expertise or practice of nurses within The Royal Marsden NHS Trust, an international cancer hospital.

A different approach has been taken to the preparation of the sixth edition of this manual: led by clinical experts, nurses in clinical practice have been involved in reviewing the latest evidence and testing the revised procedures in practice. This has provided professional development opportunities for junior staff and practical experience of identifying and then implementing evidence in practice. We hope that it has also acknowledged and recognized that important aspect of generating evidence in nursing: using the evidence that comes from practice (Kitson *et al.* 1998).

All chapters have been reviewed and some expanded to encompass new material including the legislative changes that have impacted on nursing roles. Context of care (Chapter 1) explores the concept of clinical governance in respect of clinical nursing practice, and includes an expanded section about the consent to examination and treatment in light of the NHS Reform and Health Care Professions Act (2002). A new chapter, Communication and assessment (Chapter 2), looks in depth at the process of patient assessment, emphasizing its importance in relation to carrying out clinical nursing procedures. Aseptic technique (Chapter 4) now includes a procedure for hand washing. Breast care (Chapter 6) now incorporates a section about seroma drainage. Drug administration (Chapter 9) includes an expanded section on nurse prescribing. Central venous pressure measurement has been moved to

Observations (Chapter 25); a section on peak flow measurement has also been added to this chapter.

In this edition the chapters have been reorganized, grouping together those addressing similar aspects of care: Drug administration; Elimination; Observations; Pain management and Personal hygiene, with the intention that information can be found more easily.

This edition continues the work that began 20 years ago, providing a practical resource for nursing practice. The format follows that of the preceding editions with only a few changes.

Every chapter begins with **definition**: this concisely defines the aspect of care addressed by the chapter.

This is followed by a **reference material section** consisting of a review of the literature and other relevant material. If available, the related research findings have been presented. If there is no research evidence available the procedures have been based on experience and systematic reviews.

The **procedure guidelines** begin with a list of the equipment needed, followed by a detailed step-by-step account of the procedure and the rationale for the proposed action. All relevant procedures begin with the action 'Explain and discuss the procedure with the patient', the rationale for this being 'to ensure the patient understands the procedure and gives his/her valid consent'. Gaining consent is an integral part of the person-focused approach to care, a core principle of nursing practice at The Royal Marsden Hospital. This is discussed further in Chapter 1.

Some chapters also include a **problem-solving section**. This lists the problems that may occur with a procedure, their possible causes and suggestions for their resolution and prevention.

The **references and further reading** at the end of the chapter indicate the sources from which information has been drawn to write the reference material and develop the procedures. It is also available to assist the reader if they want to study the subject in more depth. The further reading lists have been substantially revised for this edition; only publications from the past 10 years have been included, unless they are seminal texts or the only material available.

This book is intended as a reference and resource, not a replacement for practice-based education. None of the procedures in this book should be undertaken without prior instruction and subsequent supervision from an appropriately qualified and experienced professional.

We hope that *The Royal Marsden Hospital Manual of Clinical Nursing Procedures* will continue to be a resource and be a contribution to 'continually improving the overall standard of clinical care, whilst reducing variations in outcomes ... as well as ensuring that clinical decisions are based on the most up to date evidence of what is known to be effective' (NHSE 1999, p. 3).

References

Kitson, A., Harvey, G. & McCormack, B. (1998) Enabling the implementation of evidence based practice: a conceptual framework. *Qual Health Care*, **7**(3), 149–158.

NHS (2002) *NHS Reform and Health Care Professions Act*. HMSO, London.

NHSE (1999) *Clinical Governance Quality in the New NHS*. Department of Health, London.

Lisa Dougherty
Sara Lister
Editors

Context of care

Chapter contents

Introduction

'The essence of nursing at the Royal Marsden is the relationship between the nurse, the patient and their loved ones ... however, it is against this philosophical background that there is an emerging interest in ensuring that the fundamentals of nursing practice such as expertise in carrying out clinical procedures are given high priority.'

(Weir-Hughes 2000, Foreword)

The Royal Marsden Hospital Manual of Clinical Nursing Procedures is now in its twentieth year of publication with the fifth edition selling more copies than ever before. This illustrates that clinical procedures are now being given a high priority in nursing practice. This is because of some significant changes in the context of care. Today the real focus of health care is the patient: 'Every patient who is treated in the NHS wants to know that they can rely on receiving high-quality care when they need it' (NHSE 1997, para. 3.2). Clinical governance means that for the first time health care providers have a statutory duty for quality improvement to 'continually improve the overall standard of clinical care, whilst reducing variations in outcomes of, and access to, services as well as ensuring that clinical decisions are based on the most up-to-date evidence of what is known to be effective' (NHSE 1999a, p. 3).

In reality this has prompted the development of new methods of service delivery, the erosion of previous role boundaries and the rapid expansion of specialist and advanced practice roles in nursing aimed at meeting patient needs more effectively. The Chief Nurse's 'Ten Roles for Nursing' (NHSE 2000) has directly indicated the increased contribution nurses can have to overall care delivery. Patients and the public are being encouraged to be involved in defining what they want and monitoring the provision of health care they receive. There is an emphasis on developing national standards so that all patients can be partners in care and receive care which is based on the most up-to-date evidence with as little variation as possible.

So in this person-focused and quality-driven culture, clinical procedures, the fundamentals of nursing care, must be clinically effective. This means 'doing the right thing, the right way' (Kibbe *et al.* 1994, p. 181).

Evidence-based practice: doing the right thing

Historically, nursing, and specifically clinical procedures, have been very ritualistic (Walsh & Ford 1989; Ford & Walsh 1994). Nurses were taught the precise way to lay out all the items in the dressing pack; that catheters had to come out at midnight; that observations had to be done either four hourly or at least twice a day. Although nursing has been striving to become more research based since the 1970s (Briggs 1972), it has been the introduction of clinical governance and the drive towards evidence-based practice that has challenged our ways of work most recently. Clinical effectiveness can be defined as 'when specific clinical interventions do what they intend to do' (Mann 1996, p. 2); in other words, this means carrying out care that is based on procedures underpinned by the conscientious, explicit and judicious use of current best evidence (NHSE 1999a). The National Institute for Clinical Excellence (NICE) leads the work nationally on developing guidelines for health professionals about the effectiveness of particular interventions for specific client groups. What constitutes good evidence is the subject of continual debate. The best evidence in the medical context is considered to be from scientific quantitative studies (Cox & Reyes-Hughes 2002). This has contributed to a hierarchy of grades for robustness and validity (Goding & Edwards 2002) (Box 1.1).

In nursing, the nature of the evidence for practice is drawn from different sources, so there is considerable argument that nursing should not use the medical system

of grading evidence. Kitson *et al.* (1998) encourage the valuing of feedback from patients and professional experience alongside research to determine best practice. It is not losing sight of the important principle that: 'The foundation of nursing, if it has one, is surely the facilitative human relationship between patient and nurse which makes skilled biomedical nursing and technical excellence possible' (Rolfe 2001, p. 147). To develop this manual the current research has been appraised and the procedures have been updated accordingly. However, feedback from clinical experts has also been important in revising the procedures to ensure that current practice is reflected and the procedure guidelines do enable nurses to 'do the right thing'.

National guidance for care has developed and been defined at various levels. When reading and using any guidance, it is important to be aware of the context for which it was written and at what level it is intended for use. The framework in Box 1.2 explains the relationship between the many terms used to define evidence-based statements of good practice.

How do we know we have done it right?

Setting clear standards for practice is only the first step in clinical effectiveness. Clinical audit is a clinically led initiative seeking to improve the quality and outcome of patient care as clinicians examine and modify their practices, according to standards of what could be achieved, based on the best evidence available (Mann 1996) (Fig. 1.1).

Not doing the wrong thing! Clinical risk management

Another aspect of ensuring that the fundamentals of nursing practice are carried out effectively is reviewing policies and procedures for potential risks. Risk can be defined as the possibility of incurring misfortune or loss resulting in:

- Harm to patients
- Resources being diverted to provide extra treatment to correct the initial injury
- Resources being diverted to the investigation of complaints, adverse incidents and medical negligence
- Harm to the reputation of the provider because of poor performance
- Reduction in confidence of the public (adapted from Swage 2000).

Risk management is a means of reducing the risks of adverse events occurring in organizations by systematically assessing, reviewing and then seeking ways to prevent their occurrence (NHSE 1999b). When considering

---

Box 1.1 Levels of evidence (adapted from Goding & Edwards 2002).

1 Strong evidence from at least one systematic review of multiple, well-designed randomized controlled trials.
2 Strong evidence from at least one properly designed, randomized controlled trial of appropriate size.
3 Evidence from well-designed trials without randomization, single group pre–post, cohort, time series or matched case–control studies.
4 Evidence from well-designed non-experimental studies from more than one centre or research group.
5 Opinions of respected authorities, based on clinical evidence, descriptive studies or reports of expert committees.

Box 1.2 Definitions and relationships between terms used to define good practice statements (adapted from NICE NHS Modernization Agency 2003).

National Standards

Definition: *NHS standards set by or on behalf of the Department of Health. These are authoritative national statements based on research evidence and developed by multidisciplinary teams.*

Include:

- National Service Frameworks, e.g. NSF for Older People (DoH 2001a)
- NICE guidelines, e.g. Pressure Ulcer Risk Assessment and Prevention (NICE 2001)
- Strategies and good practice statements drawn up by the Department of Health, e.g. NHS Cancer Plan (DoH 2000) and Essence of Care Benchmarks (DoH 2001b)

Local Protocols

Definition: *The detailed descriptions of the steps taken to deliver care or treatment to a patient. They are sometimes called integrated care pathways. They are designed at a local level to implement national standards or to determine care provision using the best available evidence if national standards are not available.*

Include:

- Integrated care pathways, e.g. integrated care pathway for the last two days of life (Fowell *et al.* 2002)
- Discharge pathway (DoH 2002, p. 56)

Procedures

Definition: *The operational subsection of a protocol. These are used at an individual patient level and may apply in a number of protocols. They list tasks in the order in which they should be carried out and have often been developed before the protocol. They are also developed with reference to the best available evidence.*

Include:

- The procedures in *The Royal Marsden Hospital Manual of Clinical Nursing Procedures*. These are essential in the care of an individual with cancer but are also applicable to the care of patients with many other diseases or conditions, who need nursing care
- The Resuscitation Guidelines (Resuscitation Council (UK) 2000)

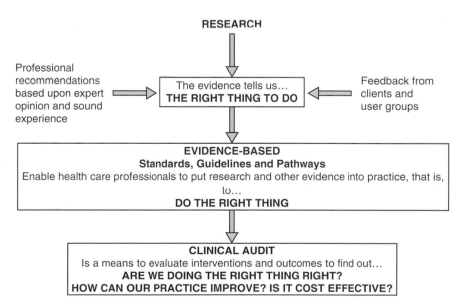

Figure 1.1 The relationship between clinical audit and clinical effectiveness (Royal Marsden Hospital Quality Assurance Department 2001).

nursing procedures the potential for adverse events may arise from:

- Malfunctioning or inappropriate equipment
- System failures – procedures that are ill defined or not followed correctly
- Procedures carried out by practitioners who are inadequately educated or trained (Wilson 1999)

Effective clinical governance should help to prevent clinical errors and encourage a commitment from all health care professionals to learn from mistakes and to share that learning with others in the environment of a 'no blame' culture. As professionals we have a responsibility to assess every patient and situation and adapt the procedures appropriately to the circumstances, always acknowledging limits of professional competence (NMC 2002).

Being competent to do it. Doing it the right way

The *Code of Professional Conduct* (NMC 2002, p. 8) states:

'6.10 As a registered nurse, midwife or health visitor, you must maintain your professional knowledge and competence

6.5 You have a responsibility to deliver care based on current evidence, best practice and, where applicable, validated research when available.'

As a qualified nurse there is an expectation that you will have the competence on qualifying to carry out fundamental procedures. It is suggested that a registered nurse should 'possess the knowledge, skills and abilities required for lawful, safe and effective practice without direct supervision' (NMC 2002, p. 8) and be able to carry out at least 75% of the procedures in this manual. Nurse training prepares practitioners to do things the 'right way'.

As the environments in which health care is delivered have diversified, so have the career opportunities and the potential roles and responsibilities of nurses. The advanced practice roles of nurse practitioner, clinical nurse specialist and nurse consultant have developed in response to a number of factors. Initially *The New Deal* for doctors (NHS Management Executive 1991) began the debate about the areas of medical practice that could be taken over by nurses, with bold statements being made about the potential cost savings (Richardson & Maynard 1995). With the publication of *The Scope of Professional Practice* (UKCC 1992) procedures previously carried out by doctors became the responsibility of nurses and new advanced practice roles have evolved. Advanced Practice is an umbrella term relating to the skills, knowledge, expertise and attitude that are firmly grounded in clinical practice, and encompasses aspects of education, research, consultation and case management (Hawkins & Holcombe 1995; NMC 1999; Royal Marsden 2003). In practice this means that nurses are undertaking procedures that are more numerous, invasive and complex than 20 years ago when the first edition of this manual was published, such as seroma drainage, the insertion of a peripherally inserted central catheter and removal of a skin-tunnelled catheter.

In seeking clinical effectiveness and wanting to do things the right way, one of the challenges has been assessing competence at this higher level of practice (Lillyman 1998). Benner's (1984) model of skill acquisition offers a framework to define the development from novice through to clinical expert. This and her subsequent work (Benner *et al.* 1996) have been used extensively to articulate the qualities that distinguish an expert nurse and to define expert nursing care. This framework has been used to develop role development profiles, tools that:

'support competence acquisition in relation to role developments … enabling individuals to take responsibility for planning, managing and evaluating learning in relation to the role development and to provide the opportunity for the individual to maintain a record of their own developing competence.'

(Royal Marsden NHS Trust 1999)

Those activities that have not previously fallen within the scope of nursing practice and for which the nurse has not received education and training may be considered to be role developments. Procedure guidelines are integral to role development and are part of the process of ensuring clinical effectiveness in 'doing the right thing the right way'.

A recent study entitled *Improving the Effectiveness of the Nursing Workforce* (Centre for Health Economics 2003) has highlighted the shift in roles at the other end of the novice-to-expert continuum, with health care assistants taking responsibility for an increasing number of procedures that historically have been the professional domain of nursing (O'Dowd 2003). There is concern that this may not be the 'right way'. If qualified nurses deliver all care there is an increased opportunity for patients to benefit from therapeutic nursing. Evidence demonstrates that this does contribute positively to the patient's experience of care (Spilsbury & Meyer 2001).

Are we doing it the right way? Patient and public involvement

Clinical governance means that the patient should be at the centre of all that is done in health care; mechanisms need to be in place so they can be involved in the broad aspects of health care delivery as well as their own individual care (Health and Social Care Act 2001, NHS Reform and Health Care Professions Act 2002). In every trust a Patient Advice and Liaison Service (PALS) has been established to provide on-the-spot help and information about health and care. This advice may cover anything from more information about a patient's condition and disease and treatment options, to information about self-help groups or specific care procedures. The mechanisms for patients with complaints have been reviewed and include the new Independent Complaints Advocacy Service (ICAS). Patient forums have been set up through which patients can be involved in the operational and strategic developments of the trust (NHSE 2000). It is important that the concept of involving patients and the public is not limited to these formal statutory methods. Establishing user groups, using surveys and facilitating focus groups will provide opportunities for patients to share their experiences of care, including such aspects as cleanliness, food and nutrition, and privacy and dignity (Kelson 2001). Involving patients in the review of written information and asking their opinion of the clarity of procedure guidelines for aspects of self-care such as self-catheterization are fundamental to person-focused care.

At another level it has been recognized that patients need to be more equal partners in their own care. The process of gaining valid consent to examination and treatment has been reviewed as part of the commitment to deliver excellence in health care, emphasizing the importance of clear and consistent information. The second section of this chapter focuses on this issue.

Consent

Medical 'consent' is a patient's agreement for a health professional to provide care (DoH 2001c). The consent process is a partnership between the patient and the health care professional involved. It is a two-way process that is dependent upon competence (of the provider and requester of consent) and information. Consent is a core clinical activity and is fundamental to patient care, best practice and clinical governance. Patients may indicate consent non-verbally (for example, by presenting their arm for their pulse to be taken), verbally or in writing (DoH 2001c). The Department of Health recently issued guidelines entitled *Reference Guide to Consent for Examination or Treatment* (DoH 2001c) as part of the *NHS Plan* reforms. These guidelines should have been applied in all NHS institutions from 1 October 2002 as part of the Good Practice in Consent initiative.

Patients have a fundamental legal and ethical right to determine what happens to their own bodies. Valid consent to treatment is therefore absolutely central in all forms of health care, from providing personal care to undertaking major surgery. Seeking consent is also a matter of common courtesy between health professionals and patients.

Human rights form the basis of ethical principles that include self-determination, privacy, anonymity and confidentiality, fair treatment and protection from discomfort and harm (Ling 1997). The ethical principle of respecting human dignity includes the patient's right to self-determination and the right to full disclosure (Polit & Hungler 1995). The right to self-determination suggests that patients should be treated as an autonomous group who are capable of controlling their own activities and destinies and have a right to elect voluntarily whether to consent to treatments, procedures, etc. (Polit & Hungler 1995).

The right to full disclosure enables patients to make informed voluntary decisions about their care. The information-giving process requires sophisticated assessment and communication skills, together with a profound respect for the rights of the individual. The health care professional, in order to demonstrate respect for a patient, must obtain that individual's consent prior to any procedure. Health professionals who do not respect this principle can be liable to both legal action by the patient and action from their professional body (DoH 2001c).

While there is no English statute setting out the general principles of consent, case law ('common law') has established that touching a patient without valid consent may constitute the civil or criminal offence of battery. Further, if health professionals fail to obtain proper consent and the patient subsequently suffers harm as a result of treatment, this may be a factor in a claim of negligence against the health professional involved. Poor handling of the consent process may also result in complaints from patients through the NHS complaints procedure or to professional bodies (DoH 2001c).

Health care professionals have unique relationships with their patients. On entering this relationship, the practitioner assumes certain special duties towards the patient, over and above those which ordinary human beings have to each other, such as a duty not to kill them, a duty to keep a promise or a duty not to tell a lie. The features of this relationship are described generally as a duty of care that contains the following:

- A duty to respect the patient as an individual
- A duty to act to minimize risk to patients
- A duty to obtain consent before giving any treatment or care (NMC 2002).

English common law identifies three components of a valid consent:

- Competency
- Information
- Voluntariness.

If an examination, procedure or treatment is carried out without these requirements being fulfilled then a civil action may be brought in the tort of battery, which protects a person from unwanted touching, or in the tort of negligence, where harm results directly from the procedure. It is the health care professional's duty to ensure that a person is competent to consent, has sufficient information on which to base their decision and that the decision is voluntary and uncoerced (DoH 2001c).

Does the patient have capacity?

For an adult's consent to be valid that person must have 'capacity to consent to the intervention in question'. The British Medical Association (1995) has set guidelines for assessing mental capacity and suggests that in order to be classed as competent, an adult should be able to:

- 'Understand, in broad terms and simple language, what the medical treatment is, its purpose and nature and why it has been proposed.'
- Understand its principal benefits, risks and alternatives.
- Understand, in broad terms, what the consequences are of not receiving the proposed treatment.
- Make a choice free from undue pressure.
- Retain the information long enough to make an effective decision (BMA 1995).

However, no single standard of decision-making competence is adequate as competence can potentially vary from day to day and from procedure to procedure (Rees 2001).

A lack of capacity to give or withhold consent may be due to communication difficulties as opposed to genuine incapacity. Appropriate colleagues should be consulted when making such assessments of incapacity, e.g. specialist learning disability teams and speech and language therapists, unless the urgency of the patient's situation prevents this. If at all possible, the patient should be assisted to make and communicate their own decision by providing information in non-verbal ways where appropriate (DoH 2001c). Patients may have capacity to consent to some interventions but not to others. Adults are always presumed to have capacity, but if any doubt exists the health professional should ensure that an assessment of the patient's capacity to make the decision in question is made. It is important that a record of this assessment and the conclusions drawn from it is made in the patient's notes (DoH 2001c).

In addition, a patient's capacity to understand may be temporarily affected by factors such as confusion, panic, shock, pain and medication. However, the existence of such factors should not be assumed automatically to render the patient incapable of consenting. Capacity should never be confused with a health professional's assessment of the reasonableness of the patient's decision. The patient is entitled to make a decision that is based on their own religious belief or value system, even if it is perceived by others to be irrational, as long as the patient understands the potential implications of their decision. An irrational decision has been defined as one that is so outrageous in its defiance of logic or of accepted moral standards that no sensible person who had applied his or her mind to the question could have arrived at it (DoH 2001c). However, if the decision which appears irrational is based on a misperception of reality, as opposed to an unusual value system (for example, a patient who, despite the obvious evidence, denies that his foot is gangrenous or a patient with anorexia nervosa who is unable to comprehend her failing physical condition) then the patient may not be able to comprehend and make use of the relevant information and hence may lack capacity to make the decision in question (DoH 2001c).

Is the consent given voluntarily?

'Informed consent is an unavoidably complicated issue.'
(Smith 1998)

'The process of obtaining consent from patients is both time consuming and requires good communication skills. Patients should feel confident that they are being treated in privacy and cannot be overheard. Similarly they shouldn't feel rushed or pressurized into giving consent.'
(Rees 2001)

The patient's participation in the decision-making process and ultimate decision regarding care must be voluntary. A choice that has been coerced, or that resulted from serious manipulation of a person's ability to make an intelligent and informed decision, is not the person's own free choice. This has long been recognized in law: consent forced by threats or induced by fraud or misrepresentation is legally viewed as no consent at all. Consent should be given without pressure or undue influence being exerted on the patient either to accept or to refuse treatment. Such pressure can come from partners or family members as well as health care professionals. Professionals should be alert to this possibility and, where appropriate, should arrange to see the patient on their own to establish that the decision is truly that of the patient.

The nature of chronic illness, the vulnerability of an individual faced with an unfamiliar and frightening environment and the disproportionate amount of power and perceived inequality between health care professional and patient may all, to varying degrees, intrude into the decision-making process.

Health professionals have several responsibilities related to the voluntary nature of decision making.

- To recognize the vulnerability of patients and to be alert to circumstances when undue influence may be exerted by colleagues or relatives.
- To gain consent for all investigations, treatment or acts of care and not to assume that 'routine' procedures can be carried out automatically.
- To communicate effectively and impartially with patients to enable them to reach a voluntary decision, and to offer support for that decision.

Consent by proxy

'Legally, as soon as people reach their legal majority, no one else has the authority to act on their behalf and give consent, whatever their mental capacity. Consent by proxy is not an acceptable method of consent for patients who have previously been deemed competent.'

(Rees 2001)

Documentation

For significant procedures, it is essential for health professionals to document clearly both a patient's agreement to the intervention and the discussions that led up to that agreement. This may be done either through the use of a consent form (with further detail in the patient's notes if necessary) or through documenting in the patient's notes that they have given oral consent.

A standard consent form should provide space for a health professional to identify what information they have provided to the patient and to sign confirming that they have done so. The health professional who provides this information must be competent to do so.

Consent is often wrongly equated with a patient's signature on a consent form. A signature on a form is *evidence* that the patient has given consent but is not *proof* of valid consent (DoH 2001c). Patients who are rushed into signing a form or are given too little information or too little time may not have given valid consent, despite the signature. Similarly, if a patient has given valid verbal consent, the fact that they are physically unable to sign the form is no bar to treatment (DoH 2001c). Patients are entitled to withdraw consent any time after signing a consent form; their signature acts only as evidence of the process of consent giving, it is not a binding contract.

It is rarely a legal requirement to seek written consent, but it is good practice to do so if any of the following circumstances apply.

- The treatment or investigative procedure is complex or involves significant risks (the term 'risk' is used throughout to refer to any adverse outcome, including those which some health professionals would describe as 'side-effects' or 'complications')(DoH 2001c).
- The procedure involves a local or general anaesthetic or sedation.
- The clinical care being provided is not the primary purpose of the procedure, e.g. photography (DoH 2001c).
- There may be significant consequences for the patient's employment, social or personal life (DoH 2001c).
- For each course of anticancer medical therapy (cytotoxic, radiotherapy, hormonal, biological or other). NB: Course = planned treatments, e.g. one treatment, six treatments or maintenance therapy.
- The treatment is part of a project or programme of research approved by a local research ethics committee.

Consent for one procedure or course of treatment does not give any automatic right to undertake any further treatment or procedure.

Table 1.1 provides an example of the standard consent arrangements for The Royal Marsden NHS Trust (i.e. whether written/oral/non-verbal consent is appropriate for specified procedures).

Once signed, completed consent forms should be filed in the patient's medical notes. If any changes are made to a form after the patient has signed it, these should be initialled and dated by both patient and health professional. Patients should be given a copy of the consent form that they have signed.

It is generally not necessary to document a patient's consent to routine and low-risk procedures, such as providing personal care or taking a routine blood sample. However, if the health care professional has any reason to believe that the consent may be disputed later or if the procedure is of particular concern to the patient (for example, if they have declined, or become very distressed about, similar care in the past), it would be appropriate to do so (DoH 2001c). The record should be put in the patient's medical notes and should specify the actual information given to the patient.

Duration of consent

When a patient has given a valid consent to an intervention, generally that consent will remain valid for an indefinite duration unless the patient withdraws it. However, if any new information becomes available regarding the proposed intervention (for example, new evidence of risks or new treatment options) between the time when consent was sought and when the intervention is undertaken, the GMC guidance (1998) states that a doctor or member of the health care team should inform the patient and reconfirm their consent (DoH

Table 1.1 Consent arrangements (Royal Marsden Hospital)

Procedures requiring informed written consent by completion of standard consent form	Procedures requiring informed verbal consent and documentation in patient record	Implied consent (procedure discussed with patient but no formal record required)

Therapeutic
 • All surgical procedures
 • Radiotherapy procedures (including those involving external beam, brachytherapy and systemic radioisotopes)
 • Chemotherapy (including instillation of chemotherapy via pleural or peritoneal aspiration; oral chemotherapy, e.g. 6 MP, methotrexate, hydroxyurea, and intrathecal chemotherapy)
 • Hormone therapy
 • Biological therapies
 • Pleural/abdominal aspiration, drainage
 • IV/sedation for any procedure requiring it
 • Insertion of any indwelling central venous access device
 • Image-guided therapeutic or interventional procedures
 • Plasma exchange
 • Peripheral blood stem cell harvest (patient or donor)
 • Leucopheresis (therapeutic)
 • Bone marrow harvest (patient or donor)
 • Autografting and allografting
 • Percutaneous nephrostomy, suprapubic catheters
 • Blood product transfusions
 	
 Diagnostic
 • Breast diagnosis
 • Percutaneous biopsy, e.g. liver, breast, stereotactic wire localization
 • CT-guided biopsies
 	
 Other
 • HIV testing and counselling
 • Photography
 • Genetic testing
	• Imaging, e.g. barium enemas/meals
	 • Contrast infusion
	 • Contrast media application for imaging procedures
	 • Female patients undergoing pelvic simulation requiring insertion of vaginal tampon
	 • Vaginal ultrasound
	 • Physio procedures (specific procedures)
	 • Complementary therapies
		• Students/visitors attendance during treatment procedure
		 • Diagnostic tests:
		  – Plain X-ray
		  – Oral contrast studies
		  – CT (no contrast)
		  – MRI (no contrast)
		  – PET
		 • Clinical examination
		 • Breast, rectal, genital examination
		 • Urinary catherization
		 • Nasogastric tube insertion
		 • Fine-needle aspiration
		 • Lumbar puncture
		 • Bone marrow aspiration
		 • Bone marrow trephine
		 • Skin biopsy
		 • Use of patient information
		 • Venepuncture
		
		 *Supported by written information

2001c). Similarly, if the patient's condition has changed significantly in the intervening time, it may be necessary to seek consent again, on the basis that the likely benefits and/or risks of the intervention may also have changed (DoH 2001c).

If consent is obtained a significant time before the undertaking of an intervention, it is considered good practice to confirm that the person who has given consent (assuming he or she retains capacity) still wishes the intervention to proceed even if no new information needs to be provided or further questions need to be answered (DoH 2001c).

Gaining consent

When should consent be sought?

Consent to a particular intervention can occur either during a single consultation or over a number of consultations, depending on the potential seriousness of the proposed treatment and the urgency of the patient's condition.

Single-stage process

In a number of situations, it will be appropriate for a procedure to commence immediately after discussing it with the patient; for example, during an ongoing episode of care a physiotherapist may suggest a particular manipulative technique and explain how it might help the patient's condition and whether there are any significant risks (DoH 2001c). If the patient is happy for this technique to be used then they can give oral consent and the procedure can be initiated immediately. However, as previously noted, a record of the conversation with the patient, including details of the treatment and risks discussed, should be documented in the patient's notes.

It is more appropriate to gain written informed consent if the planned procedure carries significant risks. Health professionals must take into consideration whether the patient has had sufficient chance to absorb the information necessary for them to make their decision (DoH 2001c). Once it is clear the patient understands the planned procedure and has given consent, the treatment may proceed.

Two or more stage process

In the majority of situations where *written* consent is being sought from patients, potential treatment options should be discussed well in advance of the planned initiation time of treatment. This could either be as a one-off consultation or even over a number of visits with different health care professionals. This consent process is therefore considered to have at least two stages: information giving and discussion of other options with an initial decision being made orally, and the second session confirming that the patient is still willing to go ahead. Consent forms should be used to document both of these stages.

It is important that patients who are due to undergo elective procedures or treatments where written consent is necessary have been informed about the details of the consent form in advance of arriving for the appointment. Patients should also have received a copy of their consent form outlining the decision-making process. Consent forms can be signed at any appropriate time

prior to the procedure, i.e. in outpatients, preadmission clinic or when the patient arrives for treatment.

When forms have been signed before arriving for treatment a member of the health care team must ascertain whether the patient has any concerns about the treatment and if their condition has changed in any way. When confirming the patient's consent and understanding, it is advisable to use a form of words which requires more than a yes/no answer from the patient: for example, beginning with 'Tell me what you're expecting to happen', rather than 'Is everything all right?' (DoH 2001c). It is appropriate for any member of the health care team (for example, a nurse admitting the patient for an elective procedure) to confirm the patient's consent, as long as they have access to appropriate colleagues to answer questions they cannot handle themselves.

NB: For consent to be valid, the patient must feel that they were able to refuse or even change their mind about the procedure in question. It will rarely be appropriate to ask a patient to sign a consent form after they have begun to be prepared for treatment (for example, by changing into a hospital gown).

Provision of information

Provision of information to patients to achieve a valid consent to examination, treatment and care requires the health care professional to use their clinical judgement in order to:

- Assess the amount of information needed by the patient and carers
- Explain the procedure clearly and accurately
- Provide honest answers to the patient's questions in a sympathetic manner.

These require considerable communication skills and, perhaps most important of all, time. It is important to remember that a patient must be given privacy when receiving information about the consent process. Any information imparted and discussed with the patient should be treated as confidential. This is outlined in the ethical principle of justice that includes patients' rights to fair treatment and a right to privacy (Polit & Hungler 1995).

The provision of information is central to the consent process (DoH 2001c). Patients need to have received comprehensible information about the risks and benefits of a proposed treatment (including the risks/benefits of doing nothing) and about their underlying condition before they can make a decision about such procedures. In addition, patients need to be informed about any other potential investigations/treatments that may be necessary as part of the procedure, e.g. a blood transfusion. Once a decision has been made to have a particular procedure, patients will also need to be given information about what will happen to them, where to go, how long they will be in hospital and how they will feel afterwards.

All patients vary in how much information they want to hear, varying from those who want to know about everything, e.g. rare risks, to patients who would rather the health care professional make the decision for them. There has to be an element of clinical judgement in determining what information should be given but the *presumption* must be that the patient wishes to be well informed about the risks and benefits of the various options (DoH 2001c).

The GMC guidance on the provision of information states that doctors should do their best to find out the patient's individual needs and priorities when providing information about treatment options and risks. The guidance also emphasizes that if the patient asks specific questions about the procedure, these should be answered truthfully (GMC 1998).

When patients make it clear either verbally or non-verbally that they do not wish to be given this level of information, this should always be documented.

Specific arrangements should be made for patients who have impaired sight and hearing to ensure that they receive adequate information and can, therefore, give valid consent.

Provision for patients whose first language is not English

It is important to ensure that patients whose first language is not English receive the information they need and are able to communicate appropriately with health care staff. It is never appropriate to use children as interpreters for family members who cannot speak English.

Where an interpreter (or family member providing interpretation) is used to provide consent information to a patient, this should be documented on the consent form and/or in the patient notes. Where a consent form is completed, the interpreter should be requested to read and sign the appropriate section.

Who is responsible for seeking consent?

'The health professional carrying out the procedure is ultimately responsible for ensuring that the patient has given valid consent for what is to be done, it is they who will be held responsible in law if this is challenged later.'

(DoH 2001c)

'Where oral or non-verbal consent is being sought at the point the procedure will be carried out, this will naturally be done by the health professional responsible. However, teamwork is a crucial part of the way the NHS operates, and where written consent is being sought it may be appropriate

for other members of the team to participate in the process of seeking consent.'

(DoH 2001c)

It is a health professional's own responsibility to ensure that when they require colleagues to seek consent on their behalf, they are confident that the colleague is competent to do so. They should always work within their own competence and not agree to perform tasks which exceed that competence (DoH 2001c). Inappropriate delegation may mean that the consent is invalid.

Withdrawal of consent

A patient with capacity is entitled to withdraw consent at any time, including during the performance of a procedure. If a patient does object during a procedure/ treatment, it is considered good practice by the practitioner, where possible, to stop the procedure, establish the patient's concerns and explain the consequences of not completing the procedure. At times an apparent objection may reflect a cry of pain rather than withdrawal of consent and appropriate reassurance may enable the practitioner to continue with the patient's consent. If stopping the procedure at that point would genuinely put the life of the patient at risk, the practitioner may be entitled to continue until this risk no longer applies. Assessing capacity during a procedure can be difficult as factors such as pain, panic and shock may diminish capacity to consent. Practitioners should try to establish whether at that time the patient still has capacity to withdraw a previously given consent. If capacity is lacking, it may sometimes be justified to continue in the patient's best interests, although this should never be used as an excuse to ignore distress (DoH 2001c).

Refusal of treatment

If the process of seeking consent is to be meaningful, refusal must be one of the patient's options. A competent adult patient is entitled to refuse any treatment, except in circumstances governed by the Mental Health Act 1983 (DoH 2001c).

If after discussing potential options a patient decides to refuse all treatment, this should be formally and clearly documented in the patient's notes. Likewise in situations when patients subsequently change their minds after initially consenting to a procedure, this should be documented on the patient's consent form.

When patients refuse a particular intervention, the health care professional involved in their care must ensure that the patient continues to receive any other appropriate care that the patient has consented to. Patients should be informed that they are free to change their minds and accept treatment if they later wish to do so. However, patients should be advised if this affects their future treatment choices.

When patients consent to only certain aspects of a procedure, the potential consequences that may arise from this decision should be explained. There is no obligation for a procedure to be performed if it is thought that it cannot be safely carried out according to the patient's stipulations. In such cases any other appropriate care should be given. If another health care professional believes they are able to safely perform the procedure under such circumstances, the patient's care may be transferred.

Examination or treatment without patient consent

Examination or treatment of a patient may proceed without obtaining the patient's consent under the following circumstances.

- For life-saving procedures where the patient is unconscious and cannot indicate his/her wishes.
- Where there is a statutory power requiring the examination of a patient, e.g. under the Public Health Act. However, an explanation should be offered and the patient's co-operation should be sought.
- In certain cases where a minor is a ward of court and the court decides that a specific treatment is in the child's best interests.
- Treatments for mental disorder of a patient liable to be detained in hospital under the Mental Heath Act.
- Treatment for physical disorder where the patient is incapable of giving consent by reason of mental disorder and the treatment is in the patient's best interests (DoH 2001c).

Clearly in emergencies, the two stages (discussion of options and confirmation that the patient wishes to go ahead) will follow straight on from each other, and it may often be appropriate to use the patient's notes to document any discussion and the patient's consent, rather than using a form. The urgency of the patient's situation may limit the quantity of information that they can be given, but should not affect its quality (DoH 2001c).

Consent for procedures

Seeking consent for anaesthesia

When patients are undergoing a general anaesthetic it is the responsibility of the anaesthetist and not the surgeon to gain consent for the anaesthetic, ensuring the risks and benefits have been explained (DoH 2001c). For elective treatments it is unacceptable for patients to only receive information about the anaesthetic at their pre-op visit from the anaesthetist, as patients will not be in a position at this time to make a truly informed decision about whether they wish to undergo the anaesthetic procedure. In such situations it is advisable that patients either receive some written information regarding the proposed anaesthetic in a preassessment clinic or outpatients, or are able to discuss the planned anaesthetic in advance of their admission. Anaesthetists should ensure that these discussions are formally documented. If the clinician involved in either procedure is also responsible for the anaesthetic, e.g. local anaesthetic or sedation, it is they who should also gain consent for this.

Consent to care by health care students (e.g. medical, nursing and allied health professions)

Care should be taken to respect the patient's wishes. It should not be assumed that a patient is available for teaching purposes or for practical experience by medical, dental or other staff under training. An explanation of the need for practical experience should be given and agreement obtained before proceeding. It should be made clear that a patient may refuse without adversely affecting his or her care.

Samples of human tissue

The legal position regarding the use of human tissue (including blood samples and other bodily fluids provided for testing) raises some difficult issues and is currently under review (DoH 2001c). Such tissues can play an important role in education and research and their use can enhance medical knowledge and thus improvements in health care for all.

Pending the outcome of the review of the law governing the use of human organs and tissue, the Department of Health believes that tissue samples may be used for quality assurance purposes without requiring specific patient consent provided there is an active policy of informing patients of such use at the time the sample is taken (DoH 2001c). If at all possible, samples used for this purpose should be anonymized.

Clinical photography and conventional or digital video/audio recordings

Photographic and video/audio recordings made for clinical purposes form part of a patient's record. Although consent to certain recordings, such as X-rays, is implicit in the patient's consent to the procedure, health professionals should always ensure that they make clear in advance if any photographic or video recording will result from that procedure (DoH 2001c).

Wherever possible, all patients should be referred to the photographic department for clinical photography requests. Exceptions to this are:

- Radiographers/physicists when planning treatment (e.g. simulation) or carrying out diagnostic procedures
- Surgeons/radiographers perioperatively and medical staff during clinical procedures, e.g. a colonoscopy using specialized equipment
- Research nurses who are required to take photographs as part of their role.

Photographic and video recordings which are made for treating or assessing a patient must not be used for any purpose other than the patient's care or the audit of that care, without the express consent of the patient or a person with parental responsibility for the patient.

Before consenting to clinical photography patients need to understand:

- Why the photographs/images are necessary
- What the procedure involves
- Where the photographs/images will be stored
- Who has access to these photographs/images
- What else the photographs/images may be used for.

All patients consenting to clinical photography should be asked to sign a consent form. This will indicate that they understand the procedure and that their records will only be used for their clinical care and will be retained in their medical records. Photographic and video recordings made for treating or assessing a patient (even if there is no possibility that the patient might be recognized) may only be used within the clinical setting for education or research purposes.

Written consent must be obtained for use of pictures for non-clinical purposes, e.g. making a photographic or video recording of a patient specifically for education, publication or research purposes. Patients should be informed that they are free to stop any recording at any time and if they so wish, they can view it before deciding whether to give consent for its use. If the patient decides that they are not happy for any recording to be used, it must be destroyed. Patients must also receive full information about any possible uses of a recording and also be informed that it is not always possible to withdraw a recording once it is in the public domain.

The situation may sometimes arise where a recording is made specifically for education, publication or research purposes, but the patient is temporarily unable to give or withhold consent because, for example, they are unconscious. In such cases it is permitted to make such a recording, but consent must be obtained as soon as the patient regains capacity. The recording must not be used until consent has been obtained for its use. If the patient does not consent to any form of use, the recording must be destroyed (DoH 2001c). If the patient is likely to be permanently unable to give or withhold consent for a recording to be made, agreement should be sought from someone close to the patient. Recordings that might be against the interests of the patient must not be used (DoH 2001c). Some institutions insist that consent is obtained both before and after any recordings have been made, thereby giving patients the opportunity to withdraw their consent after the event if they so wish.

Key recommendations for photography include the following.

- Checking that the patient does not mind being photographed by a photographer of the opposite gender. If they do, ask the patient if they would like a chaperone or to wait for another member of staff to take the picture.
- Checking whether the patient is willing to proceed. Always give the opportunity to refuse (even if written consent has been previously given).
- A record of all clinical photographs must be kept and the original negatives referenced and archived. Staff who circumvent the photographic department by using their own photographic equipment are responsible for the storage and usage of negatives and picture processing. This includes digitizing negatives for teaching CD-ROMs and/or making up slides.
- A copy of the clinical photograph, and consent form, should be placed within the patient's medical notes.

Clinical research

Informed consent is the cornerstone of ethical research and this applies not only to treatments but also to use of patient data or tissue. Clinical research on a human being cannot be undertaken without that person's full informed consent (WMA 2002). All the principles outlined above should be applied when considering or approaching a patient to enter into a clinical research study.

Ethically, an independent research ethics committee should approve any research project that is carried out on human beings. In the NHS this will be the local research ethics committee and additionally, where appropriate, the Multi-Centre Research Ethics Committee (DoH 2001c).

In general, it is not appropriate to carry out research on adults who cannot give consent for themselves, if the research can instead be carried out on adults who are able to give or withhold consent. The only exception to this rule would be where clinicians believe that it is in the person's own best interest to be involved in research.

However, there is currently no means of obtaining fully informed consent from incompetent adult patients for entry into research studies. Consent by proxy (i.e.

from relatives or carers) is valid for children but does not hold for patients over the age of 16. In the past, some studies have been done without consent from the patient following approval from local ethics committees. This is no longer an option (DoH 2001c).

Capacity

Adults previously competent but who subsequently lose the ability to consent

This section relates to adult patients who were previously competent but who have subsequently lost the ability to give consent, e.g. unconscious patients, severely ill patients in intensive care or dying patients. An assessment of the patient's capacity to give informed consent for a procedure should be made following the guidelines listed earlier (DoH 2001c).

Under English law, no one is able to give consent to the examination or treatment of an adult unable to give consent for him or herself (an 'incapable' adult) (DoH 2001c). Therefore relatives, parents or members of the health care team cannot give consent on behalf of such an adult.

In general, the refusal of an intervention made by a patient before their loss of capacity cannot be overridden if the refusal is valid and applicable to the situation, e.g. in an advance directive (DoH 2001c).

Best interests should not be confused with best medical interests. Factors such as the patient's values and preferences when competent, their psychological health, well-being, quality of life, relationships with family or other carers, spiritual and religious welfare and their own financial interests should be taken into account. Unless a patient has stated that certain individuals should not be involved in decision making, it is considered good practice for health care teams to involve those close to the patient to determine the patient's values and beliefs before their loss of capacity.

Temporary incapacity

When an adult who usually has capacity becomes temporarily incapable, e.g. whilst under a general anaesthetic or sedation or after a road accident, the law permits interventions to be made which are necessary and no more than is reasonably required in the patient's best interests pending the recovery of capacity (DoH 2001c). This includes such routine procedures as washing and assistance with feeding. This does not apply if a valid advance refusal of treatment is applicable to the circumstances. Where it is possible to delay a planned medical intervention thought to be in the patient's best interests, until the patient recovers capacity and can consent (or refuse), it should be delayed until that time.

Long-standing incapacity

Where the adult's incapacity is likely to be long-standing, it will be lawful to carry out any procedure that is in the best interests of the adult (DoH 2001c). The House of Lords has suggested that action taken 'to preserve the life, health or well-being' of a patient will be in their best interests and subsequent court judgements have emphasized that a patient's best interests go beyond their best medical interests, to include much wider welfare considerations (DoH 2001c). Routine procedures such as dressing, washing, putting to bed and assisting in the consumption of food and drink are considered to be caring for patients in their best interests.

When treatments are given to patients on the basis of best interests, a consent form for patients who are unable to give consent should be used. It should be clearly documented on the form why the treatment is thought to be in the patient's best interests.

Fluctuating capacity

It is possible for capacity to fluctuate, e.g. in cases of hypercalcaemia, sepsis and drug toxicity. In such cases, it is good practice, whilst the person has capacity, to establish their views about any clinical intervention that may be necessary during a period of incapacity and to record these views (DoH 2001c).

Patients may choose to make an advance refusal of certain aspects of treatment. If this has not happened, the treatment of the incapable patient should be in accordance with the principles for treating the temporarily incapacitated.

Legal advice

If there is an element of doubt about the patient's capacity or even their best interests, the High Court can give a ruling on these matters and also the lawfulness/unlawfulness of a planned treatment/procedure. Duty offices of the Official NHS Solicitor can advise on the appropriate procedure if necessary. The Official NHS Solicitor can be contacted through the Urgent Court Business Officer out of office hours on 020 7947 6000. This should usually be done through the legal department of the NHS body involved.

Conclusion

This chapter has discussed the current context of health care, identifying the issues that influence the use and development of nursing procedures in the delivery of patient-centred care. The procedures in this book affect the whole person. They range from those that are observational and physically non-invasive to those involving intrusion into both the physical body and the psychological persona. The intent also varies; some are diagnostic, others therapeutic and some are supportive with the aim of increasing well-being.

It is important not to forget that even if a procedure is very familiar to us and we are very confident in carrying it out, it may be new to the patient, so time must be taken to explain it and gain consent, even if this is only verbal consent. The diverse range of technical procedures that patients may be subjected to should act as a reminder not to lose sight of the unique person undergoing such procedures and the importance of individualized patient assessment (which will be discussed in the next chapter) in achieving this.

Nurses have a central role to play in helping patients to manage the demands of the procedures described in this book. It must not be forgotten that for the patient the clinical procedure is part of a larger picture, which encompasses an appreciation of the unique experience of illness.

References and further reading

Benner, P. (1984) *From Novice to Expert*. Addison Wesley, California.

Benner, P., Tanner, C.A. & Chesla, C.A. (1996) *Expertise in Nursing Practice*. Springer, New York.

BMA (1995) *Advance Statements About Medical Treatment*. BMJ Publishing, London.

Briggs, A. (1972) *Report of the Committee on Nursing*. Cmnd 5115. HMSO, London.

Centre for Health Economics (2003) *Improving the Effectiveness of the Nursing Workforce*. University of York, York.

Cox, C.L. & Reyes-Hughes, A. (2002) Clinical effectiveness, nursing diagnosis and the role of the clinical nurse specialist and nurse practitioner. In: *Clinical Effectiveness in Practice*. Palgrave, Basingstoke, pp. 1–17.

DoH (1998) *A First Class Service*. Department of Health, London.

DoH (2000) *The NHS Cancer Plan*. Department of Health, London.

DoH (2001a) *National Service Framework for Older People*. Department of Health, London.

DoH (2001b) *Essence of Care Benchmarks*. Department of Health, London.

DoH (2001c) *Reference Guide to Consent for Examination or Treatment*. Department of Health, London.

DoH (2002) *Discharge from Hospital: Pathway, Process and Practice*. Department of Health, London.

Ford, P. & Walsh, M. (1994) *New Rituals for Old*. Butterworth Heinemann, Oxford.

Fowell, A., Finlay, I., Johnstone, R. & Minto, L. (2002) An integrated care pathway for the last two days of life: Wales-wide benchmarking in palliative care. *Int J Palliat Nurs*, **8**(12), 566–73.

GMC (1998) *Seeking Patients' Consent. The Ethical Considerations*. General Medical Council, London.

Goding, L. & Edwards, K. (2002) Evidence-based practice. *Nurse Researcher*, **9**(4), 45–57.

Hawkins, J.W. & Holcombe, J.K. (1995) Titling for advanced practice nurses. *Oncol Nurs Forum*, **22**(8), 5–9.

Kelson, M. (2001) Patient involvement in clinical governance. In: *Advancing Clinical Governance* (eds M. Lugon & J. Secker-Walker). Royal Society of Medicine Press, London.

Kibbe, D.C., Kaluzny, A.D. & McLaughlin, C.P. (1994) Integrating guidelines with continuous quality improvement: doing the right thing the right way to achieve the right goals. *J Qual Improvement*, **20**(4), 181–91.

Kitson, A., Harvey, G. & McCormack, B. (1998) Enabling the implementation of evidence based practice: a conceptual framework. *Qual Health Care*, **7**(3), 149–58.

Lillyman, S. (1998) Assessing competence. In: *Advanced and Specialist Nursing Practice* (eds G. Castledine & P. McGee). Blackwell Science, Oxford.

Ling, J. (1997) Clinical trials, palliative care and the research nurse. *Int J Palliat Nurs*, **3**(4), 192–6.

Mann, T. (1996) *Clinical Audit in the NHS*. NHSE, Leeds.

NHS Management Executive (1991) *Junior Doctors: The New Deal*. NHSME, London.

NHSE (1996) *Achieving Effective Practice: A Clinical Effectiveness and Research Information Pack for Nurses, Midwives and Health Visitors*. Department of Health, Leeds.

NHSE (1997) *The New NHS: Modern, Dependable*. Department of Health, London.

NHSE (1999a) *Clinical Governance: Quality in the New NHS*. Department of Health, London.

NHSE (1999b) *Clinical Governance in London Region, Draft Template of Audit Risk Management Report for a Trust Board*. NHSE London Region (www.doh.gov.uk/ntro/risktemp.htm), London.

NHSE (2000) *The NHS Plan. A Plan for Investment, A Plan for Reform*. Department of Health, London.

NICE (2001) *Pressure Ulcer Risk Assessment and Prevention*. National Institute for Clinical Excellence, London.

NICE/NHS Modernization Agency (2003) *Protocol-Based Care* (www.modern.nhs.uk/protocolbasedcare/default.htm). Department of Health, London.

NMC (1999) *A Higher Level of Practice*. NMC, London.

NMC (2002) *The Code of Professional Conduct*. NMC, London.

O'Dowd, A. (2003) Who should perform the caring role? *Nurs Times*, **99**(10), 10–11.

Rees, E. (2001) The ethics and practicalities of consent in palliative care research: an overview. *Int J Palliat Nurs*, **7**(10), 489–92.

Resuscitation Council (UK) (2000) *Resuscitation Council Guidelines*. Resuscitation Council (UK), London.

Richardson, G. & Maynard, A. (1995) *Fewer Doctors? More Nurses? A Review of the Knowledge Base of Doctor Nurse Substitution*. Centre for Health Economics, University of Leeds, Leeds.

Rolfe, G. (2001) *Closing the Theory Practice Gap: A New Paradigm for Nursing*. Butterworth Heinemann, Oxford.

Royal Marsden Hospital (1999) *Role Development Profile*. Royal Marsden NHS Trust, London.

Royal Marsden Hospital Quality Assurance Department (2001) *The Relationship Between Clinical Audit and Clinical Effectiveness*. Royal Marsden NHS Trust, London.

Royal Marsden NHS Trust (2003) *Advanced Nursing Practice at The Royal Marsden NHS Trust 1999–2002*. Royal Marsden NHS Trust, London.

Smith, R. (1998) Informed consent: edging forwards (and backwards). Informed consent is an unavoidably complicated issue. *Br Med J*, **316**(7136), 949–51.

Spilsbury, K. & Meyer, J. (2001) Defining the nursing contribution to patient outcome: lessons from a review of the literature examining nursing outcomes, skill mix and changing roles. *J Clin Nurs*, **10**(1), 3–14.

Swage, T. (2000) *Clinical Governance in Health Care Practice*. Butterworth Heinemann, Oxford.

UKCC (1992) *Scope of Professional Practice*. UKCC, London.

Walsh, M. & Ford, P. (1989) *Nursing Rituals, Research and Rational Actions*. Heinemann Nursing, Oxford.

Weir-Hughes, D. (2000) Foreword to Fifth Edition. In: *The Royal Marsden Hospital Manual of Clinical Nursing Procedures* (eds J. Mallett & L. Dougherty). Blackwell Science, Oxford.

Wilson, J.H. (1999) Risk reviews and using a risk management strategy. In: *Clinical Risk Modification, A Route to Clinical Governance?* (eds J. Wilson & J. Tingle). Butterworth Heinemann, Oxford.

World Medical Association (2002) *Declaration of Helsinki: Ethical Principles for Medical Research Involving Human Subjects*. WMA General Assembly, Washington.

Communication and assessment

Introduction

Nursing practice encompasses a process of judgement. This facilitates identification and assessment of patients' potential needs and expectations, in order that they may be adequately and appropriately addressed before, during and after any episode of nursing care.

Effective communication is crucial to the delivery of high-quality nursing intervention. The first section of this chapter explores the knowledge and skills required to communicate with cancer patients along the cancer journey, thereby allowing patients to express their needs during the experience of illness. The second section highlights the assessment skills required to identify cancer patients' needs and the importance of regarding patients as individuals with unique expectations and problems. Although the communication issues discussed here are applied to the cancer care setting, they may be equally relevant to a wide range of different illnesses.

Communication

The effective use of communication skills is an integral and essential part of nursing practice and one of the most vital tools nurses have to support patients and their families. The need for effective communication within health care is being increasingly recognized and both *The NHS Plan* (DoH 2000a) and *The NHS Cancer Plan* (DoH 2000b) call for the development and improvement of communication skills in health care professionals. This section will consider some of the verbal and non-verbal skills required for effective communication before moving on to examine specific communication issues for patients at different stages of their cancer journey. The communication issues that arise within the areas of children with cancer and genetic counselling will also be discussed.

Verbal and non-verbal communication

Communication is a reciprocal process that involves the exchange of both verbal and non-verbal messages to convey feelings, information, ideas and knowledge (Wilkinson 1999; Wallace 2001). It is important to be aware that it is possible to give one verbal message whilst transmitting an incongruent non-verbal one. For example, a nurse may adopt an inappropriate, cheerful expression while discussing a poor prognosis. Non-verbal communication can convey much to patients who often pay close attention to the expressions and demeanour of health care professionals (Fallowfield & Jenkins 1999). It is therefore important that health care professionals are aware of the influence on communication of factors such as tone and pitch of voice, speech rate, facial expressions, eye contact, gestures, posture and touch. Touch is an important aspect of non-verbal communication that can be directed and used in a meaningful manner to offer comfort, emotional interaction and connection (Chang 2001). However, patients can vary in their interpretation and experiences of touch and it can therefore be viewed as inappropriate and non-therapeutic for some patients (Routasalo 1999; Sapir *et al.* 2000).

Skills of communication

Cancer patients and their families are often dissatisfied about their interactions with health care professionals (National Cancer Alliance 1996). Nurses' communication skills are suggested to have shown little improvement in the past 20 years (Wilkinson 1999). It has been found that nurses are often not proficient in communicating with their patients and in identifying their patients' difficulties (Wilkinson 1991; Maguire *et al.* 1996; Heaven & Maguire 1997). The following section therefore focuses on those skills that may be considered central to effective communication. Although the area of oncology is used as an example, the communication skills discussed are equally relevant to other care settings.

Basic communication skills

A central and fundamental aspect of communication is listening (Burnard 1998a). Oncology patients asked to describe what makes a nurse a good communicator have emphasized the importance of listening (Bailey & Wilkinson 1998). Listening is vital if nurses are to understand the meaning that patients attribute to their cancer (Mullally 2000). Listening is also an important tool in helping health care professionals to assess patients' problems, needs and resources (Razavi & Delvaux 1997).

Basic communication skills include the use of clarification, reflection, probing, summarizing and open questions. Clarification can be illustrated as:

Patient: 'I don't think I can cope with chemotherapy.'
Nurse: 'What is it about chemotherapy that particularly worries you?'

Here the nurse is seeking to understand more specifically what the patient means and the use of clarification gives the patient the chance to expand and amplify their previous comment (Buckman 2001).

Reflection may be used to communicate understanding, to check accuracy and to facilitate further exploration of feelings (Macleod Clark & Sims 1988). For example:

Patient: 'I'm finding things really hard at the moment since starting radiotherapy.'
Nurse: 'Really hard?'

At times probing may be employed to invite the patient to expand on a particular issue and clarify any vagueness. For example:

Nurse: 'You mentioned you were having trouble sleeping since your surgery. Can you tell me more about that?'

Summarizing helps the nurse and the patient to draw the main issues of the interaction together and allows for the clarification of mutual understanding. The use of summarizing by health care professionals has been shown to promote the disclosure of key concerns by patients (Maguire *et al.* 1996). Silence, although uncomfortable at times, can also be a powerful communication skill used to encourage the patient to reflect on what has been said.

The use of open questions can be considered one of the simplest and yet most effective means of encouraging patients to disclose their concerns and to communicate at a level comfortable for them (Burnard 1997; Wilkinson 1999). Open questions are useful in the assessment of patients' problems and their use by health care professionals has been found to facilitate disclosure of significant information (Maguire *et al.* 1996). An open question is prefixed by words such as 'When', 'What' or 'How' and will help to discourage a 'Yes' or 'No' answer.

Advanced communication skills

Some advanced skills that require more practice and self-awareness are empathy, unconditional positive regard and challenging. Confusion arises in the literature as to whether empathy is more about an attitude and an innate way of being rather than a communication skill that can be taught (Kunyk & Olson 2001; Lanceley 2001a). Empathy has been defined as 'the ability to communicate understanding of another person's experience from that person's perspective' (British Association for Counselling and Psychotherapy 2002, p. 4) and has been found to facilitate patients' disclosure of their concerns and feelings (Maguire *et al.* 1996). It differs from identification and sympathy (Hope-Stone & Mills 2001) and requires being alert to what feelings may lie behind patients' words and paying attention to what may be implied but not spoken. Deeper and more important questions may lie behind overt and obvious ones (Chauhan & Long 2000a). For example, a cancer patient asking whether they will be able to go on the holiday they have booked for next year may be indirectly asking when they will die. Unconditional positive regard (Rogers 1967) means that the patient is viewed with dignity and valued as a worthwhile human being without judgement or criticism. Finally, challenging can be described as giving an invitation to change and may involve confronting inconsistencies and picking up on what the patient has implied but is unaware of themselves. Challenges can result in patients seeing a wider perspective, deepening their perceptions or altering their point of view (Bayne *et al.* 1998).

Counselling could also be viewed as advanced practice and is frequently described in the nursing literature as an aspect of nursing work (Burnard 1998b). However, nurses using advanced communication skills may not be counselling in a formal sense but instead may be using counselling skills. For nurses to be formally counselling they have to be perceived by patients to be in that role and an agreement made with the patient to enter into a counselling relationship (Lanceley 2001a). Nurses also need to undertake a recognized training programme and have appropriate supervision if they are to work as counsellors. The British Association for Counselling and Psychotherapy (2001, p. 1) suggests that 'counselling takes place when a counsellor sees a client in a private and confidential setting to explore a difficulty the client is having'.

Communication skills training

A number of efforts have been made to improve the communication skills of health care professionals working in an oncology setting. These include formal courses, workshops and the development of guidelines, for example, around the topic of breaking bad news. However, debate exists as to whether communication skills can be taught. While it has been suggested in the past that good communicators are born and not made, studies have shown that nurses can learn and develop such skills given appropriate training (Wilkinson *et al.* 1998, 1999, 2002). It has been recommended that communication training in oncology needs to be learner centred and address attitudes, feelings and beliefs in addition to knowledge and skill development (Heaven & Maguire 1996; Booth *et al.* 1999; Fallowfield & Jenkins 1999). Nurses have been found to need most help in addressing emotionally laden

areas such as discussing diagnosis and prognosis or dealing with patients' anger (Wilkinson *et al.* 1998).

Communication along the cancer journey

Effective communication can make a huge difference to the quality of life of patients throughout the whole disease trajectory (Maguire 1999; Thorne 1999). However, it is also important to consider the specific communication needs of patients at different stages of their cancer journey and it is to this area that we now turn.

Diagnosis

How to communicate bad news is increasingly becoming a key topic. It is a topic that is relevant not only at the diagnosis stage, but throughout the cancer journey. Although nurses may not always be involved directly in giving the diagnosis, there are numerous other opportunities when effective communication skills in delivering bad news are required (Radziewicz & Baile 2001). To give some examples, nurses may be required to give explanations about diagnosis, answer questions and clarify information or may be needed to help the patient understand treatment choices. Much has been written about the way in which bad news is given and the impact that this can have on the patient's subsequent ability to cope and adjust to their disease (Lowden 1998; Chauhan & Long 2000b). For example, it has been suggested that patients who perceive that their doctor is more caring during the diagnosis consultation may have better long-term psychological adjustment to their illness (Mager & Andrykowski 2002).

Communication failures at the time of diagnosis may fuel anxiety that cancer is an unmentionable disease with an unspeakable future (Fallowfield & Jenkins 1999) and subsequently may influence patient treatment compliance and their attitude towards living with their disease (Lowden 1998). Questions such as 'What has caused my cancer?' can result in much distress if they remain undiscussed as the patient may well come to their own conclusions and perhaps view their disease as a punishment for past events (Burton & Watson 1998).

A report into NHS cancer care found that although most people felt that their diagnosis had been given in an honest, caring and sensitive manner, there were still some patients who reported negative experiences (Commission for Health Improvement 2001). Breaking bad news is clearly a very individual process and the words and manner used with one patient may not be appropriate for another (Burton & Watson 1998). Guidance has been produced on how to break bad news (Buckman 1992; Maguire 1998; Baile *et al.* 2000). Key factors include the use of clear language which avoids medical jargon or euphemisms such as 'mass' or 'blockage' (Franks 1997).

It is important to assess firstly what the patient thinks is happening and for some warning to be given that all is not well (Burton & Watson 1998). This can help in the assessment of what the patient wants to know, as it is necessary to allow patients to limit and have some control over what they are told. For example, the patient who states 'I really do not want to know the results of my scan. I assume that there is something that can be done to treat what I have?' needs to have their wishes respected. If patients do want to know their diagnosis then health care professionals need to allow the patient time in order to take in the information given and need to be empathic about how the patient might be feeling (Ptacek & Ptacek 2001).

Patients need to be allowed to disclose and discuss their feelings and concerns before health care professionals rush on to giving advice and reassurance (Maguire 1998). For example, questions such as 'I can see that this news is very upsetting for you. What concerns you most about it?' can be useful in acknowledging the patient's distress and inviting them to talk more about it. It can also be helpful to clarify what has been understood as many patients are shocked after diagnosis and cannot remember what they have been told after hearing the word 'cancer' (Burton & Watson 1998). Nurses need to be prepared to repeat information several times if required (Sawyer 2000). Audiotapes of consultations have been positively received by some patients (McClement & Hack 1999). Patients may also want to have someone with them when hearing bad news (Faulkner & Maguire 1994) and may value the provision of information on external sources of support.

It is also important to consider environmental factors in the hospital setting that inhibit therapeutic communication such as noise, interruptions and lack of privacy (Fallowfield & Jenkins 1999). If bad news is going to be given it is helpful if the patient can be seen in a private room (Maguire 1998) where an engaged sign on the door can minimize interruptions and the telephone is silenced. Screens around the patient's bed only provide visual privacy and standing in a corridor or in a busy waiting room discussing difficult and painful issues is unsatisfactory (Faulkner 1998).

Several studies have shown that the majority of patients do want to know their diagnosis and desire information about the treatment and its side-effects (Meredith *et al.* 1996; Jenkins *et al.* 2001). Cancer patients have ranked being given information on their condition and treatment as one of the most important aspects of their diagnosis consultation (Parker *et al.* 2001), and yet have reported their dissatisfaction with the information received and the manner of its delivery (Audit Commission 1993). It has been recommended that all patients should have a clear explanation of their treatment

options in order to help them make an informed choice (DoH 1991, 1995). Patients will be unable to make an informed choice if they have not been given sufficient information in the first place (Fallowfield 1997). Providing information for patients according to their own agendas may facilitate psychological adaptation and acceptance of their illness and treatment. Giving information may also help the cancer patient to regain a sense of control, enhance compliance and satisfaction, develop coping skills, decrease fear and anxiety and empower the patient to participate in their treatment (Mills & Sullivan 1999; Sawyer 2000). However, nurses need to remember that cancer patients may vary considerably in the amount of information that they want to know about their disease, and in how much they want to be involved in treatment decisions (Leydon *et al.* 2000; Drew & Fawcett 2002). Cancer patients' needs in this area may also change across their cancer trajectory (Van der Molen 1999). Whatever the information required, it needs to be communicated in a clear, simple and structured manner using short words and sentences, with the most important facts being given first (Burnard 1997).

A common problem that nurses can experience at this stage is managing the demands of friends and family for information (Woods 1998). Family and friends have high needs for information and emotional support at the diagnosis stage, as they may equally be feeling shocked, frightened and confused. Ethically, nurses should first discuss clinical information with the patient and obtain their permission before talking about it with relatives (Burton & Watson 1998). Speaking to carers separately about the diagnosis may also set up a barrier, and can be very isolating for both the carers and the patient. Instead nurses could more actively involve and support the carers of cancer patients by inviting them to consultations and arranging family meetings if the patient is in agreement (Spiece *et al.* 2000).

Several factors have been identified that may make breaking bad news to cancer patients difficult for health care professionals (Franks 1997; Radziewicz & Baile 2001). These include:

- Fear of upsetting the patient
- Fear of being blamed for the news
- Anxiety about how they will deal with the patient's reactions
- Discomfort at being around those distressed by the news
- Worry over the questions they may be asked
- Lack of training in this area.

Health care professionals may fear that patients may not be able to cope with negative information about their health and therefore try to shield patients from the reality of their diagnosis (Fallowfield 1997). It has also been suggested that nurses can hold certain illogical beliefs that may interfere with effective communication in cancer care; for example, that patients will hate them if they give them bad news (Thorne 1999). False assumptions such as the belief that patients will disclose their problems themselves may also limit effective communication. It is important to recognize that sharing bad news can also evoke a personal struggle for nurses as they walk closely alongside patients and carers on their cancer journey (Radziewicz & Baile 2001). Nurses can be left feeling vulnerable, distressed and inadequate after a patient is told bad news (Cooley 2000; Dunniece & Slevin 2000).

Treatment

The primary role of the nurse in communication at this stage of the patient pathway is to assess, identify and help to prioritize the needs of patients and families as well as facilitating their expression of feelings and building a relationship in which care can take place. Successful communication is essential if nurses are to accurately identify and assess their oncology patients' problems and plan individualized patient care to meet their differing physical, psychological, social, sexual and spiritual needs (Bailey & Wilkinson 1998; Wilkinson et al. 1999). If communication is limited then the nursing assessment may be superficial and care planned on restricted information and nurses' assumptions of need.

Effective communication skills are especially important at the time of admission for treatment as the nurse needs to create an environment of trust so that the patient feels valued, understood, involved and accepted (Kruijver et al. 2001). Oncology wards can be frightening places for patients and nurses can ask questions such as: 'How do you feel about coming into hospital for an operation?' This will give patients the opportunity to express their fears and subsequently receive information and support (Burton & Watson 1998). The treatment phase is also a vital time for nurses to follow up how their patients have adapted to the diagnosis (Faulkner & Maguire 1994). Exploratory questions such as 'What impact has your illness had on you?' and 'How supported do you feel by those around you?' can reveal much useful information for the assessment process as well as demonstrating to patients a willingness to discuss emotional issues. Indeed, the use by health care professionals of questions with a psychological focus has been found to facilitate disclosure of key concerns by patients (Maguire et al. 1996).

The organizational context may have a profound influence on the patient's opportunities for communication during treatment (Chant et al. 2002). It has been suggested that the institutional and professional culture

in which nurses work encourages them to avoid the anxiety of intimate nurse–patient relationships through practices such as task allocation and placement rotation (Menzies Lyth 1988). A task-orientated environment where talking is not considered to be working is obviously not going to encourage communication between patients and nurses. Indeed, the ward on which nurses work has been found to be a predictor of the quality of nurse–patient communication and ward sisters/charge nurses have a strong influence as role models (Wilkinson 1991). Nurses need to feel secure that they will not get into trouble for spending time communicating openly with their patients (Wilkinson et al. 1999). Indeed, it has been found that nurses who felt supported practically and psychologically by their supervisor lessened their use of blocking behaviours when communicating with patients (Booth et al. 1996).

Communication is a mutual process and it is also important to remember the influence of the patient on the communication process (Jarrett & Payne 1995). Awareness and recognition of the patient's emotional adjustment to cancer may enable nurses to communicate more effectively with them. There were initially four adjustment styles identified by Greer & Watson (1987) which indicated how patients could react to the experience of cancer and thus influence the communication process. Patients could change their adjustment styles according to their circumstances and there is a danger in assuming that patients may fall into specific categories. The adjustment styles identified were:

- Fighting spirit
- Fatalism
- Helplessness and hopelessness
- Anxious preoccupation.

Nurses can ask questions to clarify the patient's usual coping strategy and therefore gain some insight into how they are coping with the disease. For example, if helplessness is suspected an appropriate question could be: 'People diagnosed with cancer can sometimes feel very overwhelmed and helpless. How do you feel about what has happened?' (Burton & Watson 1998).

Denial is also an adjustment style and can cause much anxiety for oncology nurses who may be unsure how to manage it. Denial is a defence mechanism that may help the patient to cope by warding off anxiety (Lanceley 2001b) and it may give way when patients are more able to assimilate events or as the disease progresses. It is often not advisable therefore for health care professionals to try to break down denial by forcing patients to confront reality (Greer 1992). They can instead ensure that the patient is aware that they are available to talk if the need arises. However, if denial is resulting in negative consequences such as refusal of treatment then it may be necessary to probe further (Faulkner & Maguire 1994). This can be done gently through monitoring perceptions and exploring any inconsistencies from the patient (Faulkner 1998). For example: 'Have there been any times when you have thought that you might not beat this illness?'

There may be many other patient-led barriers to effective communication besides denial. Examples of these include (Jarrett & Payne 1995; Maguire 1999):

- Fear of appearing ignorant
- Fear of upsetting the nurse
- Reluctance to question professionals
- Reluctance to take up too much of professionals' time
- Not knowing what to ask
- Embarrassment about delicate/sensitive issues
- Fear of hearing bad news
- Fear of losing control
- Associating nurses with physical rather than psychological care.

Patients may also be socialized by their family or other patients into maintaining a brave, cheerful and non-complaining appearance or may assume that their concerns are an inevitable consequence of cancer and something that nurses can do little about (Maguire 1999). In addition, anxiety, depression or the presence of physical symptoms such as pain may impair the ability of the patient to communicate or retain information. Finally, some patients may simply not want to talk about their feelings and nurses need to recognize and respect this.

Patients with cancer have been reported to have a high prevalence of undetected psychological problems and are at risk of psychological morbidity if their concerns remain undisclosed, undetected and therefore unresolved (Parle et al. 1996; Fallowfield et al. 2001a). Patients who are given the opportunity to discuss their concerns report feeling relieved, reassured and encouraged (Bailey & Wilkinson 1998). Nurses are ideally placed to use their communication skills to assist cancer patients with any psychological problems during the treatment phase, as they are often caring for them on a 24-hour basis. Attention therefore needs to be given to eliciting and helping patients to resolve their concerns, to the detection and management of any anxiety and depression experienced and making referrals to appropriate agencies. Examples of questions that could be used to assess anxiety or depression include: 'It sounds as if you are feeling tense and on edge for much of the time. Could you tell me more about that?' or 'I am wondering how you are feeling at the moment as it sounds as if you are quite low and depressed'.

Scope also exists for improving the contribution of nurses to the care and support of families and friends of people with cancer during the treatment phase (Yates 1999). Cancer treatment seriously affects the well-being of relatives and friends as well as cancer patients themselves (Eriksson 2001). If relatives and friends are to continue to support the patient during their treatment and yet maintain their own well-being then they have considerable needs in terms of information and emotional support (Eriksson 2000). Nurses can encourage open communication between the patient and family and friends, and can also play a key role in providing information and involving family and friends in decision making (Speice et al. 2000).

Recurrence

It has been suggested that the existential crisis of having cancer is repeated every time that cancer recurs (Burton & Watson 1998), especially when patients had previously believed that they were cured or would survive for many years. However, research has shown that instead of nurses communicating openly with these patients and trying to help them cope with the anxiety of an uncertain future, nurses often used blocking behaviours in communicating with patients with recurrent cancer (Wilkinson 1991). It can be useful to remember the same basic principles described above when breaking the bad news of a recurrence and to check how the patient is managing the uncertainty by asking simple questions such as: 'How do you see things working out in the future?' Once again, some patients may benefit from detailed information about their condition and possible treatments at this stage and others may not wish to know (Faulkner & Maguire 1994). If the patient is indeed finding the uncertainty hard, it is important to acknowledge and empathize with these feelings, for example by saying: 'I imagine it is very difficult for you that we cannot be sure how things are going to work out'.

Palliative and terminal care

Effective communication has been described as a core element of palliative care (Wallace 2001). There are numerous situations within palliative care where nurses need good communication skills and the discussion above on breaking bad news at the point of diagnosis is equally relevant here. For example, nurses are often asked to confirm disease progression after the doctor has left the room and may be required to help patients come to terms with the limitations in their treatment options (Radziewicz & Baile 2001). Nurses need to establish the needs of palliative care patients and respond appropriately if they are to help them to resolve their physical, psychological, social and spiritual problems, assist them to readjust their plans and aims and make optimal use of whatever time is remaining (Booth et al. 1996). Nurses need to ask the patient how they are feeling and what they are worried about in order to ascertain fears and concerns at this stage. For example, the patient may want to talk about fears of dying in pain, choking or bleeding to death, or may have spiritual concerns about what happens after death. Unless these concerns are discussed, support and reassurance cannot be given. Failure to discuss difficult issues such as end-of-life care may also result in oncology nurses making clinical decisions that are not consistent with the preferences of their patients (Radziewicz & Baile 2001).

A key task in the palliative care setting once again may be to encourage open communication between cancer patients and their relatives and friends. The communication needs and coping strategies of patients and carers may not always match at this stage and nurses may well find themselves caught in the middle of these differences (Davy & Ellis 2000). For instance, it has been suggested that relatives may find open communication more satisfying during terminal care, whereas patients may need to escape at times into denial or avoidance of discussion of their disease outcome (Hinton 1998). Similarly, terminal patients may need to feel a degree of solitude and separateness from others as part of the dying process (Burton & Watson 1998) and it can be helpful to explain this to relatives who may be finding this withdrawal very painful. As stated previously, silence and touch can still be very useful and important ways of communicating presence and comfort.

Relatives may not want patients to be informed of disease progression or poor prognosis and may ask nurses to collude with them in this. Although it is often considered that this is based on the carers' fear and distress, it may also be requested as an act of love and a need to protect (Faulkner 1998). It can be very tempting for the nurse to agree to this request for collusion or dismiss it out of hand by telling the carer they are wrong in wanting to do so (Davy & Ellis 2000). However, it is more helpful to validate, acknowledge and normalize the relatives' feelings, to allow opportunity for further discussion in order to explore what underlies this request, and to discuss the emotional costs to relatives of hiding this news (Friedrichsen et al. 2001). It is important to explain that the patient's need for an explanation of what is happening must be met and relatives may value being informed of the fact that the patient may be aware or suspicious of the truth themselves. Relatives can also be reassured by hearing that if the patient expresses a clear wish not to be given information about what is happening, then this will be respected (Burton & Watson 1998).

Avoiding talking about death and dying with the patient does not necessarily mean that the patient will die happily in ignorance as they may well be able to see

their own deterioration for themselves (Fallowfield 1997). Glaser & Strauss (1965) studied terminally ill patients and identified four awareness contexts which may apply to patients and those close to them:

- Closed
- Suspected
- Mutual pretence
- Open awareness.

With closed and suspected awareness there is an imbalance of information as the family, nursing or medical staff act as custodians of information that the patient does not have. There is more potential for misunderstandings and distress to all parties than when the communication is open and mutual. It is important to recognize that these categories are not absolute; the patient and family may fluctuate between levels of awareness at different stages of the illness experience (Field & Copp 1999).

The patient's need for open communication may conflict with the health care professional's desire to protect their patients by retaining an optimistic message even if the prognosis is poor (Faulkner 1998). Health care professionals' use of blocking tactics with the dying have been highlighted, such as using closed questions, avoiding eye contact, ignoring cues, changing the subject, discouraging questions, giving false reassurance and selectively focusing on the physical illness symptoms (Webster 1981; Maguire 1985). Health care professionals may use distancing tactics as a means of preserving their own emotional survival if they are concerned about becoming too involved with their patients (Maguire 1985; Fallowfield & Jenkins 1999). Communicating with patients who are facing life-threatening illnesses is not simple and nurse–patient communication in oncology can be emotionally draining and a source of intense stress (Wilkinson et al. 1999; Kruijver et al. 2000). Nurses therefore may avoid communicating with patients in favour of more routine tasks in order to avoid such stress.

Although avoidance and distancing are natural defence mechanisms in stressful situations, nurses who develop increased self-awareness may recognize when this is occurring in their everyday work. Self-awareness has been described as 'the gradual and continuous process of noticing and exploring aspects of the self, whether behavioural, psychological or physical, with the intention of developing personal and interpersonal understanding' (Burnard 1997, p. 68). Self-awareness can be developed through self-monitoring and by staying aware of what one does and feels in communications with others. Good self-awareness is essential for effective communication (Wilkinson et al. 1998) and may help to deepen sensitivity and safeguard against communication blunders. Knowledge and awareness of the self can assist nurses to recognize the boundaries between their own needs and feelings and those of their patients and to discern how their own reactions may be influencing the communication process.

Communication differences

It is important to recognize the influence on communication of factors such as culture, gender, type of disease, education, age, social background, language and disability. For example, different cultures may have varying views about whether the diagnosis and prognosis are disclosed to patients (Becker 1999). A patient with head and neck cancer may have very different communication issues from a patient with breast cancer. However, communication needs to be tailored to the individual rather than based on assumptions relating to, for example, the patient's age, gender or culture. Every patient's circumstances, concerns and wishes may differ.

Interprofessional communication

It has been suggested that unless professionals communicate well with each other they are unlikely to be effective in their interactions with patients and carers (Faulkner 1998). Yet some nurses have been reported to find interacting with colleagues more challenging than with their patients (Fallowfield *et al.* 2001b). This may be due to power differences, role confusion or simply variations in communication styles and philosophies of care. One important way of resolving these difficulties is for nurses to reflect on how they influence communication and at times to try to put themselves into their colleagues' shoes and communicate using their language (Mullally 2000). Regular team meetings may also be helpful in enhancing interprofessional communication (Faulkner 1998) and in reducing stress and confusion for both oncology staff and patients.

Communicating with children with cancer

When thinking about communication with a child who has cancer, it is crucial to place them in their family context, their developmental level, their usual family communication patterns, where they are in terms of diagnosis and treatment and past experience with illness and hospitals. Communicating with children should always be seen as part of an ongoing process, based on what information they know, what they want to know, who they want to talk to and how much information they want to be given at any particular time. Checking their views, preferences and needs is paramount, in order to create the optimal environment to show respect to the child and show they are really being listened to.

Basic communication skills will involve gaining the child's confidence, showing respect and engaging the child (Pinkerton *et al.* 1994; Lansdown 1996). It will then be necessary to attend closely and listen without interruptions to what the child is saying, both verbally and nonverbally, which will facilitate the engagement process (Edwards & Davis 1997). Awareness of the child's developmental level and how their illness may affect normal development (Rowland 1989) will offer staff an insight into developmentally related communication issues and also suggest the most developmentally appropriate manner of engaging the child. It is also important to note that a child is less likely to be able to communicate if in pain, angry or frightened. It may be necessary to repeatedly attempt to engage with the child and professionals may need to accept that often it may just be the wrong time, wrong place or wrong person. At other times the circumstances are suddenly right for the child and conversation may be facilitated. Not all children can communicate verbally and with younger or regressed children who may be physically or cognitively impaired in some way, communication may need to be facilitated through non-verbal means, such as play, art or other visually creative ways. There is an additional need for flexibility when attempting communication with children (Adams & Deveau 1984; Lansdown 1996; Edwards & Davis 1997).

Children are usually part of a wider social system and any communication will usually have a family reference point. Staff therefore will need to be aware of how the child fits into the family system and how the illness becomes part of that system (Rait & Lederberg 1989; Goldenberg & Goldenberg 1996). This knowledge will enable staff to understand family communication patterns and pre-existing problems which all affect how the child copes with treatment. It will also often demonstrate the best way of interacting with the child, alone or with other family members. Potential problems can often be anticipated by the stage of the disease as different communication issues often arise at diagnosis, at the commencement of side-effects, remission, end of treatment, relapse, palliative care and bereavement (Adams & Deveau 1984; Lansdown 1996).

Communication with a minor can have its own ethical issues, concerning confidentiality, consent, spiritual and cultural issues, competency, wishes of parents and wishes of child, ethos of the treating unit and developmental appropriateness (Adams & Deveau 1984; Alderson & Montgomery 1996). Typical issues include the telling of prognosis and bad news, and conflict between family members about how much information should and could be imparted to the child patient. Often this requires the staff to act as advocates for the family members and to facilitate communication style in line with the family's wishes.

Communication with a child of an adult cancer patient

When considering communication with the child of an adult cancer patient, it is important to consider the child's developmental level and experience of illness and to see any communication as part of an ongoing dynamic process (McCue 1996). It is important to consider what has already been told, why it is being raised now, what should be told and when to tell it. In the author's experience, many parents report that they are afraid of starting the conversation because they are frightened they will say the wrong thing and cause irreparable damage. It is often a matter of guiding parents to open up conversations and find out first of all what the child already knows or fears in order to know where to pitch the conversation.

Advising parents what to say can be difficult as not only are they thinking about the needs of their child, but they are also dealing with their or their partner's illness, treatment, prognosis and related practical issues (Couldrick 1991). It may be helpful to advise the parents to think about the different issues likely to arise once the subject has been opened (Couldrick 1991) such as:

- What is cancer?
- Can children get it?
- Can it be caught?
- Will I get it?
- Are you going to leave me?
- Who can I talk to about it?
- Are you going to die?

The more a parent can feel prepared and aware of what may arise, the more confidence they will feel in facilitating communication with their child.

Genetic counselling

There are some individuals who develop cancer as the result of an inherited susceptibility. These individuals tend to develop cancer at a younger age than would be expected in the general population. Furthermore, the individual with a significant family history of other cancers has a higher risk of bilateral and/or multiple primary cancers.

The purpose of genetic counselling is to explain the realities of cancer risk and to provide appropriate screening or prevention advice. Furthermore, the individual with cancer may wish to understand more about their condition and the risk of further primary cancers. In families with high genetic risk the experiences of cancer in the family very often place a heavy emotional burden on 'healthy' relatives (Ardern-Jones 1997; Kenen *et al.* 2003).

Cancer family clinics for genetic counselling aim to collect a detailed cancer family history. It is important to collect accurate information about family members with regard to their cancer diagnosis in order to be able to assess the genetic risk. However, it is essential to have written consent from family members who are alive with regard to releasing information about their cancer diagnosis due to confidentiality regulations. Death certificates, histology departments and cancer registries provide sources of information on deceased patients.

In families where there are multiple cases of cancer at a younger age than expected and where there are known syndromes, e.g. breast/ovarian, bowel, bowel/endometrium, some family members wish to pursue the option of genetic testing as well as considering screening options. The reason for considering testing is that if there is a gene mutation in the family there is a 50/50 chance that direct relatives may not have inherited the familial mutation. If they do not have the mutation then the individual tested is at population risk of developing cancer and does not need an intensive screening programme.

The family member who has developed cancer at a younger age than expected starts off the process of genetic testing. This would involve a counselling session explaining the risks and benefits of genetic testing. It is not always possible to identify the mutation that must exist in the family because of the current limits in technology. The search for the mutation may take many months and for many families is uninformative, which can be stressful for the patient and family (Hallowell *et al.* 2002).

Communication in families may be somewhat confusing and women attending genetic counselling due to a family history of breast/ovarian cancer often put others' needs before their own (Hallowell 1999). The feeling of responsibility to be tested and to take action to balance the risk of developing cancer drives some women to consider the genetic test (Foster *et al.* 2002b).

Breast and ovarian screening is recommended for women with a high risk of a BRCA gene being present in the family (Eeles & Ardern-Jones 1999). However, the efficacy of such screening and preventive surgery in terms of saving lives in the group of patients carrying a breast/ovarian susceptibility gene is as yet unknown. Evidence is now emerging of the benefits of prophylactic surgery (Hartmann *et al.* 1999; Rebbeck *et al.* 1999). With bowel cancer families there is more evidence to suggest the efficacy of colon screening and prophylactic surgery (Tischkowitz 1999). Mutation carriers often face difficult decisions regarding screening, risk management and prophylactic surgery. Risk management includes the consideration of lifestyle factors such as choosing a time to have children, choosing whether or not to take oral contraceptive pills and in some cases choosing whether or not to undergo fertility treatment. As scientific knowledge in the area of cancer genetics is constantly changing, there is a need for gene carriers to be followed up in a specialized clinic (Ardern-Jones & Eeles 2002).

The predictive genetic test is only available to family members where the mutation is known. It is important to consider all the implications of a positive test with the person undergoing predictive testing, including the benefits of screening or surgery as well as the emotional issues (Foster *et al.* 2002a). There is no limit to the amount of time a person may need to take in this process. The specialist genetic nurse is ideally placed to support the patient throughout and after the testing. There may be considerable concerns for the 'at-risk' person who may be considering prophylactic surgery. It is recommended that a psychological counselling session or sessions should be arranged for individuals considering surgical procedures as a prevention option (Payne *et al.* 2000).

Cancer genetic counselling is a rapidly developing area of cancer medicine with many implications for family members both with and without cancer. A need for understanding and support is essential for these families who have experienced so much tragedy in their lives.

Summary

Communication with patients is not an optional issue but rather a core clinical skill which is a vital component of nursing care at whatever grade or level (Wilkinson 1999; Fallowfield *et al.* 2001b). Ineffective communication has been associated with emotional burnout, stress and poor job satisfaction in health care professionals (Wilkinson 1994; Ramirez *et al.* 1995). Conversely, effective communication with patients can help to improve satisfaction, compliance and pain control, reduce anxiety, establish trust and rapport, support and educate the patient and establish a plan for treatment (Stewart 1995; Fallowfield & Jenkins 1999).

Principles of assessment

Nursing assessment includes gathering, validating and organizing data, identifying patterns, and reporting and recording relevant data. Assessment is an ongoing dynamic process carried out by the nurse in order to identify the patient's most important needs and concerns and decide on a plan of care in collaboration with other health care professionals where appropriate. By evaluating the patient's health status and outcomes, the nurse is able to identify the patient's ongoing needs and

the effectiveness of care so that the existing care plan may be adapted (Alfaro-Lefevre 2002).

Nurses have a professional responsibility to ensure that health care records are 'an accurate account of treatment, care planning and delivery' and are viewed as 'a tool of communication within the team'. There should be 'clear evidence of the care planned, the decisions made, the care delivered and the information shared' (NMC 2002a, p. 6). The content and quality of record keeping are a measure of standards of practice relating to the skills and judgement of the nurse (NMC 2002b). Thus communication and assessment skills are integral to providing quality care.

Effective assessment of the patient will facilitate the safety, continuity and quality of patient care and fulfil nurses' legal and professional obligations. The following attributes should be considered in relation to assessment (Heartfield 1996; Allen 1998; Teytelman 2002; NMC 2002a, b; Alfaro-Lefevre 2002; White 2003).

1 Assessment is governed by the notion of patients' actual and potential needs and those of the family and friends, i.e. patient focused, and should adopt a holistic and multidisciplinary approach.
2 It should be a dynamic process, characterized by individualized care, which is relevant at any stage in the disease or treatment and should start ideally at diagnosis or before.
3 It should provide baseline information on which to plan the interventions and outcomes to be achieved, thus enabling evaluation of the care given.
4 It should be a process in which the patient ideally plays an active role.
5 It should be concerned with optimal functioning and the promotion of independence.
6 It should be concerned with quality of life.
7 It is a dimension of care influencing the patient's outcome and potential survival.
8 Assessment techniques and documentation vary according to the health care setting: day care, outpatient, inpatient, short or long stay, perioperative, critical care or rehabilitation care, acute or chronic illness, and primary care setting.

Assessment framework

Nursing models provide a framework to the assessment process enabling appropriate interventions and achievement of outcomes. A conceptual nursing model is designed as a set of concepts and statements integrated into a meaningful framework (Fawcett 1995; Christensen & Kenney 1995; Kozier *et al.* 1998). Different conceptual models have emerged over time, implying that there is a perceived value in the coexistence of a variety of perspectives. Assessment strategies and terminology are adopted from the model in question (Alfaro-Lefevre 2002). The organization of care, for example primary or team nursing, is believed to have an influence upon the decision-making process and the level of support as perceived by nurses (Waters & Easton 1999; Hansebo *et al.* 1999).

It is vital that nurses are aware of the rationale for implementing a particular nursing model for their area of practice, because this choice will largely determine the nature of patient assessment in their day-to-day work. If the model is inappropriate, the assessment data collected may be less effective than they could be (Tierney 1998; Murphy *et al.* 2000). Thus nursing models may be adapted to a particular clinical speciality to guide the overall process of care. For example, the concept of self-care, espoused by Orem (Orem *et al.* 2001), may be particularly suited to rehabilitation care but not where patients are highly dependent, such as critical care (Alfaro-Lefevre 2002). It has been suggested that nursing models have not been widely implemented in clinical practice but nurses do use them as a way to think about nursing (Griffiths 1998; Mason 1999; Wimpenny 2001).

Standardized nursing languages

Standardized nursing languages such as nursing diagnosis, nursing interventions or nursing outcomes classification systems provide nurses with a common language for communicating the nursing needs of patients (Grobe 1996; Moen *et al.* 1999; Payne 2000; Elfrink *et al.* 2001; Delaney 2001). One of the reasons for trying to structure nursing terms in a systematic way has been the need to analyse nursing information in a meaningful way from computer databases. The term 'nursing diagnosis' is not highly visible in the UK as no definitive classifications (or taxonomy) are in general use. There is a profusion of literature about nursing diagnosis from a North American perspective (Hardwick 1998) and the practicality of implementing standard language in clinical practice in the UK is currently being explored (Chambers 1998; Westbrook 2000; Lyte & Jones 2001).

'Patient problems or needs' is a common term used within nursing to facilitate communication about nursing care (Hogston 1997). As patient problems/needs may involve solutions or treatments from disciplines other than nursing, the concept of 'patient problem' is similar to but broader than nursing diagnosis. Nursing diagnosis is purely concerned with problems that may be dealt with by nursing expertise (Leih & Salentijn 1994) (see Box 2.1). Whether nursing diagnosis or problem/need identification is used in practice, the assessment data should reflect the language in use for communication, monitoring care processes and patient outcomes (Yancey *et al.* 1998;

> **Box 2.1** Characteristics of conditions labelled as nursing diagnoses (Gordon 1994)
>
> 1 Nurses can identify the condition through a process of diagnostic reasoning (assessment, problem identification).
> 2 The condition can be resolved primarily by nursing interventions.
> 3 Nurses assume accountability for patient/outcomes.
> 4 Nurses assume responsibility for research on the condition and its treatment.

Allen & Englebright 2000; Johnson 2000; Kurihara *et al.* 2001; Hensley 2002; Wenzel 2002).

Assessment skills training

The need for nurses to have the relevant knowledge and skills to ensure patient safety is fundamental to professional practice (NMC 2002a). Reorganization of health care delivery and patient pathways has meant that nurses require further training and education in assessment skills in order to respond effectively to changing patient needs. For example, more patients with acute care needs are being nursed in general wards or in the community. This has led to the development of critical care outreach teams who act as a resource and provide training for general nurses in acute patient care (McArthur-Rouse 2001; Wadsworth *et al.* 2002).

Education of staff is believed to be essential when introducing a new assessment tool or documentation and new ways of working; for example, telephone triage (Crouch *et al.* 1997; Foster & Harrison 2000; Glasper *et al.* 2000; Price *et al.* 2000; Bouvette *et al.* 2002; Kinley *et al.* 2002). In a small study and audit of patient notes, no correlation was found between the influence of cancer nursing education and the planning of care for a group of patients (Howell *et al.* 2002). However, action learning groups have been shown to be an effective way to improve symptom control for patients with cancer and to enhance interprofessional and agency working (Leslie *et al.* 2003). The use of concept mapping has been shown to help students learn about the priorities and identify the interrelationships in clinical assessment in order to effectively individualize standardized care plans. This approach has been shown to be both time saving and an effective tool for learning about clinical care planning (Schuster 2000).

Integrated care records (electronic patient records)

In the UK the development of integrated care records is fundamental to improvements to patient care (NHSE 1998). The electronic patient record provides the caring professions with the potential to use the data in a clinical nursing database for other purposes, such as care by other disciplines, quality assurance, management, policy making and research. In addition, the electronic patient record will allow collation of data across patient groups to facilitate changes in patients' needs and evaluation of interventions for patients. However, the nurse must be able to validate the data about the care process before they can be used for other purposes. From an organizational perspective, there is agreement that multidisciplinary care plans are preferred, not just a single care plan for the nurse (Goossen *et al.* 1997; Pye & Farrell 2000; Maddock 2002).

Although this era of information technology represents an exciting opportunity for nurses, there are some contentious issues surrounding the implementation of such systems. Examples of these include the potential negative influence of computer use on care delivery, lack of nursing terminology, poor involvement of nurses in decisions about systems and lack of evidence of the benefits of nursing information systems (Goossen *et al.* 1997).

Assessment process

The assessment process has five key steps: assessment, diagnosis or problem identification, planning, implementation and evaluation (see Fig. 2.1). This is an ongoing and central component of everyday care which nurses achieve by using skills of observation, critical thinking, decision making, clinical judgement and communication, and by applying relevant theoretical knowledge (Crow *et al.* 1995; O'Neill & Dluhy 1997; Kennedy 1999; Alfaro-Lefevre 2002). Decision making in nursing relates to the responsibility for the patient's nursing needs and collaboration in the medical treatment plan (Chase 1997; Junnola *et al.* 2002; Alfaro-Lefevre 2002; Hedburg & Larsson 2003).

There is an increasing emphasis on the need for nurses to think critically and creatively in relation to their practice (Daly 1998; Seymour *et al.* 2003). Critical thinking is a pivotal skill that underpins clinical judgement and decision making, and culminates in the application of knowledge and experience to clinical practice. However, many authors highlight the lack of a consensus definition around this fundamental, yet complex cognitive process (Daly 1998; Alfaro-Lefevre 1999; Clarke & Holt 2001). Based on an applied definition offered by Alfaro-Lefevre (1999, p. 9), critical thinking can be summarized as follows.

- Purposeful, outcome-directed (results-orientated) thinking.
- Driven by patient, family and community needs.
- Based on principles of nursing process and scientific method.

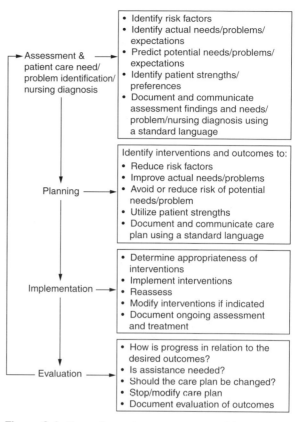

Figure 2.1 Dynamic nursing process as used by a critical thinker (adapted from Alfaro-Lefevre 1999).

- Requires knowledge, skills and experience.
- Guided by professional guidelines and ethical codes.
- Requires strategies that maximize human potential (e.g. using individual strengths) and compensate for problems created by human nature (e.g. the powerful influence of personal perspectives, values and beliefs).
- Constantly re-evaluating, self-correcting and striving to improve.

The critical thinking approach to nursing care is more than seeking a solution to a problem; it is about challenging assumptions and exploring alternatives in order to most effectively achieve a desired outcome. Critical thinking has arguably the most significant role to play in delivering a consistently high standard of nursing care with demonstrated benefits including improved documentation and enhanced clinical outcomes (Keller *et al.* 2001).

Assessment

Patients undergo different types of assessment depending on their needs and the priorities of care (see Box 2.2). A comprehensive and effective initial assessment will

---

Box 2.2 Types of assessment (Ahern & Philpot 2002; White 2003; Holmes 2003)

Mini assessment

A snapshot view of the patient based on what the nurse is told and a quick visual and physical assessment. Consider the patient's ABCs – airway, breathing and circulation – then assess the patient's mental status, overall appearance, level of consciousness and vital signs, and then focus on the patient's main problem.

Comprehensive assessment

An in-depth assessment of the patient's health status, physical examination, risk factors, psychological and social aspects of the patient's health that usually takes place on admission or transfer to a hospital or health care agency. It will take into account the patient's previous health status prior to admission.

Focused assessment

An assessment of a specific condition, problem or assessment of care; for example, continence assessment, neurological assessment following a head injury, assessment for day care, outpatient consultation for a specific condition.

Ongoing assessment

Continuous assessment of the patient's health status accompanied by monitoring and observation of specific problems identified in a mini, comprehensive or focused assessment.

---

mean that patient needs are identified at the earliest possible opportunity and that appropriate intervention is timely (Hunter 1998; Alfaro-Lefevre 2002). The gathering of appropriate data from patients, including the meanings attributed to events by the patient, is associated with greater diagnostic accuracy and thus more effective intervention (Gordon 2000; Alfaro-Lefevre 2002). The decision-making process is based upon the cues observed, analysed and interpreted and it has been suggested that expert nurses assess the situation as a whole and make decisions intuitively (King & Clark 2002; Peden-McAlpine & Clark 2002; Hedburg & Larsson 2003).

Staff should utilize an assessment approach that is useful and appropriate in their particular area of practice in order to gather relevant assessment data. It must be sensitive enough to discriminate between different clinical needs and flexible enough to be updated on a regular basis (Smith & Richardson 1996; Allen 1998). For example, a systematic assessment approach is essential for acutely ill patients in the hospital setting in order to facilitate early recognition of potential or actual deterioration in the patient's condition. By the use of a mini assessment, the nurse is then able to make a more focused assessment of the patient condition in order of priority (Ahern & Philpot 2002). In rehabilitation care the use of an occupational performance measure, in which decisions about the priorities of care are taken with the patient's involvement, allows the patient's progress to be measured on their performance (Donnelly & Carswell 2002).

Assessment data may be subjective or objective. Subjective data are based on 'what the patient says'. This may include their concerns, a description of the patient's support network, the patient's awareness and knowledge of their abilities/disabilities, disease process and prognosis, health care needs and resources. Open questions are useful to try and identify as much information as possible in a limited time (see Box 2.3). If a problem is identified then the nurse should make a focused assessment in which closed questions would be appropriate to determine the nature and extent of the problem, for example pain or continence assessment. Objective data are based upon observations and include any relevant physical assessments including vital signs, observations of the patient's support system, judgement of the patient's readiness for learning, potential ability to learn and any medical relevant information. Observation skills are related to seeing, hearing and behaviour. Answering the questions 'What did I see? What did I hear? What did the patient or I do?' and clarifying where the information was obtained from will help to ensure factual and accurate records (Coyne *et al.* 2002; Alfaro-Lefevre 2002; White 2003).

Assessment is often described as having physical, psychological, emotional, spiritual, social and cultural dimensions. In reality, however, it may not be possible to make clear distinctions between these dimensions when caring for an individual patient (Jenner 1998). Problems or needs identified in one domain may have direct effects on other domains (see Case History 2.1). Assessment should also focus on the patient's perception of their functioning in the activities of daily life and on the relevance for patient care (Ehrenberg *et al.* 1996; Horton 2002). Assessment of the patient's and family's education needs will help to plan care and maximize the patient's understanding and self-care abilities (Alfaro-Lefevre 2002).

The patient's religious, spiritual and cultural needs, emotional and psychological needs and social circumstances, including the impact of the disease and treatment on body image and sexuality, should be explored whilst respecting their privacy and dignity. It is important to be clear as to the relevance of making a specific assessment and nurses need to develop their knowledge and skills in order to plan care and make referrals as appropriate (Govier 2000; Gregory 2000; Edwards & Miller 2001; DoH 2001a, b, 2002; McSherry & Ross

---

Box 2.3 Examples of open questions (Rutenberg 2000; Leasia & Monahan 2002; Alfaro-Lefevre 2002; White 2003)

Patient's perspective	What are your main concerns or needs?
	Why did you come to hospital today?
Medical history	What is the reason for admission?
	Have you had any major illnesses or operations in the past?
	Do you have any history of X?
	Is there a family history of X?
	Are you allergic to anything?
	Are you taking any medicines?
Mental status, body systems and symptoms	What is the current pattern of X (the signs and symptoms as perceived by the patient)?
	When did the problem start?
	What makes the symptom worse?
	What helps?
	How long does it last (frequency/continuous/intermittent)?
	Do other symptoms occur?
	How much does it bother you (the severity)?
	Is X stopping you from doing what you normally do?
Activities of daily living	How do you manage day to day with X?
	What do you hope to be able to do?
Psychological needs	How do you feel?
	Do you have any worries or concerns?
	What has helped you cope in the past and what is helping at the moment?
Social circumstances	Who do you live with?
	What support do you and your family have?
	Are you a carer for anyone?
	Do you require advice on support services in the community?
	Do you require information or advice on your work, financial or accommodation situation?
Body image	How do you feel about your hair loss?
Sexuality	Has your treatment affected your relationships in any way?
Spiritual, religious and cultural needs	Do you have any specific beliefs (religious or cultural) that you would like to practise in hospital?
	What is important to you, e.g. hobbies, music?
Safety	Do you have any concerns about your safety at home?
Educational needs	What do you understand about your illness and treatment?
	Would you like any information on X?
Discharge planning	Do you have any concerns about discharge?

2001; Kuppelomaki 2002; Jolley 2002; Newell 2002a, b; Quinn 2003).

The different types of assessment needed to explore the health and social needs of older people have been highlighted in the single assessment process. This framework is being implemented nationally to facilitate a more collaborative and effective approach to assessment. The communication needs of older people are challenging and fundamental to the assessment process (Miller 2002). Referrals to other disciplines or specialists should take place according to the patient's needs with a summary of the relevant assessment details being communicated in a timely and efficient manner, minimizing duplication (DoH 2001a, b, 2002).

Assessment interview

The first assessment interview enables the nurse to obtain a baseline of information against which new and changing information can be compared. It facilitates thinking and planning ahead and consideration of the patient's likely outcome of care. However, there must be structure to the interview. It has a beginning and ending and

---

Case History 2.1

A patient with breast cancer, having chemotherapy, reports to the nurse that she is experiencing nausea and vomiting with each course of chemotherapy. Anxiety, fatigue, consequential anorexia and poor nutritional intake are also complications of this side-effect. The patient is concerned about not being able to care for her young daughter adequately due to the physical effects of treatment. She may consider not having any more treatment. Careful assessment of the patient's needs requires a holistic approach to identify the interrelated components of these complications/side-effects, to maximize any appropriate interventions and to minimize the risks of psychological morbidity. In this way, the acceptability of the treatment plan and the patient's quality of life are improved. It may therefore be more useful to view assessment as a holistic process with particular aspects demanding more focus on specific occasions.

Box 2.4 Examples of assessment tools

Waterlow Pressure Sore Risk Assessment (Waterlow 1995)

Early Warning Scoring Systems (McArthur-Rouse 2001)

Manual Handling Risk Assessment (see Ch. 23, Moving and handling)

Chemotherapy Assessment Scale (Brown *et al.* 2001).

Nutritional Screening Tool (see Ch. 24, Nutritional support)

Piper Fatigue Scale, measuring subjective fatigue in cancer patients (Piper 1997)

Oral Assessment (Eilers *et al.* 1988) (see Ch. 32, Mouth care)

Pain assessment: postoperative and chronic (see Ch. 27, Pain assessment)

Pain and Symptom Assessment Records (PSAR) (Bouvette *et al.* 2002)

Oncology patients' concerns in the outpatient setting (Dennison & Shute 2000)

---

should progress logically, ensuring meaning for the participants. It may also be the case that the information gathered is incomplete, either because the patient was not well enough to continue the interview or because it was inappropriate to examine certain physical and psychological aspects of the patient's problems at the time.

To end the interview the nurse may ask the following questions to gain an understanding of the patient's priorities for care. 'Tell me the most important things I can help you with.' 'Is there anything else you want me to know about?' In order to help the patient to feel that the nurse will be taking on ongoing interest in their needs, the nurse may for example say 'If there are any changes or you think of something else or you have any questions do let me know' (Alfaro-Lefevre 2002, pp. 54–5).

Patients and their families often see the assessment as a time to obtain clear answers to questions about their illness and treatment. It allows the nurse–patient relationship to be established on the basis of mutual concern for the patient's well-being. Some problems may not be disclosed by the patient and may only be identified when the nurse–patient relationship develops and the patient trusts the nurse. Asking patients to describe their needs and difficulties may be particularly helpful when dealing with complex problems such as anxiety and stress. Information of this kind can also be collected in a health diary, which patients can use to record their needs and experiences since their last appointment (Richardson & Wilson Barnett 1995; Burton & Watson 1998).

Efforts should be made to overcome language or cultural barriers to communication and thus patient assessment by the use of interpreters or interpreting services, for example telephone interpreting services. There may be times when it is not possible to obtain vital information from the patient directly; they may be too emotionally distressed, unconscious or unable to speak clearly, if at all. In such situations, the appropriate details will have to be obtained from relatives or friends. Note should be made in the record of the name and relationship of the person who gave the information, as conflicting information may be given by different individuals. If the patient is unconscious or unable to speak clearly the nurse has a responsibility to ensure that this does not go unrecognized and a mechanism is in place to ensure that the document is duly completed. The patient also needs to be assured of the use to which the data will be put (NHSE 2000; White 2003).

Assessment tools

The use of an assessment tool enables a baseline assessment of the patient's health status for a specific patient problem and is an aid to the assessment process. The decision-making process is facilitated by using a standardized approach to obtain specific data and referrals may be made earlier and more efficiently, especially by inexperienced staff. If the assessment tool is used as a monitoring mechanism, it will allow regular and ongoing evaluation of patient needs.

The choice of assessment tool should be based on the variable to be measured in a particular patient group, the tool's purpose, measurement framework, conceptual base, reliability, validity and sensitivity. Tools link assessment of clinical variables with measurement of clinical interventions (Frank-Stromborg & Olsen 1997). Nurse researchers and clinicians have developed a broad spectrum of tools to assess the problems frequently encountered by people with cancer (see Box 2.4).

The use of assessment tools can also assist health care professionals in practice development and research, by developing a body of knowledge concerning outcomes of intervention. An example of developing cancer nursing practice is the WISECARE project which involved European collaboration (Kearney 2001). Nurses were encouraged to develop a systematic measurement for patient outcomes such as oral problems, fatigue, pain and nausea and vomiting and this assessment was accompanied by nurse–patient interaction about patient self-care measures. Improvements in patient outcomes were demonstrated and nurses were enabled to share good practice by using information technology (Kearney 2001).

Diagnosis or problem identification

It is necessary to analyse each problem (for nursing relevance) and need in context, where possible, together with the patient and/or significant other persons in order to obtain a good understanding of the patient's situation (Ehrenberg *et al.* 1996). A diagnosis or problem should be written from the patient's need for nursing care and the aetiology or related events/factors and any relevant assessment data. The patient's care needs should be prioritized according to their severity and whether they are of major concern to the patient. It has been suggested that immediate problems (Alfaro-Lefevre 1999) are:

- *Airway* problems
- *Breathing* problems
- *Cardiac/circulation* problems
- *Signs* (vital signs).

After treating the immediate problems, the next priorities are:

- *Mental* status change
- *Acute* pain
- *Acute* urinary problems
- *Untreated* medical problems requiring immediate action
- *Abnormal* laboratory results
- *Risk* of infection, safety or security (for patient or others).

Finally other health problems should be addressed, for example eating difficulties, sleep problems or family support. The priority order may change; for example, if the abnormal laboratory results are life threatening, such as a low blood potassium result (Alfaro-Lefevre 1999). Recognizing the areas of care for which the nurse is able to take actions, and those of the multiprofessional and community teams and other agencies, is essential so that nurses make appropriate referrals (Alfaro-Lefevre 2002; White 2003).

Box 2.5 Examples of measurable and non-measurable verbs for use in outcome statements (Alfaro-Lefevre 2002, pp. 134–5)

Measurable verbs (use these to be specific)

- State; verbalize; communicate; list; describe; identify
- Demonstrate; perform
- Will lose; will gain; has an absence of
- Walk; stand; sit

Non-measurable verbs (do not use)

- Know
- Understand
- Think
- Feel

Planning

When planning care it is vital:

- To determine the immediate priorities and recognize whether patient needs and problems require nursing care or whether a referral should be made to someone else
- To identify the anticipated outcome for the patient, noting what the patient will be able to do and in what timeframe. The use of 'measurable' verbs that describe patient behaviour or what the patient says facilitates the evaluation of patient outcomes (see Box 2.5)
- To determine the nursing interventions, i.e. what nursing actions will prevent or manage the patient's problems so that the patient's outcomes may be achieved
- To record the care plan for the patient which may be written or individualized from a standardized/core care plan or a computerized care plan (Shaw 1998; Alfaro-Lefevre 2002; White 2003).

Outcomes should be patient focused and realistic, stating how the outcomes or goals are to be achieved and when the outcomes should be evaluated. Patient-focused outcomes centre on the desired results of nursing care, i.e. the impact of care on the patient, rather than on what the nurse does. Outcomes may be short, intermediate or long term, enabling the nurse to identify the patient's health status and progress (stability, improvement or deterioration) over time. Setting realistic outcomes and interventions requires the nurse to distinguish between problems that are life threatening or are an immediate risk to the patient's safety and those problems that may be dealt with at a later stage. Identifying which problems contribute to other problems (for example, difficulty breathing will contribute to the patient's ability to mobilize) will make the problem a higher priority. By dealing with the breathing difficulties, the patient's ability to mobilize will be improved.

By asking negative questions such as 'What would happen if I didn't provide this care or report this problem?', the nurse will be able to focus on what is really important. If the answer is 'Not much can happen', then the problem has a low priority. The urgency of the problem, such as loss of consciousness related to head injury, or the speed with which an outcome needs to be achieved, such as the timing of an operation or discharge of a day case patient, will also determine the priorities of care (Alfaro-Lefevre 2002, p. 128).

The nature of the patient outcomes will differ according to the specific patient group or focus of the patient's problems. For example, patient outcomes related to safety, physiological and behavioural responses are defined in the perioperative patient-focused model (Kleinbeck & McKennet 2000). However, in the community setting, patient and family outcomes relate to the knowledge, behaviour and signs and symptoms as described in the Omaha nursing classification system (Martin & Scheet 1992). Health visitors in the UK are now using this framework to demonstrate the effectiveness of care and to facilitate the assessment process and identify clients' progress (Clark *et al.* 2001). Nursing has been shown to influence patient outcomes in the hospital setting according to Lee (1999) in a review of the literature, but more research is necessary to evaluate further the interrelationship. No benefit has been identified from any studies between written manual care planning, record keeping and patient outcomes (Moloney & Maggs 1999; Currell *et al.* 2003).

It appears that the formulation of nursing interventions is dependent on adequate information collection and clinical judgement during patient assessment. As a result specific patient outcomes may be derived and appropriate nursing interventions undertaken to assist the patient to achieve those outcomes (Hardwick 1998). Nursing interventions should be specific to help the patient achieve the outcome and should be evidence based. When determining what interventions to choose for a patient problem, it may be helpful to clarify the potential benefit to the patient after an intervention has been performed, as this will help to ensure its appropriateness.

Implementation

It is important to continue to assess the patient on an ongoing basis whilst implementing the care plan. Assessing the patient's current status prior to implementing care will enable the nurse to check whether the patient has developed any new problems that require immediate action. During and after providing any nursing action, the nurse should assess and reassess the patient's response to care. The nurse will then be able to determine whether changes to the patient's care plan should be made immediately or at a later stage. If there are any patient care needs or problems that need immediate action, for example consultation or referral to a doctor, recording the actions taken is essential. Involving the patient and their family or friends will promote the patient's well-being and self-care abilities. The use of clinical documentation in nurse handover will help to ensure that the care plans are up to date and relevant (Alfaro-Lefevre 2002; White 2003).

Interventions may be nurse led or collaborative in nature, i.e. implementing interventions that involve another health care professional, for example an exercise programme from the physiotherapist or administering medication as prescribed by the doctor (White 2003). It is important to record when exceptional or critical incidents have occurred (NMC 2002a, b). Local standards for documentation may be developed to support the implementation of record keeping (see Box 2.6). In the event of a procedure being performed, document the relevant details; for example, chest drainage of pleural fluid:

- The procedure
- The equipment details
- When the procedure was performed
- Who performed the procedure
- How the procedure was performed
- How well the patient tolerated it
- Adverse reactions to the procedure
- Vital signs, e.g. respiratory status
- The nature of the drainage, i.e. amount and type
- Dressings and the patient's skin condition
- Patient and family teaching (Shaw 1998, pp. 237, 248).

Evaluation

The nurse reflects and critically analyses the patient's health status to determine whether the patient's condition is stable, has deteriorated or has improved. Seeking the patient's and family's views in the evaluation process will facilitate decision making. By evaluating the patient's outcomes the nurse is able to decide whether changes need to be made to the care plan. Questions such as:

- What are the patient's health status and self-care abilities?
- Is the patient able to do what you expected?
- If not, why not?
- Has something changed?
- Are you missing something?
- Are there new care priorities?

will help to clarify the patient's progress (Alfaro-Lefevre 2002, p. 5; White 2003). It is helpful to consider what is observed in the patient and what is measurable to indicate that the patient has achieved the outcome – this has been described as the corresponding indicators (see Table 2.1) (Alfaro-Lefevre 2002).

Box 2.6 Guidelines for nursing documentation (Royal Marsden NHS Trust 2003)

General principles

1 Records should be written legibly in black ink in such a way that they cannot be erased and are readable when photocopied.
2 Entries should be factual, consistent and accurate, and not contain jargon, abbreviations or meaningless phrases (e.g. slept well).
3 Each entry must include the date and the time (using the 24-hour clock).
4 Each entry must be followed by a signature and the name printed as well as:
   • the job role (e.g. staff nurse or clinical nurse specialist)
   • if a nurse is a temporary employee (i.e. an agency nurse) the name of the agency must be included under the signature.
5 If an error is made this should be scored out with a single line and the correction written alongside with date, time and initials. Correction fluid (e.g. Tippex) should not be used at any time.
6 All assessment and entries made by student nurses must be countersigned by a registered nurse.
7 Health care assistants:
   • can write on fluid balance and food intake charts
   • who have demonstrated achievement of the learning outcomes for observing and monitoring the patient's condition as defined in the Royal Marsden Hospital Health Assistant Role Assessment and Development Profile (2001) can write on observation charts
   • must not write on prescription charts, assessment sheets, care plans or evaluation sheets.

Assessment and care planning

1 The first written assessment and the identification of the patient's immediate needs must begin within 4 hours of admission. This must include any allergies or infection risks of the patient and the contact details of the next of kin.
2 A full assessment must be completed within 24 hours of admission and must include:
   • completion of nutritional, oral, pressure sore and manual handling risk assessments
   • other relevant assessment tools, e.g. pain and wound assessment
   • a record of all the current nursing needs and an initial discharge plan.
3 Care plans should be written wherever possible with the involvement of the patient, in terms that they can understand, and include:
   • patient-focused, measurable, realistic and achievable goals
   • nursing interventions reflecting best practice
   • relevant core care plans which are individualized, signed, dated and timed.
4 The care plan must be referred to at shift handover so it must be kept up to date and evaluated every shift. The written evaluation must correlate with the care plan and identify whether the patient's condition is stable, has deteriorated or has improved.

Reference: NMC (2002b)

The ability to develop good practice in record keeping is considered to be an area for improvement by nurses (Frank-Stromborg & Christensen 2001a, b; Rodden & Bell 2002; Wood 2003) (see Table 2.2). Record keeping is an integral part of nursing care (NMC 2002a), and the purpose of health records is to ensure that 'those coming after you can see what has been done, or not done, and why and by whom' (NHSE 1999). This will ensure not only that patient care is not compromised but also that 'any decisions made can be justified or reconsidered at a later date' (NHSE 1999).

Protocol-based care

Screening tools and specific assessment documentation or care pathways to decipher pertinent information, and to elicit the patient's and carers' perspective, have been developed in different specialities and health care settings (see Box 2.7). The need for a consistent method

Table 2.1 Example outcomes and corresponding indicators (Alfaro-Lefevre 2002, p. 132)

Example outcomes	Corresponding indicators
Will demonstrate knowledge of medication regimen by discharge	• Lists drug names, actions, doses, administration route and side-effects • Explains when drugs are to be taken, including whether to take them on an empty or full stomach, and what to do if dose is missed • Demonstrates special administration techniques (e.g. injection, if applicable) • Lists reportable signs and symptoms
Will maintain intact skin	• Skin shows no signs of discoloration or irritation • Risk factors managed (patient has adequate nutrition and hydration, repositioned hourly, skin care performed as per protocol)

Table 2.2 How to record patient care in a useful and meaningful way (Chase 1997; Castledine 1998; Price et al. 2000; Coyne et al. 2002; Alfaro-Lefevre 2002; White 2003)

Type of data	Poor standard	How to improve the standard	Good standard
Subjective assessment data	a) 'Moody today' b) 'Appears depressed'	a) Identify if it was the patient perspective b) Note the patient's behaviour and responses to support the patient's statement	a) Patient states 'feeling moody' b) 'Low in mood – unsmiling, fails to make eye contact' or patient states 'concerned about his diagnosis and how this will affect him'
Objective assessment data	a) Pale – dizzy at times	a) Be specific – indicate the signs and symptoms and actions taken in response	a) Pale. Patient states that he becomes dizzy on standing. Lying BP 130/80 and standing BP 90/70. Doctor X informed – to remain on current medication. For review tomorrow
Patient care need/ problem	a) Chest infection b) Risk of falls	a) Identify the problem from the patient's perspective and what is their need for nursing care b) Indicate the related factors to the patient problem which will help to identify the priority of the problem and the nursing interventions	a) 'Acute breathlessness related to lung cancer and chest infection' b) 'Risk of falls related to poor mobility and left-sided weakness'
Anticipated/expected outcome	a) Patient will receive 4-hourly observations b) To have bowels opened c) To prepare the patient for preoperative care and safety	a) Indicate the results of the interventions for the patient b) Indicate the timeframe for the outcome c) Be specific and indicate how the outcome will be measured	a) *For high blood pressure:* 'Patient's blood pressure will remain between 110/80 and 140/80 at all times' b) *For constipation:* 'Patient will have a soft bowel movement every other day' c) *For preoperative care:* 'Patient will have the correct surgical procedure and patient safety will be maintained throughout' and 'Patient and carer will state they have an understanding of the anaesthetic, operation and the possible complications'
Interventions	a) Assist with activities of daily living as required b) Promote comfort	a) Be specific – indicate the patient's abilities, level of assistance required, i.e. number of nurses, the equipment, the method b) Be specific	a) Turning in bed – patient able to lean forward and move up the bed, requires one nurse to move pillows and place pillow under swollen left arm b) Administer analgesia 30 minutes before leg dressing and position leg on two pillows
Progress/evaluation notes	a) 'Appears comfortable – slept well' b) 'No problems with wound' c) Patient fell d) Uncooperative and refuses help e) Very confused	a) Identify if it was the patient perspective b) Be specific c) Be specific and add the actions taken by the nurse d) Be specific e) Be specific	a) Patient states 'My pain was better last night and I slept well' b) Wound healing – no signs of infection c) Patient states 'Tried to walk, slipped and knocked knees on the table legs'. Knees examined – no signs of injury. On questioning, the patient confirmed that he did not knock any other part of his body. Falls risk assessment – no change in care plan required. d) Patient states 'I don't want to have a bath, and I don't want to eat' and refuses help from the nurse. Expresses anger by shouting and swearing at the nurses and relatives e) Patient confused in time, place and person

---

Box 2.7 Examples of specific assessments and protocols of care

---

Primary and secondary care

- Chronic obstructive pulmonary disease (Pilling & Wolstenholme 2002)
- Continuing care assessment for health and social care needs for long-term care (DoH 2001b)
- Leg ulcer management (Evans 2001)
- Mental health needs in physical care settings (Harrison 2001)
- Needs assessment using an empowerment framework within a health visitor/client interaction in the home setting (Houston & Cowley 2002)
- Older people with nursing and social care needs (McCormick 1999; DoH 2001a, 2002; Standing Nursing & Midwifery Advisory Committee 2001)
- Older people's need for registered nursing in continuing health care (Ford & McCormack 1999)
- Screening for dementia and depression in older people (Pritchard 1999; Insel & Badger 2002)
- Sexuality (Gregory 2000)
- Spiritual care (Govier 2000)
- Symptom management in people with AIDS (Coyne et al. 2002)
- Terminal restlessness (Travis et al. 2001)

Hospital setting

- Acutely ill patient on a general ward (Ahern & Philpot 2002)
- Assessing adults with leukaemia (Murphy-Ende & Chernecky 2002)
- Assessment for lung cancer patients (Scullion & Henry 1998)
- Breast disease/breast cancer pathway (De Luc 2000; Bryan et al. 2002a, b)
- Critical care patients (McArthur-Rouse 2001)
- Midwifery-led maternity service (De Luc 2000)
- Nurse-led physical assessment framework (Harris et al. 1998)
- Outpatient chemotherapy: telephone triage for symptom management (Anastasia & Blevins 1997)
- Paediatric mental health needs (Gall 2002)
- Perioperative nursing (Rothbrook & Smith 2000; Beyea 2001)
- Preoperative assessment (Kinley et al. 2002)
- Psychosocial care in day case surgery patients (Mitchell 2002)
- Self-Reporting Health History and Outpatient Oncology Record (Skinn & Stacey 1994)
- Telephone assessment and/or triage in oncology or palliative care (Korcz & Moreland 1998; Elfrink et al. 2002)

---

of assessment in order to facilitate communication between professionals in differing health care settings has influenced changes in practice (Bouvette et al. 2002; DoH 2002).

In clinical practice clinical protocols, shared documentation, patient-held records, patient self-assessment tools and care pathways have been developed to improve the patient's experience of care and service delivery (Coyle et al. 1996; Smith & Richardson 1996; Dyer et al. 1998; Harris et al. 1998; Read 1999; Selwood 2000; McEvoy 2000; Dennison & Shute 2000; Lecouturier et al. 2002; Simpson 2003). The usefulness of care plans and the difficulty in keeping care plans updated have been factors in the development of clinical protocols. The benefits of a clinical protocol are the identification of specific care for their patient population, allowing for individual variation, and that staff found them to be easier to update (O'Connell et al. 2000). A national care pathways database has been developed in the UK via the National Electronic Library for Health and protocols of care are being shared through the NHS Modernisation Agency.

Cancer nursing practice

Shortened inpatient stays and admission guidelines have markedly increased the number of outpatient and day care patients in cancer nursing practice (Smith & Richardson 1996). It is essential that assessment documentation is sensitive to the facets of a particular client group, in this case people affected by cancer, their families and friends. The assessor should possess knowledge and some understanding of the particular client group and the treatments that they are undergoing, so that diagnostic reasoning and critical thinking skills are enhanced (O'Neill & Dluhy 1997).

In the acute phase of cancer care, it has been demonstrated that certain changes in function are common, whether physical, psychosocial or spiritual. In this acute phase, accurate assessment enables appropriate and therapeutic interventions to achieve outcomes (Smith & Richardson 1996; Burton & Watson 1998; Larsson et al. 1998). Referral can then be made to specialist nurses, therapists or other professionals as appropriate, in order to continue the assessment process in more depth (Hunter 1998). Cancer is a chronic illness for many people, as more patients are living with cancer for longer. The assessment process and interventions here aim ideally to move patients out of the sick role and into effective day-to-day self-management of their illness (Davies et al. 1997; Hunter 1998). With the goal of optimal functioning, any health care professional involved in patient care will play a part in assessment.

Larsson et al. (1998, p. 863) summarized the approach to assessment in cancer care succinctly by stating that:

'Even though various tools facilitate the communication with the patient, the use of assessment tools alone is not sufficient to capture the whole spectrum of patient perceptions concerning their care.'

Ongoing assessment of patient need is particularly important when disease processes are unpredictable and characterized by repeated admissions to hospital. During these times the patient and family may experience disruption in every aspect of their life, including work and relationships. Whilst assessment schedules may allow these issues to be addressed, they must be used in a way that allows ongoing changes to be noted and regular evaluations to be taken into account (Bowling 1997; Frank-Stromborg & Olsen 1997).

Conclusion

This chapter has emphasized, and reiterated, the need for the patient to be the central focus, whatever the situation and whatever the procedure or activity. Nurses have a central role to play in helping patients to manage the demands of the procedures described in this book. Caring for a person involves respect for their rights, using communication that is open, honest and facilitative. The key to success in this role is accurate assessment of patients' needs and a commitment to meeting them with sensitivity.

Assessment is impossible without the ability to communicate, using both verbal and non-verbal skills to explore, and allow expression of, the patient's feelings. Fear of many of the procedures described here may exist – because they are unknown, because of previous experiences or because of what may be revealed. Good, clear communication may be able to allay fears, minimize discomfort and enable individual adjustment.

Assessment enables the nurse to ascertain the patient's attitudes, beliefs and values and to discover their needs, including the amount of involvement they wish to have in their care, how much information they require and what is acceptable to them, particularly as their disease experience progresses. Taking time to explore individual needs is one way of demonstrating caring in everyday practice. The diverse range of technical procedures that patients may be subjected to acts as a reminder not to lose sight of the unique person undergoing such procedures.

References and further reading

Adams, D. & Deveau, E. (1984) *Coping with Childhood Cancer*. Kinbridge Publications, Hamilton, pp. 3–39.

Ahern, J. & Philpot, P. (2002) Assessing acutely ill patients on general wards. *Nurs Stand*, **16**(47), 47–52.

Alderson, P. & Montgomery, J. (1996) Children may be able to make their own decisions. *Br Med J*, **313**(7048), 50.

Alfaro-Lefevre, R. (1999) *Critical Thinking in Nursing: A Practical Approach*, 2nd edn. W.B. Saunders, Philadelphia.

Alfaro-Lefevre, R. (2002) *Applying Nursing Process: Promoting Collaborative Care*. Lippincott, Williams & Wilkins, Philadelphia.

Allen, D. (1998) Record-keeping and routine nursing practice: the view from the wards. *J Adv Nurs*, **27**(6), 1223–30.

Allen, J. & Englebright, J. (2000) Patient-centered documentation: an effective and efficient use of clinical information systems. *J Nurs Admin*, **30**(2), 90–5.

Anastasia, P.J. & Blevins, M.C. (1997) Outpatient chemotherapy: telephone triage for symptom management. *Oncol Nurs Forum*, **24**(1, Suppl), 13–22.

Anstey, K. (1999) *Patient Assessment in Continuing Care. Nurs Times Clinical Monograph*, London.

Ardern-Jones, A. (1997) *Living with a Cancer Legacy*. Unpublished MSc Thesis, Institute of Cancer Research, London University.

Ardern-Jones, A. & Eeles, R. (2002) Forum for applied cancer education and training. Cancer genes – management of carriers of breast cancer genes who have already developed breast cancer: the carrier clinic model. *Eur J Cancer Care*, **11**(1), 64–8.

Audit Commission (1993) *What Seems to Be the Matter? Communication between Hospitals and Patients*. Stationery Office, London.

Baile, W.F., Buckman, R., Lenzi, R., Glober, G., Beale, G.A. & Kudelka, A.P. (2000) SPIKES: a six step protocol for delivering bad news: application to the patient with cancer. *Oncologist*, **5**(4), 302–11.

Bailey, K. & Wilkinson, S. (1998) Patients' views on nurses' communication skills: a pilot study. *Int J Palliat Nurs*, **4**(6), 300–305.

Bayne, R., Horton, I., Merry, T. & Noyes, E. (1998) *The Counsellor's Handbook*. Stanley Thornes, Cheltenham, pp. 41–50.

Becker, R. (1999) Teaching communication with the dying across cultural boundaries. *Br J Nurs*, **8**(14), 938–42.

Benbow, M. (1999) *Health Care Documentation. Nurs Times Clinical Monograph*, London.

Beyea, S. (ed.) (2000) *The Perioperative Nursing Data Set*. American Association of Perioperative Nurses, Denver.

Beyea, S.C. (2001) The Ideal state for perioperative nursing (data receiving and recording). *AORN J*, **73**(5), 897–901.

Booth, K., Maguire, P.M., Butterworth, T. & Hillier, V.F. (1996) Perceived professional support and the use of blocking behaviours by hospice nurses. *J Adv Nurs*, **24**(3), 522–7.

Booth, K., Maguire, P. & Hillier, V.F. (1999) Measurement of communication skills in cancer care: myth or reality? *J Adv Nurs*, **30**(5), 1073–9.

Bouvette, M., Fothergill-Bourbonnais, F. & Perreault, A. (2002) Implementation of the pain and symptom assessment record (PSAR). *J Adv Nurs*, **40**(6), 685–700.

Bowling, A. (1997) *Measuring Health – A Review of Quality of Life Measurement Scales*, 2nd edn. Open University Press, Buckingham.

British Association for Counselling and Psychotherapy (2001) *Training and Careers in Counselling*. British Association for Counselling and Psychotherapy, Rugby.

British Association for Counselling and Psychotherapy (2002) *Ethical Framework for Good Practice in Counselling and Psychotherapy*. British Association for Counselling and Psychotherapy, Rugby.

Brown, V., Sitzia, J., Richardson, A., Hughes, J., Hannon, H. & Oakley, C. (2001) The development of the Chemotherapy

Symptom Assessment Scale (C-SAS): a scale for the routine clinical assessment of the symptom experiences of patients receiving cytotoxic chemotherapy. *Int J Nurs Stud*, **38**(5), 497–510.

Bryan, S., Holmes, S., Postlethwaite, D. & Carty, N. (2002a) The role of integrated care pathways in improving the patient experience. *Prof Nurse*, **18**(2), 77–9.

Bryan, S., Holmes, S., Postlethwaite, D. & Carty, N. (2002b) A breast unit care pathway: enhancing the role of the nurse. *Prof Nurse*, **18**(3), 151–4.

Buckingham, C.D. & Adams, A. (2000) Classifying clinical decision making: a unifying approach. *J Adv Nurs*, **32**(4), 981–9.

Buckman, R. (1992) *How to Break Bad News: A Guide for Health Professionals*. Johns Hopkins University Press, Baltimore.

Buckman, R. (2001) Communication skills in palliative care: a practical guide. *Neurol Clin*, **19**(4), 989–1004.

Burnard, P. (1997) *Effective Communication Skills for Health Professionals*. Stanley Thornes, Cheltenham, pp. 48–78.

Burnard, P. (1998a) Listening as a personal quality. *J Community Nurs*, **12**(2), 32–4.

Burnard, P. (1998b) Personal qualities or skills? A report of a study of nursing students' views of the characteristics of counsellors. *Nurse Educ Today* **18**(8), 649–54.

Burton, M. & Watson, M. (1998) *Counselling People with Cancer*. John Wiley & Sons, Chichester.

Butterworth, C. (2003) Evaluating a new care planning system in nursing homes. *Nurs Times*, **99**(14), 30–2.

Casteldine, G. (1998) *Writing, Documentation and Communication for Nurses*. Redwood Books, Swindon.

Chambers, S. (1998) Nursing diagnosis in learning disabilities nursing. *Br J Nurs*, **7**(19), 1177–81.

Chang, S.O. (2001) The conceptual structure of physical touch in caring. *J Adv Nurs*, **33**(6), 820–7.

Chant, S., Jenkinson, T., Randle, J. & Russell, G. (2002) Communication skills: some problems in nursing education and practice. *J Clin Nurs*, **11**(1), 12–21.

Chase, S.K. (1997) Charting critical thinking: nursing judgements and patient outcome. *Dimens Crit Care Nurs*, **16**(2), 102–11.

Chauhan, G. & Long, A. (2000a) Communication is the essence of nursing care 2: ethical foundations. *Br J Nurs*, **9**(15), 979–84.

Chauhan, G. & Long, A. (2000b) Communication is the essence of nursing care 1: breaking bad news. *Br J Nurs*, **9**(14), 931–8.

Christensen, P.J. & Kenney, J.W. (1995) *Nursing Process Application of Conceptual Models*. Mosby, St Louis.

Clark, J., Christensen, J., Mooney, G. *et al.* (2001) Professional briefing. New methods of documenting health visiting practice. *Community Practitioner*, **74**(3), 108–12.

Clarke, D.J. & Holt, J. (2001) Philosophy: a key to open the door to critical thinking. *Nurse Educ Today*, **21**, 71–8.

Commission for Health Improvement (2001) *National Service Framework Assessments No. 1: NHS Cancer Care in England and Wales*. Commission for Health Improvement, London.

Cooley, D. (2000) Communication skills in palliative care. *Prof Nurse*, **15**(9), 603–5.

Couldrick, A. (1991) *When Your Mum or Dad Has Cancer*. Sobell Publications, Oxford.

Coyle, N., Layman Goldstein, M., Passik, S., Fishman, B. & Portenoy, R. (1996) Development and validation of a patient needs assessment tool (PNAT) for oncology clinicians. *Cancer Nurs*, **19**(2), 81–92.

Coyne, P.J., Lyne, M.E. & Watson, A.C. (2002) Symptom management in people with AIDS. *Am J Nurs*, **102**(9), 48–57.

Crouch, R., Woodfield, H., Dale, J. & Patel, D. (1997) Telephone assessment and advice: a training programme. *Nurs Stand*, **11**(47), 41–4.

Crow, R.A., Chase, J. & Lamond, D. (1995) The cognitive component of nursing assessment: an analysis. *J Adv Nurs*, **22**, 206–12.

Currell, R., Wainwright, P. & Urquhart, C. (2003) *Nursing record systems*. Cochrane Effective Practice and Organisation of Care Group. Cochrane Database of Systematic Reviews 1.

Daly, W.M. (1998) Critical thinking as an outcome of nursing education. What is it? Why is it important to nursing practice? *J Adv Nurs*, **28**(2), 323–31.

Davies, S., Laker, S. & Ellis, L. (1997) Promoting autonomy and independence for older people within nursing practice: a literature review. *J Adv Nurs*, **26**, 408–17.

Davy, J. & Ellis, S. (2000) *Counselling Skills in Palliative Care*. Open University Press, Buckingham.

De Luc, K. (2000) Care pathways: an evaluation of their effectiveness. *J Adv Nurs*, **32**(2), 485–96.

Delaney, C. (2001) Health informatics and oncology nursing. *Semin Oncol Nurs*, **17**(1), 2–6.

Dennison, S. & Shute, T. (2000) Identifying patient concerns: improving the quality of patient visits to the oncology outpatient department – a pilot audit. *Eur J Oncol Nurs*, **4**(2), 91–8.

Di Vito-Thomas, P. (2000) Identifying critical thinking behaviours in clinical judgements. *J Nurses Staff Dev*, **16**(4), 174–80.

DoH (1991) *The Patient's Charter*. Stationery Office, London.

DoH (1995) *A Policy Framework for Commissioning Cancer Services*. Stationery Office, London.

DoH (2000a) *The NHS Plan*. Stationery Office, London.

DoH (2000b) *The NHS Cancer Plan*. Stationery Office, London.

DoH (2001a) *NHS Funded Nursing Care: Practice Guide and Workbook*. Department of Health, London.

DoH (2001b) *Continuing Care: NHS and Local Councils' Responsibilities (HSC 2001/015: LAC (2001) 18)*. Department of Health, London.

DoH (2002) *The Single Assessment Process: Assessment Tools and Scales*. Department of Health, London.

Donnelly, C. & Carswell, A. (2002) Individualized outcome measures. *Can J Occup Ther*, **69**(2), 84–94.

Dowding, D. (2001) Examining the effects that manipulating information given in the change of shift report has on nurses' care planning ability. *J Adv Nurs*, **33**(6), 836–46.

Drew, A. & Fawcett, T. (2002) Responding to the information needs of patients with cancer. *Prof Nurse*, **17**(7), 443–6.

Dunniece, U. & Slevin, E. (2000) Nurses' experiences of being present with a patient receiving a diagnosis of cancer. *J Adv Nurs*, **32**(3), 611–18.

Dyer, M., Harte, J. & Brereton, J. (1998) Reducing paperwork in a medical assessment unit. *Nurs Times*, **94**(12), 50–1.

Edwards, S. (2002) Nursing knowledge: defining new boundaries. *Nurs Standard*, **17**(2), 40–4.

Edwards, M. & Davis, H. (1997) *Counselling Children with Chronic Medical Conditions*. BPS Books, Leicester, pp. 82–98.

Edwards, M. & Miller, C. (2001) Improving psychosocial assessment in oncology. *Prof Nurse*, **16**(7), 1223–6.

Eeles, R. & Ardern-Jones, A. (1999) *Breast Cancer: Sharing the Decision*. Oxford University Press, Oxford, pp. 152–64.

Ehrenberg, A., Ehnfors, M. & Thorell-Ekstrand, I. (1996) Nursing documentation in patient records: experience of the use of the VIPS model. *J Adv Nurs*, **24**, 853–67.

Eilers, J., Berger, A.M. & Petersen, M.C. (1988) Development, testing, and application of the oral assessment guide. *Oncol Nurs Forum*, **15**(3), 325–30.

Elfrink, V., Bakken, S., Coenen, A., McNeil, B. & Bickford, C. (2001) Standardised nursing vocabularies: a foundation for quality care. *Semin Oncol Nurs*, **17**(1), 18–23.

Elfrink, E.J., Van der Rijt, C.C., Van Boxtel, R. J., Elswijk-de Vries, P., Van Zuijlen, L. & Stoter, G. (2002) Problem solving by telephone in palliative care: use of a predetermined assessment tool within a program of home care technology. *J Palliat Care*, **18**(2), 105–10.

Eriksson, E. (2000) Informational and emotional support for cancer patients' relatives. *Eur J Cancer Care*, **9**(1), 8–15.

Eriksson, E. (2001) Caring for cancer patients: relatives' assessments of received care. *Eur J Cancer Care*, **10**(1), 48–55.

Evans, T. (2001) An integrated care pathway for leg ulcer management. *NT Plus*, **97**(3), X–XII.

Fallowfield, L. (1997) Truth sometimes hurts but deceit hurts more. *Ann NY Acad Sci*, **809**, 525–36.

Fallowfield, L. & Jenkins, V. (1999) Effective communication skills are the key to good cancer care. *Eur J Cancer*, **35**(11), 1592–7.

Fallowfield, L., Ratcliffe, D., Jenkins, V. & Saul, J. (2001a) Psychiatric morbidity and its recognition by doctors in patients with cancer. *Br J Cancer*, **84**(8), 1011–15.

Fallowfield, L., Saul, J. & Gilligan, B. (2001b) Teaching senior nurses how to teach communication skills in oncology. *Cancer Nurs*, **24**(3), 185–91.

Faulkner, A. (1998) The ABC of palliative care: communication with patients, families and other professionals. *Br Med J*, **316**(7125), 130–2.

Faulkner, A. & Maguire, P. (1994) *Talking to Cancer Patients and Their Relatives*. Oxford University Press, Oxford.

Fawcett, J. (1995) *Analysis and Evaluation of Conceptual Models for Nursing*, 3rd edn. F.A. Davis, Philadelphia.

Field, D. & Copp, G. (1999) Communication and awareness about dying in the 1990s. *Palliat Med*, **13**(6), 459–68.

Ford, P. & McCormack, B. (1999) Determining older people's need for registered nursing in continuing health care: the contribution of the Royal College of Nursing's Older People Assessment Tool. *J Clin Nurs*, **8**(6), 731–42.

Foster, C., Evans, D., Eeles, R. *et al.* (2002a) Predictive testing for BRCA1/2: attributes, risk perception and management in a multi-centre cohort. *Br J Cancer*, **86**(8), 1209–16.

Foster, C., Watson, M., Moynihan, C., Ardern-Jones, A. & Eeles, R. (2002b) Genetic testing for breast and ovarian cancer predisposition: cancer burden and responsibility. *J Health Psychol*, **7**(4), 469–84.

Foster, E. & Harrison, M. (2000) Setting up a collaborative care plan. *Nurs Standard*, **15**(8), 40–3.

Franks, A. (1997) Breaking bad news and the challenge of communication. *Eur J Palliat Care*, **4**(2), 61–5.

Frank-Stromborg, M. & Christensen, A. (2001a) Nurse documentation: not done or worse, done the wrong way – Part I. *Oncol Nurs Forum*, **28**(4), 697–702.

Frank-Stromborg, M. & Christensen, A. (2001b) Nurse documentation: not done or worse, done the wrong way – Part II. *Oncol Nurs Forum*, **28**(5), 841–6.

Frank-Stromborg, M. & Olsen, S.J. (1997) *Instruments for Clinical Health Care – Research*, 2nd edn. Jones and Bartlett, London.

Friedrichsen, M.J., Strang, P.M. & Carlsson, M.E. (2001) Receiving bad news: experiences of family members. *J Palliat Care*, **17**(4), 241–7.

Gall, G.B. (2002) A useful screening tool. *RN*, **65**(9), 41–3.

Glaser, B. & Strauss, A. (1965) *Awareness of Dying*. Weidenfeld and Nicolson, London.

Glasper, E.A., Lattimer, V.A., Thompson, F. & Wray, D. (2000) NHS Direct: examining the challenges for nursing practice. *Br J Nurs*, **9**(17), 1173–81.

Goldenberg, I. & Goldenberg, H. (1996) *Family Therapy. An Overview*. Brooks/Cole Publishing, Pacific Grove, pp. 41–61.

Goossen, W.T.F., Epping, P.J.M.M. & Dassen, T. (1997) Criteria for nursing information systems as a component of the electronic patient record. *Comput Nurs*, **15**(6), 307–15.

Gordon, M. (1994) *Nursing Diagnosis, Process and Application*. Mosby, St Louis.

Gordon, M. (2000) *Manual of Nursing Diagnosis*, 9th edn. Mosby, St Louis.

Govier, I. (2000) Spiritual care in nursing: a systematic approach. *Nurs Stand*, **14**(17), 32–6.

Greer, S. (1992) The management of denial in cancer patients. *Oncology*, **6**(12), 33–6.

Greer, S. & Watson, M. (1987) Mental adjustment to cancer: its measurement and prognostic importance. *Cancer Surv*, **6**(3), 439–53.

Gregory, P. (2000) Patient assessment and care planning: sexuality. *Nurs Stand*, **15**(9), 38–41.

Griffiths, P. (1998) An investigation into the description of patients' problems by nurses using two different needs-based nursing models. *J Adv Nurs*, **28**(5), 969–77.

Grobe, S.J. (1996) The nursing intervention lexicon and taxonomy. Implications for representing nursing care in automated patient records. *Holistic Nurs Pract*, **11**(1), 48–63.

Hale, C., Thomas, L., Bond, S. & Todd, C. (1997) The nursing records as a research tool to identify nursing interventions. *J Adv Nurs*, **6**, 207–14.

Hallowell, N. (1999) Doing the right thing: genetic risk and responsibility. *Sociol Health Illness*, **21**(5), 597–621.

Hallowell, N., Foster, C., Moynihan, C. *et al.* (2002) Genetic testing for women previously diagnosed with breast/ovarian cancer: examining the impact of BRCA1 and BRCA2 mutation screening. *Genet Test*, **6**(2), 79–87.

Hansebo, G., Kihlgren, M., Ljunggren, G. (1999) Review of nursing documentation in nursing home wards – changes after intervention for individualized care. *J Adv Nurs*, **29**(6), 1462–73.

Harbison, J. (2001) Clinical decision making in nursing: theoretical perspectives and their relevance to practice. *J Adv Nurs*, **35**(1), 126–33.

Hardwick, S. (1998) Clarification of nursing diagnosis from a British perspective. *Assign – Ongoing Work Health Care Studies*, **4**(2), 3–9.

Harris, R. (2002) *Physical Assessment of Patients. The Byron Physical Assessment Framework*. Whurr, London.

Harris, R., Wilson-Barnett, J., Griffiths, P. & Evans, A. (1998) Patient assessment: validation of a nursing instrument. *Int J Nurs Stud*, **35**, 303–13.

Harrison, A. (2001) The mental health needs of patients in physical care settings. *Nurs Stand*, **15**(1), 47–56.

Hartmann, L.C., Schaid, D.J., Woods, J.E. *et al.* (1999) Efficacy of bilateral prophylactic mastectomy in women with a family history of breast cancer. *N Engl J Med*, **340**(2), 77–84.

Heartfield, M. (1996) Nursing documentation and nursing practice: a discourse analysis. *J Adv Nurs*, **24**(1), 98–103.

Heaven, C. & Maguire, P. (1996) Training hospice nurses to elicit patient concerns. *J Adv Nurs*, **23**(2), 280–6.

Heaven, C. & Maguire, P. (1997) Disclosure of concerns by hospice patients and their identification by nurses. *Palliat Med*, **11**(4), 283–90.

Hedburg, B. & Larsson, U.S. (2003) Observations, confirmations and strategies – useful tools in decision-making process for nurses in practice. *J Clin Nurs*, **12**(2), 215–22.

Hensley, K. (2002) Forms and function. *Nurs Manage*, **33**(11), 38–40.

Hinton, J. (1998) An assessment of open communication between people with terminal cancer, caring relatives, and others during home care. *J Palliat Care*, **14**(3), 15–23.

Hirshfield-Bartek, J., Dow, K. & Creaton, F. (1990) Decreasing documentation time using a patient self assessment tool. *Oncol Nurs Forum*, **17**(2), 251–5.

Hogston, R. (1997) Nursing diagnosis and classification systems: a position paper. *J Adv Nurs*, **26**, 496–500.

Holland, D.E., Hanse, D.C., Matt-Hensrud, N.N., Severson, M.A. & Wenninger, C.R. (1998) Continuity of care: a nursing needs assessment instrument. *Geriatr Nurs*, **19**(6), 331–4.

Holmes, H.N. (ed.) (2003) *3-Minute Assessment*. Lippincott, Williams & Wilkins, Philadelphia, pp. 1–19, 20–32.

Hope-Stone, L.D. & Mills, B.J. (2001) Developing empathy to improve patient care: a pilot study of cancer nurses. *Int J Palliat Nurs*, **7**(3), 146–50.

Horton, R. (2002) Differences in assessment of symptoms and quality of life between patients with advanced cancer and their specialist palliative care nurses in a home care setting. *Palliat Med*, **16**(6), 488–94.

Houston, A. & Cowley, S. (2002) An empowerment approach to needs assessment in health visiting practice. *J Clin Nurs*, **11**(5), 640–50.

Howell, M., Walton, G. & Henderson, K. (2002) Does cancer nursing education influence patient care planning? *Prof Nurse*, **18**(4), 216–19.

Hunter, M. (1998) Rehabilitation in cancer care: a patient focused approach. *Eur J Cancer Care*, **7**, 85–7.

Insel, K.C. & Badger, T.A. (2002) Deciphering the 4 D's: cognitive decline, delirium, depression and dementia – a review. *J Adv Nurs*, **38**(4), 360–8.

Jarrett, N. & Payne, S. (1995) A selective review of the literature on nurse–patient communication: has the patients' contribution been neglected? *J Adv Nurs*, **22**(1), 72–8.

Jenkins, V., Fallowfield, L. & Saul, J. (2001) Information needs of patients with cancer: results from a large study in UK cancer centres. *Br J Cancer*, **84**(1), 48–51.

Jenner, E.A. (1998) A case study analysis of nurses' roles, education and training needs associated with patient focused care. *J Adv Nurs*, **27**, 1087–95.

Johnson, M., Maas, M. & Moorehead, S. (1997) *Nursing Outcomes Classification (NIC): Iowa Outcomes Project*, 2nd edn. Mosby, St Louis.

Johnson, M., Bulechek, G.M., McCloskey, J.M., Maas, M. & Moorehead, S. (2001) *Nursing Diagnosis, Outcomes, Interventions: NANDA, NIC, NOC Linkages*. Mosby, St Louis.

Johnson, T. (2000) Functional health pattern assessment on-line: lessons learned. *Comput Nurs*, **18**(5), 248–54.

Jolley, S. (2002) Taking a sexual history: the role of the nurse. *Nurs Times*, **98**(18), 39–41.

Junnola, T., Eriksson, E., Salantera, S. & Lauri, S. (2002) Nurses' decision-making in collecting information for the assessment of patients' nursing problems. *J Clin Nurs*, **11**(2), 186–96.

Kearney, N. (2001) Classifying nursing care to improve patient outcomes: the example of WISECARE. *NT Res*, **6**(4), 747–56.

Keller, C.A., Carolin, K. & Fedoronko, K. (2001) Bone marrow transplant teaching rounds: promoting excellence in nursing care. *Oncol Nurs Forum*, **28**(3), 457–8.

Kenen, R., Ardern-Jones, A. & Eeles, E. (2003) We are talking but are you listening? Communication patterns in families with a history of breast/ovarian cancer. *J Health Risk Soc (submitted)*.

Kennedy, C. (1999) Decision making in palliative nursing practice. *Int J Palliat Nurs*, **5**(3),142–6.

King, L. & Clark, J.M. (2002) Intuition and the development of expertise in surgical ward and intensive care nurses. *J Adv Nurs*, **37**(4), 322–9.

Kinley, H., Czoski-Murray, C. & George, S. (2002) Effectiveness of appropriately trained nurses in preoperative assessment: randomized controlled equivalence/non-inferiority trial. *Br Med J*, **325**(7376), 1323–6.

Kleinbeck, S. & McKennett, M. (2000) Challenges of measuring intraoperative patient outcomes. *AORN J*, **72**(5), 845–50, 853.

Korcz, I.R. & Moreland, S. (1998) Telephone prescreening. *Cancer Pract*, **6**(5), 270–5.

Kozier, B., Erb, G., Blais, K., Wilkerson, J.M. & Van Leuven, K. (1998) *Fundamentals of Nursing: Concepts, Process, and Practice*, 5th edn. Addison Wesley Longman, Menlo Park.

Kruijver, I.P.M., Kerkstra, A., Bensing, J.M. & Van de Wiel, H.B.M. (2000) Nurse–patient communication in cancer care. *Cancer Nurs*, **23**(1), 20–31.

Kruijver, I.P.M., Kerkstra, A., Bensing, J.M. & Van de Wiel, H.B.M. (2001) Communication skills of nurses during interactions with simulated cancer patients. *J Adv Nurs*, **34**(6), 772–9.

Kunyk, D. & Olson, J.K. (2001) Clarification of conceptualizations of empathy. *J Adv Nurs*, **35**(3), 317–25.

Kuppelomaki, M. (2002) Spiritual support for families of patients with cancer: a pilot study of nursing staff assessments. *Cancer Nurs*, **25**(3), 209–18.

Kurihara, Y., Kusunose, T., Okabayashi, Y. *et al.* (2001) Full implementation of a computerised nursing records system at Kochi Medical School Hospital in Japan. *Comput Nurs*, **19**(3), 122–9.

Lanceley, A. (2001a) Therapeutic strategies in cancer care. In: *Cancer Nursing: Care in Context* (eds J. Corner & C. Bailey). Blackwell Science, Oxford.

Lanceley, A. (2001b) The impact of cancer on health care professionals. In: *Cancer Nursing: Care in Context* (eds J. Corner & C. Bailey). Blackwell Science, Oxford.

Lansdown, R. (1996) *Children in Hospital*. Oxford University Press, Oxford, pp. 52–62.

Larsson, G., Widmark Peterson, V., Lampic, C. *et al.* (1998) Cancer patient and staff ratings of the importance of caring behaviours and their relations to patient anxiety and depression. *J Adv Nurs*, **27**, 855–64.

Lauri, S., Lepisto, M. & Kappeli, S. (1997) Patients' needs in hospital: nurses' and patients' views. *J Adv Nurs*, **25**, 339–46.

Leasia, M.S., Monahan, F.D. (2002) *A Practical Guide to Health Assessment*, 2nd edn. W.B. Saunders, Philadelphia, pp. 1–22.

Lecouturier, J., Crack, L., Mannix, K., Hall, R.H. & Bond, S. (2002) Evaluation of a patient-held record for patients with cancer. *Eur J Cancer Care*, **11**, 114–21.

Lee, J. (1999) Does what nurses do affect clinical outcomes for hospitalized patients? A review of the literature. *Health Services Res*, **34**(5), 1011–32.

Leih, P. & Salentijn, C. (1994) Nursing diagnosis: a Dutch perspective. *J Clin Nurs*, **3**, 313–20.

Leslie, K., Curtis, M. & Lunn, D. (2003) Education to achieve symptom control for patients with cancer. *Nurs Times*, **99**(16), 34–6.

Leydon, G.M., Boulton, M., Moynihan, C. *et al.* (2000) Cancer patients' information needs and information seeking behaviour: in depth interview study. *Br Med J*, **320**(7329), 909–13.

Lillibridge, J. & Wilson, M. (1999) Registered nurses' descriptions of their health assessment practices. *Int J Nurs Pract*, **5**(1), 29–37.

Lowden, B. (1998) The health consequences of disclosing bad news. *Eur J Oncol Nurs*, **2**(4), 225–30.

Lyte, G. & Jones, K. (2001) Developing a unified language for children's nurses, children and their families in the United Kingdom. *J Clin Nurs*, **10**, 79–85.

Macleod Clark, J. & Sims, S. (1988) Communication with patients and relatives. In: *Oncology for Nurses and Health Care Professionals*, Vol. 2 (eds R. Tiffany & P.Webb), 2nd edn. Harper and Row, Beaconsfield.

Maddock, E. (2002) The benefits of implementing an electronic patient record system. *Nurs Times*, **98**(49), 34–6.

Mager, W.M. & Andrykowski, M.A. (2002) Communication in the cancer 'bad news' consultation: patient perceptions and psychological adjustment. *Psycho-oncology*, **11**(1), 35–46.

Maguire, P. (1985) Barriers to the psychological care of the dying. *Br Med J*, **291**(6510), 1711–13.

Maguire, P. (1998) Breaking bad news. *Eur J Surg Oncol*, **24**(3), 188–91.

Maguire, P. (1999) Improving communication with cancer patients. *Eur J Cancer*, **35**(14), 2058–65.

Maguire, P., Faulkner, A., Booth, K., Elliot, C. & Hillier, V. (1996) Helping cancer patients disclose their feelings. *Eur J Cancer*, **32A**(1), 78–81.

Martin, K. & Scheet, N. (1992) *The Omaha System: A Pocket Guide for Community Health Nursing*. W.B. Saunders, Philadelphia, pp. 37–41.

Mason, C. (1999) Guide to practice or 'load of rubbish'? The influence of care plans on nursing practice in five clinical areas in Northern Ireland. *J Adv Nurs*, **29**(2), 380–7.

McArthur-Rouse, F. (2001) Critical care outreach services and early warning scoring systems: a review of the literature. *J Adv Nurs*, **36**(5), 696–704.

McClement, S.E. & Hack, T.F. (1999) Audio-taping the oncology treatment consultation: a literature review. *Patient Educ Couns*, **36**(3), 229–38.

McCloskey, J.C. & Bulechek, G.M. (eds) (2000) *Nursing Interventions Classification (NIC): Iowa Intervention Project*, 3rd edn. Mosby, St Louis.

McCormick, W. (1999) Assessment made EASY. *Nurs Stand*, **13**(22), 24–5.

McCue, K. (1996) *How to Help Children Through a Parent's Serious Illness*. St Martin's Griffin, New York, pp. 5–22.

McEvoy, M. (2000) Development of a new approach to palliative care documentation. *Int J Palliat Nurs*, **6**(6), 288–97.

McIllmurray, M.B., Thomas, C., Francis, B., Morris, S., Soothill, K. & Al-Hamad, A. (2001) The psychosocial needs of cancer patients: findings from an observational study. *Eur J Cancer Care*, **10**, 261–9.

McSherry, W. & Ross, L. (2001) Dilemmas of spiritual assessment: considerations for nursing practice. *J Adv Nurs*, **38**(5), 479–88.

Menzies Lyth, I. (1988) The functioning of social systems as a defence against anxiety. In: *Containing Anxiety in Institutions* (ed. I. Menzies Lyth). Free Association Books, London.

Meredith, C., Symonds, P., Webster, L. *et al.* (1996) Information needs of cancer patients in west Scotland: cross sectional survey of patients' views. *Br Med J*, **313**(7059), 724–6.

Miller, L. (2002) Effective communication with older people. *Nurs Stand*, **17**(9), 45–50, 53, 55.

Mills, M.E. & Sullivan, K. (1999) The importance of information giving for patients newly diagnosed with cancer: a review of the literature. *J Clin Nurs*, **8**(6), 631–42.

Mitchell, M. (2002) Guidance for the psychological care of day case surgery patients. *Nurs Stand*, **16**(40), 41–3.

Moen, A., Bakken, S., Henry, & Warren, J.J. (1999) Representing nursing judgements in the electronic record. *J Adv Nurs*, **30**(4), 990–7.

Moloney, R. & Maggs, C. (1999) A systematic review of the relationships between written manual nursing care planning, record keeping and patient outcomes. *J Adv Nurs*, **30**(1), 51–7.

Mullally, S. (2000) The Annual Robert Tiffany Memorial Lecture: June 2000. *Eur J Cancer Care*, **9**(4), 186–90.

Murphy, K., Cooney, A., Casey, D., Connor, M., O'Connor, J. & Dineen, B. (2000) The Roper, Logan and Tierney (1996) model: perceptions and operationalization of the model in psychiatric nursing within a Health Board in Ireland. *J Adv Nurs*, **31**(6), 1333–41.

Murphy-Ende, K. & Chernecky, C. (2002) Assessing adults with leukaemia. *Nurse Practitioner*, **27**(11), 49–60.

National Cancer Alliance (1996) *'Patient-Centred Cancer Services?' What Patients Say*. National Cancer Alliance, Oxford.

Newell, R. (2002a) Living with disfigurement. *Nurs Times*, **98**(15), 34–5.

Newell, R. (2002b) The fear-avoidance model: helping patients to cope with disfigurement. *Nurs Times*, **98**(16), 38–9.

NHSE (1998) *Information for Health: An Information Strategy for the Modern NHS 1998–2005. A National Strategy for Local Implementation*. NHSE, Leeds.

NHSE (1999) *For the Records: Managing Records in NHS Trusts and Health Authorities (HSC 199/53 1999)*. NHSE, London.

NHSE (2000) *Data Protection Act 1998: Protection and Use of Patient Information (HSC2000/009 2000)*. NHSE, London.

NMC (2002a) *Code of Professional Conduct*. Nursing and Midwifery Council, London.

NMC (2002b) *Guidelines for Records and Record Keeping*. Nursing and Midwifery Council, London.

North American Nursing Diagnosis Association (NANDA) (2001) *Nursing Diagnoses: Definitions and Classification. 2001–2002*. NANDA, Philadelphia.

O'Connell, B., Myers, H., Twigg, D. & Entriken. F. (2000) Documenting and communicating patient care: are nursing care plans redundant? *Int J Nurs Pract*, **6**(5), 276–80.

O'Neill, E.S. & Dluhy, N.M. (1997) A longitudinal framework for fostering critical thinking and diagnostic reasoning. *J Adv Nurs*, **26**, 825–32.

Orem, D.E., Taylor, S.G. & Renpenning, K. (2001) *Nursing: Concepts of Practice*, 6th edn. Mosby, St Louis.

Parker, P.A., Baile, W.F., De Moor, C., Lenzi, R., Kudelka, A.P. & Cohen, L. (2001) Breaking bad news about cancer: patients' preferences for communication. *J Clin Oncol*, **19**(7), 2049–56.

Parle, M., Jones, B. & Maguire, P. (1996) Maladaptive coping and affective disorders. *Psychol Med*, **26**(4), 735–44.

Payne, D., Biggs, C., Tran, K., Borgen, P. & Massie, M. (2000) Women's regrets after bilateral prophylactic mastectomy. *Ann Surg Oncol*, **7**(1), 150–4.

Payne, J. (2000) The nursing interventions classification: a language to define nursing. *Oncol Nurs Forum*, **27**(1), 99–103.

Peden-McAlpine, C. & Clark, N. (2002) Early recognition of client status changes: the importance of time. *Dimens Crit Care Nurs*, **21**(4), 144–50.

Pilling, A. & Wolstenholme, R. (2002) A nurse-led service for COPD patients. *NT Plus*, **98**(12), 53–4.

Pinkerton, C.R., Cushing, P. & Sepion, B. (1994) *Childhood Cancer Management*. Chapman and Hall, London.

Piper, B.F. (1997) Measuring fatigue. In: *Instruments for Clinical Health Care Research* (eds M. Frank-Stromborg & S.J. Olsen), 2nd edn. Jones and Bartlett, Massachusetts.

Price, C.I.M., Han, S.W. & Rutherford, I.A. (2000) Advanced nursing practice: an introduction to physical assessment. *Br J Nurs*, **9**(22), 2292–6.

Pritchard, E. (1999) Screening for dementia and depression in older people. *Nurs Stand*, **14**(5), 46–52.

Ptacek, J.T. & Ptacek, J.J. (2001) Patients' perceptions of receiving bad news about cancer. *J Clin Oncol*, **19**(21), 4160–4.

Pye, H. & Farrell, M. (2000) Using information technology to plan nursing care in a paediatric hospital setting. *Paediatr Nurs*, **12**(4), 22–5.

Quinn, B. (2003) Sexual health in cancer care. *Nurs Times*, **99**(4), 32–4.

Radziewicz, R. & Baile, W.F. (2001) Communication skills: breaking bad news in the clinical setting. *Oncol Nurs Forum*, **28**(6), 951–3.

Rait, D. & Lederberg, M. (1989) The family of the cancer patient. In: *Handbook of Psychooncology* (eds J.C. Holland & J.H. Rowland). Oxford University Press, New York.

Ramirez, A.J., Graham, J., Richards, M.A. *et al.* (1995) Burnout and psychiatric disorder among cancer clinicians. *Br J Cancer*, **71**(6), 1263–9.

Razavi, D. & Delvaux, N. (1997) Communication skills and psychological training in oncology. *Eur J Cancer*, **33**(6 Suppl), S15–21.

Read, H. (1999) Documentation in the outpatient setting. *Nurs Stand*, **13**(34), 41–3.

Rebbeck, T.R., Levin, A.M., Eisen, A. *et al.* (1999) Breast cancer risk of bilateral prophylactic oophorectomy in BRCA1 mutation carriers. *J Natl Cancer Inst*, **91**(17), 1475–9.

Richardson, A. & Wilson Barnett, J. (eds) (1995) *Nursing Research in Cancer Care*. Scutari Press, London.

Rodden, C. & Bell, M. (2002) Record keeping: developing good practice. *Nurs Stand*, **17**(1), 40–2.

Rogers, C. (1967) *On Becoming a Person*. Constable, London.

Rothbrook, J.C. & Smith, D. (2000) Selecting the perioperative patient focused model. *AORN J*, **71**(5), 1030–2, 1034, 1036–7.

Routasalo, P. (1999) Physical touch in nursing studies: a literature review. *J Adv Nurs*, **30**(4), 843–50.

Rowland, J.H. (1989) Developmental stage and adaptation: child and adolescent model. In: *Handbook of Psychooncology* (eds J.C. Holland & J.H. Rowland). Oxford University Press, New York.

Rutenberg, C. (2000) Telephone triage. *Am J Nurs*, **100**(3), 77–81.

Sapir, R., Catane, R., Kaufman, B. *et al.* (2000) Cancer patient expectations of and communication with oncologists and oncology nurses: the experience of an integrated oncology and palliative care service. *Supportive Care Cancer*, **8**(6), 458–63.

Sawyer, H. (2000) Meeting the information needs of cancer patients. *Prof Nurse*, **15**(4), 244–7.

Schuster, P.M. (2000) Concept mapping: reducing clinical care plan paperwork and increasing learning. *Nurse Educator*, **25**(2), 76–81.

Scullion, J.E. & Henry, C. (1998) A multidisciplinary approach to managing breathlessness in lung cancer. *Int J Palliat Nurs*, **4**(2), 65–9.

Selwood, K. (2000) Integrated care pathways: an audit tool in paediatric oncology. *Br J Nurs*, **9**(1), 34–8.

Seymour, B., Kinn, S. & Sunderland, N. (2003) Valuing both critical and creative thinking in clinical practice: narrowing the research–practice gap. *J Adv Nurs*, **42**(3), 288–96.

Shaw, M. (1998) *Charting Made Incredibly Easy!* Springhouse Corporation, Springhouse.

Simpson, M. (2003) Multidisciplinary patient records in a palliative care setting. *Nurs Times*, **99**(3), 33–4.

Skinn, B. & Stacey, D. (1994) Establishing an integrated framework for documentation: use of a self reporting health history and outpatient oncology record. *Oncol Nurs Forum*, **21**(9), 1557–66.

Smith, G.Sr. & Richardson, A. (1996) Development of nursing documentation for use in the outpatient oncology setting. *Eur J Cancer Care*, **5**, 225–32.

Spcice, J., Harkness, J., Laneri, H. *et al.* (2000) Involving family members in cancer care: focus group considerations of patients and oncological providers. *Psycho-oncology*, **9**(2), 101–12.

Standing Nursing and Midwifery Advisory Committee (2001) *Practice Guidance: Principles, Standards and Indicators. A Resource Tool Caring for Older People: A Nursing Priority*. Department of Health, London.

Stewart, M.A. (1995) Effective physician–patient communication and health outcomes: a review. *Can Med Assoc J*, **152**(9), 1423–33.

Teytelman, Y. (2002) Effective nursing documentation and communication. *Semin Oncol Nurs*, **18**(2), 121–7.

Thorne, S.E. (1999) Communication in cancer care: what science can and cannot teach us. *Cancer Nurs*, **22**(5), 370–8.

Tierney, A.J. (1998) Nursing models: extant or extinct? *J Adv Nurs*, **28**(1), 77–85.

Tischkowitz, M. (1999) Hereditary non polyposis colorectal cancer. *CME Oncol*, **1**(4), 103–7.

Travis, S., Conway, J., Daly, M. & Larsen, L. (2001) Terminal restlessness in the nursing facility: assessment, palliation, and symptom management. *Geriatr Nurs*, **22**(6), 308–12.

Van der Molen, B. (1999) Relating information needs to the cancer experience: 1. Information as a key coping strategy. *Eur J Cancer Care*, **8**(4), 238–44.

Wadsworth, L., Smith, A. & Waterman, H. (2002) The nurse practitioner's role in day case pre-operative assessment. *Nurs Stand*, **16**(47), 41–4.

Wallace, P.R. (2001) Improving palliative care through effective communication. *Int J Palliat Nurs*, **7**(2), 86–90.

Waterlow, J. (1995) *Pressure Sore Prevention Manual*. Newtons, Taunton.

Waters, K.R. & Easton, N. (1999) Individualized care: is it possible to plan and carry out? *J Adv Nurs*, **29**(1), 79–87.

Webster, M. (1981) Communicating with dying patients. *Nurs Times*, **77**(23), 999–1002.

Wenzel, G. (2002) Creating an interactive interdisciplinary electronic assessment. *Comput Informatics Nurs*, **20**(6), 251–60.

Westbrook, A. (2000) Learning curve. Nursing language. *Nurs Times*, **96**(14), 41.

White, L. (2003) *Documentation and the Nursing Process*. Thomson Delmar Learning, Canada.

Wilkinson, S. (1991) Factors which influence how nurses communicate with cancer patients. *J Adv Nurs*, **16**, 677–88.

Wilkinson, S. (1994) Stress in cancer nursing – does it really exist? *J Adv Nurs*, **20**(6), 1079–84.

Wilkinson, S. (1999) Communication: it makes a difference. *Cancer Nurs*, **22**(1), 17–20.

Wilkinson, S., Roberts, A. & Aldridge, J. (1998) Nurse–patient communication in palliative care: an evaluation of a communication skills programme. *Palliat Med*, **12**(1), 13–22.

Wilkinson, S., Bailey, K., Aldridge, J. & Roberts, A. (1999) A longitudinal evaluation of a communication skills programme. *Palliat Med*, **13**(4), 341–8.

Wilkinson, S., Gambles, M. & Roberts, A. (2002) The essence of cancer care: the impact of training on nurses' ability to communicate effectively. *J Adv Nurs*, **40**(6), 731–8.

Wimpenny, P. (2001) The meaning of models of nursing to practising nurses. *J Adv Nurs*, **40**(3), 346–54.

Wood, C. (2003) The importance of good record-keeping for nurses. *Nurs Times*, **99**(2), 26–7.

Woods, S. (1998) Ethics and communication: developing reflective practice. *Nurs Stand*, **12**(18), 44–7.

Yancey, R., Given, B.A., White, N.J., DeVoss, D. & Coyle, B. (1998) Computerized documentation for a rural nursing intervention project. *Comput Nurs*, **16**(5), 275–84.

Yates, P. (1999) Family coping: issues and challenges for cancer nursing. *Cancer Nurs*, **22**(1), 63–71.

Abdominal paracentesis

Chapter contents

Definition

Abdominal paracentesis is a technique used to drain an abnormal collection of ascitic fluid from the abdomen (Campbell 2001). A fenestrated catheter is inserted through the abdominal muscles into the peritoneal cavity (Kouraklis 2002). This procedure is usually done for the relief of symptoms caused by ascites.

Indications

Abdominal paracentesis is indicated under the following circumstances:

- To obtain a specimen of fluid for analysis for diagnostic purposes
- To relieve the symptoms associated with ascites, both physical and psychological
- To administer substances such as radioactive gold colloid, cytotoxic drugs (e.g. bleomycin, cisplatin) or other agents into the peritoneal cavity, to achieve regression of scrosae deposits responsible for fluid formation.

Reference material

Anatomy and physiology

The peritoneum is a semi-permeable serous membrane consisting of two separate layers.

- Parietal layer – this covers the abdominal and pelvic walls and the undersurface of the diaphragm.
- Visceral layer – this lines and supports the abdominal organs and the parietal peritoneum (Fig. 3.1).

Fluid is produced from the capillaries lining the peritoneal cavity and is drained by lymphatic vessels under the diaphragm. The fluid is collected by the right lymphatic duct which drains into the vena cava. However, in patients with malignant ascites, this bal-

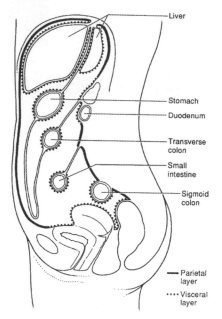

Figure 3.1 Peritoneum of female in lateral view.

ance of production and drainage is disrupted and ascitic fluid collects in the peritoneal cavity.

Functions of the peritoneum

- The peritoneum is a serous membrane which enables the abdominal contents to glide over each other without friction.
- It forms partial or complete cover for the abdominal organs.
- It forms ligaments and mesenteries which help to keep the organs in position.
- The mesenteries contain fat and act as a store for the body.
- The mesenteries can move to engulf areas of inflammation and this prevents the spread of infection.
- It has the power to absorb fluids and exchange electrolytes.

Abdominal paracentesis can be caused by non-malignant conditions such as cirrhosis of the liver, advanced congestive heart failure and chronic pericarditis or by malignant conditions such as metastatic cancer of the ovary, stomach, colon or breast. Cirrhosis of the liver is the most common cause of ascites; only 10% of ascites are related to malignancy (Runyon 1994). However, ascites occurs in up to 50% of patients with an already diagnosed malignancy (Bain 1998). It is accompanied by debilitating

symptoms of breathlessness, indigestion, alteration in bowel habit, fatigue, ankle oedema, reduced mobility, loss of appetite, nausea and vomiting, abdominal swelling, pain and change in body image (Preston 1997). For some patients, minimal ascites can cause great distress through the effect upon their body image and the meaning of the symptoms to the individual (Preston 1997).

Malignant ascites accumulates owing to a number of causes:

- Peritoneal carcinomatosis, when tumour seeds onto the peritoneum. Many tumours secrete vascular permeability factor (VPF) leading to increased permeability and leakage of protein-rich fluid into the peritoneum (Nagy *et al.* 1993).
- Liver metastases causing compression of the hepatic portal vein, leading to fluid being forced into the peritoneal cavity. If ascites is due to mechanical obstruction the ascitic fluid is often low in protein concentration (Preston 1997).
- Chylous ascites – when the lymphatics behind the peritoneum are obstructed (Campbell 2001).

In patients with advanced cancer, malignant ascites is the most likely diagnosis and often reflects end-stage disease. However, in some cases such as ovarian cancer and lymphoma, ascites can be an early presentation and efforts to obtain tumour shrinkage and prolongation of survival should be undertaken (Marincola & Schwartzentruber 2001). If a definitive diagnosis is needed to establish cause to aid staging and possible surgical intervention then a peritoneal tap and analysis of fluid will be useful (Marincola & Schwartzentruber 2001). Fentiman (2002) states that cytological confirmation of malignant cells is difficult with only a 50% chance of success. One third of patients with a known malignancy have a non-malignant cause of ascites (Runyon 1994).

Treatment for ascites may include:

- Paracentesis – the most common way of managing ascites as it gives immediate effect in 90% of cases (Marincola & Schwartzentruber 2001; Campbell 2001)
- Diuretics – useful mainly in cirrhotic-type ascites
- Peritoneovenous shunt – generally used in patients with long-term prognosis. This provides symptomatic relief in two out of three patients
- Instillation of intraperitoneal agents – cytotoxics, sclerosants and biological substances have been tried in an attempt to control the recurrence of ascites. As yet intraperitoneal agents have not been proven, unequivocally, to have a greater beneficial effect than the use of diuretics (Fentiman 2002).

Abdominal paracentesis is not undertaken lightly because of the risk of inducing hypovolaemia, hypokalaemia or hyponatraemia (Lee *et al.* 2000). Because ascitic fluid contains proteins, repeated paracentesis may cause protein depletion. The serum albumin may also be lowered substantially (Parsons *et al.* 1996). Occasional complications include perforation of the bowel, which can be reduced by ultrasound guided paracentesis (Preston 1997; Eriksonn & Redlin Frazier 1997). The introduction of infection during insertion of the ascitic drain can be reduced by following aseptic technique (Lee *et al.* 2000). Up to 13% of patients may develop an abdominal wall metastasis at the puncture site following abdominal paracentesis and, depending upon the size of the abdominal wall metastasis, radiotherapy may be required (Krutiwagen *et al.* 1996). Ascitic fluid may become loculated in the peritoneal cavity, making it difficult to drain the ascitic fluid. Other complications include haemorrhage into the peritoneal cavity, pulmonary emobli and peritonitis (Campbell 2001).

Large amounts of fluid in the peritoneal cavity cause an increase in intra-abdominal pressure. There may be pain as a result of pressure on internal structures. Gastric pressure may cause anorexia, indigestion or hiatus hernia. Intestinal pressure may result in constipation, bowel obstruction or decreased bladder capacity. Pressure on the diaphragm decreases the intrathoracic space and causes shortness of breath. The relief of these symptoms following paracentesis can be dramatic and the procedure is often justified by the relief offered.

Nursing care

Nursing care of patients with abdominal ascites is aimed at relief of the suffering caused by the symptoms. Each patient should be carefully assessed with consideration of their individual circumstances, maintaining respect for their wish to have or not have interventional treatment (Preston 1997; Campbell 2001). Optimal intervention for relief of ascites should have a minimal negative effect on quality of life and be highly effective, especially for those at the end of their life (Lee *et al.* 1998). Care of the patient undergoing abdominal paracentesis is directed at prevention of discomfort and complications. It is an invasive procedure performed at present by a doctor assisted by a nurse at the patient's bedside.

There is much debate about whether it is safe to drain large volumes of fluid rapidly from the abdomen.

Profound hypotension may follow because of the sudden release of intra-abdominal pressure and consequent possible vasodilatation.

Stephenson & Gilbert (2002), following a recent local study and literature search, suggest that several litres of fluid may be safely drained in a few hours. They also state that it is not necessary to drain the abdomen until dry. McNamara (2000) points out that the maximum relief of symptoms is achieved after the initial few litres are drained. This is supported by Moorsom (2001) who suggests that several litres can be drained on free flow over one hour. Clinical practice at The Royal Marsden Hospital reflects a drainage pattern depending on the medical condition of the patient.

In patients who have had multiple paracentesis, the ascites may become loculated. An ultrasound to locate the point of maximum fluid is recommended in these patients. It is known that prolonged drainage times can lead to catheter infection and peritonitis. It has been found that in most cases free drainage of ascites can be allowed to occur. This has been shown to be safe for up to 5 litres of ascitic fluid (Stephenson & Gilbert 2002). Intravenous fluid or albumin replacement and clamping of the drain to reduce flow are not routinely needed. Patients with renal impairment, however, may require some interventions. In all cases regular observations must be carried out to detect early signs of shock, cardiovascular compromise and infection so that the doctor can be informed and action can be taken promptly. Drainage of the fluid must be monitored regularly, volumes recorded and blockages detected and managed. Patients may require assistance to move and position themselves and may experience pain requiring careful repositioning or appropriate analgesia. The drain should be taken out when the desired amount of fluid has been removed and not left in for longer than 12 hours. The patient's renal function should be checked following this procedure.

Nursing interventions for patients undergoing abdominal paracentesis include education about the nature of the procedure, about what results can realistically be expected, and the risks and benefits. Information should also be given about postprocedure care of the puncture site and about the importance of diet and fluid intake to replace proteins and fluid lost in the ascitic fluid. Consideration must be given at this point to quality of life and what expectations the patient and their family have, with full knowledge of the course of disease (Eriksson & Redlin Frazier 1997).

Procedure guidelines: **Abdominal paracentesis**

Equipment

1 Sterile abdominal paracentesis set containing forceps, scalpel blade and blade holder, swabs, towels, suturing equipment, trocar and cannula (or other approved catheter and introducer), connector to attach to the cannula and guide fluid into the container.
2 Sterile dressing pack.
3 Sterile receiver.
4 Sterile specimen pots.
5 Local anaesthetic.
6 Needles and syringes.
7 Chlorhexidine 0.5% in 70% alcohol.
8 Adhesive dressing.
9 Large sterile drainage bag or container (with connector if appropriate to attach to cannula).
10 Gate clamps.
11 Sterile gloves.
12 Weighing scales if appropriate.
13 Tape measure if appropriate.

Procedure

Action	Rationale
1 Explain and discuss the procedure with the patient.	To ensure that the patient is involved in the decision and understands the procedure, the agreed aim, the risks and benefits. Informed consent may then be obtained.
2 Ask the patient to empty his/her bladder.	If the bladder is full there is a chance of it being punctured when the trocar is introduced.
3 Weigh patient before and after procedure and record.	To assess weight changes and the fluid loss.
4 Ensure privacy.	To maintain dignity.
5 Measure patient's girth around umbilicus before and after procedure and record.	This provides an indication of fluid shift and how much fluid has reaccumulated.
6 The patient should lie supine in bed with the head raised 45–50 cm with a back rest.	Normally the pressure in the peritoneal cavity is no greater than atmospheric pressure, but, when fluid is present, pressure becomes greater than atmospheric pressure. This position will then aid gravity in the removal of fluid and the fluid will drain of its own accord until the pressure is equalized.
7 The procedure is performed by a doctor assisted by a nurse throughout:	
(a) The abdomen is prepared aseptically and draped with sterile towels. Local anaesthetic is administered.	To reduce the risk of local and/or systemic infection. The peritoneal cavity is normally sterile.
(b) Once the anaesthetic has taken effect the doctor makes an incision.	To minimize pain during the procedure and thus maximize patient comfort and facilitate co-operation.
(c) The trocar and cannula are inserted via the incision.	
(d) The trocar is removed.	
8 Ascitic fluid is collected (20–100 ml as instructed by the doctor) and sent for cytology.	In order to diagnose the cause of ascites.
9 If the cannula is to remain in position, sutures will be inserted.	To ensure cannula remains in situ. To reduce risk of trauma to the patient.
10 A closed drainage system is now attached to the cannula using a connector if appropriate. A supportive dry dressing is applied and taped firmly in position.	A sterile container with a non-return valve is necessary to maintain sterility. To reduce local and/or systemic infection.
11 Monitor the patient's blood pressure, pulse and respirations and observe the rate and nature of the drainage. A clamp should be available on the tubing to reduce the flow of fluid if necessary.	To observe for signs of shock and/or infection, and to ensure unobstructed drainage.

*Procedure guidelines: **Abdominal paracentesis** (cont'd)*

Action	Rationale
12 Monitor the patient's fluid balance. Encourage a high-protein and high-calorie diet.	After removal of large amounts of peritoneal fluid, fluid moves from the vascular space and reaccumulates in the peritoneal cavity. Ascitic fluid contains protein in addition to sodium and potassium. Problems of dehydration and electrolyte imbalance may be present.
13 Drainage of fluid should be free flowing up to 5 litres unless adverse symptoms present.	

Procedure guidelines: **Removal of an intraperitoneal drain (short term)**

Equipment

1 Sterile dressing pack.
2 Sterile gloves.
3 Stitch cutter (if drain has a suture holding it in place).
4 Adhesive tape.
5 Transparent dressing.
6 Gauze (low linting).
7 Bactericidal alcohol handrub (if appropriate).

Procedure

This procedure is usually carried out by a member of the nursing team who has been instructed in the removal of intraperitoneal drains. Removal of the drain should be done at a maximum of 12 hours after insertion.

Action	Rationale
1 Explain and discuss the procedure with the patient.	To ensure the patient understands the procedure and is ready to proceed.
2 Establish that the patient is comfortable, and is not in pain or allergic to the tape to be used.	To reduce unnecessary discomfort and to ensure the patient will not have a local reaction to the tape.
3 Wash hands with bactericidal soap and water or bactericidal alcohol handrub.	To reduce the risk of infection.
4 Prepare equipment using aseptic technique. Apply gloves.	To minimize the risk of contamination.
5 Remove the old dressing.	To allow access to the relevant area.
6 Cut the knot from the purse-string suture (if present).	To allow mobility of the suture.
7 Cut the suture holding the drain in place if present. A second nurse may be required to hold the drain in place.	To free the drain and prevent it falling out.
8 Tie the purse-string suture loosely at skin level if present.	To enable rapid tightening of the suture when the drain is removed.
9 Instruct patient to breathe normally, explain that you are about to take the drain out and steadily pull the drain out.	To ensure that the patient is fully aware of what is about to happen so as not to cause unnecessary distress.
10 As the drain leaves the skin, tighten the purse-string suture if present and tie a firm double knot.	To prevent leakage of fluids.
11 Place gauze over the site and secure it firmly. A transparent dressing may also be used to provide a seal.	To prevent leakage of fluids.
12 Explain to the patient that the procedure is complete and that there may be some temporary leakage. In the event of this occurring, the dressing will be changed or a stoma bag may be placed over the site for a short period of time.	To reduce the risk of leakage and prevent the patient becoming distressed if there is leakage and to reduce risk of contamination to clothes.
13 Ensure the patient is comfortable and clear the equipment away.	To reduce the risk of cross-infection.
14 Wash hands with bactericidal soap and water.	To reduce the risk of cross-infection.
15 Measure fluid drained and record in appropriate document.	To provide an accurate record.

*Procedure guidelines: **Removal of an intraperitoneal drain (short term)** (cont'd)*

Action	Rationale
16 Record vital signs and document procedure done.	To ascertain that the patient is stable and to promote continuity of care and for future reference.
17 Check renal function on the following day.	

Problem solving

Problem	Cause	Suggested action
Patient exhibits shock.	Major circulatory shift of fluid or sudden release of intra-abdominal pressure, vasodilatation and subsequent lowering of blood pressure.	Clamp the drainage tube with a gate clamp to prevent further fluid loss. Record the patient's vital signs. Refer to the medical staff for immediate intervention.
Cessation of drainage of ascitic fluid.	Abdomen is empty of ascitic fluid.	Check with the total output of ascitic fluid given on the patient's fluid balance chart. Measure the patient's girth; compare this measurement with the pre-abdominal paracentesis measurement. Suggest to medical staff that the cannula should be removed. Discontinue the drainage system.
	Patient's position is inhibiting drainage.	Change the patient's position, i.e. move the patient upright or onto his/her side to encourage flow by gravity. Encourage patient to mobilize.
	The ascitic fluid has clotted in the drainage system.	'Milk' the tubing. If this is unsuccessful, change the drainage system aseptically.
Signs of local or systemic infection.	Bacterial invasion at site of abdominal paracentesis cannula.	Obtain a swab from the site of the cannula for cultural review. Apply a dry dressing. Antibiotics may be necessary and instructions to check site and clean wound until resolved. Refer to the medical staff.
Cannula becomes dislodged.	Ineffective sutures or trauma at the puncture site.	Apply a secure dry dressing. Reassure patient. Inform the medical staff.
Pain.	Pressure of ascites or position of drain.	Identify cause. Anchor drain securely to avoid pulling at insertion site or movement within abdomen. Assist patient with repositioning. Administer appropriate prescribed analgesic, monitor the patient's response and inform medical staff.

References and further reading

Aslam, N. & Marino, C.R. (2001) Malignant ascites: new concepts in pathophysiology, diagnosis and management. *Arch Intern Med*, **161**(22), 10–24.

Bain, V.G. (1998) *Oxford Book of Palliative Medicine*, 2nd edn. Oxford University Press, Oxford, pp. 557–71.

Cairns, W. & Malone, R. (1999) Octreotide as agent for the relief of malignant ascites in palliative care patients. *Palliat Med*, **13**(5), 429–30.

Campbell, C. (2001) Controlling malignant ascites. *Eur J Palliat Care*, **8**(5), 187–90.

Eriksson, J. & Redlin Frazier, S. (1997) Epithelial cancers of the ovary and fallopian tube. In: *Women and Cancer; A Gynaecologic Oncology Nursing Perspective* (ed. G.J. Moore). Prentice Hall, London, pp. 232–4.

Fentiman, I. (2002) *Oxford Text Book of Oncology*, 2nd edn. Oxford University Press, Oxford.

Kouraklis, G. (2002) Post-operative drainage in patients with malignant ascites: a safe method. *J Surg Oncol*, **79**, 124–5.

Krutiwagen, R. *et al.* (1996) Incidence and effect on survival of abdominal wall metastases at trocar of puncture sites following laparoscopy or paracentesis in women with ovarian cancer. *Gynaecol Oncol*, **60**, 233–7.

Lee, A., Lau, T.N. & Yeong, K.Y. (2000) Indwelling catheters for the management of malignant ascites. *Supportive Care Cancer*, **8**(6), 493–9.

Lee, C., Bociek, G. & Faught, W. (1998) A survey of practice in the management of malignant ascites. *J Pain Symptom Manage*, **16**(2), 96–101.

Mackey, J.R., Wood, L., Nabholtz, J.-M., Jensen, J. & Venner, P. (2000) A phase II trial of triamcinolone hexacetanide for symptomatic recurrent malignant ascites. *J Pain Symptom Manage*, **19**(3), 193–9.

Marincola, F.M. & Schwartzentruber, D.J. (2001) *Cancer Principles and Practice of Oncology*, 6th edn. Lippincott, Williams and Wilkins, Philadelphia, pp. 2745–52.

Maxwell, M.B. (1997) Malignant effusions and edemas. In: *Cancer Nursing: Principles and Practice* (eds S.L. Groenwald, M. Hansen Frogge, M. Goodman *et al.*). Jones & Bartlett, London, pp. 721–41.

McNamara, P. (2000) Paracentesis – an effective method of symptom control in the palliative care setting? *Palliat Med*, **14**, 62–4.

Moorsom, D. (2001) Paracentesis in a home care setting. *Palliat Med*, **15**, 169–70.

Nagy, J., Herzberg, K. & Dvorak, J. (1993) Pathogenesis of malignant ascites formation: initiating events that lead to fluid accumulation. *Cancer Res*, **53**, 2631–43.

Parsons, S.L., Watson, S.A. & Steele, R.J. (1996) Malignant ascites: review. *Br J Surg*, **83**, 6–14.

Preston, N. (1997) Current practice in the management of malignant ascites. *J Cancer Care*, **13**, 144–6.

Regnard, C. & Tempest, S. (1992) *A Guide to Symptom Relief in Advanced Cancer*, 3rd edn. Haigh & Hochland, Manchester.

Runyon, B.A. (1994) Care of patients with ascites. *N Engl J Med*, **330**, 337–42.

Stephenson, J. & Gilbert, J. (2002) The development of clinical guidelines on paracentesis for ascites related to malignancy. *Palliat Med*, **16**, 213–18.

Tueche, S.G. & Pector, J.C. (2000) Peritoneovenous shunt in malignant ascites. The Bordet Institute experience from 1975–1998. *Hepato-gastro-enterology*, **47**(35), 1322–4.

Verheul, H.M.W., Hoekman, K., Jorna, A.S., Smit, E.F. & Pinedo, H.M. (2000) Targetting vascular endothelial factor blockade: ascites and pleural effusion formation. *Oncologist*, **5**(1), 45–50.

Zanon, C., Grosso, M., Apra, F. *et al.* (2002) Palliative treatment of malignant refractory ascites by positioning of Denver peritoneovenous shunt. *Tumori*, **88**(2), 123–7.

Aseptic technique

Chapter contents

Definition

Aseptic technique is the effort taken to keep the patient as free from hospital micro-organisms as possible (Crow 1989). It is a method used to prevent contamination of wounds and other susceptible sites by organisms that could cause infection. This can be achieved by ensuring that only sterile equipment and fluids are used during invasive medical and nursing procedures. Ayliffe *et al.* (2000) suggest that there are two types of asepsis: medical and surgical asepsis. Medical or clean asepsis reduces the number of organisms and prevents their spread; surgical or sterile asepsis includes procedures to eliminate micro-organisms from an area and is practised by nurses in operating theatres and treatment areas.

A randomized prospective study has been undertaken to evaluate whether some procedures should be included in the medical or surgical category. Using a medical aseptic non-touch technique compared to a surgical technique when changing central venous devices, fluids or lines caused no difference in infection rates, indicating that it was safe to use the simpler non-touch medical aseptic technique (Larwood *et al.* 2000).

Indications

Patients have a right to be protected from preventable infection and nurses have a duty to safeguard the well-being of their patients (King 1998). An aseptic technique should be implemented during any invasive procedure that bypasses the body's natural defences, e.g. the skin and mucous membranes, or when handling equipment such as intravenous cannulae and urinary catheters that have been used during these procedures.

Whilst it is difficult to maintain sterility, it is important to prevent contamination of sterile equipment. Poor aseptic techniques can lead to contamination. A 22% syringe contamination rate was observed for syringes prepared by intensive care unit nurses, compared to a 1% rate for the syringes prepared by pharmaceutical technicians (Van Grafhorst *et al.* 2002).

A study to establish nurses' actions whilst carrying out aseptic techniques suggested that not all nurses followed the same actions and that the rationale for the practice of aseptic techniques is not always research based (Bree-Williams & Waterman 1996). Similar discrepancies were found amongst medical staff (Sellors *et al.* 2002). Nurses can feel uncertain about how to undertake an aseptic technique (Hallett 2000). Unfortunately some infection control practices routinely used cannot be rigorously studied for ethical or logistical reasons, for example wearing versus not wearing gloves (Mangram *et al.* 1999).

Briggs *et al.* (1996) suggest assessment of the individual patient's circumstances before each procedure. By predicting and planning for potential problems asepsis can be maintained.

Reference material

Hospital-acquired infection (HAI) (also called nosocomial infection) is defined as infection occurring in patients after admission to hospital that was neither present nor incubating at the time of admission. Infections acquired in hospital but not manifest until after the patient is discharged are included in the definition (Ayliffe *et al.* 2000). Crowe & Cooke (1998) reviewed the case definition for nosocomial infections, finding areas of consensus and variation which made comparisons of infection rates difficult.

In 1980 a national survey found that one in ten patients acquired an infection whilst in hospital (Meers *et al.* 1980). Few changes were found following a second national prevalence survey of HAI which was reported on in 1996. This survey assessed 37 111 patients from 157 centres and found a HAI prevalence rate of 9% (range 2–29%) (Emmerson *et al.* 1996). Three major sites of infection related to asepsis were highlighted: urinary tract infection 23.2% (risk increased following catheterization), surgical wound infection 10.7% and skin infection 9.6% (invasive procedures increasing the risk of skin infection).

Immunocompromised patients have an increased risk of HAI. Risk factors include underlying disease, invasive procedures, medical devices and length of hospital stay. Prevention of infection for those immunocompromised patients with multiple risk factors cannot always be achieved (Taylor *et al.* 2001). Infections acquired by neutropenic patients differ from those of general hospitalized patients. Bloodstream infections are the most common infections for neutropenic patients with haematological malignancies (Glauser & Calandra 2000) and recovery from these is often poor (Garrouste-Orgeas *et al.* 2000).

Risk factors associated with HAI include invasive procedures, indwelling devices, malignancy, a stay in intensive care or surgical department and length of hospital stay (Rojo *et al.* 1999).

The cost of infection is high, to both the patient and the hospital. HAI increase mortality and morbidity and cause an increase in pain and suffering experienced by the patients (Fagon *et al.* 1994). The patient may be inconvenienced by a prolonged period of hospitalization, which can cause economic and social hardships to the whole family: 1–4 days for urinary tract infection; 7–8.2 days for surgical site infection; 7–21 days for bloodstream infections and 6.8–30 days for pneumonia (Jarvis 1996). The hospital will have increased waiting lists and increased hospital costs. Breaks in aseptic techniques have been implicated in outbreaks of infection (Manning *et al.* 2001). It is essential when aseptic techniques are used as a method of preventing infection that these procedures are sound in theory and are carried out correctly.

Hospitals recognize the significance of nosocomial infections and employ infection control teams to:

- Reduce the likelihood of patients being exposed to infectious micro-organisms while in hospital.
- Provide adequate care for patients with communicable infections.
- Minimize the likelihood of employees, visitors and communicable contacts being exposed to infectious micro-organisms.
- Develop policies for appropriate management of patients with communicable infections.
- Provide surveillance systems which give adequate feedback to appropriate staff.
- Provide education in techniques to prevent the emergence and spread of infection.

A 10-year study in the USA found that an infection control team reduced the incidence of HAI by up to 32%. Hospitals in the study with no infection control programme experienced an increase in infection rates of up to 18% (Haley *et al.* 1985a). A 3-year study reported a reduction in the infection rate from 10.5 to 5.6% following the introduction of an infection control team (French *et al.* 1989).

A survey of factors which influence compliance with infection control procedures highlighted lack of knowledge, lack of time and shortage of staff and the standard set by senior staff including surgeons and nurses (Sherwood 1995) and overcrowding (Archibold *et al.*

Table 4.1 Surgical site infections can be further divided by surgical category

Surgical category	Infection risk
Clean (non-traumatic wound where respiratory, alimentary and genitourinary tracts were not entered)	1.5–4.2%
Clean/contaminated (non-traumatic wound in which respiratory, alimentary and genitourinary tracts were entered without significant spillage)	Less than 10%
Contaminated (fresh traumatic wound from a relatively clean source or an operative wound with gross spillage from the gastrointestinal tract or entrance into genitourinary or biliary tract in the presence of infected urine or bile)	10–20%
Dirty or infected (traumatic wound from a dirty source or delayed treatment, faecal contamination, foreign bodies, a devitalized viscus or pus)	20–30%

1997) as relevant indicators. It was suggested that greater emphasis and knowledge may motivate staff to make time for correct compliance with infection control procedures.

All staff involved in patient care must receive education and training in the prevention of HAI (DoH 2001a). Creativity is required when facilitating learning related to infection control (Ford & Koehler 2001). Feedback of infection rates can achieve changes in practice (Reilly 2002).

When cross-infection does occur the cost of investigating and controlling even a small outbreak is high. It has been estimated that an infection increases the costs of health care by more than 300% (Whitehouse *et al.* 2002), emphasizing how important it is to prevent infection. The Infection Control Standards Working Party has prepared standards for practice to make prevention, detection and control of infection in hospitals as effective as possible (Infection Control Standards Working Party 1993). Surgical wound infections are the second most common nosocomial infection in England and Wales (Mangram *et al.* 1999). Prevention of postoperative wound infections relies on flawless aseptic technique principles in the operating theatre and the wards (Clayton 1996).

The diagnosis of infection relies on classic signs of inflammation such as local redness, swelling and pain, although decreased numbers of neutrophils produce minimal or atypical clinical signs of infection (Candell & Whedon 1991). These local signs and symptoms can precede a further sequence of events, which can be lymphangitis, lymphadenitis, bacteraemia and septicaemia which, if not promptly recognized and treated, can result in death.

Some patients die each year as a result of HAI. Whilst many of these fatalities occur in patients already dying from other causes and/or in patients whose infections were not preventable, a proportion of these deaths are avoidable (DoH 1995; Taylor *et al.* 2001). The risk of death increases with the severity of the patient's underlying disease.

A study to assess nurses' adherence to aseptic techniques revealed an unanticipated high number of errors (McLane *et al.* 1983). The nurses' heavy workload was a contributing factor in poor compliance to aseptic techniques, which suggests that unnecessary time-consuming aspects of an aseptic technique should be avoided (Kelso 1989). This view is supported by Bree-Williams & Waterman's (1996) study, which highlighted that the practice of aseptic technique has become ritualistic and complex, and simpler practices are easier, cheaper and not detrimental to the patients.

Gwyther (1988) discusses how most teaching occurs on the hospital ward and questioned whether this teaching was based on knowledge of the principles of, for example, wound care, or simply on experience. Jenks & Ferguson (1994) reviewed the discrepancy between what is taught in the classroom and what nurses experience in the clinical setting. This suggested that collaboration is needed between education and service staff to integrate learning within the nursing curricula. Thomlinson (1990) emphasizes the importance of replacing infection control procedures which involve unnecessary ritual with sound, cost-efficient and environmentally responsible practices to encourage a greater understanding of the principles of asepsis. These authors highlight a continuing problem and it has been suggested that the principles of aseptic techniques need to be re-established (Lund & Caruso 1993), to ensure nurses understand the importance of prevention of infection (Davey 1997).

Principles of asepsis

Infection is caused by organisms which invade the host's immunological defence mechanisms, although susceptibility to infection may vary from person to person (Gould 1994). The risk of infection is increased if the patient is immunocompromised (Hart 1990) by:

- Age. Neonates and the elderly are more at risk because their immune systems are less efficient.
- Underlying disease. For example, those patients with severe debilitating or malignant disease.

- Prior drug therapy, such as the use of immunosuppressive drugs or the use of broad-spectrum antimicrobials.
- Patients undergoing surgery or instrumentation.

The following factors must be considered when nursing immunocompromised patients.

- Classic signs and symptoms of infection are often absent.
- Untreated infection may disseminate rapidly.
- Infections may be caused by unusual organisms or organisms which, in most circumstances, are non-pathogenic.
- Some antibiotics are less effective in immunocompromised patients.
- Repeated infections may be caused by the same organism.
- Superinfections, where a patient acquires a more pathogenic organism (of the same or different species) than the one already causing infection (Laurence *et al.* 2002), require nursing care of the highest standard, including strict adherence to aseptic technique to prevent such infections.

Sproat & Inglis (1992) suggest that a basic principle of infection control for all patients is to assess the risk of infection from one patient to another and to plan nursing care accordingly before action is taken. Haley *et al.* (1985b) add that if each patient is evaluated individually it is possible to focus more closely on those patients who are most susceptible to infection. The most usual means for spread of infection include:

- Hands of the staff involved
- Inanimate objects, e.g. instruments and clothes
- Dust particles or droplet nuclei suspended in the atmosphere.

Hand washing

Hand washing is well researched and uncontroversial, having been found to be the single most important procedure for preventing nosocomial infection as hands have been shown to be an important route of transmission of infection (DoH 2001a). Even brief contact can transmit 10 000 colony-forming units to hands (Gould 1993). However, studies have shown that hand washing is rarely carried out in a satisfactory manner (Taylor 1978a), with the most important factor inhibiting hand washing being busyness (Cohen *et al.* 2002) or inaccessible sinks (Harris *et al.* 2000). Studies have shown that up to 89% of staff miss some part of the hand surface during hand washing (Taylor 1978a) (Fig. 4.1).

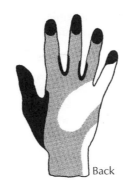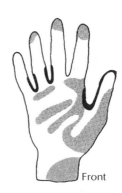

Back   Front

- ■ Most frequently missed
- ▨ Less frequently missed
- □ Not missed

Figure 4.1 Areas most commonly missed following hand washing. (Reproduced by kind permission of *Nursing Times*, where this article first appeared in 1978.)

Hands must be cleaned before and after every patient contact (DoH 2001a). Hand washing can be achieved by three methods:

- Soap and water are effective in removing physical dirt or soiling and transient micro-organisms (Grinbaums *et al.* 1995). Extrinsic contamination of non-medicated liquid soap can lead to handborne transmission of infection (Sartor *et al.* 2000).
- Antimicrobial detergent is effective in removing physical dirt and soiling and more effective in removing resident micro-organisms than soap and water.
- Alcohol-based handrub, whilst not effective in removing physical dirt or soiling, is more effective in destroying transient bacteria than more time-consuming hand-wash methods. Therefore, hands that are visibly soiled or potentially contaminated with dirt or organic matter must be washed first with liquid soap and running water before using alcohol-based handrub (DoH 2001a).

Taylor (1978b) and Phillips (1989) use Feldman's criteria for hand washing, which include the following:

1 Roll up sleeves, remove rings and wrist watches.
2 Use continuously running water.
3 Use soap.
4 Position hands to avoid contaminating arms.
5 Avoid splashing clothing or floor.
6 Rub hands together vigorously.
7 Use friction on all surfaces.
8 Rinse hands thoroughly with hand held down to rinse.
9 Dry hands thoroughly.

Hand washing should be undertaken after patient contact and before an aseptic technique is performed (DoH 2001a).

A dispenser of alcoholic handrub should be placed on the lower shelf of all trolleys used for aseptic techniques, to allow hands to be cleaned during the aseptic procedure. A nurse with 'socially clean' hands will not need to wash them during the aseptic procedure, but should use a bactericidal alcoholic handrub whenever disinfection is required, e.g. after opening the outer wrappers of dressings. It is unlikely that nurses' hands will become soiled with blood or body fluids as long as blood and body fluid precautions are adopted at all times (Hart 1991). The use of a handrub will also remove the need for the nurse to leave the patient during the procedure to wash the hands at the nearest basin, during which time contamination may occur.

Compliance with hand washing can be improved through targeted teaching (Colombo *et al.* 2002). Multiple interventions to improve compliance have been seen to be more successful than individual events, although compliance can decrease when interventions cease (Hinkin 2002).

The wearing of rings increases the number of bacteria on hands (Salisbury *et al.* 1997). Studies comparing the quantities of bacteria from under rings and watches found increased numbers of bacteria compared to the control group who were not wearing jewellery. Effective hand washing is difficult to achieve if watches and rings are not removed (Field *et al.* 1996). Artificial nails harbour microbes and cannot be cleaned as effectively as short, natural nails and must not be worn by those undertaking aseptic techniques (Porteous 2002).

Washed, wet and poorly dried hands can more easily transfer micro-organisms to other surfaces than dry hands (Patrick *et al.* 1997); the damper the hands, the greater the number of micro-organisms (Taylor *et al.* 2000). Thorough drying of hands after hand washing is essential but lapses in hand drying do occur (Chandra & Milind 2001). Electric air drying or disposable paper towels are the usual method of hand drying; the choice depends on the area where the hand washing is being undertaken and on issues such as noise and heat generation, waste disposal and the availability of a regular supply of paper towels. Research indicates that there is no significant difference between the two drying methods (Gustafson *et al.* 2000). However, if hands have not been washed thoroughly, electric air drying removes more organisms than paper towels (Ansari *et al.* 1991). Electric air dryers have been found to be ineffective for drying larger amounts of water (Merry *et al.* 2001). This suggests that the preferred method is the drying of hands with a good-quality paper towel (DoH 2001a).

No-touch technique

A no-touch technique is essential to ensure that hands, even though they have been washed, do not contaminate the sterile equipment or the patient. This can be achieved by the use of either forceps or sterile gloves (DoH 2001a). However, it must be remembered that forceps may damage tissue (David 1991) and gloves can become damaged during use (Driever *et al.* 2001). There is no direct evidence that gloves that leak result in transmission of infection (DoH 2001a). However, gloves can become contaminated during use with firm touching of the skin rather than light touching, leading to increased contamination (Kocent *et al.* 2002). Gloves must be removed carefully to prevent hands becoming contaminated during removal (DoH 2001a).

It has been reported that prolonged glove use can produce occlusion conditions which encourage the rapid growth of skin flora on nurses' hands (Pereira *et al.* 1997). It is, therefore, essential to clean hands following the removal of gloves.

Inanimate objects

All instruments, fluids and materials that come into contact with the wound must be sterile if the risk of contamination is to be reduced. Crow (1994) suggests four principles of asepsis which are: know what is sterile, and what is not sterile, keep these two types of items separate and replace contaminated items immediately. The sterile supplies department should normally provide all sterile instruments.

The Department of Health (NHSE 2000) requires that all surgical instruments are traceable to the process that washed, packed and autoclaved the pack, and on whom the pack has been used. A traceability system means that the cleaning, packing and sterilization process can be checked. This ensures that the correct procedure had been undertaken at all stages of the process. If a problem occurs either with the pack or with the patient on whom the pack has been used, the instruments can be traced. These systems involve the instrument pack being labelled to prove it has gone through a sterile process. Prior to the pack being released from the autoclave, a trained person inspects the autoclave cycle responsible for the sterilization of the pack, to ensure the autoclave cycle was completed satisfactorily (NHSE 2000). When using the pack it must be checked for conformance; this includes whether the steam indicator has changed colour, the product is in date and it is undamaged. Once the pack has been used, the label has to be removed from the pack and put in the patient's notes.

All medical devices must carry the CE (Conformité Europèene) marking which allows patients, clinicians and other users to be confident that the medical device will perform as the manufacturer intends and is safe when used as instructed (Medical Devices Agency 1997). Any faults or incidents with medical devices must be reported (Medical Devices Agency 2000).

The manufacturer's recommendations for all clinical supplies must be followed at all times. The reuse of single-use items must not occur and could result in legal, economic and ethical consequences (Medical Devices Agency 1995).

Forceps can be used to arrange the dressing pack, and then to remove the used dressing before being discarded (Kelso 1989). Alternatively the washed hands can be inserted into the polythene waste bag to arrange the pack before removing the used dressing. The bag which contains the used dressing is then inverted, before the bag is attached to the dressing trolley. Any equipment that becomes contaminated during a procedure must be discarded. On *no* account should it be returned to the sterile field. Care must also be taken to ensure that equipment and lotions are sterile and that packaging is undamaged before use.

While following aseptic technique, it is important to evaluate the whole procedure to ensure that the principles are followed throughout the whole process. Potential problems such as reusing left-over dressings or taking tape from a contaminated roll (Oldman 1991) will therefore be avoided.

The dressing trolley

Most disinfectants are not sporicidal, have a limited antimicrobial spectrum and must be used only on clean surfaces or equipment, e.g. instruments, as they may fail to penetrate blood or pus (Ayliffe *et al.* 2000). Therefore it is essential that equipment such as trolleys is cleaned daily and, when it becomes contaminated, with a detergent solution and dried carefully with paper towels. This will remove a high proportion of micro-organisms, including bacterial spores (Ayliffe *et al.* 2000). Prior to use for aseptic technique, trolleys should be wiped over with chlorhexidine in 70% ethanol alcohol using a clean paper towel (Ayliffe *et al.* 2000). Trolleys used for aseptic procedures must not be used for any other purpose.

Personal protective equipment (PPE)

PPE means all equipment which is intended to be worn to protect a person against risks to their health and that which may compromise their safety. The Personal Protective Equipment at Work Regulations (HSE 1992) require employers to carry out a formal assessment of the PPE needs of their employees. The aim of the assessment is to identify any foreseeable risks that cannot be controlled by other means and the suitable PPE available to reduce risk (Masterson & Teare 2001). All PPE must have an appropriate British Standard kitemark or European Community CE mark. Staff required to wear PPE must be provided with information, instruction and training on the hazards from which the PPE does or does not protect the wearer, and the purpose, correct use, limitations, maintenance and storage information related to the PPE. If an individual is carrying out any task that involves blood or body fluids they require PPE for the following reasons.

- To prevent the user's clothing becoming contaminated with pathogenic micro-organisms which may subsequently be transferred to other patients in their care (Callaghan 1998).
- To prevent the user's clothing becoming soiled, wet or stained during the course of their duties.
- To prevent transfer of potentially pathogenic micro-organisms from user to patient.
- To prevent the user acquiring infection from the patient (DoH 2001a).

Uniform and other protective clothing should not be taken home for laundering unless it is unavoidable (Ayliffe *et al.* 2000). In these circumstances an automatic washing machine and an automatic dryer on a hot setting should be used (Kiehl *et al.* 1997).

There is evidence that transfer of organisms can occur from one room to another on clothing (Hambraeus 1973). An impermeable apron offers better protection than a cotton gown, which allows bacteria and moisture to pass through because of the weave (Mackintosh *et al.* 1980). It is therefore recommended that a disposable plastic apron, which is impermeable to bacteria, is worn during aseptic procedures. Plastic aprons are single-use items and are worn for one procedure or episode of patient care and then removed (DoH 2001a). Gowns must be worn when undertaking invasive surgical procedures, for example when inserting central venous catheters (DoH 2001b). Reusable gowns demonstrate variations in penetrability but the disposable gown performs to a higher standard (Lankester *et al.* 2001). Reusable gowns can allow bacteria to pass through, providing a false sense of security to the wearer (Lovitt *et al.* 1992).

Surgical masks are an integral part of theatre clothing. However, it has never been shown that wearing a surgical mask decreases postoperative wound infections (Tunevall 1991). Lipp & Edwards (2002) suggest further research is required to evaluate the benefit to patients of surgical masks. The wearing of masks continues to be essential for the wearer's protection against aerosol contamination from blood and body fluids (Sharma *et al.* 1997; Edwards 2001). Masks must be worn as part of routine universal precautions when there is a risk of airborne aerosol of blood or body fluids, administration of toxic drugs or contact with patients who are smear positive with drug-resistant tuberculosis (DoH 1998). These masks must comply with The Control of Substances Hazardous to Health (COSHH) (1988) regulations. For surgical procedures undertaken on the wards masks are generally not required. There is no evidence that wearing a face mask is important in preventing catheter-related infection during central catheter insertion (DoH 2001b).

Gloves

Disposable gloves are available in latex and synthetic materials, in sterile and non-sterile form and with and without powder (O'Toole 1997). Some people are allergic to the natural proteins or the chemical additives found in latex medical gloves, resulting in allergic reactions that range from contact dermatitis to anaphylactic shock (Medical Devices Agency 1998). Some allergies are caused by the use of powdered gloves (North Thames Audit and Clinical Effectiveness in Occupational Health 2000). Non-powdered gloves made from materials other than latex must be provided (Medical Devices Agency 1998).

Latex allergy guidelines pertaining to the safety of patients and staff must be available, All health care workers must be knowledgeable about latex allergy and its related issues (Wright *et al.* 2001). Problems related to latex allergies must be reported to the Occupational Health Department immediately for early diagnosis and treatment (Medical Devices Agency 1996). Incidences of latex sensitivity are reportable to the Health and Safety Executive under RIDDOR (HSE 1995; NHSE 1999).

Boxed, clean, non-sterile, powder-free gloves made from materials other than latex are safe for routine use (Rossoff *et al.* 1993), in particular to protect hands from contamination with organic matter and microorganisms (DoH 2001a). However, boxed, clean, non-sterile gloves should not be used for aseptic techniques (Kunaratanapruk & Silpapojakul 1999; Raybould 2001) as there is insufficient evidence to justify a practice change to non-sterile gloves for aseptic techniques (St Clair & Harrabee 2002). Efforts must be made when wearing gloves to avoid glove contamination (Kocent *et al.* 2002) and glove damage (Cork *et al.* 1995).

Protective footwear

Micro-organisms can be found on the bottom of footwear (Haigh 1993). However, the risk of acquiring infection from floors (Ayliffe *et al.* 2000) and the bottom of health care workers' footwear is low (Haigh 1993). Whilst washable shoes must be kept for those entering the operating theatre (Ayliffe *et al.* 2000), footwear worn elsewhere in the hospital is chosen to comply with risk management rather than infection control.

Environmental cleanliness

The NHS requires that patients are nursed in a clean, comfortable and safe environment. The NHS Performance Assessment Framework (1999) includes a cleanliness standard. The standard can be used to monitor and improve cleaning services. The standard has five key objectives: take cleaning seriously, listen to patients, infection control, education, development and monitoring. Included in the standard are lists of elements and their cleaning requirements. These include odour control and a tidy, uncluttered, well-maintained environment (NHS 2001).

Good hospital hygiene is an integral and important component for preventing HAI. Unfortunately extensive contamination of the hospital environment is known to occur (Oie *et al.* 2002). The patient area must be visibly clean, free of dust and soilage before an aseptic technique is commenced. Therefore thorough cleaning, clean laundry, safe collection of waste and food hygiene and pest control are essential (DoH 2001a).

Routine cleaning of the environment is the responsibility of the hospital domestic staff. Cleaning must be suspended during aseptic techniques (Ayliffe *et al.* 2000).

Patient hygiene

Most surgical site infections are caused by microorganisms from the patient's own commensal flora (Lauwers & de Smet 1998). People who shower with chlorhexidine detergent have a significant reduction in skin flora (Paulson 1993). During surgery, studies indicate that preoperative showering with chlorhexidine reduces intraoperative wound contamination, although there was no significant difference in bacterial counts at the end of surgery between preoperative bathing with chlorhexidine or plain soap (Byrne *et al.* 1991a). Concerns regarding the colonization of the skin with potential pathogens of the patients who had preoperative chlorhexidine were unfounded (Byrne *et al.* 1991b). A large prospective study to establish whether showering or bathing was more efficient in reducing skin flora found that showering decreased levels by 93.55% and bathing by 70.98% (Byrne *et al.* 1990).

Studies have established that it is not detrimental for stitches of surgical wounds to get wet, as healing is not delayed and there is no increase in the incidence of infections (Noe *et al.* 1988).

A protective dressing should be worn whilst showering or bathing to protect the wound and stitches. After showering any non-waterproof dressing should be changed immediately. The use of a transparent film dressing allows continuous inspection and more secure anchorage as well as protecting against wetting during showering (Ward *et al.* 1997).

Airborne contamination

The spread of airborne infection is most likely to occur following procedures such as bed making (Shiomori *et al.* 2002) and cleaning, which can disperse organisms into the air. Airborne contamination of sterile goods can occur (Dietze *et al.* 2001). Ideally such activities should cease 30 minutes before a dressing is to be undertaken. To reduce further the risk of airborne contamination of open wounds the wound should be exposed for as short a time as possible (Ayliffe *et al.* 2000). Dirty dressings should be placed carefully in a yellow clinical waste bag, which is sealed before disposal (Lowbury *et al.* 1981). Clean wounds should be dressed before contaminated wounds. Colostomies and infected wounds should be dressed last of all to minimize environmental contamination and cross-infection.

Air movement should be kept to a minimum during the dressing. This means that adjacent windows should be closed and the movement of personnel within the area discouraged.

Procedure guidelines: **Aseptic technique**

Equipment

1 Sterile dressing pack* containing gallipots or an indented plastic tray, low-linting swabs and/or medical foam, disposable forceps, gloves, sterile field, disposable bag.
2 Fluids for cleaning and/or irrigation.
3 Hypo-allergenic tape.
4 Appropriate dressing (see Ch. 47, Wound management).
5 Appropriate hand hygiene preparation.
6 Any other material will be determined by the nature of the dressing: special features of a dressing should be referred to in the patient's nursing care plan.
7 Any extra equipment that may be needed during procedure, e.g. sterile scissors.
8 Chlorhexidine in 70% spirit and paper towels for cleaning trolley.
9 Total traceability system for surgical instruments and patient record form.

Procedure

Action	Rationale
1 Explain and discuss the procedure with the patient.	To ensure that the patient understands the procedure and gives his/her valid consent.
2 Clean hands with bactericidal alcohol rub.	Hands must be cleaned before and after every patient contact and before commencing the preparations for aseptic technique, to prevent cross-infection.
3 Clean trolley with chlorhexidine in 70% spirit with a paper towel.	To provide a clean working surface.
4 Place all the equipment required for the procedure on the bottom shelf of a clean dressing trolley.	To maintain the top shelf as a clean working surface.
5 Take the patient to the treatment room or screen the bed. Position the patient comfortably so that the area to be dealt with is easily accessible without exposing the patient unduly.	To allow any airborne organisms to settle before the sterile field (and in the case of a dressing, the wound) is exposed. Maintain the patient's dignity and comfort.
6 If the procedure is a dressing and the wound is infected or producing copious amounts of exudate, put on a disposable plastic apron.	To reduce the risk of cross-infection.
7 Take the trolley to the treatment room or patient's bedside, disturbing the screens as little as possible.	To minimize airborne contamination.
8 Loosen the dressing tape.	To make it easier to remove the dressing.
9 Clean hands with a bactericidal alcohol handrub.	To reduce the risk of wound infection.

*Procedure guidelines: **Aseptic technique** (cont'd)*

Action	Rationale
10 Check the pack is sterile (i.e. the pack is undamaged, intact and dry. If autoclave tape is present, check that it has changed colour from beige to beige and brown lines), open the outer cover of the sterile pack and slide the contents onto the top shelf of the trolley.	To ensure that only sterile products are used.
11 Open the sterile field using only the corners of the paper.	So that areas of potential contamination are kept to a minimum.
12 Check any other packs for sterility and open, tipping their contents gently onto the centre of the sterile field.	To prepare the equipment and, in the case of a wound dressing, reduce the amount of time that the wound is uncovered. This reduces the risk of infection and a drop in temperature of the wound which will delay wound healing (Stronge 1984).
13 Clean hands with a bactericidal alcohol rub.	Hands may become contaminated by handling outer packets, etc.
14 Place hand in disposable bag, arrange contents of dressing pack.	To maintain sterility of pack.
15 Remove used dressing with hand covered with the disposable bag, invert bag and stick to trolley.	To minimize risk of contamination, by containing dressing in bag.
16 Where appropriate, swab along the 'tear area' of lotion sachet with chlorhexidine in 70% spirit/swab saturated with 70% isopropyl alcohol. Tear open sachet and pour lotion into gallipots or on indented plastic tray.	To minimize risk of contamination of lotion.
17 Put on sterile gloves, touching only the inside wrist end.	To reduce the risk of infection. Gloves provide greater sensitivity than forceps and are less likely to cause trauma to the patient.

Carry out procedure

18 Make sure the patient is comfortable.	
19 Dispose of waste in yellow plastic clinical waste bags.	To prevent environmental contamination. Yellow is the recognized colour for clinical waste.
20 If necessary, draw back curtains or, if appropriate, help the patient back to the bed area and ensure the patient is comfortable.	
21 Check that the trolley remains dry and physically clean. If necessary, wash with liquid detergent and water and dry throughly with a paper towel.	To reduce the risk of spreading infection.
22 Clean hands with bactericidal alcohol handrub.	To reduce the risk of spreading infection.
23 Place sterility label from the outside of any surgical instrument packs used during the procedure on the patient record form which is to be placed in the patient's notes.	Provides a record, as the sterility label proves the pack has gone through a sterile process and that prior to release has been inspected by a trained person in the Sterile Services Department.

*Please note that for some procedures it may be more appropriate to use different types of sterile packs (e.g. intravenous packs). Since usage of these will vary locally reference is generally made to 'sterile dressing pack'.

Procedure guidelines: **Hand washing**

Hands must be cleaned before and after each patient contact, and after any task that may have resulted in the hands becoming contaminated. There is substantial evidence to indicate that hand washing is the single most important action to reduce the incident of hospital-acquired infection (DoH 2001a).

Procedure guidelines: **Hand washing** *(cont'd)*

Equipment and facilities

Wrist/knee/elbow or automatic taps should be used in all clinical areas in order to prevent dirty hands contaminating the taps, which could lead to cross-contamination of the next person who uses the taps. Hand basins should be located conveniently near to where they are required. They must be maintained in good working order and always kept stocked with a plentiful supply of paper towels and liquid soap in disposable containers. This ensures the soap containers are not topped up from a larger container. Soap containers can become contaminated (Ayliffe *et al.* 2000) and by renewing them on a regular basis, a potential source of infection is removed. It is important that the design of the paper towel dispenser allows for easy removal of the paper towel without contaminating the remaining towels. Contaminated paper towels could lead to cross-infection.

Procedure

	Action	Rationale
1	Remove rings, bracelets and wristwatch.	Jewellery inhibits good hand washing. Dirt and bacteria can remain beneath jewellery after hand washing.
2	Roll up sleeves.	Long sleeves prevent washing of wrists.
3	Cover cuts and abrasions on hands with waterproof dressing.	Cuts and abrasions can become contaminated with bacteria and cannot be easily cleaned. Repeated hand washing can increase the injury.
4	Remove nail varnish and artificial nails. Nails must also be short and clean.	Long nails and false nails can be a source of infection by harbouring dirt and bacteria. Nail varnish can become cracked, which could lead to contamination if the nail polish fell into a patient's wound. Nail polish can also inhibit effective hand washing by potentially harbouring bacteria in microscopic imperfections of nail varnish.
5	Hands that are visibly or potentially soiled or contaminated with dirt or organic material should be washed with liquid soap from a dispenser and running hand-hot water.	Liquid soap is very effective in removing dirt, organic material and any loosely adherent transient flora, but has little antimicrobial activity. Liquid soap must be used, as tablets of soap can become contaminated.
	(a) Turn on the taps using wrist/elbow or foot and direct the water flow away from the plughole. Run the water at a flow rate that prevents splashing.	Plugholes are often contaminated with micro-organisms that could be transferred to the environment or the user if splashing occurs.
	(b) Run the water until hand hot.	Hand-hot water to be used to ensure that the skin of hands is not damaged by cold water. Water that is too hot could cause scalding. Soap is more effective in breaking down dirt and organic matter when used with hand-hot water.
	(c) Wet the surface of hands and wrists.	Soap applied directly onto dry hands may damage the skin. The water will also quickly mix with the soap to speed up hand washing.
	(d) Apply liquid soap and water to all surfaces of the hands.	To ensure all surfaces of the hands are cleaned.
	(e) Rub hands together for a minimum of 10–15 seconds, with particular attention to between the fingers and the tips of fingers and thumbs.	To ensure all surfaces of the hands are cleaned. Areas that are missed can be a source of cross-infection.
	(f) Nail brushes should not be used.	Nail brushes can damage the skin and result in increased shedding of bacteria from the hands.
	(g) Rinse soap thoroughly off hands.	A residue of soap can lead to irritation and damage to the skin. Damaged skin does not provide a barrier to infection for the health care worker and can become colonized with potentially pathogenic bacteria, leading to cross-infection.
	(h) Care must be taken not to contaminate the taps, sink or nozzle of the soap dispenser with dirt or organic material that is washed off hands.	Contamination of the nozzle of the soap dispenser can result in contamination of the liquid soap, leading to cross-infection.

Procedure guidelines: Hand washing (cont'd)

Action	Rationale
(i) Dry hands thoroughly with a good-quality disposable paper towel from a towel dispenser.	Damp hands encourage the multiplication of bacteria and can potentially become sore.
(j) Dispose of used paper towels in a black bag on a foot-operated stand.	Black is the colour coding for paper waste. Using a foot-operated waste bag stand prevents contamination of the hands.
6 Hands that are visibly clean and not soiled or contaminated with dirt, organic material or toxic substances can be cleaned using an alcoholic handrub.	The antimicrobial activity of alcohol is due to its ability to denature proteins. Alcoholic handrub solutions are a quick convenient method of cleansing clean hands of Gram-negative, Gram-positive vegetative bacteria, tuberculosis and a variety of fungi, but have poor activity against bacterial spores and cannot remove dirt, organic material or toxic substances such as drugs or radioactivity. Alcoholic handrub comes in a variety of solutions, gels and foams with an emollient (which reduces the drying effect of the alcohol).
(a) Follow the manufacturer's instructions for the amount of handrub to be used.	The instructions must be followed so that the correct amount of handrub is used to ensure effective hand cleaning. Too much will cause delays and leave hands sticky, too little will not clean hands adequately.
(b) Rub an alcoholic handrub into **all** areas of the hands, until the hands are dry.	To ensure all areas of the hands are cleaned. Alcohol is a rapid-acting disinfectant, with the added advantage that it evaporates, leaving the hands dry. This prevents contamination of equipment, whilst facilitating the application of unpowdered gloves.
7 Hand washing for surgical procedures outside the operating theatre to be undertaken using a bactericidal detergent.	Rapid multiplication of bacteria occurs under surgical gloves if hands are washed with a non-bactericidal soap. The use of bactericidal soap reduces the resident skin flora. Bactericidal detergents have a persistent activity, which means that following use the bacteria appear to reproduce slowly on hands.
(a) Turn on the taps using wrist/elbow or foot and direct the water flow away from the plughole. Run the water at a flow rate that prevents splashing.	Plugholes are often contaminated with micro-organisms that could be transferred to the environment or the user if splashing occurs.
(b) Run the water until hand hot.	Hand-hot water to be used to ensure that the skin of hands is not damaged by cold water. Water that is too hot could cause scalding. Soap is more effective in breaking down dirt and organic matter when used with hand-hot water.
(c) Wet hands with hand-hot water.	Applying bactericidal detergent direct onto dry hands increases the risk of skin damage/irritation.
(d) Apply the amount of bactericidal detergent advised by the manufacturer.	The correct amount of detergent must be used to ensure effective hand cleaning.
(e) The following washing/rubbing actions should be undertaken five times: • Rotational rubbing of wrists • Palm to palm • Right palm to back of left hand • Left palm to back of right hand • Palm to palm, fingers interlaced • Back of fingers of one hand to palm of other hand with fingers interlaced • Rotational rubbing of right thumb in left palm and left thumb in right palm • Rotational rubbing of fingers in clasped palm of opposite hand.	All surfaces of hands must be thoroughly washed for effective hand washing to have taken place.

Procedure guidelines: Hand washing (cont'd)

Action	Rationale
(f) Holding hands upright, rinse them and wrists under hand-hot running water to remove soap.	Soap residue can cause skin damage. Hands must be held upright to ensure water splashes from unwashed areas of arm do not run down onto clean hands.
(g) Dry hands carefully using a good-quality paper towel.	Wet hands can encourage the growth of bacteria and may lead to sore hands.
8 Hand washing for surgical procedures in theatre. The routine is the same as above but the forearms are included. The hand washing is extended to 2 minutes during which time repeated applications of the bactericidal detergent are required. Hands are dried using a sterile disposable paper towel.	The optimal length of the hand washing is unknown. The important factor is that all areas have been effectively cleaned and rinsed. To prevent contamination from unsterile paper towels.

References and further reading

Ansari, S.A., Springthorpe, V.S., Sattar, S.A. *et al.* (1991) Comparison of cloth, paper, and warm air drying in eliminating viruses and bacteria from washed hands. *Am J Infect Control*, **19**(5), 243–9.

Archibold, L.K., Manning, M.L., Bell, L.M., Banerjee, S. & Jarvis, W.R. (1997) Patient density, nurse-to-patient ratio and nosocomial infection risk in a pediatric cardiac intensive care unit. *Pediatr Infect Dis*, **16**(11), 1045–8.

Ayliffe, G.A.J., Fraise, A.P., Geddes, A.M. & Mitchell, K. (2000) *Control of Hospital Infection. A Practical Handbook*, 4th edn. Arnold, London.

Bree-Williams, E.J. & Waterman, H. (1996) An examination of nurses' practices when performing aseptic technique for wound dressing. *J Adv Nurs*, **23**, 48–54.

Briggs, M., Wilson, S. & Fuller, A. (1996) The principles of aseptic technique in wound care. *Prof Nurse*, **11**(12), 805–8.

Byrne, D.J., Napier, A. & Cuschieri, A. (1990) Rationalizing whole body disinfection. *J Hosp Infect*, **15**(2), 183–7.

Byrne, D.J., Phillips, G., Napier, A. & Cuschieri, A. (1991a) The effect of whole body disinfection on intraoperative wound contamination. *J Hosp Infect*, **18**(2), 145–8.

Byrne, D.J., Napier, A., Phillips, G. & Cuschieri, A. (1991b) Effects of whole body disinfection on skin flora in patients undergoing elective surgery. *J Hosp Infect*, **17**(3), 217–22.

Callaghan, I. (1998) Bacterial contamination of nurses' uniforms: a study. *Nurs Stand*, **13**(1), 37–42.

Candell, K.A. & Whedon, M.B. (1991) Haematopoietic complications found in bone marrow transplantation. In: *Principles, Practices and Nursing Insight* (ed. M.B. Whedon). Jones & Bartlett, Boston, pp. 135–57.

Centers for Disease Control (1986) Guidelines for handwashing and hospital environmental control. *Infect Control*, **7**(4), 233–5.

Chandra, P.N. & Milind, K. (2001) Lapses in measures recommended for preventing hospital-acquired infection. *J Hosp Infect*, **47**(3), 218–22.

Clayton, J.L. (1996) Decontamination, sterilization, and disinfection. *Surg Nurs*, **10**(1), 13–20.

Cohen, H.A., Kitai, E., Levy, I. & Ben-Amitai, D. (2002) Hand-washing patterns in two dermatology clinics. *Dermatology*, **205**(4), 358–61.

Colombo, C., Giger, H., Grote, J. *et al.* (2002) Impact of teaching intervention on nurse compliance with hand disinfection. *J Hosp Infect*, **51**(1), 69–72.

Cork, R.C., Wood, D., Evans, B., DeLanzac, K. & Naraghi, M. (1995) Leak rate of latex gloves after tearing adhesive tape. *Am J Anesthesiol*, **22**(3), 133–7.

Crow, S. (1989) Asepsis: an indispensable part of the patient's care plan. *Crit Care Nurse Quart*, **11**(4), 11–15.

Crow, S. (1994) Asepsis: a prophylactic technique. *Semin Perioper Nurs*, **3**(2), 93–100.

Crowe, M.J. & Cooke, E.M. (1998) Review of case definition for nosocomial infection – towards a consensus. Presentation by nosocomial infection surveillance unit to hospital infection liaison group, subcommittee of Federation of Infection Societies. *J Hosp Infect*, **39**(1), 3–11.

Davey, J.G. (1997) Discovering nursing students' understanding about aseptic technique. *Int J Nurs Pract*, **3**(2), 105–10.

David, J. (1991) Letters. *Wound Manage*, **1**(2), 15.

Dietze, B., Rath, A., Wendt, C. & Martiny, H. (2001) Survival of MRSA on sterile goods packaging. *J Hosp Infect*, **49**(4), 255–61.

DoH (1995) *Hospital Infection Control: Guidance on the Control of Infection in Hospitals*. Department of Health, London.

DoH (1998) *Prevention and Control of Tuberculosis in the United Kingdom*. Department of Health (HSC 1998/196), London.

DoH (2001a) Standard principles for preventing hospital-acquired infection. *J Hosp Infect*, **47**(Suppl), S21–37.

DoH (2001b) Guidelines for preventing infections associated with the insertion and maintenance of central venous catheters. *J Hosp Infect*, **47**(Suppl), S49–67.

Driever, R., Beie, M., Schmitz, E. *et al.* (2001) Surgical glove perforation in cardiac surgery. *Thorac Cardiovasc Surg*, **49**(6), 328–30.

Edwards, P. (2001) Contamination of the surgical field. *J Periop Nurs*, **11**(12), 543–6.

Emmerson, A.M., Enstone, J.E. & Griffin, A. (1996) The second national prevalence survey of infection in hospital – overview of the results. *J Hosp Infect*, **32**(3), 175–90.

Fagon, J.Y., Novara, A., Stephan, F., Girou, E. & Safar, M. (1994) Mortality, attributable to nosocomial infection in the ICU. *Infect Control Hosp Epidemiol*, **15**(7), 428–34.

Field, E.A., McGowan, P., Pearce, P.K. & Martin, M.V. (1996) Rings and watches: should they be removed prior to operative dental procedures? *J Dent*, **24**(1), 65–9.

Ford, D.A. & Koehler, S.H. (2001) A creative process for reinforcing aseptic technique practices. *AORN J*, **73**(2), 446–50.

French, G.L. *et al.* (1989) Repeated prevalence surveys for monitoring effectiveness of hospital infection control. *Lancet*, **11**, 1021–3.

Garrouste-Orgeas, M., Chevret, S., Mainardi, J.L., Timsit, J.F., Misset, B. & Carlet, J. (2000) A one-year prospective study of nosocomial bacteraemia in ICU and non-ICU patients and its impact on patients outcome. *J Hosp Infect*, **44**(3), 206–13.

Glauser, M.P. & Calandra, T. (2000) Infections in patients with hematologic malignancies. In: *Management of Infections in Immunocompromised Patients* (eds M.P. Glauser & P.A. Pizzo). W.B. Saunders, London.

Gould, D. (1993) Assessing nurses' hand decontamination performance. *Nurs Times*, **89**(25), 47–50.

Gould, D. (1994) Understanding the nature of bacteria. *Nurs Stand*, **8**(28), 29–31.

Grinbaums, R.S., de Mendonca, J.S. & Cardo, D.M. (1995) An outbreak of handscrubbing-related surgical site infections in vascular surgical procedures. *Infect Control Hosp Epidemiol*, **16**(4), 198–202.

Gustafson, D.R., Vetter, E.A., Larson, D.R. *et al.* (2000) Effects of 4 hand-drying methods for removing bacteria from washed hands: a randomized trial. *Mayo Clin Proc*, **75**(7), 705–8.

Gwyther, J. (1988) Skilled dressing. *Nurs Times*, **84**(19), 60–1.

Haigh, C. (1993) A study of micro-organism levels on nurses' footwear. *Br J Nurs*, **2**(22), 1109–12.

Haley, R.W. *et al.* (1985a) The efficiency of infection surveillance and control programmes in preventing nosocomial infections in US hospitals. *Am J Epidemiol*, **121**, 182–205.

Haley, R.W. *et al.* (1985b) Identifying multivariate index of patients' susceptibility and wound contamination. *Am J Epidemiol*, **121**(2), 206–15.

Hallett, C.E. (2000) Infection control in wound care: a study of fatalism in community nursing. *J Clin Nurs*, **9**(1), 103–9.

Hambraeus, A. (1973) Transfer of *Staphylococcus aureus* via nurses' uniform. *J Hyg*, **71**, 799–814.

Harris, A.D., Samore, M.H., Nafziger, R. *et al.* (2000) A survey on handwashing practices and opinions of health care workers. *J Hosp Infect*, **45**(4), 318–21.

Hart, S. (1990) The immunosuppressed patient in infection control. In: *Guidelines for Nursing Care* (eds M.A. Worsley *et al.*). Surgikos Ltd, pp. 15–20.

Hart, S. (1991) Blood and body precautions. *Nurs Stand*, **5**(25), 25–8.

Hinkin, J. (2002) Hand decontamination: what interventions improve compliance? *J Eur Dialysis Tranplant Nurs Assoc*, **28**(3), 134–7.

HSE (1992) *Personal Protective Equipment at Work Regulations.* Department of Health, London.

HSE (1995) *Reporting of Injuries, Diseases and Dangerous Occurrences Regulations (RIDDOR).* Department of Health, London.

Infection Control Standards Working Party (1993) *Standards in Infection Control in Hospitals.* HMSO, London.

Jarvis, W.R. (1996) Selected aspects of the socioeconomic impact of nosocomial infections, morbidity, cost and prevention. *Infect Control Hosp Epidemiol*, **17**(8), 552–7.

Jenks, A.M. & Ferguson, K.E. (1994) Intergrating what is taught with what is practised in the nursing curriculum, a multidimensional model. *J Adv Nurs*, **20**, 687–95.

Kelso, H. (1989) Alternative technique. *Nurs Times*, **85**(23), 68–72.

Kiehl, E., Wallace, R. & Warren, C. (1997) Tracking perinatal infection: is it safe to launder your scrubs at home? *Am J Matern Child Nurs*, **22**(4), 195–7.

King, S. (1998) Decontamination of equipment and the environment. *Nurs Stand*, **12**(52), 57–63.

Kocent, H., Corke, C., Alajeel, A. & Graves, S. (2002) Washing of gloved hands in antiseptic solution prior to central line insertion reduces contamination. *Anaes Intens Care*, **30**(3), 338–40.

Kunaratanapruk, S. & Silpapojakul, K. (1999) Unnecessary hospital infection control practices in Thailand: a survey. *J Hosp Infect*, **40**(1), 55–9.

Lankester, B.J.A., Bartlett, G.E., Garnet, N., Blom, A.W., Bowker, K.E. & Bannister, G.C. (2001) Direct measurement of bacterial penetration through surgical gowns: a new method. *J Hosp Infect*, **50**(4) 281–5.

Larwood, K.A., Anstey, C.M. & Dunn, S.V. (2000) Managing central venous catheters: a prospective randomised trial of two methods. *Aust Crit Care*, **13**(2), 44–50.

Laurence, J., Clark, L., Hart, S. *et al.* (2002) *Antibiotic Resistance: Theory and Practice.* Infection Control Nurses Association Pharmacia, Edinburgh.

Lauwers, S. & de Smet, F. (1998) Surgical site infections. *Acta Clin Belg*, **53**(5), 303–10.

Lipp, A. & Edwards, P. (2002) Disposable surgical face masks for preventing surgical wound infection in clean surgery. *Cochrane Database Syst Rev*, CD002929.

Lovitt, S.A., Nichols, R.L., Smith, J.W., Muzik, A.C. & Pearce, P.F. (1992) Isolation gowns: a false sense of security. *Am J Infect Control*, **20**(4), 185–91.

Lowbury, E.J. *et al.* (1981) *Control of Hospital Infection – A Practical Handbook*, 2nd edn. Chapman & Hall, London.

Lund, C. & Caruso, R. (1993) Nursing perspective: aseptic technique in wound care. *Dermatol Nurs*, **5**(3), 2215–16.

Mackintosh, C.A. *et al.* (1980) The evaluation of fabric in relation to their use as protective garments in nursing and surgery. *J Hyg*, **85**, 393–403.

Mangram, A.J., Horan, T.C., Pearson, M.L., Silver, L.C. & Jarvis, W.R. (1999) Guideline for prevention of surgical site infection, 1999. Centers for Disease Control and Prevention [CDC] Hospital Infection Practices Advisory Committee. *Am J Infect Control*, **27**(2), 97–132.

Manning, M.L., Archibald, L.K., Bell, L.M., Banerjee, S.N. & Jarvis, W.R. (2001) *Serratia marcescens* transmission in a pediatric intensive care unit: a multifactorial occurrence. *Am J Infect Control*, **29**(2), 115–19.

Masterson, R.G. & Teare, E.L. (2001) Clinical governance and infection control in the United Kingdom. *J Hosp Infect*, **47**(1), 25–31.

McLane, C. *et al.* (1983) A nursing practice problem: failure to observe aseptic techniques. *Am J Infect Control*, **11**(5), 178–82.

Medical Devices Agency (1995) *The Reuse of Medical Devices Supplied for Single Use Only*. DB 9501. Department of Health, London.

Medical Devices Agency (1996) *Latex Sensitivities in Health Care Setting (Use of Latex Gloves)*. MDA DB 9601. Medical Devices Agency, London.

Medical Devices Agency (1997) *Advice leaflet. Products You Can Have Confidence In*. Medical Devices Agency, London.

Medical Devices Agency (1998) *Latex Medical Gloves (Surgeons and Examination) Powdered Latex Medical Gloves*. MDA SN9825. Medical Devices Agency, London.

Medical Devices Agency (2000) *Equipped to Care. The Safe Use of Medical Devices in the 21st Century*. Medical Devices Agency, London.

Meers, P.D., Ayliffe, G.A.J. & Emmerson, A.M. (1980) Report of the national survey of infection in hospitals 1980. *J Hosp Infect*, **2**(Suppl), 23–8

Merry, A.F., Miller, T.E. & Findon, G. *et al.* (2001) Touch contamination levels during anaesthetic procedures and their relationship to hand hygiene procedures: a clinical audit. *Br J Anaes*, **87**(2), 291–4.

NHSE (1999) *Latex Medical Gloves and Powdered Latex Medical Gloves*. Department of Health, London.

NHSE (2000) *Decontamination of Medical Devices*. Department of Health, London.

NHSE (2001) *National Standards of Cleanliness for the NHS*. Department of Health, London.

Noe, J.M. *et al.* (1988) Can stitches get wet? *Plast Reconstruct Surg*, **81**(1), 82–4.

North Thames Audit and Clinical Effectiveness in Occupational Health (2000) *Report on Latex Gloves Policies and Procedures*. Royal Free Hampstead Centre, London.

Oie, S., Hosokawa, I. & Kamiya, A. (2002) Contamination of room handles by methicillin-sensitive/methicillin-resistant *Staphylococcus aureus*. *J Hosp Infect*, **51**(2), 140–3.

Oldman, P. (1991) A sticky situation – microbiological study of adhesive tape used to secure IV cannulae. *Prof Nurse*, February 265–9.

O'Toole, S. (1997) Disposable gloves. *Prof Nurs*, **13**(3), 184–90.

Patrick, D.R., Findon, G. & Miller, T.E. (1997) Residual moisture determines the level of touch-contact-associated bacterial transfer following hand washing. *Epidemiol Infect*, **119**(3), 319–25.

Paulson, D.S. (1993) Efficacy evaluation of a 4% chlorhexidine gluconate as a full body shower wash. *Am J Infect Control*, **21**(4), 205–9.

Pereira, L.J., Lee, G.M. & Wade, K.J. (1997) An evaluation of five protocols for surgical handwashing in relation to skin condition and microbial counts. *J Hosp Infect*, **36**, 49–65.

Phillips, C. (1989) Hand hygiene. *Nurs Times*, **85**(37), 76–9.

Porteous, J. (2002) Artificial nails: very real risk. *Can Oper Room Nurs*, **20**(3), 16–17, 20–1.

Raybould, L.M. (2001) Disposable non sterile gloves: a policy for appropriate usage. *Br J Nurs*, **10**(17), 1135–41.

Reilly, J. (2002) Changing surgical practice through feedback of performance data. *J Adv Nurs*, **38**(6) 607–14.

Rojo, D., Pinedo, A., Clavijo, E., Garcia-Rodriguez, A. & Garcia, V. (1999) Analysis of risk factors associated with nosocomial bacteraemias. *J Hosp Infect*, **42**(2), 135–41.

Rossoff, L.J., Lam, S., Hilton, E., Borenstein, M. & Isenberg, H.D. (1993) Is the use of boxed gloves in an intensive care unit safe? *Am J Med*, **94**(6), 602–7.

Salisbury, D.M., Hutfilz, P., Treen, L.M. *et al.* (1997) The effect of rings on microbial load of health care workers' hands. *Am J Infect Control*, **25**(1), 24–7.

Sartor, C., Jacomo, V., Duvivier, C., Tissot-Dupont, H., Sambuc, R. & Drancourt, M. (2000) Nosocomial *Serratia marcescens* infection associated with extrinsic contamination of a liquid non-medicated soap. *Infect Control Hosp Epidemiol*, **21**(3), 196–9.

Sellors, J.E.I., Cyna, A.M.I. & Simmons, S.W.I. (2002) Aseptic precautions for inserting an epidural catheter: a survey of obstetric anaesthetists. *Anaesthesia*, **57**(6), 593–6.

Sharma, J.B., Ekoh, S., McMillan, L., Hussain, S. & Annan, H. (1997) Blood splashes to the masks and goggles during caesarean section. *Br J Obstet Gynaecol*, **104**(2), 1450–6.

Sherwood, E. (1995) Motivation, the key factor. *Nurs Times*, **91**(20), 65–6.

Shiomori, T., Miyamoto, H., Makishima, K. *et al.* (2002) Evaluation of bed making-related airborne and surface methicillin resistant *Staphylococcus aureus* contamination. *J Hosp Infect*, **50**(1), 30–5.

Sproat, L.J. & Inglis, T.J.J. (1992) Preventing infection in the intensive care unit. *Br J Intens Care*, September, 277–85.

St Clair, K. & Larrabee, J.H. (2002) Clean versus sterile gloves; which to use for postoperative dressing changes? *Outcome Management*, **6**(1), 17–21.

Stronge, V.L. (1984) Principles of wound care. *Nursing*, **2**(26), Suppl, 7–10.

Taylor, J.H., Brown, K.L., Toivenen, J. & Holah, J.T. (2000) A microbiological evaluation of warm air hand driers with respect to hand hygiene and the washroom environment. *J Appl Microbiol*, **89**(6), 910–19.

Taylor, K., Plowman, R. & Roberts, J.A. (2001) *The Challenge of Hospital Acquired Infection*. National Audit Office, London.

Taylor, L. (1978a) An evaluation of handwashing techniques 1. *Nurs Times*, **74**(2), 54–5.

Taylor, L. (1978b) An evaluation of handwashing techniques 2. *Nurs Times*, **74**(3), 108–10.

Thomlinson, D. (1990) Time to dispense with the rituals. *Prof Nurse*, May, 421–4.

Tunevall, T.G. (1991) Postoperative wound infections and surgical masks: a controlled study. *World J Surg*, **15**(3), 383–7.

Van Grafhorst, J.P., Foudraine, N.A., Nooteboom, F., Crombach, W.H.J., Oldenhof, N.J.J. & Van Doore, H. (2002) Unexpected high risk of contamination with staphylococci species attributable to standard preparation of syringes for continuous intravenous drug administration in a simulation model in intensive care units. *Crit Care Med*, **30**(4), 833–6.

Ward, V., Wilson, J., Taylor, L. *et al.* (1997) *Preventing Hospital Acquired Infection. Clinical Guidelines*. Public Health Laboratory Service, London, pp. 19–21.

Whitehouse, J.D., Friedman, N.D. & Kirkland, K.B. *et al.* (2002) The impact of surgical-site infections following orthopaedic surgery at a community hospital and a university hospital: adverse quality of life, excess length of stay and extra cost. *Infect Control Hosp Epidemiol*, **23**(4), 183–9.

Wright, L., Spickett, G. & Stoker, S. (2001) Latex allergy awareness among hospital staff. *NT Plus*, **97**(38), 49–52.

Barrier nursing: nursing the infectious or immunosuppressed patient

Chapter contents

Barrier nursing

Definition

Barrier nursing is the use of infection control practices aimed at controlling the spread of, and eradicating, pathogenic organisms. These practices may require the setting up of mechanical barriers to contain pathogenic organisms within a specified area.

Indications

Barrier nursing includes:

- Source isolation to segregate infected patients in single rooms to prevent the spread of infection.
- Cohort source isolation to segregate a number of patients with the same infection in one ward when there are inadequate number of single rooms, to prevent the spread of infection (Working Party 1998).
- Protective isolation (reverse barrier nursing) to segregate immunosuppressed patients (individuals with impaired immunity due to disease or treatment) to protect them from acquiring an exogenous infection.
- Strict source isolation to segregate patients infected with a serious contagious disease, e.g. viral haemorrhagic fever, in isolation units to prevent the spread of infection (DoH 1998a).

Reference material

Nine per cent of hospitalized patients in the UK will develop a hospital-acquired infection (HAI) (Taylor *et al.* 2001). This means more than 300 000 infections per year, with as many as 5000 inpatient deaths directly attributed to HAI. HAI costs the NHS a billion pounds. The main sites of infections are: urinary 23.2%, lower respiratory tract 22.9%, surgical wounds 10.7%, skin 9.6%, blood 6.2%, others 27.4% (Taylor *et al.* 2001).

Treatment and care of infected patients cost on average 2.9 times more than those patients without infections. Additional inpatient hospital care related to HAI costs the hospital sector as much as £930 million a year (Plowman *et al.* 1999).

Neutropenic patients with haematological malignancies are at increased risk of infectious morbidity and mortality (Tsiodras *et al.* 2000). The incidence of HAI in neutropenic patients is significantly higher (up to 25.3%) than in immune-competent patients (Engelhard *et al.* 2002). The incidence of infection is directly related to the neutrophil count, with the probability that 25% of patients with a neutrophil count less than $100/mm^3$ for one week will develop an infection. Bloodstream infections are the most common type of infection (Glauser & Calandra 2000).

The risk of infection also depends on the patient's ability to respond to infection, rather than the number of neutrophils in the peripheral blood (Dale *et al.* 1998). A careful patient medical history and physical examination provide an initial assessment of the patient's susceptibility to infection.

Most precautions against transferring infection demand more effort, take more time and cost more when neutropenic patients are cared for, than the comparable procedures in normal circumstances. However, the cost of an outbreak of infection can be far more (Wilcox & Dane 2000).

For the infected patient the consequences can be considerable and may include:

- Delayed or prevented recovery
- Increased pain, discomfort and anxiety
- Extended hospitalization, which has implications for the patient, the family and the hospital
- Psychological stress as a result of long periods spent in isolation (Knowles 1993).

One study of the psychological effects of hospitalization and source isolation found that isolated patients were significantly more anxious and depressed than other hospitalized patients. The fear of the unknown, of further spread and contamination to others and feelings of guilt were linked to uncertainty and loss of control as patients experienced lack of clarity, ambiguity and lack of information from staff (Gammon 1998).

A recent study showed that a number of patients associated barrier nursing with being dirty or unclean (Madeo & Owen 2002).

Sources of infection

Self-infection (endogenous infection)

Self-infection results when tissues become infected from other sites in the patient's body. The normal microbial flora of the human body consists largely of the organisms in the alimentary tract, upper respiratory tract and female genital tract and on the skin. This flora may include versatile pathogens (e.g. *Staphylococcus aureus*) that may cause disease in almost any tissue, as well as others (e.g. micrococcus species and diphtheroids) which are usually of very low pathogenicity, and rarely cause infection. Many organisms exist with capabilities between these extremes, with most surgical site infections (Lauwers & de Smet 1998) and infections acquired by immunosuppressed patients being caused by the patient's own microbial flora (Glauser & Calandra 2000).

Cross-infection (exogenous infection)

Cross-infection may be caused by infection from patients, hospital staff or visitors who are suffering from the relevant disease (cases) or who are symptomless carriers. Food and the environment may also be factors in cross-infection (Ayliffe *et al.* 2000).

Routes and reservoirs of infection

A reservoir of infection is anywhere where organisms can survive and multiply. For infection to occur there has to be a route of transmission between the reservoir and the susceptible host.

The health care environment is a secondary reservoir for organisms with the potential for infecting patients. It is essential that all plans for new or renovated health care buildings are designed to ensure that health care-associated infection is reduced (NHS Estates 2002). Routes of spread include the following.

Direct contact

Organisms can be transmitted directly to susceptible people by the hands of health care workers and by contaminated equipment. Therefore it is essential that all equipment is cleaned following each and every episode of use (Medical Devices Agency 2002). Hand washing has been shown to reduce the spread of infection, so hands must be washed before and after every patient contact and contact with contaminated equipment (DoH 2001a). However, studies of hand washing by nurses and others have shown that this procedure is generally not carried out efficiently (Cohen *et al.* 2002). Teaching interventions (Colombo *et al.* 2002) and feedback on performance (Naikoba & Hayward 2001) can improve compliance with hand-washing requirements. Washing with soap removes transient micro-organisms, whilst the use of bactericidal soap removes both transient and resident skin micro-organisms (DoH 2001a).

In clinical areas washing in running water is essential. Basins should be deep enough to contain any splashing water and should be plugless. Taps should not be operated by hand but by remote control, elbow, knee or foot, as appropriate.

A quick, convenient and effective disinfectant for clean hands, without the use of soap and water, is an alcoholic handrub which can remove organisms such as MRSA from visibly clean hands (Kampf *et al.* 1998), is less drying to hands and well liked if introduced following educational initiatives (Girard *et al.* 2001). Alcoholic handrubs are not effective on hands which are visibly soiled or potentially contaminated with dirt or organic matter. In such circumstances washing with soap and running water, followed by careful drying with a good-quality paper towel, is required (DoH 2001a).

Airborne

Organisms can be transmitted in dust or skin scales carried by air. This is likely to occur during procedures such as bed making, when particles may land directly on open wounds or puncture sites. The hospital ward environment must be visibly clean, free from dust and soilage and acceptable to patients, their visitors and staff (DoH 2001a). Sites most likely to fail a ward cleaning inspection are the toilets and kitchen (Griffith *et al.* 2000). Airborne infection may also occur through droplets. Water from nebulizers or humidifiers may be contaminated by *Pseudomonas* species (Ayliffe *et al.* 2000). Fine droplet spray from ventilation cooling towers or showers contaminated with *Legionella pneumophila* has also been shown to be a hazard (Jansa *et al.* 2002).

Food borne

Food poisoning occurs when contaminated foods are ingested, with *Salmonella* species being one of the most common causes. This is particularly associated with contaminated eggs and chicken (Mason *et al.* 2001; Capita *et al.* 2003). Prevention includes good infection control practices (Maguire *et al.* 2001). Statutory requirements related to food hygiene must be met (DoH 2001a). Hand washing, thorough cooking, storage, segregation of cooked and uncooked food, clean environment and equipment are essential. Hot food must be kept hot and cold food must be kept chilled. As some organisms such as *Listeria* can multiply in low temperatures, ideally ward refrigerators should be kept below 3°C (Ayliffe *et al.* 2000). Food products must also be obtained from reputable suppliers (Ejidokun *et al.* 2000).

Blood borne

Blood, or blood-stained material, is potentially hazardous, transmitting infection through inoculation accidents, existing breaks in the skin, gross contamination of mucous membranes, sexual activity or, prenatally, from mother to baby (UK Health Department 2002a).

Vector borne (an insect or animal carrier/transmitter of disease)

International movement of people and products is associated with the emergence of infectious diseases (Ostroff & Kozarsky 1998) by introducing infectious agents into areas in which they had previously been absent (Gratz 1999). Research on vaccines, environmentally safe insecticides, vector control and training programmes for health care workers can assist in disease control (Gubler 1998). Although disease transmitted by biting insects is not a major problem in the UK, insects such as cockroaches can carry pathogenic organisms on their bodies and in their digestive tracts. This may infect the hospital environment, which includes food and sterile supplies (Wilson 2001). Storage of supplies in dry, clean, well-ventilated areas is therefore essential. Statutory requirements related to pest control must also be met (DoH 2001a).

Types of barrier nursing

1 Source isolation
2 Protective isolation

Source isolation is designed to prevent the spread of pathogenic micro-organisms from an infected patient to other patients, hospital personnel and visitors. The need for isolation is determined by the ease with which the disease can be transmitted in hospital and, if it is transmittable, by its severity. As infectious diseases are transmitted by different routes, isolation procedures must, in order to be effective, provide appropriate barriers to the route of transmission. In addition, the procedures imposing these barriers must be adhered to universally by all hospital staff entering the isolation unit. Risk assessment of the patient to evaluate the risk of cross-infection to other patients must be undertaken, to ensure the most appropriate restrictions are implemented (Beaujean *et al.* 2001).

Protective isolation protects the patient from the hospital environment. Protective isolation techniques have also been referred to as reverse barrier nursing and reverse isolation, and include the use of high-efficiency particulate air (HEPA) filters (Wilson 2001) (see 'Protective isolation', below).

Source isolation

Definition

Source isolation is a process of care whereby an infectious patient and any material that has been in contact with them or eliminated by them are isolated from others to prevent the spread of infection.

Indications

The decision to isolate a patient will be influenced by the availability of facilities as well as by the physical condition of the area where the isolation is to take place. In determining the most suitable area, a number of criteria need to be met. Among these are the relative cleanliness of the ward, the standard of domestic services support, the microbiological infectious or the immune status of the other patients and the anticipated length of the isolation.

A British study demonstrated that on average 2.2% of patients require source isolation nursing (Beaujean *et al.* 2001). It appears that many hospitals have few or no isolation beds, often relying on side-rooms not designed and not always available for the isolation of infectious patients (Barlow *et al.* 2002).

Reference material

Source isolation may be achieved by:

1 Purpose-built infectious disease wards.
   Advantages:
   (a) decrease risk of cross-infection
   (b) less disruption to general wards
   (c) nurses often more informed and motivated
   (d) improved, supervised cleaning.
   Disadvantages:
   (a) increased costs
   (b) when full, similar patients have to remain on general wards
   (c) when there are no infectious patients requiring admission, beds are closed to the admission of patients without a contagious infection
   (d) inadvisable to admit immunosuppressed patient who would be at significant risk of morbidity and mortality if cross-infection were to occur with virulent infections such as drug-resistant tuberculosis
   (e) problem of staff recruitment
   (f) staff may not be conversant with patients' underlying clinical conditions (Chattopadhyay 2001).
2 Negative pressure plastic isolator used for dealing with patients who have highly contagious infections such as Ebola virus infection (Bruce & Brysiewiez 2002).
   Advantages:
   (a) provides a high degree of protection to those in contact with patient
   (b) said to be comfortable and acceptable to patients (Trexler *et al.* 1977).
   Disadvantages:
   (a) not freely available
   (b) expensive to obtain and maintain

   (c) limited experienced health care workers to provide required care.
3 Single rooms on general wards.
   Advantages:
   (a) allows patients to remain on ward, which provides continuity of care
   (b) will reduce cross-infection (Eveillard *et al.* 2001)
   (c) en-suite single rooms provide greater privacy and are preferred by many patients (NHS Estates 2002)
   (d) some patients suggest barrier nursing in a single room allows greater freedom for visitors and from routine (Newton *et al.* 2001).
   Disadvantages:
   (a) some patients report a negative experience of barrier nursing, with feelings of being 'a leper' (Newton *et al.* 2001)
   (b) shortage of suitable single rooms.
4 Cohort barrier nursing: when a group of patients have the same infection, it may be necessary to cohort barrier nurse these patients in a small bay.
   Advantage:
   (a) undertaken correctly can successfully control and contain infection (Zafar *et al.* 1998).
   Disadvantage:
   (a) restrictions on admissions to these beds.

Transmission rates of bacteria causing infections have been seen to be transmitted more easily between patients in the same ward compared to those patients in separate single rooms (Fryklund *et al.* 1997). The bed around infected patients can often be contaminated with the infecting organism (Green *et al.* 1998), particularly following bedmaking (Shiomori *et al.* 2002).

Effective source barrier nursing practice is achieved most easily by isolating the patient in a single room with the following:

- An anteroom area for protective clothing
- Hand-washing facilities
- Toilet facilities.

However, with good technique, an area in the ward away from especially vulnerable patients can be used. In some instances where cross-infection has occurred it may be more appropriate to cohort nurse these patients together in a small ward with designated staff, so containing the infection to one area, rather than using side rooms on different wards (NHS Estates 2002). Uninfected patients must not be admitted into this area until all the infected patients have been discharged and the area has been thoroughly cleaned.

General principles of source isolation

The main emphasis for successful source isolation nursing procedures is on hand washing and protection of clothes; both have been seen to reduce cross-infection (Eveillard *et al.* 2001). Several general principles need to be adhered to if effective barrier nursing is to occur. Every effort must be made to ensure that instructions are kept simple and realistic. Regular assessment and evaluation of the situation must take place to ascertain whether barrier nursing continues to remain the most appropriate form of care.

Protective clothing

Gowns or aprons

The wearing of a plastic apron is an accepted part of barrier nursing technique to prevent the spread of micro-organisms from one patient to the next on clothing (Callaghan 1998a).

When there is a risk of extensive contamination a full body fluid-repellent gown must be worn (DoH 2001a). Wearing a gown and gloves has been shown to reduce the transmission of micro-organisms such as vancomycin-resistant enterococci (VRE) (Srinivasan *et al.* 2002). However, another study found that gowns did not prevent infection in patients undergoing bone marrow transplantation (Duquette-Petersen *et al.* 1999).

Disposable plastic aprons are cheap, impermeable to bacteria and water, are easy to put on, protect the probable area of maximum contamination and are preferable to cotton gowns, which provide increased cover but are readily penetrated by moisture and bacteria (Belkin 2002). Another investigation found that uniforms and plastic aprons were heavily contaminated with bacteria (Callaghan 1998a) and the author recommended that nurses are provided with a clean uniform each day (Callaghan 1998b).

Doctors should also be encouraged to change their white coats regularly as it has been shown that a white coat can easily be contaminated and that the design should be modified in order to facilitate hand washing (Loh *et al.* 2000).

Caps

Although the wearing of disposable head covering while nursing infected patients is still practised, hair that is clean and tidy has not been implicated in cross-infection. Therefore, unless heavy contamination or splashing is present, the wearing of caps is not justified. However, head covering continues to be required in the operating theatre, as its use has been shown to reduce wound infections (Friberg *et al.* 2001).

Masks

Masks are sometimes worn to protect the patient, for example when a large burn is being dressed. Studies indicate that masks are generally of little value outside the operating theatre (McCluskey 1996) (see Ch. 30, Perioperative care). Masks can also be worn to protect the wearer, for example when caring for patients with untreated meningococcal meningitis. The organism which causes meningococcal meningitis is found at the back of the throat, and can be passed from person to person by droplet spread from the mouth and nose. Within a hospital, staff would be at risk following very close contact, for example following mouth-to-mouth resuscitation (Ayliffe *et al.* 2000). This procedure should not be undertaken, unless an aid such as a face mask is used. Masks should be worn by all persons providing regular and prolonged close contact with patients suspected or confirmed to be tuberculosis smear positive, particularly during bronchoscopy and other cough-inducing procedures (Interdepartmental Working Group on Tuberculosis 1998). Masks must be worn during all procedures likely to cause splashing of body substances into the face (DoH 2001a). If a mask needs to be worn it must be a filter type and fit the face closely (Ayliffe *et al.* 2000).

Eye protection

Eye protection must be worn to prevent contamination by blood and body fluids (DoH 2001a). One study found that 12% of goggles were contaminated with blood during caesarean section (Sharma *et al.* 1997).

Overshoes

The floors of hospital wards become easily contaminated by large numbers of bacteria (Ayliffe *et al.* 2000). However, the wearing of overshoes has little value (Duquette-Petersen *et al.* 1999) and there could even be an increased risk of cross-infection by contaminating the hands while putting on overshoes, making it necessary for the hands to be washed after putting them on or taking them off (Jones *et al.* 1988).

Gloves

Gloves must conform to Conformité Europèene (CE) standards, be of an acceptable quality and be available in all clinical areas (DoH 2001a). Gloves should be unpowdered (Medical Devices Agency 1998) and not be made of latex (Medical Devices Agency 1996; NHSE 1999a), as latex allergies have serious implications for patients and health care workers (Wright *et al.* 2001).

Boxed, clean non-sterile gloves are adequate for routine non-invasive nursing care (Rossoff *et al.* 1993). Clean gloves must be worn when handling blood or body fluids, or cleaning (DoH 2001a), but are not a substitute for hand washing, as gloved hands can become contaminated during as many as 13% of all contacts with patients' mucous membranes (Bolsen *et al.* 1993). Gloves must be changed between patients, and hands must be washed with bactericidal soap and water or bactericidal alcohol handrub after removing gloves.

Cleaning

Thorough cleaning of the environment is essential as dust from floors and surfaces contains organisms that, if transferred to patients, can cause infection (Dancer *et al.* 2002). All furniture must be damp dusted to remove organisms dispersed into the air from bed making. The floor must be either vacuum cleaned with a machine fitted with a filter or damp mopped with hot, soapy water (the mop head must be laundered daily). Dry dusting or the use of a broom should be forbidden as studies have shown this method of cleaning simply redisperses the organisms into the air (Ayliffe *et al.* 2000). The cleaning equipment must be kept for this patient's sole use.

Patient hygiene

The numbers of micro-organisms on the skin will be reduced by using an antiseptic detergent for skin and hair washing (Byrne *et al.* 1991) and this has been shown to be effective in eradicating the carriage of MRSA (Duckworth 1990). The antiseptic should be applied directly to the flannel and rinsed off thoroughly.

It is essential that baths are cleaned and dried between patients with a non-abrasive cleaning agent, ideally incorporating a hypochlorite, as viable organisms can survive in bath scum (Ayliffe *et al.* 2000). Bathing and showering are preferable to bed baths, as organisms can be redistributed over the body during bed bathing (Greaves 1985). If bed bathing is unavoidable the patient should be supplied with their own bowl which is washed and dried after use and stored at the bedside to prevent cross-infection.

Waste

Waste is divided into two categories: domestic (to be placed in black bags) and clinical (to be placed in yellow bags). The segregation, labelling, handling and subsequent incineration of clinical waste must conform to Health and Safety Commission (1992) requirements and local recommendations (London Waste Regulation Authority 1994).

Within a source barrier nursing room all waste other than sharps or unused drugs must be put into the yellow clinical waste bag, sealed securely in the room, labelled with ward, hospital and date and sent for incineration.

Sharps and unused drugs must be placed in disposal boxes (that conform to UN3291 and BS7320) at the point of use. These boxes must not be overfilled. When full, the container must be shut, labelled with ward, hospital and date and sent for incineration. Containers must not be left on the floor in public areas (DoH 2001a).

Linen

Infected linen must be placed in a red alginate polythene bag. The bag is tied shut and then placed in a red linen bag to be sent in a safe manner to the laundry for barrier washing. This entails placing the full alginate bag in the washing machine where it dissolves, allowing the hot water to wash and disinfect the linen. In this way staff and the environment are protected from contamination.

Cutlery and crockery

Crockery and cutlery can become contaminated with pathogenic organisms. Hands must be washed after handling utensils used by patients (NHSE 1995). All crockery must be machine washed in a dishwasher with a final rinse of 80°C for one minute to disinfect it. Disposable crockery and cutlery are needed only when gross contamination has occurred or if a dishwasher is not available.

Urine, faeces and vomit

These must be disposed of immediately and carefully to prevent contamination of the environment. This may be by using a bedpan washer or macerator. Hands must be washed following disposal of blood and body fluids (DoH 2001a).

Notification of infection

If a patient develops signs and symptoms of infection or if bacteriological analysis identifies an organism which necessitates barrier nursing, swift communication and action are needed to instigate this. Any problems may be discussed with the infection control team.

Informing the patient and visitors

Giving careful explanation to the patient is essential so that they can co-operate fully with the restrictions (Ayliffe *et al.* 2000). The nurse should be sensitive to the psychological implications of being labelled 'infectious' and of being confined in isolation (Gammon 1999). Rees *et al.* (2000) examined the psychological effects of being admitted to a barrier nursing room, and found that patients were unlikely to have significant psychological problems unless there was a previous history of mental illness. Fortunately, many patients in fact preferred a single room, and adapted well to any subsequent loneliness and boredom. Other research has indicated that patients' needs are sometimes neglected when they are barrier nursed (Knowles 1993). The patient's visitors must also be told why the barrier nursing restrictions are necessary. Visitors will generally be allowed into the room at the discretion of the infection control team. They must be taught to observe the correct procedures for entering and leaving the room. As children are more susceptible to infection than adults, any visit by a child should be discussed with the infection control team.

Domestic staff

The domestic manager must be informed as soon as barrier nursing is commenced. He or she will then provide the ward domestic with written instructions.

The ward domestic staff must understand clearly why barrier nursing is required and should be instructed on the correct procedure. The nursing staff must check that the ward domestics understand and are following their instructions correctly. If the patient is in a single room, a mop (laundered daily), bucket (washed and dried after use), cleaning fluid and disposable cloths should be used solely for this patient's use. If the patient is in a general ward, special care must be taken with the cleaning so that potentially infectious material is not transferred from the area around the infected patient to other patient areas. The infected patient's area must be cleaned last and separately.

Staff allocation

A minimum number of staff should be involved with an infected patient. The nurse concerned with the infected patient should not also attend to other susceptible patients. If barrier nursing is for an infectious disease such as chicken pox, it is important that only personnel who have already had the disease should attend this patient.

The protection of staff against the risk of infection is one of the main functions of the occupational health department. This department offers an immunization and counselling service.

Procedure guidelines: **Source isolation**

Equipment

1 Isolation suite if possible.
2 All items required to meet the patient's nursing needs during the period of isolation, e.g. instruments to assess vital signs.

3 Protective clothing.
4 Alcoholic handrub.

Procedure

Preparation of the isolation room

Action	Rationale
1 Place a barrier nursing sign outside the door.	To inform anyone intending to enter the room of the situation.
2 List requirements for personnel before entering and after leaving the isolation area.	To decrease entries and exits to the room.
3 Remove all non-essential furniture. The remaining furniture should be easy to clean and should not conceal or retain dirt or moisture either within or around it.	To minimize the risk of furniture harbouring microbial spores or growth colonies.
4 Stock the hand basin with a suitable bactericidal soap preparation and paper towels for staff use.	Facilities for hand washing within the infected area are essential for effective barrier nursing.
5 Place yellow clinical waste bag in the room on a foot-operated stand. The bag must be sealed before it is removed from the room.	For containing contaminated rubbish within the room. Yellow is the recognized colour for clinical waste.
6 Place a container for 'sharps' in the room.	To contain contaminated 'sharps' within the infected area.
7 When the 'sharps' container is two-thirds full it must be firmly shut and sent for incineration.	To minimize the risk of leakage from the 'sharps' container.
8 Keep the patient's personal property to a minimum. Advise him/her to wear hospital clothing. All belongings taken into the room should be washable, cleanable or disposable.	The patient's belongings may become contaminated and cannot be taken home unless they are washable or cleanable. Anything else may have to be destroyed.

*Procedure guidelines: **Source isolation** (cont'd)*

Action	Rationale
9 Provide the patient with his/her own thermometer and sphygmomanometer, and all items necessary for attending to personal hygiene.	Equipment used regularly by the patient should be kept within the infected area to prevent the spread of infection.
10 Keep dressing solutions, creams and lotions, etc., to a minimum and store them within the room.	All partially used materials must be discarded when barrier nursing ends (sterilization is not possible), therefore unnecessary waste should be avoided.
11 Set up a trolley outside the door to hold plastic aprons and bactericidal alcoholic handrub (this is contraindicated if the trolley causes an obstruction or is a hazard to staff and others).	Staff are more likely to use the equipment if it is readily available.

Entering the room

Action	Rationale
1 Collect all equipment needed.	To avoid entering and leaving the infected area unnecessarily.
2 Roll up long sleeves to the elbow.	To allow hand washing to take place.
3 Put on a disposable plastic apron.	A plastic apron is inexpensive, quick to put on and protects the front of the uniform, which is the most likely area to come in contact with the patient.
4 Put on a disposable, impermeable gown 'when heavy contamination is anticipated'.	To protect clothing from contamination to shoulders, arms and back. Cotton gowns are an ineffective barrier against bacteria, particularly when wet.
5 Put on a disposable well-fitting mask if there is a risk of airborne contamination, i.e. (a) Meningococcus meningitis (b) Blood and body fluids (c) Tuberculosis.	To reduce the risk of inhaling organisms and to comply with safe techniques and practices.
6 Safety glasses, visors and goggles should be put on when it is likely that aerosolized droplets of blood or body fluids are present in the air.	To give protection to the conjunctiva from blood and body fluid splashes.
7 Rinse hands with bactericidal alcoholic handrub.	Hands must be cleaned before and after patient contact to reduce the risk of cross-infection.
8 Put on disposable gloves only if you are intending to deal with blood, excreta or contaminated material.	To reduce the risk of hand contamination.
9 Enter the room, shutting the door behind you.	To reduce the risk of airborne organisms leaving the room.

Attending to the patient

Action	Rationale
1 *Meals.* Meals only need to be served on disposable crockery and eaten with disposable cutlery if deemed necessary by the infection control team. Disposables and uneaten food should be discarded in the appropriate bag.	Contaminated crockery is a potential disease vector.
2 *Non-disposable crockery and cutlery* must be washed in a dishwasher with a hot disinfecting cycle.	Water at 80°C for 1 minute in a dishwasher will disinfect crockery and cutlery.
3 *Excreta.* Ideally, a toilet should be kept solely for the patient's use. If neither this nor disposable items are available, a separate bedpan or urinal and commode should be left in the patient's room. Gloves must be worn by staff when dealing with excreta. Bedpans and urinals should be bagged in the isolation room, emptied and then washed in a bedpan washer, then	To minimize the risk of infection being spread from excreta, e.g. via a toilet seat or a bedpan.

Procedure guidelines: **Source isolation** *(cont'd)*

Action	Rationale
dried and returned immediately to the patient's room. On discharge of the patient, bedpans/urinals must be sent to the sterile supplies department (SSD) for disinfection.	
4 *Accidental spills*. Any suspected contaminated fluids must be mopped up immediately and the area cleaned with disinfectant.	Damp areas encourage microbial growth and increase the risk of spread of infection.
5 *Bathing*. An infected patient must be bathed last on the ward. Clean and dry the bath after the previous patient and after the infected patient.	Leaving the bath dry after disinfection reduces the risk of microbes surviving and infecting others. Bacteria will not easily grow on clean, dry surfaces.
6 *Dressings*. Aseptic technique must be used for changing all dressings. Waste materials and dirty dressings should be discarded in the appropriate yellow clinical waste bag. Used lotions, creams, etc., must be kept in the room and not used for other patients (Dietze *et al.* 2001). Sterile packs must be stored safely to protect them from contamination and damage.	Aseptic procedure minimizes the risk of cross-infection. Lotions and creams can become easily contaminated. Micro-organisms can survive on unopened sterile packs.
7 *Linen*. Place infected linen in a red alginate polythene bag, which must be secured tightly before it leaves the room. Just outside the room, place this bag into a red linen bag which must be secured tightly and not used for other patients. These bags should await the laundry collection in a safe area.	Placing infected linen in a red alginate polythene bag confines the organisms and allows staff handling the linen to recognize the potential hazard.
8 *Waste*. Yellow clinical waste bags should be kept in the room for disposal of all the patient's rubbish. The bag's top should be sealed and labelled with the name of the ward or department before it is removed from the room.	Yellow is the international colour for clinical waste.

Leaving the room

Action	Rationale
1 If wearing gloves, remove and discard them in the yellow clinical waste bag. Clean hands with bactericidal alcoholic handrub.	To remove pathogenic organisms acquired during contact with patient before removing gown, so preventing contamination of uniform.
2 Remove apron and discard it in the appropriate bag. Clean hands with bactericidal alcoholic handrub.	Hands may be contaminated by a dirty gown.
3 Used gowns should not be reused.	To reduce the risk of cross-infection by contaminated uniforms, as staff find it hard to distinguish the inside/outside of a gown. If the gown is worn inside out, uniforms can be contaminated.
4 Leave the room, shutting the door behind you.	To reduce the risk of airborne spread of infection.
5 Rub hands with a bactericidal alcoholic handrub.	To remove pathogenic organisms acquired from such items as the door handle (Oie *et al.* 2002).

Cleaning the room

Action	Rationale
1 Domestic staff must understand why barrier nursing is required and should be instructed on the correct procedure.	To reduce the risk of mistakes and to ensure that barrier nursing is maintained.
2 The area where barrier nursing is being carried out must be cleaned last.	To reduce the risk of the transmission of organisms.

*Procedure guidelines: **Source isolation** (cont'd)*

Action	Rationale
3 Separate cleaning equipment must be kept for this area.	Cleaning equipment can easily become infected. Cross-infection may result from shared cleaning equipment.
4 Members of the domestic services staff must wear gloves and plastic aprons.	To reduce the risk of cross-infection.
5 *Floor* (hard surface). This must be washed daily with a disinfectant as appropriate. All excess water must be removed.	Daily cleaning will keep bacterial count reduced. Organisms, especially Gram-negative bacteria, multiply quickly in the presence of moisture (Scott & Bloomfield 1990) and on equipment (Wilson 2001).
6 Cleaning solutions must be freshly diluted and the spray container emptied, cleaned and dried daily.	Cleaning fluid can easily become contaminated (Dharan *et al.* 1999).
7 After use, the bucket must be cleaned and dried.	Bacteria will not easily survive on clean, dry surfaces.
8 Mop heads should be laundered in a hot wash daily.	Mop heads become contaminated easily.
9 *Floor* (carpet). An infected patient may have been admitted into a room with a carpet. A vacuum cleaner should be used which is fitted with an efficient filter. After use the dust bag must be changed and the brush head washed and dried.	Vacuum cleaning reduces the dust, thus reducing organisms (Trakumas *et al.* 2001).
10 On discharge, the carpet must be steam cleaned.	Bacteria can survive in dust trapped in the carpet fibres. The heat of the steam will kill these bacteria.
11 Furniture and fittings should be damp dusted using a disposable cloth and a detergent solution or a disinfectant if appropriate.	To remove any organisms.
12 The toilet, shower and bathroom area must be cleaned at least once a day using a non-abrasive hypochlorite powder or cream. A disinfectant will only be required if soiling of the area has occurred.	Non-abrasive powders or creams preserve the integrity of the surfaces. These areas recontaminate rapidly after cleaning and routine chemical disinfection is of little value and should be saved for terminal cleaning following discharge of the patient.

Transporting infected patients outside the source isolation area

Action	Rationale
1 Inform the department concerned about the diagnosis.	To allow other departments time to make their own arrangements.
2 Arrange for the patient to have the last appointment of the day.	The department concerned, the hospital corridors, lifts, etc., will be less busy and will allow more time for special cleaning and disinfecting.
3 Any porters involved must be instructed carefully. The trolley or chair should be cleaned after use.	Protection and reassurance of porters are necessary to allay fear and to minimize the risk of the infection being spread to them.
4 It may be necessary for the nurse to escort the patient.	To ensure the necessary precautions are maintained.
5 In some circumstances, for example meningococcus meningitis and tuberculosis, the patient should wear a mask when leaving the room.	To prevent airborne cross-infection.

Discharging the patient

Action	Rationale
1 Inform the infection control team when the patient is due for discharge.	The infection control team 'may need to provide advice' on any special precautions.
2 The room should be stripped. All textiles must be changed and curtains sent to the laundry.	Curtains readily become colonized with bacteria.
3 Impervious surfaces, e.g. lockers, stools and blinds, should be washed with soap and water.	Wiping of surfaces is the most effective way of removing contaminants. Relatively inaccessible places, e.g. ceilings,

*Procedure guidelines: **Source isolation** (cont'd)*

Action	Rationale
	may be omitted; these are not generally relevant to any infection risk.
4 The floor must be washed and dried thoroughly.	To remove any organisms present.
5 The room can be reused as soon as it has been correctly and thoroughly cleaned.	Most organisms will survive in the environment for long periods of time. Effective cleaning will remove these organisms. Once cleaning has been completed, the room is ready to admit another patient.

Protective isolation

Definition

Protective isolation is a process of care which provides a safe environment for patients who are susceptible to infection by isolating them as far as possible from the risk of infection from all exogenous sources.

Indications

Protective isolation can be an appropriate form of care for many patients, e.g. burns patients, children with immunodeficiency disease and patients receiving bone marrow transplantation. The aim of protective isolation is to prevent and treat infection until the period of immunosuppression has passed.

Immunosuppression is a generalized depression of the immune system, which increases the risk of acquiring an infection. This necessitates protecting immunosuppressed patients from micro-organisms carried in the environment, on health care workers providing care, on visitors and on other patients.

Present-day treatments have increased the number of immunosuppressed patients, owing to their underlying disease and intensive treatment regimens. This is particularly noticeable with oncology and transplant patients. At the same time changes have occurred in the organisms associated with infection (Wingard 1999), particularly the emergence of antimicrobial-resistant micro-organisms (Glauser & Pizzo 2000). Concurrently difficulties related to factors such as recruitment and retention of health care workers (Newman *et al.* 2002), achieving high standards of cleanliness, decontamination and sterilization have occurred (Taylor *et al.* 2001).

Immunosuppressed patients can become infected with pathogens that can infect people with normal immune responses, as well as with opportunistic micro-organisms that do not usually cause disease in healthy persons (Gerberding 1998). Traditionally protective isolation has been used to eliminate sources of infection to protect the immunosuppressed patient during their hospital stay, so increasing their chances of recovery (Maertens *et al.* 2001).

Immunosuppression can be caused by many factors including:

- Primary disease such as leukaemia, lymphoma, acquired immune deficiency syndrome (AIDS) and severe combined immunodeficiency disease (SCID)
- Secondary disease, such as diabetes, which may complicate primary disease
- Drugs, in particular cytotoxic drugs and corticosteroids
- Antimicrobial therapy causing changes in the patient's microbial flora
- Irradiation therapy: the degree of immunosuppression is related directly to the area being treated
- Trauma and burns
- Age (Taylor *et al.* 2001).

On admission a detailed clinical history of the patient's past and current health status must be obtained. This initial assessment, along with ongoing physical examination, is essential to assess for any complications that may affect the patient's recovery. Prior to commencing high-dose chemotherapy, a risk assessment to evaluate the patient's immune status must be undertaken to assess their risk of acquiring an infection (Dales & Liles 1998). These risks include: underlying cause of immune defect, expected extent and duration of planned immunosuppression treatment, presence of invasive devices and damage to skin and mucous membranes, such as mucositis (Van Burik & Weisdorf 1999). This assessment will also ensure that practical measures can be adopted to reduce the risk of infection (Farrington & Pascoe 2001; Masterton & Teare 2001).

The risk of infection will be increased by breaches in the body's natural defence mechanisms, for example:

- Skin by, for example, indwelling catheters, repeated venepuncture, pressure ulcers
- Mucous membranes, from oral ulceration

- Body cavities by urinary catheters or endotracheal tubes (Calandra 2000).

Immunosuppressed patients are at increased risk of HAI and for those most at risk HAI cannot always be prevented (Taylor *et al.* 2001). The likelihood of developing an infection is related to the neutrophil count. This risk is greatest:

- The lower the count
- With a rapidly falling count
- If the length of neutropenia is extended (Glauser & Calandra 2000).

The recovery from HAI by immunosuppressed patients is often poor (Garrouste-Orgeas *et al.* 2000), making infection the leading cause of death amongst allogeneic bone marrow transplant immunosuppressed patients (Working Group 2000).

Immunosuppressed patients are at risk of infections that affect immunocompetent patients, as well as from opportunistic micro-organisms. Antibiotic-resistant infections are of particular concern. Prompt diagnosis of infection is essential (Gillespie & Masterton 1998). All signs and symptoms of infection or deteriorating health must be considered significant and swiftly investigated. Once microbiological samples have been obtained, antibiotics should be commenced as soon as possible (Bodey & Rolston 2001). These will generally be broad-spectrum antibiotics (Viscoli 1998) administered via the intravenous route to ensure speed of delivery since recovery is improved with early treatment (ICNA/Pharmacia 2002).

Some patients have an increased risk of infection due to a combination of immunosuppressive factors (Yuen *et al.* 1998). For example, a patient with leukaemia who is undergoing bone marrow transplantation and who develops graft-versus-host disease (GVHD) may require treatment with increased doses of immunosuppressive drugs (Marr *et al.* 2002).

In the 1970s and 1980s trials to evaluate the effectiveness of protective isolation were undertaken. For example a study by Yates *et al.* (1973) found no difference in infection rates in the first 21 days following admission. However, after this time patients experienced fewer infections if they were being cared for in protective isolation rooms. Others have demonstrated that protective isolation with topical and non-absorbable antibiotics and low microbial diet significantly reduced the number of infections, but did not affect long-term survival (Levine *et al.* 1973; Ribas-Mundom *et al.* 1981). It has also been suggested that protective isolation reduces the incidence of GVHD in patients with aplastic anaemia (Storb *et al.* 1983), although in contrast a study by

Petersen *et al.* (1987) suggested that the incidence of GVHD was not affected. Nevertheless, the results of Petersen's project indicated that infection rates were significantly reduced in patients in protective isolation compared to those patients in conventional hospital rooms. The Centers for Disease Control in the USA (Garner & Simmons 1983) highlight that expensive isolation precautions do not prevent endogenous infections and therefore do not appear to be warranted for most compromised patients. This view is supported by Russell *et al.* (2000), who point out that the majority of infections will be endogenous and will have very little to do with the environment. However, Johnson *et al.* (2000) suggest that the incidence of systemic fungal infections in immunosuppressed patients is increasing and some preventive measures such as air filtration, hand washing and exclusion of items such as flowers known to be contaminated will be worthwhile. A survey of 91 bone marrow transplantation units in the USA found that while all units used some type of protective environment practice, these varied between units. The researchers recommended that national standards for protective isolation need to be compiled, which could be used to rationalize nursing care (Poe *et al.* 1994). A later study in Italy found that more than 60% of bone marrow transplant centres used complex and multiple measures to prevent infection (Errico *et al.* 1999).

Immunosuppressed patients require skilled nursing care (Radwin 2000). To prevent infection, all staff must receive infection control education, training and supervision (DoH 2001a).

The British Committee for Standards in Haematology (BCS 1995) defines four levels of care required for the management of adult patients with haematological malignancies and bone marrow failure as:

1 Level 1 for patients with transient severe neutropenia. This involves rooms designated for neutropenic patients, which have skilled staff over the 24-hour period. Expert advice and support are available from a nurse specialist.

2 Level 2 for patients requiring induction chemotherapy for leukaemia.

3 Level 3 for patients undergoing autologous transplantation. Levels 2 and 3 management require single rooms with en-suite facilities. Level 2 requires experienced nurses with recognized certificates in haematology. The view of the British Committee for Standards in Haematology (BSC 1995) is supported by the Croner's Health Service Risk Management and Practice special report (1998) which suggests that immunosuppressed patients require cubicle facilities and en-suite toilet facilities.

4 Level 4 for patients undergoing related allogeneic and autologous transplantation. Care at level 4 requires single rooms, en-suite facilities, laminar airflow or positive filtered air conditioning and a designated kitchen area. Levels 3 and 4 require nurses who are experienced, with at least 25% of nurses having certificates in haematology or oncology. The BSC (1995) highlights the stresses experienced by nurses caring for bone marrow transplantation (BMT) patients and recommends the provision of staff support.

Reference material

Protective isolation may be achieved by:

- Purpose-built units
- Plastic isolators
- Single rooms on a general ward
- Shared rooms within a controlled environment on a general ward
- Bioclean room, which is a new technology where a dust-free aseptic environment is created by circulating air containing ultra-fine water droplets with negative air ions which collect and facilitate the removal of airborne organisms (Shinjo *et al.* 2002).

Purpose-built units

A purpose-built unit will include:

- Positive pressure filtered air supply which is required for immunosuppressed patients in protective isolation (NHS Estates 2002). This will ensure airborne micro-organisms outside the protective isolation ward do not enter the room.
- Single rooms with integral toilet, shower, a hatch system for the aseptic transfer of equipment into the room, and an entry area for visitors and staff where protective clothing can be donned and hands washed
- Facilities to provide pathogen-free food
- Gastrointestinal decontamination.

These units are expensive to build, maintain and staff.

Plastic isolators

An isolator consists of a framework erected around a bed from which a PVC tent is suspended (Trexler 1975). The tent has an air supply attached which keeps the whole apparatus inflated. A positive air pressure is usually maintained within the isolator. In some cases, for example when nursing patients with Lassa fever, the pressure within the isolator is slightly below atmospheric pressure, which prevents the escape of any infected particles. Although patients may feel a strong sense of containment within the isolator, this system does have the advantage of achieving high standards of bacteriological control, and it can be assembled and dismantled rapidly.

Single rooms and shared rooms in general wards

Immunosuppressed patients are at risk of acquiring an infection from environmental micro-organisms (Kusne & Krystofiak 2001). Therefore the decision to isolate a patient will be influenced by the availability of facilities coupled to the general condition of the ward area where the isolation is to take place. In determining the most suitable area, a number of criteria need to be met. Among these are the relative cleanliness of the ward, the standard of domestic services support, the microbiological status of the other patients and the anticipated length of the isolation. This less vigorous method of protective isolation is unlikely to greatly reduce the acquisition of potential pathogens, as only person-to-person transfer of infection is prevented, since facilities such as clean air and pathogen-free food are not usually available on general wards.

When shared facilities are used, it is essential that all patients are carefully screened to ensure that those with infections are excluded.

Protective isolation environment

The prevention of exogenous transmission of infection is important and can be achieved by careful monitoring of the environment to remove items which could predispose to infection, for example plants, flowers and dried flower arrangements, which are known to harbour *Aspergillus* species. Whilst they have never been implicated in cross-infection, they should not be kept in the room (Johnson *et al.* 2000). Scrupulous cleaning with special attention to furniture and equipment within the room will also prevent transmission (Boden 1999). All surfaces must be cleanable, especially items such as electric fans, air cooling systems and chairs (Custovic *et al.* 1998), with excess equipment removed to make the cleaning process easier and more effective (King 1998). The patient area must be well maintained. This was highlighted by Loach (1997), who discussed how her experience of protective isolation was badly affected by a shower being broken. In addition, contaminated plumbing can be an infection risk, which can be reduced by routine servicing (Ferroni *et al.* 1998).

Patient hygiene

Studies have highlighted the overwhelming fatigue experienced by patients with leukaemia and lymphoma. Fatigue hinders patients' ability to take care of themselves and demonstrates the importance of expert nursing intervention and assessment (Persson *et al.* 1997).

The limiting of endogenous transmission of infection, which is the major cause of infection in immunosuppressed patients, is difficult but good patient hygiene and restriction of invasive devices and procedures are essential (Errico *et al.* 1999).

Infection

In the early period of immunosuppression, respiratory, gastrointestinal, skin, mucosa bacterial and fungal flora may cause infection. These include: *Staphylococccus aureus* and *epidermidis*, Streptococci, Candida, enterococci and Gram-negative bacteria such as *Escherichia coli* and Pseudomonas. Later reactivation of latent infections or new infections such as herpes simplex, zoster, cytomegalovirus, Epstein–Barr virus, *Pneumocystis carinii*, Aspergillus and toxoplasmosis may occur (Working Group 2000). Unfortunately, signs and symptoms of infection are often absent in immunosuppressed patients (Viscoli 1998). Progression of infection in the immunosuppressed patient may be rapid and widespread, and the earliest signs of infection must be looked for (see Ch. 25, Observations). When fever appears, diagnostic and therapeutic measures must be instigated immediately (Barber 2001). Patient survival depends upon prompt recognition of problems and instigation of medical and nursing intervention (Shaffer & Wilson 1993). Investigations to establish the cause of infection include chest X-ray, bacteriological and viral culture of blood, urine and sputum and swabs obtained from any suspicious lesion. Riley (1998) discusses the value of surveillance cultures in predicting causative organisms of infection, suggesting they should be limited to weekly samples from nose, throat and stool samples (see Ch. 39, Specimen collection).

Hand washing

Immunosuppressed patients are at increased risk of nosocomial infection, and bacteria that cause infection are particularly easily disseminated by health care workers' hands. Strict hand washing before and after patient contact can reduce rates of infection (see Ch. 4, Aseptic technique). Hand washing can be said to be the most important means of infection control (DoH 2001a). Compliance with hand washing can be poor; one study found that only 56% of clinicians and 86% of nurses complied with hand-washing policy requirements (Lai *et al.* 1998). The use of an alcohol handrub to cleanse clean hands improves compliance with hand-cleaning policies (Hugonnet *et al.* 2002).

Diet

Food is a potential source of infection (Meier & Lopez 2001) and good food hygiene practice is essential (Food Safety (General Food Hygiene) Regulations 1995a). Generally, if non-absorbable gut antibiotics are prescribed, pathogen-free food must be provided (Patterson 1993). This includes thoroughly cooked foods, canned foods and foods known to be pathogen free such as cereal. Reheated food is not likely to be pathogen free and should not be used. If pathogen-free food is unavailable the diet should consist only of food that has been well cooked, with foods known to have high bacterial counts avoided. Foods known to have an increased risk of being contaminated, for example fresh cream, shellfish, raw or lightly cooked eggs (Ejidokun *et al.* 2000), soft cheeses (Gillespie *et al.* 2001), pâté, raw vegetables, salads and fruit, must be eliminated from the diet. Infection from ice can also occur from contamination within the ice maker or from staff, patients or visitors. Surveys of hospital ward ice machines demonstrated a wide range of potentially opportunistic pathogenic micro-organisms (Wilson *et al.* 1997). Ice for immunosuppressed patients should be made by putting drinking water into single-use ice makers, then into a conventional freezer (NHS Estates 2002). It should be noted that microwave cookers have been found to be an unreliable means of heating food (George 1997) and therefore should not be used in these circumstances.

Well-nourished people undergoing BMT have a better survival rate and shorter hospital stay than undernourished patients (Henry 1997). A survey of bone marrow transplant units in Canada indicated that most hospitals acknowledge the potential for food to cause infection amongst immunosuppressed patients (French *et al.* 2001). Food provided for patients must be prepared following recognized food safety regulations (General Food Hygiene Regulations 1995a), including thorough hand washing. Food cooked and brought in from home must be avoided as this may not have been prepared according to good food hygiene practices (Gilbert *et al.* 2000). Visitors should be encouraged to bring in prepackaged food such as biscuits and crisps or tinned items (McCulloch 1998) which will have been manufactured to the necessary food hygiene standards. A review of practice related to clean diets found evidence of a move away from stringent sterile diets towards more relaxed regimens with rational, justifiable food hygiene guidelines (Patterson 1993).

Psychological issues

Protective isolation can cause increased stress for patients (Cohen *et al.* 2001), and they should be prepared before they enter isolation (Heiney *et al.* 1994). Nurses can reduce anxiety by assisting patients to learn about their situation and about health-promoting activities (Ward

2000). Research has shown that the overriding concern of patients in isolation was a desire to receive information about their disease and reassurance regarding their treatment (Campbell 1999). It is important that health care workers are aware of the impact of protective isolation on patients (Gaskill *et al.* 1997), and it has been suggested that patients should only be offered a BMT if anticipated physical and psychological benefits outweigh the risk (Collins *et al.* 1989). Other studies suggest that patients view protective isolation as a temporary inconvenience rather than a stressor (Zerbe *et al.* 1994). A study of long-term adult BMT survivors found that despite lingering side-effects these patients were leading full and meaningful lives (Haberman *et al.* 1993). However, one patient's view of isolation highlighted the stifling confined environment, loss of bodily freedom and the shock of physical deterioration (Loach 1997).

Nursing care

The value of nursing care has been emphasized in improving the care of patients undergoing BMT (Thain & Gibbon 1996). Therefore orientation, education and training for new and existing staff are essential (Rees *et al.* 2000), to allow nurses to keep up with developments and to ensure optimum patient care (Porter 1998). A study by Larson *et al.* (1993) describes the lack of nurses' perception of the patient's distress during hospitalization for BMT. Other studies highlight the importance of BMT nurses' training, which should include specific psychosocial strategies to delineate psychosocial needs of patients and families (Winters *et al.* 1994).

It is suggested that nursing on a protective isolation unit, particularly with patients undergoing BMT, increases the stress suffered by nurses themselves (Kelly *et al.* 2000). This can result in burn-out, producing symptoms such as fatigue, anxiety, depression and poor concentration (Stordeur *et al.* 1999), which can be detrimental to nurses, their colleagues and the patients in their care. Nursing managers of intensive care units such as protective isolation units need to be aware of this risk and provide support and a treatment plan if burn-out does occur (Kiss 1994).

Nurses must recognize the factors which increase the risk of infection and must not contribute to this risk (McCulloch 1998). Pettinger & Nettleman's (1991) study investigating compliance with isolation precautions found that non-compliance with protective isolation procedures was widespread, although visitors were more compliant than health care workers.

Discharge home

Discharge planning should start early (see Ch. 8). Risk assessment of the home should be undertaken to ensure the home is clean and well maintained, with a well-equipped kitchen for food preparation, storage and cooking (Bloomfield 2002). Caution should be taken when in contact with domestic pets, which may be carriers of infection. For example, dogs can be infected with a wide range of infections including Cryptosporidium (Fayers *et al.* 2001) which can cause serious infection in an immunosuppressed person (Robinson & Pugh 2002).

Procedure guidelines: **Nursing the neutropenic patient**

Procedure

Preparation of the room and maintenance of general cleanliness

	Action	Rationale
1	A single room or a designated shared room should be used if possible.	To reduce airborne transfer of micro-organisms.
2	A toilet to be kept for the sole use of the patient.	To reduce the risk of cross-infection.
3	Area to be cleaned meticulously before the patient is admitted.	To reduce the risk of infection.
4	Equipment and supplies to be kept for the sole use of the patient. (This must also include any cleaning equipment used by domestic staff.)	To reduce the risk of cross-infection. Cleaning equipment can easily become colonized with micro-organisms which may cause cross-infection.
5	Surfaces and furniture to be damp dusted daily using disposable cleaning cloths and detergent solution.	Damp dusting and mopping remove micro-organisms without distributing them into the air.
6	Floor to be mopped daily using soap and water.	To reduce the risk of cross-infection.
7	Mop head to be laundered daily.	As above.
8	Bucket and mop handle to be cleaned and dried.	As above.

*Procedure guidelines: **Nursing the neutropenic patient** (cont'd)*

Nursing procedure

Entering room

	Action	Rationale
1	Clean hands with bactericidal alcoholic handrub.	Hands are regarded as the principal source of transfer of micro-organisms. (For further information see Ch. 4, Aseptic technique.)
2	A disposable plastic apron to be worn when in contact with the patient.	To protect staff clothing from becoming contaminated, which could transfer organisms to the other patients in their care.
3	Door of room to be kept closed. Ideally the air in the room should be under slightly positive pressure. The air flow should be from the room into the corridor.	To reduce the risk of airborne transmission of infection from other areas of the ward.

Visitors

	Action	Rationale
1	The patient should be asked to nominate close relatives and friends who may then, after instruction, visit freely. The patient or his or her representative should inform casual acquaintances or non-essential visitors that they should avoid visiting during the period of neutropenia.	The incidence of infection increases in proportion to the number of people visiting. Large numbers of visitors are difficult to screen and educate. Unlimited visiting by close relatives and friends diminishes the sense of isolation that the patient may experience.
2	Any visitor with an infection or who has been in contact with infection should be excluded.	Neutropenic patients are susceptible to infection.
3	Children, unless very close relatives, should be discouraged.	Children are more likely to have been in contact with infectious diseases which can have serious consequences if transmitted to a neutropenic patient.

Diet

	Action	Rationale
1	Educate the patient to choose only cooked food from the hospital menu and eliminate raw fruit, salads and uncooked vegetables from the diet.	Uncooked foods are often heavily colonized by micro-organisms, particularly Gram-negative bacteria.
2	Food brought into the hospital by visitors must be restricted and: (a) Obtained from well-known, reliable firms (b) In undamaged, sealed tins and packets (c) Within the expiry date.	Correctly processed and packaged foods are more likely to be of an acceptable food hygiene standard.
3	Filtered water to be used.	Tap water is safe to drink but can become colonized by organisms, particularly Gram-negative organisms found in the plughole of sinks or overflow outlet when the water is being filled.
4	Sealed packets of fruit juice (long shelf-life varieties, particularly those rich in vitamins) are suitable. Juice should be poured directly into a clean jug and drunk the same day.	These juices have been pasteurized and remain pathogen free until they are opened.

Discharging the patient

	Action	Rationale
1	Crowded areas, for example shops, cinemas, pubs and discos, should be avoided.	Although the patient's white cell count is usually high enough for discharge, the patient remains immunocompromised for some time.

*Procedure guidelines: **Nursing the neutropenic patient** (cont'd)*

Action	Rationale
2 Pets should not be allowed to lick the patient, and new pets should not be obtained.	Pets are known carriers of infection (Mims *et al. 1993*).
3 Certain foods, for example take-away meals, soft cheese and pâté, should continue to be avoided.	Take-away meals are subject to handling by a large number of individuals and are stored for longer periods, both of which increase the likelihood of contamination.
4 Salads and fruit should be washed carefully, dried and, if possible, peeled.	To remove as many pathogens as possible.
5 Any sign or symptoms of infection should be reported immediately to the patient's general practitioner or to the discharging hospital.	Any infection may continue to have serious consequences if left unlocated.

Acquired immune deficiency syndrome (AIDS)

Definition

Acquired immune deficiency syndrome (AIDS) is a state of immunosuppression caused by the human immunodeficiency viruses 1 (HIV 1) and 2 (HIV 2), which causes a chronic, progressive disruption of the immune system. Due to mutation and recombination HIV 1 has diversified. There are now at least 24 circulating genetic forms including 11 subtypes (subtype A, B, C and so on) and 13 circulating recombinant forms (Thomson *et al.* 2002). In order to map the genetic variation of HIV 1, scientists have classified different strains of the virus into three groups: M (main), O (outlier) and N (non-M, non-O) (WHO 2002a). As no overall description can be made for AIDS, an internationally agreed case definition has been made. This definition provides uniform, simple criteria for categorizing HIV conditions to facilitate evaluation of treatment and care of persons with HIV (Centers for Disease Control 1992).

HIV infection is divided into four groups:

- Primary HIV infection (often associated with a rash and fever; Hecht *et al.* 2002)
- Asymptomatic phase
- Persistent generalized lymphadenopathy
- Symptomatic infection, which is further subdivided. Some patients' symptoms may be classified as AIDS-defining conditions (Mindel & Tenant-Flowers 2001).

AIDS-defining conditions include:

- Certain opportunistic infections
- Certain cancers
- Wasting syndrome
- Encephalopathy.

AIDS-defining cancers include:

- Kaposi's sarcoma, which is decreasing in prevalence
- Primary CNS lymphoma
- Non-Hodgkin's lymphoma (Burkitt's or immunoblastic)
- Invasive cervical cancer (Lucas 2002).

The outlook for the latter three cancers is poor. Goedert *et al.* (1998) investigated the relationship of HIV and cancer and found that AIDS leads to immunological failure which predisposes to a significant increase in the risk of cancers; this risk increases with longer survival.

Reference material

Since 1989 several investigators have independently reported cases of unexplained severe immunodeficiency without evidence of infection with HIV 1 or 2 (Pankhurst & Peakman 1989; Jowitt *et al.* 1991; Laurence *et al.* 1992). A relatively small number of people claim that HIV does not cause AIDS. Ellison and colleagues (1995) state that the disease is caused by 'lifestyle'. This explanation has been discounted by others (Weiss 2001).

Approximately 5 million new HIV infections occurred in 2001, 800 000 of them affecting children. At least 20 million people have died of AIDS in the world. Sub-Saharan Africa is the worst affected region in the world, with approximately 3.5 million new infections occurring in 2001, bringing the total to 28.5 million. Of these, fewer than 30 000 people receive antiretroviral drugs (www.unaids.org). In the UK 14 205 new cases of HIV were reported; this had increased by 62% by the end of 2000 and it is expected to have increased by 139% by the end of 2005 (McHenry *et al.* 2002). The prevalence of HIV infection in pregnant women continues to rise. The majority of infected women are born abroad; for example, 85% of HIV-infected women in London were born in sub-Saharan Africa (DoH 2001b).

The epidemiology of HIV and AIDS is changing and although HIV is still incurable despite the introduction of new treatments, the increased uptake of antiretroviral therapy has reduced the need for HIV-positive patients to be admitted to hospital (Rogers *et al.* 2000). However, although therapy delays the development of AIDS, the median survival time from the diagnosis of AIDS to death remains about 19.3 months. The exceptions to this would be patients whose HIV infection was diagnosed late, those who had the opportunity to receive treatment before the diagnosis of AIDS and those whose treatment has failed.

Unfortunately the emergence of HIV drug resistance in patients receiving antiretroviral therapy is common. One study estimates that the transmission of resistant HIV strains was 27% in people infected with HIV during 2000. This high figure is thought to be due to the increased use of antiretroviral drugs and because unprotected sex among those at most risk of acquiring HIV persists (Little *et al.* 2002).

Antibody and antigen serological tests are used to diagnose HIV infection and to monitor the disease process (Saville *et al.* 2001). Concerns have been raised related to the reliability of the enzyme linked immunosorbent assay (ELISA) blood test, used for first line screening for HIV, as other illnesses can produce a false positive test (Harrison & Corbett 1999), and newer tests continue to produce false positive results (Weber *et al.* 2002a). Other limitations of the antibody tests include absence of antibody in the early stages of seroconversion and changing levels of virus which may be missed by the antigen tests (Saville *et al.* 2001). The Department of Health and Social Security (DHSS 1996a) recommended that patients should not be tested for HIV antibodies without their consent, and that counselling should be offered to the patient before and after the test. During this counselling the patient should be informed about how HIV is transmitted and the significance of a negative and positive test. In 1996 further Department of Health guidelines provided a framework for counselling as there was a lack of consistency in the content of pre-test counselling. Hospitals involved in anonymous HIV antibody screening must ensure that patients are aware of the ongoing research project. No post-test counselling is possible in these circumstances.

The major disadvantage of diagnosis based on serology is the window period before immunoglobulin G (IgG) antibodies are produced in response to the HIV infection. Earlier diagnosis can be obtained by the use of IgM antibody screening. The presence of IgM indicates recent infection, which will help narrow the window period. Diagnosis can also be aided by the use of the HIV p24 antigen assay (Saville *et al.* 2001). p24 antigen is present in serum samples prior to and following seroconversion, when the antibody screening test is negative or indeterminate (Weber *et al.* 1998). p24 antigen tests can be used for diagnosis of HIV from the time of seroconversion until late stages of disease (Hashida *et al.* 1996). Viral load in peripheral blood can be measured and used for diagnostic, prognostic and monitoring of antiviral therapy purposes (Erb & Matter 1998).

Early diagnosis of HIV infection is important as it can improve patient outcomes by providing the patient with early treatment and care. An additional benefit is that if a person knows that they are HIV antibody positive, they can take steps to reduce transmission of HIV to others (Suarez *et al.* 2001).

Transmission

HIV has been isolated in the blood, semen, tears and saliva, breast milk, genital secretions of women, cerebrospinal fluid and the brain.

Currently in the UK HIV appears to affect younger adults, with 76% aged 15–39 years at diagnosis. During 2001, HIV was found to be predominantly transmitted by sex between men and women (55%), closely followed by sex between men (32%), less commonly by injecting drug misuse (2%), mother to infant (2%), blood products (rare), blood/tissue transfer (rare) and other undetermined routes (8%) (Communicable Disease Surveillance Centre 2002). Whilst transmission of HIV by blood and blood products is rare and HIV is known to have been transmitted via a platelet donation; in this case the donor was HIV antibody negative at the time of donation but was later found to be HIV antigen positive (Kopko *et al.* 2001). A similar incident occurred where three recipients received blood products from a donor who at the time of donation tested HIV negative, but who since has tested HIV positive (Martlew *et al.* 2000). Whilst the risk of transfusion infection in the UK is very small (Regan *et al.* 2000), initiatives such as donor deferrals for at-risk behaviours and the introduction of more sensitive viral screening assays should reduce the risk of blood and blood product transmission of HIV even further (Strong & Katz 2002).

A resurgence of risky sexual behaviours is causing concern as complacency related to HIV prevention appears to exist (Nicholl & Harmer 2002). Educational interventions to promote safer sex amongst gay man led to an increased uptake of hepatitis B vaccine and HIV testing but no significant decrease in unsafe sex (Flowers *et al.* 2002), with unsafe sex more likely to occur following the use of marijuana or inhaled nitrites (Clutterbuck *et al.* 2001). The first national strategy for sexual health and HIV in England has been produced, to deal with the increasing public health problem of HIV (Adler *et al.* 2002). Postexposure prophylaxis, which is available following unprotected sex with a known HIV partner, has increased (Giele *et al.* 2002). Partner notification of HIV exposure has also been seen to be effective and useful for early diagnosis of HIV infection (Mir *et al.* 2001).

Worldwide there have been two reports of possible transmission of HIV from infected health care workers to patients during exposure-prone procedures (EPP). All health care workers have an ethical and legal responsibility to protect the health and safety of their patients. All health care workers who believe they may have been exposed to HIV have to seek and follow confidential professional advice. Those known to be HIV positive are not to undertake EPP. If it is thought that any EPP have been performed by an HIV-positive person, the Consultant in Communicable Diseases has to be informed. An appraisal of the EPP will be made and if necessary, a decision about whether a patient notification of exposure to HIV needs to be taken. This process is included in the Department of Health guidance for HIV-infected health care workers (DoH 2002a).

World-wide there are up to 300 reports (102 confirmed) of occupational transmission of HIV to health care workers (McCarthy *et al.* 2002). The risk of surgeons acquiring HIV occupationally during EPP has been estimated as 1 in 2 000 000 to 1 in 200 000 depending on the surgery. This would be reduced to 1 in 10 000 000 and 1 in 1 000 000 if postexposure prophylaxis was given (Goldberg *et al.* 2000).

The use of antiretroviral drugs for postexposure prophylaxis needs to be fully explained to all health care workers exposed to blood and body fluids to ensure they respond quickly and correctly following such exposure (Scoular *et al.* 2000).

It is expected that heat treatment of blood products, and increased risk awareness through donation and donor screening, will virtually eliminate new infections through blood products transfusion and transplantation (Mortimer & Spooner 1997). These factors, coupled with more conservative use of blood, should result in a decrease in the transmission of HIV infection by blood transfusion (Lackritz 1998). However, debate continues with regard to the value of including viral antigen tests in the screening tests applied to all blood donations (Korelitz *et al.* 1996).

Unusual HIV transmissions have occurred, for example by fighting, removal of bleeding bodies from railway lines and deliberate self-inoculation with known HIV-positive blood (Gilbert *et al.* 1998). However, studies of prolonged social contact with HIV infection have failed to show that transmission has occurred, unless the transmission routes already mentioned are present (Jason *et al.* 1986). There have been exceptions to this, including from a child to a mother who was providing health care (Centers for Disease Control 1986), and transmission between children living in the same house (Centers for Disease Control 1993).

HIV is not a notifiable disease, although partner notification is encouraged. Most patients do co-operate in notifying some of their sex partners, who are generally receptive to being notified although they are often unaware of the HIV risks; these sex partners are often found to have high rates of HIV infection (West & Stark 1997).

Women and children

Studies on the transmission of HIV infection in Britain found that risk factors for HIV were:

1 Women heterosexually infected:
   • resident in London
   • widowhood
   • being a young black woman.
2 Women who shared needles:
   • resident in London or Scotland
   • large number of sexual partners
   • termination of pregnancy.

These differences need to be considered when prevention and control policies are being planned (Boisson & Rodrigues 2002).

Most antenatal units offer HIV testing to all women, and most HIV units offer antiretroviral therapy in pregnancy (Brook *et al.* 2000). Antiretroviral therapy generally involves the use of zidovudine prior to and during birth and then to the neonate for 6 weeks. In developed countries this should be given in conjunction with caesarean section delivery and no breast feeding (Bhana *et al.* 2002). Babies born of mothers with advanced disease have a poorer prognosis and failure to thrive is a significant clinical sign (Chearskul *et al.* 2002).

Perinatal transmission of HIV from mother to foetus can occur during intrauterine, intrapartum and postpartum periods. During the postpartum period it is mainly through breast feeding, as HIV has been found in both colostrum and breast milk, which internationally accounts for one third to one half of all transmissions from mother to child (Fowler & Newell 2002). The risk of the transmission of HIV via breast milk has to be balanced against the effect of early weaning on infant mortality, morbidity and maternal fertility (Pronczuk *et al.* 2002). The incidence of vertical transmission varies in different continents and is more likely to occur in

Africa (Kotler 1998). Risk factors for transmission include: obstetric risk factors; long duration of ruptured membranes; factors such as bleeding during pregnancy and amniocentesis; maternal drug use during pregnancy; and the presence of sexually transmitted diseases (Nourse & Butler 1998). High viral load is also associated with premature delivery (O'Shea *et al.* 1998). These research findings can be used to reduce the risk of transmission for infants born of HIV 1 infected women (Goedert *et al.* 1991).

The emphasis for the management and care of children with HIV is on prevention, early recognition and treatment (Sharland *et al.* 1997), with the advances in and the use of antiretroviral therapy being beneficial in slowing the progression of HIV disease (Doerholt *et al.* 2002).

AZT, given during pregnancy, has been seen to decrease vertical transmission of HIV (Brocklehurst & Volmink 2002). No problems have been identified from AZT taken during pregnancy (Sperling *et al.* 1998).

Clinical presentation

Following HIV infection a period occurs during which an HIV antibody test will be negative. Following seroconversion and the production of HIV antibodies, the test will be positive and the incubation period begins. The progression to AIDS disease will occur following an increase in plasma viral load and a fall in the CD4 count. These are factors which will determine when treatment should be started (Weller & Williams 2001).

It is clear that an AIDS diagnosis increases mortality significantly (Stover & Way 1998). Prognostic factors can be used to predict survival times of people with advanced disease (Chene *et al.* 1997). Those patients with good performance status will have a longer survival rate (Apolonio *et al.* 1995), while those patients with low body weight and neurological manifestations will have a reduced survival rate (Gerard *et al.* 1996).

Treatment

Combination antiretroviral therapies have considerably improved survival and quality of life of HIV-positive persons (Rogers *et al.* 2000). This improvement has led to the patients having fewer opportunistic infections, fewer hospital admissions and a reduction in mother-to-baby transmission of HIV. Most of these drugs have the added advantage of penetrating the CSF (Wynn *et al.* 2002). However, there are a number of disadvantages, including short- and long-term side-effects, lifelong commitment to treatment, food and diet restrictions and pill burden, all of which are difficult to incorporate

into the patient's lifestyle and are constant reminders of illness and confidentiality issues.

Drug-resistant strains of HIV have now developed (Velasco-Hernandez *et al.* 2002). In the USA it has been estimated that 1–11% of newly infected persons have a drug-resistant strain of HIV (Little *et al.* 2002). To reduce the risk of resistance, monotherapy is rare and treatment with three or even four drugs is common, including nucleoside/nucleotide analogues, nonnucleoside reverse transcriptase inhibitors and protease inhibitors (Pillay 1998). New drugs may soon be available for patients with HIV who have become resistant to existing treatments (Vass 2002).

Antiretroviral therapy has dramatically reduced the number of common opportunistic infections associated with HIV (Samuel *et al.* 2002), Kaposi's sarcoma (Ives *et al.* 2001) and cervical cancer (Robinson & Freeman 2002). Improvements have also occurred in diagnosis, prevention and treatment of infections (Kaplan *et al.* 2002).

The decision on which drugs to choose and when to commence treatment depends not only on the patient's clinical picture but also on their lifestyle and when they feel ready (Johnson 2002). In some cases, for example in injecting drug users, antiretroviral therapy is provided at the same time as directly observed methadone maintenance therapy (Clarke *et al.* 2002).

A survey of HIV clinics in the London area found that most units provided dose-dispensing boxes and alarms arranging early follow-up and continuing support to encourage compliance with drug regimens, although lack of motivation, high drug burden and drug side-effects led to suboptimal adherence (Brook *et al.* 2001).

Approximately a third of HIV-positive people in the world also have tuberculosis; 70% of these live in sub-Saharan Africa (Colebunder & Lambert 2002). Treatment involves conventional drugs for extended periods of time. Drug-resistant tuberculosis is on the increase, is more difficult to treat and the few alternative drugs available are less effective and more often associated with side-effects than standard drug regimens (DoH 1998b).

HIV-related cancer remains a significant problem (Boshoff & Weiss 2002), in particular Kaposi's sarcoma, non-Hodgkin's lymphoma and cervical cancer (Spano *et al.* 2002). One study found that antiretroviral therapy increased the survival of non-Hodgkin's lymphoma (Baiocchi *et al.* 2002). Radiotherapy has been seen to moderately improve the prognosis of HIV-related primary cerebral lymphoma (Khoo *et al.* 2000), although only about 10% of patients survive beyond 1 year (Sparano 2001). Kaposi's sarcoma remains the most common HIV tumour but fortunately antiretroviral regimens decrease the incidence of new Kaposi's sarcoma and the size of existing lesions (Dezube 2002).

Vaccine

Containment of HIV will require an effective vaccine (Ho & Huang 2002). Such a vaccine will need to be preventive to protect HIV-negative people and therapeutic to reduce infectivity in those already found to be HIV positive. Considerable effort is now being focused on evaluating different approaches in developing a vaccine (Baltimore & Heilman 1998). Unfortunately the genetic variability of HIV will make the development of a vaccine difficult. There is a need to discover aspects of the virus that are consistent enough for a vaccine to produce an effective immune response against multiple variants of HIV (WHO 2002a). Vaccine formation will need to take into consideration the special needs and problems of the developing world (Smith *et al.* 1998a), since lack of resources and the ability to vaccinate large numbers of people in developing countries create particular difficulties.

It is thought that a single vaccine is unlikely to achieve all of this (Van der Ryst 2002). Recent animal and human experiments highlight the difficulty in producing an effective HIV vaccine (McMicheal *et al.* 2002; Alving 2002).

Confidentiality

HIV/AIDS raises many ethical issues (Gruskin & Tarantola 2001). Confidentiality related to testing, treatment and care is essential. Persons with HIV have raised confidentiality as one of five main concerns and prefer to receive care at a genitourinary medicine clinic which provides a strict confidentiality service (Petchey *et al.* 2000). A UK investigation of primary care policies and procedures related to confidentiality found that a review of practices needed to be undertaken (Petchey *et al.* 2001).

Psychological support

Anxiety is a universal problem for people with AIDS (Phillips & Morrow 1998). Katz's (1997) study explored the feelings of HIV-positive people and highlighted the enormous stress of an HIV diagnosis. The study found that disclosure to family and friends was considered traumatic, although family members generally overcame these feelings and provided valuable help and support. This suggested that the initial emotional distress at the time of disclosure was worthwhile. Depression is not an inevitable consequence of HIV disease, being neither

common nor expectable (Rabkin 1997), and feelings of unhappiness, anger, grief or diminished future expectations are often accompanied by or intermingled with positive emotions and a fighting spirit. AIDS counsellors have been identified as the main source of psychosocial help for people with HIV/AIDS (Burnard 1992).

Counselling should include: pre- and post-test counselling, importance of risky behaviour reduction, natural history of HIV disease, family and relationships, and bereavement discussions. Telephone hotlines, outreach contacts and crisis intervention should also be provided. Crisis intervention should include a structured support programme and support groups (Chippindale & French 2001).

HIV palliative care offers disease-specific therapy and comfort with symptom-oriented treatment throughout the clinical course of the disease, not just at the end of life. Issues such as treatment choices and resuscitation need to be discussed early and whenever physical status changes.

Infection control

There is a legal requirement for employers under the general duties of the Health and Safety at Work etc. Act 1975, Management of Health and Safety at Work Regulations 1992 and the Control of Substances Hazardous to Health Regulations 1999 to safeguard employees and others against occupational risk. This includes risk posed by blood-borne infection (Wilcox 1997). Strategies must be in place to reduce the incidence of exposure to HIV (McKee 1996). The risk of HIV infection in health care workers can be reduced by strict adherence to universal precautions (Reyes & Legg 1997). Employees have a responsibility to adopt universal precautions for all patients (Ward *et al.* 1997). Factors such as fatigue, stress, levels of training, skill and experience affect safe practices. If nurses are willing to care for infected patients they are entitled to the safest environment that can reasonably be created (Hanrahan & Reutter 1997).

HIV infection alone does not affect a person's ability to continue with regular employment (Department of Employment – Health and Safety Executive 1987), unless injury to the worker could result in blood contaminating a patient's open tissues (DoH 1991).

The risk of acquiring HIV infection following a needlestick injury is 3 per 1000 injuries. The risk of acquiring HIV through mucous membrane exposure is even less at 1 in 1000 (DoH 1997). As many as 300 reports of occupationally acquired HIV infection in the world have been received (Public Health Laboratory Service AIDS and STD Centre 1997). In the UK, to June

1997, four people were known to have developed HIV following a documented accident, with eight others who may have occupationally acquired HIV (Local Collaborators 1998). The Chief Medical Officer's Expert Advisory Group on AIDS advises that postexposure prophylaxis is offered following exposure to a patient known or strongly suspected to be infected with HIV; accidents leading to exposure include percutaneous injury, contamination of broken skin and exposure of mucous membrane including the eye (DoH 1997).

Concerns have been raised related to the possibility of drug-resistant HIV being transmitted to health care workers who have received a significant inoculation accident (Veenstra *et al.* 1995), to sexual partners (Carlon *et al.* 1994) or by vertical transmission (Frenkel *et al.* 1995).

The risk of patients acquiring HIV from HIV-positive health care workers is low. Patients may be at risk by inadequate infection control practices, an example being child transmission through exposure to HIV-positive needles in a sharps bin (Public Health Laboratory Service AIDS and STD Centre 1997). Postexposure to HIV prophylaxis is now available following high-risk unprotected anal or vaginal intercourse (Katz & Gerberding 1997).

In 2001 the first successful prosecution for the sexual transmission of HIV occurred in the UK, when a man was convicted of recklessly injuring his former girlfriend by infecting her with HIV (Chalmers 2002).

Nursing care

Nursing problems associated with HIV include pain, confusion, depression, anxiety, fatigue, fever, dyspnoea, nausea and vomiting, diarrhoea, wasting and dehydration (Kemp & Stepp 1995). Nutrition is a significant issue; early detection and intervention can decrease problems (Davidhizar & Dunn 1998). Good care is essential for persons with HIV/AIDS, although surveys have indicated that patients are not universally satisfied with the care they are receiving (Jones *et al.* 2002). A recent study found that health care workers' knowledge related to the care of HIV antibody-positive patients was good but further education, training and support were identified as necessary (Duffy & Moore 2000).

The Public Health (Infectious Diseases) Regulations (1985) make certain provisions to safeguard public health related to a person with AIDS. It is stressed that these provisions are to be used only in exceptional circumstances where transmission of HIV may occur. One study has indicated that HIV remains viable for a considerable time in a cadaver. It is important, therefore, that careful procedures to avoid contamination are

maintained after the death of an infected person (Ball *et al.* 1991).

Prevention of HAI relies on the availability of resources for cleaning and, where necessary, sterilization of both equipment and the environment. Patients' accommodation can be vacuum cleaned and washed with hot soapy water (Ayliffe *et al.* 2000), unless contamination with blood or body fluids has occurred. In these circumstances, the statutory regulations require cleaning with fresh hypochlorite solution or granules (Health and Safety Commission 1999). When non-disposable equipment is used, autoclaving is the method of choice for sterilization. Equipment likely to be damaged by autoclaving can be disinfected (Ayliffe *et al.* 2000).

Nurses must keep up to date with improved, earlier diagnosis of AIDS with better treatments and the increased use of prophylaxis. They must be ready to adapt to these changes and be prepared and able to provide good care. This process will be achieved only by good education (Hall & Sutton 2002) and management support.

Human immunodeficiency virus 2 (HIV 2)

Definition

HIV 2 is closely related to HIV 1 but is antigenically distinct and demonstrates distinct replication and cytopathic characteristics (Albert *et al.* 1990).

Reference material

HIV 2 was first recognized in 1986 (Clavel *et al.* 1986), although evidence existed that HIV 2 infections were present in many West Africans as far back as 1966 (Karamura *et al.* 1989). Serological evidence supporting the existence of a second HIV was published in 1985 (Barin *et al.* 1985).

A more recent retrospective study of sera in West Africa proves that HIV 2 was circulating in West Africa at the beginning of the 1980s (Piedade *et al.* 2000). HIV 2 infections are predominantly found in Africa (CDC 2002). Current studies show low levels of HIV 2 infection in Thailand (Chanbancherd *et al.* 2000) and India (Solomon *et al.* 1998). High levels have been found in Nigeria (Esu-Williams *et al.* 1997) which are increasing (Odaibo *et al.* 1998), with some patients being infected with both HIV 1 and HIV 2 (Schim Van der Loeff *et al.* 2002). Infection with HIV 2 does not protect against HIV 1 (Van der Loeff *et al.* 2001).

HIV 2 appears less virulent than HIV 1 possibly due to the lower levels of HIV 2 virus compared to HIV 1 (Berry *et al.* 1998). An early study suggested that mortality in HIV 2-infected African adults was only twice as high as that in uninfected African adults (Poulsen *et al.* 1997).

In the UK, screening of blood donors and people attending genitourinary medicine clinics shows that the occurrence of HIV 2 infection is rare.

Transmission of HIV 2 follows the same pattern as HIV 1 (CDC 2002), although the rate of vertical transmission from mother to child is uncertain. HIV 2 seems to be less transmissible from an infected mother to her child (CDC 2002), with high maternal plasma viral load a risk factor for maternal transmission of HIV 2 (O'Donovan *et al.* 2000). More children born to HIV 1-infected mothers died in comparison with those born to HIV 2-infected mothers. This was said to be due to the higher viral load amongst the HIV 1-infected mothers (Ota *et al.* 2000).

Studies have shown that HIV 2-infected patients with CD4 cell counts of 500 cells/μl and greater had a significantly lower mortality rate than patients with a similar count who were infected with HIV 1 (Schim Van der Loeff *et al.* 2002). However, a high HIV 2 viral load indicates disease progression (Ariyoshi *et al.* 2000). Generally a low and stable level of HIV 2 characterizes

HIV 2 infection in West African communities (Berry *et al.* 2002).

There are differences in clinical manifestation observed in AIDS patients infected with HIV 2 and HIV 1, with chronic diarrhoea and diarrhoea caused by bacterial infections more common in HIV 2-infected persons (Ndour *et al.* 2000). There are also fewer cases of Kaposi's sarcoma seen in patients infected with HIV 2 (Ariyoshi *et al.* 1998).

Little is known about the best approach to the clinical treatment and care of patients with HIV 2. This is due to the slower development and the limited clinical experience with HIV 2 (CDC 2002).

In May 1989 the AIDS laboratory diagnostic working group advised combined screening in diagnostic laboratories in the UK (Evans *et al.* 1991). In July 1990, combined anti-HIV 1/HIV 2 testing of all donations of blood was introduced in the UK Blood Transfusion Service. Of the first 250 000 donations, only one HIV 2 infected donor was detected.

Since there is no difference in the method of transmission and symptoms between HIV 1 and HIV 2, prevention and nursing care are the same.

Procedure guidelines: **Acquired immune deficiency syndrome in a general ward**

Procedure

Action	Rationale
1 All staff should read and be familiar with government guidelines on AIDS and their own hospital's codes of practice.	To ensure all staff are aware of, and take, the necessary precautions.
2 Hospital staff should cover any broken skin with a waterproof dressing.	To prevent the entry of infectious material.
3 Immunocompromised staff, either through illness or therapy, should not nurse patients who are HIV antibody positive.	HIV antibody positive patients who present with generalized infection could put this category of staff at risk.
4 Staff suffering from eczema should not nurse patients who are HIV antibody positive.	Any break in staff members' skin should be covered with a waterproof dressing to prevent entry of HIV. This would be difficult to accomplish with eczema lesions and would exacerbate the eczema.
5 Accidental inoculations must be avoided at all cost.	Serious inoculation accidents have been seen to be a means of transmission of HIV.
6 In the event of gross contamination of intact skin the affected area must be washed thoroughly with soap under warm water. A scrubbing brush must not be used.	Intact skin is a natural barrier against infection. By thorough washing the infectious material can be removed. Scrubbing brushes can cause skin damage which allows infection to enter.
7 Puncture wounds or cuts must be made to bleed freely and washed under hot running water.	To flush out infectious material.
8 A waterproof dressing must be applied and medical advice sought for large wounds.	To prevent further infection to the wound.

*Procedure guidelines: **Acquired immune deficiency syndrome in a general ward** (cont'd)*

Action	Rationale
9 An accident form must be completed immediately and taken to bacteriology, the occupational health physician or other medical advisor as appropriate.	It is important to have accurate records of all accidents and incidents in order to monitor events.
10 HIV postexposure prophylaxis should be considered for all significant exposure to HIV.	HIV postexposure prophylaxis antiviral therapy has been shown to prevent seroconversion following significant exposure to HIV (DoH 1997).

Low-risk, HIV-positive individuals (i.e. patients who are not bleeding, incontinent, confused or infected with a contagious disease)

Nursing assessment of the risk of contamination of the environment with pathogenic organisms, blood or body fluids from a patient known to be HIV antibody positive allows care to be more accurately planned.

Action	Rationale
1 If the patient is not bleeding, incontinent, confused or infected with a contagious disease, he/she is considered to be of low risk of transmitting infection to others and can be nursed on an open ward using all the patients' facilities as normal.	HIV cannot be transmitted by social contact that occurs in hospital wards.
2 If a low-risk, HIV-positive individual develops an infection, is undergoing invasive procedures or becomes incontinent nursing care will commence as for high-risk, HIV-positive persons.	Incontinent, bleeding HIV antibody-positive patients have the potential risk of transmitting the HIV virus to others.

Increased risk, HIV-positive individuals

Action	Rationale
1 Known or strongly suspected HIV antibody-positive patients who are bleeding, incontient, infected with a contagious disease or receiving invasive procedures should be nursed in a single room with its own toilet and hand-washing facilities.	To minimize the risk of transmitting infection. HIV can be transmitted via blood and body fluid.

Entering the room

Action	Rationale
1 When the patient is not bleeding, coughing, incontinent or receiving procedures, protective clothing is not required.	Transmission of HIV is not possible from general contact in the absence of blood and blood-stained body fluids.
2 When the patient is incontinent, bleeding or undergoing invasive procedures, disposable well-fitting gloves and a plastic apron are needed.	Transmission of HIV is possible from body fluids.
3 If there is a possibility of airborne contamination, a correctly fitting mask and safety spectacles should be worn.	Transmission of HIV is possible if contaminated material is allowed to contaminate mucous membranes.

Liquid waste

Action	Rationale
1 All liquid waste from HIV-positive patients must be disposed of in a bedpan washer immediately, taking care to avoid splashing.	To prevent contamination of the environment.
2 Areas without bedpan washers will need to use the slop hopper. Great care must be taken to pour waste slowly and carefully down the hopper to avoid splashing.	To prevent contamination of the environment.

colonization. The researchers concluded that surveillance results may indicate when prompt treatment or more aggressive prophylaxis may be required (Richardson *et al.* 2000).

Clostridium difficile

Definition

Clostridium difficile is a slender, Gram-positive anaerobic rod which is spore forming and motile and is capable of surviving in the environment for prolonged periods (Cunha 1998). Bacteria of this type may be a normal component of gut flora and flourish when other gut organisms are eradicated by antibiotics (Zadik & Moore 1998).

Reference material

Clostridium difficile causes gastrointestinal infection ranging from symptomless colonization to severe diarrhoea, with toxin-producing strains causing pseudomembranous colitis (Spencer 1998). It is now one of the most commonly detected enteric pathogens and an important cause of nosocomial infection in nursing homes and hospitals (Zadik & Moore 1998) and a common cause of mortality and morbidity in hospitalized patients (Yousuf *et al.* 2002).

Diarrhoea can be caused by disruption of the normal flora of the gut by antibiotics which allow *C. difficile* to multiply. The colonic mucosa becomes covered with a characteristic fibrinous pseudomembrane. Signs and symptoms can be relatively mild, resolving when antibiotics are discontinued, or more severe, as in cases of pseudomembranous colitis (Szczesny *et al.* 2002) which may require surgical resection of parts of the colon and is associated with a significant mortality rate (Spencer 1998).

About 5% of healthy adults carry *C. difficile* in their faeces, usually in small numbers. The elderly are at particular risk and appear to develop more serious symptoms compared with younger patients (Melillo 1998). This causes considerable mortality and morbidity among elderly people, costing the Health Service millions of pounds each year (Brazier & Duerden 1998). During an outbreak in Ireland 9.6% of elderly patients died (Kyne *et al.* 1998). Infants are more likely to carry the organisms but are less likely to develop colitis (Fekety & Shah 1993).

Diagnosis

Diagnosis is based on clinical findings, endoscopy and laboratory evaluation. Clinical findings range from profuse, watery, green, foul smelling or bloody diarrhoea, with cramping abdominal pains, tenderness and high fever, to hypovolaemic shock and overwhelming sepsis. Endoscopy may reveal effects similar to those seen in non-specific colitis, or may show the yellow–white raised plaques which go on to form a membrane on the intestinal mucosa (Kofsky *et al.* 1991).

Laboratory diagnosis

Clostridium difficile is difficult to isolate in ordinary culture because of overgrowth by other organisms. To overcome this a selective culture medium is used. The presence of *C. difficile* in culture is not by itself an indication of infection, it simply marks the organism's presence. Infection or disease is indicated by the presence of toxins produced by the organism which can be identified using screening tests (Moyenuddin *et al.* 2002). Pathogenic strains of *C. difficile* produce two protein exotoxins, toxin A (enterotoxin) and toxin B (cytotoxin) (Brazier 1998). *Clostridium difficile* toxin A induces detachment of human epithelial cells from the basement membrane and subsequent death by apoptosis (Mahida *et al.* 1998). This process may be asymptomatic or cause mild diarrhoea or it can lead to pseudomembranous colitis (Kelly & LaMont 1998). Recurrence is common (Do *et al.* 1998), ranging from 5 to 42% of patients (Zimmerman *et al.* 1997).

Typing of *Clostridium difficile* isolates allows for investigation of outbreaks of infection (Brazier 1998).

Treatment

Initial treatment involves discontinuing antibiotics and providing supportive care (Spencer 1998). However, significant infection can be treated with metronidazole or vancomycin (Moyenuddin *et al.* 2002). In extreme cases of pseudomembranous colitis surgery will be required, which may include resectional or diversion procedures (Viswanath & Griffiths 1998), but death can occur even when diagnosis is made early and appropriate therapy is given (Kavan *et al.* 1998). Patients susceptible to *C. difficile* reinfection need to be protected from exposure until their bowel flora recovers (Barbut & Petit 2001).

Studies using probiotics, which are live organisms that improve the microbial balance of the host, are ongoing (D'Souza *et al.* 2002).

Transmission

Pseudomembranous colitis develops from overgrowth of *C. difficile* already present in the gut, or from exogenous organisms acquired via person-to-person contact or the faecal-oral route. *Clostridium difficile* leads to increased costs associated with increased length of hospital stay (Kyne *et al.* 2002), and outbreaks in hospital have resulted in the deaths of a number of elderly people (Duerden *et al.* 1994). Bignardi (1998) identified nine risk factors which appear to influence the chance of acquiring *C. difficile*; these were increasing age, severity of underlying disease, non-surgical gastrointestinal procedures, presence of nasogastric tube, antiulcer medication, stay in ITU, duration of hospital stay, duration of antibiotic therapy and administration of multiple antibiotics.

Antibiotic use was shown to be statistically significantly associated with both diarrhoea and carriage of *C. difficile*. Risks include type of antibiotic, route of administration and dose. Accurate identification of risk factors allows for appropriate decisions to be made to reduce risk and thereby reduce incidence. High-risk patients can be monitored closely to facilitate early detection of infection, commencement of treatment and infection control precautions.

Prevention of spread and management of infection

Reducing the risk of an outbreak of *C. difficile* relies on restriction of the use of those antibiotics associated with the highest risk (Aziz *et al.* 2001), reducing the duration of antibiotic courses and the length of stay in hospital (Bignardi 1998). Prevention of epidemics relies on careful hand washing (Worsley 1998), environmental decontamination (Surawicz 1998) and isolation of symptomatic patients (Wilcox *et al.* 1998). Cross-infection has been seen to be reduced by thorough cleaning of the environment and the use of clean equipment for each patient (Worsley 1998). For example, the use of tympanic thermometers instead of oral and rectal thermometers appears to reduce the incidence of *C. difficile* (Brooks *et al.* 1998). Johnson *et al.* (1990) demonstrated a decrease in the incidence of infection following the introduction of gloves for staff in contact with patients infected with *C. difficile*. When an infected patient is discharged, the ward must be thoroughly cleaned before other patients are allowed into the area.

Nursing care

Careful barrier nursing is required for all patients with toxin-producing *C. difficile* or unexplained diarrhoea. Segregation from other patients must continue until stool cultures are clear of infectious organisms. Healthy staff and visitors who are not receiving antibiotics are not at risk (Sanderson 1999).

Cryptosporidiosis

Definition

Cryptosporidium is a protozoan coccidian parasite, first isolated in 1907. Human infection is usually caused by *Cryptosporidium parvum* (DoH 1990).

Reference material

Cryptosporidium species are a major cause of diarrhoea infections in both immunocompetent and immunosuppressed persons (Hunter & Nichols 2002) and can cause life-threatening infections in the latter (Chalmers & Elwin 2000), resulting in deaths (Willocks *et al.* 2000). However, in otherwise healthy persons usually only a self-limiting illness occurs (Holley & Thiers 1986).

Transmission

Cryptosporidium has a worldwide distribution (Mead 2002) and can infect livestock, particularly calves and lambs, whose faecal matter infects water supplies, which then can infect humans (Hunter & Syed 2002). Based on epidemiological evidence, consumption of certain foods (especially undercooked sausages, offal and unpasteurized milk) appears to be a risk factor (Casemore 1987). Infection can also occur following direct contact with animals (Fayer *et al.* 2001; Robinson & Pugh 2002) by hand-to-mouth route, and is easily transmitted from one person to another (Chalmers & Elwin 2000). This latter route is probably the main mode of transmission in urban populations. Only a small inoculum of organism appears to be required to cause infection.

Outbreaks of cryptosporidiosis traceable to swimming baths have been reported, which are difficult to control (Puech *et al.* 2001). Prevention relies on the efficacy of cleaning, filtration and disinfection procedures (Fournier *et al.* 2002).

Cryptosporidium is unaffected by chlorine in the concentrations that can be used in the treatment of drinking water, and is inactivated only by being frozen or heated to temperatures of 65–85°C for 5–10 minutes or by exposure to boiling water. Prevention relies on compliance with safe practices by water companies and health authorities in water treatment processes.

Routine water disinfection by chlorination is ineffective in controlling the organism except in small numbers. Therefore all domestic water supplies are filtered to remove harmful pathogens. As 30% of all public water supplies in England and Wales comes from ground water, contamination of the water supply generally occurs when heavy rains follow drought (Peeters *et al.* 1989), causing leakage of effluent or slurry into treated water. The public water supplies in the UK are generally of a very high standard (Casemore 1998), with outbreaks of cryptosporidiosis due to contamination of mains tap water in the UK being uncommon, although outbreaks can occur (Hunter & Syed 2002). Infection can also be acquired from ice cubes and contaminated drinking water, eating food that has been cleaned and inadequately cooked in contaminated water and from milk (Ravin *et al.* 1991).

The time from ingestion of oocysts to the development of symptoms can range from 5 to 28 days (Ungar 1995). *Cryptosporidium* infection in the immunocompetent person generally causes a self-limiting gastroenteritis. Symptoms include watery stools, vomiting and weight loss (Casemore *et al.* 1994), fever, nausea, vomiting and weakness (Ungar 1995). Recovery involves an intact humoral and cellular immune response. Excretion of oocysts can continue after symptoms have ceased (Ungar 1995). During an outbreak involving water in 1991, 85 immunocompetent cases were involved, 10% of the cases required hospital admission and symptoms lasted an average of 13 days (Aston *et al.* 1991). For severely immunocompromised patients, particularly those with AIDS and bone marrow transplant recipients, infection is protracted, severe and sometimes life threatening (Gardner 1994). Severity reflects the level of immunosuppression (Petersen 1992). Symptoms include a debilitating cholera-like diarrhoea and vomiting which, when found in terminal AIDS patients, is particularly distressing. Remission and relapse of cryptosporidiosis probably reflect fluctuation in immune status (Casemore *et al.* 1994).

Respiratory tract involvement has been caused either through aspiration of oocysts during vomiting or through haematogenous spread. Coughing can result in aerosol transmission of oocysts to others. Rare presentations include cholecystitis, hepatitis, pancreatitis and reactive arthritis (Ungar 1995).

Prevention

Immunocompetent people who swim in or drink water may be regularly exposed to infection, and may have higher levels of immunity to infection. The Third Report of the Group of Experts on *Cryptosporidium* in Water Supplies (1998) states that there is a strong correlation between outbreaks of infection and inadequacy in the treatment of water supplies or where there is overloading of the treatment process. This group and others recommend that immunocompromised persons should:

1 Boil or filter all tap and bottled water used for drinking.
2 Avoid contact with infected animals and people (Heathcock *et al.* 1998).

3 Avoid contaminated water during recreational activities (Kramer *et al.* 1998).
4 Avoid uncooked food that may have been washed in contaminated water.
5 Avoid exposure to young farm animals and pets, and avoid acquiring new young pets, as young animals are particularly susceptible to crytosporidiosis (Current 1987).
6 Filter domestic water supplies. Currently water companies regularly monitor water supplies; increased continuous sampling is being considered (Casemore 1998). If contamination occurs users are informed and told to boil all drinking water; supplies are not turned off as water is needed for flushing toilets and fighting fires, etc. Unfortunately, during outbreak situations when all drinking water has to be boiled, compliance is often poor (Willocks *et al.* 2000).
7 Refrain from swimming whilst immunosuppressed.

Diagnosis

Microbiological testing of stools, using conventional staining microscopy and molecular techniques, provides a diagnosis as well as epidemiology data in outbreak situations (Chalmers & Elwin 2000; Bialek *et al.* 2002).

Treatment

The host immune response prevents initial infection and facilitates clearance of infection; prolonged infection is seen in immunocompromised persons. There is no reliable curative treatment for cryptosporidiosis (Mead 2002).

Nursing care

Oocysts are shed in large numbers during infection and only a small number of oocysts are required to cause infection. Strict barrier nursing is required while diarrhoea persists, with segregation from other patients continuing until clear specimens of stool cultures are obtained.

Special attention to hand washing is essential. Nurses were found to develop infection from a very ill, demented patient who had severe diarrhoea and vomiting. In this instance infection control practices were good, however it was thought that cross-infection occurred by both the faecal–oral and aerosol routes (O'Mohony *et al.* 1992). Any sign of cross-infection must be pursued vigorously to prevent further spread. This will include close co-operation with health and local authorities, with the appropriate water companies and between the outbreak control team and the authority.

Hepatitis

Hepatitis may be caused by a variety of agents including viruses and certain chemicals, and it may be secondary to other illnesses. Nurses need to be aware of the epidemiology, modes of transmission and prevention of hepatitis.

Hepatitis A

Definition

Hepatitis A virus (HAV) is an enterically transmitted positive strand RNA virus classified as a hepavirus, a member of the Picornaviridae family, which causes an acute, self-limiting infection of the liver (Gunn 2002).

Reference material

HAV is a small, symmetrical RNA virus (enterovirus type 72) (Melnick 1982). The virus is unusually stable, resisting heat at 60°C for 1 hour, at 25°C for 3 months, indefinite cold storage (5°C), acidic conditions (pH 3) and non-ionic detergents (Siegl *et al.* 1984; Sorbey *et al.* 1988). It can survive for several months in sewage and the environment. However, HAV can be inactivated after 4 minutes at 70°C, after 5 seconds at 80°C and instantly at 85°C (Battegay *et al.* 1995).

HAV is spread predominantly by the faecal–oral route. Following infection, the virus enters the bloodstream from unknown sites in the gastrointestinal tract. It can then infect liver cells when passing via the biliary tract to the intestine and into the faeces (Gunn 2002). Viral replication probably occurs in the jejunum before transmission via the portal vein to the liver (Siegl 1988). HAV has been associated with the following:

- Contaminated water, milk and food. Any uncooked food and drink could be responsible for infection. However, particular problems are due to contamination at the time of harvesting and packaging of uncooked frozen foods which are then thawed and used (Ramsey *et al.* 1989). Large outbreaks of hepatitis A can be due to contamination of uncooked or cooked food (Kingsley *et al.* 2002), by one infected food handler or infected food source (Koopmans *et al.* 2002).
- Poor general hygiene and low economic status (Pebody *et al.* 1998), contact with children in day centres (Hanna *et al.* 2001) and intensive care units (Hanna *et al.* 1996). Outbreaks of HVA at school were associated with lack of toilet paper, soap and hand towels (Rajaratnam *et al.* 1992) and poor hygiene in school toilets (Leoni *et al.* 1998).

- Foreign travel to countries where HAV is endemic (Colak *et al.* 2002; Vaidya *et al.* 2002).
- Blood transfusions (Kocazeybek *et al.* 2002). Documented evidence that HAV has been transmitted by factor VIII concentrate (Soucie *et al.* 1998).
- Contact with a case of hepatitis A in the home (Maguire *et al.* 1995) or in hospital (Petrosillo 2002) due to breaches in infection control measures.
- Sexual contact. HAV can be reduced among homosexual men by HAV vaccination (Centers for Disease Control 1998).
- Perinatal transmission of hepatitis A is extremely uncommon (Duff 1998a), although an instance of an infant being infected by his mother before or during birth has been reported (Renge *et al.* 2002).
- Intravenous drug misusers. Needle-sharing practices contribute to the spread of HAV (O'Donovan *et al.* 2001).

The incidence of hepatitis A infection in England and Wales has fallen (Morris *et al.* 2002).

Following ingestion of hepatitis A virus, multiplication occurs as the virus moves through the stomach, small intestine and large intestine. The virus eventually reaches the liver after leaving the alimentary system via the blood. Further replication occurs in the liver before being released into bile (Cuthbert 2001).

Diagnosis of acute HAV infection is usually confirmed serologically, by detecting immunoglobulin M (IgM) antibodies to HA antigen (Ag) which appear in serum 2–7 weeks after oral inoculation, and may persist for some time, occasionally for more than a year. Evidence of past infection, and therefore immunity which can persist for life, is obtained by detecting serologically the presence of IgG antibody to HAAg. HAV can be detected by a variety of immunological and molecular techniques including blood and stool (Cuthbert 2001), urine (Joshi *et al.* 2002) and saliva (Ang 2000).

HAV has an incubation period of 2–7 weeks. HAAg can be detected in stools early in the course of illness (DoH 1996). HAAg levels decline rapidly with the onset of symptoms but can remain detectable for up to 2 weeks after the onset of clinical hepatitis (Ciocca 2000).

HAV usually causes a minor illness in children and young adults, with as few as 5% of cases being symptomatic (Eddleston 1990). The illness often presents as an upper respiratory infection with the following signs and symptoms: anorexia, malaise, weight loss, pyrexia, diarrhoea and vomiting (Gunn 2002), dark urine and jaundice. Complications of HAV include cholestasis, prolonged or relapsing disease, extrahepatic disease and fulminant hepatitis (Battegay *et al.* 1995).

Control and prevention of HAV rely on provision of good sanitation facilities, clean drinking water and supervision of food handlers. Careful personal hygiene (Crowcroft *et al.* 2001) and the use of condoms (Brook 1998) will limit person-to-person spread. Passive immunization with intramuscular normal pooled immunoglobulin (HNIg) gives protection against clinical hepatitis for about 3 months in most people. Post-exposure prophylaxis is advisable for household contacts during outbreaks of HAV infection (DoH 1996c).

Hepatitis A vaccine is available and immunization has been seen to be effective (Werzberger *et al.* 1998). One dose provides protection for one year, a booster dose at 6–12 months provides immunity for up to 10 years. The vaccine should be administered to those travelling in developing countries (Dick 1998), in areas of moderate or high HAV endemicity, particularly where sanitation and food hygiene are poor, but it is not an alternative to preventive behaviours (Birthistle 1998). The Department of Health (1996c) has recommended that sewage workers, military personnel and foreign diplomats should be considered for vaccination. In institutions for the care of the mentally ill, and in children's centres where the children are not toilet trained, vaccination policy should be formulated according to local circumstances (DoH 1996c). However a study by Maguire *et al.* (1995) showed no clear evidence that health care workers are at increased occupational risk of acquiring hepatitis A. Response to hepatitis A vaccine takes about 12–15 days (Irwin & Millership 2001).

A combined hepatitis A and B vaccine is also available (Zuckerman 1998) which increases convenience and compliance and reduces costs whilst providing prolonged dual protection (Koff 2002). Human normal immunoglobulin (HNIG) offers short-term protection for up to 4 months and can be given to people who have been in close contact with infected cases and to those travelling to areas where the disease is endemic (DoH 1996c).

HAV infection does not generally require hospital treatment. Strict barrier nursing in a single room with en-suite toilet would be required (Pearse 1992). Two outbreaks of HVA among health care workers were attributed to inadequate hand washing and eating on the ward (Doebbeling *et al.* 1993; Hanna *et al.* 1996).

Procedure guidelines: **Hepatitis A**

Outpatient

Action	Rationale
1 It is not usually necessary to admit the individual to hospital.	Self-limiting disease.
2 Patient education is essential and must include advice on good personal hygiene and careful hand washing.	Limits the spread of the virus. Careful hand washing removes contamination from hands.
3 Separate soap, flannel and towel must be provided.	To minimize the risk of infection being spread via equipment used for hygiene purposes.
4 Meticulous cleaning of bath, wash basin and toilet with a cream cleaner and hot water.	To remove contamination.
5 Bath and wash basin must be allowed to dry after use.	Viruses will not survive on clean dry surfaces.
6 Soiled bed linen and underclothing should be washed.	To remove contamination.
7 Patient should refrain from intimate kissing and sexual intercourse while symptoms are present.	To reduce risk of cross-infection.
8 People with hepatitis A should avoid contact with susceptible people, i.e. very young or old or those with debilitating illness.	To reduce the likelihood of infection.
9 Crockery and cutlery must be washed and rinsed in hot water.	Heat destroys the virus.
10 Close contacts of the infected person should seek medical advice from their general practitioner.	To enable the GP to assess whether the contact person should receive human normal immunoglobulin (HNIG) prophylaxis.

Procedure guidelines: Hepatitis A (cont'd)

Inpatient

Action	Rationale
1 Whenever possible, the patient should have medical or surgical treatment postponed until he/she is symptom free.	Medical and surgical treatment will debilitate the patient further and recovery will be slower.
2 Ideally, the patient should be discharged.	Cross-infection is less likely to occur at home.
3 A single room with separate toilet should be made available for the patient, although barrier nursing is not necessary.	In general patients are no longer excreting the virus once they have become symptomatic, however there are always exceptions.
4 Blood, secretions and excreta (particularly faeces) must be disposed of immediately in a heat-disinfecting bedpan washer.	To prevent cross-infection.
5 Careful hand washing after patient contact.	To prevent cross-infection.

Hepatitis B

Definition

Hepatitis B is a serious infectious disease caused by the hepatitis B virus (HBV), which produces an inflammatory condition of the liver leading to acute and in some cases chronic infection (Hsu *et al.* 1995).

Reference material

HBV is a 42 nm double-shelled particle, inside which is a 27 nm inner core particle which contains the viral nucleic acid and represents the intact infectious virion (Lau & Wright 1993). HBV was termed initially 'Dane particle' after its discoverer (Dane *et al.* 1970).

Of the two billion people who have been infected with the HBV, more than 350 million have chronic lifelong infections.

Hepatitis B is one of the major diseases of humans and is a serious global public health problem. In sub-Saharan Africa and most of Asia and the Pacific as many as 8–10% of the general population are chronically infected with liver cancer caused by HBV, one of the three main causes of death from cancer in men. In the Middle East and Indian subcontinent about 5% are chronically infected. Infection is less common in Western Europe and North America where less than 1% of people are chronically infected (WHO 2000). It is not known how many people are infected with HBV in the UK. A study of drug users in Edinburgh and rural southeast England found that 44% and 20.4% respectively were HBV positive (Peat *et al.* 2000; Edeh & Spalding 2000), whilst in a small study of fit people attending a conception clinic in London, 1.4% of people were HBV positive (Hart *et al.* 2001). However, HBV is more common in persons living in the UK who were born in areas where HBV infection is endemic (Aweis *et al.* 2001). Outbreaks continue to occur in developing countries due to inadequate infection control policies (Singh *et al.* 1998). Prevention of HBV includes vaccination, prophylaxis and improved infection control and safer sex practices (Alexander 1998).

Epidemiology

HBV may be found in virtually all body secretions and excreta of patients with acute hepatitis B and carriers of the virus. Blood, semen and vaginal fluids are mainly implicated in the transmission of infection, which occurs by:

- Sexual transmission, both vaginal and anal
- Accidental inoculation of blood following, for example, a sharps injury, or by drug addicts sharing used needles and syringes
- Contamination of mucous membranes, eye, nose or mouth
- Contamination of non-intact skin
- Perinatal route at or about the time of birth
- Blood transfusion. Two studies investigating the risk of transfusion-acquired hepatitis B in the UK found that in 26 032 blood donations no evidence of hepatitis B infection was found (Howell *et al.* 2000; Regan *et al.* 2000). The risk of acquiring hepatitis B from a blood transfusion abroad would depend on the country. For example, 3.44% of blood donors in India were found to be hepatitis B positive (Garg *et al.*

2001) whilst a review of European donors suggests the risk is very low at 96 per 10 million red blood cell transfusions (Weusten *et al.* 2002).

HBV infection acquired during infancy and early childhood has a high likelihood of progressing to chronic infection, which can lead to chronic hepatitis, cirrhosis and primary hepatocellular carcinoma (Hsu *et al.* 2002). Vaccination would reduce this risk (Strine *et al.* 2002).

Clinical response

HBV infection is clinically extremely variable, with the incubation period varying from 4 weeks to as long as 6 months.

Symptoms of acute HBV infection include jaundice of skin and eyes, dark urine, fatigue, nausea, vomiting and abdominal pain. Recovery can take several months to a year. Chronic infection can predispose the infected person to develop cirrhosis or cancer of the liver. HBV reactivation can occur in patients following allogeneic bone marrow transplantation and has been reported as 20.5% of cases (Dhedin *et al.* 1998). Ter-Borg *et al.* (1998) suggest this is due to enhanced immunological responses to hepatocytes harbouring reactivated HBV.

Infectivity

The progress of HBV can be monitored by serological testing. HBsAg is detected in the blood approximately 3–4 weeks after exposure, with antibodies to hepatitis B core (HBc) antigen (HBcAg) developing about 2 weeks after HBsAg occurs. Anti-HBc will eventually be replaced by anti-HBs, the antibody to HBsAg, which marks the end of high infectivity and the development of immunity to subsequent HBV infection (Lau & Wright 1993). The antigen HBeAg is an internal component of the core of HBs and is an indicator of high infectivity; it will be replaced eventually by anti-HBe, which correlates with loss of viral replication (Tedder 1980). HBV is capable of surviving for at least 1 week in the environment (Trevelyan 1991).

Diagnosis

Diagnosis is confirmed by a virological blood test with regular monitoring of antigen and antibody status to evaluate progress (Teo 1992).

Screening policy for HBsAg

Screening of the entire hospital patient population would be an effective way to identify hepatitis B infection, but this would be costly and time consuming in terms of the benefits derived.

In general, the best compromise is to test those patients belonging to groups in which there is a high prevalence of hepatitis B. These include the following people:

- All new admissions who currently live or were born in countries where there is a high prevalence of hepatitis B
- Drug addicts
- Institutionalized people with learning difficulties
- All patients acutely or recently jaundiced.

HBV is not transmitted by normal daily contact including coughing, sneezing, hugging, holding hands or sharing bathrooms and toilets, cups and crockery with an HBV-positive person (DoH 2002b).

Transmission of HBV in the health care setting

Transmission of HBV to health care workers can be substantially reduced by vaccination and adoption of universal safe precautions (Moloughney 2001).

Unfortunately not all health care workers exposed to blood and body fluids are vaccinated. A study in Greater Manchester found that 10% of injured staff had never been vaccinated and 27% of those vaccinated had no HBV immunity. The reasons for the lack of immunity were loss of immunity with time, failure of checks on vaccine respond, failure to complete vaccine courses and failure to respond to the vaccine (Alzahrani *et al.* 2000). Following all accidents involving inoculation or exposure to mucous membranes or non-intact skin, the patient should be tested for HBV, with the incident fully evaluated by the Occupational Health Unit and appropriate care provided. Health care workers who are involved in an incident can experience considerable distress and anxiety (Molonghney 2001).

Transmission of HBV from infected health care workers to their patients has occurred. This is generally during exposure-prone procedures in theatre or dental practice (Bell *et al.* 1995). The Department of Health (2000d) requires that HBeAg-positive staff are not to undertake exposure-prone procedures. Those staff who are HBeAg negative must have additional testing to establish viral load. Those persons with HBV DNA levels exceeding 10^3 genome equivalents per ml cannot undertake exposure-prone procedures. These whose viral load is below this figure have to be retested yearly (DoH 2000b).

Immunization and vaccination

Passive protection against hepatitis B
Specific hepatitis B immunoglobulin (HBIG), prepared from pooled plasma with a high titre of hepatitis B

surface antibody, is available for passive protection and is usually used in combination with hepatitis B vaccine to confer passive/active immunity under certain defined conditions (DoH 1996c), including:

- Persons who have an inoculation, ingestion or splashing accident with HBsAg-infected blood
- Babies of mothers with hepatitis B. In these cases babies should receive HBIG no later than 48 hours after birth
- Sexual partners and, in some cases, family contacts judged to be high risk, or individuals suffering from acute hepatitis B and who are seen within one week of onset of jaundice.

Active immunization

Active immunization is by hepatitis B vaccine. Hepatitis B vaccine is a genetically engineered vaccine. The basic regimen consists of three doses of vaccine over 6 months, with a booster dose every 5 years. An accelerated schedule of three doses over 3 months with a booster at 12 months and then every 5 years can be given when rapid acquisition of immunity is required. Approximately 80–90% of vaccinated individuals respond to the vaccine.

Risk groups which include health care workers who have direct contact with blood and body fluids are recommended to be immunized against HBV. Their response to the vaccine must be checked: levels of 100 IU/ml and above indicate immunity; levels of 10–100 IU/ml indicate the need for a booster dose of vaccine; levels below 10 IU/ml indicate no response. Between 10 and 20% of those receiving vaccine will not respond at all to hepatitis B vaccine. Lack of response is more common in people aged 40 years and over and in people who are immunocompromised (DoH 1996c).

Health care workers involved in exposure prone procedures (EPP), including theatre nurses, are required to be immunized against HBV. This means theatre nurses will have to provide evidence of HBV vaccination prior to employment. Those who fail to respond to vaccine have to be tested for HBV every 6 months to prove their continuing non-carrier status (Fox 1996).

Indications for immunization include:

- Personnel including teaching, training and nursing staff directly involved over a period of time in patient care where there is a high prevalence of HBV or where blood and blood products are handled regularly
- Laboratory workers
- Dentists and dental personnel
- Medical and surgical personnel
- Health care personnel on secondment to work in areas of the world where there is a high prevalence of HBV

- Patients on entry to residential institutions where there is a high prevalence of HBV
- Patients treated by maintenance haemodialysis
- Sexual contacts of patients with acute HBV or carriers of HBV
- Infants born to mothers who are HBsAg positive
- Health care workers who receive an inoculation accident from a needle used on a patient who is HBsAg positive, either used alone or in combination with hepatitis B immunoglobulin.

In addition, HBV vaccine is offered to selected high-risk populations; this includes homosexual men attending genitourinary clinics, as studies indicate they are at the greatest risk of acquiring HBV. A combined HBV and HAV vaccine is now available (Zuckerman 1998) which has been seen to be safe and well tolerated (Levie *et al.* 2002).

Prevention of hepatitis B in health care workers

It is important that health care workers adopt safe techniques when in contact with blood and body fluids of all patients, regardless of their hepatitis status.

Avoiding inoculation accidents and contamination of mucous membranes and skin is an essential component of safe techniques. Resheathing needles accounts for 15–41% of all needlestick injuries and must not be undertaken (McCormick *et al.* 1981). Resheathing commonly occurs as a result of trying to ensure safe transit to a disposal sharps bin (Edmond *et al.* 1990), suggesting that sharps bins should be either attached to trolleys or placed at the bedside (Hart 1990).

Vickers *et al.* (1994) reviewed an outbreak of hepatitis B which involved three volunteers at a residential drug trial unit where blood samples were taken by staff who did not wash their hands after each patient contact, and whose hands, gloves, and equipment were visibly contaminated with blood. Such incidents demonstrate the importance of written policies that are regularly reviewed and updated.

Death of patients with hepatitis B

When infected patients die, their bodies are no more hazardous than when they were alive, providing that appropriate precautions against contamination with blood and body fluids are maintained (Young & Healing 1995). Guidelines recommend that bodies of patients known to be infected with hepatitis should be placed in a body bag. Relatives and significant others should be permitted to view, touch and spend time with the deceased person. However, embalming should not be undertaken (Healing *et al.* 1995). The first fatal outcome resulting from transmission of hepatitis B from surgeon to patient was reported in 1996 (Sundkvisst *et al.* 1998).

Patient education

The DHSS (1996c) recommends that individuals found to be HBsAg carriers should be educated about the ways in which hepatitis B may spread and the precautions which can be taken to reduce the risk to others. It is stressed that unnecessary restrictions and precautions may cause distress and should be avoided.

Antiviral therapy

Treatment including interferon-alpha and drugs such as lamivudine, tenofovir or famciclovir is available for HBV infection (Marques *et al.* 1998).

Only 3–5% of adults in the UK with acute HBV infection will progress to chronic HBV; these are the patients who have the highest risk of acquiring cirrhosis and hepatocellular cancer. Therapy includes interferon-alpha and lamivudine. Seroconversion occurs in 30–40% of those patients receiving interferon, with treatment often limited by drug toxicity. The seroconversion is 15–20% for patients receiving lamivudine. Treatment is well tolerated but resistance can occur. Combination treatment is therefore often the treatment of choice (Matthews & Nelson 2001). Care should include education on preventing cross-infection and on improving general health, for example by reducing alcohol intake.

Excellent long-term results have been achieved following liver transplantation of those persons who are HBV positive (Steinmuller *et al.* 2002). Prophylactic therapy is necessary following transplantation to prevent reactivation of HBV (Starkel *et al.* 2002).

Procedure guidelines: **Hepatitis B**

Procedure

	Action	Rationale
1	The patient may be nursed on an open ward using all the patients' facilities as normal unless there is a high risk of blood contamination of the ward environment.	If adequate precautions can be adhered to on an open ward, there is no need to isolate the patient.
2	The patient must be assessed daily to establish accurately any sites of bleeding. Changes in the patient's condition should be recorded in the care plan.	Sites of bleeding must be identified in order that the appropriate precautions can be taken.
3	Used sharps must be correctly disposed of in a sharps bin.	Contaminated sharps are a potential inoculation hazard to others, so particular caution must be taken in handling them. Overloaded sharps containers may cause needles to pierce the walls of the container or even protrude through the top.
4	A yellow clinical waste bag should be kept on a regular holder with a lid for the patient's disposable waste. When full this should be securely closed, and sent for incineration.	To confine potentially contaminated material, e.g. blood-stained tissues. Yellow is the internationally recognized colour for clinical waste.
5	The patient's personal hygiene equipment must be kept at the bedside.	To prevent accidental use of equipment by others.
6	Used linen that is not bloodstained is placed in the white linen bags in the usual way.	Linen free from blood stains is not contaminated and may be dealt with in the normal manner.
7	During venepuncture or other procedures likely to cause bleeding, furniture, bedding and clothing in the adjacent area should be protected with polythene sheeting.	To prevent contamination of the environment with spilled blood.
8	All staff involved with the patient should cover any cuts or grazes on their hands with waterproof dressings.	Broken skin provides a portal of entry for the hepatitis virus in the event of contact with the patient's blood.
9	Routine daily cleaning procedures may be carried out as normal. As part of universal safe technique and practices, domestic staff will be aware of the potential hazard associated with any blood contamination.	Education is necessary so the domestic staff can understand the hazards involved.

Procedure guidelines: **Hepatitis B** *(cont'd)*

Accidental inoculation or spillage of blood

Action	Rationale
1 Any accident involving skin penetration or heavy contamination of abraded skin or mucosal surfaces of staff should be recorded on an accident form and this taken to bacteriology immediately. Occupational health must be informed, who will make an assessment for the need of HBV vaccine or HBV IgG.	To protect personnel. To comply with legal and/or hospital requirements.
2 Blood spillage onto unbroken skin should be washed off with soap and running water. A scrubbing brush should not be used as this could break the skin. Complete an accident form, as above, and inform occupational health.	To remove the source of potential contamination. To comply with legal and/or hospital requirements.
3 Accidental inoculation sites should be cleaned under running water, encouraged to bleed freely and then covered with waterproof plaster. Complete an accident form, as above.	Bleeding helps to expel the inoculated virus from the site. To comply with legal and/or hospital requirements.
4 Blood spilled on hard surfaces must be wiped up immediately with paper towels and the area washed well with a solution such as hypochlorite.	To prevent viral spread. Dried blood remains infectious for several days.
5 Linen stained with blood should be treated as infected linen and placed in a red alginate polythene bag before being placed in a red linen bag.	Bloodstained linen is highly infectious. All linen in red alginate polythene bags will be washed in a barrier wash at the laundry.

Precautions if bleeding is present

Action	Rationale
1 If bleeding is present in the mouth: (a) Use disposable crockery and cutlery and, with any contaminated food, dispose of as clinical waste. (b) Keep a personal food tray and water jug at the bedside. (c) Disposable mouth-care equipment, sputum pot and tissues should be kept at the bedside.	The sputum may be contaminated with blood from the mouth, therefore precautions must include avoiding contact with the patient's sputum.
2 If haematuria or melaena is present: (a) Wear plastic gowns and gloves when handling excreta. (b) Keep a toilet and handbasin for the patient's sole use, if practicable. (c) If a toilet is not available for the patient's sole use, bedpans or urinals must be used. These should be washed in the usual manner in the bedpan washer. Disposable bedpans are dealt with in the routine manner.	Blood present in the urine or faeces makes the patient's excreta a potential source of hepatitis B contamination.
3 If the patient has a wound or a break in the skin: (a) Cover the area adequately so that there is no seepage. (b) Used dressings should be sealed securely in a plastic bag before being disposed of as clinical waste.	To prevent the spread of the virus from dried or fresh blood. Dried blood can remain infectious for several days.

*Procedure guidelines: **Hepatitis B** (cont'd)*

Action	Rationale
(c) All tapes, lotions and creams are kept solely for the patient's use.	
(d) The dressing trolley must be cleaned carefully before reuse.	
(e) Non-disposable equipment should be emptied and wiped clean, placed in a central sterile supplies department bag, securely stapled shut and sent to the sterile supplies department in a safe manner, to be resterilized.	

Other hospital departments

Action	Rationale
1 All departments and staff who will be undertaking invasive procedures to the patient must be made aware of the patient's hepatitis B diagnosis.	To allow them to make their own precautionary arrangements.
2 All request cards to be labelled appropriately.	To alert the receiving department of the diagnosis.
3 All specimens to be labelled appropriately and correctly bagged. (For further information on specimen collection see Ch. 39.)	To alert the receiving department of the diagnosis and prevent contamination of the environment.
4 If a patient who is bleeding has to be transported elsewhere, a nurse must accompany the patient and the porter involved should be provided with the following: (a) Disposable gloves and aprons (b) Cleaning equipment for the trolley or chair before use by the next patient.	To prevent the contamination of the porter or other patients.

Discharging the patient

Action	Rationale
1 The majority of precautions can cease.	Discharge normally implies that the risk of cross-infection is no longer present.
2 The patient should be advised not to share razors, toothbrushes or similar personal property likely to be contaminated by blood.	To reduce the risk of cross-infection.
3 If bleeding occurs, the patient clears up the blood himself/herself and disposes safely of such items as contaminated tissues by burning or flushing down the toilet. If regular persistent bloodstained waste is generated, the health authority must be requested to make special collections.	To reduce the risk of cross-infection.
4 If emergency treatment or dental care is required, the patient must inform the health care worker of the fact that he/she has a recent history of hepatitis B infection.	To allow the correct precautions to be taken.

Death of a patient with hepatitis B

Action	Rationale
1 There should be minimal handling of the body. However, routine last offices can be undertaken (see Ch. 21).	To reduce the risk of infecting the nursing staff.

*Procedure guidelines: **Hepatitis B** (cont'd)*

	Action	Rationale
2	Nurses should wear disposable plastic aprons and gloves when handling the body.	
3	The body should be totally enclosed in a body bag specifically designed for infected patients.	To reduce the risk of infecting the nursing staff.
4	The mortuary staff should be informed of the diagnosis.	To ensure that all staff are aware of the infection risk.
5	If the relatives want to view the body, they must be supervised. The body bag can be opened by a nurse to allow viewing.	To prevent contamination.

Non-A non-B hepatitis

Definition

Due to major advances in knowledge concerning hepatitis, hepatitis A, B, C, D, E, F, G and H have been distinguished. There remains the theoretical possibility of further hepatitis types being reported. Until this time, the hepatitis virus non-A non-B (NANB) is the term given to all clinical hepatitis that does not fall into the above-mentioned categories (Editorial 1990). The aetiology of non-A non-B hepatitis remains unclear (Fukai *et al.* 1998).

Reference material

There are no accepted serological tests for NANB. Diagnosis is achieved by excluding infections associated with NANB (Main *et al.* 1992). These include symptoms associated with hepatitis A, B and C, cytomegalovirus, Epstein–Barr virus, toxic and drug-induced liver injury (including alcoholic liver disease), circulatory abnormalities, shock, sepsis, biliary tract disease and metabolic liver disease (Dienstag 1983; Hsu *et al.* 1995). As new hepatitis viruses are discovered, studies involving retesting patients previously diagnosed as NANB hepatitis continue to highlight patients who fall into none of the known hepatitis categories (Wejstal *et al.* 1997). A search for yet another hepatitis virus continues (Crow & Ng 1997).

NANB hepatitis has been shown to occur in patients who have received:

- Blood transfusions (Dienstag *et al.* 1977)
- Clotting factors for coagulation disorders
- Haemodialysis

as well as

- Outbreaks of epidemics in tropical areas (Wong *et al.* 1980)
- Sporadic cases with no identifiable cause.

Transmission appears to be similar to that of hepatitis B, i.e. principally through blood and blood products. There is an increased incidence in drug addicts due to the sharing of contaminated needles and syringes (Bamber *et al.* 1983). There is evidence, however, of sporadic cases with no obvious contributory factors (Farrow *et al.* 1981).

The incubation period is estimated at 6–8 weeks followed by clinical features similar to hepatitis B, although as a rule acute illness tends to be less severe. A study by Rochling *et al.* (1997) found that patients with NANB hepatitis have been seen to have a more acute illness than those with HCV infection. Despite its relatively mild, often asymptomatic and anicteric presentation during acute infection, approximately 20% of people infected with NANB will develop cirrhosis and may die from hepatic-related death such as hepatocellular carcinoma (Lefkowitch *et al.* 1987). Assessment of treatment protocols for chronic NANB hepatitis has been hindered by the lack of viral markers (Ellis 1990).

A further non-specific hepatitis is autoimmune hepatitis, which is a chronic inflammation of the liver often associated with abnormal liver function tests, tiredness, lethargy, weight loss, anorexia, jaundice, dark urine and pale stools. It is caused by the lymphocytes damaging the liver cells which, if left untreated, can lead to cirrhosis and liver failure (Medina *et al.* 2003). The cause is unknown. Diagnosis is by history, clinical examination, blood tests and liver biopsy. Treatment involves corticosteroids, plus an immunosuppressant such as azathioprine, plus the appropriate treatment of the symptoms of the disease (Obermayer-Straub *et al.* 2000).

It is essential that safe techniques are used at all times when in contact with blood and body fluids. Human immunoglobulin should be given prophylactically following a previous history of needlestick injuries.

Procedure guidelines: **Non-A non-B hepatitis**

The procedure should be as for hepatitis B (see p. 106).

Hepatitis C

Definition

Hepatitis C is an acute infectious disease caused by hepatitis C virus (HCV), which is a single-stranded RNA virus, and a member of the Flaviviridae (Forns & Bukh 1998).

Reference material

HCV was discovered in 1989, and is a major health problem. It is estimated that the global prevalence of HCV ranges from 0.1 to 5% in different countries (Consensus Statement 1999), with about 180 million chronic HCV carriers throughout the world. The prevalence of hepatitis C in the UK is uncertain but is estimated at 0.5% of the general population of England (DoH 2002b). HCV is now emerging as a major health problem (Mohsen & Group 2001) and a national HCV register will provide data towards establishing the natural history of HCV in the UK (Harris *et al.* 2000). HCV is transmitted primarily through contact with blood and blood products (Crowe 1994). One important means of transmission is misuse of intravenous drugs and sharing of needles (Hope *et al.* 2001).

Other routes of transmission include mother to child, sexually (Bird *et al.* 2001), from infected health care worker to patients during exposure-prone procedures (Cody *et al.* 2002) and from sharing personal property such as razors (Sawayama *et al.* 2000).

Clinical response

The incubation period following infection varies from 6 to 8 weeks (Teo 1992). The clinical manifestations of hepatitis C infection are non-specific and include fatigue, malaise and nausea, with only about 5% of patients developing acute jaundice (Girakar *et al.* 1993). The disease may be mild and go unnoticed by the infected person (Griffiths-Jones 1994), with patients recovering spontaneously and completely (Smith 1993). However, up to 50% of patients develop chronic active hepatitis and some progress to cirrhosis. Infection with hepatitis C also appears to be associated with cancer of the liver (Kao & Chen 2002) and an increased risk of death from liver disease (Harris *et al.* 2002). Alcohol misuse presents an increased risk of hepatic complications associated with HCV (Booth 1998).

The Department of Health (2002c) has compiled an HCV strategy for England. Included in the strategy are six action points.

- Keeping people healthy
- Reducing health inequalities
- Shaping services around patients, their families and carers
- Working with others
- Providing a comprehensive service
- Responding to the needs of different populations and continuously improving services.

Transmission

Transfusion services in the UK began to screen for antibodies to HCV in September 1991 (DoH 1995). The screening programme was estimated to have a considerable positive effect on the prevention of post-transfusion HCV infection (Teo 1992).

Diagnosis

Diagnosis of acute hepatitis C infection is established by the presence of antibodies to hepatitis C (anti-HCV IgG) in the blood. Results are confirmed by recombinant immunoblot assay (DoH 1995b).

Treatment

Cases should be referred to a specialist in liver disease for evaluation, close observation and care (Consensus Statement 1999). This may involve liver biopsy and liver function tests. Treatment includes combination therapy with interferon-alpha and ribavirin (Shepherd *et al.* 2000). Relapses do occur (Angelico *et al.* 1995).

Nursing care

Since there is no vaccine for HVC it is critical for health care workers to work safely to prevent exposure to HCV (Lanphear 1997). Watson's (1997) survey of nurses' knowledge of HCV found that their understanding of HCV was poor and that the majority felt that they were not provided with adequate protection against HCV while at work.

The Department of Health (2002d) has produced advice for HCV-infected health care workers undertaking or planning to undertake exposure-prone procedures, to ensure patients are not put at risk, and the action to be taken when a health care worker is occupationally exposed to HCV. Currently there is no post-exposure prophylaxis for HCV, but early treatment may prevent chronic HCV developing.

Nursing care for the patient infected with hepatitis C is the same as for patients with hepatitis B (see Procedure guidelines: Hepatitis B, p. 111).

Hepatitis D

Definition

Hepatitis D virus (HDV), also referred to as delta virus, is a very small RNA virus (Ellett 1999). HDV is always associated with HBV and causes both fulminant hepatitis and the accelerated progression of pre-existing HBV hepatitis (Taylor 1999). HDV can only multiply in a cell which is infected with hepatitis B as it is dependent on HBV for its surface antigens (Zar *et al.* 2001).

Reference material

Hepatitis D is uncommon in the UK and USA, but common in parts of South America and Africa and is usually associated with intravenous drug use and sexually transmitted infections (Smith *et al.* 1992). HDV is transmitted in the same way as HBV (Crowe 1994). Huang & Wu (1998) evaluated the correlation of HDV antibody levels, in particular IgM with HDV viraemia, and found that an anti-HDV titre of 100 or over could be considered to be a marker for acute HDV. Chronic HDV is defined as HDV viraemia for more than 6 months (Huang & Wu 1998).

HDV has a relatively short incubation period of 3–6 weeks (Teo 1992). Infection with HBV and HDV results in a more severe and symptomatic illness than infection with HBV alone (Crowe 1994).

Diagnosis

Diagnosis relies on the detection of HDV antibody in serum (Centers for Disease Control 1990a).

Prevention

Prevention is based on vaccination (Baker 1994) as HBV vaccine is also effective against HDV (Duff 1998).

Treatment

It has been suggested that high-dose interferon-alpha may be beneficial in chronic HDV infection, although relapses can occur (Lau *et al.* 1999). Children with HBV and associated HDV progress to liver cirrhosis within 15–20 years. Treatment involves interferon-alpha therapy with or without lamivudine for at least a year (Wolters *et al.* 2000). Liver transplantation for delta cirrhosis has proved to be a successful treatment for HDV cirrhosis, with few reinfections of the grafted liver (Hadziyannis 1997).

Presenting symptoms and nursing care are the same as for hepatitis B (see hepatitis B, p. 111).

Hepatitis E

Definition

Hepatitis E is caused by an acute icteric virus leading to self-limiting disease. Hepatitis E virus (HEV) is a member of the Calicivirus family (Balayan 1997).

Reference material

HEV is a faeco-orally transmitted hepatitis virus which has many features similar to HAV (Skidmore 1997). Major outbreaks have occurred due to consumption of contaminated food and water (Clayson *et al.* 1998), although person-to-person transmission is rarely seen (Rab *et al.* 1997). Travelling to endemic areas carries a risk of HEV infection (Wu *et al.* 1998). HEV is widely spread in many tropical and subtropical countries (Balayan 1997), and is also found in sewage in Spain. This has implications for contamination of the environment and shellfish (Pina *et al.* 1998). Cases of HEV have been seen in England, but have been associated with patients returning from the Indian subcontinent (Hussaini *et al.* 1997).

Experimental data suggest HEV may be a zoonosis as HEV is pathogenic for some domestic and wild animals (Balayan 1997). Pigs in the USA have been found to be infected with swine HEV, which is closely related to human HEV; there is experimental evidence that cross-species infection with swine HEV can occur (Meng *et al.* 1998). Parenteral (Duff 1998), intrauterine and perinatal routes of spread, while uncommon, have been implicated in the spread of HEV (Irshad 1997).

The incubation period ranges between 2 and 9 weeks, with an average of 6 weeks (Teo 1992). The virus is eliminated from the body on recovery, which prevents carriage of the virus (Mims *et al.* 1993). HEV has been associated with other hepatotropic viruses and can induce fulminant hepatitis with or without the simultaneous presence of other viruses (Irshad 1997). In areas with endemic HEV acute liver failure is found secondary to HEV infection (Hamid *et al.* 2002). HEV is common in pregnancy and associated with a mortality rate of up to 20% (Hussaini *et al.* 1997).

Chauhan *et al.* (1998) investigated the effectiveness of HEV antibodies in humans and found they offered little protection from further infection. In India preparations of immune serum globulin were evaluated in pregnant women; some patients went on to develop HEV (Arankalle *et al.* 1998).

Diagnosis

Diagnosis is made by detecting HEV antibody in serum (Usuda *et al.* 2000). Serological tests for HEV vary in different laboratories (Ghabrah *et al.* 1998).

Vaccination

There is no vaccine for HEV prevention (Moyer & Mast 1998).

Nursing care

Barrier nursing is necessary for patients with hepatitis E infection.

Hepatitis B genotype F

Definition

Hepatitis B genotype F is the name given to a recently discovered virus causing hepatitis (Mbayed *et al.* 2001). This virus is commonly referred to as HBV genotype F (Norder *et al.* 1994), as immunodiffusion experiments show that this virus is a serotype of HBV (Magnius & Norder 1995).

Reference material

HBV genotype F is regarded as indigenous to the American Indian population of the New World (Arauz-Ruiz *et al.* 1997). It appears to cause acute and chronic liver disease (Uchida *et al.* 1994) and is associated with serious disease, with outbreaks of hepatitis B genotype F causing significant morbidity and mortality (Casey *et al.* 1996). Polymerase chain reaction (PCR) tests are now able to distinguish and identify hepatitis F virus (Moraes *et al.* 1999). Much remains to be learned about this virus, although the studies of hepatitis F viruses suggest a subgenome of genotype F has been isolated, which is being referred to as genotype H (Arauz-Ruiz *et al.* 2002). Nursing care is as for hepatitis B.

Hepatitis G

Definition

Hepatitis G virus (HGV) is a recently identified member of the Flaviviridae family (Guilera *et al.* 1998), and is a positive, single-stranded RNA virus, distantly related to HCV (Miyakawa & Mayumi 1997). HGV causes acute and chronic liver disease (De Medina *et al.* 1998) and fulminant hepatitis (Sheng *et al.* 1998).

Reference material

HGV was first described in Egypt and Indonesia, but has also been found in the Americas, Europe and Australia (Corwin *et al.* 1997). HGV route of transmission includes blood donation (Roth *et al.* 1997), sexual transmission, with transmission from male to female more efficient than vice versa (Lefrere *et al.* 1999), mother to child (Lefrere *et al.* 2000), blood-sucking insects (Ribeiro-Dos-Santos *et al.* 2002) and by needlestick injury (Shibuya *et al.* 1998). Diagnosis is by PCR serology tests (Kato *et al.* 2001). HGV RNA levels are suppressed but not eradicated by interferon-alpha and are unaffected by ribavirin treatment. Spontaneous loss of HGV RNA occurs over time in a proportion of patients (Marrone *et al.* 1997). Much remains to be learned about HGV. Nursing care is as for hepatitis B.

The herpes viruses

There are four human herpes viruses which cause infection. These are detected more frequently in immunocompromised people than in immunologically intact individuals (Kedzierski 1991). The four types are:

- Cytomegalovirus (CMV)
- Epstein–Barr virus (EBV)
- Herpes simplex virus (HSV)
- Varicella zoster virus (VZV).

Cytomegalovirus

Definition

Cytomegalovirus (CMV) is a member of the herpes virus family.

Reference material

Primary CMV infection in a immunocompetent person causes a transient infectious mononucleosis-like illness, often in childhood (Horowitz *et al.* 1986), but it can occur throughout life in a non-immune person. Following primary infection CMV persists in a latent state in leucocytes (Jarvis & Nelson 2002) where they can reactivate later in life, particularly when a person is immunosuppressed. Secondary CMV infection occurs when a previously immune person is infected with a new strain of CMV or through reactivation with the person's latent endogenous strain of CMV (Prentice *et al.* 1998). Clinical disease can occur from both primary and secondary infection, although primary infection appears to cause more severe infection (Ho 1995). In the immunosuppressed, e.g. immature neonate, patients who are receiving a transplant and in HIV-positive patients primary CMV causes significant infection (Ho 1995).

CMV is distributed widely throughout the world. There are many strains of CMV, with identical strains found in individuals connected with one another. Babies born with congenital CMV infection, for example, have the same strain as their mother (Griffiths 1991).

CMV infection can be acquired by intrauterine (Bale *et al.* 2002) and perinatal routes (Diosi 1997), sexual transmission (Numazaki *et al.* 2000), blood transfusions (Vrielink & Reesink 1998) and during transplantation (Peggs & Mackinnon 2001). Approximately 50% of the population in the UK carry the antibody to CMV. Consequently, many people are capable of transmitting the infection through blood donation. Those most recently infected appear to be more likely to transmit the virus (Vancikova & Dvorak 2001).

During primary infection, the virus can be isolated from saliva (Fidouh-Houhou *et al.* 2001), tears (Yamamoto *et al.* 1994), urine (Halwachs-Baumann *et al.* 2002), breast milk (Bryant *et al.* 2002), blood (Guertler 2002), semen (Aynaud *et al.* 2002) and cervical secretions (Mostad *et al.* 1999). After initial infection the virus establishes a latent infection thought to be in the lymphocytes. The latent infection may subsequently reactivate with production of infectious virions. Reactivation is generally controlled by the host's cell-mediated immune response. Hence CMV infection is common in immunocompromised people, particularly patients with AIDS (Leach *et al.* 2002). Approximately 1% of all babies have congenital CMV infection, and 90–95% of these infants are asymptomatic. Some infants with asymptomatic symptoms at birth may have sensorineural hearing loss (Rivera *et al.* 2002) and others may have mild learning disabilities (Hanshaw *et al.* 1976). Clinical manifestation of congenital infection includes jaundice, hepatosplenomegaly, rash and multiple organ involvement including the central nervous system. CMV-associated morbidity has been seen in both full-term and preterm infants (Maeda *et al.* 1994). Postnatally acquired CMV infection is less acute and multiple organ infection is rare. However, the diagnosis of CMV infection should be considered in all children with persistent jaundice (Liberek *et al.* 2002).

Patients with malignancies, or those receiving chemotherapeutic therapies, transplantation of kidney heart (Foti *et al.* 2002) or bone marrow (Meyers 1988) have a high risk of contracting CMV disease.

Studies related to risk factors for patients who have received allogeneic stem cell transplants found that acute graft-versus-host disease and stem cells from seronegative donors to CMV-seropositive recipients increased the risk of CMV infection (Lin *et al.* 2002).

Infection in healthy adults is mild and the prognosis is good. However, infection in the immunosuppressed can be severe and be a major cause of mortality and morbidity, with interstitial pneumonitis, hepatitis, Guillain–Barré syndrome, meningoencephalitis, myocarditis, colitis, thrombocytopenia and haemolytic anaemia, plus retinitis in patients with AIDS (Ho 1995).

Patients with acute leukaemia treated with high-dose chemotherapy and bone marrow transplantation are at high risk of CMV infection (Reusser 1998). The incidence of CMV infection among allogeneic bone marrow transplants was significant higher in patients who received HLA matched unrelated donations compared to those from human histocompatibility complex (HLA) matched sibling donors (Takenaka *et al.* 1997). A significant increase in the incidence of graft-versus-host disease has been noted in the CMV-positive group compared to the CMV-negative group (Matthes-Martin *et al.* 1998). The use of CMV-free blood is recommended for CMV-seronegative patients with newly diagnosed malignant disease, for whom a bone marrow transplant is a future treatment option (Preiksaitis *et al.* 2002). CMV infection should be suspected if CMV seropositive patients with leukaemia have unexplained fever, drop in blood count, lung infiltrates or gastrointestinal symptoms (Singhal *et al.* 1997). Treatment should be commenced early and the disease monitored.

Patients with HIV infection have an increased risk of CMV infection, with between 70% and 100% of AIDS patients developing ocular lesions often due to CMV infection (Verma & Kearney 1996). HIV-positive patients with CMV infection have an increased risk of death independently of CD4 cell counts (Chaisson *et al.* 1998). The use of HIV protease inhibitors in combination antiretroviral therapy has been associated with a marked increase in the survival of patients with CMV retinitis, with median survival increasing from 256 days before 1995 to 720 days in 1996 (Walsh *et al.* 1998).

Diagnosis

The diagnosis of CMV requires laboratory confirmation and cannot be made on clinical evidence alone. Laboratory tests include demonstration of the virus or serological antibody screening, using PCR assays (Cunha *et al.* 2002). CMV is readily found in urine, mouth swabs and buffy coat of blood (Ho 1995), bronchoalveolar lavage fluid, biopsy and autopsy specimens (Prentice *et al.* 1998).

Despite the considerable progress in the diagnostic techniques for CMV infection, there continues to be a need for improved tests that can provide quantitative methods for early detection of viral activity (De la Hoz *et al.* 2002).

Treatment

Antiviral treatment with ganciclovir and foscarnet (Limaye 2002) has been seen to reduce mortality from CMV infection (Anders *et al.* 1998). Antiviral drug resistance to CMV is an emerging problem (Limaye 2002). Newer antiviral drugs continue to be evaluated and may be active against certain strains of virus resistant CMV (Kendle & Fan-Havard 1998; Reusser 1996). Continuing CMV viraemia after seven to ten ganciclovir treatments suggests drug resistance; foscarnet is the drug of second choice. Intravenous antibiotics have been safely administered in the community, which has significantly reduced length of hospital stay as well as improving patient satisfaction (Kayley *et al.* 1996).

Despite the progress in diagnosis and treatment of CMV, infection remains a significant cause of morbidity and mortality among immunosuppressed patients (De la Hoz *et al.* 2002; Saavedra *et al.* 2002).

Prevention

Prevention relies on decreasing the risk of virus acquisition and reactivation. Therefore, blood products used should either derive from CMV seronegative donors or be free from viable leucocytes, which can be achieved by irradiating or washing the blood product (Pamphilon *et al.* 1999).

Prophylactic ganciclovir has been seen to effectively prevent large numbers of CMV infection when given during treatments such as bone marrow transplantation (Boeckh *et al.* 2002).

Studies to establish the risks of CMV infection among health care workers have found that the prevalence of antibodies to CMV among the general population and health care workers does not differ. This suggests that the risk of transmission is no greater for those health care workers in contact with CMV infections (De Schryver *et al.* 1999) and that pregnant health care workers are not at increased risk of acquiring CMV (Sobaszek *et al.* 2000). Routine blood and body fluid precautions are essential to avoid CMV transmission among health care workers (Boussemart *et al.* 1998).

Patients with CMV infection generally do not require barrier nursing as they feel ill and do not mix closely with other patients. Therefore, patient-to-patient transmission is unlikely.

Epstein–Barr virus

Definition

Epstein–Barr virus (EBV) is a herpes virus which causes infectious mononucleosis. EBV is generally a self-limiting infection characterized by fever, malaise, headache, anorexia, pharyngitis and adenopathy, which resolves spontaneously in 2 to 3 weeks (Peter & Ray 1998). However pathological changes can occur (Epstein 2001) which can cause complications that include lymphoid and epithelial malignancies (Dantuma & Masucci 2003) and Guillain–Barré syndrome (Winer 2001).

Reference material

EBV primary infection in childhood is usually asymptomatic, although occasional cases have been seen to resemble chronic active hepatitis (Cruchley *et al.* 1997). In adolescence, approximately 50% of cases are accompanied by fever, malaise, pharyngitis and lymphadenopathy, while in adults over the age of 40, fever, jaundice and hepatomegaly can commonly occur (Longnecker 2000).

EBV can persist in the host and reactivate at a later time, particularly during immunosuppression (Niedobitek *et al.* 2001), commonly following transplantation (Pearlman 2002) or in people with cancer or leukaemia (Crawford 2001). Immunosuppression decreases EBV specific immune function, which results in increased EBV load in peripheral blood and in the oropharynx (Haque *et al.* 1997). Initially, EBV replication appears to take place in epithelial cells of the nasopharynx (Sixbey *et al.* 1984) followed by infection of B lymphocytes. The incubation period between exposure and clinical manifestation in normal people varies from 30 to 50 days.

EBV is found in the saliva (Madar *et al.* 2002) and on the cervix (Lanham *et al.* 2001), and can be transmitted by kissing and sexual contact, and rarely by blood transfusion (Van Baarle *et al.* 2000; Crawford *et al.* 2002; Tattevin *et al.* 2002). Diagnosis relies on serological methods that detect the presence of IgG and IgM antibodies to EBV viral capsid antigen (Wielaard *et al.* 1988).

EBV infection in healthy people is generally self-limiting with spontaneous recovery. Management consists of basic supportive care (Peter & Ray 1998) as the use of antiviral agents and corticosteroids in the treatment of EBV remains limited (Holmes & Sokol 2002). Barrier nursing is not necessary for EBV infection, but the patient should avoid kissing and sexual contact while symptoms persist. The patient's personal hygiene articles must not be shared.

Herpes simplex virus

Definition

Herpes simplex virus (HSV) is a herpes virus which causes a range of infections, from painful vesicular lesions (cold sores) to life-threatening illness in the immunocompromised patient (Darville *et al.* 1998). It has an affinity for the skin and nervous system.

Reference material

HSV has two presentations:

1 HSV 1 infections (oral herpes or cold sores) tend to occur on the face or lips. However, primary infection can occur in the conjunctiva, where it causes conjunctivitis and keratitis; in the fingers, where it causes herpetic whitlow; and in the mouth, where it causes herpes gingivomatitis (Arvin & Prober 1991). The HSV 1 incubation period is 2–12 days.
2 HSV 2 infections (herpes genitalis or genital herpes) are usually limited to the genital region (DiCarlo & Martin 1997). However, both types of herpes can be contracted either genitally or orally. The HSV 2 incubation period is 2–7 days.

The incidence of HSV 1 infection in childhood is falling (Vyse *et al.* 2000), while HSV-2 is a common infection affecting about 20% of sexually active people (Coyle *et al.* 2003). The incidence of HSV 2 infection appears to be increasing (Snoeck & De Clercq 2002).

Herpes simplex infections are worldwide in distribution. HSV 1 usually infects children between the ages of 2 and 10 years. Latent infection is then lifelong. Transmission is primarily by contact with oral secretions. HSV 1 is chiefly responsible for perioral, ocular and encephalitic infections in adults (McIntyre 2001). HSV 2 is spread by genital contact and is one of the most common sexually transmitted diseases (Tetrault & Boivin 2000). HSV 2 is the major cause of penile vesicular lesions, cervicovaginitis and proctitis, as well as neonatal disseminated disease (Patel 2002).

Recurrent infection occurs frequently, generally as a result of reactivation of the virus, since HSV 1 may become latent within the trigeminal sensory nerve ganglion, and HSV 2 within the corresponding sacral ganglion (Siegel 2002). Infection or reactivation in the normal host tends to be a mild, self-limiting disease.

The reactivated disease tends to be less severe than the primary infection (Dwyer & Cunningham 2002). In most cases there are prodromal symptoms such as burning and tingling sensations before blisters appear (Goodall 1992). Patients often become aware of a trigger factor that leads to reactivation and infection (Scott *et al.* 1997).

Individuals who are immunocompromised are susceptible to more severe presentations of HSV infections, which include pneumonia, hepatitis and/or encephalitis (Darville *et al.* 1998), with HSV infection the most frequent cause of corneal blindness in the USA (Fillet 2002). Deaths can also occur (Pinna *et al.* 2002).

HSV transmission can occur both from asymptomatic and symptomatic excretors (Woolley 1997). One means of minimizing the risk of infection is to avoid contact with infected lesions. Gloves are essential for all health care staff in direct contact with lesions. The use of condoms is advisable to minimize the risk of transmission during sexual intercourse (Casper & Wald 2002).

Neonatal herpes simplex infections result in serious morbidity and mortality, and can be due to asymptomatic cervical shedding of the virus. If active infection is present at delivery, a caesarean section should be performed (Rudnick & Hoekzema 2002).

Diagnosis

Prompt diagnosis is essential in order to allow appropriate treatment to be given (Smith & Nathan 2002).

The oral presentation of blisters and inflammation of HSV 1 is easily recognizable. With HSV 2, inflammation at the site of infection, general feeling of being unwell and symptoms of burning when passing urine are common, followed by blisters or sores which are characteristic of infection. Reactivation is often accompanied by warning symptoms of itching, tingling or pain in the genital regions followed by blisters. Confirmation of diagnosis is obtained by isolation of the virus in cell culture, and by an increase in antibody levels using PCR or ELISA (Rogers *et al.* 1991).

Treatment

The majority of infections in normal hosts resolve spontaneously. For the immunocompromised patient, prompt treatment with antiviral chemotherapy reduces morbidity and the risk of serious complications. Oral, intravenous and topical preparations are available.

Therapy includes aciclovir, ganciclovir and foscarnet (Gilbert *et al.* 2002). Therapy for children will depend on the severity and time of acquisition (Whitley 2002). Resistance to therapy is being seen (Reusser 1996;

Darville *et al.* 1998) which is often associated with prolonged antiviral therapy (Gilbert *et al.* 2002). Newer drugs appear to be successful in reducing the severity and frequency of recurrence (Yeung-Yue *et al.* 2002). For immunocompromised patients, antiviral therapy during immunosuppression can prevent reactivation of HSV (Fillet 2002).

Nursing care

Barrier nursing is essential in cases of extensive infection with herpes virus. Counselling (Kinghorn 1993) and psychological support may also be required (Williams 1994). Studies have shown that 50% of people with recurrent herpes infection experience depression, 15% have suicidal thoughts and 10% avoid sexual relationships (Chandiok 1992). Goodall (1992) suggests that these effects may be a result of insufficient information and understanding of the true nature of HSV infection.

Postherpetic neuralgia (PHN) is a common problem, which is reduced by antiviral therapy. However, adequate analgesia must also be administered (Fillet 2002).

Varicella zoster virus

Definition

Initial infection with varicella zoster virus (VZV) causes varicella (chicken pox). Following clinical recovery, the virus persists in the latent form in the dorsal root ganglia of nerves; reactivation of the latent VZV causes zoster (shingles) (Gershon 1996). Viral reactivation appears as cellular immunity wanes (Weller 1996). Between 80 and 90% of adults in the UK have had chicken pox (Jones *et al.* 1997), but there is a constant immigration of non-immune adults who will be susceptible to acquiring varicella from a person with varicella or zoster infection (Weller 1996).

Reference material

Varicella

Varicella is a common disease. By the age of 40 years, the blood of 97% of the population of England will test positive for varicella zoster antibodies, providing evidence of past varicella infection (Ross & Fleming 2000).

The varicella incubation period is 11–21 days. Varicella is characterized by fever, viraemia and scattered vesicular lesions of the skin. Neuralgia often precedes the onset of herpes zoster (shingles), which is a localized, painful, vesicular rash involving one or adjacent dermatomes (Arvin 1996). Chronic pain may persist after the rash has healed and is referred to as PHN, which can often be severe and refractory to many forms of treatment. In elderly patients the incidence of PHN varies from 27 to 68% (Schmader 1998). PHN is probably related to neuronal inflammation induced by the replicating VZV (Wood 1991). VZV viraemia occurs in patients with varicella and zoster (Mainka *et al.* 1998).

VZV is a highly infectious virus; transmission is by airborne route for chicken pox, and via infected vesicle fluid in shingles. People who have not been infected with VZV can acquire varicella from individuals infected with varicella or zoster. However, there is little evidence to support the view that in healthy people zoster can be contracted by exposure to zoster or varicella (Dolin *et al.* 1978). A person is infectious 2–3 days before the chicken pox rash appears and until the lesions crust (Jones & Reeves 1997). Immunosuppressed patients have been known to develop chicken pox when they are within 20–30 m of an infected patient (Jones *et al.* 1997). Air samples from hospital rooms of patients with VZV found that the virus was detectable 1.2–5.5 m from the bed and for up to 6 days following the onset of the rash (Sawyer *et al.* 1994).

Following local replication, the virus will be carried by the bloodstream to other sites (Arvin 1996). It is thought that infected lymphocytes persist in the circulation and can go on to carry virus to major organs, causing pneumonia, hepatitis or other life-threatening complications (Arvin *et al.* 1996). Both chicken pox and shingles can lead to neurological infection and disease (Gnann 2002). The virus reaches the nervous system either through the bloodstream or by direct spread from sensory ganglia. The most frequent manifestations include cerebral ataxia, neuralgia, acute encephalitis, aseptic meningitis and myelitis (Echevarria *et al.* 1997). Recovery from varicella in a fit adult is usually spontaneous and without sequelae but can result in serious life-threatening complications in healthy children (Phuah *et al.* 1998).

Immunocompromised patients with VZV infection are at greater risk for dissemination and development of complications than the immunocompetent person (Rolston *et al.* 1998), and can be associated with serious morbidity and significant mortality (Stover & Bratcher 1998). In the immunocompromised adult or child, a much more serious presentation occurs, with a high mortality rate for untreated varicella (Rowland *et al.* 1995). In the immunocompromised patient visceral involvement involving the lung usually occurs 3–7 days after the onset of skin lesions. Neurological complications occur less commonly and generally present 4–8 days after the onset of rash, and often indicate a poor prognosis. The liver is less commonly involved (Ziebold *et al.* 2001).

Emphasis must be placed on early diagnosis, prophylaxis and treatment of varicella infection in immunosuppressed persons to reduce morbidity and mortality associated with herpesvirus infections (Taplitz & Jordan 2002).

Pregnant women who contract varicella may develop complications such as pneumonia. Pregnant women who smoke and have multiple lesions are more likely to develop varicella pneumonia (Harger *et al.* 2002a). Varicella can be transmitted from mother to foetus, which can cause congenital varicella or perinatal infection (McCarter-Spaulding 2001). Fortunately the frequency of congenital varicella is very low (Harger *et al.* 2002b).

Zoster

It is thought that zoster appears when cell-mediated immunity fails to curtail virus reactivation. This may happen as a result of age, the side-effects of drugs or disease. The virus reactivates randomly in the nerve ganglion and spreads down the peripheral nerve producing vesicular skin lesions at the site supplied by the affected neurons (Mims *et al.* 1993). Cancer patients are particularly susceptible to zoster, which is more common during advanced stage disease and develops more frequently at areas of regionalized tumour and/or localized radiotherapy. Most cases of zoster occur within the first year after the diagnosis of cancer, although no single chemotherapeutic regimen or agent has been consistently implicated (Dolin *et al.* 1978).

Patients with AIDS or AIDS-related complex (ARC) appear to be at increased risk of zoster; the incidence of zoster in an HIV antibody-positive person appears to be a sign for the development of AIDS (Melbye *et al.* 1987). VZV is particularly severe in patients with AIDS (Stewart 1995). Rapidly progressive VZV herpetic retinal necrosis can occur (Ormerod *et al.* 1998). Clinical presentation includes mild to moderate ocular or periorbital pain, foreign body sensation and a red eye; visual symptoms include hazy vision, floaters and decreased vision. If left untreated permanent damage can result (Spires 1992). Early diagnosis and aggressive therapy may enable return of useful vision (Lee *et al.* 1998).

Premature babies are at risk of developing varicella zoster infections, as they will not have received the protective maternal antibodies to varicella infection during the third trimester of pregnancy (Van der Zwet *et al.* 2002). Immunocompetent children who develop varicella during the first year of life are at increased risk of developing herpes zoster, whilst immunosuppressed children have a more than 80% risk of developing herpes zoster within 2 years of being diagnosed as having cancer (Takayama *et al.* 2000).

Diagnosis

The diagnosis of chicken pox can usually be made from the characteristic pattern of vesicles (Chen *et al.* 2002). Confirmation is possible by culture of vesicle fluid or by serological antibody tests (Whitley 1995). Neuralgia often proclaims the onset of zoster and can occur several days before skin signs occur. Erythematous patches are the first sign. They progress to macules then to papules and finally to vesicles. New outbreaks of vesicles continue in untreated persons for some time (Couillard-Getreuer 1982). Fever, headaches and malaise can accompany the rash (Mims *et al.* 1993). The vesicles generally correspond in distribution to one or more sensory nerves. Secondary bacterial infection of the lesions can develop (Hirsch 1988). To minimize the risk of infection, care must be taken not to break the vesicles. Daily hygiene must be meticulous. Dissemination of zoster in an immunosuppressed patient generally occurs 6–10 days after the onset of localized lesions and is usually limited to cutaneous involvement, with occasional involvement of the central nervous system (CNS), lung, heart or gastrointestinal tract (Jemsek 1983).

Treatment

Treatment of varicella is normally only necessary for immunosuppressed patients (Chen *et al.* 2002), and involves the use of antiviral agents such as acyclovir, (Arvin 2002) which reduces the time of new lesion formation, fever and visceral complications. The sequential use of intravenous followed by oral acyclovir has been shown to be effective and results in reduction of intravenous therapy and hospitalization (Carcao *et al.* 1998). Oral acyclovir administered to healthy people who have been exposed to varicella can effectively prevent or modify clinical varicella (Lin *et al.* 1997). Failure to respond to 7–10 days of acyclovir suggests drug resistance (Pillay 1998); in such cases foscarnet (Wutzler 1997) or ganciclovir would be the drug of choice (Reusser *et al.* 1996).

Prevention

Pregnant women who have not had chicken pox should be counselled to avoid contact with people with chicken pox (Chapman 1998), as infants born to women who acquire varicella during or shortly after pregnancy are at high risk of infection (Weller 1996). Varicella embryopathy is rare, occurring in 1–2% of maternal infections, particularly in the first half of pregnancy. Varicella of the newborn is a life-threatening illness which may occur when birth is within 5 days of the onset of maternal illness, or due to postdelivery exposure to varicella (Chapman 1998).

Immunosuppressed patients without a history of varicella and, in some cases, patients with a history of varicella, but who are currently on high-dose chemotherapy, should receive varicella zoster immunoglobulin (VZIg) when exposed to varicella or zoster. To be effective, VZIg must be administered as soon after exposure as possible (Wisnes 1978), which will give protection for approximately 4 weeks. Second cases of chicken pox in healthy people are extremely rare. However, among the immunosuppressed, second cases have been seen to occur and are often referred to as atypical disseminated zoster or varicelliform zoster. They do not have dermatomal distribution (Dolin *et al.* 1978).

A varicella vaccine is available and has been seen to be safe and effective (Stover & Bratcher 1998). Studies evaluating the costs and benefits of vaccinating varicella susceptible health care workers suggest there are cost benefits (Tennenberg *et al.* 1997). Health care workers should be screened for VZV immunity (Weber *et al.* 1996). Non-immune health care workers exposed to varicella infection should be removed from patient contact during the 10–21 day incubation period to prevent them infecting patients if they were to develop chicken pox (Swinker 1997).

Nursing care

Nurses must identify those patients at increased risk of VZV infection, and plan and implement interventions to decrease this risk to prevent outbreaks of VZV among patients (Kavaliotis *et al.* 1998). Only staff who have had varicella should have contact with patients with varicella or zoster. Source isolation is essential (see the beginning of this chapter). The door of the room must be kept closed to minimize airborne transmission of the virus (Josephson & Gombert 1988).

Legionnaire's disease

Definition

Legionnaire's disease is an acute bacterial pneumonia caused by infection with *Legionella pneumophila*. This is responsible for about 90% of infection caused by the *Legionella* family. *Legionella* is a Gram-negative, aerobic, non-spore-forming unencapsulated bacillus (Yu 1995).

Reference material

In the summer of 1976 an outbreak of pneumonia occurred among about 5000 people who had attended an American Legion convention in Philadelphia. There were 182 cases and 29 deaths. The epidemic aroused enormous public interest. Epidemiological investigations showed that the focus was the lobby of a famous hotel, but the cause remained unidentified for months until a small Gram-negative organism was found, which subsequently became known as *Legionella pneumophila* (Fraser *et al.* 1977).

There are more than 40 species of the *Legionella* family, with more than 50 serotypes (Fields *et al.* 2002) which have been isolated from a range of environmental sites including lakes, rivers, soils and man-made water systems such as cooling towers and water distribution systems (Cooper 1991). The latter two sites have been responsible for numerous outbreaks of legionnaire's disease which have occurred mainly during June to October (Centers for Disease Control 1978). Half of the reported cases of legionnaire's disease in the UK are associated with travel abroad. Since 1987, countries in Europe have collaborated in surveillance of legionnaire's disease. Over 50 clusters of travel related disease have been reported. Many cases are associated with Mediterranean countries, reflecting the large numbers of holidaymakers from across Europe who visit the area (Public Health Laboratory Service Communicable Disease Surveillance Centre 1994). Even though thousands of people go abroad and stay in hotels, the risk of getting legionnaire's disease for most people is extremely small and the number of cases remains low.

Up to 30% of sporadic cases of hospital-acquired pneumonia are caused by *Legionella* (Hart & Makin 1991). The pattern of infection is unique. The outbreaks are site specific and associated with factors which predispose to infection, including water systems contaminated with the organism. *Legionella pneumophila* is a thermophile which flourishes at temperatures from 25 to 42°C and can survive a range of temperatures from 5 to 58°C. However, it is unusual for this organism to proliferate in temperatures of below 20°C (Health and Safety Executive 1991). The most critical temperature is 36°C. Every effort should be made to avoid stagnant water conditions and to store and supply water outside this critical temperature (Harper 1986). The quality of cold water can be improved by a dedicated supply direct from the incoming mains, and circulating hot water should be kept at a temperature of 60°C (Patterson *et al.* 1997).

Legionella is ubiquitous in surface water. The major route of infection is by aerosol dispersion and inhalation of the bacteria from, for example, shower heads or more commonly from air conditioning systems. Contaminated shower heads and tap water aerosolize low numbers of the organisms during use. The aerosols are small enough to penetrate the lower respiratory system and cause infection (Sabria & Yu 2002). Unusual causes of infection have been seen; for example, water birth pools (Franzin *et al.* 2001) and a whirlpool (Boshuizen *et al.* 2001) have both been implicated in infections. Effective maintenance of water systems is essential to minimize the risk of *Legionella* infection (NHSE 1994). Removal of 'dead legs' in plumbing systems where sludge has formed, which predisposes to proliferation of the organisms, plus regular flushing of water systems not in regular use, reduce Legionellae to below detectable levels (Makin & Hart 1990). Water systems incorporating cooling towers and evaporation condensers pose particular problems, as their mode of operation produces conditions for microbial growth, deliberately creating sprays and aerosols which can disperse the organisms over wide areas if not controlled properly. When water from this source evaporates, droplets containing *Legionella* may be drawn into the air intakes of the building or fall on people passing by (Health and Safety Executive 1991).

Legionnaire's disease is not a notifiable disease, but since 1977 the Communicable Disease Surveillance Centre has maintained a surveillance programme of cases reported voluntarily by medical microbiologists. On average there are approximately 200–250 reported cases of legionnaire's disease each year in the UK, half of which are associated with travel abroad (Local Authority Circular 2002).

Virulence is coupled to a susceptible host. The disease tends to affect males, by a factor of 2 or 3 to 1. Those who smoke or consume excess alcohol, people who are already immunocompromised and the elderly are all predisposed to infection (Stout 1987).

The incubation period is about 2–10 days following first exposure. The signs and symptoms include malaise, general aches and headache, diarrhoea and vomiting, followed by high temperature, cough, rigors and respiratory distress. Immunosuppressed patients may have fever without any other symptoms of infection despite radiographic abnormalities (Muder & Yu 1995). Some patients do not develop pneumonia but progress to profound septicaemia with symptoms of diplopia and mental confusion (Potterton 1985). Pneumonia is the most common presentation of *Legionella* infection, but wound infections have followed immersion in contaminated water (Brabender *et al.* 1993). Fatality rates are about 10% (Rowbotham 1998). Postinfection symptoms of ill health, in particular fatigue, can persist for as long as 1.5 years (Lettinga *et al.* 2002).

Diagnosis

Diagnosis relies on laboratory diagnosis by:

1 Isolation of the causative organism

2 Demonstration of the presence of the organism, its antigen or its products in the patient's body fluids or tissues (Harrison 1985)

3 Demonstration of specific antibodies directed against the organism, its antigens or its products (Dominguez *et al.* 2001).

The above are coupled to the clinical picture and chest X-ray findings.

Treatment

Historically, treatment has included the antibiotic erythromycin (Centers for Disease Control 1978), although newer antibiotics are being used (Yu 1995). Supportive therapy is also required for complications as they arise, which may include pulmonary failure, shock and acute renal failure. Person-to-person spread has never been demonstrated (Hart & Makin 1991) and therefore barrier nursing is not required. However, careful disposal of sputum and encouraging patients to cover their mouth and nose when coughing are necessary precautions.

Prevention

The Approved Code of Practice (2000) provides a basic framework for preventing outbreaks of disease, as well as identifying and assessing risk. In the event of an outbreak of legionnaire's disease, the outbreak committee is convened to protect public health and prevent further infections by identifying and controlling infection risks (Local Authority Circular 2002).

Prevention relies on regular inspection and maintenance of the water system, including planning, installation and commissioning (Finch 1988). Discovery of a single case of hospital-acquired legionnaire's disease is an important sign of additional undiscovered cases, therefore each case must be investigated fully (Sabria & Yu 2002).

Listeriosis

Definition

Listeriosis is an infectious disease caused by *Listeria monocytogenes*, a Gram-negative bacterium, and is a serious life-threatening infection (Crum 2002).

Reference material

Listeria has a widespread distribution in the environment, including in soil, dust and vegetation (Watkins *et al.* 1981). It also inhabits the gastrointestinal tract of animals and humans who may remain symptomless

(Botsen-Moller 1972). The genus *Listeria* includes many types which are non-pathogenic to humans (Raybourne 2002). *Listeria monocytogenes* is recognized as being the cause of listeriosis in humans (Lamont *et al.* 1988). Infection in immunocompromised adults varies from a mild, chill-like illness to bacteraemia, septicaemia and meningitis (Limaye *et al.* 1998). *Listeria* was initially isolated and described in 1992 (Low & Donachie 1997), with most cases arising from ingestion of contaminated food (Low & Donachie 1997). A US study found that at least one food specimen in the refrigerators of infected patients grew *Listeria* (Pinner *et al.* 1992). Gilot *et al.* (1997), however, suggest that most cases of listeriosis occur sporadically and can rarely be linked with consumption of a specific food.

Listeria has the ability to survive and multiply in low temperatures including 0°C (Taormina & Beuchat 2001), which means that it can survive in food stored in a refrigerator. Contact with chlorinated water reduces the growth and survival of *Listeria* (Delaquis *et al.* 2002), whilst mild heating of food facilitates the growth of *Listeria* species (Li *et al.* 2002).

Whilst the incidence of foodborne disease remains high, a decrease in the number of infected people needing to be admitted to hospital or dying from listeriosis has been seen (Adak *et al.* 2002). A total of 543 cases of listeriosis were reported to the Public Health Laboratory Service during 1995 to 1999. Of these, a high number were patients with major medical conditions (72%) or those receiving immunosuppressive therapy (31%) (Smerdon *et al.* 2001).

Transmission, particularly among immunocompromised patients (Hung *et al.* 1995) and pregnant women (Gilbert 2002), causes bacteraemia and meningitis, and in pregnant women premature delivery and often foetal death (Armstrong 1995). Maternal symptoms are often absent, and neonatal listeriosis presents as meningitis or occasionally as septicaemia (Gill 1988). In cases where the mother presented with decreased foetal movement, diagnosis was made by ultrasound examination (Quinlivan *et al.* 1998; Miyakoshi *et al.* 1998). Abortion and stillbirths due to listeriosis have been reported (Smerdon *et al.* 2001).

Treatment

Early diagnosis and prompt administration of appropriate antibiotics are essential (Jones & MacGowan 1995); even so deaths will still occur (Chang *et al.* 1995). Ampicillin or penicillin is usually regarded as the drug of choice (Trautman *et al.* 1985), often in combination with gentamicin (Azimi *et al.* 1979). However, even with prompt antibiotic therapy, mortality may be as high as 30% in patients with other serious underlying conditions (Rouquette & Berche 1996).

Transmission

Contaminated food is the most important vehicle of spread (McLaughlin & Gilbert 1990). There are increasing reports of *Listeria* found in raw meat, fruit and vegetables which predispose to contamination of, for example, coleslaw. Prepared mixed salads have a much higher rate of contamination than individual salad ingredients, probably because prepared salads are contaminated during the chopping, mixing and packaging process (Valani & Robert 1990). Contaminated sandwiches have also caused infections (Graham *et al.* 2002).

Prevention entails scrupulous preparation of cooked food for immunocompromised people and the avoidance of uncooked foods. Person-to-person transmission during normal contact is unlikely. However, careful disposal of blood and body fluids and thorough hand washing after contact with the patient are essential.

Pneumocystosis

Definition

Pneumocystosis is an infection caused by the organism *Pneumocystis carinii* (PC), which is closely related to fungi (Wakefield 2002).

Reference material

Pneumocystis carinii was first discovered in 1909 and was associated with outbreaks of pneumonia in people subjected to malnutrition and overcrowding (Radman 1973). Molecular epidemiological studies identified more than 50 strains of PC (Kovacs *et al.* 2001). PC is an organism that is widely distributed in the environment and most children demonstrate that they have been harmlessly exposed to PC at an early age (Walzer 1995). PC can be detected in hospital and community areas with and without infected patients being present (Bartlet *et al.* 1997). It had been thought that *Pneumocystis carinii* pneumonia (PCP) was a result of reactivation of latent infection but more recent data suggest PCP is caused by acquisition of the organisms from the environment or person-to-person transmission (Morris *et al.* 2002a).

The organism has been recognized as being an important cause of pneumonia in the immunocompromised host for over 20 years. Three types of patients have been particularly affected:

1 Patients of all ages receiving immunosuppressive agents for the treatment of cancer and during organ

transplantation (Kruger *et al.* 1999), particularly if chronic graft-versus-host reaction is present (Chen *et al.* 2003). Deaths from PCP continue to occur (Okamoto *et al.* 2002).

2 Children and infants with primary immunodeficiency disorders, particularly severe combined immunodeficiency (SCID) (Berrington *et al.* 2000), with severe malnutrition (Russian & Levine 2001) or malignancy (Neville *et al.* 2002).

3 Patients with AIDS, particularly in patients whose blood CD4 T lymphocytes are below 200/mm³ of blood (Phair *et al.* 1990). PC remains the most frequently reported serious opportunistic infection in AIDS patients and the second highest cause of mortality among people with AIDS (Morris 2002a). In addition, the occurrence of PC is significantly associated with the death of HIV-positive people (Chaisson *et al.* 1998). PC is commonest among those who are unaware of their HIV-positive status or who have declined prophylaxis despite knowing they are HIV positive (Miller 1998). The incidence of PC among intravenous drug misusers, heterosexual and homosexual men is very similar, while subsequent survival is lowest among intravenous drug misusers, possibly due to the lower uptake of antiretrovirals in this group (Laing *et al.* 1997). PC prophylaxis for HIV-positive patients has been seen to be cost effective (Goldie *et al.* 2002). Studies evaluating efficacy and toxicity rates for prophylaxis regimens are ongoing (Wynia *et al.* 1998). PC may still occur despite appropriate prophylaxis (Massie *et al.* 1998).

Most epidemiological studies have focused on clusters of cases within hospitals, orphanages or private clinics. All have common denominators of overcrowding, protein calorie malnutrition, prematurity or immunosuppressive disease, predisposing to PCP. These studies give the impression of outbreaks of infection, when no spread has actually occurred; rather the disease probably occurred from reactivation of latent infection triggered by immunosuppression (Dutz 1970).

PC infections associated with deprivation in children are reported to be slow and insidious in onset, with initial non-specific signs of restlessness, lethargy, poor feeding over a period of weeks, resulting in tachypnoea, severe dyspnoea, use of accessory muscles for breathing, marked cyanosis and exhausting non-productive cough (Perera *et al.* 1970). Children and adults with underlying disease such as neoplasm often experience an abrupt onset of illness, with high lever, tachypnoea and cough, which can progress to a fatal outcome even with treatment (Walzer 1970).

Diagnosis

It is possible, using PCR tests, to detect PC in specimens containing low numbers of PC where conventional microscopic staining failed to do so (Lundgren & Wakefield 1998).

Fibreoptic bronchoscopy or bronchial washings are valuable in diagnosing PCP (Huaringa 2000). Survival is related directly to the aggressiveness with which the diagnosis is pursued in the early stages of disease and with the early institution of appropriate therapy (Young 1984).

Treatment

Advances in prevention and treatment of PCP have led to a decrease in the incidence and improved outcomes (Santamauro *et al.* 2002).

Trimethoprim–sulphamethoxazole is the treatment of choice (Kovacs *et al.* 2001), but can be toxic and may fail, resulting in treatment changes. Alternative drugs may include alovaquone or dapsone (Goldie *et al.* 2002). PCP prophylaxis includes trimethoprim–sulphamethoxazole, dapsone (Souza *et al.* 1999) or aerosolized pentamidine (Vasconcelles *et al.* 2000). HIV-infected patients who develop PCP and are receiving antiretroviral therapy have an improved overall survival rate (Morris 2002b). Aerosolized pentamidine prophylaxis has significantly improved the prognosis for patients with AIDS (Miller *et al.* 1989). Therefore, patients receiving aerosolized prophylaxis must be monitored carefully for signs of disseminated disease (Dubé & Sattler 1993).

Nursing care

Hospitalized patients who develop PCP may well be cared for in areas where there are large concentrations of immunosuppressed patients. Owing to reports of clustering of this disease and the difficulty of identifying whether this represents person-to-person spread, patients with a productive cough should be placed in a single room until the cough improves. Precautions other than careful hand washing following patient contact are unnecessary.

Tuberculosis

Definition

Tuberculosis (TB) is a destructive infectious disease caused by *Mycobacterium tuberculosis*, which is an acid-fast bacillus. Other species of *Mycobacterium* which cause infection are referred to as 'atypical' mycobacteria.

Reference material

Mycobacterium tuberculosis is defined as an acid-fast bacillus because of a waxy material in the cell wall, which resists simple laboratory staining techniques unless treated with hot carbol fuchsin, which allows impregnation by the dye. This is retained despite attempts to decolourize it with acid or alcohol. Mycobacteria are distributed widely throughout the world, but only a few species are pathogenic to humans. These include *M. tuberculosis*, whose main host is humans, and *M. bovis* (the bovine type of tubercle bacillus), which is pathogenic to humans as well as to cattle (Sales *et al.* 2001). Outbreaks of infection in humans due to *M. bovis* have been reported (Guerrero *et al.* 1997), *M. bovis* has been found in milk samples (Perez *et al.* 2002).

There are also atypical mycobacteria associated with patients who are severely immunocompromised due to HIV infection. These are *M. avium intracellulare* (MAC), *M. malmoense, M. xenopi* and *M. kansasii* (Lamden *et al.* 1996). A significant decrease in MAC infections has now been seen amongst HIV-positive patients receiving antiretroviral therapy (Ives *et al.* 2001). In the past, these types rarely caused disease in humans, but now cause a disease which quickly disseminates to most organs in the body (Young 1996), and do not respond as readily to established tuberculosis drugs (Chaisson 1993). Atypical mycobacteria are not highly adapted to humans like *M. tuberculosis* and are not transmitted from person to person, but can survive in the environment and pass to human hosts.

TB causes characteristically chronic granulamatous lesions, mainly in the lungs, but the glands, bones, joints, brain and meninges and other internal organs may be affected. An increase in cutaneous TB has been seen among patients with HIV (Barbagallo *et al.* 2002). However, with the exception of pulmonary TB, the numbers remain small; for example, over a 20-year period, Great Ormond Street Hospital only identified 38 children with CNS TB (Farinha *et al.* 2000). Infection in immunocompromised adults varies from a mild, chill-like illness to bacteraemia, septicaemia and meningitis.

Mycobacterium tuberculosis is a pathogenic organism because of its ability to reside in and restrict the ability of the host macrophages (Russell 2001), as well as being able to adhere to, invade and multiply within respiratory epithelial cells (Reddy & Hayworth 2002).

Epidemiology

One third of the world's population is currently infected with TB, with approximately 3 million deaths occurring each year. In the UK there are about 6500 new

notifications of TB each year (DoH 2002e) and London has seen the largest increase. Risk factors include young age (0–19 years), black Caribbean ethnic group and alcohol dependency (Maguire *et al.* 2002). Clustering of cases is more common amongst those persons known to be HIV positive (Hayward *et al.* 2002).

Over 50% of cases of TB in the UK are in people born overseas. Screening of 53 911 political asylum seekers arriving at Heathrow airport found 241 per 100 000 persons had active TB. It is estimated that 101 political asylum seekers with active TB enter the UK every year (Callister *et al.* 2002). Clusters of TB infection have occurred (Kumar *et al.* 2000). Outbreaks in extended families and church contacts has been seen in the UK (Cook *et al.* 2000), as well as in a hostel for homeless men (Kearns 2000). The Centers for Disease Control (1998b) outline how linguistic, cultural and health service barriers impeded the provision of TB preventive therapy. The effects of poverty, homelessness and the HIV epidemic also account for the increase in infections (Mangtani *et al.* 1995; WHO 2002b). Some authors suggest badgers infect cattle in the UK (Mairtin *et al.* 1998).

Certain conditions predispose to the development of TB, including general physical debilitation and lowered resistance due to disease, immunosuppressive drugs and alcoholism (Washington & Miller 1998). Among 4360 patients with AIDS, 200 were reported to have TB in 1991 (Watson *et al.* 1993). TB has the potential to cause progression of HIV disease (Perneger *et al.* 1995), with HIV-positive people being more likely to progress to active disease than an immunocompetent person (DoH 1998).

Transmission

The mode of spread for TB is occasionally by ingestion, for example by drinking infected milk, but principally by inhalation of small droplets produced by coughing. These droplets are probably the most effective vehicle of spread since they dry rapidly in the air to yield droplet nuclei of less than 5 nm in diameter which, when inhaled, can reach the alveoli. PCR-based assays provide a rapid and simple means of identification for TB (Parsons *et al.* 2002). The organism can survive in moist or dried sputum for up to 6 weeks, but is killed by a few hours' exposure to direct sunlight (Loudon *et al.* 1969).

Special attention must be given to equipment contaminated with *Mycobacterium* species. Thorough cleaning followed by autoclaving is the sterilization method of choice. As certain equipment such as endoscopes can be damaged by autoclaving, disinfection must be used. The use of antiretroviral therapy for HIV-positive patients, which restores the immune response, has been seen to improve the outcome of antituberculosis therapy (Schluger *et al.* 2002). An audit of the disinfection of fibreoptic bronchoscopes showed that many units do not adhere to guidelines related to disinfection procedures and staff safety (Honeybourne & Neumann 1997). Transmission of TB has occurred due to inadequately cleaned bronchoscopes (Michele *et al.* 1997).

Diagnosis

TB should be suspected in all people with a cough with or without cause, which lasts more than 3 weeks, with or without weight loss, anorexia, fever, night sweats or haemoptysis (DoH 1998b). A provisional diagnosis can be based on microscopic findings of acid-fast bacilli in, for example, sputum, tissue, urine or cerebrospinal fluid. This is termed 'smear positive'. Confirmation and species identification by culture may take several weeks and is termed 'culture positive' (Kremer & Besra 2002). Newer methods are now available which reduce the time required for identification.

Patients with smear-positive pulmonary disease are infectious, those with smear-negative or non-pulmonary disease are not. Once appropriate combination chemotherapy has commenced (Joint Tuberculosis Committee of the British Thoracic Society 1994) smear-positive people are considered non-infectious after 2 weeks of treatment (Subcommittee of the Joint Tuberculosis Committee of the British Thoracic Society 1990) and when three consecutive good quality sputum samples are found to be smear negative (DoH 1998b).

Treatment

Until the 1960s, treatment included bed rest and attention to diet, but chemotherapy is now the preferred treatment. It involves the use of combination drugs designed to reduce viable bacteria as rapidly as possible in order to minimize the risk of ineffective treatment in those patients infected by drug-resistant bacteria (Cooke 1985). A 3–6 month regimen with four standard drugs in the initial phase, for all forms of TB excluding meningitis (which may need to be treated for a longer period (Ormerod 1998)), supervised by physicians with full training and care provided by nurse specialists, is recommended in the UK (Joint Tuberculosis Committee of the British Thoracic Society 1998).

The UK mycobacterial resistance network (mycobnet) had 25 217 reports of TB in the UK between 1993 and 1999: 1523 (6.1%) of isolates were resistant to one or more drugs, 1397 (5.6%) were resistant to isoniazid and 299 (1.2%) were multidrug resistant (Djuretic *et al.* 2002).

An increase in multidrug-resistant TB (MDR-TB) is a major cause for concern. Outbreaks of hospital-acquired MDR-TB have been associated with mortality rates of 72–89% (Beck-Sage *et al.* 1992). Deaths have occurred among health care staff in the USA who are believed to have contracted TB at work (Di Perri *et al.* 1992). Resistance to drugs in the UK remains low but is rising. Alternative drugs are available but are less effective and are more often associated with side-effects than standard drug regimens (DoH 1998b). If the resistant pattern is extensive there may be no suitable treatment that the patient can tolerate. Outbreaks of MDR-TB have occurred in London; one involved seven HIV-positive patients where the index case and two contacts died. Cross-infection was due to the index patient being cared for in a positive pressure single room (Breathnach *et al.* 1998).

European evaluation of treatment outcomes is ongoing (Veen *et al.* 1998). Transmission of MDR-TB to health care workers has been seen (Centers for Disease Control 1990b). Respiratory protection is an important element of TB infection control, especially important during procedures such as bronchoscopy and autopsy (Nicas 1998). The recent increase in MDR-TB has meant that health care workers should wear a dust/mist respirator mask rather than a surgical mask (McCullough *et al.* 1997) when caring for smear-positive TB patients where there is a risk of MDR-TB (Chen *et al.* 1994).

Coker (1998) explains how failure of treatment compliance is the basis of a drug-resistant TB epidemic. This means that patients remain infectious, relapses are more frequent and drug resistance flourishes. Vagrants, alcoholics and patients with learning difficulties would be among those expected to be non-compliant patients. Simple urine tests are available to check for the patient's adherence to treatment (Ormerod 1998). Improvements will only be seen if services are more patient centred, more accessible and adapted to the population at risk, ensuring that people with infection comply with their treatment regimens (DoH 2002e).

TB continues to be a notifiable disease (DoH 1995). It is the responsibility of the Medical Officer for Environmental Health to follow up all contacts of infected people. Contact tracing involves identifying the index case, plus those who may have become infected. As transmission requires prolonged close contact with a smear-positive case, contact tracing is generally limited to those from the same household or equivalent. If transmission is shown to have occurred among this close contact group a wider contact tracing may be required, including family, friends and work colleagues (DoH 1998b). TB is found in 1% of contacts; about 10% of notified cases each year are found through contact tracing (Ejidokun *et al.* 1998). Only contacts of smear-positive TB-infected persons are followed up as the transmission from smear-negative persons is very low. One study evaluated 85 young children who had been closely and regularly in contact with a smear-negative child care assistant, and no evidence of transmission was found (Millership *et al.* 1998). The infection control doctor with the consultant in communicable disease will evaluate whether hospital contacts will be followed up; generally this will only involve immunocompromised patients and health care workers. Contact tracing is likely to start from the date one month before the patient became symptomatic. In cases without symptoms it may be necessary to look back over 3 months (DoH 1998b). Advice on handling outbreaks of TB is available (DoH 1998b).

The World Health Organization recognizes that TB persists as a global health problem and has prepared guidance on TB control to reduce mortality, morbidity and transmission of the disease, whilst preventing drug resistance (WHO 2002b).

Prevention

The priorities for TB control are early detection of cases, examination of contacts, barrier nursing if appropriate and immunization of people with a negative tuberculin skin test, with bacille Calmette-Guérin (BCG) vaccine. BCG vaccine contains a live attenuated strain derived from *M. bovis* (Mustafa 2001). Since 1953, children are immunized before they leave school. The vaccine has been shown to be 70–80% effective in protecting against TB, with protection lasting at least 15 years. Efficacy of BCG varies in different populations, but the precise mechanism for failure is not known (Brandt *et al.* 2002). It is recommended that all health care workers who have not had BCG and may have contact with infectious patients or specimens are immunized with BCG. A tuberculin skin test must be carried out before BCG immunization. The test assesses the person's sensitivity to tuberculin protein – the greater the reaction the more likely the individual is to have active disease. Those with a strongly positive test need to be referred to a chest clinic for assessment (DoH 1996b). BCG is less effective in HIV-positive persons and, being a live vaccine, is not recommended in the UK. Any immunity from a previous BCG can be expected to reduce as the CD4 count falls (DoH 1998b).

Certain professions, for example those working in hospitals, prisons, care of older people homes and schools, should be screened on employment. This may include a tuberculin test and chest radiography for staff who have not received a BCG vaccination in the past. TB can be transmitted from patients to health care workers, but in areas of low incidence where infection control practices are good the risk of transmission is negligible (Riley *et al.* 1997). Transmission from health care worker to patient rarely occurs (Menzies *et al.* 1995). There are four recorded incidences of hospital staff being diagnosed with smear-positive pulmonary TB. All relevant patients and staff who had had close contact were followed up, but no cases of TB were found (National Health Service Executive 1998). However, outbreaks involving children in a hospital nursery where infection and active disease developed relatively quickly have been seen (Nivin *et al.* 1998).

Staff in contact with untreated, smear-positive patients for a week or more should be reported to the occupational health department, and a chest X-ray arranged for 6 months' time. However, if the employee develops suspicious symptoms such as an unexplained cough lasting longer than 3 weeks, persistent fever or weight loss, then a full examination must be undertaken.

The World Health Organization advises that control of TB relies on consideration of the type of TB, presence of concomitant infection with HIV and patient characteristics (Maher & Nunn 1998). Van Buynder (1998) suggests that control in developed countries must focus on the groups at risk of TB, which include ethnic minorities, the homeless and those with impaired immunity. Singleton *et al.* (1997) state that patients with TB who are non-adherent to therapy or who have complicated medical and social problems pose a threat to public health. Therefore, specialized medical management for patients to complete therapy in a safe and supportive environment is essential. Patients infected with HIV are predisposed to develop TB (Haramati & Jenny-Avital 1998). Preventive treatment against TB in adults infected with HIV has been seen to reduce the incidence of infection (Wilkinson *et al.* 1998). TB is more likely to be diagnosed in patients unaware of their HIV diagnosis and therefore not offered prophylaxis (Porter *et al.* 1996). Early diagnosis and effective treatment of TB among HIV-infected patients are critical for curing and minimizing the negative effects of TB on HIV progression (Centers for Disease Control 1998c), as TB increases the risk of death among HIV-positive persons independently of CD4 cell counts (Chaisson *et al.* 1998).

Nursing care

High awareness of the disease is essential (DoH 2002e). Patients do not necessarily require admission to hospital but can be investigated and treated on an outpatient basis. Generally, home contacts will have already been exposed and will be routinely contacted and investigated (DoH 1998b). Segregation while undergoing tests or routine visits to the outpatient department is required to prevent more people being exposed. Adequate resources and an appropriately skilled workforce, including specialist nurses and outreach workers, are necessary (DoH 2002e).

Evaluation of infectivity will be necessary. Sputum smear-positive people are considered infectious and those whose results are not yet known are treated as potentially positive. People who have smear-negative culture-positive pulmonary disease, plus non-pulmonary disease, are considered not to be infectious (DoH 1998). Infectious and potentially infectious patients should be cared for in a single room with the door closed. Patients being cared for with immunocompromised persons must be placed in a negative pressure room which is continuously and automatically monitored. All patients with known or suspected MDR-TB must be placed in a negative pressure single room with the door closed. If the patient is HIV antibody positive this room should be near, but physically separated from, the HIV ward (DoH 1998b).

Patients require careful explanation to ensure they and their visitors comply with the barrier nursing precautions. Initially visitors should be restricted to those who have already had contact. Visitors who themselves are immunocompromised should only visit after careful discussion with and agreement by their own physician. Paediatric facilities and restrictions should be the same as the adults' (Kellerman *et al.* 1998).

Patients must be taught to cover their mouths when coughing to prevent droplet spread, and to wash their hands after coughing. Patients must expectorate into sputum pots with tight fitting lids, and the pots must be changed frequently. As compliance to therapy can be poor, patients must be encouraged and, if necessary, supervised to ensure compliance with the drug treatment. Unconscious patients will need to have their drugs administered via a nasogastric tube, intravenously or intramuscularly (Ormerod 1996).

Legislation

Patients with TB who are non-adherent to therapy or who have complicated medical and social problems may pose a threat to others (Singleton *et al.* 1997). Sections 37 and 38 of the Public Health (Control of Disease Act) 1984 provide legal powers to control infected patients who refuse to comply with treatment and pose a threat to public health. The Control of Substances Hazardous to Health (COSHH) Regulations 1999 include issues such as TB and disinfectants. These guidelines requires a risk assessment, and the provision of adequate information, instruction and training to be carried out where an employee is exposed to substances hazardous to health.

Transmissible spongiform encephalopathies

Definition

Transmissible spongiform encephlopathies (TSEs), also referred to as prion diseases, are fatal degenerative brain diseases which occur in humans and some animal species. A common feature of all TSEs is the appearance of microscopic holes in the grey matter of the brain, giving it a sponge-like appearance, from which the conditions derive their names. TSE is very rare (Advisory Committee on Dangerous Pathogens Spongiform Encephalopathy 1998).

Reference material

There are several TSEs. In humans these are:

- Creutzfeldt–Jakob disease (CJD), including classic, sporadic, familial, iatrogenic and new variant (vCJD)
- Gerstmann–Straussler–Scheinker syndrome
- Fatal familial insomnia
- Kuru.

In animals these are:

- Scrapie, bovine spongiform encephalopathy (which may be transmitted to humans by eating infected animal tissue) (Dealler & Lacey 1991)
- Transmissible mink encephalopathy
- Chronic wasting disease
- Feline spongiform encephalopathy in domestic cats and captured exotic felines and ungulates.

TSEs are caused by an infectious agent, thought to be an infectious protein called a prion. Prions are not uniformly spread in the tissues, but high levels are thought to be in neural tissue, less in spinal fluid and lymphoreticular tissue, with very little in blood and other body fluids and tissue. CJD has been found to be transmitted by the reuse of experimental brain electrodes, neurosurgery, dura mater and corneal grafts, pituitary growth hormones and gonadotrophins (Dealler 2002).

Of major concern is that TSEs exhibit a high resistance to conventional chemical and physical decontamination methods and are not affected by disinfectants or autoclaving at conventional times and temperatures. The Department of Health (2001c) allocated £200 million to modernize NHS decontamination and sterilization facilities in order to minimize the risk of vCJD.

TSEs have a preclinical phase that lasts for years, followed by a rapid progressive dementia, loss of memory and intellect, personality changes, progressive unsteadiness and clumsiness. In CJD involuntary muscular jerking is common. There is no known treatment or prophylaxis and all TSEs are fatal within a few months, with the exception of vCJD where survival may be up to 2 years, once clinical signs appear (DoH 2000c).

Risk assessment

The risk related to vCJD was raised when it was found in tonsillar tissue of people who had died of vCJD. In 1999 the NHSE provided guidance on minimizing the risk of transmission of vCJD. Advice included:

- Single-use kits for all lumbar punctures
- Using single-use instruments whenever possible
- Properly cleaned and sterilized surgical instruments to be used at all times
- Instruments and equipment used in the care of patients with confirmed CJD should not be reused but disposed of by incineration
- Instruments used on patients suspected of having CJD should be quarantined pending confirmation of diagnosis. Certain patients should be regarded as at particular risk, e.g. recipients of dura mater grafts (DoH 2001c).

Concerns have been raised about the risk to workers from being exposed to the agent of CJD. Lists of workers with unintentional exposure to CJD have to be compiled and kept for 40 years after the last known exposure (NHSE 1999).

The Department of Health (2001d) issued a risk assessment related to the transmission of vCJD via used surgical instruments. An effort was made to clarify the most important factors affecting this risk. The assessment suggests that the risk of surgical transmission of vCJD from instruments used on a patient with vCJD cannot be ruled out, even when the instruments have been decontaminated and sterilized following government guidelines. This poses a risk to public health (DoH 2001c).

Blood transfusions

Concerns have been raised related to the potential risk of CJD being transmitted by blood transfusion. There is little evidence to support these fears (Turner 2001). However, the importance of improving safety of blood and maintaining a sufficient blood supply is becoming an increasing issue (Reynolds *et al.* 2001) (see Ch. 42, Transfusion of blood).

Nursing care

The nursing care for patients with known or suspected CJD infection is the same as for any patient with an infection carried by blood and body fluids (see AIDS section of this chapter).

Safe techniques and practices need to be maintained at all times, and care must be taken to avoid contamination or needlestick injuries. If an accident occurs routine first aid care must be given and the occupational health department informed.

The patient must be carefully assessed. If there is no evidence or likelihood of blood or body fluid contamination no restrictions are necessary, although close observations will have to be undertaken for bleeding or incontinence, particularly if dementia is a problem.

All specimens must be labelled with a biohazard sticker, double bagged and taken to the laboratory in a safe manner. If the patient is being referred for an invasive procedure they should be told in advance of the restrictions.

Patients requiring an operation must be last on the theatre list to allow for thorough cleaning of the theatre at the end of the operation. Disposable instruments should be used whenever possible and non-disposable instruments sent for incineration.

When the patient is ready for discharge, discharge planning must be negotiated with the community staff, as standard infection control procedures should be continued to prevent transmission of infection in the community. General guidelines for the control of infection in residential and nursing homes are available (DoH 1996b).

Legislation

Legislation, guidance, local safety policies, codes of practice, accident reporting and health surveillance must be used to reduce the risk of vCJD. These include:

- The Health and Safety at Work, etc. Act 1974
- Management of Health and Safety at Work Regulations 1992
- Genetically Modified Organisms (Contained Use) Regulations 1992
- Control of Substances Hazardous to Health Regulations 1999
- Reporting of Incidents, Diseases and Dangerous Occurrences Regulations 1995 (RIDDOR).

Nursing care for patients infected or suspected of being infected with TSEs is the same as for those infected with HIV and hepatitis B. Advice should be sought from the Infection Control Team.

References and further reading

Adak, G.K., Long, S.M. & O'Brien, S.J. (2002) Trends in indigenous foodborne disease and deaths, England and Wales 1992–2000. *Gut*, **51**(6), 832–41.

Adler, M.W., French, P., McNab, A. *et al.* (2002) The national strategy for sexual health and HIV: implications for genitourinary medicine. *Sex Transm Infect*, **78**(2), 83–6.

Advisory Committee on Dangerous Pathogens Spongiform Encephalopathy Advisory Committee (1998) *Transmissible Spongiform Encephalopathy Agents. Safe Working and the Prevention of Infection*. Department of Health, London.

Albert, J. *et al.* (1990) Replicative capacity of HIV-2 like HIV-1, correlates with severity of immunosuppression. *AIDS*, **4**(4), 291–5.

Alberti, C., Bouakline, A., Ribaud, P. *et al.* (2001) Relationship between environmental fungal contamination and the incidence of invasive aspergillosis in haematology patients. *J Hosp Infect*, **48**(3), 198–206.

Alexander, I.M. (1998) Viral hepatitis: primary care diagnosis and management. *Nurse Pract*, **23**(10), 13–14.

Alving, C.R. (2002) Design and selection of vaccine adjuvants: animal models and human trials. *Vaccine*, **20**(Suppl 3), S56–64.

Alzahrani, A.J., Vallely, P.J. & Klapper, P.E. (2000) Needlestick injuries and hepatitis B virus vaccination in health care workers. *Commun Dis Public Health*, **3**(3), 217–18.

Anaissie, E. (1992) Opportunistic mycoses in the immunocompromised host: experience at a cancer centre and review. *Clin Infect Dis*, **14**(Suppl 1), S43–53.

Anders, H.J. *et al.* (1998) Ganciclovir and foscarnet efficacy in AIDS related CMV polyradiculopathy. *J Infect*, **36**(1), 29–33.

Ang, L.H. (2000) Outbreak of hepatitis A in a special needs school in Kent 1999. *Comm Dis Public Health*, **3**(2), 139–40.

Angelico, M., Gandin, C., Pescarmona, E. *et al.* (1995) Recombinant interferon-alpha and ursodeoxycholic acid versus interferon-alpha alone in the treatment of chronic hepatitis C: a randomized clinical trial with long term follow up. *Am J Gastroenterol*, **90**(2), 263–9.

Anteby, I. *et al.* (1997) Necrotizing choroiditis-retinitis as presenting symptom of disseminated aspergillosis after lung transplantation. *Eur J Ophthalmol*, **7**(3), 294–6.

Apolonio, E.G. *et al.* (1995) Prognostic factors in HIV positive patients with CD4+ lymphocyte count below 50 microlitres. *J Infect Dis*, **171**(4), 829–36.

Arankalle, V.A. *et al.* (1998) Role of immune serum globulin in pregnant women during an epidemic of hepatitis E. *J Viral Hepat*, **5**(3), 199–204.

Arauz-Ruiz, P. *et al.* (1997) Genotype F prevails in HBV infected patients of hispanic origin in Central America and may carry the precore stop mutant. *J Med Virol*, **51**(4), 305–12.

Arauz-Ruiz, P., Norder, H., Robertson, B.H. & Magnius, L.O. (2002) Genotype H: a new Amerindian genotype of hepatitis B virus revealed in central America. *J Gen Virol*, **83**(8), 2059–73.

Ariyoshi, K., Van der Schim, M., Loeff, P. *et al.* (1998) Kaposi's sarcoma in the Gambia. *J Hum Virol*, **1**(3), 193–9.

Ariyoshi, K., Jaffar, S., Alabi, A.S. *et al.* (2000) Plasma RNA viral load predicts the rate of CD4 T cell decline and death in HIV-2 infected patients in West Africa. *AIDS*, **14**(4), 339–44.

Armstrong, D. (1995) *Listeria monocytogenes*. In: *Principles and Practice of Infectious Diseases* (eds G.L. Mandell, J.E. Bennett &

R. Dolin). Churchill Livingstone, New York, Vol. 2, Chap. 185, pp. 1880–5.

Arnow, P.M. *et al.* (1978) Pulmonary aspergillosis during hospital renovation. *Am Rev Respir Dis*, **118**, 49–53.

Arvin, A.M. (1996) Varicella-zoster virus. *Clin Microbiol Rev*, **9**(3), 361–81.

Arvin, A.M. (2002) Antiviral therapy for varicella and herpes zoster. *Semin Pediatr Infect Dis*, **13**(1), 12–21.

Arvin, A.M. & Prober, C.G. (1991) Herpes simplex viruses. In: *Manual of Clinical Microbiology*, 5th edn (eds A. Balows *et al.*) American Society for Microbiology, Washington DC, pp. 822–8.

Arvin, A.M., Moffat, J.F. & Redman, R. (1996) Varicella-zoster virus: aspects of pathogenesis and host response to natural infection and varicella vaccine. *Adv Virus Res*, **46**, 263–309.

Aston, R., Mawer, S. & Casemore, D. (1991) *Report of the Outbreak Control Group to Coordinate the Investigation and Control of the Outbreak of Cryptosporidiosis in North Humberside*. Formal report to the local authorities of Beverley and Kingston-upon-Hull, UK.

Aucken, H.M., Ganner, M., Murchan, S., Cookson, B.D. & Johnson, A.P. (2002) A new strain of epidemic methicillin resistant *Staphylococcus aureus* (EMRS 17) resistant to multiple antibiotics. *J Antimicrob Chemother*, **50**(2), 171–5.

Aweis, D., Brabin, B.J., Beeching, N.J. *et al.* (2001) Hepatitis B prevalence and risk factors for HBs Ag carriage amongst Somali households in Liverpool. *Commun Dis Public Health*, **4**(4), 247–52.

Ayliffe, G.A.J., Fraise, A.P., Eddes, A.M. & Mitchell, K. (2000) *Control of Hospital Infection. A Practical Handbook*. Arnold, London.

Aynaud, O., Poveda, J.D., Huynh, B. *et al.* (2002) Frequency of herpes simplex virus, cytomegalovirus and human papillomavirus DNA in semen. *Int J STD AIDS*, **13**(8), 547–50.

Azimi, P.H. *et al.* (1979) *Listeria monocytogenes*. Synergistic effects of ampicillin and gentamicin. *Am J Clin Pathol*, **72**, 974–7.

Aziz, E.E., Ayis, S., Gould, F.K. & Rawlins, M.D. (2001) Risk factors for the development of *Clostridium difficile* toxin-associated diarrhoea: a pilot study. *Pharmacoepidemiol Drug Saf*, **10**(4), 303–8.

Baiocchi, O.C., Colleoni, G.W., Navajas, E.V. *et al.* (2002) Impact of highly active antiretroviral therapy in the treatment of HIV-infected patients with systemic non-Hodgkins lymphoma. *Acta Oncol*, **41**(2), 192–6.

Baker, S.A. (1994) Hepatitis: protecting BMETs & CEs. *J Clin Eng*, **19**(6), 446–51.

Balayan, M.S. (1997) Epidemiology of hepatitis E virus infection. *J Viral Hepat*, **4**(3), 155–65.

Bale, J.F., Miner, L. & Patheram S.J. (2002) Congenital cytomegalovirus infection. *Curr Treat Options Neurol*, **4**(3), 225–30.

Ball, J. *et al.* (1991) Long lasting viability of HIV after patient's death. *Lancet*, **338**, 63.

Baltimore, D. & Heilman, C. (1998) HIV vaccine: prospects and challenges. *Sci Am*, **279**(1), 98–103.

Bamber, M. *et al.* (1983) Acute type A, B and non-A non-B hepatitis in a hospital population in London: clinical and epidemiological features. *Gut*, **24**(6), 561–4.

Barbagallo, J., Tager, P., Ingleton, R., Hirsch, R.J. & Weinberg, J.M. (2002) Cutaneous tuberculosis: diagnosis and treatment. *Am J Clin Dermatol*, **3**(5), 319–28.

Barbara, J. (1990) Microbiology in the national blood transfusion service. *Public Health Lab Serv Microbiol Dig*, **7**(1), 4–7.

Barber, F.D. (2001) Management of fever in neutropenic patients with cancer. *Nurs Clin North Am*, **36**(4), 631–44.

Barbut, F. & Petit, J.C. (2001) Epidemiology of *Clostridium difficile*-associated infections. *Clin Microbiol Infect*, **7**(8), 405–10.

Barin, F. *et al.* (1985) Serological evidence for virus related to Simian T-lymphotropic retrovirus III in residents of West Africa. *Lancet*, **ii**, 1387–9.

Barlow, G., Sachdev, N. & Nathwani, D. (2002) The use of adult isolation facilities in a UK infectious disease unit. *J Hosp Infect*, **50**(2), 127–32.

Barrett, S.P., Mummery, R.V. & Chattopadhyay, B. (1998) Trying to control MRSA causes more problems than it solves. *Hosp Infect*, **39**, 85–93.

Bartlet, M.S. *et al.* (1997) Detection of *Pneumocystis carinii* DNA in air samples: likely environmental risk to susceptible persons. *J Clin Microbiol*, **35**(10), 2511–13.

Bates, J. (1997) Epidemiology of vancomycin resistant enterococci in the community and the relevance of farm animals to human infection. *J Hosp Infect*, **37**, 89–101.

Battegay, M., Gust, I.D. & Feinstone, S.M. (1995) Hepatitis A virus. In: *Principles and Practice of Infectious Diseases*, 4th edn (eds G.L. Mandell, J.E. Bennett & R. Dolin). Churchill Livingstone, New York, Vol. 2, Chap. 150, pp. 1636–66.

Beaujean, D., Blok, H., Gigengack, A. *et al.* (2001) Five year surveillance of patients with communicable diseases nursed in isolation. *J Hosp Infect*, **47**, 210–17.

Beck-Sage, C. *et al.* (1992) Hospital outbreak of multidrug resistant *Mycobacterium tuberculosis* infection: factors in transmission to staff and HIV-infected patients. *JAMA*, **268**, 1280–6.

Belkin, N.L. (2002) A historical review of barrier materials. *AORN J*, **76**(4), 648–53.

Bell, D.M., Shapiro, C.N., Ciesielski, C.A. & Chamberland, M.E. (1995) Preventing bloodborne pathogen transmission from health care worker to patient. The CDC perspective. *Surg Clin North Am*, **75**(6), 1189–203.

Bennett, J.F. (1995) *Aspergillus* species. In: *Principles and Practice of Infectious Diseases*, 4th edn (eds G.L. Mandell, J.E. Bennett & R. Dolan). Churchill Livingstone, New York, Chap. 238, pp. 2306–11.

Berrington, J.E., Flood, Y.J., Albinun, M., Galloway, A. & Cant, A.J. (2000) Unsuspected *Pneumocystis carinii* pneumonia at presentation of severe primary immunodeficiency. *Arch Dis Child*, **82**(2), 144–7.

Berry, N., Ariyoshi, K., Jaffar, S. *et al.* (1998) Low peripheral blood viral HIV-2 RNA in individuals with high CD4 percentage differentiates from HIV-2 infection. *J Hum Virol*, **1**(7), 457–68.

Berry, N. *et al.* (2002) Low level viremia and high CD4 % predict normal survival in a cohort of HIV type 2 infected villagers. *AIDS Res Hum Retroviruses*, **18**(16), 1167–73.

Bhana, N., Ormrod, D., Perry, C.M. & Figgitt, D.P. (2002) Zidovudine: a review of its use in the management of vertically acquired pediatric HIV infection. *Paediatr Drugs*, **4**(8), 515–53.

Bialek, R., Binder, N., Dietz, K. *et al.* (2002) Comparison of fluorescence, antigen and PCR assays to detect *Cryptosporidium parvum* in fecal specimens. *Diagn Microbiol Infect Dis*, **43**(4), 283–8.

Bignardi, G.E. (1998) Risk factors for *Clostridium difficile* infection. *J Hosp Infect*, **40**, 1–15.

Bird, S.M., Goldberg, D.J. & Hutchinson, S.J. (2001) Projecting severe sequelae of injection-related hepatitis C virus epidemic in the UK. Part 1: critical hepatitis C and injector data. *J Epidemiol Biostat*, **6**(3), 243–65.

Birthistle, K. (1998) New combined hepatitis A and B vaccine. New vaccine is an adjunct, not an alternative to preventive behaviors. *Br Med J*, **316**(7140), 1317.

Boden, M. (1999) Contamination in moving and handling equipment. *Prof Nurse*, **14**(7), 484–7.

Bodey, G.P. & Rolston, K.V. (2001) Management of fever in neutropenic patients. *J Infect Chemother*, **7**(1), 1–9.

Boeckh, M., Leisenring, W., Riddell, S.R. *et al.* (2002) Late cytomegalovirus disease and mortality in allogeneic hematopoietic stem cell transplant recipients: importance of viral load and T-cell immunity. *Blood*, **101**(2), 407–14.

Boisson, E.V. & Rodrigues, L.C. (2002) Factors associated with HIV infection are not the same for all women. *J Epidemiol Commun Health*, **56**(2), 103–8.

Bolsen, R.J. *et al.* (1993) Examination gloves as barriers to hand contamination in clinical practice. *JAMA*, **270**(3), 350–3.

Bonten, M.J. *et al.* (1998) The role of 'colonization pressure' in the spread of vancomycin resistant enterococci: an important infection control variable. *Arch Intern Med*, **158**(10), 1127–32.

Booth, J.C. (1998) Chronic hepatitis C: the virus, its discovery and the natural history of the disease. *J Viral Hepat*, **5**(4), 213–22.

Boshoff, C. & Weiss, R. (2002) Aids-related malignancies. *Nat Rev Cancer*, **2**(5), 373–82.

Boshuizen, H.C., Neppelenbroek, S.E., Va Vliet, H. *et al.* (2001) Subclinical Legionella infection in workers near the source of a large outbreak of Legionnaires disease. *J Infect Dis*, **184**(4), 515–18.

Botsen-Moller, J. (1972) Human listeriosis, diagnostic epidemiological and clinical studies. *Acta Pathol Microbiol Scand*, **229**(Suppl), 1–57.

Boussemart, T., Baudon, J.J., Garbarg-Chenon, A. *et al.* (1998) Cytomegalovirus, pregnancy and occupational risk. *Arch Pediatr*, **5**(1), 24–6.

Bow, E.J., Laverdiere, M., Lussier, N. *et al.* (2002) Antifungal prophylaxis for severely neutropenic chemotherapy recipients: a meta analysis of randomized-controlled clinical trials. *Cancer*, **94**(12), 3230–46.

Bowden, R., Chandrasekar, P., White, M.H. *et al.* (2002) A double blind randomized controlled study of amphotericin B colloidal dispersion versus amphotericin B treatment of invasive aspergillosis in immunocompromised patients. *Clin Infect Dis*, **35**(4), 367–9.

Bowler, I.C.J.W. *et al.* (1998) Guidelines for the management of patients colonised or infected with vancomycin resistant enterococci. *J Hosp Infect*, **39**, 75–82.

Boyce, J.M. (2001) MRSA patients: proven methods to treat colonization and infection. *J Hosp Infect*, **48**(Suppl A), S9–14.

Boyce, J.M. *et al.* (1997) Environmental contamination due to methicillin resistant *Staphylococcus aureus*: possible infection control implications. *Infect Control Hosp Epidemiol*, **18**(9), 622–7.

Brabender, W., Hinthorn, D.R. & Asher, M. (1993) *Legionella pneumophila* wound infection. *JAMA*, **250**, 3091–5.

Bradley, C.R. & Fraise, A.P. (1996) Heat and chemical resistance of enterococci. *J Hosp Infect*, **34**, 191–6.

Brandt, L., Feino-Cunha, J., Weinreich-Olsen, A. *et al.* (2002) Failure of the *Mycobacterium bovis* BCG vaccine: some species of environmental mycobacteria block multiplication of BCG and induction of protective immunity to tuberculosis. *Infect Immun*, **709**(2), 672–8.

Branger, C. *et al.* (1997) Epidemiology typing of extended-spectrum beta-lactamase producing *Klebsiella* pneumoniae isolates responsible for five outbreaks in a university hospital. *J Hosp Infect*, **36**(1), 23–36.

Brazier, J.S. (1998) The diagnosis of *Clostridium difficile* associated disease. *J Antimicrob Chemother*, **41**(Suppl C), 29–40.

Brazier, J.S. & Duerden, B.I. (1998) Guidelines for optimal surveillance of *Clostridium difficile* infection in hospitals. *Commun Dis Public Health*, **1**(4), 229–30.

Breathnach, A.S. *et al.* (1998) An outbreak of multi drug resistant tuberculosis in a London teaching hospital. *J Hosp Infect*, **39**(2), 111–17.

Brennen, C., Wagener, M.M. & Muder, R.R. (1998) Vancomycin resistant *Enterococcus faecium* in a long term care facility. *Am Geriatr Soc*, **46**(2), 157–60.

British Committee for Standards in Haematology (BSC) (1995) Guidelines on the provision of facilities for the care of adult patients with haematological malignancies (including leukaemia and lymphoma and severe bone marrow failure). *Clin Lab Haem*, **17**, 3–10.

Brocklehurst, P. & Volmink, J. (2002) Antiretrovirals for reducing the risk of mother-to-child transmission of HIV infection. *Cochrane Database Syst Rev*, (2), CD003510.

Brook, M.G., Taylor, G.P., Dale, A., Lyall, E.G. & Tomlinson, D. (2000) Management of HIV and pregnancy in England's North Thames region 1999: a survey of practice in 21 hospitals. *HIV Med*, **1**(3), 143–7.

Brook, M.G., Dale, A., Tomlinson, D., Waterworth, C., Daniels, D. & Forster, G. (2001) Adherence to highly active antiretroviral therapy in the real world: experience of twelve English HIV units. *AIDS Patient Care STDs*, **15**(9), 491–4.

Brooks, M.G. (1998) Sexual transmission and prevention of the hepatitis viruses A–E and G. *Sex Transm Infect*, **74**(6), 395–8.

Brooks, S. *et al.* (1998) Reduction in vancomycin resistant enterococcus and *Clostridium difficile* infections following change to tympanic thermometers. *Infect Control Hosp Epidemiol*, **19**(5), 333–6.

Broomfield, S.F. (2002) Preventing infection in the home. *Br J Infect Control*, **3**(3), 14–17.

Bruce, J. & Brysiewicz, P. (2002) Ebola fever: the African emergency. *Int J Trauma Nurs*, **8**(2), 36–41.

Bryant, P., Morley, C., Garland, S. & Curtis, N. (2002) Cytomegalovirus transmission from breast milk in premature babies: does it matter? *Arch Dis Child Fetal Neonatal Ed*, **87**(2), F75–7.

Burke, J.P. & Pestotnik, S.L. (1996) Breaking the chain of antibiotic resistance. *Curr Opin Infect Dis*, **9**, 253–5.

Burnard, P. (1992) Nurse training needs in AIDS counselling. *Nurs Stand*, **6**(34), 34–9.

Burnie, J.P. & Loudon, K.W. (1997) Ciprofloxacin resistant *Staphylococcus epidermidis* and hands. *Lancet*, **349**, 649–50.

Butler, J.C. *et al.* (1999) Pneumococcal vaccines: history, current status, and future directions. *Am J Med*, **107**(1), 69–76S.

Byers, K.E. *et al.* (1998) Disinfection of hospital rooms contaminated with vancomycin resistant *Enterococcus faecium*. *Infect Control Hosp Epidemiol*, **19**(4), 261–4.

Byrne, D.J., Phillips, G., Napier, A. & Cschieri, A. (1991) The effect of whole body disinfection on intraoperative wound contamination. *J Hosp Infect*, **1**(2), 45–8.

Calandra, T. (2000) Practical guide to host defence mechanisms and the predominant infections encountered in immunocompromised patients. In: *Management of Infections in Immunocompromised Patients* (eds M.P. Glauser & P.A. Pizzo). W.B. Saunders, London.

Callaghan, I. (1998a) Bacterial contamination of nurse's uniform: a study. *Nurs Stand*, **13**(1), 37–42.

Callaghan, I. (1998b) Implementing change: influencing the process. *Nurs Stand*, **13**(2), 37–42.

Callister, M.E., Barringer, J., Thanabalasingam, S.T., Gair, R. & Davidson, R.N. (2002) Pulmonary tuberculosis among political asylum seekers screened at Heathrow airport London 1995–1999. *Thorax*, **57**(2), 152–6.

Campbell, T. (1999) Feelings of oncology patients about being nursed in protective isolation as a consequence of cancer chemotherapy treatment. *J Adv Nurs*, **30**(2), 439–47.

Capita, R., Alvarez-Astorga, M., Alonso-Calleja, C. *et al.* (2003) Occurrence of Salmonellae in retail carcasses and their products in Spain. *Int J Food Microbiol*, **81**(2), 169–73.

Carcao, M.D. *et al.* (1998) Sequential use of intravenous and oral acyclovir in the therapy of varicella in immunocompromised children. *Pediatr Infect Dis J*, **17**(7), 626–31.

Carlon, C.P., Klenerman, P., Edwards, A. *et al.* (1994) Heterosexual transmission of HIV type 1 variants associated with zidovudine resistance. *J Infect Dis*, **169**, 411–15.

Carter, C.D. & Barr, B.A. (1997) Infection control issues in construction and renovation. *Infect Control Hosp Epidemiol*, **18**(8), 587–96.

Casemore, D.P. (1987) Cryptosporidiosis PHLS. *Microbiol Dig*, **4**, 1–5.

Casemore, D.P. (1998) *Cryptosporidium* and the safety of our water supplies. *Commun Dis Public Health*, **1**(4), 218–19.

Casemore, D.P., Gardner, C.A. & O'Mahony, C.O. (1994) Cryptosporidial infection, with special reference to nosocomial transmission of *Cryptosporidium parvum*: a review. *Folia Parasitol*, **41**, 17–21.

Casewell, M.W. (1982) The role of multiply resistant coliforms in hospital acquired infection. *Recent Adv Infect*, **2**, 31–50.

Casewell, M.W. (1995) New threats to the control of methicillin-resistant *Staphylococcus aureus*. *J Hosp Infect*, **30**(Suppl), 465–71.

Casey, J.L. *et al.* (1996) Hepatitis B virus (HBV)/hepatitis D virus coinfection in outbreaks of acute hepatitis in the Peruvian Amazon basin: the role of HDV genotype III and HBV genotype F. *J Infect Dis*, **174**(5), 920–6.

Casper, C. & Wald, A. (2002) Condom use and the prevention of genital herpes acquisition. *Herpes*, **9**(1), 10–14.

Centers for Disease Control (1978) Legionnaires' disease, diagnosis and management. *Ann Intern Med*, **88**, 363–5.

Centers for Disease Control (1986) Apparent transmission of human T-lymphotropic type 111/lymphadenopathy associated virus from a child to a mother providing health care. *MMWR Morb Mortal Wkly Rep*, **35**, 76–9.

Centers for Disease Control (1990a) Protection against viral hepatitis. *MMWR Morb Mortal Wkly Rep*, **39**(RR2), 1–26.

Centers for Disease Control (1990b) Nosocomial transmission of multi-drug resistant tuberculosis to health care workers and

HIV positive patients in an urban hospital – Florida. *MMWR Morb Mortal Wkly Rep*, **39**, 718–22.

Centers for Disease Control (1992) Revised classification system for HIV infection and expanded surveillance case definition for AIDS among adolescents and adults. *MMWR Morb Mortal Wkly Rep*, **41**, 1–19.

Centers for Disease Control (1993) HIV transmission between children at home. Public Health Laboratory Service Communicable Disease Surveillance Centre, London. *Commun Dis Rep*, **3**(52), 1.

Centers for Disease Control (1998a) Hepatitis A vaccination of men who have sex with men. Atlanta Georgia, 1996–1997. *MMWR Morb Mortal Wkly Rep*, **47**(34), 708–11.

Centers for Disease Control (1998b) Recommendations for prevention and control of tuberculosis among foreign-born persons. Report of the working group on tuberculosis among foreign born persons. *MMWR Morb Mortal Wkly Rep*, **47**(RR-16), 1–29.

Centers for Disease Control (1998c) Prevention and treatment of tuberculosis among patients infected with HIV: principles of therapy and revised recommendations. *MMWR Morb Mortal Wkly Rep*, **47**(RR-20), 1–51.

Centers for Disease Control (2002) *Human Immunodeficiency Virus Type 2*. National Center for HIV, STD and TB Prevention, Washington DC.

Chaisson, R. (1993) Mycobacterial infections and AIDS. *Curr Opin Infect Dis*, **6**, 237–43.

Chaisson, R.E. *et al.* (1998) Impact of opportunistic disease on survival in patients with HIV infection. *AIDS*, **12**(1), 29–33.

Chalmers, J. (2002) The criminalisation of HIV transmission. *J Med Ethics*, **28**(3), 160–3.

Chalmers, R. & Elwin, K. (2000) Implications and importance of genotyping cryptosporidium. *Commun Dis Public Health*, **3**(3), 155–8.

Chanbancherd, P. *et al.* (2000) HIV-2 infection in Thailand. *Asian Pac J Allergy Immunol*, **18**(4), 245–8.

Chandiok, S. (1992) The GP's role in the management of viral STDs. *J Sex Health*, **1**(1), 32–3.

Chang, J. *et al.* (1995) Listeriosis in bone marrow transplant recipients: incidence, clinical features, and treatment. *Clin Infect Dis*, **21**(5), 1289–90.

Chapman, S.J. (1998) Varicella in pregnancy. *Semin Perinatol*, **22**(4), 339–46.

Chattopadhyay, B. (2001) Control of infection wards: are they worthwhile? *J Hosp Infect*, **47**(2), 88–90.

Chauhan, A. *et al.* (1998) Role of long-persisting human hepatitis E virus antibodies in protection. *Vaccine*, **16**(7), 755–6.

Chearskul, S., Chotpitayasunondh, T., Simonds, R.J. *et al.* (2002) Survival disease manifestations and early predictors of disease progression among children with perinatal human immunodeficiency virus infection in Thailand. *Pediatrics*, **110**(2 pt 1) 25.

Chen, S.K. *et al.* (1994) Evaluation of single use mask and respirators for protection of health care workers against mycobacterial aerosols. *Am J Infect Control*, **22**(2), 65–74.

Chen, T.M., George, S., Woodruff, C.A. & Hsu, S. (2002) Clinical manifestations of varicella-zoster virus infection. *Dermatol Clin*, **20**(2), 267–82.

Chene, G. *et al.* (1997) Long term survival in patients with advanced immunodeficiency. *AIDS*, **11**(2), 209–16.

Chippindale, S. & French, L. (2001) HIV counselling and the psychosocial management of patients with HIV or AIDS. *Br Med J*, **322**(7301), 1533–5.

Chomarat, M. (2000) Resistance of bacteria in urinary tract infections. *Int J Antimicrob Agents*, **16**(4), 483–7.

Ciocca, M. (2000) Clinical course and consequences of hepatitis A infection. *Vaccine* **18**(Suppl 1), 71–4.

Clarke, S., Keenan, E., Ryan, M., Barry, M. & Mulcahy, F. (2002) Directly observed antiretroviral therapy for injecting drug users with HIV infection. *AIDS Read*, **12**(7), 312–16.

Clavel, F. *et al.* (1986) Isolation of a new human retrovirus from West African patients with AIDS. *Science*, **233**, 343–6.

Clayson, E.T. *et al.* (1998) Association of hepatitis E virus with an outbreak of hepatitis at a military training camp in Nepal. *J Med Virol*, **54**(3), 178–82.

Clutterbuck, D.J., Gorman, D., McMillan, A., Lewis, R. & Macintyre, C.C. (2001) Substance use and unsafe sex amongst homosexual men in Edinburgh. *AIDS Care*, **13**(4), 527–35.

Cody, S.H., Nainan, O.V., Garfein, R.S. *et al.* (2002) Hepatitis C virus transmission from an anethesiologist to a patient. *Arch Int Med*, **162**(3), 345–50.

Cohen, H.A., Kitai, E., Levy, I. & Ben-Amitai, D. (2002) Handwashing patterns in two dermatology clinics. *Dermatology*, **205**(4), 358–61.

Cohen, M.Z., Ley, C. & Tarzian, A.J. (2001) Isolation in blood and marrow transplantation. *West J Nurs Res*, **23**(6), 592–609.

Coker, R. (1998) Lessons from New York's tuberculosis epidemic, *Br Med J*, **317**, 616.

Colak, D., Ogunc, D., Gunseren, F., Velipasaoglu, S., Aktekin, M.R. & Gultekin, M. (2002) Seroprevalence of antibodies to hepatitis A and E viruses in pediatric groups in Turkey. *Acta Microbiol Immunol Hung*, **49**(1), 93–7.

Colebunders, R. & Lambert, M.L. (2002) Management of co-infection with HIV and TB. *Br Med J*, **324**(7341), 802–3.

Collins, C., Upright, C. & Aleksich, J. (1989) Reverse isolation: what patients perceive. *Oncol Nurse Forum*, **16**(5), 675–9.

Colombo, C., Giger, H., Grote, J. *et al.* (2002) Impact of teaching interventions on nurse compliance with hand disinfection. *J Hosp Infect*, **51**(1), 69–72.

Communicable Disease Report (CDR) (2002) First report of the Department of Health's mandatory MRSA Bacteremia Surveillance Scheme in acute NHS Trusts in England April to September 2001. *CDC Weekly*, **12**(6), 1–15.

Communicable Disease Surveillance Centre (2002) *HIV and AIDS in the UK in 2001*. Public Health Laboratory Service, London.

Consensus Statement (1999) EASL international consensus conference on hepatitis C. *J Hepatol*, **30**, 956–61.

Cook, S.A., Blair, I. & Tyers, M. (2000) Outbreak of tuberculosis associated with a church. *Commun Dis Public Health*, **3**(3), 181–3.

Cooke, N.J. (1985) Treatment of tuberculosis. *Br Med J*, **291**, 497–8.

Cookson, B. (1997) How to resist? *Health Serv J*, 30 October, 9–11.

Cooper, J. (1991) Positive discrimination. *Lab Pract*, **40**(1), 16–17.

Corwin, A.L. *et al.* (1997) Short report: evidence of worldwide transmission of hepatitis G virus. *Am J Trop Med Hyg*, **57**(4), 455–6.

Cotterill, S., Evans, R. & Fraise, A.P. (1996) An unusual source of an outbreak of methicillin resistant *Staphylococcus aureus* on an intensive therapy unit. *J Hosp Infect*, **32**(3), 207–16.

Couillard-Getreuer, D.L. (1982) Herpes zoster in the immunocompromised patient. *Cancer Nurs*, **10**, 361–70.

Cox, R.A. & Conquest, C. (1997) Strategies for the management of health care staff colonized with epidemic methicillin resistant *Staphylococcus aureus*. *J Hosp Infect*, **35**(2), 117–27.

Cox, R.A. et al. (1995) A major outbreak of methicillin-resistan *Staphylococcus aureus* caused by a new phage-type (EMRSA 16). *J Hosp Infect*, **29**, 87–106.

Coyle, P.V. et al. (2002) Emergence of herpes simplex type 1 as the main cause of recurrent genital ulcerative disease in women in Northern Ireland. *J Clin Virol*, **27**(1), 22–9.

Crawford, D.H. (2001) Biology and disease association of Epstein–Barr virus. *Phil Trans R Soc Lond B Biol Sci*, **356**(1408), 461–73.

Crawford, D.H., Swerdlow, A.J., Higgins, C. et al. (2002) Sexual history and Epstein–Barr virus infection. *J Infect Dis*, **186**(6), 731–6.

Croner's Health Service Risk Management and Special Report (1998) *Infection Control Isolation Precautions*. Croner Publications, London.

Crow, W.C. & Ng, H.S. (1997) Hepatitis C, E and G virus – three new viruses identified by molecular biology techniques in the last decade. *Ann Acad Med Singapore*, **26**(5), 682–6.

Crowcroft, N. et al. (1996) Methicillin resistant *Staphylococcus aureus*: investigations of a hospital outbreak using a case–control study. *J Hosp Infect*, **34**, 301–9.

Crowcroft, N.S. & Catchpole, M. (2002) Mortality from methicillin resistant *Staphylococcus aureus* in England and Wales: analysis of death certificates. *Br Med J*, **325**(7377), 1390–1.

Crowcroft, N.S., Walsh, B., Davison, K.L. & Gungabissoon, U. (2001) Guidelines for the control of hepatitis A virus infection. *Commun Dis Public Health*, **4**(3), 213–27.

Crowe, H.M. (1994) Forum: perspective on hepatitis. *Asepsis*, **16**(2), 13–17.

Cruchley, A.T., Williams, D.M., Niedobitek, G. & Young, L.S. (1997) Epstein–Barr virus: biology and disease. *Oral Dis*, 3(Suppl 1), S156–63.

Crum, N.F. (2002) Update on *Listeria monocytogenes* infection. *Curr Gastroenterol Rep*, **4**(4), 287–96.

Cunha, A.A., Marin, L.J., Aquino, V.H. & Figueiredo, L.T. (2002) Diagnosis of cytomegalovirus infections by qualitative and quantitative PCR in HIV infected patients. *Rev Inst Med Trop Sao Paulo*, **44**(3), 127–32.

Cunha, B.A. (1998) Nosocomial diarrhoea. *Crit Care Clin*, **14**(2), 329–38.

Current, W.L. (1987) *Cryptosporidium*: its biology and potential for environmental transmission. *CRC Crit Rev Environ Control*, **17**, 21–51.

Custovic, A. et al. (1998) Domestic allergens in public places. *Clin Exp Allergy*, **28**(1), 53–9.

Cuthbert, J.A. (2001) Hepatitis A: old and new. *Clin Microbiol Rev*, **14**(1), 38–58.

Dales, D.C. & Liles, C. (1998) How many neutrophils are enough? *Lancet*, **351**(9118), 1752–3.

Dance, D.A.B. (1987) A hospital outbreak caused by a chlorhexidine and antibiotic resistant *Proteus mirabilis*. *J Hosp Infect*, **10**, 10–16.

Dancer, S., Raeside, J. & Boothman, M. (2002) Environmental organisms from different hospital wards. *Br J Infect Control*, **3**(94), 10–14.

Dane, D.S. et al. (1970) Virus-like particle in serum of patients with Australian antigen-associated hepatitis. *Lancet*, **i**, 695–8.

Dantuma, N.P. & Masucci, M.G. (2003) The ubiquitin/proteasome system in Epstein–Barr virus latency and associated malignancies. *Semin Cancer Biol*, **13**(1), 69–76.

Darville, J.M., Ley, B.E., Roome, A.P. & Foot, A.B. (1998) Acyclovir-resistant herpes simplex virus infections in a bone marrow transplant population. *Bone Marrow Transplant*, **22**(6), 587–9.

Davidhizar, R. & Dunn, C. (1998) Nutrition and the client with AIDS. *J Pract Nurs*, **48**(1), 16–25.

De la Hoz, R.E., Stephens, G. & Sherlock, C. (2002) Diagnosis and treatment approaches of CMV infections in adult patients. *J Clin Virol*, **25**(Suppl 2), S1–12.

De Medina, M. et al. (1998) Prevalence of hepatitis C and G virus infection in chronic hemodialysis patients. *Am J Kidney Dis*, **31**(2), 224–6.

De Schryver, A., Glazemakers, J., De Bacquwe, D. et al. (1999) Risk of cytomegalovirus infection among educators and health care personnel serving mentally disabled children. *J Infect*, **38**(1), 36–40.

Dealler, S. (2002) Prevention of cross infection in variant Creutzfeldt Jakob Disease [v CJD]. *Br J Infect Control*, **2**(1), 5–8.

Dealler, S. & Lacey, R. (1991) Beef and bovine spongiform encephalopathy: the risk persists. *Nutr Health*, **7**(3), 117–33.

DeBock, R. & Middelheim, A.Z. (2000) Febrile neutropenia in allogeneic transplantation. *Int J Antimicrob Agents*, **16**(2), 177–80.

Deinhardt, F.D. et al. (1985) Immunization against hepatitis B. Report of a WHO meeting on viral hepatitis in Europe. *J Med Virol*, **17**, 209–17.

Delaquis, S., Stewart, S., Cazaux, S. et al. (2002) Survival and growth of *Listeria monocytogenes* and *Escherichia coli* 0157:H7 in ready to eat iceberg lettuce washed in warm chlorinated water. *J Food Prot*, **65**(3), 459–64.

Dennesen, P.J., Bonten, M.J. & Weinstein, R.A. (1998) Multi-resistant bacteria as a hospital epidemic problem. *Ann Med*, **30**(2), 176–85.

Department of Employment – Health and Safety Executive (1987) *AIDS and Employment*. Central Office of Information, London.

Deshpande, L.M., Fix, A.M., Pfaller, M.A. & Jones, R.N. (2002) Emerging elevated mupirocin resistance rates among Staphylococcus isolates in the SENTRY Antimicrobial Surveillance Program[2000]: correlation of results from disk diffusion, Etest and reference dilution methods. *Diagn Microbiol Infect Dis*, **42**(4), 283–90.

Dezube, B.J. (2002) Management of AIDS-related Kaposi's sarcoma: advances in target discovery and treatment. *Expert Rev Anticancer Ther*, **2**(2), 193–200.

Dharan, S., Mourouga, P., Copin, P. et al. (1999) Routine disinfection of patients' environment surfaces. Myth or reality? *J Hosp Infect*, **42**(2), 113–17.

Dhedin, N. et al. (1998) Reverse seroconversion of hepatitis B after allogeneic bone marrow transplantation: a retrospective study of 37 patients with pretransplant anti HBs and anti HBc. *Transplantation*, **66**(5), 616–19.

DiCarlo, R.P. & Martin, D.H. (1997) The clinical diagnosis of genital ulcer disease in men. *Clin Infect Dis*, **25**(2), 292–8.

Dick, L. (1998) Travel medicine: helping patients prepare for trips abroad. *Am Fam Physician*, **58**(2), 383–98.

Dietze, B., Rath, A., Wendt, C. & Martiny, H. (2001) Survival of MRSA on sterile goods packaging. *J Hosp Infect*, **49**(4), 255–61.

Dienstag, J.L. (1983) Non-A non-B hepatitis recognition epidemiology and clinical features. *Gastroenterology*, **85**, 439–62.

Dienstag, J.L. *et al.* (1977) Non-A non-B post transfusion hepatitis. *Lancet*, **i**, 560–2.

Diosi, P. (1997) Cytomegalovirus (CMV) in cervical secretions and breast milk. A thirty year perspective. *Roum Arch Microbiol Immunol*, **56**(3–4), 165–78.

Di Perri, G. *et al.* (1992) Transmission of HIV associated tuberculosis of health care workers. *Lancet*, **340**(8820), 682.

Djuretic, T., Herbert, J., Drobniewski, F. *et al.* (2002) Antibiotic resistant tuberculosis in the United Kingdom 1993–1999. *Thorax*, **57**(6), 477–82.

Do, A.N. *et al.* (1998) Risk factors for early recurrent *Clostridium difficile* associated diarrhoea. *Clin Infect Dis*, **26**(4), 954–9.

Doebbeling, B.N., Li, N. & Wenzel, R.P. (1993) An outbreak of hepatitis A among health care workers: risk factors for transmission. *Am J Public Health*, **83**(12), 1679–84.

Doerholt, K., Sharland, M., Ball, C. & DuMont, G. (2002) Paediatric antiretroviral therapy audit in South London. *HIV Med*, **3**(1), 44–8.

DoH (1985) *The Public Health (Infectious Diseases) Regulations 1985 (HC(85)17) (LAC(85)10)*. Stationery Office, London.

DoH (1990) *Advisory Committee on Dangerous Pathogens. HIV. The Causative Agent of AIDS and Related Conditions. Second Revision of Guidelines HN(90)4*. Stationery Office, London.

DoH (1990) *Report of the Group of Experts on* Cryptosporidium *in Water Supplies* (Chairman Sir John Badenock). Stationery Office, London.

DoH (1991) *AIDS and HIV-Infected Health Care Workers: Occupational Guidance for Health Care Workers, their Physicians and Employers*. Stationery Office, London.

DoH (1993) *AIDS-HIV Infected Health Care Workers: Practical Guidance on Notifying Patients*. Stationery Office, London.

DoH (1995a) *General Food Hygiene Regulations*. Stationery Office, London.

DoH (1995b) *Hepatitis C and Blood Transfusion Look Back. PL CMO (95)1*. Stationery Office, London.

DoH (1995c) *Hospital Infection Control. Guidance on the Control of Infection in Hospitals*. Lancashire Health Publications Unit, 2383 IP 25K, February 1995.

DoH (1996a) *Guidelines for Pre-Test Discussion on HIV Testing*. Stationery Office, London.

DoH (1996b) Guidelines on the control of infection in residential and nursing homes. Stationery Office, London.

DoH (1996c) *Immunisation Against Infectious Disease*. Stationery Office, London.

DoH (1997) *Guidelines on Post-Exposure Prophylaxis for Health Care Workers Occupationally Exposed to HIV*. PL/CO[97]. Stationery Office, London.

DoH (1998a) *Management and Control of Viral Haemorrhagic Fevers. Summary of Guidance from the Advisory Committee on Dangerous Pathogens*. 12491 HP 14k 1P Mar 98 (MUL). Stationery Office, London.

DoH (1998b) *The Prevention and Control of Tuberculosis in the United Kingdom. HSC 1998/196*. Stationery Office, London.

DoH (2000a) *United Kingdom Antimicrobial Resistance Strategy and Action Plan*. Department of Health, London.

DoH (2000b) *Further Background Information for Occupational Health Departments*. Department of Health, London.

DoH (2000c) *Creutzfeldt–Jakob Disease. Guidance for Health Care Workers*. Department of Health, London.

DoH (2000d) *Hepatitis B Infected Health Care Workers*. Department of Health, London.

DoH (2001a) Standard principles for preventing hospital-acquired infections. *J Hosp Infect*, **47**(Suppl), S21–37.

DoH (2001b) *Prevalence of HIV and Hepatitis Infections in the United Kingdom 2000*. Department of Health, London.

DoH (2001c) *Further Advice on vCJD, Tonsillectomy and Issues Relating to the Introduction of Single Use Instruments*. Department of Health, London.

DoH (2001d) *Risk Assessment for Transmission of vCJD via Surgical Instruments. A Modelling Approach and Numerical Scenarios*. Department of Health, London.

DoH (2002a) *HIV Infected Health Care Workers. A Consultative Paper on the Management and Patient Notification*. Department of Health, London.

DoH (2002b) *Guidance for Clinical Health Care Workers. Protection against Infection with Bloodborne Viruses*. Department of Health, London.

DoH (2002c) *Hepatitis C for England Strategy*. HMSO, London.

DoH (2002d) *Hepatitis C Infected Health Care Workers*. HMSO, London.

DoH (2002e) *Getting Ahead of the Curve. A Strategy for Combatting Infectious Diseases (Including Other Aspects of Health Promotion)*. HMSO, London.

Dolin, R. *et al.* (1978) Herpes zoster-varicella infection in immunosuppressed patients. *Ann Intern Med*, **89**, 375–88.

Dominguez, J., Gali, N., Blanco, S. *et al.* (2001) Assessment of a new test to detect legionella urinary antigen for the diagnosis of Legionnaires disease. *Diag Microbiol Infect Dis*, **41**(4), 199–203.

D'Souza, A.L., Rajkumar, C., Cooke, J. & Bulpitt, C.J. (2002) Probiotics in prevention of antibiotic diarrhoea: meta-analysis. *Br Med J*, **324**(7350), 1361–7.

Dubé, M. & Sattler, F.R. (1993) Prevention and treatment of opportunistic infections. *Curr Opin Infect Dis*, **6**, 230–6.

Duckworth, G. (1990) Revised guidelines for the control of epidemic methicillin-resistant *Staphylococcus aureus*. *J Hosp Infect*, **16**, 351–77.

Duerden, B.I. *et al.* (1994) Report of the PHLS *Clostridium difficile* working party. *Public Health Lab Serv Microbiol Dig*, **11**(1), 22–4.

Duff, P. (1998) Hepatitis in pregnancy. *Semin Perinatal*, **22**(4), 277–83.

Duffy, T. & Moore, C. (2000) Health visitors' knowledge and attitudes relating to HIV and AIDS. *Br J Commun Nurs*, **5**(9), 422–30.

Duquette-Petersen, J., Francis, M.E., Dohnalek, L., Skinner, R. & Dudas, P. (1999) The role of protective clothing in infection prevention in patients undergoing autologous bone marrow transplantation. *Oncol Nurs Forum*, **26**(8), 1319–24.

Dutz, W. (1970) *Pneumocystis carinii* pneumonia. *Path Ann*, **5**, 309.

Dwyer, D.E. & Cunningham, A.L. (2002) Herpes simplex and varicella-zoster virus infections. *Med J Aust*, **177**(5), 267–73.

Echevarria, J.M., Casas, I. & Martinez-Martin, A. (1997) Infection of the nervous system caused by varicella zoster virus: a review. *Intervirology*, **40**(2–3), 72–84.

Eddleston, A. (1990) Modern vaccines. Hepatitis. *Lancet*, **335**, 1142–5.

Edeh, J. & Spalding, P. (2000) Screening for HIV, HBV and HCV markers among drug users in treatment: I. Rural south-east England. *J Public Health*, **22**(4), 531–9.

Editorial (1990) The A to F of viral hepatitis. *Lancet*, **336**, 1158–60.

Edmond, M. *et al.* (1990) Effects of bedside needle disposal units on needle recapping frequency and needlestick injury. *Can Intraven Nurs Assoc J*, **6**(1), 10–11.

Ejidokun, O.O., Ramaiah, S. & Sandhu, S. (1998) A cluster of tuberculosis cases in a family. *Commun Dis Public Health*, **1**(4), 259–62.

Ejidokun, O.O., Killalea, D., Cooper, M. *et al.* (2000) Four linked outbreaks of *Salmonella enteritidis* phage type 4 infection: the continuing egg threat. *Commun Dis Public Health*, **3**(2), 95–100.

Ellett, M.L. (1999) Hepatitis A, B, and D. *Gastroenterol Nurs*, **22**(6), 236–44.

Ellis, M.E. (1990) Non-A non-B hepatitis; quandaries in serological testing and treatment. *J Infect*, **21**, 235–40.

Ellison, B.J., Downey, A.B. & Duesberg, P.H. (1995) HIV as a surrogate marker for drug use: a re-analysis of the San Francisco Men's Health Study. *Genetica*, **95**(1–3), 165–71.

Engelhart, S., Glasmacher, A., Exner, M. & Kramer, M.H. (2002a) Surveillance for nosocomial infections and fever of unknown origin among adult hematology–oncology patients. *Infect Control Hosp Epidemiol*, **23**(5), 244–8.

Engelhart, S., Loock, A., Skutlarek, D. *et al.* (2002b) Occurrence of toxigenic *Aspergillus versicolor* isolates and sterigmatocystin in carpet dust from damp indoor environment. *Appl Environ Microbiol*, **68**(8), 3886–90.

Epstein, M.A. (2001) Reflections on Epstein–Barr virus: some recently resolved old uncertainties. *J Infect*, **43**(2), 111–15.

Erb, P. & Matter, L. (1998) HIV diagnosis 1998. *Ther Umsch*, **55**(5), 279–84.

Erjavec, Z. & Verweij, P.E. (2002) Recent progress in the diagnosis of fungal infections in the immunocompromised host. *Drug Resist Update*, **5**(1), 3–10.

Errico, A., Rasero, L., Bertelli, A. & Tellarini, G. (1999) Survey of measures for the prevention of infection in bone marrow transplantation centers. *Assist Inferm Ric*, **18**(2), 80–6.

Esu-Williams, E., Mulango-Kabeya, C., Takena, H. *et al.* (1997) Seroprevalence of HIV-1, HIV-2 and HIV-1 group 0 in Nigeria: evidence for a growing increase of HIV infection. *J AIDS Hum Retroviral*, **16**(3), 204–10.

Evans, B.G. *et al.* (1991) HIV 2 in the United Kingdom. A review. *Commun Dis Rep*, **1**(2), R19–232.

Evans, H.S. *et al.* (1998) General outbreaks of infectious intestinal disease in England and Wales, 1995–1996. *Commun Dis Public Health*, **1**(3), 165–71.

Eveillard, M., Tramier, B., Schmit, J.L. *et al.* (2001) Evaluation of the contribution of isolation precautions in prevention and control of multi-resistant bacteria in a teaching hospital. *J Hosp Infect*, **47**(2), 116–24.

Eveillard, M., Ernst, C., Cuviller, S. *et al.* (2002) Prevalence of methicillin resistant *Staphylococcus aureus* carriage at the time of admission in two acute geriatric wards. *J Hosp Infect*, **50**(2), 122–6.

Farinha, N.J., Razli, K.A., Holzel, H., Morgan, G. & Novelli, V.M. (2000) Tuberculosis of the central nervous system in children: a 20 year survey. *J Infect*, **41**(1), 61–8.

Farrington, M. & Pascoe, G. (2001) Risk management and infection control – time to get our priorities right in the United Kingdom. *J Hosp Infect*, **47**(1), 19–24.

Farrington, M., Trundle, C., Redpath, C. & Anderson, I. (2000) Effects of nursing workload on different methicillin resistant *Staphylococcus aureus* control strategy. *J Hosp Infect*, **46**(2), 118–22.

Farrow, L.J. *et al.* (1981) Non-A non-B hepatitis in west London. *Lancet*, **i**, 982–4.

Fayer, R., Trout, J.M., Xiao, L. *et al.* (2001) *Cryptosporidium canis* n. sp. from domestic dogs. *J Parasitol*, **87**(6), 1415–22.

Fekety, R. & Shah, A.B. (1993) Diagnosis and treatment of *Clostridium difficile* colitis. *JAMA*, **269**(1), 71–5.

Ferroni, A. *et al.* (1998) Outbreak of nosocomial urinary tract infections due to *Pseudomonas aeruginosa* in a paediatric surgical unit associated with tap water contamination. *J Hosp Infect*, **39**, 301–7.

Fidouh-Houhou, N., Duval, X., Bissuel, F. *et al.* (2001) Salivary cytomegalovirus (CMV) shedding, glycoprotein B genotype distribution, and CMV disease in human immunodeficiency virus-seropositive patients. *Clin Infect Dis*, **33**(8), 1406–11.

Field, B.S., Benson, R.F. & Besser, R.E. (2002) Legionella and Legionnaires disease: 25 years of investigation. *Clin Microbiol Rev*, **15**(3), 506–26.

Fillet, A.M. (2002) Prophylaxis of herpesvirus infections in immunocompetent and immunocompromised older patients. *Drugs Aging*, **19**(5), 343–54.

Finch, R. (1988) Minimizing the risk of Legionnaires' disease. *Br Med J*, **296**, 1343–5.

Flaherty, J.P. & Weinstein, R.A. (1996) Nosocomial infection caused by antibiotic-resistant organisms in the intensive-care unit. *Infect Control Hosp Epidemiol*, **17**(4), 236–48.

Flowers, P., Hart, G.J., Williamson, L.M., Frankis, J.S. & Der, G.J. (2002) Does bar-based, peer-led sexual health promotion have a community-level effect amongst gay men in Scotland? *Int J STD AIDS*, **13**(2), 102–8.

Forns, X. & Bukh, J. (1998) Methods for determining the hepatitis C virus genotype. *Viral Hep Rev*, **4**(1), 1–19.

Foti, G., Hyeraci, M., Kunkar, A. *et al.* (2002) Cytomegalovirus infection in the adult. *Minerva Med*, **93**(2), 109–17.

Fournier, S., Dubrou, S., Liguory, O. *et al.* (2002) Detection of microsporidia, cryptosporidia and Giardia in swimming pools: a one-year prospective study. *FEMS Immunol Med Microbiol*, **33**(3), 209–13.

Fowler, M.G. & Newell, M.L. (2002) Breast-feeding and HIV-1 transmission in resource-limited settings. *J AIDS*, **30**(2), 230–9.

Fox, J.A. (1996) Hepatitis B and the theatre nurse. *Br J Theatre Nurse*, **6**(7), 26–9.

Franzin, L., Scolfaro, C., Cabodi, D., Valera, M. & Povo, P.A. (2001) Legionella pneumophila pneumonia in a newborn after water birth: a new mode of transmission. *Clin Infect Dis*, **33**(9), 103–4.

Fraser, D.W. *et al.* (1977) Legionnaires' disease: description of an epidemic of pneumonia. *N Engl J Med*, **297**, 1189–97.

French, G. *et al.* (1990) Hong Kong strains of methicillin resistant and methicillin sensitive *Staphylococcus aureus* have similar virulence. *J Hosp Infect*, **15**, 117–25.

French, G.L. (1998) Enterococci and vancomycin resistance. *Clin Infect Dis*, **27**(Suppl 1), S75–83.

French, M.R., Levy-Milne, R. & Zibrik, D. (2001) A survey of the use of a low microbial diet in pediatric bone marrow transplant programs. *J Am Diet Assoc*, **101**(10), 1194–8.

Frenkel, L.M. *et al.* (1995) Effects of zidovudine use during pregnancy on resistance and vertical transmission of HIV type 1. *Clin Infect Dis*, **20**, 1321–6.

Friberg, B., Friberg, S., Ostensson, R. & Burman, L.G. (2001) Surgical area contamination comparable bacterial counts using disposable head and mask and helmet aspirator system, but dramatic increase upon omission of head-gear: an experimental study in horizontal laminar air-flow. *J Hosp Infect*, **47**(2), 110–15.

Fryklund, B. *et al.* (1997) Transmission of urinary bacterial strains between patients with indwelling catheters nursing in the same room and in separate rooms compared. *J Hosp Infect*, **36**, 147–53.

Fukai, K., Yokosuka, O., Fujiwara, K. *et al.* (1998) Etiologic considerations of fulminant non-A/non-B viral hepatitis in Japan: analysis by nucleic acid amplification method. *J Infect Dis*, **178**(2), 325–33.

Gammon, J. (1998) Analysis of the stressful effects of hospitalization and source isolation on coping and psychological constructs. *Int J Nurs Pract*, **4**, 84–96.

Gammon, J. (1999) The psychological consequences of source isolation: a review of the literature. *J Clin Nurs*, **8**(1), 13–21.

Gardner, C. (1994) An outbreak of hospital acquired cryptosporidiosis. *Br J Nurs*, **3**(4), 154–8.

Garg, S., Mathur, D.R. & Garg, D.K. (2001) Comparison of seropositivity of HIV, HBV, HCV and syphilis in replacement and voluntary blood donors in western India. *Indian J Pathol Microbiol*, **44**(4), 409–12.

Garner, J.S. & Simmons, B.P. (1983) CDC guidelines for isolation precautions in hospital. *Infect Control*, **4**(4), 325.

Garrouste-Orgeas, M., Chevret, S., Mainardi, J.L. *et al.* (2000) A one year prospective study of nosocomial bacteraemia in ICU and non ICU patients and its impact on patient outcome. *J Hosp Infect*, **44**(3), 206–13.

Gaskill, D., Henderson, A. & Fraser, M. (1997) Exploring the everyday world of the patient in isolation. *Oncol Nurse Forum*, **24**(4), 695–700.

Gedded, A.M. (1996) Antiviral drug resistance. *Br Med J*, **313**, 503–4.

George, R.H. (1997) Killing activity of microwaves in milk. *J Hosp Infect*, **35**, 319–26.

Gerard, L. *et al.* (1996) Life expectancy in hospitalised patients with AIDS: prognostic factors on admission. *J Palliat Care*, **12**(1), 26–30.

Gerberding, J.L. (1998) Nosocomial transmission of opportunistic infections. *Infect Control Hosp Epidemiol*, **19**(8), 574–7.

Gershon, A.A. (1996) Epidemiology and management of post-herpetic neuralgia. *Semin Dermatol*, **15**(Suppl 1), 8–13.

Ghabrah, T.M. *et al.* (1998) Comparison tests for antibody to hepatitis E virus. *J Med Virol*, **55**(2), 134–7.

Giele, C.M., Maw, R., Carne, C.A. *et al.* (2002) Post-exposure prophylaxis for non-occupational exposure to HIV: current clinical practice and opinions in the UK. *Sex Transm Infect*, **78**(2), 130–2.

Gilbert, C., Bestman-Smith, J. & Boivin, G. (2002) Resistance of herpesviruses to antiviral drugs: clinical impact and molecular mechanisms. *Drug Resist Update*, **5**(2), 88–114.

Gilbert, G.L. (2002) Infections in pregnant women. *Med J Aust*, **176**(5), 236.

Gilbert, R.J., de Louvois, J., Donavan, T. *et al.* (2000) Guidelines for the microbiological quality of some ready to eat foods sampled at the point of sale. PHLS Advisory Committee for food and dairy products. *Commun Dis Public Health*, **3**(3), 163–7.

Gilbert, V.L. *et al.* (1998) Unusual HIV transmission through blood contact: analysis of cases reported in the UK. To December 1997. *Commun Dis Public Health*, **1**(2), 108–13.

Gill, P. (1988) Is listeriosis often a food-borne illness? *J Infect*, **17**, 1–5.

Gillespie, I.A., Adak, G.K., O'Brien, S.J. *et al.* (2001) General outbreak of infectious intestinal disease associated with fish and shell fish, England and Wales, 1992–1999. *Commun Dis Public Health*, **4**(2), 117–23.

Gillespie, T. & Masterton, R.G. (1998) Investigation of infection in the neutropenic patient. *J Hosp Infect*, **38**(2), 77–91.

Gilot, P. *et al.* (1997) Sporadic case of listeriosis associated with the consumption of a *Listeria monocytogenes*-contaminated 'Camembert' cheese. *J Infect*, **35**(2), 195–7.

Girakar, A. *et al.* (1993) Hepatitis C virus: when to suspect, how to detect. *J Crit Illness*, **8**, 1287–95.

Girard, R., Amazian, K. & Fabry, J. (2001) Better compliance and better tolerance in relation to a well-conducted introduction to rub in hand disinfection. *J Hosp Infect*, **47**(2), 131–7.

Glauser, M.P. & Calandra, T. (2000) Infections on patients with hematologic malignancies. In: *Management of Infections in Immunocompromised Patients* (eds M.P. Glauser & P.A. Pizzo). W.B. Saunders, London.

Glauser, M.P. & Pizzo, P.A. (2000) *Management of Infections in Immunocompromised Patients*. W.B. Saunders, London.

Gnann, J.W. (2002) Varicella-zoster virus: atypical presentation and unusual complications. *J Infect Dis*, **186**(Suppl 1), S91–8.

Goedert, J.J. *et al.* (1998) Spectrum of AIDS associated malignant disorders. *Lancet*, **351**, 1833–9.

Goedert, J.J. *et al.* (1991) High risk of HIV-1 infection for first born twins. The international registry of HIV exposed twins. *Lancet*, **338**, 1471–5.

Goldberg, D., Johnson, J., Cameron, S. *et al.* (2000) Risk of HIV transmission from patients to surgeons in the era of post-exposure prophylaxis. *J Hosp Infect*, **44**(2), 99–105.

Goldie, S.J., Kaplan, J.E., Losina, E. *et al.* (2002) Prophylaxis for human immunodefiency virus-related *Pneumocystis carinii* pneumonia: using simulation modelling to inform clinical guidelines. *Arch Intern Med*, **162**(8), 921–8.

Goldrick, B. (2002) First reported case of VRSA in the United States. *Am J Nurs*, **102**(11), 17.

Goodall, B. (1992) A recurring problem. *Nursing*, **5**(5), 23–4.

Gopal Rao, G., Ojo, F. & Kolokithas, D. (1997) Vancomycin resistant gram positive cocci: risk factors for faecal carriage. *J Hosp Infect*, **35**, 63–9.

Grabs, A.J. & Lord, R.S. (2002) Treatment failure due to methicillin-resistant *Staphylococcus aureus* (MRSA) with reduced susceptibility to vancomycin. *Med J Aust*, **176**(11), 563.

Graham, J.C., Lanser, S., Bignardi, G., Pedler, S. & Hollyoak, V. (2002) Hospital-acquired listeriosis. *J Hosp Infect*, **51**(2), 136–9.

Granzebrook, J. (1986) Counting the cost of infection. *Nurs Times*, **83**(6), 24–6.

Gratz, N.G. (1999) Emerging and resurging vector-borne diseases. *Annu Rev Entomol*, **44**, 51–75.

Green, J. *et al.* (1998) The role of environmental contamination with small round structured viruses in a hospital outbreak investigated by reverse transcriptase polymerase chain reaction assay. *J Hosp Infect*, **39**, 39–45.

Griffith, C.J., Cooper, R.A., Gilmore, J., Davies, C. & Lewis, M. (2000) An evaluation of hospital cleaning regimes and standards. *J Hosp Infect*, **45**(1), 19–28.

Griffiths, P.D. (1991) Advances in the prevention and treatment of cytomegalovirus infection in hospital patients. *J Hosp Infect*, **18**(Suppl A), 330–4.

Griffiths-Jones, A. (1994) Hepatitis revisited. *Nurs Times*, **90**(46), 54–62.

Groll, A.H. & Walsh, T.J. (2001) Caspofungin: pharmacology, safety and therapeutic potential in superficial and invasive fungal infections. *Expert Opin Invest Drugs*, **10**(8), 1545–58.

Gruskin, S. & Tarantola, D. (2001) HIV/AIDS and human rights revisited. *Can HIV AIDS Policy Law Rev*, **6**(1–2), 24–9.

Gubler, D.J. (1998) Resurgent vector borne diseases as a global health problem. *Emerg Infect Dis*, **4**(3), 442–50.

Guerrero, A. *et al.* (1997) Nosocomial transmission of *Mycobacterium bovis* resistant to 11 drugs in people with advanced HIV-1 infection. *Lancet*, **350**(9093), 1738–42.

Guertler, L. (2002) Virus safety of human blood, plasma, and derived products. *Thromb Res*, **107**(Suppl 1), S39.

Guilera, M., Saiz, J.C., Lopez-Labrador, F.X. *et al.* (1998) Hepatitis G virus infection in chronic liver disease. *Gut*, **42**(1), 107–11.

Gunn, K. (2002) Dealing with hepatitis A. *NT Plus*, **98**(23), 50–1.

Haberman, M. *et al.* (1993) Quality of life of adult long term survivors of bone marrow transplantation: a quantitative analysis of narrative data. *Oncol Nurs Forum*, **20**(10), 1545–53.

Hadziyannis, S.J. (1997) Review: hepatitis delta. *J Gastroenterol Hepatol*, **12**(4), 289–98.

Hall, J. & Sutton, A. (2002) Non-HIV nurses' knowledge of HIV therapy. *Nurs Stand*, **16**(43), 33–6.

Halwachs-Baumann, G., Genser, B., Pailer, S. *et al.* (2002) Human cytomegalovirus load in various body fluids of congenitally infected newborns. *J Clin Virol*, **25**(Suppl 3), 81–7.

Hamid, S.S., Atiq, M., Shehzad, F. *et al.* (2002) Hepatitis E virus superinfection in patients with chronic liver disease. *Hepatology*, **36**(2), 474–8.

Hamilton-Miller, J.M. (2002) Vancomycin-resistant *Staphylococcus aureus*: a real and present danger. *Infection*, **30**(3), 118–24.

Hanna, J.N., Loewenthal, J.L., Hills, S.L. *et al.* (2001) Recognising and responding to outbreaks of hepatitis A associated with child care centres. *Aust NZ J Public Health*, **25**(6), 525–8.

Hanna, J.N., Loewenthal, M.R., Negel, P. *et al.* (1996) An outbreak of hepatitis A in an intensive care unit. *Anaesth Intens Care*, **24**(4), 440–4.

Hanrahan, A. & Reutter, L. (1997) A critical review of the literature on sharps injuries: epidemiology, management of exposure and prevention. *J Adv Nurs*, **25**, 144–54.

Hanshaw, J.B. *et al.* (1976) School failure and deafness after silent congenital cytomegalovirus infection. *N Engl J Med*, **295**, 468–70.

Haque, T. *et al.* (1997) A prospective study in heart and lung transplant recipients correlating persistent Epstein–Barr virus infection with clinical events. *Transplantation*, **64**(7), 1028–34.

Haramati, L.B. & Jenny-Avital, E.R. (1998) Approach to the diagnosis of pulmonary disease in patients infected with the human immunodeficiency virus. *J Thorac Imaging*, **13**(4), 247–60.

Harger, J.H., Ernest, J.M., Thurnau, G.R. *et al.* (2002a) Risk factors and outcome of varicella-zoster virus pneumonia in pregnant women. *J Infect Dis*, **185**(4), 422–7.

Harger, J.H., Ernest, J.M., Thurnau, G.R. *et al.* (2002b) Frequency of congenital varicella syndrome in a prospective cohort of 347 pregnant women. *Obstet Gynecol*, **100**(2), 260–5.

Harper, D. (1986) Legionnaires' disease: prevention better than cure. *Health Safety Work*, March, 41–6.

Harris, H.E., Ramsay, M.E., Heptonstall, J., Soldan, K. & Eldridge, K.P. (2000) The HCV national register: towards informing the natural history of hepatitis C infection in the UK. *J Viral Hepat*, **7**(6), 420–7.

Harris, H.E., Ramsay, M.E., Andrews, N. & Eldridge, K.P. (2002) Clinical course of hepatitis C virus during the first decade of infection: cohort study. *Br Med J*, **324**(7335), 450–3.

Harrison, R. & Corbett, K. (1999) Screening of pregnant women for HIV: the case against. *Practis Midwife*, **2**(7), 24–9.

Harrison, T.G. (1985) A nasty family from Philadelphia. *Med Lab World*, September, 19–23.

Hart, C.A. & Makin, T. (1991) Legionella in hospitals: a review. *J Hosp Infect*, **18**(Suppl A), 481–9.

Hart, R., Khalaf, Y., Lawson, R., Bickerstaff, H., Taylor, A. & Braude, P. (2001) Screening for HIV, hepatitis B and C infection in an inner London hospital. *Br J Obstet Gynaecol*, **108**(6), 654–6.

Hart, S. (1990) Clinical hepatitis B; guidelines for infection control. *Nurs Stand*, **4**(45), 24–7.

Hashida, S. *et al.* (1996) Shortening of the window period in diagnosis of HIV-1 infection by simultaneous detection of p24 antigen and antibody IgG to p17 and reverse transcriptase in serum with ultrasensitive enzyme immunoassay. *J Virol Method*, **62**(1), 43–53.

Hauggaard, A., Ellis, M. & Ekelund, L. (2002) Early chest radiography and CT in the diagnosis management and outcome of invasive pulmonary aspergillosis. *Acta Radiol*, **43**(3), 292–8.

Hayward, A.C., Goss, S., Drobniewski, F. *et al.* (2002) The molecular epidemiology of tuberculosis in inner London. *Epidemiol Infect*, **128**(2), 175–84.

Healing, T.D. *et al.* (1995) The infection hazards of human cadavers. *Commun Dis Rep*, **5**, R61–9.

Health and Safety Commission (1992) *The Safe Disposal of Clinical Waste*. HMSO, London.

Health and Safety Commission (1999) *Control of Substances Hazardous to Health (COSHH) Approved Code of Practice*. Stationery Office, London.

Health and Safety Executive (1991) *The Control of Legionellosis including Legionnaires' Disease*. Stationery Office, London.

Heathcock, R. *et al.* (1998) Survey of food safety awareness among HIV positive individuals. *AIDS Care*, **10**(2), 237–41.

Hecht, F.M., Busch, M.P., Rawal, B. *et al.* (2002) Use of laboratory tests and clinical symptoms for identification of primary HIV infection. *AIDS*, **16**(8), 1119–29.

Heiney, S.P., Neuberg, R.W., Myers, D. & Bergman, L.H. (1994) The aftermath of bone marrow transplant for parents of pediatric patients: a post traumatic stress disorder. *Oncol Nurs Forum*, **21**(5), 843–7.

Heinz, T. *et al.* (1996) Soft-tissue fungal infections: surgical management of 12 immunocompromised patients. *Plast Reconstr Surg*, **97**(7), 1391–9.

Henry, L. (1997) Immunocompromised patients and nutrition. *Prof Nurse*, **12**(9), 655–9.

Hirsch, M.S. (1988) Herpes group virus infections in the compromised host. In: *Clinical Approach to Infection in the Compromised Host*, 2nd edn (eds R.H. Rubin & L.S. Young). Plenum Medical Books, New York, pp. 347–66.

Ho, D.D. & Huang, Y. (2002) The HIV-1 vaccine race. *Cell*, **110**(2), 135–8.

Ho, M. (1995) Cytomegalovirus. In: *Principles and Practice of Infectious Disease*, 4th edn (eds G.L. Mandell, J.E. Bennett & R. Dolin). Churchill Livingstone, New York, Vol. 2, Chap. 117, pp. 1351–64.

Hobson, R.P., MacKenzie, F.M. & Gould, I.M. (1996) An outbreak of multiple resistant *Klebsiella pneumoniae* in the Grampian region of Scotland. *J Hosp Infect*, **33**(4), 249–62.

Hodgson, M.J. *et al.* (1998) Building associated pulmonary disease from exposure to *Stachybotrys chartarum* and *Aspergillus versicolor*. *J Occup Environ Med*, **40**(3), 241–9.

Holley, H.P. & Thiers, B.H. (1986) Cryptosporidium in a patient receiving immunosuppressive therapy. Possible activation of latent infection. *Dig Dis Sci*, **31**(9), 1004–7.

Hollis, R.J. *et al.* (1995) Familial carriage of methicillin resistant *Staphylococcus aureus* and subsequent infection in a premature neonate. *Clin Infect Dis*, **21**(2), 328–32.

Holmes, R.D. & Sokol, R.J. (2002) Epstein–Barr virus and post-transplant lymphoproliferative disease. *Pediatr Transplant*, **6**(6), 456–64.

Honeybourne, D. & Neumann, C.S. (1997) An audit of bronchoscopy practice in the United Kingdom: a survey of adherence to national guidelines. *Thorax*, **52**(8), 709–13.

Hope, V.D., Judd, A., Hickman, M. *et al.* (2001) Prevalence of hepatitis C among injection drug users in England and Wales: is harm reduction working? *Am J Public Health*, **91**(1), 38–42.

Hospital Infection Control Practice Advisory Committee (HIC-PAC) (1995) Recommendations for preventing the spread of vancomycin resistance. *Infection Control Hosp Epidemiol*, **16**(2), 105–13.

Howell, D.R., Webster, M.H. & Barbara, J.A. (2000) Retrospective follow-up of recipients and donors of blood donations reactive for anti-HBc or for single HCV. *Transfus Med*, **10**(4), 265–9.

Hsu, H.Y. *et al.* (1995) Precore mutant of hepatitis B virus in childhood fulminant hepatitis B: an infrequent association. *J Infect Dis*, **171**(4), 776–81.

Hsu, Y.S., Chien, R.N., Yeh, C.T. *et al.* (2002) Long term outcome after spontaneous HbeAg seroconversion in patients with chronic hepatitis B. *Hepatology*, **35**(6), 1522–7.

Huang, Z.S. & Wu, H.N. (1998) Identification and characterization of the RNA chaperone activity of hepatitis delta antigen peptides. *J Biol Chem*, **273**(41), 26455–61.

Huaringa, A.J., Leyva, F.J., Signes-Costa, J. *et al.* (2000) Bronchoalveolar lavage in the diagnosis of pulmonary complications of bone marrow patients. *Bone Marrow Transplant*, **25**(9), 975–9.

Hudome, S.M. & Fisher, M.C. (2001) Nosocomial infections in the neonatal intensive care unit. *Curr Opin Infect Dis*, **14**(3), 303–7.

Hugonnet, S., Perneger, T.V. & Pittet, D. (2002) Alcohol-based handrub improves compliance with hand hygiene in intensive care units. *Arch Intern Med*, **162**(9), 1037–43.

Hung, C.C. *et al.* (1995) Antibiotic therapy for *Listeria monocytogenes* bacteremia. *J Formos Med Assoc*, **94**(1–2), 19–22.

Hunt, C.P. (1998) The emergence of enterococci as a cause of nosocomial infection. *Br J Biomed Sci*, **55**, 149–56.

Hunt, D.A. *et al.* (1994) Cryptosporidiosis associated with a swimming pool complex. *Commun Dis Rep*, **4**(2), R20–22.

Hunter, P.R. & Nichols, G. (2002) Epidemiology and clinical features of Cryptosporidium infection in immunocompromised patients. *Clin Microbial Rev*, **15**(1), 145–54.

Hunter, P.R. & Syed, Q. (2002) A community survey of self-reported gastroenteritis undertaken during an outbreak of cryptosporidiosis strongly associated with drinking water after much press interest. *Epidemiol Infect*, **128**(3), 433–8.

Huovinen, P. & Cars, O. (1998) Control of antimicrobial resistance: time for action. *Br Med J*, **317**, 613.

Hussaini, S.H. *et al.* (1997) Severe hepatitis E infection during pregnancy. *J Viral Hepat*, **4**(1), 51–4.

Interdepartmental Working Group on Tuberculosis (1998) *The Prevention and Control of Tuberculosis in the United Kingdom*. Stationery Office, London.

Infection Control Nurses Association (ICNA) in partnership with Pharmacia (2002) *Antibiotics Resistance Theory and Practice*. Edinburgh: Fitwise.

Irshad, M. (1997) Hepatitis E virus: a global view of its seroepidemiology and transmission pattern. *Trop Gastroenterol*, **18**(2), 45–9.

Irwin, D.J. & Millership, S. (2001) Antibody responses to hepatitis A vaccine in healthy adults. *Commun Dis Public Health*, **4**(2), 139–40.

Ives, N.J., Gazzard, B.G. & Easterbrook, P.J. (2001) The changing pattern of AIDS defining illnesses with the introduction of highly active retroviral therapy [HAART] in a London clinic. *J Infect*, **42**(2), 134–9.

Jaffe, H.W. *et al.* (1980) Identity and interspecific transfer of gentamicin resistant plasmids in *Staphylococcus aureus* and *Staphylococcus epidermidis*. *J Infect Dis*, **141**, 738.

Jang, T.N., Kuo, B.I., Shen, S.H. *et al.* (1999) Nosocomial Gram-negative bacteremia in critically ill patients: epidemiologic characteristics and prognostic factors in 147 episodes. *J Formos Med Assoc*, **98**(7), 465–75.

Jansa, J.M., Cayla, J.A., Ferrer, D. *et al.* (2002) An outbreak of legionnaires' disease in an inner city district: importance of the first 24 hours in the investigation. *Int J Tuberc Lung Dis*, **6**(9), 831–8.

Jarrett, W.A., Ribes, J. & Manaligot, J.M. (2002) Biofilm formation on tracheostomy tubes. *Ear Nose Throat J*, **81**(9), 659–61.

Jarvis, M. & Nelson, J. (2002) Human cytomegalovirus persistence and latency in endothelial cells and macrophages. *Curr Opin Microbiol*, **5**(4), 403–7.

Jason, J.M. *et al.* (1986) HTLV III/LAV antibody and immune status of household contacts and sexual partners of persons with haemophilia. *JAMA*, **155**, 212.

Jemsek, J. (1983) Herpes zoster-associated encephalitis: clinico-pathologic report of 12 cases and review of the literature. *Medicine*, **62**(2), 81–97.

Jensen, P.A. *et al.* (1993) Evaluation and control of workers exposed to fungi in a beet sugar refinery. *Am Ind Hyg Assoc J*, **54**, 742–8.

Jevons, M.P. (1961) Celberin resistant staphylococci. *Br Med J*, **1**, 124–5.

Johnson, A.P. (1998) Antibiotic resistance among clinically important Gram positive bacteria in the UK. *J Hosp Infect*, **40**, 17–26.

Johnson, A.P. *et al.* (1996) Prevalence of antibiotic resistance and serotype in pneumococci in England and Wales: results of observational surveys in 1990 and 1995. *Br Med J*, **312**, 1454–6.

Johnson, D. (2002) Therapeutic management of HIV. *Oral Dis*, **8**(Suppl 2), 17–20.

Johnson, E., Gilmore, M., Newman, J. & Stephens, M. (2000) Preventing fungal infections in immunocompromised patients. *Br J Nurs*, **9**(17), 1154–64.

Johnson, S. *et al.* (1990) Prospective controlled study of vinyl glove use to interrupt *Clostridium difficile* transmission. *Am J Med*, **88**, 137–40.

Joint Tuberculosis Committee of the British Thoracic Society (1994) Control and prevention of tuberculosis in the United Kingdom: Code of Practice 1994. *Thorax*, **49**, 1193–200.

Joint Tuberculosis Committee of the British Thoracic Society (1998) Chemotherapy and management of tuberculosis in the United Kingdom. *Thorax*, **53**(7), 536–48.

Jones, E.M. & MacGowan, A.P. (1995) Antimicrobial chemotherapy of human infection due to *Listeria monocytogenes*. *Eur J Clin Microbiol Infect Dis*, **14**(3), 165–75.

Jones, E.M. & Reeves, D.S. (1997) Controlling chickenpox in hospital. *Br Med J*, **314**, 4–5.

Jones, E.M. *et al.* (1997) Control of varicella-zoster infection on renal and other specialist units. *J Hosp Infect*, **36**, 133–40.

Jones, M. *et al.* (1988) Over-estimating overshoes. *Nurs Times*, **84**(41), 66–71.

Jones, R.N. (2001) Resistance patterns among nosocomial pathogens: trends over the past few years. *Chest*, **119**(2 Suppl), 397–404S.

Jones, S.G., Messmer, P.R., Charron, S.A. & Parns, M. (2002) HIV positive women and minority patients' satisfaction with inpatient hospital care. *AIDS Patient Care*, **16**(3), 127–34.

Josephson, A. & Gombert, M. E. (1988) Airborne transmission of nosocomial varicella from localized zoster. *J Infect Dis*, **158**(1), 238–41.

Joshi, M.S., Chitambar, S.D., Arankalle, V.A. & Chadha, M.S. (2002) Evaluation of urine as a clinical specimen for diagnosis of hepatitis A. *Clin Diag Lab Immunol*, **9**(4), 840–5.

Jowitt, S.N. *et al.* (1991) CD4 lymphocytopenia without HIV in patients with cryptococcal infection. *Lancet*, **337**, 500–1.

Kampf, G., Jarosch, R. & Ruden, H. (1998) Limited effectiveness of chlorhexidine based hand disinfectants against methicillin-resistant *Staphylococcus aureus* (MRSA). *J Hosp Infect*, **38**(4), 297–303.

Kao, J.H. & Chen, D.S. (2002) Recent research progress in hepatocellular carcinoma. *J Formos Med Assoc*, **101**(4), 239–48.

Kaplan, J.E., Masur, H. & Holmes, K.K. (2002) Guidelines for preventing opportunistic infections among HIV infected persons. 2002 Recommendations of the US Public Health Service and the Infectious Disease Society of America. *MMWR Recomm Rep*, **51**(RR8), 1–52.

Karamura, M. *et al.* (1989) HIV 2 in West Africa in 1966. *Lancet*, **i**, 385.

Karas, J.A., Barker, C., Hawtin, L. & Hoadley, M. (2002) Turning a blind eye to vertical blinds in hospital wards. *J Hosp Infect*, **51**(1), 75.

Kato, H., Orito, E., Sugauchi, F. *et al.* (2001) Determination of hepatitis B virus genotype G by polymerase chain reaction with hemi-nested promers. *J Virol Methods*, **98**(2), 153–9.

Katz, A. (1997) 'Mom, I have something to tell you'. Disclosing HIV infection. *J Adv Nurs* **25**, 139–43.

Katz, M.H. & Gerberding, J.L. (1997) Postexposure treatment of people exposed to HIV through sexual contact or injection–drug use. *N Engl J Med*, **336**, 1097–100.

Kavaliotis, J. *et al.* (1998) Outbreak of varicella in a pediatric oncology unit. *Med Pediatr Oncol*, **31**(3), 166–9.

Kavan, P. *et al.* (1998) Pseudomembraneous clostridium after autologous bone marrow transplantation. *Bone Marrow Transplant*, **21**(5), 521–3.

Kayley, J. *et al.* (1996) Safe intravenous antibiotic therapy at home: experience of a UK based programme. *J Antimicrob Chemother* **37**(5), 1023–9.

Kearnes, A.M., Freeman, R. & Lightfoot, N.F. (1995) Nosocomial enterococci; resistance to heat and sodium hypochlorite. *J Hosp Infect*, **30**, 193–9.

Kearns, A.M., Barrett, A., Marshall, C. *et al.* (2000) Epidemiology and molecular typing of an outbreak of tuberculosis in a hostel for homeless men. *J Clin Pathol*, **53**(2), 122–4.

Keating, M.R. *et al.* (1996) Transmission of invasive aspergillosis from a subclinically infected donor to three different organ transplant recipients. *Chest*, **109**(4), 119–24.

Kedzierski, M. (1991) Understanding virology. *Prof Nurse*, **7**(2), 99–102.

Kellerman, S.E. *et al.* (1998) APIC and CDC survey of *Mycobacterium tuberculosis* isolation and control practices in hospitals caring for children. Part 2: environmental and administrative controls. *Am J Infect Control*, **26**(5), 483–7.

Kelly, C.P. & LaMont, J.T. (1998) *Clostridium difficile* infection. *Annu Rev Med*, **49**, 375–90.

Kelly, D., Ross, S., Gray, B. & Smith, P. (2000) Death, dying and emotional labour: problematic dimensions of the bone marrow transplant nursing role. *J Adv Nurs*, **32**(4), 952–60.

Kemp, C. & Stepp, L. (1995) Palliative care for patients with acquired immunodeficiency syndrome. *Am J Hosp Palliat Care*, **12**(6), 14, 17–27.

Kendle, J.B. & Fan-Havard, P. (1998) Cidofovir in the treatment of CMV. *Ann Pharmacother*, **32**(11), 1181–92.

Kennedy, P. & Hamilton, L.R. (1997) Psychological impact of the management of methicillin resistant *Staphylococcus aureus* (MRSA) in patients with spinal cord injury. *Spinal Cord*, **35**(9), 617–9.

Khoo, V.S., Wilson, P.C., Sexton, M.J. & Liew, K.H. (2000) Acquired immunodeficiency syndrome-related primary cerebral lymphoma response to irradiation. *Aust Radiol*, **44**(2), 178–84.

Kibbler, C.C., Quick, A. & O'Neil, A.M. (1998) The effect of increased bed numbers on MRSA transmission in acute medical wards. *J Hosp Infect*, **39**, 213–19.

King, S. (1998) Decontamination of equipment and the environment. *Nurs Stand*, **12**(52), 57–63.

Kinghorn, G.R. (1993) Genital herpes natural history and treatment of acute episodes. *J Med Virol* (Suppl), **1**, 33–8.

Kingsley, D.H., Meade, G.K. & Richards, G.P. (2002) Detection of both hepatitis A virus and Norwalk-like virus in imported clams associated with food borne illness. *Appl Environ Microbiol*, **68**(8), 3914–8.

Kiss, A. (1994) Support of the transport team. *Support Care Cancer*, **2**(1), 56–60.

Klein, G., Pack, A. & Reuter, G. (1998) Antibiotic resistance patterns of enterococci and occurrence of vancomycin-resistant enterococci in raw minced beef and pork in Germany. *Appl Environ Microbiol*, **64**(5), 1825–30.

Knowles, H.E. (1993) The experience of infectious patients in isolation. *Nurs Times*, **89**(30), 53–6.

Kocazeybek, B., Arabaci, U. & Sezgic, M. (2002) Investigation of transfusion transmitted viruses in cases clinically suspected of post transfusion hepatitis with undetermined etiology. *Transfus Apheresis*, **26**(3), 157–65.

Koff, R.S. (2002) Hepatitis A, hepatitis B, and combination hepatitis vaccines for immunoprophylaxis: an update. *Dig Dis Sci*, **47**(6), 1183–94.

Kofsky, P. et al. (1991) *Clostridium difficile*: a common and costly colitis. *Dis Colon Rectum*, **34**(3), 244–8.

Kopko, P.M., Fernando, L.P., Bonney, E.N., Freeman, J.L. & Holland, P.V. (2001) HIV transmission from a window period platelet donation. *Am J Clin Pathol*, **116**(5), 562–6.

Korelitz, J.J., Busch, M.P. & Williams, A.E. (1996) Antigen testing for HIV and the magnet effect: will the benefit of a new HIV test be offset by the number of higher risk, test seeking donors attracted to blood centers? Retrovirus Epidemiology Donor Study. *Transfusion*, **36**(3), 203–8.

Kotler, D.P. (1998) HIV in pregnancy. *Gastroenterol Clin North Am*, **27**(1), 269–80.

Kovacs, J.A., Gill, V.J., Meshnick, S. & Masur, H. (2001) New insight into transmission, diagnosis, and drug treatment of *Pneumocystis carinii* pneumonia. *JAMA*, **286**(190), 2450–60.

Kramer, M.H. et al. (1998) First reported outbreak in the United States of cryptosporidiosis associated with a recreational lake. *Clin Infect Dis*, **26**(1), 27–33.

Kremer, L.S. & Besra, G.S. (2002) Current status and future development of antitubercular chemotherapy. *Expert Opin Invest Drugs*, **11**(8), 1033–49.

Kruger, W., Russmann, B., Kroger, N. et al. (1999) Early infections in patients undergoing bone marrow or blood stem cell transplantation: 7-year single centre investigation of 409 cases. *Bone Marrow Transplant*, **23**(6), 589–97.

Kumar, D., Saunders, N.A., Watson, J.M. et al. (2000) Clusters of new tuberculosis in north-west London: a survey from three hospitals based on IS6110 RFLP typing. *J Infect*, **40**(2), 132–7.

Kumari, D.N. et al. (1998) Ventilation grilles as a potential source of methicillin resistant *Staphylococcus aureus* causing an outbreak in an orthopaedic ward at a district general hospital. *J Hosp Infect*, **39**(2), 127–33.

Kusne, S. & Krystofiak, S. (2001) Infection control issues after bone marrow transplantation. *Curr Opin Infect Dis*, **14**(4), 427–31.

Kyne, L. et al. (1998) Simultaneous outbreak of two strains of toxigenic *Clostridium difficile* in a general hospital. *J Hosp Infect*, **38**(2), 101–12.

Laa Poh, C. & Yeo, C.C. (1993) Recent advances in typing *Pseudomonas aeruginosa*. *J Hosp Infect*, **24**, 175–81.

Lacey, S., Flaxman, J., Scales, J. & Wilson, A. (2001) The usefulness of masks in preventing transient carriage of epidemic MRSA by health care workers. *J Hosp Infect*, **48**(4), 308–11.

Lackritz, E.M. (1998) Prevention of HIV transmission by blood transfusion in the developing world: achievements and continuing challenges. *AIDS*, **12**(Suppl A), S81–6.

Laing, R., Brettle, R., Leen, C. et al. (1997) Features and outcome of *Pneumocystis carinii* pneumonia according to risk category for HIV infection. *Scand J Infect Dis*, **29**(1), 57–61.

Lam, T. et al. (1998) Prophylactic use of itraconazole for the prevention of invasive pulmonary aspergillosis in high risk neutropenic patients. *Leuk Lymphoma*, **30**(1–2), 163–74.

Lamden, K. et al. (1996) Opportunist mycobacteria in England and Wales 1982–1994. *Commun Dis Rep CDR Rev*, **6**(11), R147–51.

Lamont, R.J. et al. (1988) *Listeria monocytogenes* and its role in human infection. *J Infect*, **17**, 7–28.

Lanham, S., Herbert, A., Basarab, A. & Watt, P. (2001) Detection of cervical infections in colposcopy clinic patients. *J Clin Microbiol*, **39**(8), 2946–50.

Lanphear, B.P. (1997) Transmission and control of blood borne viral hepatitis in health care workers. *Occup Med*, **12**(4), 717–30.

Larson, P.J. et al. (1993) Comparison of perceived symptoms of patients undergoing bone marrow transplant and the nurses caring for them. *Oncol Nurs Forum*, **20**(1), 81–8.

Lau, D.T., Kleiner, D.E., Park, Y., Bisceglie, A.M. & Hoofnagle, J.H. (1999) Resolution of chronic delta hepatitis after 12 years of interferon alfa therapy. *Gastroenterology*, **117**(5), 1229–33.

Lau, J.Y.N. & Wright, T.L. (1993) Molecular virology and pathogenesis of hepatitis B. *Lancet*, **342**, 1335–9.

Laurence, J. et al. (1992) AIDS without evidence of infection with HIV-1 and 2. *Lancet*, **340**, 273–4.

Laurichesse, H., Romaszko, J.P., Nguyen, L.T. et al. (2001) Clinical characteristics and outcome of patients with invasive pneumococcal disease. Puy-de-Dome, France, 1994–1998. *Eur J Clin Microbiol Infect Dis*, **20**(5), 299–308.

Lauwers, S. & de Smet, F. (1998) Surgical site infections. *Acta Clin Belg*, **53**(5), 303–10.

Leach, C.T. et al. (2002) Human herpes virus 6 and cytomegalovirus infections in children with human immunodeficiency virus infection and cancer. *Pediatr Infect Dis*, **21**(2), 125–1232.

Lee, M.S. et al. (1998) Varicella zoster virus retrobulbar optic neuritis preceding retinitis in patients with acquired immune deficiency syndrome. *Ophthalmology*, **105**(3), 467–71.

Lefkowitch, J.H. et al. (1987) Liver cell dysplasia and hepatocellular carcinoma in non-A non-B hepatitis. *Arch Pathol Lab Med*, **III**, 170–3.

Lefrere, J.J., Roudot-Thoraval, F., Morand-Joubert, L. et al. (1999) Prevalence of GB virus type C/Hepatitis G virus. *Transfusion*, **39**(1), 83–94.

Lefrere, J.J., Sender, A., Mercier, B. et al. (2000) High rates of GB virus type C/HGV transmission from mother to infant: possible implications for the prevalence of infection in blood donors. *Transfusion*, **40**(5), 602–7.

Lettinga, K.D., Verbon, A., Nieuwkerk, P.T. et al. (2002) Health-related quality of life and posttraumatic stress disorder among survivors of an outbreak of Legionnaires disease. *Clin Infect Dis*, **35**(1), 11–17.

Levie, K., Beran, J., Collard, F. & Nguyen, C. (2002) Long term[24 months] follow up of a hepatitis A and B vaccine. Comparing a two and three dose schedule in adolescents aged 12–15 years. *Vaccine*, **20**(19–20), 257–8.

Levine, A.S., Siegal, S.E. & Schrieber, A.D. (1973) Protected environment and prophylactic antibiotics. A perspective controlled study of their utility in the therapy of acute leukaemia. *N Engl J Med*, **288**, 477–83.

Levy, R., Hindley, D.T., Burman, R. *et al.* (1995) Unusual cause of pseudomonal infection. *Br Med J*, **310**(6974), 258.

Levy, S.B. (1998) The challenge of antibiotic resistance. *Sci Am*, **278**(3), 46–53.

Levy, S.B. (2001) Antibiotic resistance: consequences of inaction. *Clin Infect Dis*, **33**(Suppl 3), S124–9.

Li, Y., Brackett, R.E., Chen, J. & Beuchat, L.R. (2002) Mild heat treatment of lettuce during subsequent storage at 5 degrees C or 15 degrees C. *J Appl Microbiol*, **92**(2), 269–75.

Liberek, A., Rytlewska, M., Szlagatys-Sidorkiewicz, A. *et al.* (2002) Cytomegalovirus disease in neonates and infants – clinical presentation, diagnostic and therapeutic problem – own experience. *Med Sci Monit*, **8**(12), CR815–20.

Limaye, A.P. (2002) Antiviral resistance in cytomegalovirus: an emerging problem in organ transplant recipients. *Semin Respir Infect*, **17**(4), 265–73.

Limaye, A.P., Perkins, J.D. & Kowdley, K.V. (1998) Listeria infection after liver transplantation: report of a case and review of the literature. *Am J Gastroenterol*, **93**(10), 1942–4.

Lin, T.S., Zahrieh, D., Weller, E., Alyea, E.P., Antin, J.H. & Soiffer, R.J. (2002) Risk factors for cytomegalovirus reactivation after CD6 + T-cell-depleted allogeneic bone marrow transplantation. *Transplantation*, **74**(1), 49–54.

Lin, T.Y. *et al.* (1997) Oral acyclovir prophylaxis of varicella after intimate contact. *Pediatr Infect Dis*, **16**(12), 1162–5.

Little, S.J., Holte, S., Routy, J.P. *et al.* (2002) Antiretroviral-drug resistance among patients recently infected with HIV. *N Engl J Med*, **347**(6), 385–94.

Loach, L. (1997) Blue days. *Nurs Times*, **93**(32), 31–2.

Local Authority Circular (2002) *Legionnaires' Disease*. Health and Safety Executive/Local Authorities Enforcement Liaison Committee, London.

Local Collaborators (1998) Occupational acquisition of HIV infection among health care workers in the UK: data to June 1997. *Commun Dis Public Health*, **1**(2), 103–7.

Loh, W., Ng, V.V. & Holton, J. (2000) Bacterial flora on the white coats of medical students. *J Hosp Infect*, **45**(1), 65–8.

London Waste Regulation Authority (1994) *Guidelines for the Segregation, Handling and Disposal of Clinical Waste*. London Waste Regulation Authority, London.

Longnecker, R. (2000) Epstein–Barr virus latency: LMP2, a regulator or a means for Epstein–Barr virus persistence? *Adv Cancer Res*, **79**, 175–200.

Loudon, K.W. *et al.* (1996) Kitchens as a source of *Aspergillus niger* infection. *J Hosp Infect*, **32**, 191–8.

Loudon, R.G. *et al.* (1969) Cough frequency and infectivity in patient with pulmonary tuberculosis. *Am Rev Respir Dis*, **99**, 109–11.

Low, J.C. & Donachie, W. (1997) A review of *Listeria monocytogenes* and listeriosis. *Vet*, **153**(1), 9–29.

Lucas, S. (2002) The pathology of HIV infection. *Lepr Rev*, **73**(1), 64–71.

Lundgren, B. & Wakefield, A.E. (1998) PCR for detecting *Pneumocystis carinii* in clinical or environmental samples. *Immunol Med Microbiol*, **22**(1–2), 97–101.

Macarter-Spaulding, D.E. (2001) Varicella infection in pregnancy. *Obstet Gynecol Neonatal Nurs*, **30**(6), 667–73.

MacKinnon, M.M. & Allen, K.D. (2000) Longterm MRSA carriage in hospital patients. *J Infect Control*, **46**(3), 216–21.

MacMillan, M.L., Goodman, J.L., DeFor, T.E. & Weisdorf, D.J. (2002) Fluconazole to prevent yeast infections in bone marrow transplantation patients: a randomized trial of high dose versus reduced dose and determination of the value of maintenance therapy. *Am J Med*, **112**(5), 369–79.

Madar, R., Straka, S. & Baska, T. (2002) Detection of antibodies in saliva – an effective auxiliary method in surveillance of infectious diseases. *Bratisl Lek Listy*, **103**(1), 38–41.

Madeo, M. & Owen, E. (2002) Isolation: a patient satisfaction and compliance survey. *Br J Infect Control*, **3**(3), 18–20.

Maeda, A., Sata, T., Sata, Y. & Kurata, T. (1994) A comparative study of congenital and postnatally acquired human cytomegalovirus infection in infants: lack of expression of viral immediate early protein in congenital cases. *Virchows Arch*, **424**(2), 121–8.

Maertens, J., Vrebos, M. & Boogaerts, M. (2001) Assessing risk factors for systemic fungal infections. *Eur J Cancer Care*, **10**(1), 56–62.

Magnius, L.O. & Norder, H. (1995) Subtype, genotypes and molecular epidemiology of the hepatitis B virus reflected by sequence variability of the S-gene. *Intervirology*, **38**(1–2), 24–34.

Maguire, H., Pharoah, P., Walsh, B. *et al.* (2001) Hospital outbreak of salmonella virchow possibly associated with a food handler. *J Hosp Infect*, **44**(4), 261–6.

Maguire, H., Dale, J.W., McHugh, T.D. *et al.* (2002) Molecular epidemiology of tuberculosis in London 1995–1997 showing low rates of transmission. *Thorax*, **57**(7), 617–22.

Maguire, H.C. *et al.* (1995) A collaboration case control study of sporadic hepatitis A in England. *Commun Dis Rep*, **5**(3), R33–40.

Maher, D. & Nunn, P. (1998) Evaluation and determinants of outcome of tuberculosis treatment. *Bull World Health Organ*, **76**(3), 307–8.

Mahida, Y.R. *et al.* (1998) Effect of *Clostridium difficile* toxin A on human colonic lamina propria cells: early loss of macrophages followed by T cell apoptosis. *Infect Immunol*, **66**(11), 5462–9.

Main, J. *et al.* (1992) The diagnosis and management of viral hepatitis. *Commun Dis Rep*, **2**(10), R117–20.

Mainka, C. *et al.* (1998) Characterization of viremia at different stages of varicella-zoster virus infection. *J Med Virol*, **56**(1), 91–8.

Mairtin, D.O. *et al.* (1998) The effect of a badger removal programme on the incidence of tuberculosis in an Irish cattle population. *Pre Vet Med*, **34**(1), 47–56.

Makin, T. & Hart, C.A. (1990) The efficacy of control measures for eradicating Legionellae in showers. *J Infect Control*, **16**(1), 1–7.

Mangtani, P. *et al.* (1995) Socioeconomic deprivation and notification rates for tuberculosis in London during 1987–1991. *Br Med J*, **310**, 963–6.

Manuel, R.J. & Kibbler, C.C. (1998) The epidemiology and prevention of aspergillosis. *J Hosp Infect*, **39**(2), 95–109.

Marques, A.R. *et al.* (1998) Combination therapy with famciclovir and interferon-alpha for the treatment of chronic hepatitis B. *J Infect Dis*, **178**(5), 1483–7.

Marr, K.A., Carter, R.A., Boeckh, M., Martin, P. & Corey, L. (2002) Invasive aspergillosis in allogeneic stem cell transplant recipients: changes in epidemiology and risk factors. *Blood*, **100**(13), 4358–66.

Marrone, A. *et al.* (1997) Prevalence of hepatitis G virus in patients with hepatocellular carcinoma. *J Viral Hepat*, **4**(6), 411–14.

Marshall, B. *et al.* (1998) Environmental contamination of a new general surgical ward. *J Hosp Infect*, **39**(3), 242–3.

Martlew, V.J., Carey, P., Tong, C.Y. *et al.* (2000) Post-transfusion HIV infection despite donor screening: a report of three cases. *J Hosp Infect*, **44**(2), 93–7.

Maslow, J.N., Brecher, S. & Gunn, J. (1995) Variation and persistence of methicillin resistant *Staphylococcus aureus* strains among individual patients over extended periods of time. *Eur J Clin Microbiol Infect Dis*, **14**, 282–90.

Mason, B.W., Williams, N., Salmon, R.L. *et al.* (2001) Outbreak of Salmonella Indiana associated with egg mayonnaise sandwiches at a NHS hospital. *Commun Dis Public Health*, **4**(4), 300–4.

Massie, R.J. *et al.* (1998) *Pneumocystis carinii* pneumonia: pitfalls of prophylaxis. *J Paediatr Child Health*, **43**(5), 477–9.

Masterton, R.G. & Teare, E.L. (2001) Clinical governance and infection control in the United Kingdom. *J Hosp Infect*, **47**(1), 25–31.

Matthes-Martin, S. *et al.* (1998) CMV-viraemia during allogenic bone marrow transplantation in paediatric patients: association with survival and graft-versus-host disease. *Bone Marrow Transplant*, **21**(Suppl 2), S53–6.

Matthews, G.V. & Nelson, M.R. (2001) The management of chronic hepatitis B infection. *Int J STD AIDS*, **12**(6), 353–7.

Mbayed, V.A., Barbini, L., Lopez, J.L. & Campos, R.H. (2001) Phylogenetic analysis of the hepatitis B virus (HBV) genotype F including Argentine isolates. *Arch Virol*, **146**(9), 1803–10.

McCarter-Spaulding, D.E. (2001) Varicella infection in pregnancy. *J Obstet Gynecol Neonatal Murs*, **30**(6), 667–73.

McCarthy, G.M., Ssali, C.S., Bednarsh, H. *et al.* (2002) Transmission of HIV in the dental clinic and elsewhere. *Oral Dis*, **8**(Suppl 2), 126–35.

McCluskey, F. (1996) Does wearing a face mask reduce bacterial wound infection? A literature review. *J Hosp Infect*, **6**(5), 18–20.

McCormick, R.D. *et al.* (1981) Epidemiology of needlestick injuries in hospital personnel. *Am J Med*, **70**, 928–32.

McCulloch, J. (1998) Infection control: principles for practice. *Nurs Stand*, **13**(1), 49–52.

McCullough, N.V. *et al.* (1997) Collection of three bacterial aerosols by respirator and surgical mask filters under varying conditions of flow and relative humidity. *Ann Occup Hyg*, **41**(6), 677–90.

McHenry, A., Evans, B.G., Sinka, K., Shaheem, Z., Macdonald, N. & DeAngelis, D. (2002) Numbers of adults with diagnosed HIV infection: 1996–2005 adjusted totals and extrapolations for England, Wales and Northern Ireland. *Commun Dis Public Health*, **5**(2), 97–100.

McIntyre, G.T. (2001) Viral infections of the oral mucosa and perioral region. *Dent Update*, **28**(4), 181–6.

McKee, J.M. (1996) Human immunodeficiency virus. Healthcare workers' safety issues. *J Intraven Nurs*, **19**(3), 132–40.

McLaughlin, J. & Gilbert, R.J. (1990) Listeria in food. *Public Health Lab Serv Microbiol Dig*, **7**(3), 54–5.

McMichael, A. *et al.* (2002) Design and tests of an HIV vaccine. *Br Med Bull*, **62**(1), 87–98.

McNeil, S.A., Mody, L. & Bradley, S.F. (2002) Methicillin-resistant *Staphylococcus aureus*. Management of asymptomatic colonization and outbreaks of infection in long-term care. *Geriatrics*, **57**(6), 16–27.

Mead, J.R. (2002) Cryptosporidiosis and the challenges of chemotherapy. *Drug Resist Update*, **5**(1), 47–57.

Medical Devices Agency (1996) *Latex Sensitisation in the Health Care Setting*. Department of Health, London.

Medical Devices Agency (1998) *Latex Medical Gloves*. Department of Health, London.

Medical Devices Agency (2002) *Sterilization, Disinfection and Cleaning of Medical Equipment*. Department of Health, London.

Medina, J., Garcia-Buey, L. & Moreno-Otero, R. (2003) Immunopathogenetic and therapeutic aspects of autoimmune hepatitis. *Aliment Pharmacol Ther*, **17**(1), 1–16.

Meers, P.D. & Matthews, R.B. (1978) Multiple-resistant pneumococcus. *Lancet*, **ii**, 219.

Meier, J. & Lopez, L. (2001) Listeriosis: an emerging food-borne disease. *Clin Lab Sci*, **14**(3), 187–92.

Melbye, M. *et al.* (1987) Risk of AIDS after herpes zoster. *Lancet*, **i**, 728–31.

Melillo, K.D. (1998) *Clostridium difficile* and older adults: what primary care providers should know. *Nurse Pract*, **23**(7), 25–6.

Melnick, J.-L. (1982) Classification of hepatitis A virus as enterovirus type 72 and of hepatitis B virus as hepadnovirus type 1. *Intervirology*, **18**, 105–6.

Mendoza, M.C. (1985) Evidence for the dispersion and evolution of R. plasmids from *Serratia marcescens* in hospital. *J Hosp Infect*, **6**, 147–53.

Meng, X.J. *et al.* (1998) Genetic and experimental evidence for cross-species infection by swine hepatitis E virus. *J Virol*, **72**(12), 9714–21.

Menzies, D. *et al.* (1995) Review article: Current concepts: tuberculosis among health care workers. *N Engl J Med*, **332**, 92–8.

Meyer, I.D. (1986) Infection in bone marrow transplant recipients. *Am J Med*, **81**, 27–8.

Meyers, J.D. (1988) Management of cytomegalovirus infection. *Am J Med*, **85**(2A), 102–6.

Michele, T.M. *et al.* (1997) Transmission of *Mycobacterium tuberculosis* by a fiberoptic bronchoscope. Identification by DNA fingerprinting. *JAMA*, **278**(13), 1093–5.

Miller, M.A., Dascal, A., Portnoy, J. *et al.* (1996) Development of mupirocin resistance among methicillin resistant *Staphylococcus aureus* after widespread use of nasal mupirocin ointment. *Infect Control Hosp Epidemiol*, **17**(12), 811–13.

Miller, R. (1998) Clinical aspects of pneumocystis pneumonia in HIV infected patients 1997. *Immunol Med Microbiol*, **22**(1–2), 103–5.

Miller, R.F. *et al.* (1989) Nebulized pentamidine as treatment for *Pneumocystis carinii* pneumonia in the acquired immunodeficiency syndrome. *Thorax*, **44**, 565–9.

Millership, S., Roberts, C.M. & Irwin, D.J. (1998) Screening child playgroup contacts of an adult with smear negative tuberculosis. *Commun Dis Public Health*, **1**(4), 283–4.

Mims, C.A. *et al.* (1993) *Medical Microbiology*. Mosby, London.

Mindal, A. & Tenant-Flowers, M. (2001) Natural history and management of early HIV infection. *Br Med J*, **322**(7297), 96.

Mir, N., Scoular, A., Lee, K. *et al.* (2001) Partner notification in HIV-1 infection: a population based evaluation of process and outcome in Scotland. *Sex Transm Infect*, **77**(3), 187–9.

Miyakawa, Y. & Mayumi, M. (1997) Hepatitis G virus. A true hepatitis virus or an accidental tourist? *N Engl J Med*, **336**(11), 795–6.

Miyakoshi, K., Tanaka, M., Miyazaki, T. *et al.* (1998) Prenatal ultrasound diagnosis of small bowel torsion. *Obstet Gynecol*, **91**(5, Part 2), 802–3.

Moellering, R.C. (1998a) Antibiotic resistance: lesson for the future. *Clin Infect Dis Suppl*, **1**, S135–40.

Moellering, R.C. (1998b) Vancomycin resistant enterococci. *Clin Infect Dis*, **26**(5), 1196–9.

Mohsen, A.H. & Group, T.H. (2001) The epidemiology of hepatitis C in the UK health regional population of 5.12 million. *Gut*, **48**(5), 707–13.

Moloughney, B.W. (2001) Transmission and post exposure management of blood borne virus infections in the health care setting: where are we now? *CAMJ*, **165**(4), 445–51.

Monnet, D.L. (1998) Methicillin resistant *Staphylococcus aureus* and its relationship to antimicrobial use: possible implications for control. *Infect Control Hosp Epidemiol*, **19**(8), 552–9.

Moraes, M.T., Niel, C. & Gomes, S.A. (1999) A polymerase chain reaction-based assay to identify genotype F of hepatitis B virus. *Braz J Med Biol Res*, **32**(1), 45–9.

Morris, A., Beard, C.B. & Huang, L. (2002a) Update on the epidemiology and transmission of *Pneumocystis carinii*. *Microbes Infect*, **4**(1), 95–103.

Morris, A., Creasman, J., Turner, J., Luce, J.M., Wachter, R.M. & Huang, L. (2002b) Intensive care of human immunodeficiency virus-infected patients during the era of highly active antiretroviral therapy. *Am J Respir Crit Care Med*, **166**(3), 262–7.

Morris, G., Kokki, M.H., Anderson, K. & Richardson, M.D. (2000) Sampling of Aspergillus spores in air. *J Hosp Infect*, **44**(2), 81–92.

Morris, M.C., Gay, N.J., Hesketh, L.M., Morgan-Capner, P. & Miller, E. (2002) The changing epidemiological pattern of hepatitis A in England and Wales. *Epidemiol Infect*, **128**(3), 457–63.

Mortimer, J.Y. & Spooner, R.J.D. (1997) HIV infection transmitted through blood product treatment, blood transfusion, and tissue transplantation. *CDR Rev*, **7**(9), R130–2.

Mostad, S.B., Kreiss, J.K., Ryncarz, A.J. *et al.* (1999) Cervical shedding of cytomegalovirus in human immunodeficiency virus type 1 infected women. *J Med Virol*, **59**(4), 469–73.

Moyenuddin, M., Williamson, J.C. & Ohl, C.A. (2002) *Clostridium difficile*-associated diarrhea: current strategies for diagnosis and therapy. *Curr Gastroenterol Rep*, **4**(4), 279–86.

Moyer, L.A. & Mast, E.E. (1998) Hepatitis A through E. *J Intraven Nurs*, **21**(5), 286–90.

Muder, R.R. & Yu, V.L. (1995) Other legionella species. In: *Principles and Practices of Infectious Disease*, 4th edn (eds G.L. Mandell, J.E. Bennett & R. Dolin). Churchill Livingstone, New York, Vol. 2, Chap. 212, pp. 2097–103.

Mustafa, A.S. (2001) Biotechnology in the development of new vaccines and diagnostic reagents against tuberculosis. *Curr Pharm Biotechnol*, **2**(2), 157–73.

Naikoba, S. & Hayward, A. (2001) The effectiveness of interventions aimed at increasing handwashing in healthcare workers – a systematic review. *J Hosp Infect*, **57**, 173–80.

National Health Service Executive (1993) *Public Health: Responsibilities of the NHS and the Roles of Others. HSG (93) 56*. Stationery Office, London.

National Health Service Executive (1994) *The control of legionellae in Health Care Premises*, Health Technical Memorandum 2040, Code of Practice NHS Estates. Stationery Office, London.

National Health Service Executive (1995) *Hospital Infection Control: Guidance on the Control of Infection in Hospitals. HSG (95) 10 1995*. Stationery Office, London.

National Health Service Executive (1998) *Communicable Disease Control in the Thames Regions in 1997*. Department of Health, London, pp. 8–11.

National Health Service Executive (1999a) *Latex Medical Gloves and Powdered Latex Medical Gloves*. Department of Health, London.

National Health Service Executive (1999b) *Variant Creutzfeldt–Jakob Disease (vCJD). Minimising the Risk of Transmission*. Department of Health, London.

Ndour, M., Sow, P.S., Coll-Seck, A.M. *et al.* (2000) AIDS caused by HIV1 and HIV2 infection: are there clinical differences? Results of AIDS surveillance 1986–1997 at Fann Hospital in Dakar, Senegal. *Trop Med Int Health*, **5**(10), 687–91.

Neely, A.N. & Maley, M.P. (2000) Survival of enterococci and staphylococci on hospital fabrics and plastic. *J Clin Microb*, **38**(1), 724–6.

Neville, K., Renbarger, J. & Dreyer, Z. (2002) Pneumonia in the immunocompromised pediatric cancer patient. *Semin Respir Infect*, **17**(1), 21–32.

Newman, K., Maylor, U. & Chansarkar, B. (2002) The nurse satisfaction, service quality and nurse retention chain: implications for management of recruitment and retention. *J Manage Med*, **16**(4–5), 271–91.

Newton, J.T., Constable, D. & Senior, V. (2001) Patients' perceptions of methicillin-resistant *Staphylococcus aureus* and source isolation: a qualitative analysis of source isolated patients. *J Hosp Infect*, **48**(4), 275–80.

NHS Estates (2002) *Infection Control in the Built Environment*. Department of Health, London.

Nicas, M. (1998) Assessing the relative importance of the components of an occupational tuberculosis control program. *J Occup Environ Med*, **40**(7), 648–54.

Nicoll, A. & Hamers, F.F. (2002) Are trends in HIV, gonorrhoea and syphilis worsening in western Europe? *Br Med J*, **324**(7349), 27.

Niedobitek, G., Meru, N. & Delecluse, H.J. (2001) Epstein–Barr virus infection and human malignancies. *Int J Exp Pathol*, **82**(3), 149–70.

Nishijima, S. & Kurikawa, I. (2002) Antimicrobial resistance of *Staphylococcus aureus* isolated from skin infections. *Int J Antimicrob Agents*, **19**(3), 241–3.

Nivin, B. *et al.* (1998) A continuing outbreak of multidrug-resistant tuberculosis, with transmission in a hospital nursery. *Clin Infect Dis*, **26**(2), 303–7.

Norder, H. *et al.* (1994) Complete genomes, phylogenetic relateness, and structural proteins of six strains of the hepatitis B virus, four of which represent two new genotypes. *Virology*, **198**(2), 489–503.

Noskin, G.A., Stosor, V., Cooper, I. & Peterson, L.R. (1995) Recovery of vancomycin-resistant enterococci on fingertips and environmental surfaces. *Infect Control Hosp Epidemiol*, **16**(10), 577–81.

Nourse, C.B. & Butler, K.M. (1998) Perinatal transmission of HIV and diagnosis of HIV infection in infants: a review. *Irish J Med Sci*, **167**(1), 28–32.

Numazaki, K., Fujikawa, T. & Chiba, S. (2000) Relationship between seropositivity of husbands and primary cytomegalovirus infection during pregnancy. *J Infect Chemother*, **6**(2), 104–6.

Obermayer-Straub, P., Strassburg, C.P. & Manns, M.P. (2000) Autoimmune hepatitis. *J Hepatol*, **32**(Suppl 1), 181–97.

Odaibo, G.N., Olaleye, O.D. & Tomori, O. (1998) Human immunodeficiency virus types 1 and 2 infection in some rural areas of Nigeria. *Rom J Virol*, **49**(1–4), 89–95.

O'Donovan, D., Ariyoshi, K., Milligan, P. *et al.* (2000) Maternal plasma viral RNA levels determine marked differences in mother-to-child transmission rates of HIV-1 and HIV-2 in the Gambia. *AIDS*, **14**(4), 441–8.

O'Donovan, D., Cooke, R.P., Joce, R. *et al.* (2001) An outbreak of hepatitis A amongst injecting drug users. *Epidemiol Infect*, **127**(3), 469–73.

Offner, F. *et al.* (1998) Impact of previous aspergillosis on the outcome of bone marrow transplantation. *Clin Infect Dis*, **26**(5), 1098–103.

Oie, S., Hosokawa, I. & Kamiya, A. (2002) Contamination of room door handles by methicillin resistant *Staphylococcus aureus*. *J Hosp Infect*, **51**(2), 140–3.

Okamoto, S., Watanabe, R., Takahashi, S. *et al.* (2002) Long term follow-up of allogeneic bone marrow transplantation after reduced-intensity conditioning in patients with chronic myelogenous leukaemia in the chronic phase. *Int J Hematol*, **75**(5), 493–8.

Oldman, T. (1998) Isolated cases. *Nurs Times*, **94**(11), 67–71.

O'Mohony, C., Gardner, C. & Casemore, D.P. (1992) Hospital acquired cryptosporidiosis. *Public Health Lab Serv Commun Dis Rep*, **3**(2), R18–19.

Ormerod, L.D. *et al.* (1998) Rapidly progressive herpetic retinal necrosis: a blinding disease charcteristic of advanced AIDS. *Clin Infect Dis*, **26**(1), 34–45.

Ormerod, L.P. (1996) Tuberculosis and immigration. *Br J Hosp Med*, **56**(5), 209–12.

O'Shea, S. *et al.* (1998) Maternal viral load, CD4 count and vertical transmission of HIV-1. *J Med Virol*, **54**(2), 113–17.

Ostroff, S.M. & Kaozarsky, P. (1998) Emerging infectious diseases and travel medicine. *Infect Dis Clin North Am*, **12**(1), 231–41.

Ota, M.O., O'Donovan, D., Alabi, A.S. *et al.* (2000) Maternal HIV-1 and HIV-2 infection and child survival in the Gambia. *AIDS*, **14**(4), 435–9.

Overberger, P.A., Wadowsky, R.M. & Schaper, M.M. (1995) Evaluation of airborne particulates and fungi during hospital building renovation. *Am Ind Hyg Assoc J*, **56**(7), 706–12.

Pamphilon, D.H. *et al.* (1999) Prevention of tranfusion – transmuted cytomegalovirus infection. *Transfus Med*, **9**(2), 115–23.

Pankhurst, C. & Peakman, M. (1989) Reduced CD4 T-cells and severe candidiasis in absence of HIV infection. *Lancet*, **i**, 672.

Parsons, M.L., Brosch, R., Cole, S.T. *et al.* (2002) Rapid and simple approach of identification of *Mycobacterium tuberculosis* complex isolates by PCR based genomic deletion analysis. *J Clin Microbiol*, **40**(7), 2339–45.

Patel, R. (2002) Progress in meeting today's demands in genital herpes: an overview of current management. *J Infect Dis*, **186**(Suppl 1), S47–56.

Patterson, A.J. (1993) Review of current practices in clean diets in the UK. *J Hum Nutr Diet*, **6**, 3–11.

Patterson, R., Sommers, H. & Fink, J.N. (1974) Farmer's lung following inhalation of *Aspergillus flavus* growing in mouldy hay. *Clin Allergy*, **4**, 79–86.

Patterson, W.J. *et al.* (1997) Colonization of transplant unit water supplies with legionella and protozoa: precautions required to reduce the risk of legionellosis. *J Hosp Infect*, **37**(1), 7–17.

Payne, D.N., Gibson, S.A. & Lewis, R. (1998) Antiseptics: a forgotten weapon in the control of antibiotic resistant bacteria in hospital and community setting. *J R Soc Health*, **118**(i), 18–22.

Pearlman, L.S. (2002) Post transplant viral syndromes in pediatric patients: a review. *Proc Transplant*, **12**(2), 116–24.

Pearse, J. (1992) Infection control. Nursing management of a patient with hepatitis A and B. *Nurs RSA*, **7**(5), 28–9.

Peat, M., Budd, J., Burns, S.M. & Robertson, R. (2000) Audit of bloodborne virus infections in injecting drug users in general practice. *Commun Dis Public Health*, **4**(3), 244–6.

Pebody, R.G., Leino, T., Ruutu, P. *et al.* (1998) Foodborne outbreaks of hepatitis A in a low endemic country: an emerging problem. *Epidemiol Infect*, **120**(1), 55–9.

Peeters, J.E. *et al.* (1989) Effects of disinfection of drinking water with ozone or chlorine dioxide on survival of *Cryptosporidium parvum* oocysts. *Appl Microbiol*, **55**(6), 1519–22.

Peggs, K.S. & Mackinnon, S. (2001) Cytomegalovirus infection and disease after autologous peripheral blood stem cell transplantation. *Br J Haematol*, **115**(4), 1032–3.

Perea, S. & Patterson, T.F. (2002) Invasive aspergillus infections in hematologic malignancy patients. *Semin Respir Infect*, **17**(2), 99–105.

Perera, D.R. *et al.* (1970) *Pneumocystis carinii* pneumonia in a hospital for children. *JAMA*, **214**, 1074–8.

Perez, A., Reniero, A., Forteis, A., Meregalli, S., Lopez, B. & Ritacco, V. (2002) Study of *Mycobacterium bovis* in milk using bacteriological methods and polymerase chain reaction. *Rev Argent Microbiol*, **34**(1), 45–51.

Perez-Fontan, M., Rosales, M., Rodriguez-Carmona, A., Falcon, T.G. & Valdes, F. (2002) Mupirocin resistance after long-term use of *Staphylococcus aureus* colonization in patients undergoing chronic peritoneal dialysis. *Am J Kidney Dis*, **39**(2), 337–41.

Perneger, T.V. *et al.* (1995) Does the onset of tuberculosis in AIDS predict shorter survival? Results of a cohort study in 17 European countries over 13 years. *Br Med J*, **311**, 1468–71.

Persson, L., Hallberg, I.R. & Ohlsson, O. (1997) Survivors of acute leukaemia and highly malignant lymphoma – retrospective views of daily life problems during treatment and when in remission. *J Adv Nurs*, **25**, 68–78.

Petchey, R., Farnsworth, W. & Williams, J. (2000) 'The last resort would be to go to the GP'. Understanding the perceptions and use of general practitioner services among people with HIV/AIDS. *Soc Sci Med*, **50**(2), 233–45.

Petchey, R., Farnsworth, W. & Heron, T. (2001) The maintenance of confidentiality in primary care: a survey of policies and procedures. *AIDS Care*, **13**(2), 251–6.

Peter, J. & Ray, C.G. (1998) Infectious mononucleosis. *Pediatr Rev*, **19**(8), 276–9.

Petersen, C. (1992) *Cryptosporidium* in patients infected with HIV. *Clin Infect Dis*, **15**, 903–9.

Petersen, F.B. *et al.* (1987) Infectious complications in patients undergoing marrow transplantation: a prospective randomized study of the additional effects of contamination and laminar air flow isolation among patients receiving prophylactic systemic antibiotics. *Scand J Infect Dis*, **19**(5), 559–67.

Petrosillo, N., Raffaele, B., Martini, L. *et al.* (2002) A nosocomial and occupational cluster of hepatitis A virus infection in a pediatric ward. *Infect Control Hosp Epidemiol*, **23**(6), 343–5.

Pettinger, A. & Nettleman, M.D. (1991) Epidemiology of isolation precautions. *Infect Control Hosp Epidemiol*, **12**(5), 303–7.

Phair, J. *et al.* (1990) The risk of *Pneumocystis carinii* pneumonia among men infected with human immune deficiency virus type 1. *N Engl J Med*, **322**, 161–5.

Phillips, K.D. & Morrow, J.H. (1998) Nursing management of anxiety in HIV infection. *Issues Ment Health Nurs*, **19**(4), 375–97.

Phuah, H.K. *et al.* (1998) Complicated varicella zoster infection in eight paediatric patients and review of literature. *Singapore Med J*, **39**(3), 115–20.

Piedade, J., Venenno, T., Prieto, E. *et al.* (2000) Longstanding presence of HIV-2 infection in Guinea-Bissau (West Africa). *Acta Trop*, **76**(2), 119–24.

Pillay, D. (1998) Emergence and control of resistance to antiviral drugs in resistance in herpes viruses, hepatitis B virus and HIV. *Commun Dis Public Health*, **1**(1), 5–13.

Pina, S. *et al.* (1998) Characterization of a strain of infectious hepatitis E virus isolated from sewage in an area where hepatitis E is not endemic. *Appl Environ Microbiol*, **64**(11), 4485–8.

Pinna, A.D., Rakela, J., Demetris, A.J. & Fung, J.J. (2002) Five cases of fulminant hepatitis due to herpes simplexvirus in adults. *Dig Dis Sci*, **47**(4), 750–4.

Pinner, R.W. *et al.* (1992) Role of food in sporadic listeriosis. Microbiologic and epidemiologic investigation. The listeria study group. *JAMA*, **267**(15), 2046–50.

Pitten, F.A. *et al.* (2001) Transmission of multiresistant *Pseudomonas aeruginosa* strain at a German University Hospital. *J Hosp Infect*, **47**(2), 125–30.

Plowman, R., Graves, N., Griffin, M. *et al.* (1999) *The Socio-Economic Burden of Hospital Acquired Infection*. Public Health Laboratory Service, London.

Poe, S.S. *et al.* (1994) A national survey of infection prevention practices on bone marrow transplant units. *Oncol Nurs Forum*, **21**(10), 1687–93.

Porter, H. (1998) Nursing management in the BMT unit. In: *The Clinical Practice of Stem-Cell Transplantation* (eds J. Barrett & J. Treleaven). ISIS Medical Media, Oxford, **2**(59), 879–89.

Porter, K. *et al.* (1996) AIDS: defining disease in the UK. The impact of PCP prophylaxis and twelve years of change. *Int J STD AIDS*, **7**(4), 252–7.

Potterton, D. (1985) Mystery of the organism. *Nurs Times*, **82**(22), 20–1.

Poulsen, A.G. *et al.* (1997) 9-year HIV-2 associated mortality in an urban community in Bissau, west Africa. *Lancet*, **349**(9056), 911–14.

Preiksaitis, J.K., Sandhu, J. & Strautman, M. (2002) The risk of transfusion-acquired CMV infection in seronegative solid-organ transplant recipients receiving non-WBC-reduced blood components not screened for CMV antibody (1984 to 1996): experience at a single Canadian center. *Transfusion*, **42**(4), 396–402.

Prentice, G., Grundy, J.E. & Kho, P. (1998) Cytomegalovirus. In: *The Clinical Practice of Stem Cell Transplantation* (eds J. Barrett & J. Treleaven). ISIS Medical Media, Oxford, **2**(44), 698–707.

Prester, E., Mueller-Uri, P., Grisold, A., Georgopoulos, A. & Graninger, W. (2001) Ciprofloxacin and methicillin resistant *Staphylococcus aureus* susceptible to moxifloxacin, levofloxacin, teicoplanin, vancomycin and linezolid. *Eur J Clin Microbiol Infect Dis*, **20**(7), 486–9.

Pronczuk, J., Akre, J., Moy, G. & Vallenas, C. (2002) Global perspectives in breast milk contamination: infection and toxic hazards. *Environ Health Perspect*, **110**(6), A349–51.

Public Health Laboratory Service AIDS and STD Centre (1997) *Occupational Transmission of HIV*. PHLS, London.

Public Health Laboratory Service Communicable Disease Surveillance Centre (1994) European surveillance of legionnaires' disease associated with travel. *Commun Dis Rep*, **4**(6), 25.

Puech, M.C., McAnulty, J.M., Lesjak, M. *et al.* (2001) A statewide outbreak of cryptosporidiosis in New South Wales associated with swimming at public pools. *Epidemiol Infect*, **26**(3), 389–96.

Quale, J. *et al.* (1996) Experience with a hospital-wide outbreak of vancomycin resistant enterococci. *Am J Infect Control*, **24**(5), 372–9.

Quinlivan, J.A., Newnham, J.P. & Dickinson, J.E. (1998) Ultrasound features of congenital listeriosis. A case report. *Prenat Diag*, **18**(10), 1075–8.

Rab, M.A. *et al.* (1997) Water-borne hepatitis E virus epidemic in Islamabad, Pakistan: a common source outbreak traced to the malfunction of a modern water treatment plant. *Am J Trop Med Hyg*, **57**(2), 151–7.

Rabaud, C. & Mauuary, G. (2001) Infection and/or colonization by methicillin-resistant *Staphylococcus epidermidis* (MRSE). *Pathol Biol (Paris)*, **49**(10), 812–14.

Rabkin, J. (1997) Meeting the challenge of depression in HIV. *Treatment Issues*, **11**(10), 6–11.

Radman, J.C. (1973) *Pneumocystis carinii* pneumonia in an adopted Vietnamese infant. *J Am Med Assoc*, **230**, 1561–3.

Radwin, L. (2000) Oncology patients' perception of quality nursing care. *Res Nurs Health*, **23**(3), 179–90.

Rae, G.G. (1998) Risk factors for the spread of antibiotic-resistant bacteria. *Drugs*, **55**(3), 323–30.

Rajaratnam, G. *et al.* (1992) An outbreak of hepatitis A: school toilets as a source of transmission. *J Public Health Med*, **14**(1), 72–7.

Ramsey, C.N. *et al.* (1989) Hepatitis A and frozen raspberries. *Lancet*, **i**, 43–4.

Ravin, P., Lundgren, J.D. & Kjaeldgaard, P. (1991) Nosocomial outbreak of *Cryptosporidium* in AIDS patients. *Br Med J*, **302**, 277–80.

Raybourne, R.B. (2002) Virulence testing of *Listeria monocytogenes*. *J Assoc Official Analyt Chem*, **85**(2), 516–23.

Reddy, V.M. & Hayworth, D.A. (2002) Interaction of *Mycobacterium tuberculosis* with human respiratory epithelial cells (Hep-2). *Tuberculosis (Edinb)*, **82**(1), 31–6.

Redpath, C. & Farrington, M. (1997) Dispose of disposables. *J Hosp Infect*, **35**, 313–17.

Rees, J., Davies, H.R., Birchall, C. & Price, J. (2000) Psychological effects of course isolation nursing (2): patient satisfaction. *Nurs Stand*, **14**(29), 32–6.

Regan, F.A.M., Hewitt, P., Barbara, J.A.J. & Contreras, M. (2000) Prospective investigation of transfusion transmitted infection in recipients of over 20 000 units of blood. *Br Med J*, **320**(7232), 403–6.

Renge, R.L., Danoi, V.S., Chitambar, S.D. & Arankalle, V.A. (2002) Vertical transmission of hepatitis A. *Indian J Pediatr*, **69**(6), 535–6.

Reusser, P. (1996) Herpesvirus resistance to antiviral drugs: a review of the mechanisms. Clinical importance and therapeutic options. *J Hosp Infect*, **33**(4), 235–48.

Reusser, P. (1998) Current concepts and challenges in the prevention and treatment of viral infections in the immunocompromised cancer patients. *Support Care Cancer*, **6**(1), 39–45.

Reusser, P. *et al.* (1996) European survey of herpes virus resistance to antiviral drugs in bone marrow transplant recipients. Infectious Diseases Working Party of the European Group for Blood and Marrow Transplantation (EBMT). *Bone Marrow Transplant*, **17**(5), 813–17.

Reyes, E.M. & Legg, J.J. (1997) Prevention of HIV transmission. *Prim Care*, **24**(3), 469–77.

Reynolds, E., Wickenden, C. & Oliver, A. (2001) The impact of improved safety on maintaining a sufficient blood supply. *Transfus Clin Biol*, **8**(3), 235–9.

Rhame, F.S. (1991) Prevention of nosocomial aspergillosis. *J Hosp Infect*, **18**(Suppl A), 466–72.

Ribas-Mundom, M., Granena, A. & Rozman, C. (1981) Evaluation of a protective environment in the management of granulocytopenic patients. A comparative study. *Cancer*, **48**, 419–24.

Ribeiro-Dos-Santos, G., Nishiya, A.S., Nascimento, C.M. *et al.* (2002) Prevalence of GB virus C (hepatitis G virus) and risk factors for infection in Sao Paulo, Brazil. *Eur J Clin Mirobiol Infect Dis*, **21**(6), 438–43.

Richardson, M.D., Rennie, S., Marshall, I. *et al.* (2000) Fungal infection of an open haematology ward. *J Hosp Infect*, **45**(4), 288–92.

Riley, M. *et al.* (1997) Tuberculosis in health care service employees in Northern Ireland. *Respir Med*, **91**(9), 546–50.

Riley, U. (1998) Bacterial infections. In: *The Clinical Practice of Stem Cell Transplantation* (eds J. Barrett & J. Treleaven). Isis Medical Media, Oxford, **2**(43), 690–7.

Rivera, L.B. *et al.* (2002) Predictors of hearing loss in children with symptomatic congenital cytomegalovirus infection. *Pediatrics*, **110**(4), 762–7.

Robinson, R.A. & Pugh, R.N. (2002) Dogs, zoonoses and immunosuppression. *J R Soc Health*, **122**(2), 95–8.

Robinson, W.R. & Freeman, D. (2002) Improved outcome of cervical neoplasia in HIV infected women in the era of highly active antiretroviral therapy. *AIDS Patient Care STDs*, **16**(2), 61–5.

Rochling, F.A., Jones, W.F., Chau, K. *et al.* (1997) Acute sporadic non-A, non-B, non-C, non-D, non-E hepatitis. *Hepatology*, **25**(2), 478–83.

Rogers, B.B., Josephson, S.L. & Mak, S.K. (1991) Detection of herpes simplex virus using polymerase chain reaction followed by endonuclease cleavage. *Am J Pathol*, **139**(1), 1–6.

Rogers, P.A., Sinka, K.J., Molesworth, A.M., Evans, B.G. & Allardice, G.N. (2000) Survival after diagnosis of AIDS among adults resident in the United Kingdom in the era of multiple therapies. *Commun Dis Public Health*, **3**(3), 188–94.

Rolston, K.V. *et al.* (1998) Ambulatory management of varicella-zoster virus infection in immunocompromised cancer patients. *Support Care Cancer*, **6**(1), 57–62.

Romero-Vivas, J. *et al.* (1995) Mortality associated with nosocomial bacteraemia due to methicillin resistant *Staphylococcus aureus*. *Clin Infect Dis*, **21**, 1417–23.

Ronals, N. & Jones, M.D. (2001) Resistance patterns among nosocomial pathogens. *Chest*, **119**(2 Suppl 3), 97–404S.

Ross, A.M. & Fleming, D.M. (2000) Chickenpox increasingly affects pre-school children. *Commun Dis Public Health*, **3**(3), 213–14.

Rossoff, L.J. *et al.* (1993) Is the use of boxed gloves in an intensive care unit safe? *Am J Med*, **94**, 602–7.

Roth, W.K., Waschk, D., Marx, S. *et al.* (1997) Prevalence of hepatitis G virus and its strain variant, the GB agent, in blood donations and their transmission to recipients. *Transfusion*, **37**(6), 569–72.

Rouquette, C. & Berche, P. (1996) The pathogenesis of infection by *Listeria monocytogenes*. *Microbiologia*, **12**(2), 245–58.

Rowbotham, T.J. (1998) Legionellosis associated with ships 1977–1997. *Commun Dis Public Health*, **1**(3), 146–51.

Rowland, P. *et al.* (1995) Progressive varicella presenting with pain and minimal skin involvement in children with acute lymphoblastic leukemia. *J Clin Oncol*, **13**(7), 1697–703.

Rudnick, C.M. & Hoekzema, G.S. (2002) Neonatal herpes simplex virus infections. *Am Fam Physician*, **65**(6), 1138–42.

Russell, D.G. (2001) *Mycobacterium tuberculosis*: here today and here tomorrow. *Nat Rev Mol Cell Biol*, **2**(8), 569–77.

Russell, J.A., Chaudhry, A., Booth, K. *et al.* (2000) Early outcomes after allogeneic stem cell transplantation for leukemia and myelodysplasia without protective isolation: a 10 year experience. *Biol Blood Marrow Transplant*, **6**(2), 109–14.

Russian, D.A. & Levine, S.J. (2001) *Pneumocystis carinii* pneumonia in patients with HIV infection. *Am J Med Sci*, **321**(1), 56–65.

Saavedra, S., Jarque, I., Sanz, G.F. *et al.* (2002) Infectious complications in patients undergoing unrelated donor bone marrow transplantation: experience from a single institution. *Clin Microbiol Infect*, **8**(11), 725–33.

Sabria, M. & Yu, V.L. (2002) Hospital acquired legionellosis: solutions for a preventable infection. *Lancet Infect Dis*, **ii**(6), 368–73.

Safdar, N. & Maki, D.G. (2002) The commonality of risk factors for nosocomial colonization and infection with antimicrobial-resistant *Staphylococcus aureus*, enterococcus, Gram negative bacilli, *Clostridium difficile* and Candida. *Ann Intern Med*, **136**(11), 834–44.

Sales, M.P., Taylor, G.M., Hughes, S. *et al.* (2001) Genetic diversity among *Mycobacterium bovis* isolates: a preliminary study of strains from animals and human sources. *Clin Microbiol*, **39**(12), 4558–62.

Samuel, R., Bettiker, R.L. & Suh, B. (2002) AIDS related opportunistic infections. Going but not gone. *Arch Pharm Res*, **25**(3), 215–28.

Sande, M.A. & Mandell, G.L. (1980) Chemotherapy of microbial diseases. In: *The Pharmacological Basis of Therapeutics* (eds L.S. Goodman *et al.*). Macmillan, London.

Sanderson, P.J. (1999) What should we do about patients with *Clostridium difficile*? *J Hosp Infect*, **43**(4), 251–3.

Santamauro, J.T., Aurora, R.N. & Stover, D.E. (2002) *Pneumocystis carinii* pneumonia in patients with and without HIV infection. *Comp Ther*, **28**(2), 96–108.

Saraceno, J.L. *et al.* (1997) Chronic necrotizing pulmonary aspergillosis: approach to management. *Chest*, **112**(2), 542–8.

Saville, R.D., Constantine, N.T., Farley, R. *et al.* (2001) Fourth-generation enzyme linked immunosorbent detection of human immunodeficiency virus antigen and antibody. *J Clin Microbiol*, **39**(7), 2518–24.

Sawayama, Y., Hayashi, J., Kakuda, K. *et al.* (2000) Hepatitis C virus infection in institutionalized psychiatric patients: possible role of transmission by razor sharing. *Dig Dis Sci*, **45**(2), 351–6.

Sawyer, M.H. *et al.* (1994) Detection of varicella-zoster virus DNA in air samples from hospital rooms. *J Infect Dis*, **169**, 91–4.

Schim van der Loeff, M.F. *et al.* (2002) Mortality of HIV-1 and HIV-1/HIV-2 dually infected patients in a clinic-based cohort in the Gambia. *AIDS*, **16**(13), 1775–83.

Schluger, N.W., Perez, D. & Liu, Y.M. (2002) Reconstitution of immune responses to tuberculosis in patients with HIV infection who receive antiretroviral therapy. *Chest*, **122**(2), 597–602.

Schmader, K. (1998) Post-therapeutic neuralgia in immunocompetent elderly people. *Vaccine*, **16**(18), 1768–70.

Scott, D.A., Coulter, W.A. & Lamey, P.J. (1997) Oral shedding of herpes simplex virus type 1: a review. *J Oral Pathol Med*, **26**(10), 441–7.

Scott, E. & Bloomfield, S.F. (1990) Investigations of the effectiveness of detergent washing, drying and chemical disinfection on contamination of cleaning cloths. *J Appl Bacteriol*, **68**(3), 279–83.

Scoular, A., Watt, A.D., Watson, M. & Kelly, B. (2000) Knowledge and attitudes of hospital staff to occupational exposure to bloodborne viruses. *Commun Dis Public Health*, **3**(4), 247–9.

Sefton, A.M. (2002) Mechanisms of antimicrobial resistance: their clinical relevance in the new millennium. *Drugs*, **62**(4), 557–66.

Shaffer, S. & Wilson, J.N. (1993) Bone marrow transplantation. Critical care nurses. *Clin North Am*, **5**(3), 531–50.

Sharland, M., Gibb, D., Tudor-Williams, G. *et al.* (1997) Paediatric HIV infection. *Arch Dis Child*, **76**(4), 293–7.

Sharma, J.B., Ekoh, S., McMillan, L., Hussain, S. & Annan, H. (1997) Blood splashes to the masks and goggles during caesarean section. *Br J Obstet Gynaecol*, **104**(12), 1405–6.

Sheng, L. *et al.* (1998) Hepatitis G virus infection in acute fulminant hepatitis: prevalence of HGV infection and sequence analysis of a specific viral strain. *J Viral Hepat*, **5**(5), 301–6.

Shepherd, J., Waugh, N. & Hewitson, P. (2000) Combination therapy (interferon alfa and ribavirin) in the treatment of chronic hepatitis C: a rapid and systematic review. *Health Technol Assess*, **4**(33), 1–67.

Shibuya, A., Takeuchi, A., Sakurai, K. & Saigenji, K. (1998) Hepatitis G virus infection from needlestick injuries in hospital employees. *J Hosp Infect*, **40**(2), 287–90.

Shinjo, K., Takeshita, A., Yanagi, Y. *et al.* (2002) Efficacy of the Shinki bioclean room for preventing infection in neutropenic patients. *J Adv Nurs*, **37**(3), 227–33.

Shiomori, T., Miyamoto, H., Makishima, K. *et al.* (2002) Evaluation of bedmaking-related airborne and surface methicillin-resistant *Staphylococcus aureus* contamination. *J Hosp Infect*, **50**(1), 30–5.

Siegel, G. *et al.* (1984) Stability of hepatitis A virus. *Intervirology*, **22**, 218–26.

Siegel, M.A. (2002) Diagnosis and management of recurrent herpes simplex infections. *J Am Dent Assoc*, **133**(9), 1245–9.

Siegl, G. (1988) Virology of hepatitis. In: *Viral Hepatitis and Liver Disease* (ed. A.J. Zuckerman). Alan R. Liss, New York, pp. 3–7.

Singh, J. *et al.* (1998) Outbreak of viral hepatitis B in rural community in India linked to inadequately sterilized needles and syringes. *Bull World Health Organ*, **76**(1), 93–8.

Singh, N. *et al.* (1997) Invasive aspergillosis in liver transplant recipients in the 1990s. *Transplantation*, **64**(5), 716–20.

Singhal, S. *et al.* (1997) Cytomegaloviremia after autografting for leukemia: clinical significance and lack of effect on engraftment. *Leukemia*, **11**(6), 835–8.

Singleton, L. *et al.* (1997) Long term hospitalization for tuberculosis control. Experience with a medical-psychosocial inpatient unit. *JAMA*, **278**(10), 838–42.

Sixbey, J.W. *et al.* (1984) Epstein–Barr virus replication in oropharyneal epithelial cells. *N Engl J Med*, **310**(19), 1225–30.

Skidmore, S.J. (1997) Tropical aspects of viral hepatitis: hepatitis E. *Trans R Soc Trop Med Hyg*, **91**(2), 125–6.

Smerdon, W.J., Jones, R., McLauchlin, J. *et al.* (2001) Surveillance of listeriosis in England and Wales 1995–1999. *Commun Dis Public Health*, **4**(3), 188–93.

Smith, H.M., Alexander, G.J., Webb, G., McManua, T., McFarlane, I.G. & Williams, R. (1992) Hepatitis B and delta virus infection among 'at risk' population in south east London. *J Epidemiol Comm Health*, **46**(2), 144–7.

Smith, J.P. (1993) Hepatitis C: a major public health problem. *J Adv Nurs*, **18**(3), 503–6.

Smith, T.L. & Nathan, B.R. (2002) Central nervous system infections in the immune-competent adult. *Curr Treat Options Neurol*, **4**(4), 323–32.

Smith, T.L., Van Rensburg, E.J. & Engelbrecht, S. (1998a) Neutralization of HIV-1 subtypes: implication for vaccine formations. *J Med Virol*, **56**(3), 264–8.

Smith, T.L., Iwen, P.C., Olson, S.B. *et al.* (1998b) Environmental contamination with vancomycin-resistant enterococci in an outpatient setting. *Infect Control Hosp Epidemiol*, **19**(7), 515–18.

Snoeck, R. & De Clercq, E. (2002) New treatment for genital herpes. *Curr Opin Infect Dis*, **15**(1), 49–55.

Sobaszek, A., Fantoni-Quinton, S., Frimat, P. *et al.* (2000) Prevalence of cytomegalovirus infection among health care workers in pediatric and immunosuppressed adult units. *J Occup Environ Med*, **42**(11), 1109–14.

Solomon, S. *et al.* (1998) Prevalence and risk factors of HIV-1 and HIV-2 in urban and rural areas in Tamil Nadu, India. *Int J STD AIDS*, **9**(2), 98–103.

Sorbey, M.D. *et al.* (1988) Survival and persistence of hepatitis A virus in environmental samples. In: *Viral Hepatitis and Liver Disease* (ed. A.J. Zuckerman). Alan R. Liss, New York, pp. 121–4.

Soubani, A.O. & Chandrasekar, P.H. (2002) The clinical spectrum of pulmonary aspergillosis. *Chest*, **121**(6), 1988–99.

Soucie, J.M. *et al.* (1998) Hepatitis A virus infection associated with clotting factor concentrate in the United States. *Transfusion*, **38**(6), 573–9.

Souza, J.P., Boeckh, M., Gooley, T.A., Flowers, M.E. & Crawford, S.W. (1999) High rates of *Pneumocystis carinii* pneumonia in allogeneic blood and marrow transplant recipients receiving dapsone prophylaxis. *Clin Infect Dis*, **29**(6), 1467–71.

Spano, J.P., Atlan, D., Breau, J.L. & Farge, D. (2002) AIDS and non AIDS related malignancies. A new vexing challenge in HIV positive patients. Part 1: Kaposi's sarcoma, non Hodgkins lymphoma and Hodgkins lymphoma. *Eur J Int Med*, **13**(3), 170–9.

Sparano, J.A. (2001) Clinical aspects and management of AIDS-related lymphoma. *Eur J Cancer*, **37**(10), 1296–305.

Spencer, T.C. (1998) Clinical impact and associated costs of *Clostridium difficile* associated disease. *J Antimicrob Chemother*, **41**(Suppl C) 5–12.

Sperling, R.S. *et al.* (1998) Safety of the maternal–infant zidovudine regimen utilized in the pediatric AIDS Clinical Trial Group 076 study. *AIDS*, **12**(14), 1805–13.

Spires, R. (1992) Acute retinal necrosis syndrome. *J Ophthal Nurs Technol*, **11**(3), 103–8.

Srinivasan, A., Song, X., Ross, T., Merz, W., Brower, R. & Perl, T.M. (2002) A prospective study to determine whether cover gowns in addition to gloves decrease nosocomial transmission of vancomycin-resistant enterococci in an intensive care unit. *Infect Control Hosp Epidemiol*, **23**(8), 420–3.

Stacey, A. *et al.* (1998) Contamination of television sets by methicillin resistant *Staphylococcus aureus* (MRSA). *J Hosp Infect*, **39**(3), 243–4.

Standing Medical Advisory Committee (1998) *The Path of Least Resistance*. Department of Health, Wetherby.

Starkel, P., Cicarelli, O., Lerut, J., Goubau, P., Rahier, J. & Horsmans, Y. (2002) Limited lamivudine and long-term hepatitis B immunoglobulin immunoprophylaxis for prevention of hepatitis B recurrence after liver transplantation. *Transplantation*, **74**(3), 408–10.

Steinmuller, T., Seehofer, D., Rayed, N. *et al.* (2002) Increasing applicability of liver transplantation for patients with hepatitis B related liver disease. *Hepatology*, **35**(6), 1528–35.

Stewart, J.A. *et al.* (1995) Herpesvirus infection in persons infected with HIV. *Clin Infect Dis*, **21**(Suppl 1), S114–20.

Strine, T.W., Barker, L.E., Mokdad, A.H., Luman, E.T., Sutter, R.W. & Chu, S.Y. (2002) Vaccination coverage of foreign born children 19 to 35 months of age: findings from the national immunization survey 1999–2000. *Pediatrics*, **110**(2 pt 1), 15.

Storb, R. *et al.* (1983) GVHD and survival in patients with aplastic anaemia treated by bone marrow grafts with HLA identifiable siblings. *N Engl J Med*, **308**, 302–7.

Stordeur, S., Vandenberghe, C. & D'hoore, W. (1999) Prediction of nurses' professional burnout: a study in a university hospital. *Rech Soins Infirm*, (59), 57–67.

Stout, J.E. (1987) Legionnaires' disease acquired within the homes of two patients. *JAMA*, **257**(9), 1215–17.

Stover, B.H. & Bratcher, D.F. (1998) Varicella-zoster virus: infection, control and prevention. *Am J Infect Control*, **26**(3), 369–81.

Stover, J. & Way, P. (1998) Projecting the impact of AIDS on mortality. *AIDS*, **12**, Suppl 1, S29–39.

Strom, T.B. (1990) Immunosuppression in graft rejection. In: *Organ Transplantation – Current Clinical and Immunological Concepts* (eds L. Brent & R. Sells). Baillière Tindall, Eastbourne, pp. 44–56.

Strong, D.M. & Katz, L. (2002) Blood-bank testing for infectious disease: how safe is blood transfusion? *Trends Mol Med*, **8**(7), 355–8.

Suarez, A.A., Sokol-Anderson, M.L., Creer, M., Taylor, J.F. & Ritter, D. (2001) Case report. Diagnosis of early HIV-1 infection. *AIDS Patient Care STDs*, **15**(5), 237–41.

Subcommittee of the Joint Tuberculosis Committee of the British Thoracic Society (1990) Control and prevention of tuberculosis in Britain: an updated code of practice. *Br Med J*, **300**, 995–9.

Subira, M., Martino, R., Franquet, T. *et al.* (2002) Invasive pulmonary aspergillosis in patients with hematologic malignancies: survival and prognostic factors. *Haematologica*, **87**(5), 528–34.

Sundkvisst, T. *et al.* (1998) Fatal outcome of transmission of hepatitis B from an e antigen negative surgeon. *Commun Dis Public Health*, **1**(1), 48–50.

Surawicz, C.M. (1998) *Clostridium difficile* disease: diagnosis and treatment. *Gastroenterologist*, **6**(1), 60–5.

Swinker, M. (1997) Occupational infection in health care workers: prevention and intervention. *Am Fam Physician*, **56**(9), 2291–300.

Szczesny, A., Kanski, A. & Martirosian, G. (2002) Incidence of pseudomembranous colitis after vancomycin treated MRSA infection. *Clin Microbiol Infect*, **8**(1), 58–9.

Szewczyk, E.M., Piotrowski, A. & Rozalska, M. (2000) Predominant staphylococci in the intensive care unit of a paediatric hospital. *J Hosp Infect*, **45**(2), 145–54.

Takayama, N., Yamada, H., Kaku, H. *et al.* (2000) Herpes zoster in immunocompetent and immunosuppressed Japanese children. *Pediatrics*, **42**(3), 275–9.

Takenaka, K. *et al.* (1997) Increased incidence of CMV infection and CMV associated disease after allogeneic bone marrow transplantation from unrelated donors. The Fukuoko bone marrow transplantation group. *Bone Marrow Transplant*, **19**(3), 241–8.

Taormina, P.J. & Beuchat, L.R. (2001) Survival and heat resistance of *Listeria monocytogenes* after exposure to alkali and chlorine. *Appl Environ Microbiol*, **67**(6), 2555–63.

Taplitz, R.A. & Jordan, M.C. (2002) Pneumonia caused by herpesviruses in recipients of hematopoietic cell transplants. *Semin Respir Infect*, **17**(2), 121–9.

Tattevin, P., Cremieux, A.C., Descamps, D. & Carbon, C. (2002) Transfusion-related infectious mononucleosis. *Scand J Infect*, **34**(10), 777–8.

Taylor, J.M. (1999) Hepatitis delta virus. *Intervirology*, **42**(2–3), 173–8.

Taylor, K., Plowman, R. & Roberts, J.A. (2001) *The Challenge of Hospital Acquired Infection*. National Audit Office, London.

Tedder, R.S. (1980) Hepatitis B in hospitals. *Br J Hosp Med*, **23**(3), 266–79.

Tennenberg, A.M. *et al.* (1997) Varicella vaccination for health care workers at a university hospital: an analysis of costs and benefits. *Infect Control Hosp Epidemiol*, **18**(6), 405–11.

Tenover, F.C., Biddle, J.W. & Lancaster, M.V. (2001) Increasing resistance to vancomycin and other glycopeptides in *Staphylococcus aureus*. *Emerg Infect Dis*, **7**(21), 13.

Teo, C.G. (1992) The virology and serology of hepatitis: an overview. *Commun Dis Rep*, **2**(10), R109–13.

Ter Borg, F. *et al.* (1998) Recovery from life threatening, corticosteroid-unresponsive, chemotherapy-related reactivation of hepatitis B associated with lamivudine therapy. *Dig Dis Sci*, **43**(10), 2267–70.

Tetrault, I. & Boivin, G. (2000) Recent advances in management of genital herpes. *Can Fam Physician*, **46**, 1622–9.

Thain, C.W. & Gibbon, B. (1996) An exploratory study of recipients' perceptions of bone marrow transplantation. *J Adv Nurs*, **23**(3), 528–35.

Thio, C.L., Smith, D., Merz, W.G. *et al.* (2000) Refinement of environmental assessment during an outbreak investigation of invasive aspergillosis in a leukemia and bone marrow transplant unit. *Infect Control Hosp Epidemiol*, **21**(1), 18–23.

Third Report of the Group of Experts (1998) Cryptosporidium *in Water Supplies*. Department of the Environment, Transport and the Regions, and Department of Health, London.

Thomson, M.M., Perez-Alvarez, L. & Najera, R. (2002) Molecular epidemiology of HIV-1 genetic forms and its significance for vaccine development and therapy. *Lancet*, **ii**(8), 461–71.

Thornsberry, C. (1995) Trends in antimicrobial resistance among today's bacterial pathogens. *Pharmacotherapy*, **15**(1 Part 2), 3–8S.

Trakumas, S., Willeke, K., Grinshpun, S.A. *et al.* (2001) Particle emission characteristics of filter-equipped vacuum cleaners. *Am Ind Hyg Assoc J*, **62**(4), 482–93.

Trautman, M. *et al.* (1985) Listeria meningitis: report of 10 cases and review of current therapeutic recommendations. *J Infect*, **10**, 107–14.

Trevelyan, J. (1991) Hepatitis B – who is at risk? *Nurs Times*, **87**(5), 26–9.

Trexler, P.C. (1975) Microbial isolators for use in the hospital. *Biomed Eng*, **10**(2), 63–7.

Trexler, P.C., Emond, R.T. & Evans, B. (1977) Negative pressure plastic isolator for patients with dangerous infections. *Br Med J*, **ii**(6086), 559–61.

Tsiodras, S., Samonis, G., Keating, M.J. & Kontoyiannis, D.P. (2000) Infection and immunity in chronic lymphocytic leukemia. *Mayo Clin Proc*, **75**(10), 1039–54.

Turner, M.L. (2001) Variant Creutzfeldt–Jakob disease and blood transfusions. *Curr Opin Hematol*, **8**(6), 372–9.

Uchida, T. *et al.* (1994) Pathology of livers infected with silent hepatitis B virus mutant. *Liver*, **14**(5), 251–6.

UK Health Department (2002a) AIDS/HIV infected health care workers: guidance on the management of infected health care workers and patient notification, UK Health Department.

UK Health Department (2002b) Guidance for clinical health care workers. Protection against infection with blood borne viruses. UK Health Department.

Ungar, B.L.P. (1995) *Cryptosporidium*. In: *Principles and Practices of Infectious Disease*, 4th edn (eds G.L. Mandell, J.E. Bennett & R. Dolan). Churchill Livingstone, New York, Vol. 2, Chap. 262, pp. 2500–10.

Usuda, S., Okamoto, H., Tanaka, T. *et al.* (2000) Differentiation of hepatitis B virus genotype D and E by ELISA using monoclonal antibodies to epitopes on the preS2-region product. *J Virol Methods*, **87**(1–2), 81–9.

Vaidya, S.R., Chitambar, S.D. & Arankalle, V.A. (2002) Polymerase chain reaction-based prevalence of hepatitis A, hepatitis E and TT viruses in sewage from an endemic area. *J Hepatol*, **37**(1), 131–6.

Valani, S. & Robert, D. (1990) *Listeria monocytogenes* and other *Listeria* spp. in pre-packed mixed salads and individual salad ingredients. *Public Health Lab Serv Microbiol Dig*, **8**(1), 21–2.

Van Baarle, D., Hovenkamp, E., Dukers, N.H. *et al.* (2000) High prevalence of Epstein–Barr virus type 2 among homosexual men is caused by sexual transmission. *J Infect Dis*, **181**(6), 2045–9.

Van Burik, J.A. & Weisdorf, D.J. (1999) Infections in recipients of blood and marrow transplantation. *Hematol Oncol Clin North Am*, **13**(5), 1065–89.

Van Buynder, P. (1998) Enhanced surveillance of tuberculosis in England and Wales: circling the wagons. *Commun Dis Public Health*, **1**(4), 219–20.

Vandecasteele, S.J., Van Wijngaerden, E., Van Eldere, J. & Peetermans, W.E. (2000) New insights in the pathogenesis of foreign body infections with coagulase negative staphylococci. *Act Clin Belg*, **55**(3), 148–53.

Van de Ryst, E. (2002) Progress in HIV vaccine research. *Oral Dis*, **8**(Suppl 2), 21–6.

Van der Loeff, M.F., Aaby, P., Aryioshi, K. *et al.* (2001) HIV-2 does not protect against HIV-1 infection in a rural community in Guinea-Bissau. *AIDS*, **15**(17), 2303–10.

Van Der Zwet, W.C., Vanderbroucke-Grauls, C.M., Van Elburg, R.M. *et al.* (2002) Neonatal antibody titers against varicella-zoster virus in relation to gestational age, birth weight, and maternal titer. *Pediatrics*, **109**(1), 79–85.

Vancikova, Z. & Dvorak, P. (2001) Cytomegalovirus infection in immunocompetent and immunocompromised individuals – a review. *Curr Drug Targets Immune Endocr Metabol Disord*, **1**(2), 179–87.

Vasconcelles, M.J., Bernardo, M.V., King, C., Weller, E.A. & Antin, J.H. (2000) Aerosolized pentamidine as pneumocystis prophylaxis after bone marrow transplantation is inferior to other regimens and is associated with decreased survival and an increased risk of other infections. *Biol Blood Marrow Transplant*, **6**(1), 35–43.

Vass, A. (2002) Hopes rise for patients with drug resistant HIV. *Br Med J*, **325**(7355), 62.

Veen, J. *et al.* (1998) Standardized tuberculosis treatment outcome monitoring in Europe. *Eur Respir J*, **12**(2), 505–10.

Veenstra, J. *et al.* (1995) Transmission of zidovudine-resistant HIV type 1 variants following deliberate injection of blood from a patient with AIDS. Characteristics and natural history of the virus. *Clin Infect Dis*, **21**, 536–60.

Velasco-Hernandez, J.X., Gershengorn, H.B. & Blower, S.M. (2002) Could widespread use of combination antiretroviral therapy eradicate HIV epidemic? *Lancet*, **ii**(8), 487–93.

Verma, N. & Kearney, J. (1996) Ocular manifestations of AIDS. *Postgrad Med J*, **39**(3), 196–9.

Verschraegen, C.F. *et al.* (1997) Invasive *Aspergillus* sinusitis during bone marrow transplantation. *Scand J Infect Dis*, **29**(4), 436–8.

Vickers, V. *et al.* (1994) Hepatitis B outbreak in a drug trials unit: investigations and recommendations. *Commun Dis Rep*, **4**(1), R1–4.

Viscoli, C. (1998) The evolution of the empirical management of fever and neutropenia in cancer patients. *J Antimicrob Chemother*, **41**(Suppl D), 56–80.

Viswanath, Y.K. & Griffiths, C.D. (1998) The role of surgery in pseudomembranous enterocolitis. *Postgrad Med J*, **74**(870), 216–19.

Von Eiff, C., Proctor, R.A. & Peters, G. (2001) Coagulase-negative staphylococci. Pathogens have a major role in nosocomial infections. *Postgrad Med*, **110**(4), 63–76.

Von Eiff, C., Peters, G. & Heilmann, C. (2002) Pathogenesis of infections due to coagulase negative staphylococci. *Lancet Infect Dis*, **ii**(11), 677–85.

Vrielink, H. & Reesink, H.W. (1998) Transfusion-transmissible infections. *Curr Opin Hematol*, **5**(6), 396–405.

Vyse, A.J. *et al.* (2000) The burden of infection with HSV-1 and HSV-2 in England and Wales: implications for the changing epidemiology of genital herpes. *Sex Transm Infect*, **76**(3), 183–7.

Wagenvoort, J.H., Sluijsmans, W. & Penders, R.J. (2000) Better environmental survival of outbreaks vs. sporadic MRSA isolates. *J Hosp Infect*, **45**(3), 231–4.

Wakefield, A.E. (2002) *Pneumocystis carinii. Br Med Bull*, **6**(1), 184–8.

Walsh, J.C. *et al.* (1998) Increasing survival in AIDS patients with CMV retinitis treated with combination antiretroviral therapy including HIV protease inhibitors. *AIDS*, **12**(6), 613–18.

Walzer, P.D. (1970) *Pneumocystis carinii* infection. Review article. *South Med J*, **70**(11), 1330–3.

Walzer, P.D. (1995) *Pneumocystis carinii*. In: *Principles and Practices of Infectious Diseases*, 4th edn (eds G.L. Mandell, J.E. Bennett & R. Dolin). Churchill Livingstone, New York, Vol. 2, Chap. 258, pp. 2475–86.

Wang, J.T., Chang, S.C., Ko, W.J. *et al.* (2001) Hospital-acquired outbreak of methicillin resistant *Staphylococcus aureus* infection initiated by a surgeon carrier. *J Hosp Infect*, **47**(2), 104–9.

Ward, D. (2000) Infection control: reducing the psychological effects of isolation. *Br J Nurs*, **9**(3), 162–70.

Ward, V., Wilson, J. & Taylor, L. (1997) Guidelines for routine blood and body substances precautions. In: *Preventing Hospital Acquired Infection. Clinical Guidelines*. Public Health Laboratory Service, London, pp. 11–16.

Warren, R.E. *et al.* (1982) Clinical manifestations and management of aspergillosis in the compromised patient. In: *Fungal Infections in the Compromised Patient* (eds D.W. Warnock & M.D. Richardson). John Wiley, New York, pp. 119–53.

Washington, L. & Miller, W.T. (1998) Mycobacterial infection in immunocompromised patients. *J Thorac Imag*, **13**(4), 271–81.

Watkins, J. *et al.* (1981) Isolation and enumeration of *Listeria monocytogenes* from sewage, sewage study and river water. *J Appl Bacteriol*, **5**, 1–9.

Watson, C. (1997) Hepatitis C: it's in the blood. *Nurs Times*, **93**(19), 68–9.

Watson, J.M. *et al.* (1993) Tuberculosis and HIV estimates of the overlap in England and Wales. *Thorax*, **48**, 199–203.

Weber, B. *et al.* (1998) Reduction of diagnostic window by new fourth-generation HIV screening assays. *J Clin Microbiol*, **36**(8), 2235–9.

Weber, B., Berger, A., Rabenau, H. & Doerr, H.W. (2002a) Evaluation of a new combined antigen and antibody human immunodeficiency virus screening assay, VIDAS HIV DUO ULTRA. *J Clin Microbiol*, **40**(4), 1420–6.

Weber, B., Gurtler, L. & Thorstensson, R. (2002b) Multicenter evaluation of a new automated fourth-generation human immunodeficiency virus screening assay with a sensitive antigen detection module and high specificity. *J Clin Microbiol*, **40**(6), 1938–48.

Weber, D.J., Rutala, W.A. & Hamilton, H. (1996) Prevention and control of varicella-zoster infections in healthcare facilities. *Infect Control Hosp Epidemiol*, **17**(10), 694–705.

Weinbren, M. & Struthers, K. (2002) Emergence of *Staphylococcus aureus* (MRSA) with reduced susceptibility to teicoplanin during therapy. *J Antimicrob Chemother*, **50**(2), 306–7.

Weiss, R.A. (2001) Natural and iatrogenic factors in human immunodeficiency virus transmission. *Phil Trans R Soc Lond B Biol Sci*, **356**(1410), 947–53.

Wejstal, R., Norkrans, G. & Widell, A. (1997) Chronic non-A, non-B, non-C: is hepatitis G/GBV-C involved? *Scand J Gastroenterol*, **32**(10), 1046–51.

Weller, I.V.D. & Williams, I.G. (2001) Antiretroviral drugs. *Br Med J*, **322**(7299), 412.

Weller, T.H. (1996) Varicella: historical perspective and clinical overview. *J Infect Dis*, **174**(Suppl 3), S306–9.

Wendt, C. *et al.* (1998) Survival of vancomycin-resistant and vancomycin-susceptible enterococci on dry surfaces. *J Clin Microbiol*, **36**(12), 3734–6.

Werzberger, A., Kuter, B. & Nalin, B. (1998) Six years following after hepatitis A vaccination. *N Engl J Med*, **338**(16), 1160.

West, G.R. & Stark, K.A. (1997) Partner notification for HIV prevention: a critical reexamination. *AIDS Educ Prev*, **9**(Suppl 3), 68–78.

Weusten, J.J., Van Drimmelen, H.A. & Lelie, P.N. (2002) Mathematic modelling of the risk of HBV, HVC and HIV transmission by window-phase donation not detected by NAT. *Transfusion*, **42**(5), 537–48.

White, D.A. & Santamauro, J.T. (1995) Pulmonary infections in immunosuppressed patients. *Curr Opin Pulm Med*, **1**(3), 202–8.

Whitley, R. (1995) Varicella-zoster virus. In: *Principles and Practice of Infectious Diseases*, 4th edn (eds G.L. Mandell, J.E. Bennett & R. Dolin). Churchill Livingstone, New York, Vol. 2, Chap. 116, pp. 1345–50.

Whitley, R.J. (2002) Herpes simplex virus in children. *Curr Treat Options Neurol*, **4**(3), 231–7.

Wielaard, F. *et al.* (1988) Development of an antibody-capture IgM enzyme-linked immunosorbent assay for diagnosis of acute Epstein–Barr virus infection. *J Virol Methods*, **21**, 105–15.

Wilcox, M.H. (1997) Bloodborne viruses. *Croner's Health Service Risks*, **9**, 2–7.

Wilcox, M.H. & Dane, J. (2000) The cost of hospital-acquired infection and the value of infection control. *J Hosp Infect*, **45**(2), 81–4.

Wilcox, M.H. *et al.* (1998) Recurrence of symptoms in *Clostridium difficile* infection; relapse or reinfection? *J Hosp Infect*, **38**(2), 93–100.

Wilkinson, D., Squire, S.B. & Garner, P. (1998) Effect of preventive treatment for tuberculosis in adults infected with HIV. *Br Med J*, **317**(7159), 625–9.

Williams, K. (1994) Fact or fiction? *Nur Times*, **90**(3), 38–41.

Willocks, L.J., Sufi, F., Wall, R. *et al.* (2000) Compliance with advice to boil drinking water during an outbreak of cryptosporidiosis. *Commun Dis Public Health*, **3**(2), 137–8.

Wilson, I.G., Hogg, G.M. & Barr, J.G. (1997) Microbiological quality of ice in hospital and community. *J Hosp Infect*, **36**, 171–80.

Wilson, J. (2001) *Infection Control in Clinical Practice*. Baillière Tindall, London.

Winer, J.B. (2001) Guillain Barre syndrome. *World J Gastroenterol*, **54**(6), 381–5.

Wingard, J.R. (1999) Opportunistic infections after blood and marrow transplantation. *Transpl Infect Dis*, **1**(1), 3–20.

Winters, G. *et al.* (1994) Provisional practice: the nature of psychosocial bone marrow transplant nursing. *Oncol Nurs Forum*, **21**(7), 1147–54.

Wise, R. *et al.* (1998) Antimicrobial resistance. *Br Med J*, **317**, 609–10.

Wisnes, R. (1978) Efficacy of zoster immunoglobulin in prophylaxis of varicella in high-risk patients. *Acta Paediatr Scand*, **67**, 77–82.

Wolters, L.M., Van Nunen, A.B., Honkoop, P. *et al.* (2000) Lamivudine-high dose interferon combination therapy for chronic hepatitis B patients co-infected with the hepatitis D virus. *J Viral Hepat*, **7**(6), 428–34.

Wong, O.C. *et al.* (1980) Epidemic and endemic hepatitis in India: evidence for a non-A non-B hepatitis virus aetiology. *Lancet*, **ii**, 876–8.

Wood, M.J. (1991) Herpes zoster and pain. *Scand J Infect Dis Suppl*, **80**, 53–61.

Woolley, P. (1997) Genital herpes: recognizing the problem. *Medscape Women's Health*, **2**(5), 2.

Working Group (2000) Guidelines for preventing opportunistic infections among hematopoietic stem cell transplant recipients. *Biol Blood Marrow Transplant*, **6**(6A), 7–83.

Working Party (1998) Revised guidelines for the control of methicillin resistant *Staphylococcus aureus* infection in hospitals. *J Hosp Infect*, **39**, 253–90.

World Health Organization (2000) *Hepatitis B Fact Sheet*. World Health Organization, Geneva.

World Health Organization (2002a) *AIDS Epidemic Update*. UNAIDS, Geneva.

World Health Organization (2002b) *Framework for Effective Tuberculosis Control*. World Health Organization, Geneva.

Worsley, M.A. (1998) Infection control and prevention of *Clostridium difficile* infection. *J Antimicrob Chemother*, **41**(Suppl C), 59–66.

Wright, L., Spickett, G. & Stoker, S. (2001) Latex allergy awareness among hospital staff. *NT Plus*, **97**(38), 4–8.

Wu, J.C. *et al.* (1998) The impact of traveling to endemic areas on the spread of hepatitis E virus infection: epidemiological and molecular analyses. *Hepatology*, **27**(5), 1415–20.

Wutzler, P. (1997) Antiviral therapy of herpes simplex and varicella-zoster virus infections. *Intervirology*, **40**(5–6), 343–56.

Wynia, M.K., Ioannidis, J.P. & Lau, J. (1998) Analysis of life-long strategies to prevent *Pneumocystis carinii* pneumonia in patients with variable HIV progression rates. *AIDS*, **12**(11), 1317–25.

Wynn, H.E., Brundage, R.C. & Fletcher, C.V. (2002) Clinical implications of CNS penetration of antiretroviral drugs. *CNS Drugs*, **16**(9), 595–609.

Yamamoto, S., Shimomura, Y., Kinashita, S. *et al.* (1994) Detection of herpes simplex virus DNA in human tear film by the polymerase chain reaction. *Am J Ophthalmol*, **117**(2), 160–3.

Yates, J.W. *et al.* (1973) A controlled study of isolation and endogenous microbial suppression in acute myelocytic leukaemia patients. *Cancer*, **32**, 1490–8.

Yeung-Yue, K.A., Brentjens, M.H., Lee, P.C. & Tyring, S.K. (2002) Herpes simplex viruses 1 and 2. *Dermatol Clin*, **20**(2), 249–66.

Young, L.S. (1984) Clinical aspects of pneumocystosis in man. In: Pneumocystis carinii *Pneumonia* (ed. L.S. Young). Marcel Dekker, New York, pp. 139–74.

Young, L.S. (1996) Mycobacterial infection in immunocompromised patients. *Curr Opin Infect Dis*, **9**, 240–5.

Young, S.E.J. & Healing, T.D. (1995) The management of the deceased with known or suspected infectious disease. *Commun Dis Rep*, **5**, R69–73.

Yousuf, K., Saklayen, M.G., Markert, R.J., Barde, C.J. & Gopalswamy, N. (2002) *Clostridium difficile* associated diarrhoea and chronic renal insufficiency. *South Med J*, **95**(7), 681–3.

Yu, V.L. (1995) *Legionella pneumophila* (Legionnaires' disease). In: *Principles and Practices of Infectious Disease,* 4th edn (eds G.L. Mandell, J.E. Bennett & R. Dolin). Churchill Livingstone, New York, Vol. 2, Chap. 211, pp. 2087–97.

Yuen, K.Y. *et al.* (1998) Unique risk factors for bacteraemia in allogeneic bone marrow transplant recipients before and after engraftment. *Bone Marrow Transplant*, **21**(11), 1137–43.

Zadik, P.M. & Moore, A.P. (1998) Antimicrobial association of an outbreak of diarrhoea due to *Clostridium difficile*. *J Hosp Infect*, **39**(3), 189–93.

Zafar, A.B., Gaydos, L.A., Furlong, W.B. *et al.* (1998) Effectiveness of infection control program in controlling nosocomial *Clostridium difficile*. *Am J Infect Control*, **26**(6), 588–93.

Zanotti, S., Kumar, A. & Kumar, A. (2002) Cytokine modulation in sepsis and septic shock. *Expert Opin Invest Drugs*, **11**(8), 1061–75.

Zar, T., Sharar, Z., Mughal, M. & McClintock, C. (2001) Severe hepatitis due to HBV–HDV coinfection. *Conn Med*, **65**(11), 649–52.

Zerbe, M.B., Parkerson, S.G. & Spitzer, T. (1994) Laminar air flow versus reverse isolation: nurses' assessment of moods, behaviours, and activity levels in patients receiving bone marrow transplants. *Oncol Nurs Forum*, **21**(3), 565–8.

Ziebold, C., Von Kries, R., Lang, R. *et al.* (2001) Severe complications of varicella in previously healthy children in Germany: a 1 year survey. *Pediatrics*, **89**(435), 17–21.

Zimmerman, M.J., Bak, A. & Sutherland, L.R. (1997) Review article: treatment of *Clostridium difficile* infection. *Aliment Pharmacol Ther*, **11**(6), 1003–12.

Zuckerman, J.N. (1998) New combined hepatitis A and B vaccine. Risks of viral hepatitis related to travel. *Br Med J*, **316**(7140), 1317.

Breast aspiration and seroma drainage

Breast aspiration

Definition

Breast aspiration is the insertion of a needle into the breast to obtain cells for cytological examination or to remove fluid to drain a cyst. It is usually carried out using a fine needle and so is often referred to as fine-needle aspiration or FNA.

Reference material

Anatomy and physiology

The breast is a glandular organ designed to produce milk in women (Fig. 6.1). Each breast contains 12–20

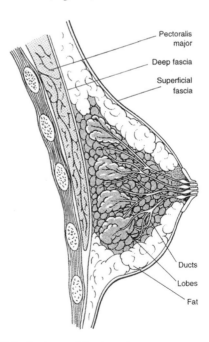

Figure 6.1 Anatomy of the breast.

lobes, each of which branches into hundreds of tiny lobules where milk is produced when a woman breast feeds (Chaplin 1996). The lobules are connected to the nipple by a ductal system. Male and female breasts have a similar rudimentary duct system until puberty. The female breast develops further after puberty due to hormonal influences, whereas the male breast remains unchanged (Tucker 1993). The entire breast is enclosed by two layers of fibrous tissue called the fascia. The superficial fascia is thinner and lies between the breast and the skin. The deep fascia, the thicker layer, lies underneath the breast, separating it from the pectoralis major and the pectoralis minor (the muscles of the chest wall) (Berger & Bostwick 1998). Most of the normal breast is composed of fat. Less than 5% is made up of duct epithelial cells. The vast majority of breast cancers and most benign conditions arise in these cells (Dixon 2000).

Breast tissue in women is highly sensitive to hormonal changes that occur naturally, for example during the menstrual cycle or in pregnancy. Hormonal control of normal physiological change is largely determined by oestrogen and progesterone. As a result of their influence, the breasts are subject to constant change that may result in the development of nodularity. This nodularity or lumpiness is attributed to increased interlobular oedema and cell proliferation, most notably in the luteal phase (second half) of the menstrual cycle, and is more pronounced in some women than in others (Berger & Bostwick 1998; Osborne 2000). Cyclical nodularity is so common that it can be regarded as physiological rather than pathological. Focal breast nodularity or lumpiness is the most common cause of a breast lump and is seen in women of all ages (Dixon 2000).

Breast cancer

Breast cancer is a disease that affects 38 000 women in the UK every year (Cancer Research UK 2002). Invasive ductal carcinoma is the most common type of breast cancer accounting for over 70% of cases. Invasive lobular carcinoma forms the next biggest group, although only 9% are of this histological type. The remainder are made up of less common tumours such as Paget's disease, inflammatory carcinoma, mucinous carcinoma, medullary carcinoma, tubular carcinoma and very rare types such as lymphomas or sarcomas of the breast (Dixon & Sainsbury 1997; Brogi & Harris 1999; Diab *et al.* 1999; Pederson *et al.* 1999). Most breast cancers are invasive, i.e. the cells have spread through the linings of the ducts into surrounding tissues, but a few may be non-invasive or in situ. Some breast cancers may never become invasive and those that do may disseminate at

different points in their development, dependent on their individual nature, varying from weeks in some, to years or never in others (Pointon & Day 1998).

Most lumps in the breast are found by patients themselves and these are far more likely to represent a benign condition such as a cyst or a fibroadenoma. Nine out of every ten breast lumps investigated in the hospital setting are benign (DoH 1993; Galea 1994). Consequently the majority of women are undergoing investigations to exclude malignancy. It is therefore important to find a simple, non-invasive test that can determine malignancy within given resources at minimal inconvenience to the patient.

Ideally less than 10% of all new patients with breast symptoms should be required to attend the hospital on more than two occasions for *diagnostic* purposes (British Association of Surgical Oncologists 1998).

Diagnostic methods

When a lump is found in the breast it is necessary to differentiate between benign and malignant disease in order to provide the appropriate treatment and care. Historically, where breast cancer was suspected diagnosis was made by surgical excision of a tumour (known as excision biopsy) under general anaesthetic and then examination of the tumour by a histopathologist. The patient was given the results and subsequently, if positive, needed further excision requiring a second anaesthetic. Alternatively, histopathological examination was carried out rapidly using a frozen section of the tumour while the patient was anaesthetized. Where the tumour was shown to be malignant, further excision or even mastectomy was carried out at the time. While this had the advantage of giving the patient only one anaesthetic, the disadvantage was that patients frequently went to theatre not knowing whether they had cancer or indeed whether they would undergo mastectomy. Nowadays diagnosis is facilitated by triple assessment, a correlation of clinical examination, mammogram and/or ultrasound and FNA cytology. Combining all three is recommended as the standard assessment approach and leads to a marked improvement in diagnostic accuracy (National Cancer Institute 1997; British Association of Surgical Oncologists 1998; Wilson *et al.* 2001) and enables a definitive diagnosis to be made in the vast majority of patients (Dixon & Sainsbury 1997). Consequently patients will know the diagnosis prior to any surgical intervention and can be prepared and informed beforehand. Health care professionals are also less reliant on surgery in the first instance, at a time when chemotherapy and endocrine therapy are increasingly used as primary treatments for breast cancer.

An alternative method of biopsy is trucut biopsy. This is where an incision is made in the breast under local anaesthetic and a wide bore needle used to take a core of breast tissue. This also gives the patient the diagnosis before surgery, but is more invasive and more painful than FNA. However, unlike tissue removed by FNA, tissue gathered using this method can be used to distinguish between invasive and non-invasive tumours. Many other prognostic markers can now be measured from FNAs. In conjunction with immunocytochemistry it is possible to measure oestrogen receptor, progesterone receptor and other markers such as the p53 enzyme and HER2/neu (McManus & Anderson 2001), although currently these are still more commonly performed on histological material. Such markers indicate the likely growth mechanisms of the cancer and which medical treatments may be appropriate.

Fine-needle aspiration cytology

Accuracy

Although aspiration cytodiagnosis has been possible since the nineteenth century, the first report of its widespread use (3479 patients) was in 1968 in Scandinavia (Franzen & Zajicek 1968). It is now possible to obtain very high accuracy rates in diagnosing breast cancer with FNA cytology. Both sensitivity (the number of cancers reported as cancer) and specificity (the number of benign lesions reported as benign) with this technique are reported as between 90 and 98% (Dixon 2000; Rocha et al. 1997; Arisio et al. 1998). Recent data suggest that most centres report false positive rates (i.e. mistaken diagnosis of cancer) of less than 0.5% (Dixon 2000) and false negative rates of about 5% (Layfield et al. 1993). False negative readings can occur when insufficient cells are obtained for analysis or when cancer cells are missed. Therefore accuracy is largely dependent on the expertise of the individuals performing the aspiration and interpreting the results (Shumate 1996; McKenzie & Dalrymple 1998). It is essential that people undertaking this procedure are adequately trained, have been assessed as competent (Koss 1993) and practise several times a week to ensure consistent results (Ljung et al. 1994).

Application

Advantages of FNA are that it is quick, relatively noninvasive and can be performed in the outpatient department. It also enables solid and cystic lesions to be differentiated. If the lump is a cyst then the fluid will drain out on aspiration and the lump will disappear. Therefore FNA has a therapeutic role in the symptomatic relief of a painful cyst, as well as a diagnostic role in the presence of a solid lesion. Clear fluid aspirated from breast cysts need not have cytological examination unless the lump has not disappeared. Discoloured or cloudy fluid, either blood stained or green, should be sent to the laboratory for examination as carcinoma can, on rare occasions, be associated with a cyst (Trott 1991).

A limitation with the application of FNA to breast diagnosis is that it may not be possible to reliably distinguish between in situ and invasive carcinoma, due to the lack of structural information derived from cells (McManus & Anderson 2001) when compared with that derived from tissues (histology).

Preparation of sample

Once obtained the aspirate is expressed onto microscope slides and sent to the cytology department. Two main staining techniques are used for the visualization of the slides. The Papanicolaou stain technique requires fixing in spirit (95% ethanol) before it dries, so it is suitable for a thick smear of cells. The Romanovsky staining technique, using the May-Grunwald Giemsa stain, requires the cells to dry almost instantaneously in order to achieve good staining and therefore is better when the smear is scanty. Ideally both stains should be made for each specimen as different lesions are more easily identifiable using the different techniques (Trott 1991). Special preparation of material may be required for measuring prognostic markers, for example cytospins. This technique is more costly but enables high quality preparations to be made (National Cancer Institute 1997). The cytologist will also find it useful to be given a description of what is felt in the breast when the needle is inserted. Cancers often feel more gritty and benign lesions feel more rubbery.

Reporting

Reports are usually descriptive and have a numerical score or 'C score' (standing for cytology): C5 confirms malignancy; C4 indicates the cells are highly suspicious for malignancy (70–90% of these will eventually turn out to be malignant); C3 is reported when atypical cells are seen, but the majority of these will still be benign; C2 indicates benign cells only with no atypical features; C1 is usually reported when only scanty material has been obtained, which is insufficient for a diagnosis to be made (Dixon & Sainsbury 1997; McManus & Anderson 2001).

The patient's experience

Many patients undergoing this procedure may be highly anxious due to concern over the possible diagnosis of cancer. Anxiety may increase the perceived pain of the procedure and if the patient is restless due to anxiety they may move when the needle is inserted. If the patient moves then the FNA may not be accurate and the chances of pneumothorax and haematoma are increased. It is hypothetically possible to pierce the lung and cause pneumothorax so care should be taken when performing aspiration in those areas of the breast where there is little breast tissue. However, the risk from this is considered negligible (Trott 1991). Tumours are often vascular so there is a risk of haematoma formation if care is not taken. This in turn can cause distortion of a mammogram and therefore difficulty in interpretation, which may delay the time a patient has to wait to receive a definitive diagnosis and perpetuates further anxiety.

The process of aspiration can be uncomfortable or even painful for some, although notably greater discomfort is reported if 21 gauge needles are used rather than 23 gauge (Daltrey & Kissin 2000). Local anaesthetic is not normally used because this may distort the area to be needled and decrease the accuracy. From general experience most people find the administration

of the local anaesthetic to be as painful as the FNA itself.

It is essential that patients receive explanations about each step of the procedure and are given a chance to discuss it or ask questions as required. Information delivered at a pace and in a language the patient can understand may result in decreased anxiety, decreased pain levels and improved compliance (Meissner *et al.* 1990; Schapiro *et al.* 1992; Poroch 1995).

Summary

FNA of the breast is cost effective, rapid and accurate (McManus & Anderson 2001) and causes less discomfort and emotional distress than open biopsy (Layfield *et al.* 1993). With the proviso that experienced personnel undertake the procedure and examination of cells, for the majority of centres this is now the preferred method of diagnosis in breast cancer.

Procedure guidelines: **Breast aspiration**

Equipment

1 70% isopropyl alcohol swabs.
2 Sterile syringes (10 or 20 ml).
3 Sterile needles (21 or 23 G).
4 Microscope slides.
5 Universal container.
6 Slide tray.
7 Fixative (ethanol).
8 Low-linting gauze.
9 Plaster/surgical tape.
10 Sharps container.
11 Cytology request form.
12 Microscope slide holders.

Procedure

Action	Rationale
1 Place the patient lying down on a couch in a position that facilitates access to the site on the breast requiring aspiration. This may require them to roll slightly on their side or to lift their arm above the head.	To ensure the patient is comfortable and to ensure safety should the patient feel faint during the procedure.
2 Explain and discuss the procedure with the patient.	To ensure that the patient understands the procedure and gives his/her valid consent.
3 Place slides on a tray.	In preparation for breast aspirate.
4 Prepare syringe by introducing 2 ml of air into the barrel.	To prevent aspirated material being sucked into the syringe.
5 Choose appropriate size needle and attach to the syringe.	Preferably 23 G, but for a large breast or deep lesion 21 G may be necessary (Walker 1998; Daltrey & Kissin 2000).
6 Clean area of patient's skin with single-use sterile swab saturated with 70% isopropyl alcohol.	To reduce the risk of infection.
7 Firmly fix breast lump or area of clinical interest between the fingers of one hand.	To stabilize the area before introducing the needle to ensure the correct area sampled.
8 Warn the patient that a needle is about to be inserted.	To reduce the risk of the patient moving.
9 Push the needle tip into the centre of the lump or area of clinical interest. Note consistency (Fig. 6.2).	To obtain specimen from appropriate area. Consistency can be a diagnostic indicator, i.e. gritty (malignant) or rubbery (benign). This information is of use to the cytologist.

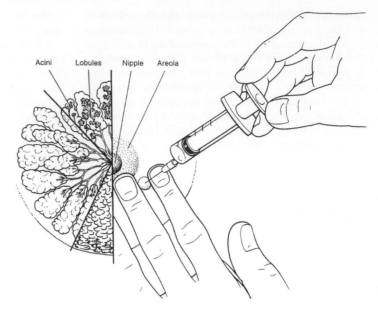

Figure 6.2 Performing fine-needle aspiration of the breast.

*Procedure guidelines: **Breast aspiration** (cont'd)*

Action	Rationale
10 If the lump is thought to be cystic be careful not to move the needle whilst withdrawing fluid. Withdraw the needle when no further fluid appears in the syringe. If the fluid is discoloured send for cytological examination.	The needle must be kept in place in the cyst sack whilst withdrawing fluid to enable complete drainage of the cyst and reduce chances of it refilling. Clear fluid is indicative of a cyst only. Anything else should be sent to the laboratory to exclude malignancy.
11 Aspirate a solid lesion or area of clinical interest using the maximum amount of suction moving the tip of the needle back and forth and in different directions without withdrawing the needle through the skin.	To enable sampling of different areas and to obtain an adequate sample for transferring to the slide. There is no evidence that tumour cells can be disseminated along the needle tract.
12 After aspiration, allow the barrel of the syringe to return to 2 ml before withdrawing the needle to eliminate any negative pressure in the syringe.	To avoid the contents of the needle being sucked into the syringe.
13 After withdrawal of the needle from the breast, express the aspirate on to the slides. If the aspirate is thick then more slides will be required. Smear the cells evenly on the slides, with a second slide.	To prepare the cells for cytodiagnosis. A monolayer is required because if the smear is blood stained or there is too much material on the slide, staining can be a problem and the cytologist cannot make a diagnosis.
14 Low linting swab should be placed over the puncture site and pressure applied for at least one minute or until bleeding has stopped.	To reduce the risk of haematoma formation.
15 Leave one slide to dry in the air and add fixative to the other as required by the cytologist. Label appropriately.	When such a small amount of material is available the cytologist will require different staining techniques for accurate diagnosis.
16 If the aspirate is lost into the barrel of the needle 5 ml of 0.9% sodium chloride should be drawn into the syringe through the same needle and the resultant suspension placed in a universal container.	So that the sample can be recovered by centrifugation and then stained as normal. A large percentage of the cells will still be lost.
17 Dispose of needle and syringe in sharps container.	To reduce risk of injury and infection to staff.
18 Label slides with name, number and which breast.	To ensure correct identification of specimen.

*Procedure guidelines: **Breast aspiration** (cont'd)*

Action	Rationale
19 Apply a plaster or non-allergenic dressing to puncture site.	To protect clothing.
20 Complete cytology forms with full details.	To ensure correct identification and most accurate information for diagnosis.
21 Place slides in slide holder. Slide holder and cytology forms to be placed in plastic specimen bag.	To ensure safe transfer to laboratory.

Seroma drainage

Definition

A seroma is defined as a clinically identifiable collection of serous fluid within any *surgical* cavity (Woodworth *et al.* 2000).

Possible causes of seroma formation after breast surgery

There are no proven causes of seroma formation. However, the likelihood appears to be dependent on the median yield of axillary lymph nodes excised and the surgical level of axillary dissection performed. There is no relationship between seroma formation and the patient's age, tumour size, grade or body mass index (Woodworth *et al.* 2000).

Effects of seroma formation on the patient

Seroma formation, if recurrent, can cause a delay in the initiation of adjuvant therapy. Patients will commonly experience pain and discomfort, which may in turn prevent them from performing postoperative arm exercises which are recommended to restore mobility and minimize the risk of lymphoedema. In more extreme circumstances, if a seroma is left untreated, the patient is at risk of infection and also skin flap necrosis if they have undergone breast reconstruction (Miller 1998).

Indications for seroma drainage

The following list indicates when it is appropriate for a nurse to undertake the procedure of seroma drainage.

- A seroma is visible to the naked eye, is located under skin in the axilla, chest wall or back, has a 'water-bed' consistency when depressed and released and the area is free from infection.
- A seroma is causing pain, discomfort or pressure/tightness.

- A seroma is causing the patient restricted mobility, i.e. they are unable to maintain their exercise regime or daily activities.
- The patient has been adequately informed and is physically and psychologically prepared to undergo the procedure.
- The individual nurse has attained a level of proficiency and is competent to drain seromas independently.

Contraindications for seroma drainage

The following list indicates when it is inappropriate for a nurse to undertake the procedure of seroma drainage.

- An infection is clinically evident or suspected.
- The presence of a haematoma is suspected.
- The patient has a breast implant in situ (secondary to breast reconstruction), unless the seroma is located on the back as a result of autologous tissue transfer.
- The seroma is not causing discomfort or pain and is not affecting the patient's ability to continue their postoperative exercise regime or daily activities.
- The individual nurse has not attained a level of proficiency to be competent to drain seromas independently.

Potential complications arising during or following seroma drainage

Table 6.1 is a list of complications and subsequent actions required if they are suspected.

Summary

Seroma drainage is a relatively quick and atraumatic procedure that can relieve pain and discomfort and improve mobility and healing, with the proviso that it is conducted by proficient and appropriately trained nurses who ensure their competence is kept up to date by regularly incorporating it into their practice.

Table 6.1

Complication	Action required
• Suspected pneumothorax on insertion of needle	• Withdraw needle and call medical staff for assistance immediately
• Suspected local infection (characterized by inflammation and erythema at wound site but with nil exudate) (Miller 1998)	• Continue with seroma drainage, referring to medical staff if the symptoms do not resolve after drainage as the patient may require antibiotic therapy
• Suspected systemic infection (characterized by the patient feeling unwell and feverish with a pyrexia of 38°C or greater and inflammation and exudate present at the wound site) (Miller 1998)	• Discontinue seroma drainage, referring to medical staff as the patient will require antibiotic therapy and may need further investigations
• Drainage fails to resolve the seroma	• Refer to medical staff for advice and assistance
• Fluid aspirated is suspected to contain blood or pus in addition to or instead of serous fluid	• Send fluid sample to microbiology for culture and sensitivity and inform the medical staff
• The seroma is recurrent, filling again in excess of five times with the amount of fluid removed remaining static or increasing .	• Drain the seroma and refer to medical staff for advice on any further action required, such as insertion of a wound drain

Procedure guidelines: **Seroma drainage**

Equipment

1 Sterile dressing pack containing indented plastic tray, low linting gauze swabs, disposable gloves, sterile field and disposable bag.
2 Sterile syringes (30 and 50 ml).
3 Sterile needles (21 G).
4 Chlorhexidine in 70% alcohol solution (or equivalent).
5 Sterile dressing (non-adherent, 5 × 7 cm) or hypo-allergenic tape and gauze.
6 Sharps container.
7 Universal container.

Procedure

Action	Rationale
1 Place the patient lying down on a couch in a position that facilitates access to the seroma.	To ensure the patient is comfortable and the seroma is visible and accessible.
2 Explain and discuss the procedure with the patient.	To ensure that the patient understands the procedure and gives valid consent and co-operation.
3 Open dressing pack on a clean trolley and lay out equipment, adhering to an aseptic technique as stated in Ch. 4, p. 57.	To ensure no equipment is missing and to maintain asepsis.
4 Clean identified puncture site for drainage of seroma with chlorhexidine-soaked gauze and allow to dry.	To prevent infection and minimize 'stinging' when the needle is inserted.
5 Insert needle at a 45° angle towards seroma fluid.	To minimize discomfort and optimize the seroma drainage.
6 Gently draw back on the syringe. If the syringe becomes full, disconnect and discard in a yellow waste bag. Connect a new syringe and repeat.	To drain the fluid from the seroma and to ensure safe disposal of waste products.
7 When fluid ceases to flow, remove both the needle and the syringe together (do not disconnect them). Dispose both immediately in a sharps container.	To ensure the safe disposal of sharps and to minimize the risk of needle-stick injury.
8 Apply pressure with gauze over the puncture site for at least one minute, after removal of the needle.	To reduce the risk of leakage and to allow the puncture site to close.
9 If infection is suspected, expel 10–20 ml of aspirated fluid gently into the universal container. Send to microbiology with the appropriate form.	To identify infection present and to enable appropriate intervention.
10 Apply a non-adherent dressing or non-allergenic tape and gauze over the puncture site. Instruct the patient to remove this 24 hours from the time of drainage.	To protect the patient's clothing and the puncture site, and to reduce the risk of infection.

Procedure guidelines: Seroma drainage (cont'd)

Action	Rationale
11 Ensure the patient understands what to do in the event of reaccumulation of the seroma.	To maximize patient education and to ensure the safe discharge of the patient.
12 Complete the appropriate paperwork.	To ensure accurate record keeping and to promote continuity of patient care.

References and further reading

Arisio, R., Cuccorese, C., Accinelli, G. *et al.* (1998) Role of fine-needle aspiration biopsy in breast lesions: analysis of a series of 4110 cases. *Diagn Cytopathol*, **18**(6), 462–7.

Berger, K. & Bostwick, J. (1998) Breast anatomy and physiology. In: *A Woman's Decision: Breast Care, Treatment and Reconstruction*, 3rd edn. Quality Medical Publishing, Missouri, pp. 7–12.

British Association of Surgical Oncologists (1998) Guidelines for surgeons in the management of symptomatic breast disease in the UK (revision). *Eur J Surg Oncol*, **24**, 464–76.

Brogi, E. & Harris, N. (1999) Lymphomas of the breast: pathology and clinical behaviour. *Semin Oncol*, **26**(3), 357–64.

Cancer Research UK (2002) *About Cancer: Statistics – Incidence and Mortality*. www.cancerresearchuk.org/

Chaplin, B. (1996) Breast cancer: knowledge for practice. *Nurs Times*, Prof Dev Suppl, **92**(10), 1–4.

Daltrey, I.R. & Kissin, M.W. (2000) Randomised controlled trial of the effect of needle gauge and local anaesthetic on the pain of breast fine needle aspiration cytology. *Br J Surg*, **87**, 777–9.

Diab, S., Clark, G., Osborne, C. *et al.* (1999) Tumour characteristics and clinical outcome of tubular and mucinous breast carcinomas. *J Clin Oncol*, **17**(5), 1442–8.

Dixon M. (2000) Symptoms, assessment and guidelines for referral. In: *ABC of Breast Diseases*, 2nd edn (ed. M. Dixon). BMJ Books, London.

Dixon, M. & Sainsbury, R. (1997) *Handbook of Diseases of the Breast*, 2nd edn. Churchill Livingstone, London.

DoH (1993) *Breast Cancer*. Stationery Office, London.

Franzen, S. & Zajicek, J. (1968) Aspiration biopsy in diagnosis of palpable lesions of the breast: critical review of 3479 consecutive biopsies. *Acta Radiol*, **7**, 241–62.

Galea, M. (1994) Breast disease. *Matern Child Health*, 386–91.

Koss, L. (1993) The palpable breast nodule: a cost-effectiveness analysis of alternate diagnostic approaches. *Cancer*, **72**(5), 1499–502.

Layfield, L. *et al.* (1993) The palpable breast nodule: a cost-effectiveness analysis of alternate diagnostic approaches. *Cancer*, **72**(5), 1642–51.

Ljung, B.-M. *et al.* (1994) Fine needle aspiration techniques for the characterization of breast cancers. *Cancer*, **74**, 1000–5.

McKenzie, J.G. & Dalrymple, J. (1998) Fine needle aspiration. In: *Early Breast Cancer: From Screening to Multidisciplinary Management* (eds M. Morgan, R. Warren, G. Querci Della Rovere). Harwood Academic Publishers, Canada.

McManus, D.T. & Anderson, N.H. (2001) Fine needle aspiration cytology of the breast. *Curr Diagnost Pathol*, **7**, 262–71.

Meissner, H., Anderson, D. & Odenkirchen, J. (1990) Meeting information needs of significant others and the use of the cancer information service. *Patient Educ Counsel*, **15**(2), 171–9.

Miller, M. (1998) How do I diagnose and treat wound infection? *Br J Nurs*, **7**(6), 335–8.

National Cancer Institute (1997) The uniform approach to breast fine needle aspiration biopsy. *Am J Surg*, **174**(4), 371–85.

Online Management of Breast Diseases (1997) *Anatomy of the Breast and Axilla: Standard Axillary Lymphadenectomy*. www.breastdiseases.com

Osborne, M.P. (2000) Breast anatomy and development. In: *Diseases of the Breast*, 2nd edn (eds J.R. Harris, M.E. Lippman, M. Morrow & C.K. Osborne). Lippincott, Williams and Wilkins, London.

Pederson, L., Holck, S., Mouridsen, H. *et al.* (1999) Prognostic comparison of three classifications for medullary carcinoma of the breast. *Histopathology*, **34**(2), 175–8.

Pointon, L.J. & Day, N.E. (1998) The background of screening for breast cancer. In: *Early Breast Cancer: From Screening to Multidisciplinary Management* (eds M. Morgan, R. Warren & G. Querci Della Rovere). Harwood Academic Publishers, Canada.

Poroch, D. (1995) The effect of preparatory patient education on the anxiety and satisfaction of cancer patients receiving radiation therapy. *Cancer Nurs*, **18**(3), 206–14.

Rocha, P., Nadkarni, N. & Menezes, S. (1997) Fine needle aspiration biopsy of breast lesions and histopathological correlation. An analysis of 837 cases in 4 years. *Acta Cytol*, **41**(3), 705–12.

Schapiro, D., Boggs, R., Melamed, B. *et al.* (1992) The effect of varied physician effect on recall, anxiety and perceptions in women at risk for breast cancer: an analogue study. *Health Psychol*, **11**(1), 61–6.

Shumate, C. (1996) Surgical evaluation and treatment of breast cancer. In: *Diagnosis and Management of Breast Disease* (eds R. Blackwell & J. Grotting). Blackwell Science, Massachusetts.

Soo, M.S. & Williford, M.E. (1995) Seromas in the breast: imaging findings. *Crit Rev Diagnost Imag*, **36**(5), 385–440.

Steering Committee on Clinical Practice Guidelines for the Care and Treatment of Breast Cancer (1998) Axillary dissection. *Can Assoc Radiat Oncol*, **158**(3), 22–6.

Trott, P. (1991) Aspiration cytodiagnosis of the breast. *Diag Oncol*, **1**, 79–87.

Tucker, A.K. (1993) *Textbook of Mammography*. Churchill Livingstone, London.

Walker, S. (1998) A randomized controlled trial comparing a 21G needle with a 23G needle for fine needle aspiration of breast lumps. *J R Coll Surg*, **43**(5), 322–3.

Wilson, R., Asbury, D., Cooke, J., Michell, M. & Patnick, J. (2001) *Clinical Guidelines for Breast Cancer Screening Assessment*. NHS Cancer Screening Programmes, Sheffield.

Woodworth, P.A., McBoyle, M.F., Helmer, S.D. & Beamer, R.L. (2000) Seroma formation after breast cancer surgery: incidence and predicting factors. *Am J Surg*, **66**(5), 444–50.

Cardiopulmonary resuscitation

Chapter contents

Definition

The term cardiac arrest implies a sudden interruption of cardiac output. It may be reversible with appropriate treatment (Handley 1999). The patient will collapse, lose consciousness, stop breathing and will be pulseless (Jevon 2001a).

The four arrhythmias that cause cardiac arrest are:

- Asystole
- Ventricular fibrillation (VF)
- Pulseless ventricular tachycardia (VT)
- Pulseless electrical activity (PEA).

For the purposes of resuscitation guidelines these rhythms are divided into two groups by their treatment.

- VF and pulseless VT – that require defibrillation
- Non-VF/VT – that do not require defibrillation (Resuscitation Council UK (RCUK) 2000a).

Indications

The patient is unconscious, has absent or gasping respiration and has no pulse. Other clinical features such as pupil size, cyanosis and pallor are unreliable and so the practitioner should not waste time looking for them (Skinner & Vincent 1997).

Reference material

Principles

Failure of the circulation for 3–4 minutes will lead to irreversible cerebral damage (Docherty & Hall 2002). Basic life support (BLS) acts to slow down the deterioration of the brain and the heart until defibrillation and/or advanced life support (ALS) can be provided (RCUK 2000b).

Resuscitation is the emergency treatment of any condition in which the brain fails to receive enough oxygen.

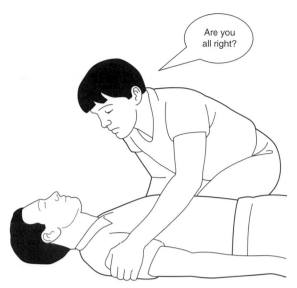

Figure 7.1

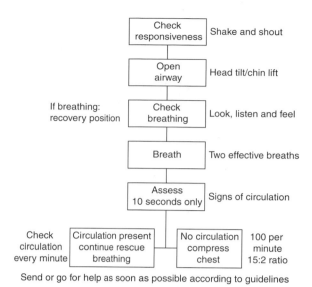

Figure 7.2 Basic life support algorithm.

The basic technique involves a rapid simple assessment of the patient followed by the ABC of resuscitation.

Assessment

There are two stages of assessment.

1 An immediate assessment by the rescuer to ensure that cardiopulmonary resuscitation may safely proceed (i.e. checking there is no immediate danger to the rescuer from any hazard, for example electrical power supply).
2 Assessment by the rescuer of the likelihood of injury sustained by the patient, particularly injury to the cervical spine. Although there may be no external evidence of injury, the immediate situation may provide the necessary evidence. For example, trauma to the cervical spine should be suspected in an accelerating/decelerating injury such as a road traffic accident with a motorbike travelling at speed.

Check the patient's level of consciousness by gently shaking his shoulders and asking loudly if he is all right (Fig. 7.1). If there is no response the rescuer should commence the BLS assessment (Fig. 7.2) immediately.

Note: if the arrest is witnessed or monitored, and a defibrillator is not immediately to hand, a single precordial thump should be administered. If delivered within 30 seconds after cardiac arrest, a sharp blow with a closed fist on the patient's sternum may convert VF back to a perfusing rhythm (RCUK 2000b).

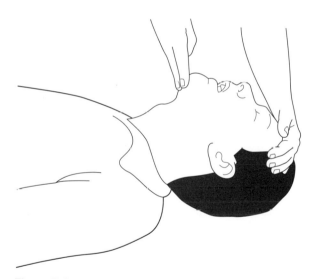

Figure 7.3 Head tilt/chin lift manoeuvre.

Basic life support

Basic life support is sometimes known as the 'ABC'.

Airway

The rescuer should look in the mouth and remove any visible obstruction (leave well-fitting dentures in place). The most likely obstruction in an unconscious person is the tongue. The head tilt/chin lift manoeuvre (Fig. 7.3), which removes the tongue from occluding the oropharynx, is an effective method of opening an airway and

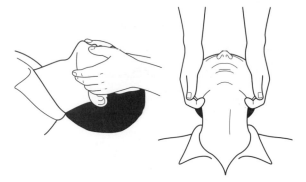

Figure 7.4 Jaw thrust.

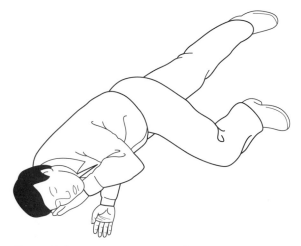

Figure 7.5 The recovery position.

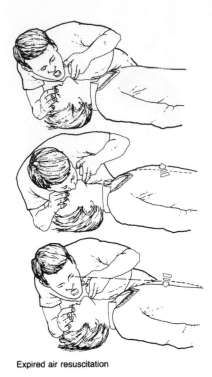

Expired air resuscitation

Figure 7.6 If patient is not breathing, expired air resuscitation must be started immediately. (Courtesy of Colqhoun, M., Handley, A.J. & Evans, T.R. (1999) *ABC of Resuscitation*, 4th edn. BMJ Publishing Group.)

relieving obstruction in 80% of patients (Simmons 1999).

Note: if there is any suspicion of cervical spine injury (see above) try to avoid head tilt. Jaw thrust (Fig. 7.4) is the technique of choice (RCUK 2000b). Particular care must be taken during handling and resuscitation to maintain alignment of the head, neck and chest in a neutral position.

Breathing

Keeping the airway open, the rescuer should look, listen and feel for breathing (more than an occasional gasp or weak attempts at breathing) for up to 10 seconds. If the patient is breathing they should be turned into the recovery position (Fig. 7.5). If the adult patient is not breathing and there is no suspicion of trauma or drowning, an immediate call for the cardiac arrest team should be made. Artificial ventilation must then be commenced and maintained. If there are no aids to ventilation available then direct mouth-to-mouth ventilation should be used (Fig. 7.6). When cardiac arrest occurs in hospital,

the RCUK (2000b) recommend the use of adjuncts such as the pocket mask or the bag mask unit. They can be used to avoid direct person-to-person contact and some devices may reduce the risk of cross-infection between patient and rescuer (RCUK 2000b).

One of the most easily learnt aids is the 'mouth to face mask' method. This is where a valved exhaled air ventilation mask with an oxygen attachment valve is used. The mask directs the patient's exhaled air and any fluid away from the rescuer and the oxygen port allows attachment of oxygen with enrichment up to 45%.

If the operator is skilled in airway management an Ambu bag and mask may be used. When the bag is attached to oxygen, high levels, of up to 85%, can be obtained. However it should be emphasized that to manipulate the head tilt, and hold on a face mask while squeezing a bag is a procedure that requires practice (Hodgetts & Castle 1999).

The most effective method of airway management is to use an endotracheal tube, thus enabling the application of 100% oxygen (Bossaert *et al.* 1998). This method of airway management is included in the advanced life support section.

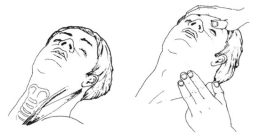

Figure 7.7 If patient does not have a pulse in a major artery (carotid), or if there is a neck injury, the femoral artery may be felt. Circulation must then be established with compression. (Courtesy of Colqhoun, M., Handley, A.J. & Evans, T.R. (1999) *ABC of Resuscitation*, 4th edn. BMJ Publishing Group.)

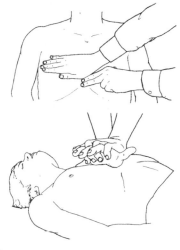

Figure 7.8 Establishing circulation with compression. Note fingers are clear of chest wall. (Courtesy of Colqhoun, M., Handley, A.J. & Evans, T.R. (1999) *ABC of Resuscitation*, 4th edn. BMJ Publishing Group.)

Circulation

As soon as the rescuer has delivered two slow effective breaths (i.e. the chest is seen to rise) the patient should be assessed for signs of a circulation. If following five attempts by the rescuer two effective breaths have still not been achieved, they should proceed to assess the circulation.

Circulation is assessed by looking for any signs of movement, including swallowing or breathing. If trained to do so, a check should also be made for the carotid pulse (Fig. 7.7) for up to 10 seconds. If no circulation is detected it must be maintained by compressions. The correct place to compress is in the centre of the lower half of the sternum (Fig. 7.8). The rescuer should position themselves vertically above the patient with arms straight and elbows locked. The sternum should be pressed down to depress it by 4–5 cm. This should be repeated at a rate of about 100 times a minute. After 15 compressions two rescue breaths are given, continuing compressions and rescue breaths in a ratio of 15:2 (RCUK 2000a).

Potentially reversible causes of a cardiopulmonary arrest

During cardiac arrest, potential causes or aggravating factors for which specific treatment exists should be considered. For ease of memory there are eight common causes of arrest, four of which begin with the letter H and four with the letter T (RCUK 2000b).

Hypoxia

There are many reasons why a patient may become severely hypoxic (see Ch. 25, Observations and Ch. 37, Respiratory therapy), the most common being the following:

- Acute respiratory failure
- Airway difficulties

- Acute lung injury
- Severe anaemia
- Neuromuscular disorders.

For healthy cell metabolism the body requires a constant supply of oxygen. When this is interrupted for more than 3 minutes in most situations (except when there is severe hypothermia) cell death occurs, followed by lactic acidosis and very rapidly a cardiorespiratory arrest. The risk of hypoxia is minimized by ensuring that the patient's lungs are ventilated adequately with 100% oxygen (RCUK 2000b).

Hypovolaemia

Hypovolaemia in adults that results in PEA is usually due to severe blood loss. While it is not the nurse's role to make a medical diagnosis, they may be aware of significant factors in the history of a patient that may have led to PEA.

The most common causes of severe blood loss are:

- Trauma
- Surgical procedure
- Gastrointestinal mucosa erosion
- Oesophageal varices
- Peripheral vessel erosion (by tumour usually)
- Clotting abnormality.

Note: blood loss, although usually overt, can be covert such as a gastrointestinal bleed which may only become apparent when the patient collapses.

The treatment for hypovolaemia is identifying and stopping the source of fluid or blood loss, and replacing the circulating volume with the appropriate fluid. Fluid resuscitation is normally started with a crystalloid, e.g. 0.9% sodium chloride, and/or colloid, e.g. Haemacel (depending on local protocols). Blood is likely to be required if the blood loss exceeds 1500–2000 ml in an adult (RCUK 2000b).

Hypothermia

Hypothermia should be suspected in any submersion or immersion injury. During a prolonged resuscitation attempt, a patient who was normothermic at the onset of cardiac arrest may become hypothermic (RCUK 2000b). A low reading thermometer, which can often be located in the Accident and Emergency Department, should be used if available.

Hypo/hyperkalaemia and other metabolic disorders

Because potassium is so closely linked with muscle and nerve excitation any imbalance will affect both the nervous conduction and the muscular working of the heart. Therefore a severe rise or fall in potassium can cause arrest arrhythmias. The causes of hypokalaemia are:

- Gastrointestinal fluid losses
- Urinary fluid loss
- Drugs that affect cellular potassium, e.g. antifungal agents such as amphotericin.

The immediate treatment for hypokalaemia which has resulted in an arrest is to give concentrated boluses of potassium while carefully monitoring the serial potassium measurements. Most ITU/A&E departments and coronary care units will have an arterial blood gas analyser that enables the potassium to be measured in one minute.

The patients who are most at risk of hyperkalaemia are those with renal failure or Addison's disease. The immediate treatment for hyperkalaemia is to give intravenous calcium. This binds to the potassium and removes it from the cell. However the patient may still require some form of renal replacement therapy post arrest as although the potassium has been removed from the cell it will return to the cell unless it has been removed from the body.

Thromboembolism

The commonest cause of thromboembolic or mechanical circulatory obstruction is a massive pulmonary embolus. Options for definitive treatment include thrombolysis or, if available, cardiopulmonary bypass and operative removal of the clot (RCUK 2000b).

Tension pneumothorax

A tension pneumothorax is the sudden collapse of a lung, usually under pressure, which results in a severe change in intrathoracic pressure and cessation of the heart as a pump. The most common causes are:

- Trauma
- Acute lung injury
- Mechanical ventilation of the newborn.

The immediate treatment is the insertion of a large-bore cannula into the second intercostal space at the midclavicular line of the affected side (RCUK 2000b). Arrangements should be made for the insertion of a formal chest tube and underwater seal drain (see Ch. 20, Intrapleural drainage).

Tamponade

This is where there is an acute effusion of fluid in the pericardial space and as it enlarges, the heart is splinted and finally cannot beat. The fluid is usually blood but can be malignant or infected fluid. The most common cause for a sudden tamponade is trauma. The immediate treatment is catheter or surgical drainage of the fluid. After drainage, the cause of the tamponade should be sought and corrected where possible, for example with appropriate antibiotic therapy for a bacterial aetiology or surgical repair of a myocardial laceration (Shoemaker 2000).

Toxicity – poisoning and drug intoxication

Poisoning rarely leads to cardiac arrest but it is a leading cause of death in patients less than 40 years old. Self-poisoning with therapeutic or recreational drugs is the main reason for hospital admission (RCUK 2000b). There are few specific therapeutic measures for poisons that are useful in the immediate situation. The emphasis must be on intensive supportive therapy, with correction of hypoxia, acid/base balance and electrolyte disorders. Specialist help can be obtained by telephoning one of the regional National Poisons Information Service Centres (RCUK 2000b).

Drugs

Only a few drugs are indicated during the immediate management of a cardiac arrest and there is only limited scientific evidence supporting their use. Drugs should be considered only after a sequence of shocks has been delivered (if indicated) and chest compressions and ventilation started (RCUK 2000b). Central venous access is optimum as it allows for drugs to be delivered rapidly. However, this is dependent on the skills available. If a peripheral intravenous cannula is already in place it should be used first (RCUK 2000b). Selected drugs – epinephrine, atropine, naloxone and lidocaine – can be administered down the endotracheal tube but the dose of the drug should be increased to 2–3 times the intravenous dose (AHA/ILCOR 2000). It is also possible to administer drugs using the intraosseous route, which is used commonly in the resuscitation of children.

The drugs used in the treatment of cardiac arrest are:

1 Epinephrine (adrenaline) 1 mg (10 ml of a 1:10 000 solution) given intravenously. The main purpose of adrenaline is to utilize its inotropic effect to maintain coronary and cerebral perfusion during a prolonged resuscitation attempt. It is the first drug used in cardiac arrest of any aetiology. Epinephrine is included in the ALS universal algorithm for use after each 3 minutes of CPR (RCUK 2000a).

2 Atropine 3 mg given intravenously once only reduces cardiac vagal tone, increases the rate of discharge of the sinoatrial node and increases the speed of conduction through the atrioventricular node. Its use is advocated in asystolic cardiac arrest and bradycardic PEA of less than 60 beats per minute.

   Note: although there is no conclusive evidence that atropine is of value in asystole during a cardiac arrest, there are anecdotal accounts of success following its administration (RCUK 2000b).

3 Amiodarone (300 mg in 20 ml) should be considered if VF or pulseless VT persists after the first three shocks. It increases the duration of the action potential in the atrial and ventricular myocardium. Thus the QT interval is prolonged.

   Note: lidocaine can still be considered if amiodarone is not available (RCUK 2000b).

4 Calcium chloride (10 ml of 10%) is only given during resuscitation when specifically indicated, i.e. for the treatment of PEA caused by hyperkalaemia, hypocalcaemia or overdose of calcium channel blocking drugs (RCUK 2000b). Although it plays a vital role in the cellular mechanisms underlying myocardial contraction there are very few data supporting any beneficial action for calcium following most cases of cardiac arrest (RCUK 2000b).

5 Sodium bicarbonate 8.4% is only used in prolonged cardiac arrest or according to serial blood gas analyses. Potential adverse effects of excessive sodium bicarbonate administration include hypokalaemia, exacerbation of respiratory acidosis and increased affinity of haemoglobin for oxygen. The high concentration of sodium can also exacerbate cerebral oedema. Other adverse effects are increased cardiac irritability and impaired myocardial performance. Sodium bicarbonate is usually given in 25–50 mmol aliquots and repeated as necessary. It can also be given in the special circumstances of tricyclic overdose or hyperkalaemia (Winser 2001).

6 Magnesium sulphate. Magnesium (4–8 mmol of 50%) should be given in cardiac arrest where there is a suspicion of hypomagnesaemia as this may precipitate refractory VF/VT (Winser 2001). The normal value for magnesium is 0.8–1.2 mmol/l (Wakeling & Mythen 2000).

Defibrillation

Defibrillation causes a simultaneous depolarization of the myocardium and aims to restore normal rhythm to the heart. This is the definitive treatment for VF/pulseless VT. It has been suggested that 80–90% of adults who collapse because of non-traumatic cardiac arrest are found to be in VF when first attatched to a monitor (Varon *et al.* 1998). In hospital cardiac arrest is more likely to present as non-VF/VT. Early defibrillation is a vital link in the chain of survival and developments in public access defibrillation and first responder defibrillation by ward nurses in hospitals are focusing firmly on this link. Delay in defibrillation decreases the chances of success by 7–10% each minute (Bossaert *et al.* 1998). Nurses are often first on the scene at a cardiac arrest, highlighting the obvious need for nurse-led defibrillation at ward level. While not all nurses are trained in defibrillation, they should understand why it is necessary and how it is done and be able to assist in an emergency (Austin & Snow 2000).

Please see Figure 7.9 for the universal ALS algorithm for the management of cardiac arrest in adults.

Cardiopulmonary resuscitation standards and training

The Resuscitation Council (UK), formed in 1981, aims to promote the education of lay and professional personnel in the most effective methods of resuscitation appropriate to their needs. In its report *CPR Guidance for Clinical Practice and Training in Hospitals* (RCUK 2000c), the Council made a number of recommendations relating to the provision of a resuscitation service in hospital.

- A resuscitation committee. This should comprise medical and nursing staff who advise on the role and composition of the cardiac arrest team, resuscitation equipment and resuscitation training equipment.
- A Resuscitation Training Officer (RTO), who should be responsible for training in resuscitation, equipment maintenance and the auditing of resuscitation/clinical trials.
- Resuscitation training. Hospital staff should receive at least annual resuscitation training appropriate to their level and role. Medical and nursing staff should receive basic resuscitation training and should be encouraged to recognize patients who are at risk of

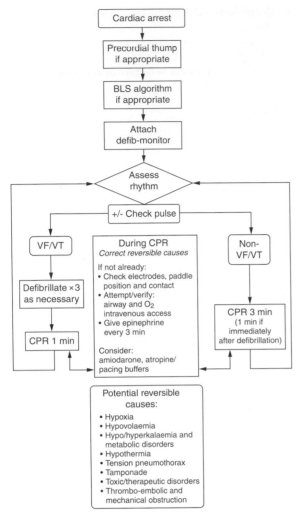

Figure 7.9 The ALS universal algorithm for the management of cardiac arrest in adults. (Courtesy of Resuscitation Council UK (2000c) *Advanced Life Support: Provider Manual*, 4th edn. RCUK, London.)

having a cardiac arrest and call for appropriate help early. This is the most effective method of improving outcome (Jevon 2002). All medical staff should have advanced resuscitation training and senior nurses and doctors working in acute specialities (CCU, ITU, A&E) should hold a valid Resuscitation Council (UK) ALS certificate.

- A cardiac arrest team. Each hospital should have a team of about five people including a minimum of two doctors (physician and anaesthetist), an ALS trained nurse, the RTO and a porter when possible. Clear procedures should be available for calling the cardiac arrest team. The Resuscitation Council has

recommended the development of a medical emergency team who recognize patients who are at risk of having a cardiac arrest and initiate the most appropriate clinical intervention to prevent it (Jevon 2002).
- Resuscitation equipment. Ideally this should be standardized throughout the hospital (see Guidelines). Defibrillators should also be standardized. The widespread deployment of automated or shock advisory defibrillators is a realistic strategy to reduce mortality from cardiac arrests related to ischaemic heart disease (Jevon 2002). Bossaert (1997) believes that defibrillation should be a basic skills requirement of all nurses. With the advent of automated external defibrillators (AEDs) this may become a possibility in the near future.
- Audit and reporting of standards. All resuscitation attempts should be audited, ideally using a nationally recognized template such as Utstein template (recommended for use by the Resuscitation Council UK).
- Decisions relating to CPR. Every hospital should have a 'Do not attempt resuscitation' (DNAR) policy based on national guidelines (BMA *et al*. 2001; Jevon 2001a).

If these recommendations are implemented the standards in resuscitation and resuscitation training should improve (Jevon 2002).

Ethics

The increase in skills, knowledge, technology and pharmacological support has proved effective in prolonging quality of life for many patients. Countless thousands of patients have good reason to be thankful for CPR and the numbers rise daily (RCUK 2000b). Resuscitation attempts in the mortally ill, however, do not enhance the dignity that most people hope for in death. Ideally, resuscitation should only be attempted in patients who have a high chance of successful revival for a good quality of life (i.e. as deemed acceptable by the individual patient). There are many important factors which need to be considered when deciding whether or not to resuscitate a patient.

- The patient's own wishes.
- The views of relatives or close friends, who may be aware of the wishes of a patient who cannot communicate.
- The patient's disease and prognosis.
- The quality of life of the patient and expected quality should resuscitation be 'successful'.

Decision making: do not attempt resuscitation

In an attempt to reduce the number of futile resuscitation attempts many hospitals have introduced formal DNAR policies, which can be applied to individual patients in specific circumstances. Health care professionals must be able to show that their decisions relating to CPR are compatible with the human rights set out in the Human Rights Act 1998 implemented on 2 October 2000 (e.g. the right to life, be free from inhuman or degrading treatment and freedom of expression) (BMA 2000).

The following guidelines are based on those provided in a joint statement by the British Medical Association, the Royal College of Nursing and the Resuscitation Council (UK) (2001).

Note: where no decision has been made and the express wishes of the patient are unknown, CPR should be performed without delay.

- Sensitive advance discussion between experienced medical/nursing staff and patients regarding attempting CPR should be encouraged, but not forced. Where patients lack competence to participate, people close to them can be helpful in reflecting their views. (Note: in England, Wales and Northern Ireland, no person is legally entitled to give consent to medical treatment on behalf of another adult.) Information about CPR needs to be realistic. Written information explaining CPR should be available for patients and those close to them to read.
- Patients are entitled to refuse CPR even when there is a reasonable chance of success.
- Some patients may ask that no DNAR order be made. Patients cannot demand treatment which the health care team judges to be inappropriate, but all efforts should be made to accommodate their wishes and preferences.
- An advance DNAR order should only be made after consideration of the likely clinical outcome, the patient's wishes and the patient's human rights. It

should be considered on an individual patient basis where:

1 Attempting CPR will not start the patient's heart and breathing
2 There is no benefit in restarting the patient's heart and breathing
3 The expected benefit is outweighed by the burdens (RCUK 2000b).

- The overall responsibility for decisions about CPR and DNAR orders rests with the consultant in charge of the patient's care. Issues should, however, be discussed with other members of the health care team, the patient and people close to the patient where appropriate.
- There are exceptional cases where resuscitation discussions with a patient may be inappropriate, e.g. where senior members of the medical and nursing team consider that CPR would be futile and that such a discussion would cause the patient unnecessary distress and anguish. This could apply to patients in the terminal phase of their illness.
- The most senior members of the medical and nursing team available should clearly document any decisions made about CPR in the patient's medical and nursing notes. The decision should be dated and the reasons for it given. This information must be communicated to all other relevant health care professionals. Unless it is against the wishes of the patient, their family should also be informed.
- The DNAR order should be reviewed on each admission or in light of changes in the patient's condition (BMA *et al.* 2001).

Finally, it should be noted that a DNAR order applies only to CPR and should not reduce the standard of medical or nursing care.

Procedure guidelines: **Cardiopulmonary resuscitation**

Equipment

All hospital wards and appropriate departments, e.g. theatre, CT scanning, should have a standardized cardiac arrest trolley or box. Resuscitation equipment should be checked on a daily basis (RCUK 2000c) by the staff on the wards or clinical areas responsible for it and a record of this check should be maintained. Below is a list of the minimum equipment recommended by the Resuscitation Council for the management of an adult cardiac arrest.

Airway management

- Pocket masks with oxygen port
- Self-inflating resuscitation bag with oxygen reservoir and tubing
- Clear face masks in sizes 4, 5 and 6
- Oropharyngeal airways in sizes 2, 3 and 4
- Yankauer suckers × 2

Additional items

- ECG electrodes
- Defibrillation gel pads
- Clock
- Gloves/goggles/aprons
- A sliding sheet or similar device should be available for safe handling

*Procedure guidelines: **Cardiopulmonary resuscitation** (cont'd)*

- Endotracheal suction catheters × 10
- Laryngeal mask airway (size 4) or Combitube (small)
- McGill forceps
- Endotracheal tubes – oral, cuffed, sizes 6, 7 and 8
- Gum elastic bougie
- Lubricating jelly
- Laryngoscopes × 2 – normal and long blades
- Spare laryngoscope bulbs and batteries
- 1 inch ribbon gauze/tape
- Scissors
- Syringe – 20 ml
- Clear oxygen mask with reservoir bag
- Oxygen cylinders × 2 (if no wall oxygen)
- Cylinder key

Circulation equipment

- Intravenous cannulae – 18 gauge × 3, 14 gauge × 3
- Hypodermic needles – 21 gauge × 10
- Syringes – 2 ml × 6, 5 ml × 6, 10 ml × 6, 20 ml × 6
- Cannula fixing dressings and tapes × 4
- Seldinger wire central venous catheter kits × 2
- 12 gauge non-Seldinger central venous catheter × 2
- Intravenous administration sets × 3
- 0.9% sodium chloride – 1000 ml bags × 2

Drugs

Immediately available prefilled syringes of:

- Atropine – 3 mg × 1
- Amiodarone – 300 mg × 1
- Epinephrine/adrenaline – 1 mg 1:10 000) × 4

Other readily available drugs

- Epinephrine/adrenaline – 1 mg (1:10 000) × 4
- Sodium bicarbonate 8.4% – 50 ml × 1
- Calcium chloride 10% – 10 ml × 2
- Lidocaine/lignocaine – 100 mg × 2
- Atropine – 1 mg × 2
- 0.9% sodium chloride – 10 ml ampoules × 10
- Naloxone – 400 µg × 2
- Epinephrine/adrenaline 1:1000 × 2
- Amiodarone – 150 mg × 4
- Magnesium sulphate 50% solution – 2 g (4 ml) × 1
- Potassium chloride 40 mmol × 1
- Adenosine – 6 mg × 10
- Hydrocortisone – 200 mg × 1
- Glucose 10% – 500 ml × 1

Procedure

Action	Rationale
1 Note time of arrest, if witnessed.	Lack of cerebral perfusion for approximately 3–4 minutes can lead to irreversible brain damage.
2 Give patient precordial thump.	This may restore cardiac rhythm, which will give a cardiac output.
3 Summon help. If a second nurse is available, he/she can call for the cardiac arrest team, bring emergency equipment and screen off the area.	Maintain patient's privacy and dignity. Cardiopulmonary resuscitation is more effective with two rescuers. One is responsible for inflating the lungs, and the other for chest compressions. Continue until medical help arrives.
4 Lie patient flat on a firm surface/bed. If on a chair, lower the patient to the floor, ensuring that the head is supported.	Effective external cardiac massage can be performed only on a hard surface.
5 If patient is in bed, remove bed head, and ensure adequate space between back of bed and wall.	To allow easy access to patient's head in order to facilitate intubation.
6 Ensure a clear airway. If cervical spine injury is excluded, extend, not hyperextend, the neck (thus lifting the tongue off the posterior wall of the pharynx). This is best achieved by lifting the chin forwards with the finger and thumb of one hand while pressing the forehead backwards with the heel of the other hand (see Fig. 7.3). If this fails to establish an airway, there may be obstruction by a foreign body. Try to remove the obstruction if visible.	To establish and maintain airway, thus facilitating ventilation.
Do not remove well-fitted dentures.	They help to create a mouth to mask seal during ventilation.
7 Insert airway, and place mask over patient's mouth and nose, making sure a seal is created.	To ventilate lungs, and avoid escape of air around face mask. It avoids contact with patient's mouth, thus minimizing risk of disease transmission.

*Procedure guidelines: **Cardiopulmonary resuscitation** (cont'd)*

Action	Rationale
8 Locate the base of the sternum, then place one hand the width of two fingers above this point over the lower third of the sternum, midline. Ensure that only the heel of the dominant hand is touching the sternum.	To ensure accuracy of external cardiac compression.
Place the other hand on top, straighten the elbows and make sure shoulders are directly over the patient's chest.	
The sternum should be depressed sharply by 4–5 cm. The cardiac compressions should be forceful, and sustained at a rate of 100 per minute.	This produces a cardiac output by applying direct downward force and compression (Smith 2000).
9 Compress the Ambu-bag in a rhythmical fashion: the bag should be attached to an oxygen source. In order to deliver 85% oxygen, a reservoir may be attached to the Ambu-bag. If, however, oxygen is not immediately available, the Ambu-bag will deliver ambient air.	Room air contains only 21% oxygen. In shock, a low cardiac output, together with ventilation–perfusion mismatch, results in severe hypoxaemia. The importance of providing a high oxygen gradient from mouth to vital cells cannot be exaggerated and so oxygen should be added during CPR as soon as it is available (80–100% is desirable) (Simmons 1999).
10 Maintain cardiac compression and ventilation at a ratio of 15:2. This rate can be achieved effectively by counting out loud 'one and two', etc. There should be a slight pause to ensure that the delivered breath is sufficient to cause the patient's chest to rise. This must continue until cardiac output returns and the patient has a palpable blood pressure.	Counting aloud will ensure co-ordination of ventilation and compression ratio. To maintain circulation and oxygenation, thus reducing risk of damage to vital organs.
11 When the cardiac arrest team arrives, it will assume responsibility for the arrest in liaison with the ward staff.	To ensure an effective expert team co-ordinates the resuscitation.
12 Attach patient to ECG monitor using three electrodes or defibrillation patches/paddles.	To obtain adequate ECG signal. Accurate recording of cardiac rhythm will determine the appropriate treatment to be initiated.

Intubation

Action	Rationale
13 Continue to ventilate and oxygenate the patient before intubation.	The risks of cardiac arrhythmias due to hypoxia are decreased.
14 Equipment for intubation should be checked before handing to appropriate medical/nursing staff: (a) Suction equipment is operational. (b) The cuff of the endotracheal tube inflates and deflates. (c) The endotracheal tube is well lubricated. (d) That catheter mount with swivel connector is ready for use.	
15 During intubation, the anaesthetist may request cricoid pressure. This involves compressing the oesophagus between the cricoid ring and the sixth cervical vertebra.	To prevent the risk of regurgitation of gastric contents and the consequent risk of pulmonary aspiration.
16 Recommence ventilation and oxygenation once intubation is completed.	Intubation should interrupt resuscitation only for a maximum of 16 seconds (Handley *et al*. 1997) to prevent the occurrence of cerebral anoxia.
17 Once the patient's trachea has been intubated, chest compressions, at a rate of 100 per minute, should continue uninterrupted (except for defibrillation and pulse check when indicated) and ventilation should continue at approximately 12 breaths per minute.	Uninterrupted compression results in a substantially higher mean coronary perfusion pressure (RCUK 2000b). A pause in chest compressions allows the coronary perfusion pressure to fall. On resuming compressions, there is some delay before the original coronary perfusion pressure is restored.

*Procedure guidelines: **Cardiopulmonary resuscitation** (cont'd)*

Intravenous access

Action	Rationale
18 Venous access must be established through a large vein as soon as possible.	To administer emergency cardiac drugs and fluid replacement.
19 Asepsis should be maintained throughout.	To prevent local and/or systemic infection.
20 The correct rate of infusion is required.	To ensure maximum drug and/or solution effectiveness.
21 Accurate recording of the administration of solutions infused and drugs added is essential.	To maintain accurate records, provide a point of reference in the event of queries and prevent any duplication of treatment.

Defibrillation

Used to terminate ventricular fibrillation or ventricular tachycardia.

Post-resuscitation care

After cardiac arrest, return of spontaneous circulation is just the first phase in a continuum of resuscitation. To return the patient to a state of normal cerebral function with no neurological deficit, a stable cardiac rhythm and normal haemodynamic function requires further resuscitation tailored to each patient's individual needs (RCUK 2000b).

Action	Rationale
1 Check patient by assessing airway, breathing, circulation, blood pressure and urine output.	To ensure a clear airway, adequate oxygenation and ventilation and aim to maintain normal sinus rhythm and a cardiac output adequate for perfusion of vital organs. To ensure adequacy of ventilation and oxygenation.
2 Check arterial blood gases.	To ensure correction of acid/base balance.
3 Check full blood count and biochemistry.	To exclude anaemia as a contributor to myocardial ischaemia. To assess renal function and electrolyte balance (K^+, Mg^{2+} and Ca^{2+}). To ensure normoglycaemia. To commence serial cardiac enzyme assay.
4 Monitor patient's cardiac rhythm and record 12-lead ECG.	Normal sinus rhythm is required for optimum cardiac function (RCUK 2000b). An assessment of whether cardiac arrest has been associated with a myocardial infarction should be made, as the patient may be suitable for coronary angioplasty or thrombolytic therapy.
5 A chest X-ray should be taken.	To establish correct siting of tracheal tube, gastric tube and central venous catheter. To exclude left ventricular failure, pulmonary aspiration and pneumothorax. To establish size and shape of heart.
6 Continue respiratory therapy.	Hypoxia and hypercarbia both increase the likelihood of a further cardiac arrest (RCUK 2000b).
7 Assess patient's level of consciousness. This can be done by use of the Glasgow Coma Scale. Although this is intended primarily for head injury, it is clinically relevant. It contains five levels of consciousness: (a) Conscious and alert (b) Drowsy but responsive to verbal commands (c) Unconscious but responsive to minimal painful stimuli (d) Unconscious and responsive to deep painful stimuli (e) Unconscious and unresponsive. See Ch. 26, Observations: neurological.	Once a heart has been resuscitated to a stable rhythm and cardiac output, the organ that influences an individual's survival most significantly is the brain (RCUK 2000c). Initial assessment and regular monitoring will alert the nurse to any changes in function.

*Procedure guidelines: **Cardiopulmonary resuscitation** (cont'd)*

Action	Rationale
8 The patient should be made comfortable and nursed in the appropriate position, i.e. upright or in the recovery position. Avoid nursing supine as this physiologically hinders cardiac output and respiration. Careful explanation and reassurance is vital at all times, particularly if the patient is conscious and aware.	
9 Following stabilization of the patient's condition, consideration should be given to moving them to an appropriate critical care environment. All established monitoring should continue during transfer.	To facilitate a safe transfer of the patient between the site of resuscitation and an appropriate place of definitive care.
A critical care outreach service, if available, may contribute to the care of the patient during stabilization and transfer.	To export the expertise of critical care to the patient and enhance the skills and understanding of ward staff in the delivery of critical care (Ridley 2002).

Please note: whether the resuscitation attempt was successful or not, the patient's relatives will require considerable support. Equally, the pastoral needs of all those associated with the arrest should not be forgotten (RCUK 2000b).

References and further reading

American Heart Association (AHA)/International Liaison Committee on Resuscitation (ILCOR) (2000) Guidelines 2000 for CPR and emergency care: an international consensus on science. *Resuscitation* **46**(1), 73–92, 109–14.

Austin, R. & Snow, A. (2000) Defibrillation. In: *Resuscitation: A Guide for Nurses* (ed. A. Cheller). Harcourt, London, pp. 141–57.

BMA (2000) *The Impact of the Human Rights Act on Medical Decision-Making*. BMA, London.

BMA, RCN, Resuscitation Council UK (2001) *Decisions Relating to Cardiopulmonary Resuscitation: A Joint Statement*. Resuscitation Council UK, London.

Bossaert, L. (1997) Fibrillation and defibrillation of the heart. *Br J Anaesth*, **79**(2), 203–13.

Bossaert, L., Handley, A., Marsden, A. *et al.* (1998) European Resuscitation Council Guidelines for adult advanced life support. *Resuscitation*, **37**(1), 81–94.

Docherty, B. & Hall, S. (2002) Basic life support and AED. *Prof Nurse* **17**(12), 705–6.

Handley, A. (1999) Basic life support. In: *ABC of Resuscitation*, (eds M. Colgohoun, A. Handley & T. Evans), 4th edn. BMJ Books, London.

Hodgetts, T. & Castle, N. (1999) *Resuscitation Rules*. BMJ Books, London.

Jevon, P. (2001a) Cardiopulmonary resuscitation. Initial assessment. *Nurs Times* **97**(42), 41–2.

Jevon, P. (2001b) A matter of life and death. *Nurs Times* **97**(37), 32–4.

Jevon, P. (2002) Resuscitation in hospital: Resuscitation Council (UK) recommendations. *Nurs Stand* **16**(33), 41–4.

Resuscitation Council UK (2000a) *CPR Guidance for Clinical Practice and Training in Hospital*. Resuscitation Council UK, London.

Resuscitation Council UK (2000b) *Resuscitation Guidelines 2000*. Resuscitation Council UK, London.

Resuscitation Council UK (2000c) *Advanced Life Support: Provider Manual*, 4th edn. RCUK, London.

Ridley, S. (2002) Critical care – modality, metamorphosis and measurement. In: *Outcomes in Critical Care*. Butterworth-Heinemann, Oxford.

Shoemaker, W.C. (2000) Pericardial tamponade. In: *Oxford Textbook of Critical Care* (eds A. Webb, M. Shapiro, M. Singer & P. Suter). Oxford University Press, London.

Simmons, R. (1999) The airway at risk. In: *ABC of Resuscitation* (eds M. Colgohoun, A. Handley & T. Evans), 4th edn. BMJ Books, London.

Skinner, D. & Vincent, R. (1997) *Cardiopulmonary Resuscitation*. Oxford University Press, London.

Smith, D. (2000) Basic life support. In: *Resuscitation: A Guide for Nurses* (ed. A. Cheller). Harcourt, London.

Varon, J., Marik, P.E. & Fromm, R.E. Jr (1998) Cardiopulmonary resuscitation: a review for clinicians. *Resuscitation* **36**(2), 133–45.

Wakeling, H.G. & Mythen, M.C. (2000) Hypomagnesemia. In: *Oxford Textbook of Critical Care* (eds A. Webb, M. Shapiro, M. Singer & P. Suter). Oxford University Press, London.

Winser, H. (2001) An evidence base for adult resuscitation. *Prof Nurse*, **16**(7), 1210–13.

Discharge planning

Chapter contents

Definition

Discharge planning is the process through which patients' needs are identified and plans are written to facilitate continuity of health care from one environment to another (Jackson 1994). Hospital discharge arrangements are based upon legislation and guidance, and government initiatives have attempted to focus attention and resources away from acute hospital services to primary and preventive care (for example, DoH 1989, 1998).

Reference material

Discharge from hospital can be a major life event for both patient and carer(s). It also has substantial implications for the use of health and social care resources. Good quality discharge should not be a matter of chance (DoH 1994). This places a responsibility on all health and social care professionals involved to work together to assess, plan and meet the needs of people leaving hospital (Henwood & Wistow 1994). Strategic health authorities (SHAs) have to ensure that health care is provided in their local areas, whereas primary care trusts (PCTs) are responsible for co-ordinating services and ensuring they are run properly (Shamash 2002). One of the key elements of the Clinical Governance agenda is improved quality and effectiveness (DoH 1998).

Therefore all hospitals should have a discharge policy which is developed, agreed and ideally jointly published with all the relevant local health and social service agencies. Standards should be applicable to the planning and delivery of care at all stages: preadmission and admission; the period as an inpatient; predischarge; the discharge process and postdischarge (Health Services Accreditation 1996). Patient admission clinics are an ideal opportunity to assess care required on discharge.

Your Guide to the NHS (NHSE 2001, p. 30) states that from the moment a patient arrives:

'Arrangements for discharging you from hospital will begin, and your discharge plan will be agreed with you, taking account of your needs and wants. When you are ready to leave hospital, the nurses and doctors will talk to you about what will happen to you during your recovery and you will be told who to contact in an emergency.

If you need ongoing care at home, your GP, midwife, health visitor, community nurse or social services department will be there to help you.

If you need any medical equipment for your return home, the NHS and your social services department will aim to provide it promptly. If you need your home to be adapted in any way, your social services department will assess your needs.'

All patients, whether short- or long-stay, those with few needs or those with complex needs, should receive comprehensive discharge planning.

Community liaison nurses

Community liaison nurses are specialist nurses who have both hospital and community experience. Their role is to advise and help with planning the care patients may need when leaving hospital, particularly when the nursing and care needs are complex. McKenna *et al.* (2000) cite poor communication between hospital and community and to this end Nixon *et al.* (1998) have endorsed the value of liaison nurses in a climate of shorter hospital stays and early patient discharge.

As an alternative to community liaison nurses, discharge progression officers may be appointed in some trusts. However, they may not necessarily be trained nurses and their role is to ensure the effective use of beds, rather than discharge planning.

For complex discharges, it is helpful if a key worker or co-ordinator is appointed to manage the discharge and, where appropriate, for family meetings/case conferences to take place to include the patient/carer, multidisciplinary and primary health care team and representatives (Health Services Accreditation 1996; Salter 1996).

Effective, safe discharge planning needs to be patient and carer focused and seamless. Therefore it is dependent on a multidisciplinary approach and the sharing of good practice (Martin 2001). The multidisciplinary approach, where all staff have a clear understanding of their roles and responsibilities, will also help to prevent inappropriate readmissions and delayed discharges (Stewart 2000) and promote the highest possible level of independence for the patient, their partner and family by encouraging appropriate self-care activities.

Discharge planning is a complex process which cannot be examined in isolation from what has occurred before or separated from the consequences that follow (Armitage 1990). Healthy individuals have sufficient self-care abilities to enable them to meet their needs with assistance from either a nurse or personal carers from social services, or they may be dependent upon someone to meet their needs for them until they are capable of resuming that self-care. In certain circumstances their needs may fluctuate owing to their disease process and so self-care may not be a realistic goal. Discharge planning is therefore a vital procedure to assist these individuals who require help to maintain their self-care or to assist them with care needs when they leave one care environment for another (Jackson 1994).

Ineffective discharge planning has been shown to have detrimental effects on a patient's psychological and physical well-being and their illness experience (Smith 1996; Nazarko 1998). Planning care, providing adequate information and involving patients, families and health care professionals, will keep disruption to a minimum.

Aims of discharge planning

- To prepare the patient and family physically and psychologically for transfer home or to an agreed environment.
- To provide the patient and carers with written and verbal information to meet their needs on discharge.
- To facilitate a smooth transfer, by ensuring that all necessary health care facilities are prepared to receive the patient.
- To promote the highest possible level of independence for the patient, partner and family by, where appropriate, encouraging self-care activities.
- To provide continuity of care between the hospital and the agreed environment by facilitating effective communication.

Principles of good discharge planning

When planning discharge from one care environment to another, certain principles should be followed. These include:

- Discharge planning should be a multidisciplinary process, by which resources to meet the needs of patients and carers are put in place (Salter 1996).
- Discharge procedures should be of a consistently high standard for all patients.
- Carers' needs should also be assessed (DoH 1995).
- Patients should be discharged to a safe and adequate environment.
- Continuity of care between environments should be paramount.

- Discharge planning should commence on the initial contact with patients.
- Information about discharge arrangements should be disseminated between professionals and patients/carers, with the latter being provided with written information of ongoing care.
- Patients' beliefs and cultural needs should be considered when planning discharge.

The discharge planning process and the primary/secondary care interface

The discharge planning process can be initiated by a member of the primary health care team (PHCT) or social services staff in the patient's home, prior to admission, in preadmission clinics or on hospital admission (Health Services Accreditation 1996). Importance is attached to developing a primary care-led NHS, reinforced by the government's white paper, 'The New NHS: Modern, Dependable' and the establishment of primary care groups (PCGs) and primary care trusts (PCTs) that came into force in April 1999 (DoH 1998). The focus on quality, patient-centred care and services closer to where people live will be dependent on primary, secondary and tertiary professionals working together (Davis 1998). To this end, the trigger questions shown in Fig. 8.1 are a useful tool for screening patients who may have high social needs.

However, it is important to note that the Community Care (Delayed Discharges) Bill (DOH 2003b) introduced a system of reimbursement to NHS bodies from Social Services Departments (SSD) for delays caused by the failure of SSDs to provide timely assessment and/or services for a patient being discharged from an acute hospital bed.

The discharge planning process takes into account a patient's physical, psychological, social, cultural and economic needs. It involves not only patients but can involve families, friends, carers, the hospital multi-disciplinary team and the community health/social services teams (Nixon *et al.* 1998), with the emphasis on health and social services departments working jointly.

In recent years the reduction in hospital beds has resulted in an increasing emphasis on shorter inpatient stays (Stewart 2000). Therefore the notion of a seamless service may be idealistic because of increasing time constraints and the complex care needs of high-dependency patients (Smith 1996). Despite well-documented concerns about the quality of procedures for the discharge of patients from hospital, shortcomings persist.

Occasionally the discharge process may not proceed as planned; a discharge may be delayed for a number of reasons and a system should be in place to record this (see Fig. 8.2). Patients may take their own discharge against medical advice and this should be documented accordingly (see Fig. 8.3). Some patients receiving news of a poor prognosis may prefer to go home to die and plans would need to be set up at short notice (see Fig. 8.6).

The role of informal carers

Patients and their carers/advocates should be actively involved at all stages of the planning and discharge

---

The Royal Marsden Hospital

These trigger questions are designed for use by nursing staff to screen patients with potentially high social care needs whose eligibility for community care services has to be assessed in more detail by a hospital-based social worker. Discussion with the social services team should be initiated regarding appropriate assessment of patient and/or their family's needs.

Patient's name: Hospital no.:   Ward: Estimated date of discharge:

Care needs
1 Significant change in ability to care for self due to the effects of treatment or the debilitating symptoms of
   progressive disease.   ☐
2 Patient has, and is aware of, limited prognosis, requiring a complex package of palliative and community care. ☐
3 Patient appears to have very high social and nursing care needs which suggest a residential or nursing home as a
   placement option.   ☐
4 Patient appears to be in need of health-funded continuing care.   ☐

Social network
5 High dependency on a carer for all or most aspects of physical care.   ☐
6 Carer shows signs of stress, or questions own ability to continue caring.   ☐
7 Patient is carer for partner, vulnerable adult dependant and/or children under 18.   ☐

Environment
8 Housing unsuitable, access problems or inadequate heating, electricity, water supplies.   ☐
9 Patient is homeless or threatened by homelessness.   ☐

Signature of referrer: Job title: Date of referral:

Figure 8.1 Trigger questions for social services referrals.

The Royal Marsden Hospital

Definition
A discharge delay is when a patient remains in hospital beyond the date agreed by the multidisciplinary team and beyond the time when they are medically fit to leave.

Monitoring
For every patient who is 'delayed' the ward nurse will complete a 'delayed discharge' form and return it to the clinical nurse specialist (CNS), community liaison. The CNS, community liaison will monitor all 'delays' of 7 days or more.

Procedure
Any patient who is 'delayed' for 7 days or more for reasons other than medical need will be discussed at a multidisciplinary meeting that includes medical staff, where appropriate. A discharge plan should be formulated and documented in the multidisciplinary care plan.

If there is no resolution at the meeting the community liaison nurse or social worker will contact their manager. If a long 'delay' is anticipated even when a discharge plan has been agreed, the community liaison nurse or the social worker should inform their manager.

All details of the reasons for the delay and actions taken must be documented in the multidisciplinary care plan.

Source: The Royal Marsden Hospital's Discharge Delay Policy/Procedure (2003).

DISCHARGE DELAY MONITORING FORM
Name of patient:
Hospital number:
Ward:
Expected date of discharge:
Reason for delay:
Signature.

Figure 8.2 Discharge delays.

The Royal Marsden Hospital

Nursing staff responsibility
If a patient wishes to take his/her own discharge the ward sister/co-ordinator should contact:

1 A member of the medical team.
2 The manager on call.
3 The clinical nurse specialist (CNS), community liaison.

The CNS, community liaison, will inform social services if appropriate.

Out of hours, following a risk assessment, the manager on call will contact the local social services department, if felt appropriate, and inform the hospital social services department the following day.

Medical staff responsibility
The doctor, following consultation with the patient, should complete the appropriate form prior to the patient leaving the hospital. The form must be signed by the patient and the doctor and filed in the medical notes.

The doctor must immediately contact the patient's GP.

Figure 8.3 Patients taking discharge against medical advice. (*Source:* The Royal Marsden Hospital's Discharge Policy/Procedure 2003.)

---

process (The Royal Marsden Hospital Discharge and Policy Procedure 2003). Studies indicate that the greater the level of patient and family involvement in the discharge planning process, the more patients perceive themselves ready for discharge (Nixon *et al.* 1998). The DoH (1989) white paper 'Caring for People' explicitly acknowledged that the majority of care is provided by informal carers and that carers need help and support to fulfil that role. A critical time to help carers is during hospital discharge when community care plans are being set up (George 1995). However, in Henwood's (1998) study, 7 out of 10 carers said they did not receive a copy of the discharge plan. Half the carers felt that they had not been informed of the type of care they were expected to give at home and more than a third did not feel their concerns were taken into consideration by the staff planning the

discharge. Policy guidance has suggested that carers' needs should be seen as being just as important as those of service users (Social Services Inspectorate 1998). The Carer's (Recognition and Services) Act (DoH 1995) gives carers a statutory right to request an assessment of their ability to provide care (Henwood 1998). Carers' needs should be acknowledged so that health care professionals adopt a proactive approach to addressing such needs. Assessment of carers' needs must be requested at the same time as that of the patient, as the assessments must be undertaken together; carers will not be assessed separately. Voluntary services play a key role in supporting patients and carers at home (Daly 1999).

Communication and discharge planning

Laminated pocket guides have been produced at the Royal Marsden Hospital for (a) doctors and (b) nurses (Fig. 8.4) to ensure liaison between these disciplines. Additionally, a complex discharge flowchart (Fig. 8.5) highlights the communication required with the multidisciplinary team.

Single Assessment Process

Referred to in *The NHS Plan* (2000) and reinforced in the National Service Framework (NSF) for Older people (DoH 2001a), the Single Assessment Process is designed to replace fragmented assessments carried out by different agencies with one seamless procedure (Hunter 2001). The aim is to produce a single, centrally

---

Guide to discharge planning for nursing staff

YOUR RESPONSIBILITIES:

The aim of this guide is to make discharge planning more effective. It should be used in conjunction with the Royal Marsden's 'Discharge Policy and Procedure'

- Within 24 hours of each admission, make every effort to complete the full nursing assessment and discharge planning section of the care plan.
- It is essential to negotiate with medical staff to set and document a discharge date. This must be reviewed daily.
- Regularly discuss discharge with the patient and/or carers as appropriate.
- Please ensure that all complex discharges are discussed at ward multidisciplinary meetings.

AS APPROPRIATE:

- Refer to other members of the Multidisciplinary Team.
- Complete Social Services Referral Forms and forward to Social Services Dept.
- Refer to District Nursing Service/Specialist Community Nurses (*try to give 48 hours notice*).
- Request nursing equipment for use in the community (it can take a week to obtain).
- Refer to Community Palliative Care Team and specify if urgent. Ensure completed green sticker (as shown) is inserted on the inside cover of medical notes.
- Fax Community Care Referral Form to all Community Nursing Services.

- Document all referrals made to community services with: **DATE, CONTACT NAME, TELEPHONE & FAX NUMBERS**
- Give written details of services arranged to patient and/or carer.

DISCHARGE DELAYS:
Definition of a delayed discharge at the Royal Marsden:

'Patients who no longer need clinical care in a comprehensive cancer centre, but who stay in the hospital because of delayed or lack of appropriate community/social care services or internal failures to plan the discharge properly'.

- All delayed discharges must be discussed at ward multidisciplinary meetings.
- Discharge Delay Monitoring Form to be completed for every delay by the ward sister or designated deputy and forwarded to the Community Liaison Office.

For further information or advice on discharge planning please contact the Clinical Nurse Specialists, Community Liaison.

Example of Green Sticker for Hospice Referrals

Patient under care of **H**ospice/**C**ommunity **P**alliative **C**are Team	Referral agreed by patient
Name/Address...	
Tel:...................................... Fax......................................	Yes ☐
PLEASE SEND COPIES OF APPROPRIATE CORRESPONDENCE	No ☐
PRINT name of staff making referral..	
Signed .... Date..................	

Figure 8.4 Guide to discharge planning for nursing staff.

held, electronic summary/tool containing all the information needed to assess, and in turn provide for, an older person's health and social care needs. The end result will be a comprehensive 'individual care plan' that will lay out their full needs and entitlements (Hunter 2001). Examples of health care professionals who may be involved in contributing to the Single Assessment Process are nurses and doctors, occupational therapists, physiotherapists, dietitians and speech therapists.

Continuous assessment of patients' needs and early liaison with the primary health care team are essential if appropriate care and a safe environment are to be provided in the community (Tierney 1993).

Intermediate care

The NHS Plan (DoH 2000) signalled the development of intermediate care as one of the major initiatives for services in the future. It is recognized that older people are best cared for at home if at all possible. To aid the transition period from hospital to home, intermediate care teams may provide a period of intensive care/rehabilitation following a hospital stay.

Residential care

Residential care (whether it be in the form of a residential or nursing home) requires careful thought as for many patients the concept and planning of giving up their own home is one of the most traumatic events that the older person has to consider and that has serious repercussions if a wrong decision is made (Macabee 1994). When a patient is transferred from an inpatient palliative care service to a nursing home, a specific prognosis may not be given, although there is an expectation that death is not imminent, or a nursing home placement, as a longer term facility, would not have been considered. The present government was concerned about the transfer of frail, elderly patients between hospitals and care homes, and such transfers may be stopped or severely restricted if the results of an investigation support the Health Secretary's impression that too many old people die as a result of being moved. Alternatives such as nurse-led 'hospital at home' schemes (Busby 1995) or 'immediate response/discharge teams' (usually local authority led) may well enable a person to remain in their own home.

HELPFUL HINTS ON ARRANGING A COMPLEX DISCHARGE HOME
NB: This is not an exhaustive list and MUST BE DISCUSSED with the Community Liaison Nurse

Complex discharge definition:

- A high level of nursing care required on discharge
- A large package of care involving different agencies
- The patient's needs have changed since admission, with different services requiring co-ordination
- The family/carer requires intensive input into discharge planning considerations (e.g. psychological interventions)

1. **Comprehensive assessment by nurse on admission and document care accordingly**

a. Provisional discharge date set	• THIS WILL ONLY BE APPROXIMATE, depending on care needs, equipment etc. • Regularly review with multidisciplinary team • DISCHARGE SHOULD **NOT** BE ARRANGED FOR A FRIDAY OR WEEKEND
b. Referrals to relevant members of multi-disciplinary team	e.g. Occupational Therapist, Physiotherapist, Social Services
c. Referral to Community Health Services (in liaison with multidisciplinary team)	e.g. District Nurse (who may be able to arrange for night sitters), Community Palliative Care Team
d. Request equipment from District Nurse and discuss with family	e.g. hoist, hospital bed, pressure-relieving mattress/cushion, commode, nebulizer • **If oxygen required,** SHO to liaise with GP re: cylinders, tubing, nasal specs/face mask • If continuous O_2 – confirm arrangements with community liasion nurse

2. **Discuss at ward multidisciplinary meeting, and arrange family meeting/case conference as required,** and invite all appropriate health care professionals, including community staff

a. Appoint discharge co-ordinator at the multidisciplinary meeting	• To act as co-ordinator for referrals and point of contact for any discharge concerns • To plan and prepare the family meeting/case conference and to arrange a chairperson and minute-taker for the meeting • Primary Team Nurse to liaise with discharge co-ordinator
b. Formulate a discharge plan at meeting	At the meeting, formulate a discharge plan in conjuction with patient, carers, and all hospital and community personnel involved and agree a discharge date – an Occupational Therapist home visit may be required.
c. Ascertain discharge address	• Liaise with services accordingly • It is important to agree who will care for patient/where the patient will be cared for, e.g. ground/first floor • Ascertain type of accommodation patient lives in so that the equipment ordered will fit in appropriately • NB. IF NOT RETURNING TO OWN HOME, A GP WILL BE REQUIRED TO TAKE PATIENT ON AS A TEMPORARY RESIDENT
d. Confirm PROVISIONAL discharge date	• This will depend on when community services and equipment can be arranged • This must be agreed with the patient and family/informal carer/s

3. **Ascertain whether district nurse is able to undertake any necessary clinical procedures** in accordance with their Primary Care Trust policy, e.g. care of skin-tunnelled catheters. Consider alternative arrangements if necessary.

a. Confirm equipment agreed and delivery date	NB. FAMILY must be informed of delivery date and also requested to contact ward to inform that this has been received
b. Confirm start date for care	e.g. Social Services/District Nurse/Community Palliative Care Team
c. Confirm with patient/family agreed discharge date	• Liaise with community liaison nurse for 'Community Services Arrangements' form (see example) • Check community services able to enter patient home as necessary

4. **48 hours prior to discharge,** Fax and telephone district nurse with Community Care Referral Form and discuss any special needs of patient, e.g. syringe driver, oxygen, wound care, intravenous therapy, MRSA or other infection status. Give written information and instructions.

a. Arrange transport and assess need for escort/oxygen during transport	
b. Ongoing review	• Should be in place for any change in patient's condition/treatment plan • IF THERE IS A CHANGE, notify/liaise with MD Team and Community Services
c. If NO change within 24 hours of discharge, confirm that:	• Patient is medically fit for discharge • All Community Services are in place as agreed above
• Patient has TTOs & next appointment	• Ensure patient has drugs to take out with written and verbal instructions • Next in/outpatient appointment as required
• Access to home, heating and food are checked	• Check arrangements for patient to get into home (front door key), heating, food and someone there to welcome them home, as appropriate

5. **Hospital equipment:** e.g. syringe drivers – ensure clearly marked and arrangements made for return
6. **After discharge,** follow-up phone call to patient by ward nurse or community liaison nurse as agreed to ensure all services in place

Figure 8.5 Guide to arranging a complex discharge home and quick reference flowchart.

COMPLEX DISCHARGE GUIDELINES 'QUICK REFERENCE' FLOWCHART

1.   **Assessment by ward nurse → patient identified as having complex discharge needs**

   Complex discharge definition:

   - a high level of nursing care required on discharge
   - a large package of care involving different agencies
   - the patient's needs have changed since admission, with different services requiring co-ordination
   - the family/carer requires intensive input into discharge planning considerations, e.g. psychological interventions

↓

2.   **Notify Community Liaison Nurse/refer to multidisciplinary team for assessments**

↓

3.   **Appoint Discharge Co-ordinator**

   - ascertain discharge address/whether patient to be cared for upstairs or ground floor and liaise with services accordingly
   - IF PATIENT BEING DISCHARGED TO RELATIVE'S HOME OUT OF AREA, SHE/HE WILL NEED TO BE A TEMPORARY RESIDENT WITH LOCAL GP

↓

4.   **Provisional discharge date set, in liaison with patient, carers, MDT and Community Services (NB it may be necessary to arrange a case conference – invite community staff)**

   - order equipment required from district nurse (e.g. hospital bed, hoist, pressure-relieving mattress, commode) NB oxygen cylinders, face mask/nasal specs should be requested from GP by SHO
   - confirm when equipment has been delivered
   - confirm care package agreed by all Community Agencies

↓

5.   **Review and confirm discharge date with patient/carers and MD team/Community Services, with 48 hours' notice of discharge given**

   - assess need for oxygen on journey home and check arrangements for oxygen/transport/escort are made

↓

6.   **Ongoing review should take place for any change in patient's condition:**

   - If there is a change, notify MD team and Community Services
   - If no change, within 24 hours of discharge confirm that:
     - ➤ patient is medically fit for discharge
     - ➤ all Community Services are in place as agreed
     - ➤ patient has drugs to take out with written/verbal instructions and next in/outpatient appointment as required
     - ➤ patient has a front door key, heating, food, and someone to welcome them home, as appropriate

↓

7.   **Day after discharge, follow-up phone call by ward nurse/community liaison nurse to ascertain all services are in place as agreed by nursing staff**

Refer to ward resource discharge folder or nursing intranet for more detailed information

Figure 8.5 Guide to arranging a complex discharge home and quick reference flowchart (*continued*).

Continuing care

Continuing care (or long-term care) is a general term that describes the care that people need over an extended period of time as the result of disability, accident or illness to address both physical and mental health needs. It may require services from the NHS and/or social care.

Government guidance (DoH 2001b) required health and local authorities to agree new joint continuing health and social care for the above groups of people. It can be provided in a range of settings from a NHS hospital or care home to care in people's own homes. Continuing NHS health care describes a package of care arranged and

This form has been designed to assist with planning an urgent discharge home for terminal care. It should be used as a trigger in conjunction with the discharge policy. Please document all relevant comments in the Multidisciplinary Care Plan.

Emergency Discharge Plan   Date of discharge: ....

(Tick when arranged or cross if not appropriate)
1 Plan agreed and discussed with patient and carers.   ☐
2 Patient and family fully aware of condition and prognosis.   ☐
3 Transport booked   ☐
   Date and time: ....
   Oxygen/suction requested   ☐
   Paramedic crew requested   ☐
   Stretcher   ☐
   Escort (family/nurse)   ☐
4 Oxygen ordered through GP and delivery date organized for ....   ☐
5 Patient/carer given list of contact numbers of community services   ☐
6 Block bed for 24–48 hour period   Yes/No

Nursing issues
1 Contact district nurse (DN) and discuss   ☐
   (a) Patient needs   ☐
   (b) Planned date and time of DN's first visit ....   ☐
   (c) Night nursing service   ☐
       • Starting ....
       • Contact numbers ....
   (d) Marie Curie provision   ☐
       • Starting ....
   (e) Return of RMH syringe driver   ☐
   (f) Delivery of equipment   ☐
       • Hospital bed (adjustable height)   ☐
       • Pressure relieving equipment   ☐
       • Commode/urinal   ☐
       • Hoist   ☐
       • Backrest/mattress variator   ☐
       • Other (please state) ....
2 Contact hospice home care team   ☐
   Planned date and time of first visit ....
3 Nursing letter for DN and hospice home care team   ☐
4 Medical letter of authorization for drugs to be administered by community nurses   ☐

5 List of medication to go with patient   ☐
6 Provide 3–4 days' supply of:
   (a) Dressing and continence aids   ☐
   (b) Syringe driver giving sets   ☐
   (c) Winged infusion devices/cannulae and dressings to secure   ☐
7 Convert syringe driver to a 24-hour pump and aim for it to be changed every morning   ☐

Medical issues
1 Medical team contact GP to discuss:
   (a) Patient needs   ☐
   (b) Drugs prescribed on discharge   ☐
   (c) Need to review patient in community   ☐
2 Prescribe adequate supply of TTOs (include diluent used in syringe driver)   ☐
   (Consider prognosis)
3 Crisis pack for use in the event of an emergency, including diamorphine, midazolam and instructions for use   ☐
4 Medical summary faxed to GP, copy with patient   ☐
5 Medical proforma for ambulance crew stating resuscitation status (signature of consultant/senior registrar)   ☐

If you have any queries please contact the community liaison team or the palliative care team.

Figure 8.6 Emergency discharge plan checklist.

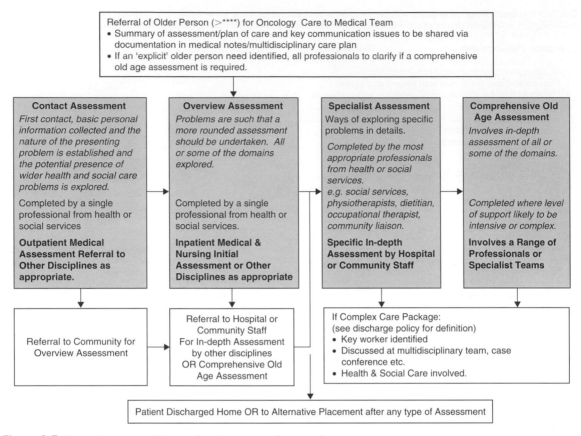

Figure 8.7 Single Assessment Process for older people (flowchart).

funded solely by the NHS. It does not include the provision by local councils of any social services.

Longer-term health care needs and eligibility criteria

The NHS (1997) survey comments in some detail on the implications of allowing health authorities to set local criteria for eligibility to receive free, NHS funded, long-term care. The NHS argued that these local criteria might create inequity, with individuals in some parts of the country receiving free NHS care, while others in identical circumstances elsewhere contribute towards the cost of care commissioned by local authorities. The NHS called for the national framework to include national eligibility criteria 'to define what the NHS, as a national service … always provide' (NHS 1997, para. 8). There will, of course, always have to be a judgement made as to what is the level of care above which domiciliary care packages cease to be realistically affordable, bearing in mind the equally valid needs of other people in the community.

Care homes

October 2001 saw important changes for those aged 18 and over requiring registered nursing care in nursing homes in England. All those over the age of 18 needing the skills and knowledge of a registered nurse to meet all or certain elements of their care needs will have that care paid for by the NHS. The amount of funding, paid directly to the nursing home, is dependent on a comprehensive assessment of the patient's care needs by a registered nurse, who will usually be employed by the local PCT. These changes also apply to short periods of respite care. However, periods of intermediate care for short-term treatment or rehabilitation, lasting no longer than 6 weeks, remain free of charge (DoH 2001b).

Audit and the discharge process

It is the responsibility of health authorities, in collaboration with social services departments, to monitor the way in which discharges from hospitals are being undertaken and, if problems occur, to establish the reasons so that any necessary changes are made to address the local needs, for example, monitoring discharge failures (DoH 1989a). Similarly, the United Kingdom Central Council for Nurses, Midwives and Health Visitors (Registrar's letter 18/1995) emphasizes that every ward should have at least a basic system of audit and quality control of discharge practice and procedures.

Patients with particular care needs

The following categories of patients were identified as having particular care needs. These include patients who:

- Live alone
- Are frail and/or elderly
- Have care needs which place a high demand on carers and carers who find difficulty coping
- Have a limited prognosis

- Have serious illnesses and will be returning to hospital for further treatments
- Have continuing disability
- Have learning difficulties
- Have mental illness or dementia
- Have dependants
- Have limited financial resources
- Are homeless or live in poor housing
- Do not have English as their first language
- Have been in hospital for an 'extended stay'
- Require aids/equipment at home.

(Adapted from DoH 1989.)

Conclusion

From the patient's and carer's perspective, discharge may be one of the most important events of the hospital stay. It is essential, therefore, that discharge planning is considered as an integral part of care.

Procedure guidelines: **Discharge planning**

Procedure

Action	Rationale
Initial assessment (within first 24–48 hours of admission)	
1 The admitting nurse is responsible for ensuring that an initial assessment is completed when the patient is admitted and is documented in the multidisciplinary care plan. Assessment should be ongoing and regularly reviewed with the multidisciplinary team.	To enable the physical, psychological and social care needs of the patient and carers to be identified at an early stage.
2 An expected date of discharge should be established.	To ensure planning for discharge commences.
3 Clarify whether the patient has dependants, e.g. elderly relatives, children or a disabled partner who is unwell. If so, establish who is looking after them and whether they receive any services.	Arrangements may need to be made for alternative carer or an increase in services. Notification may need to be made to, e.g. school nurse/teacher if patient has children at school.
4 Establish who else is involved in giving care/support and the type of help given, e.g. local support group, voluntary agency, church.	To assess the support that the patient and carers may require at home so that appropriate services can be mobilized. To establish social network in order to co-ordinate care between voluntary and statutory agencies.
5 Ascertain the type of accommodation the patient is living in, e.g. flat, bungalow (council or privately owned), residential or nursing home, sheltered housing.	To identify early potential housing problems which may entail social work intervention. To identify need for occupational therapy intervention (for equipment to aid independence).
6 Ascertain the names and telephone numbers of sheltered housing wardens or officers in charge of homes.	To enable contact to be made and to establish that an appropriate degree of care and support can continue to be provided, once the patient is discharged from hospital.
7 Ensure that the home address and telephone number of the patient are documented accurately in the care plan. Establish where the patient will be going on discharge and document the discharge address if different from the permanent address.	Personal information may not have been updated on previous nursing or medical records. It is crucial that this information is accurate when making referrals to community services, to ensure appropriate service provision.

*Procedure guidelines: **Discharge planning** (cont'd)*

Action	Rationale
8 Ensure that the patient is registered permanently with a general practitioner (GP) and with a GP on a temporary basis if going to a different address on discharge. Check the names, addresses and telephone numbers with the patient.	Community nursing services arc unable to accept the patient without medical support. Accurate information is required to establish which district nurse will have responsibility for patient care. It is important for the patient that medical care can be provided at home.
9 Establish whether any statutory community health or social services have been involved before the patient's admission. Include the health visitor when the patient has children under the age of 5 years.	To enable contact for exchange of information. Valuable information can be obtained from community services to assist in assessing potential needs on discharge.

Referrals

Action	Rationale
10 Assess the patient's ability to carry out activities of daily living at home prior to admission, e.g. was she/he able to climb stairs? Consider patient's current level of functioning and whether this will change as a result of treatment and/or rehabilitation.	To establish at an early stage whether an occupational therapy assessment is required. Home assessment may be required by occupational therapy prior to discharge which may involve complex planning and preparation.
11 Refer to other hospital personnel as soon as potential needs are recognized, e.g. occupational therapist, physiotherapists, dietitian. Referral as soon as possible after admission is essential – do not wait until treatment is completed and discharge is imminent.	To ensure multidisciplinary planning and co-ordination. Considerable time may be needed to arrange community services and early referral helps to prevent discharge delays.
12 Patients identified as requiring local authority social services support are referred to the social services department. Some hospitals use a 'trigger' form as an aid to assessment, an example of which can be found in Fig. 8.1.	To ensure early and appropriate referral to the social services department for assessment.
13 A discharge planning 'area of care' should be commenced in the care plan; all members of the multidisciplinary team should document in the care plan their assessment, plans and action taken.	To facilitate multidisciplinary planning, co-ordination and communication.
14 Where there is a designated community liaison nurse/adviser, she/he can act as a resource offering support and education to the ward team in the preparation of discharge plans, especially for those patients requiring a complex package of care.	To facilitate effective discharge planning and utilize expertise appropriately.
15 Formulate a discharge plan in conjunction with patient and carers and all involved hospital and community personnel and agree a discharge date.	To collate information and co-ordinate planning.
16 For complex discharges a discharge planning meeting should be held.	To co-ordinate continuity of care planning.
17 The ward-based nurse is responsible for arranging and co-ordinating community nursing services (including Macmillan/hospice home care nurse) in consultation with the community liaison nurse if applicable.	To facilitate continuity of care between hospital and community.
18 Refer to the community nursing services with a minimum of 48 hours' notice. If a complex package of care is being organized more notice will be required. Invite community nurses to visit the ward where appropriate.	Community nurses may wish to assess the patient's nursing care needs and ensure preparation of the home prior to discharge. They need time to liaise with other agencies to co-ordinate care and to obtain any equipment required.
19 Ascertain whether district nurses are able to carry out necessary clinical procedures in accordance with their health authority policy, e.g. care of skin-tunnelled catheters. Consider alternative arrangements if necessary. Give written information and instructions.	District nurses may not have been trained in certain procedures or may be unfamiliar with particular equipment.

Procedure guidelines: Discharge planning (cont'd)

Action	Rationale
20 Details of patient's MRSA status (or other infections) must be given to community personnel and written in referral details.	To reduce risk of cross-infection. The district nurse requires full knowledge of the patient's history and nursing requirements.
21 Complete the community care referral form or update letter. The form/letter should be completed and signed and a copy provided for the Macmillan/hospice home care team.	Provide information for community staff to ensure that they have accurate information.
22 Ensure any essential medical/nursing aids or equipment have been obtained before discharge by community services, e.g. oxygen, nebulizers, commode, pressure-relieving mattress, hoist. Home assessment may be required by occupational therapy prior to discharge.	Some equipment may not be available or may take a long time to obtain. Equipment may be loaned from the community or from hospital and appropriate legislation procedures must be followed for safety reasons.
23 Patients requiring community nursing, physiotherapy, occupational therapy, stoma care, speech therapy and/or dietetic support on discharge will be referred by the appropriate hospital-based health care professional to their equivalent in the community.	To ensure continuity of specialist care.

Leaving hospital

Action	Rationale
24 Medical staff are responsible for assessing the patient's medical fitness for discharge and for liaising with other members of the multidisciplinary team regarding arrangements for meeting the patient's care needs in the community.	To ensure that both health and social care needs are taken into consideration when formulating discharge plans.
25 Notify the sheltered housing wardens or officer in charge of the nursing/residential home of discharge date.	To ensure preparation of accommodation.
26 Ensure that patient and, with his/her agreement, carers have full information regarding the patient's medical condition and care required.	To prepare carers and to enable patient and carers to support each other.
27 Teach the patient and carers any necessary skills, allowing sufficient time to practise before discharge. This should include information on the safe use of equipment, e.g. a hoist.	To enable the patient to be as independent as possible and promote an understanding of self-care techniques.
28 Ensure that the patient has a door key and can gain entrance to their residence. Wherever possible, ensure that someone is at home to receive the patient.	The patient may have left their key with a neighbour. It is helpful for someone to be available to welcome the patient and attend to any immediate needs.
29 Book transport if required with 48 hours' notice, using relevant form. Specify if patient needs a stretcher or chair, or requires escort. Ensure that transport is also booked for return clinic appointment if necessary.	The patient may not have private transport facilities and may be too weak to use public transport.
Cancel transport if discharge date or outpatients department appointment is altered.	To prevent a waste of resources.
30 Patients should be given an appropriate supply of medication and, where necessary, a supply of wound management dressings or medical equipment.	To ensure the safe and continuous administration of medication and use of equipment at home. Time is needed to obtain items in the community.
31 Discharge plans should not be altered without consultation with all the hospital personnel who have been involved in the planning, e.g. occupational therapist, social worker, community liaison nurse and also patient/family carers.	If there is no consultation this causes considerable confusion and stress for the patient, family and friends, and all involved services. It may result in the patient being unsupported at home.
32 If discharge is cancelled or postponed, or if the patient dies, ensure that all relevant community services are informed.	To avoid distress to relatives. To avoid wasted visits and promote good community relations.

*Procedure guidelines: **Discharge planning** (cont'd)*

Action	Rationale
33 Weekend discharge: patients who require a high level of health services and social services support should not be discharged home on a Friday or Saturday or a public holiday. This applies particularly to patients who were previously unknown to community services. *Note*: assessment and planning for weekend leave are as important as for final discharge	All community services will be operating at a reduced level and emergency medical back-up may be difficult to obtain.

Patient information

Action	Rationale
34 Inform the patient and carers of potential side-effects of treatment and management.	To alleviate anxiety and to promote patient comfort, knowledge and safety.
35 Ensure that patient and carers have information on local support groups or national specialist organizations as appropriate.	Some patients may benefit from the kind of support offered by the organizations.
36 Reinforce any special instructions with written information or by giving an approved education booklet, e.g. one of the Royal Marsden Hospital series.	To promote an understanding of disease and treatment. To confirm arrangements made. To enable the patient to contact the appropriate services.
37 Information on community services arranged, including names and telephone numbers and expected date of first visit, should be given to the patient and carers prior to discharge. This information should also be documented in the patient's care plan.	To confirm arrangements made. To enable the patient to contact the appropriate services.
The social worker informs the patient and carers of local authority arrangements upon discharge, provides them with a summary of their care plan and gives contact names, including the care manager or equivalent in the patient's local social services department.	To confirm with patient and carers arrangements made upon discharge.
38 Ensure that arrangements have been made to provide patient with food at home on discharge and that there will be adequate heating.	To supply immediate needs.
39 Ensure that the patient and carers are given verbal and written information on the dosage, route, frequency and side-effects of any medication and how to obtain further supplies.	Lack of information makes it difficult for the GP to provide the medical care required.

After discharge

Action	Rationale
40 A follow-up phone call should be made to establish how the patient is managing.	To ensure services are in place.

References and further reading

Armitage, S. (1990) *Liaison and Continuity of Nursing Care. Executive Summary*. Welsh Office, Cardiff.

Daly, N. (1999) Campaigning for carers. *Commun Care*, 18–24 February, 1260.

Davis, S. (1998) *Primary secondary care interface*. Proceedings of conference, 25 March. NHS Executive, June, Issue 2.

DoH (1989) *Discharge of Patients from Hospital*. Health Circular (89) 5. Stationery Office, London.

DoH (1994) *The Hospital Discharge Workbook: A Manual on Hospital Discharge Practice*. Stationery Office, London.

DoH (1995) *Carer's (Recognition and Services) Act*. Stationery Office, London.

DoH (1998) *A First Class Service: Quality in the New NHS*. NHSE, London.

DoH (1998) *The New NHS: Modern, Dependable*. Stationery Office, London.

DoH (2000) *The NHS Plan*. Stationery Office, London.

DoH (2001a) *The Single Assessment Process*. Stationery Office, London.

DoH (2001b) *NHS Funded Nursing Care in Nursing Homes: What It Means for You*. Stationery Office, London.

DoH (2003a) *Discharge from Hospital: Pathway, Process and Practice*. Stationery Office, London.

DoH (2003b) *Delayed Transfers of Care: Planning for Implementation of Reimbursement and Improving Hospital Discharge Practice*. Stationery Office, London.

George, M. (1995) Collaborative nursing. *Nurs Stand*, **12**(46), 22–3.

George, M. (1998) Gentle persuasion. *Commun Care*, 1–7 October, 30–1.

Haywood, K. (1998) Patient-held oncology records. *Nurs Stand*, **12**(35), 44–6.

Health Services Accreditation (1996) *Service Standards for Discharge Care*. NHS, East Sussex.

Henwood, M. (1993) Key task 2, residential and nursing homes. *Commun Care*, 21 January, 17.

Henwood, M. (1998) Helping the helpers. *Commun Care*, 13–19 August, 13–15.

Henwood, M. & Wistow, G. (1994) *Hospital Discharge and Community Care: Early Days*. Stationery Office, London.

Hunter, M. (2001) Will social services suffer in new regime? *Commun Care*, **13**(87), 10–11.

Jackson, M. (1994) Discharge planning: issues and challenges for gerontological nursing. A critique of the literature. *J Adv Nurs*, **19**, 492–502.

Jupp, M. & Simms, S. (1986) Going home. *Nurs Times*, **83**(33), 40–42.

Kline, R. (1998) Opportunity knocks. *Nurs Times*, **94**(35), 10.

Martin, J. (2001) Benchmarking – how do you do it? *Nurs Times*, **97**(42), 30–1.

McKenna, H., Keeney, S., Glenn, A. & Gordon, P. (2000) Discharge planning: an exploratory study. *J Adv Nurs*, **9**, 594–601.

National Audit Office (2003) *Ensuring the Effective Discharge of Older Patients from NHS Acute Hospitals*. Stationery Office, London.

Nazarko, L. (1998) Improving discharge: the role of the discharge co-ordinator. *Nurs Stand*, **12**(49), 35–7.

NHSE (2001) *Your Guide to the National Health Service*. HMSO, London.

Nixon, A., Whitter, M. & Stitt, P. (1998) Audit in practice: planning for discharge from hospital. *Nurs Stand*, **12**(26), 35–8.

Royal Marsden Hospital Discharge Policy and Procedure (2003) (unpublished).

Salter, M. (1996) Nursing the patient in the community. In: *Nursing the Patient with Cancer* (ed. V. Tschudin). Prentice Hall, Hemel Hempstead.

Salter, M. (1998) Future planning of care. In: *Neuro Oncology for Nurses* (ed. D. Guerrero). Whurr, London.

Salter, M. (2001) Planning for a smooth discharge. *Nurs Times*, **97**(34), 32–4.

Shamash, J. (2002) What are strategic health authorities? *Nurs Times*, **98**(27), 10–11.

Smith, S. (1996) Discharge planning: the need for effective communication. *Nurs Stand*, **10**(38), 39–41.

Social Services Inspectorate (1998) *A Matter of Chance for Carers?* Stationery Office, London.

Stewart, W. (2000) Development of discharge skills: a project report. *Nurs Times*, **96**(41), 37.

UKCC (1995) *Annexe One to Registrar's Letter (18/1995). Discharge of Patients from Hospital*. UKCC, London.

Young, L. (1998) Understanding primary care groups. *Prim Health Care*, **8**(3).

9

Drug administration: general principles

Chapter contents

Definition

Drug administration can be defined as the way medicines are selected, procured, delivered, prescribed, administered and reviewed to optimize the contributions that medicines make to producing informed and desired outcomes of patient care (Audit Commission 2001). The professional role of the nurse in medicines management is the safe handling and administration of medicines, including a responsibility for making sure that patients understand what medicines they are taking and why, including the likely side-effects (Luker & Wolfson 1999). Medicinal products are defined as 'substances sold or supplied for administration to humans (or animals) for medicinal purposes' (Medicines Act 1968).

Indications

Drugs can be administered for the following purposes.

- Diagnostic purposes, e.g. assessment of liver function or diagnosis of myasthenia gravis.
- Prophylaxis, e.g. heparin to prevent thrombosis or antibiotics to prevent infection.
- Therapeutic purposes, e.g. replacement of fluids or vitamins, supportive purposes (to enable other treatments, such as anaesthesia), palliation of pain and cure (as in the case of antibiotics).

Reference material

Drug administration has been one of the most common clinical procedures a nurse has undertaken for at least the past 50 years (Shepherd 2002a). With changes in legal, professional and cultural boundaries in health care, the role of the nurse has broadened to one of medicines management.

The legal and professional context

Medicines management and specifically drug administration require thought and professional judgement (Luker & Wolfson 1999); it is not a 'mechanistic task to be performed in strict compliance with the written prescription of a medical practitioner'(NMC 2002a). All aspects of a medicine's use must be managed with a multidisciplinary approach to ensure it is supported by a strong evidence base and the safety and well-being of the patient remain paramount (NMC 2002a; Shepherd 2002a).

Legislation

Legislative frameworks, government guidelines and professional regulations govern medicines management in the United Kingdom. The two pieces of primary legislation of importance are the Medicines Act 1968 and the Misuse of Drugs Act 1971.

The Medicines Act 1968

The Medicines Act 1968 establishes a licensing system for medicines for human use, controlling the manufacture and distribution, regulating who can lawfully supply and be in possession of medicines and how they should be packaged and labelled. The Medicines and Health Care Products Regulatory Agency (MHRA) in the UK and the European Medicines Evaluation Agency (EMEA) are responsible for issuing the product licences. The availability of products is restricted by defining which of the following legal categories they are in:

- Prescription-only medicines (POM)
- Pharmacy medicines (P)
- General sales list (GSL) medicines.

Different requirements apply to the sale, supply and labelling of medicines in each category. In NHS hospitals, adherence to the Act means that a pharmacist supervises the purchasing and supply of medicines, and that supply or administration to a patient is only on a doctor's prescription. Sections 9, 10 and 11 of the Act exempt doctors, dentists, pharmacists and nurses, respectively, from many restrictions otherwise imposed by the Act on the general public, and thus allow them to supply and use drugs in the practice of their respective professions.

The Misuse of Drugs Act 1971

For reasons of public safety the Misuse of Drugs Act (1971) controls the import, export, production, supply, possession and manufacture of controlled drugs to prevent abuse as most are potentially addictive or habit forming. Other regulations of the Act govern safe storage, destruction and supply to known addicts.

The level of control to be exercised is related to the potential for abuse or misuse of the substances concerned. Under the current (1985) regulations, controlled drugs are classified into five schedules, each representing a different level of control. The requirements of the Act as they apply to nurses working in a hospital with a pharmacy department are described in Table 9.1.

Implications of the Act for nursing practice

Hospital wards and departments are authorized to hold a stock of controlled drugs. These should be stored in a suitably secure cupboard which is kept locked and to which access is restricted to registered nurses and pharmacy staff. Controlled drugs are obtained by the use of a special duplicate order form signed by the nurse in charge who is then responsible for them.

They may be administered only to a patient in that ward or department when prescribed by a doctor. A prescription must be written in the doctor's handwriting. To write a prescription for a controlled drug a doctor must be resident in the UK and the pharmacist must know their signature. In the hospital setting this excludes locum doctors from writing prescriptions for controlled drugs. The Aitken Report (1958) recommends that two nurses check all controlled drug entries. Appropriate records of their use must be maintained. There is no legal requirement for the nurse in charge or acting in charge of a ward or department to keep a record of Schedule 1 or 2 controlled drugs obtained or supplied. However, the Aitken Report (1958) recommended that this should be done and in practice a controlled drug register is usually kept according to the following guidelines.

- Each page should be clearly headed to indicate the drug and preparation to which it refers.
- Entries should be made as soon as possible after the relevant transaction has occurred and always within 24 hours.
- No cancellations or obliteration of an entry should be made. Corrections should be made by means of a note in the margin or at the foot of the page and this should be signed, dated and cross-referenced to the relevant entry.
- All entries should be indelible.
- The register should be used for controlled drugs only and for no other purposes.
- Completed registers and copies of orders should be kept for 2 years.

Unwanted drugs should normally be destroyed in the pharmacy but may, under some circumstances, be disposed of on the ward under the supervision of a

Table 9.1 Summary of legal requirements for handling of controlled drugs (CDs) as they apply to nurses in hospitals with a pharmacy

	Schedule 1: CDs Home Office Licence	Schedule 2: CDs subject to full controls	Schedule 3: CDs with no register entry	Schedule 4: CDs anabolic steroids/benzodiazepines	Schedule 5: CDs needing invoice retention
Drugs in the schedule	Cannabis + derivatives but excluding nabilone, LSD (lysergic acid diethylamide)	Most opioids in common use including: alfentanil; amphetamines; cocaine; diamorphine; methadone; morphine papaveretum; fentanyl; phenoperidine. Pethidine; codeine; Dihydrocodeine } Injections Pentazocine	Minor stimulants Barbiturates (but excluding hexobarbitone, thiopentone) Diethylpropion Buprenorphine Temazepam†	Part 1: anabolic steroids Part 2: benzodiazepines	Some preparations containing very low strengths of: cocaine; codeine; morphine; pholcodine; and some other opioids
Ordering	Possession and supply permitted only by special licence from the Secretary of State issued (to a doctor only) for scientific or research purposes	A requisition must be signed in duplicate by the nurse in charge. The requisition must be endorsed to indicate that the drugs have been supplied. Copies should be kept for 2 years	As Schedule 2	No requirement*	No requirement*
Storage	Must be kept in a suitable locked cupboard to which access is restricted	As Schedule 1	Buprenorphine and diethylpropion: as Schedule 1 drugs All other drugs no requirement	No requirement*	No requirement*
Record keeping	Controlled drug register must be used	As Schedule 1	No requirement	No requirement*	No requirement*
Prescription	Prescription must include: • the name and address of patient • the drug, the dose, the form of preparation • the total quantity of drug or the total number of dosage units to be supplied. This quantity must be stated in words and figures The prescription must be written indelibly in the prescriber's own handwriting	As Schedule 1	As Schedule 1 Except for phenobarbitone (this includes all preparations of phenobarbitone and phenobarbitone sodium). Because of its use as an antiepileptic, it does not need to be written in the prescriber's own handwriting	No requirement*	
Administration to patients	Under special licence only A doctor or dentist or anyone acting on their instructions may administer these drugs to anyone for whom they have been prescribed	A doctor or dentist or anyone acting on their instructions may administer these drugs to anyone for whom they have been prescribed	A doctor or dentist or anyone acting on their instructions may administer these drugs to anyone for whom they have been prescribed	No requirement*	No requirement*

*'No requirement' indicates that the Misuse of Drugs Act 1971 imposes no legal requirements additional to those imposed by the Medicines Act 1968.
†Temazepam preparations are exempt from record keeping and prescription requirements, but are subject to storage requirements.

pharmacist. An appropriate entry should then be made in the ward register.

Regulations and directives from the European Union

In January 1999 EU Directive 92/27/EEC was published. This creates a responsibility to provide patients with printed information leaflets with all dispensed medicines.

Storage of medicines

The Duthie Report (DoH 1988) requires NHS trusts to establish, document and maintain procedures to ensure and demonstrate that medicines are stored and handled in a safe and secure manner. Under the Duthie Report the nurse in charge of a ward or clinical area is responsible for the safe storage of all medicines. Some of these duties may be delegated, such as the ordering of additional medicines, but the responsibility remains with the nurse in charge.

The storage of medicines is governed by the following principles.

Security

All drugs should be stored in locked cupboards with separate storage for internal medicines, external medicines, controlled drugs and medicines needing refrigeration or storage in a freezer.

Diagnostic reagents, intravenous and topical agents should also be kept separately.

Stability

No medicinal preparation should be stored where it may be subject to substantial variations in temperature, e.g. not in direct sunlight. The normal temperature ranges for storage are 'a cool place', normally interpreted as meaning between 1° and 15°C; 'refrigerated' at a temperature between 2° and 8°C; 'room temperature' between 15° and 25°C.

Labelling

The wording of labels is chosen carefully to convey clearly all essential information. Printed labels should always be used.

Containers

The type of container used may have been chosen for specific reasons. Medicinal preparations should never be transferred (in bulk) from one container to another except in the pharmacy.

Stock control

A system of stock rotation must be operated (e.g. first in, first out) to ensure that there is no accumulation of old stocks.

Storage requirements of specific preparations

- *Aerosol containers* should not be stored in direct sunlight or over radiators – there is a risk of explosion if they are heated.
- *Creams* may deteriorate rapidly if subjected to extremes of temperature.
- *Eye drops and ointments* may become contaminated with micro-organisms during use and thus pose a danger to the recipient. Therefore in hospitals, eye preparations should be discarded 7 days after they are first opened. For use at home this limit is extended to 28 days.
- *Mixtures* may have a relatively short shelf-life. Most antibiotic mixtures require refrigerated storage and even then have a shelf-life of only 7–14 days. Always check the label for details.
- *Tablets and capsules* are relatively stable but are susceptible to moisture unless correctly packed. They should be stored only in the containers in which they were supplied by the pharmacy.
- *Vaccines* and similar preparations usually require refrigerated storage and may deteriorate rapidly if exposed to heat.

Patient's own drugs

If a patient brings medications into hospital they should neither be disposed of without the patient's consent nor used for other patients. They should be stored according to local policy.

Types of medicinal preparations of drugs

Preparations for oral administration

Tablets

These come in a great variety of shapes, sizes, colours and types. The formulation may be very simple and result for instance in a plain, white, uncoated tablet, or complex and designed with specific therapeutic aims. Sugar coatings are used to improve appearances and palatability. In cases where the drug is a gastric irritant or is broken down by gastric acid, an enteric coating may be used. This is designed to allow the tablet to remain intact in the stomach and to pass unchanged into the small bowel where the coating dissolves and hence the drug is released and absorbed. Tablets may be formulated specifically to achieve control of the rate of release of drug from the tablet as it passes through the alimentary tract. Terms such as 'sustained-release', 'controlled-release' and 'modified-release' are used by manufacturers to describe these preparations. Tablets may also be formulated specifically to dissolve readily ('soluble' or 'effervescent'), to be chewed or to be held under the tongue ('sublingual') or placed between the gum and inside of the mouth ('buccal'). Unscored or coated tablets should not be crushed or broken, nor should most 'slow-release' or 'sustained action' tablets, since this can alter the rate of release of drug from the tablet.

Capsules

These offer a useful method of formulating drugs which are difficult to make into a tablet or are particularly unpalatable.

The capsule shells are usually made of gelatin and the contents of the capsules may be solid, liquid or of a paste-like consistency. The contents do not cause deterioration of the shell. The shell, however, is attacked by the digestive fluids and the contents are then released. Delayed-release capsule formulations also exist. Gastro-resistant capsules are delayed-release capsules that are intended to resist the gastric fluid and to release their active substance or substances in the intestinal fluid (British Pharmacopoeia 2002). If for any reason the capsule is unsuitable, the contents should not routinely be removed from the shell without first seeking advice from a pharmacist. Removing contents from the capsule could destroy their properties and cause gastric irritation or premature release of the drug into an incompatible pH (Downie *et al.* 2000).

Lozenges and pastilles

Lozenges and pastilles are solid, single-dose preparations intended to be sucked to obtain a local or systemic effect to the mouth and/or throat (British Pharmacopoeia 2002).

Elixirs, linctuses and syrups
Elixirs

These are clear, flavoured oral liquids containing one or more active ingredients dissolved in a vehicle that usually contains a high proportion of sucrose.

Linctuses

These are viscous oral liquids that may contain one or more active ingredients; the solution usually contains a high proportion of sucrose. Linctuses are intended for use in the treatment or relief of cough (British Pharmacopoeia 2002).

Syrups

These do not contain active ingredients and many are used as vehicle ingredients for their flavouring and sweetening.

Mixtures

These are flavoured solutions or suspensions of drugs used mainly when patients cannot swallow a tablet or the drug is not available as a tablet. It is particularly important that suspensions are thoroughly mixed by shaking before each dose is measured. This ensures that the measured volume always contains the correct amount of drug.

Rectal and vaginal preparations
Enemas

These are solutions which are instilled into the rectum as laxatives or to obtain other localized therapeutic effects, or for diagnostic purposes.

Suppositories

These are solid wax pellets for rectal administration. They may either melt at body temperature or dissolve or disperse in the mucous secretions of the rectum. They may be used to obtain local effect (e.g. as laxatives) or for systemic therapy. Many drugs, such as the opioids, are well absorbed when administered this way. Suppositories sometimes offer a useful alternative to injections for very sick patients unable to take drugs orally.

Pessaries

These are solid pellets for vaginal administration and are usually designed to have a local therapeutic action.

Topical preparations
Creams

Creams are emulsions of oil and water and are generally well absorbed into the skin. They are usually more cosmetically acceptable than ointments because they are less greasy and easy to apply (BMA & RPS 2003). They may be used as a 'base' in which a variety of drugs may be applied for local therapy (BMA & RPS 2003).

Ointments

Ointments are greasy preparations, which are normally anhydrous and insoluble in water, and are more occlusive than creams (BMA & RPS 2003). They are absorbed more slowly into the skin and leave a greasy residue. They have similar uses to creams, and are particularly suitable for dry, scaly lesions (BMA & RPS 2003).

Transdermal patches

A number of drugs such as hyoscine to prevent motion sickness, oestrogens for hormone replacement therapy and fentanyl for pain control are now available in 'transdermal patches'. A very small volume of drug solution is contained in a reservoir which is stuck on the skin. Drug molecules diffuse at a constant rate through a semipermeable membrane which is in direct contact with the skin when the patch is applied. The drug is absorbed through the skin and into the capillary blood supply from where it enters the systemic circulation. Advantages include a constant rate of drug administration over several days which may reduce the incidence of side-effects and improve patient compliance.

Wound products
See Ch. 47, Wound management.

Injections

Injections are sterile solutions, emulsions or suspensions. They are prepared by dissolving, emulsifying or suspending the active ingredient and any added substances in water for injections, in a suitable non-aqueous liquid or in a mixture of these vehicles (British Pharmacopoeia 2002).

Single-dose preparations
The volume of the injection in a single-dose container is sufficient to permit the withdrawal and administration of the nominal dose using a normal technique.

Multidose preparations
Multidose aqueous injections contain a suitable antimicrobial preservative at an appropriate concentration except when the preparation itself has adequate antimicrobial properties. When it is necessary to present a preparation for parenteral use in a multidose container, the precautions to be taken for its administration and more particularly for its storage between successive withdrawals are given.

Parenteral infusions

Parenteral infusions are sterile, aqueous solutions or emulsions with water; they are free from pyrogens and are usually made isotonic with blood. They are principally intended for administration in large volume. Parenteral infusions do not contain any added antimicrobial preservative (British Pharmacopoeia 2002).

Inhalations

Two techniques – nebulization and aerosolization – permit the inhalation of a range of drugs with the aim of a localized therapeutic effect.

Nebulization involves the passage of air or oxygen driven through a solution of a drug. The resulting fine mist is then inhaled via a face mask (Trounce & Gould 2000). Some antibiotics and bronchodilators may be given in this way.

Aerosolization involves the use of a solution of drug in an inert diluent. Passing a metred volume of this solution through a valve under pressure allows the delivery to the patient of a measured dose of drug in a very fine spray of controlled particle size. Bronchodilators and steroids are administered commonly in this way. Although a very small total dose of drug is administered, the concentration achieved at the site of action is high.

Rapid and effective control of symptoms is achieved but without the side-effects commonly associated with an equivalent systemic (oral or parenteral) dose of the drug(s).

Many patients can be taught to use aerosol inhalers effectively but some patients, particularly the elderly and small children, may find it difficult to use them. Spacer devices can help such patients because they remove the need to co-ordinate actuation with inhalation (BMA & RPS 2003). For those who cannot co-ordinate aerosol inhalation, alternative methods of administration include breath-actuated inhalers or dry powder inhalers which merely require the patient to breathe in. No co-ordination of hand movement and breathing is required. Some dry powder inhalers occasionally cause coughing due to irritation of the throat and trachea by the dry powder (Downie *et al.* 2000).

Administration

The effective and safe administration of drugs to patients demands a partnership between the various health professionals concerned, i.e. doctors, pharmacists and nurses. A medicine is an active chemical or biological substance with diagnostic, curative or preventive purposes. The manner in which it is administered determines the extent to which a patient gains any clinical benefit and whether any adverse effect is experienced. One of the main factors that determines whether or not a medicine will reach its intended site of action in the body is how it is given (Shepherd 2002a). Nurses are responsible for the correct administration of prescribed drugs to patients in their care at all times, being guided by the Nursing and Midwifery Council *Guidelines for the Administration of Medicines* (NMC 2002a).

Medicine administration should ensure that the correct patient receives:

- The appropriate medicine
- In the appropriate formulation
- By the appropriate route
- At the appropriate dose
- At the appropriate time
- At the appropriate rate
- For the appropriate duration of therapy
- With the appropriate monitoring to ensure safety and efficacy of therapy
- With the appropriate reporting of adverse drug reactions (Sexton 1999, p. 240).

To achieve this the nurse must have a sound knowledge of the use, action, usual dose and side-effects of the drugs being administered. Institutional policies and procedures also assist the nurse to administer drugs safely and a sound knowledge of local procedures is essential. The importance of reporting errors to the appropriate authority should never be underestimated as research suggests that many undeclared medication errors are made by nurses. The immediate and honest disclosure that an error has occurred results in the patient receiving the required emergency treatment. Organizational policies therefore need to reflect a culture that encourages disclosure and in which the management of medication errors is viewed as a learning process as opposed to a punitive act (Martin 1994; Gladstone 1995).

It must be recognized, however, that errors in drug administration can have traumatic consequences for the individual nurse involved and that disciplinary procedures invoke fear in most nurses (Arndt 1994). The NMC, when giving guidance to managers dealing with medication errors, states that there should be a distinction made between errors which result from a serious pressure of work and those which are a result of reckless practice (NMC 2002b).

Administration in hospital

All medicines administered in hospital must be considered prescription only. This is because in the hospital setting administration, whether by a nurse or by a patient to themselves, may only take place where:

- An instruction is recorded in writing by a doctor on an official prescription chart or
- There is a Patient Group Direction (PGD).

Single nurse administration of medicines

In the majority of hospitals it is policy that medicines administration is carried out by a single qualified nurse. It is thought that single nurse administration of medicines will result in greater care being given since the nurse will be aware that she or he is solely responsible and accountable.

Those nurses who wish or need to have their administration supervised will retain the right to do so until such time as all parties agree that the requested level of proficiency has been achieved. This is in keeping with the principles of the *Code of Professional Conduct* (NMC 2002b).

Self-administration of medicines

With evidence that between 30% and 70% of patients are non-compliant with taking prescribed medication (Royal Pharmaceutical Society 1997), the self-administration of medicines in hospitals is encouraged. Non-adherence to medication regimens is a significant problem in older patients (McGraw & Drennan 2001). Self-administration of medicines is recommended by the National Service Framework for Older People (DoH

2001) as a strategy to address this major issue. All patients benefit significantly from the opportunity to adjust to the responsibility of self-administration while still having access to professional support (NMC 2002b). It has also been found that patients who had administered their own medications in hospital were more like to report that their overall care was excellent and that they were satisfied with the discharge process than patients who had not (Deeks & Byatt 2000). Bird (1990) suggests that for the majority of hospital patients, self-administration of drugs would appear to be a more appropriate method than the conventional system. Self-administration is not merely the process of patients taking their own drugs; it can also help clients retain or regain control over their health.

The safety and success of a self-administration system in hospital are based upon the nursing assessment of the patient and the subsequent teaching (Shepherd 2002b). The nursing assessment should include a measure of the patient's ability to interpret and participate in the prescribed treatment regimen and seek to determine whether the patient already takes prescribed treatment at home and how they manage that and whether they can understand the medicine labels and the dosage instructions (Shepherd 2002b). Teaching patients to take their own medication correctly forms part of their programme of rehabilitation, which should begin with the first multidisciplinary assessment on their arrival in hospital. Patients taught to self-administer their drugs in hospital are encouraged to regain independence and to participate in their own care. Self-administration also provides an opportunity to identify additional education needs and improve compliance. Importantly, it also raises awareness of those patients who are unable to self-administer and will need additional support on discharge (Shepherd 2002b).

Although, by definition, self-administration of medicines shifts the balance of responsibility for this part of care towards the patient, it in no way diminishes the fundamental professional duty of care. It is therefore essential that local policies, procedures and records are adequate to ensure that this duty is, and can be shown to be, discharged.

Even if a patient is self-administering their medication, continual assessment of this aspect of their care while they are in hospital is important. The nurse must continually be aware of the patient's capability to self-administer and the action of the drugs the patient is taking No drug produces a single effect. The combined effect of two or more drugs taken together may be different from the effects when taken separately. The effectiveness of any drug should be noted and any signs of resistance or dependence reported.

Covert drug administration

Some vulnerable groups of patients, for example those who are confused, may refuse to take medication. Traditionally in some places, medication has therefore been hidden or disguised in food. The NMC (2001a,b) offered the following position statement.

> 'As a general principle, by disguising medication in food or drink, the patient or client is being led to believe that they are not receiving medication when in fact they are. The registered nurse, midwife or health visitor will need to be sure that what they are doing is in the best interests of the patient or client and be accountable for this decision.'
>
> (NMC 2001a, p.1)

Disguising medication in food and drink is acceptable under exceptional circumstances in which covert administration may be considered to prevent a patient, who is incapable of informed consent, from missing out on essential treatment (NMC 2001b). The following principles should be followed when making such a decision.

- The medication must be considered essential for the patient's health and well-being.
- The decision to administer medication covertly should be considered only as a contingency in an emergency, not as regular practice.
- The registered practitioner must make the decision only after discussion and with the support of the multiprofessional team and, if appropriate, the patient's relatives, carers or advocates.
- The pharmacist must be involved in these decisions as adding medication to food or drink can alter its pharmacological properties and thereby affect its performance.
- The decision and action taken must be fully documented in the patient's care plan and regularly reviewed.
- Regular attempts should continue to be made to encourage the patient to take the medication voluntarily (Treloar *et al.* 2000; NMC 2001b).

Nurse prescribing and Patient Group Directions

As nurses have undertaken increasingly specialized roles the need for them to have powers to prescribe has become more apparent. *The Report of the Advisory Committee on Nurse Prescribing* (DoH 1989) initially recommended a limited nurses' formulary for district nurses and health visitors. The *Nurse Prescribing Act* (1992) granted the statutory authority for this to occur. The Crown Report (DoH 1989) also recommended that doctors and nurses collaborate in drawing up local protocols for the administration of medicines in situations that would benefit specific groups of patients, for example those requiring vaccinations.

The practice of prescribing under group protocols became widespread across the NHS. At the Royal Marsden Hospital they were used to support initiatives such as nurse-led clinics (Mallett *et al.* 1997; Laverty *et al.* 1997). The legality of this practice was questioned. Section 58 of the *Medicines Act* stipulates that 'no person shall administer (other than to himself) any such medicinal products unless he is an appropriate practitioner or a person acting in accordance with the directions of an appropriate practitioner'. The terms *direction* and *administration* were open to interpretation and how they were used varied across the country (McHale 2002).

Nurse prescribing was therefore reviewed and two further reports were published:

- *Review of Prescribing, Supply and Administration of Medicines. A Report on the Supply and Administration of Medicines under Group Protocols* (DoH 1998)
- *Review of Prescribing, Supply and Administration of Medicines. Final Report* (DoH 1999).

The first specifically offered guidance about group protocols, including changing the name to Patient Group Directions (PGDs). The subsequent publication of HSC 2000/26 (NHSE 2000) clarifies the legal definition: 'written instructions for the supply or administration of medicines to groups of patients who may not be individually identified before presentation for treatment' (SI 2000 No. 1919). The HSC advises that the majority of medication 'should be prescribed and administered on an individual patient specific basis' but that it is appropriate to use PGDs for the supply and administration of medicines in situations where this offers an advantage for patient care. Shepherd (2002b) suggests that this means, 'where medical staff are either inaccessible or unavailable'. The coincidental introduction of nurse prescribing has led to confusion and the potential, nationally, for inconsistencies; the flowchart in Figure 9.1 aims to assist practitioners in deciding the appropriate system for the prescription, supply or administration of medicines.

The second report looked at the existing arrangements for prescribing, supply and administration of medicines and suggested the introduction of a new form of prescribing to be undertaken by non-medical health professionals (DoH 2003a). Following the successful piloting of prescribing by district nurses and health visitors, the report proposed:

- The introduction of a new framework of prescribing, supply and administration of medicines whereby the

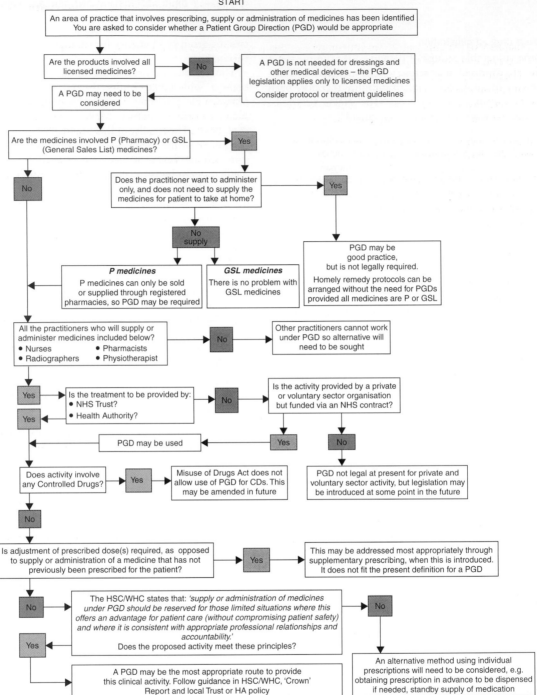

Figure 9.1 Patient Group Directions (PGDs) flowchart. This guide has been prepared in response to the many queries that are now being raised both locally and nationally about the implementation of HSC 2000/026 (in England) (WHC (2000) 116 in Wales), on Patient Group Directions. The coincidental introduction of nurse prescribing (and its likely extension to new groups of nurses) has confused many practitioners, and there is a danger that inconsistencies may develop as the implementation of both initiatives continues. Practitioners and their managers who wish to formalize or set up new systems for prescribing by nurses, or alternatively the supply or administration of medicines, are faced with a range of different methods and need to select the most appropriate route in each case. The diagram above takes the practitioner through a logical process that aims to assist decision making. **The majority of clinical care should still be provided on an individual, patient-specific basis.**

majority of patients would continue to receive medicines on an individual patient-specific basis.

- The prescribing authority of doctors, dentists, district nurses and health visitors would continue.
- Prescribing authority would be extended to include new groups of health care professionals (NPC 2003a).

As prescribing has been extended, two new categories of prescriber have been introduced.

- *Independent nurse prescribers* who are responsible for the initial assessment of the patient and drawing up the treatment plan. Independent prescribers also have authority to prescribe all medications that are on the general sales list and pharmacy items prescribable by doctors as well as a list of prescription-only medicines. This is continually being reviewed to ensure patients get quicker access to medicines.
- *Supplementary prescribers* who are authorized to prescribe for patients whose condition has been diagnosed or assessed by an independent prescriber within an agreed treatment plan. Supplementary prescribing has been defined as:

'A voluntary prescribing partnership between an independent prescriber and a supplementary prescriber to implement an agreed patient specific clinical management plan with the patient's agreement' (DoH 2003a).

The key principles that underpin supplementary prescribing are:

- The importance of communication between prescribing partners
- The need for access to shared patient records
- The patient is treated as a partner in their care and is involved at all stages in decision making, including whether part of their care is delivered via supplementary prescribing (NPC 2003a).

Preparation for both extended nurse prescribing and supplementary prescribing is at least 26 days in length and must follow the standards set out in NMC Circular 25/2002 (NMC 2001c). Any preparation must enable nurse prescribers and supplementary prescribers to reach the competencies outlined in *Maintaining Competency in Prescribing: An Outline Framework to Help Nurse Prescribers* (NPC 2001) and the additional guidance in *Maintaining Competency in Prescribing: An Outline Framework to Help Nurse Supplementary Prescribers* (NPC 2003b).

Amendments to the Prescription Only Medicines Order and changes to NHS regulations to allow the introduction of supplementary prescribing came into force on 4 April 2003. It is the responsibility of primary care trusts, NHS trusts and workforce development confederations to take steps to implement them (DoH 2003b).

Intravenous administration

Intravenous therapy is now an integral part of the majority of nurses' professional practice (RCN 2003). The nurse's role has progressed considerably since being able to add drugs to infusion bags (DHSS 1976) to now assessing patients and inserting the appropriate vascular access devices prior to drug administration (Hamilton & Fermo 1998).

Any nurse administering intravenous drugs must be competent in all clinical aspects of intravenous therapy and have validated competency in clinical judgement and practice in accordance with the NMC *Code of Conduct* (2002b), i.e. to maintain knowledge and skills (Scales 1996; Hyde 2002; RCN 2003). Training and assessment should comprise both a theoretical component and practical procedures and include legal and professional issues, fluid balance, pharmacology, drug administration, local and systemic complications, infection control issues, use of equipment and risk management (Cole 1999; Lonsway 2001; Hyde 2002; RCN 2003; Taxis & Barber 2003).

The nurse's responsibilities in relation to intravenous drug administration include:

1 Knowing the therapeutic use of the drug or solution to be administered, its normal dosage, side-effects, precautions and contraindications
2 Preparing the drug aseptically and safely, checking the container and drug for faults, using the correct diluent and only preparing immediately prior to administration
3 Being able to identify the patient and checking allergy status
4 Checking the prescription chart
5 Checking and maintaining patency of the vascular access device
6 Inspecting the site of the vascular access device and managing/reporting complications where appropriate
7 Controlling the flow rate of infusion and/or speed of injection
8 Monitoring the condition of the patient and reporting changes
9 Make clear and immediate records of all drugs administered (NMC 2002a; RCN 2003).

Injections and infusions

Injections can be described as the act of giving medication by use of a syringe and needle, and an infusion is defined as an amount of fluid in excess of 100 ml designated for parenteral infusion because the volume must be administered over a long period of time. However, medications may be given in small volumes (50–100 ml) or over a shorter period (30–60 minutes) (Weinstein 2000).

There are a number of routes for injection or infusion. The selection may be predetermined as in intra-arterial, intra-articular, intracardiac, intralesional and intrathecal injections. The choice of the remaining routes will normally depend on the desired therapeutic effect and the patient's safety and comfort.

Intra-arterial

This special technique allows the delivery of a high concentration of drug to the tissues supplied by a particular artery. This route can be used for the administration of chemotherapy and vasodilators and for diagnostic purposes. Injection of drugs into an artery is a rare and hazardous procedure. The introduction of the cannula or catheter must be performed with care as the vessel may go into spasm, causing pain and occlusion. This could result in necrosis of an organ or part of a limb. Injection of irritant chemicals increases the risk of spasm and its sequelae (see Ch. 44, Vascular access devices: insertion and management). In patients with some forms of cancer, however, arterial catheterization is occasionally performed when it is desirable to deliver a high concentration of a drug to a tumour mass (see Ch. 10, Drug administration: cytotoxic drugs). The most common procedures are catheterization of the hepatic artery and isolated limb perfusion.

Intra-articular

In inflammatory conditions of the joints, corticosteroids are given by intra-articular injection to relieve inflammation and increase joint mobility (Downie *et al.* 2000).

Intrathecal

It may be necessary to administer some drugs intrathecally if they have poor lipid solubility and, as a result, do not pass the blood–brain barrier (Downie *et al.* 2000). A drug specially prepared for the intrathecal route should be used; doses should be carefully calculated and are usually much smaller than would be given by intramuscular or intravenous injection. In the treatment of meningitis, water-soluble antibiotics are administered by the intrathecal route to achieve adequate concentrations in the cerebrospinal fluid (CSF). In addition, antifungal agents, opioids, cytotoxic therapy and radio-opaque substances (used in the diagnosis of spinal lesions) are sometimes administered by this route (Downie *et al.* 2000).

Intradermal

The intradermal route provides a local, rather than systemic effect, and is used primarily for diagnostic purposes such as allergy or tuberculin testing. It can also be used for the administration of local anaesthetics (Workman 1999). Observation of an inflammatory reaction is a priority, so the best sites are those that are highly pigmented, thinly keratinized and hairless. Chosen sites are the inner forearms and the scapulae. The injection site most commonly used is the medial forearm area. The injections are best performed using a 25 G needle inserted at a 10–15° angle, bevel up, just under the epidermis. Volumes of 0.5 ml or less should be used (Workman 1999).

Subcutaneous

Subcutaneous injections

These are given beneath the epidermis into the fat and connective tissue underlying the dermis. Injections are usually given using a 25 G needle, at a 45° angle. However, following the introduction of shorter needles the recommendation for insulin injections is at an angle of 90° (Burden 1994). Infusions require the insertion of a 25 G winged infusion set or a 24 G cannula. These may be inserted at an angle of 45° and secured with a transparent dressing (Springhouse Corporation 1999). The skin should be gently pinched into a fold to elevate the subcutaneous tissue which lifts the adipose tissue away from the underlying muscle (Workman 1999). It is no longer necessary to aspirate after the needle has been inserted, as it has been shown that piercing a blood vessel during a subcutaneous injection is rare (Peragallo-Dittko 1997; Workman 1999). It has also been noted that aspiration of heparin increases the risk of haematoma formation (Springhouse Corporation 1993). The maximum volume tolerable using this route for injection is 2 ml and drugs should be highly soluble to prevent irritation (Workman 1999).

Injection sites
Chosen sites are the lateral aspects of the upper arms and thighs, the abdomen in the umbilical region, the back and lower loins. Absorption from these sites through the capillary network is slower than that of the intramuscular route. Rotation of these sites decreases the likelihood of irritation and ensures improved absorption. Subcutaneous injections given in the upper arm are thought to be less painful since there are fewer large blood vessels and less painful sensations in those areas.

Subcutaneous infusions of fluids (hypodermoclysis)
The administration of fluids by the subcutaneous route is a safe, reliable and minimally invasive method of

assisting the control of delirium, nausea and thirst in end-stage chronic disease and the elderly (Constans *et al.* 1991; Donnelly 1999; Cerchietti *et al.* 2000). It is not recommended for emergency rehydration but it may have a limited benefit in dying patients who are distressed by lack of fluid (Donnelly 1999). It may also be useful in patients who have difficulty in taking fluids orally, such as those who have dysphagia which results in decreased oral intake and symptom distress (Fainsinger *et al.* 1994; Ellershaw *et al.* 1995; Fainsinger & Bruera 1997).

Cerchietti *et al.* (2000) evaluated the use of fluids administered subcutaneously over a 48-hour period in patients with end-stage cancer. They concluded that this method does not control symptoms when used in addition to pharmacological treatments but it can have a benefit in improving chronic nausea.

Owing to the relative ease in setting up and administering subcutaneous fluids, the procedure can be carried out in the home setting by district nurses, relatives or carers. There is a reduction in the risk of infection when compared with intravenous fluids and it has very few side-effects. However, one study did indicate that prolonged use with large volumes of fluid in a 24-hour period can lead to localized pain and oedema (Lipschitz *et al.* 1991). Caution is required in patients who have preexisting oedema (as swelling at the site would not be easily observed) and any clotting disorders (which may predispose the patients to bleeding at cannula sites).

Research has demonstrated that there is less phlebitis associated with the use of peripheral cannulae when compared with steel winged infusion devices (Dawkins *et al.* 2000; Ross *et al.* 2002). Therefore the administration of subcutaneous infusions is recommended via a plastic cannula (e.g. Insyte 24 G; 0.7 × 19 mm).

The volume of fluid administered subcutaneously in a 24-hour period ranges from 1000 to 2000 ml with a limit of up to 500 ml in an hour (Fainsinger & Bruera 1997). It may be given as a:

- 24-hour infusion
- 12-hour infusion
- Bolus.

Noble-Adams (1995) recommends the use of electrolyte replacement fluids (sodium chloride 0.9% and dextrose saline) for subcutaneous infusion.

It is possible and advisable to use more than one infusion site if the patient requires more than one litre to be infused (Bruera *et al.* 1990; Ferrand & Campbell 1996). If medications are required it is advisable to administer them via a syringe driver which allows easier control of the rate of delivery.

Hyaluronidase is an enzyme which increases the rate of subcutaneous absorption of fluids. It is usually used if more than one litre is to be infused at one site (Noble-Adams 1995). It can cause discomfort and local irritation when used for prolonged periods of time (Ferrand & Campbell 1996; Hypodermoclysis Working Group 1998). A randomized double-blind study compared the absorption and side-effect profile of administering subcutaneous fluids with or without hyaluronidase. It found that there was no significant difference in the infusion rate of the fluids or the amount or degree of side-effects caused by its use. However, it did show that on measuring the limb around the site of the infusion, those with hyaluronidase in the fluid showed a decrease in limb size compared to those without hyaluronidase (Constans *et al.* 1991).

In the context of single drug infusions, instability is not a clinically significant problem. The drug simply has to be:

- Available in injectable form
- Suitable for subcutaneous administration
- Stable in solution for the duration of the infusion (usually 12–48 hours).

Problems of drug instability and incompatibility arise when higher drug concentrations and combinations of two or more drugs are used. There is a paucity of pharmaceutical data available regarding compatibility of combining drugs and most information remains anecdotal (David 1992) although there is a growing number of small studies (from clinical situations and the laboratory) that show drug compatibility data (Dickman *et al.* 2002). Where drug compatibility is doubtful or unknown, and more than two drugs are required for adequate control of symptoms, a second syringe driver may be a reasonable option. Exposure of drug solutions to direct light and increased storage temperatures (up to 32°C) also results in drug instability.

Where drug combinations (commonly an analgesic and an antiemetic) are used, further criteria must be met:

- The drugs must be compatible with each other.
- The diluents must be compatible with each other.
- Each drug must be compatible with the diluent(s) of the other drug(s) in the combination (Dickman *et al.* 2002) (see Ch. 11, Drug administration: delivery (infusion devices)).

Infusion sites

The best sites to use for continuous infusion of drugs or fluids are the lateral aspects of the upper arms and thighs, the abdomen, the anterior chest below the clavicle and, occasionally, the back (Mitten 2001). This is because these sites usually have adequate amounts of subcutaneous tissue and will not interfere with the patient's mobility. Areas that should not be used for cannula placement are:

- Lymphoedematous limbs: the rate of absorption from a skin site would be adversely affected. A cannula breaches skin integrity, thus increasing the risk of infection in a limb that is already susceptible.
- Sites over bony prominences: the amount of subcutaneous tissue will be diminished, impairing the rate of drug absorption.
- Previously irradiated skin area: radiotherapy can cause sclerosis of small blood vessels, thus reducing skin perfusion.
- Sites near a joint: excessive movement may cause cannula displacement and patient discomfort (Hirsch & Faull 2000).

Preparation of the skin
The infusion site should be renewed when there is evidence of inflammation (erythema) or poor absorption (a hard subcutaneous swelling). The time taken for this to occur can vary from hours to over 3 weeks, dependent on the patient and the drug(s) being infused. There would appear to be a relationship between the concentration of drug(s) being infused and the duration of a skin site (Twycross *et al.* 1998).

If skin sites break down rapidly, suggestions include:

- Further dilute the drug infused or change the diluent.
- Change the infusion device.
- Use a different site cleanser.
- Change the site dressing.
- Add 0.5 mg dexamethasone to the pump (this is currently being researched).

Intramuscular

Intramuscular injections should be given into the densest part of the muscle. The injectable volume will depend on the muscle bed. In children, injectable volumes should be halved because muscle mass is less (Workman 1999). Current research evidence suggests that there are five sites that can be utilized for the administration of intramuscular injections (Workman 1999; Rodger & King 2000). These sites (Fig. 9.2) are described below.

1 The mid-deltoid site (Fig. 9.2a). This site has the advantage of being easily accessible whether the patient is standing, sitting or lying down. Owing to the small area of this site, the number and volume of injections which can be given into it are limited. Drugs such as narcotics, sedatives and vaccines, which are usually small in volume, tend to be administered into the deltoid site (Workman 1999). Rodger & King (2000) state that the maximum volume that should be administered at this site is 1 ml.

2 The dorsogluteal site (Fig. 9.2b) is used for deep intramuscular and Z-track injections. The gluteus muscle has the lowest drug absorption rate. The muscle mass is also likely to have atrophied in elderly, non-ambulant and emaciated patients. This site carries with it the danger of the needle hitting the sciatic nerve and the superior gluteal arteries (Workman 1999). The Z-track method involves pulling the skin downwards or to one side of the injection site and inserting the needle at a right angle to the skin, which moves the cutaneous and subcutaneous tissues by approximately 1–2 cm (Workman 1999). The injection is given and the needle withdrawn, while releasing the retracted skin at the same time. This manoeuvre seals off the puncture tract. In adults up to 4 ml can be safely injected into this site (Rodger & King 2000).

3 The rectus femoris site (Fig. 9.2c) is used for antiemetics, narcotics, sedatives, injections in oil, deep intramuscular and Z-track injections. The rectus femoris is the anterior quadriceps muscle, which is rarely used by nurses, but is easily accessed for self-administration of injections or for infants (Workman 1999).

4 The vastus lateralis site (Fig. 9.2c) is used for deep intramuscular and Z-track injections. One of the advantages of the vastus lateralis site is its ease of access but more importantly, there are no major blood vessels or significant nerve structures associated with this site. Up to 5 ml can be safely injected (Rodger & King 2000).

5 The ventrogluteal site (Fig. 9.2d) is used for antibiotics, antiemetics, deep intramuscular and Z-track injections in oil, narcotics and sedatives. This is the site of choice for intramuscular injections (Rodger & King 2000). Up to 2.5 ml can be safely injected into the ventrogluteal site (Rodger & King 2000).

Skin preparation

There are many inconsistencies regarding skin cleaning prior to subcutaneous or intramuscular injections. Previous studies have suggested that cleaning with an alcohol swab is not always necessary, does not result in infections and may predispose the skin to hardening (Dann 1969; Koivistov & Felig 1978; Workman 1999).

Dann (1969), in a study over a period of 6 years involving more than 5000 injections, found no single case of local and/or systemic infection. Koivistov & Felig (1978) concluded that whilst skin preparations did reduce skin bacterial count, they are not necessary to prevent infections at the injection site. Some trusts

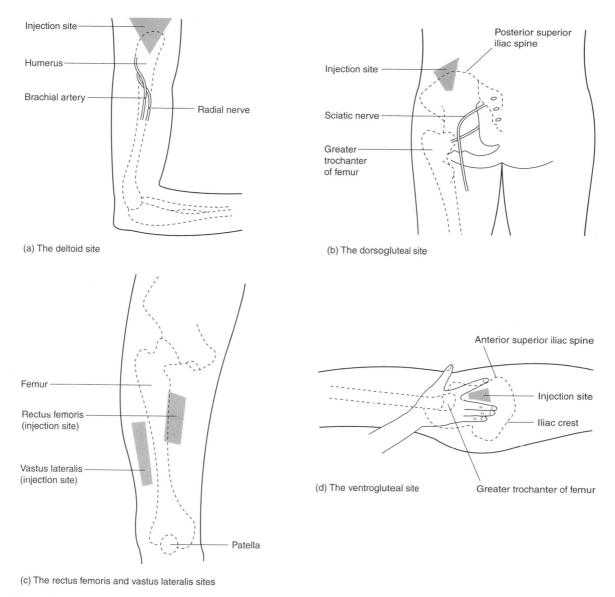

(a) The deltoid site

(b) The dorsogluteal site

(c) The rectus femoris and vastus lateralis sites

(d) The ventrogluteal site

Figure 9.2 Intramuscular injection sites. (Taken from Rodger & King 2000.)

accept that if the patient is physically clean and the nurse maintains a high standard of hand hygiene and asepsis during the procedure, skin disinfection is not necessary (Workman 1999).

In the immunosuppressed patient, the skin should be cleaned as such patients may become infected by inoculation of a relatively small number of pathogens (Downie *et al.* 2000). The practice at the Royal Marsden Hospital is to continue to clean the skin prior to injection in order to reduce the risk of contamination from the patient's skin flora. The skin should be cleaned using

an 'alcohol swab' (containing 70% isopropyl alcohol) for 30 seconds and then allowed to dry. If the skin is not dry before proceeding, skin cleaning is ineffective and the antiseptic may cause irritation by being injected into the tissues (Downie *et al.* 2000).

Needle bevel

Three categories of needle bevel are available:

1 *Regular*: for all intramuscular and subcutaneous injections.

2 *Intradermal*: for diagnostic injections and other injections into the epidermis.

3 *Short*: rarely used.

Intramuscular needle gauge size and length

Needles should be long enough to penetrate the muscle and still allow a quarter of the needle to remain external to the skin (Workman 1999). The most common sizes are 21 or 23 G and 2.5–5 cm long. Lenz (1983) states that when choosing the correct needle length for intramuscular injections it is important to assess the muscle mass of the injection site, the amount of subcutaneous fat and the weight of the patient. Without such an assessment, most injections intended for gluteal muscle are deposited in the gluteal fat. The following are suggested by the author as ways of determining the most suitable size of needle to use.

Deltoid and vastus lateralis muscles
The muscle to be used should be grasped between the thumb and forefinger to determine the depth of the muscle mass or the amount of subcutaneous fat at the injection site.

Gluteal muscles
The layer of fat and skin above the muscle should be gently lifted with the thumb and forefinger for the same reasons as before. Use the patient's weight to calculate the needle length required. Lenz (1983) recommends the following guide:

31.5–40 kg	2.5 cm needle
40.5–90 kg	5–7.5 cm needle
90 kg	10–15 cm needle.

Intramuscular injections and pain

Patients are often afraid of receiving injections because they perceive the injection will be painful (Workman 1999). Torrence (1989) listed a number of factors that cause pain:

• The needle
• The chemical composition of the drug/solution
• The technique
• The speed of the injection
• The volume of drug.

Workman (1999) listed a number of techniques that could be utilized to reduce pain and discomfort experienced by the patient such as adequate preparation of the patient, using ice or freezing spray to numb the skin, correct choice of site and technique and positioning of the patient so that the muscles are relaxed. Field (1981) attempts to answer the question of what it is like to give an injection, and goes on to explore the meaning and use of language relating to injections, the feelings involved in preparing and administering injections, and the meaning of the patient's response to the nurse.

Intravenous

Advantages of using the intravenous route

1 An immediate, therapeutic effect is achieved owing to rapid delivery of the drug to its target site, which allows a more precise dose calculation and therefore more reliable treatment.

2 Pain and irritation caused by some substances when given intramuscularly or subcutaneously are avoided.

3 The vascular route affords a route of administration for the patient who cannot tolerate fluids or drugs by the gastrointestinal route.

4 Some drugs cannot be absorbed by any other route; the large molecular size of some drugs prevents absorption by the gastrointestinal route, while other drugs, unstable in the presence of gastric juices, are destroyed.

5 The intravenous route offers the facility for control over the rate of administration of drugs; prolonged action can be provided by administering a dilute infusion intermittently or over a prolonged period of time (Campbell 1996; Weinstein 2000).

Disadvantages of using the intravenous route

1 There is an inability to recall the drug and reverse its action. This may lead to increased toxicity or a sensitivity reaction.

2 Insufficient control of administration may lead to speed shock or circulatory overload. This is characterized by a flushed face, headache, congestion, tightness in the chest, etc.

3 Additional complications may occur, such as the following:
   (a) Microbial contamination (extrinsic or intrinsic)
   (b) Vascular irritation, e.g. chemical phlebitis
   (c) Drug incompatibilities and interactions if multiple additives are prescribed (Campbell 1996; Weinstein 2000).

4 Needle phobia.

5 Altered body image, especially with central vascular access devices (Daniels 1995).

6 Time taken for administration (Hockley *et al.* 1995).

Principles to be applied throughout preparation and administration

Asepsis and reducing the risk of infection
Microbes on the hands of health care personnel contribute to hospital-associated infection (Weinstein 2000).

Therefore aseptic technique must be adhered to throughout all intravenous procedures (see Ch. 4, Aseptic technique). The nurse must employ good hand washing and drying techniques using a bactericidal soap or a bactericidal alcohol handrub. If asepsis is not maintained, local infection, septic phlebitis or septicaemia may result (Nystrom *et al.* 1983; Maki 1992; Springhouse Corporation 1999).

The insertion site should be inspected at least once a day for complications such as infiltration, phlebitis or any indication of infection, e.g. redness at the insertion site of the device or pyrexia (RCN 2003). These problems may necessitate the removal of the device and/or further investigation (Nicol 1999).

It is desirable that a closed system of infusion is maintained wherever possible, with as few connections as is necessary for its purpose (Speechley 1986). This reduces the risk of bacterial contamination. Any extra connections within the administration system increase the risk of infection. Three-way taps have been shown to encourage the growth of micro-organisms. They are difficult to clean due to their design, as micro-organisms can become lodged and are then able to multiply in the warm, moist environment (Nicol 1999). This reservoir for micro-organisms may then be released into the circulation.

The injection sites on administration sets or bungs should be cleaned using an alcohol-based antiseptic, allowing time for it to dry. Connections should be cleaned before changing administration sets and manipulations kept to a minimum. Administration sets should be changed according to use (intermittent/continuous therapy), type of device and type of solution, and the set must be labelled with the date and time of change (DoH 2001; RCN 2003).

To ensure safe delivery of intravenous fluids and medication:

- Replace all tubing when the vascular device is replaced (DoH 2001).
- Replace solution administration sets and stopcocks used for continuous infusions every 72 hours unless clinically indicated, e.g. if drug stability data indicate otherwise (DoH 2001; RCN 2003). Research has indicated that routine changing of administration sets (used for infusing solutions) every 48–72 hours instead of every 24 hours is not associated with an increase in infection and could result in considerable savings for hospitals (DoH 2001; RCN 2003).
- Replace solution administration sets used for lipid emulsions and parenteral nutrition at the end of the infusion or within 24 hours of initiating the infusion (DoH 2001; RCN 2003). Certain intravenous fluids including lipid emulsions, blood and blood products are more likely than other parenteral fluids to support microbial growth if contaminated and therefore replacement of the intravenous tubing is required more frequently than 48–72 hours (DoH 2001).
- Replace blood administration sets at least every 12 hours and after every second unit of blood (McClelland 2001).
- All solution sets used for intermittent infusions, e.g. antibiotics, should be discarded immediately after use and not allowed to hang for reuse (RCN 2003).

Inspection of fluids, drugs, equipment and their packaging must be undertaken to detect any points where contamination may have occurred during manufacture and/or transport. This intrinsic contamination may be detected as cloudiness, discoloration or the presence of particles (Perucca 1995; Weinstein 2000; BMA & RPS 2003). Infusion bags should not be left hanging for longer than 24 hours. In the case of blood and blood products this is reduced to 5 hours (RCN 2003; McClelland 2001).

Safety

All details of the prescription and all calculations must be checked carefully in accordance with hospital policy in order to ensure safe preparation and administration of the drug(s). The volume required can be calculated using the following calculation:

$$\frac{\text{Strength required}}{\text{Stock strength}} \times \text{Volume of stock solution}$$
$$= \text{Volume required}$$

(Pelletier 1995; Hutton 1998; Pickstone 1999; Weinstein 2000). The nurse must also check the compatibility of the drug with the diluent or infusion fluid. The nurse should be aware of the types of incompatibilities, and the factors which could influence them. These include pH, concentration, time, temperature, light and the brand of the drug. If insufficient information is available, a reference book (e.g. *The British National Formulary*) or the product data sheet must be consulted. If the nurse is unsure about any aspect of the preparation and/or administration of a drug, they should not proceed and should consult with a senior member of staff (NMC 2002a). Constant monitoring of both the mixture and the patient is important. The preferred method and rate of intravenous administration must be determined.

Drugs should never be added to the following: blood; blood products, i.e. plasma or platelet concentrate; mannitol solutions; sodium bicarbonate solution, etc. (Springhouse Corporation 1999). Only specially prepared additives should be used with fat emulsions or amino acid preparations.

Accurate labelling of additives and records of administration are essential (RCN 2003).

Any protective clothing which is advised should be worn, and vinyl gloves should be used to reduce the risk of latex allergy (Springhouse Corporation 1999). Health care professionals who use gloves frequently or for long periods face a high risk of allergy from latex products. All health care facilities should develop policies and procedures that determine measures to protect staff and patients from latex exposure and outline a treatment plan for latex reactions (Dougherty 2002).

It has been suggested that needle-free systems can increase the risk of bloodstream infections (Danzig *et al.* 1995). However most studies have found no difference in microbial contamination when comparing conventional and needle-free systems (Brown *et al.* 1997; Luebke *et al.* 1998; Mendelson *et al.* 1998). It appears that an increased risk is only associated where there is lack of compliance with cleaning protocols or changing of equipment (Arduino *et al.* 1997; Cookson *et al.* 1998; Hanchett & Kung 1999).

Preventing needlestick injuries should be key in any health and safety programme. Basic rules of safety include not resheathing needles, disposal of needles immediately after use into a recognized sharps bin and convenient location of sharps bins in all areas where needles and sharps are used (Springhouse Corporation 1999; Dougherty 2002; ICNA 2003; RCN 2003).

Comfort
Both the physical and psychological comfort of the patient must be considered. Comprehensive explanation of the practical aspects of the procedure together with information about the effects of treatment will contribute to reducing anxiety (Wilson-Barnett & Batehup 1992) and will need to be tailored to each patient's individual needs.

Methods of administering intravenous drugs
There are three methods of administering intravenous drugs: continuous infusion, intermittent infusion and intermittent injection.

Continuous infusion
Continuous infusion may be defined as the intravenous delivery of a medication or fluid at a constant rate over a prescribed time period, ranging from 24 hours to days to achieve a controlled therapeutic response. The greater dilution also helps to reduce venous irritation (Pickstone 1999; Weinstein 2000).

A continuous infusion may be used when:

- The drugs to be administered must be highly diluted.
- A maintenance of steady blood levels of the drug is required.

Preprepared infusion fluids with additives such as those containing potassium chloride should be used whenever possible. This reduces the risk of extrinsic contamination, which can occur during the mixing of drugs (Weinstein 2000). Only one addition should be made to each bottle or bag of fluid after the compatibility has been ascertained. More additions can increase the risk of incompatibility occurring, e.g. precipitation (Pickstone 1999; Sani 1999; Weinstein 2000; Trissel 2003). The additive and fluid must be mixed well to prevent a layering effect which can occur with some drugs (Sani 1999). The danger is that a bolus injection of the drug may be delivered. To safeguard against this, any additions should be made to the infusion fluid and the container inverted a number of times to ensure mixing of the drug and prevent a bolus of the drug being infused, before the fluid is hung on the infusion stand. The infusion container should be labelled clearly after the addition has been made. Constant monitoring of the infusion fluid mixture (Sani 1999; Weinstein 2000) for cloudiness or presence of particles should occur, as well as checking the patient's condition and intravenous site for patency, extravasation or infiltration.

Intermittent infusion
Intermittent infusion is the administration of a small-volume infusion, i.e. 50–250 ml, over a period of between 20 minutes and 2 hours. This may be given as a specific dose at one time or at repeated intervals during 24 hours (Pickstone 1999).

An intermittent infusion may be used when:

- A peak plasma level is required therapeutically.
- The pharmacology of the drug dictates this specific dilution.
- The drug will not remain stable for the time required to administer a more dilute volume.
- The patient is on a restricted intake of fluids.

Delivery of the drug by intermittent infusion may utilize a system such as a 'Y' set, if the primary infusion is of a compatible fluid, or a burette set with a chamber capacity of 100 or 150 ml. This is when the drug can be added to the burette and infused while the primary infusion is switched off. A small-volume infusion may also be connected to a cannula specifically to keep the vein open, and maintain patency.

All the points considered when preparing for a continuous infusion should be taken into account here, e.g. preprepared fluids, single additions of drugs, adequate mixing, labelling and monitoring.

Direct intermittent injection
Direct intermittent injection (also known as intravenous push or bolus) involves the injection of a drug from a

syringe into the injection port of the administration set or directly into a vascular access device. Most are administered anywhere from 3 to 10 minutes depending upon the drug (Sani 1999; Weinstein 2000).

A direct injection may be used when:

- A maximum concentration of the drug is required to vital organs. This is a 'bolus' injection which is given rapidly over seconds, as in an emergency, e.g. adrenaline.
- The drug cannot be further diluted for pharmacological or therapeutic reasons or does not require dilution. This is given as a controlled 'push' injection over a few minutes.
- A peak blood level is required and cannot be achieved by small-volume infusion.

Rapid administration could result in toxic levels and an anaphylactic-type reaction. Manufacturers' recommendations of rates of administration (i.e. millilitres or milligrams per minute) should be adhered to. In the absence of such recommendations, administration should proceed slowly, over 5–10 minutes (Dougherty 2002).

Delivery of the drug by direct injection may be via the cannula through a resealable needleless bung, extension set or via the injection site of an administration set.

- If a peripheral device is in situ the bandage and dressing must be removed to inspect the insertion of the cannula, unless a transparent dressing is in place.
- Patency of the vein must be confirmed prior to administration and the vein's ability to accept an extra flow of fluid or irritant chemical must also be checked.

Administration into the injection site of a fast-running drip may be advised if the infusion in progress is compatible in order to dilute the drug further and reduce local chemical irritation (Dougherty 2002). Alternatively, a stop–start procedure may be employed if there is doubt about venous patency. This allows the nurse to constantly check the patency of the vein and detect early signs of extravasation. If the infusion fluid is incompatible with the drug, the administration set may be switched off and a compatible solution may be used as a flush.

If a number of drugs are being administered, 0.9% sodium chloride must be used to flush in between each drug to prevent interactions. In addition, 0.9% sodium chloride should be used at the end of the administration to ensure that all of the drug has been delivered. The device should then be flushed to ensure patency is maintained (see Ch. 44, Vascular access devices: insertion and management).

Summary

The nurse is responsible for the administration of drugs by a variety of methods. The NMC (2002a) *Guidelines for the Administration of Medicines* emphasize that this 'is not solely a mechanistic task to be performed in strict compliance with the written prescription of a medical practitioner.' Shepherd (2002b) maintains that the administration of a medicine is arguably the most common clinical procedure that a nurse will undertake. He goes on to state that it is the manner in which a medicine is administered that determines to some extent whether or not the patient gains any clinical benefit and whether any adverse effect is experienced.

The nurse is accountable for the safe administration of drugs. In order to do this the nurse requires a thorough knowledge of the principles and their application, and a responsible attitude, which ensures that medications are not given without full knowledge of immediate and late effects, toxicities and nursing implications. The nurse must also be able to justify any actions taken and be accountable for the action taken (NMC 2002b).

Procedure guidelines: **Self-administration of drugs**

Procedure

	Action	Rationale
1	Discuss medication history with the patient on his/her admission. This should include an assessment of the patient's ability to self-administer medication using the following criteria. • Is the patient willing to participate in self-administration? • Is the patient confused or forgetful? • Does the patient have a history of drug/alcohol abuse/self-harm?	To ensure an accurate record of: all medicines being taken (prescribed or otherwise); dietary supplements, e.g. multivitamins, herbal remedies, complementary therapies; allergies or hypersensitivities; understanding of current medicines; possible problems with self-administration.

*Procedure guidelines: **Self-administration of drugs** (cont'd)*

Action	Rationale
• Does the patient self-administer medicines at home? • Can the patient read the labels on the medicines? • Can the patient open the medicine containers? • Can the patient open the locker where the medicines are stored while they are in hospital? • Does the patient know what his/her medicines are for, their dosage, instructions and potential side-effects? (Shepherd 2002b) Document this assessment in the patient's nursing records.	
2 Review proposed (inpatient) prescription in liaison with pharmacist and compare with details given by patient and medicines in his/her possession.	If frequent changes of drug or dose are expected, immediate self-administration may be undesirable and/or impractical. Appropriate medicines already in the patient's possession may be used, subject to local policy and agreement with the pharmacist.
3 Consider whether there are any constraints on self-administration, and if so, how they might be overcome. Discuss this with appropriate members of the multidisciplinary team.	To promote successful and safe self-administration and ensure that medicines are dispensed and labelled appropriately for the patient's needs. Constraints such as physical or visual handicap must be addressed. Changes in performance status may result from the underlying condition or its treatment, and must be allowed for. If a compliance aid such as a 'dosette' box is to be used, responsibility for filling and labelling the aid, especially whilst used on the ward, must be agreed and documented in local policies.
4 Regularly discuss with the patient his/her medication and any problems they may be having with the regimen. Document discussions in the care plan. Teach any special skills required, e.g. correct use of aerosol inhalers.	To promote the informed commitment and involvement of patients in their own care, where appropriate. To ensure that treatment is received as intended.
5 Check that drugs are taken as intended, and that the necessary records are kept.	To discharge the nurse's overall responsibility for patient care and well-being. To maintain a record of responsibilities undertaken. Particular care with record keeping is needed in the period of gradual transition from nurse administration to self-administration. Any problems encountered must be addressed. The detail and format of the record may vary according to: the patient's needs and performance status; the complexity of treatment; and local circumstances and policy.
6 Monitor changes in the patient's prescription.	To ensure that: changes are put into effect promptly; drugs are properly relabelled or redispensed; any discontinued drugs are retrieved from the patient.
7 Check when drug supplies are expected to run out and make arrangements for resupply. Order TTOs (drugs 'to take out') as far in advance as possible.	To ensure that drugs are represcribed and dispensed in time to allow uninterrupted treatment and to facilitate planned discharge.
8 Evaluate the effectiveness of the self-administration teaching programme and record any difficulties encountered and interventions made.	To identify further learning and teaching needs and modify care plan accordingly.

Procedure guidelines: **Oral drug administration**

Procedure

Action	Rationale
1 Wash hands with bactericidal soap and water or bactericidal alcohol handrub.	To minimize the risk of cross-infection.
2 Before administering any prescribed drug, check that it is due and has not already been given. Check that the information contained in the prescription chart is complete, correct and legible.	To protect the patient from harm.
3 Before administering any prescribed drug, consult the patient's prescription chart and ascertain the following:	
(a) Drug (b) Dose (c) Date and time of administration (d) Route and method of administration (e) Diluent as appropriate (f) Validity of prescription (g) Signature of doctor (h) The prescription is legible.	To ensure that the patient is given the correct drug in the prescribed dose using the appropriate diluent and by the correct route. To protect the patient from harm. To comply with NMC (2002a) *Guidelines for the Administration of Medicines.*
4 Select the required medication and check the expiry date.	Treatment with medication that is outside the expiry date is dangerous. Drugs deteriorate with storage. The expiry date indicates when a particular drug is no longer pharmacologically efficacious.
5 Empty the required dose into a medicine container. Avoid touching the preparation.	To minimize the risk of cross-infection. To minimize the risk of harm to the nurse.
6 Take the medication and the prescription chart to the patient. Check the patient's identity by asking the patient to state their full name and date of birth. If patient unable to confirm details then check patient identity band against prescription chart.	To ensure that the medication is administered to the correct patient.
7 Evaluate the patient's knowledge of the medication being offered. If this knowledge appears to be faulty or incorrect, offer an explanation of the use, action, dose and potential side-effects of the drug or drugs involved.	A patient has a right to information about treatment.
8 Administer the drug as prescribed.	
9 Offer a glass of water, if allowed.	To facilitate swallowing the medication.
10 Record the dose given in the prescription chart and in any other place made necessary by legal requirement or hospital policy.	To meet legal requirements and hospital policy.
11 Administer irritant drugs with meals or snacks.	To minimize their effect on the gastric mucosa.
12 Administer drugs that interact with food, or that are destroyed in significant proportions by digestive enzymes, between meals or on an empty stomach.	To prevent interference with the absorption of the drug.
13 Do not break a tablet unless it is scored and appropriate to do so. Break scored tablets with a file or a tablet cutter. Wash after use.	Breaking may cause incorrect dosage, gastrointestinal irritation or destruction of a drug in an incompatible pH. To reduce risk of contamination between tablets.

*Procedure guidelines: **Oral drug administration** (cont'd)*

Action	Rationale
14 Do not interfere with time-release capsules and enteric coated tablets. Ask patients to swallow these whole and not to chew them.	The absorption rate of the drug will be altered.
15 Sublingual tablets must be placed under the tongue and buccal tablets between gum and cheek.	To allow for correct absorption.
16 When administering liquids to babies and young children, or when an accurately measured dose in multiples of 1 ml is needed for an adult, an oral syringe should be used in preference to a medicine spoon or measure.	An oral syringe is much more accurate than a measure or a 5 ml spoon. Use of a syringe makes administration of the correct dose much easier in an uncooperative child. Oral syringes are available and are designed to be washable and reused for the same patient. However, in the immunocompromised patient single use only is recommended. Oral syringes must be clearly labelled for oral or enteral use only.
17 In babies and children especially, correct use of the syringe is very important. The tip should be gently pushed into and towards the side of the mouth. The contents are then *slowly* discharged towards the inside of the cheek, pausing if necessary to allow the liquid to be swallowed. In difficult children it may help to place the end of the barrel between the teeth.	To prevent injury to the mouth and eliminate the danger of choking the patient. To get the dose in and to prevent the patient spitting it out.

Controlled drugs

Action	Rationale
1 Consult the patient's prescription chart, and ascertain the following: (a) Drug (b) Dose (c) Date and time of administration (d) Route and method of administration (e) Diluent as appropriate (f) Validity of prescription (g) Signature of doctor.	To ensure that the patient is given the correct drug in the prescribed dose using the appropriate diluent and by the correct route.
2 Select the correct drug from the controlled drug cupboard.	
3 Check the stock against the last entry in the ward record book. (At the Royal Marsden Hospital, a second person is required to check the stock level and both nurses are required to sign the controlled drugs book.)	To comply with hospital policy.
4 Check the appropriate dose against the prescription chart.	
5 Return the remaining stock to the cupboard and lock the cupboard.	
6 Enter the date, dose and the patient's name in the ward record book.	
7 Take the prepared dose to the patient, whose identity is checked.	To prevent error and confirm patient's identity.
8 Administer the drug after checking the prescription chart again. Once the drug has been administered, the prescription chart is signed by the nurse responsible for administering the medication.	

*Procedure guidelines: **Oral drug administration** (cont'd)*

Action	Rationale
9 Record the administration on appropriate charts.	To maintain accurate records, provide a point of reference in the event of any queries and prevent any duplication of treatment.

Procedure guidelines: **Administration of injections**

Equipment

1 Clean tray or receiver in which to place drug and equipment.
2 21 G needle(s) to ease reconstitution and drawing up, 23 G if from a glass ampoule.
3 21, 23 or 25 G needle, size dependent on route of administration.
4 Syringe(s) of appropriate size for amount of drug to be given.
5 Swabs saturated with isopropyl alcohol 70%.
6 Sterile topical swab, if drug is presented in ampoule form.

7 Drug(s) to be administered.
8 Patient's prescription chart, to check dose, route, etc.
9 Recording sheet or book as required by law or hospital policy.
10 Any protective clothing required by hospital policy for specified drugs, such as antibiotics or cytotoxic drugs (see Ch. 10, Drug administration: cytotoxic drugs).

Procedure

Action	Rationale
1 Collect and check all equipment.	To prevent delays and enable full concentration on the procedure.
2 Check that the packaging of all equipment is intact.	To ensure sterility. If the seal is damaged, discard.
3 Wash hands with bactericidal soap and water or bactericidal alcohol handrub.	To prevent contamination of medication and equipment.
4 Prepare needle(s), syringe(s), etc., on a tray or receiver.	
5 Inspect all equipment.	To check that none is damaged; if so, discard.
6 Consult the patient's prescription chart, and ascertain the following: (a) Drug (b) Dose (c) Date and time of administration (d) Route and method of administration (e) Diluent as appropriate (f) Validity of prescription (g) Signature of doctor.	To ensure that the patient is given the correct drug in the prescribed dose using the appropriate diluent and by the correct route.
7 Check all details with another nurse if required by hospital policy.	To minimize any risk of error.
8 Select the drug in the appropriate volume, dilution or dosage and check the expiry date.	To reduce wastage. Treatment with medication that is outside the expiry date is dangerous. Drugs deteriorate with storage. The expiry date indicates when a particular drug is no longer pharmacologically efficacious.
9 Proceed with the preparation of the drug, using protective clothing if advisable.	
10 Evaluate the patient's knowledge of the medication being offered. If this knowledge appears to be faulty or incorrect, offer an explanation of the use, action, dose and potential side-effects of the drug or drugs involved.	A patient has a right to information about treatment.

*Procedure guidelines: **Administration of injections** (cont'd)*

Action	Rationale
11 Administer the drug as prescribed.	
12 Record the administration on appropriate charts.	To maintain accurate records, provide a point of reference in the event of any queries and prevent any duplication of treatment.

Single-dose ampoule: solution

Action	Rationale
1 Inspect the solution for cloudiness or particulate matter. If this is present, discard and follow hospital guidelines on what action to take, e.g. return drug to pharmacy.	To prevent the patient from receiving an unstable or contaminated drug.
2 Tap the neck of the ampoule gently.	To ensure that all the solution is in the bottom of the ampoule.
3 Cover the neck of the ampoule with a sterile topical swab and snap it open. If there is any difficulty a file may be required.	To minimize the risk of contamination. To prevent aerosol formation or contact with the drug which could lead to a sensitivity reaction. To reduce the risk of injury to the nurse.
4 Inspect the solution for glass fragments; if present, discard.	To minimize the risk of injection of foreign matter into the patient.
5 Withdraw the required amount of solution, tilting the ampoule if necessary.	To avoid drawing in any air.
6 Replace the sheath on the needle and tap the syringe to dislodge any air bubbles. Expel air. *Note*: replacing the sheath should **not** be confused with resheathing used needles. An alternative to expelling the air with the needle sheath in place would be to use the ampoule or vial to receive any air and/or drug.	To prevent aerosol formation. To ensure that the correct amount of drug is in the syringe.
7 Change the needle, and discard used needle into appropriate sharps container.	To reduce the risk of infection. To avoid tracking medications through superficial tissues. To ensure that the correct size of needle is used for the injection. To reduce the risk of injury to the nurse.

Single-dose ampoule: powder

Action	Rationale
1 Tap the neck of the ampoule gently.	To ensure that any powder lodged here falls to the bottom of the ampoule.
2 Cover the neck of the ampoule with a sterile topical swab and snap it open. If there is any difficulty a file may be required.	To minimize the risk of contamination. To prevent contact with the drug which could cause a sensitivity reaction. To prevent injury to the nurse.
3 Inject the correct diluent slowly into the powder within the ampoule.	To ensure that the powder is thoroughly wet before agitation and is not released into the atmosphere.
4 Agitate the ampoule.	To dissolve the drug.
5 Inspect the contents.	To detect any glass fragments or any other particulate matter. If present, continue agitation or discard as appropriate.
6 When the solution is clear withdraw the prescribed amount, tilting the ampoule if necessary.	To ensure the powder is dissolved and has formed a solution with the diluent. To avoid drawing in air.
7 Replace the sheath on the needle and tap the syringe to dislodge any air bubbles. Expel air.	To prevent aerosol formation. To ensure that the correct amount of drug is in the syringe.
8 Change the needle, and discard used needle into appropriate sharps container.	To reduce the risk of infection. To avoid tracking medications though superficial tissues. To ensure that the correct size of needle is used for the injection. To reduce the risk of injury to the nurse.

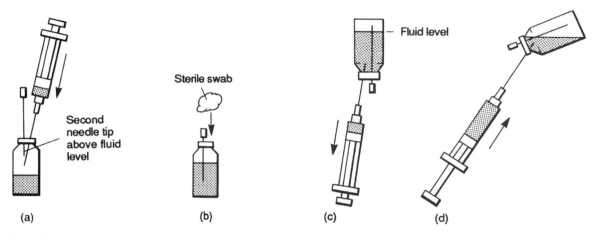

Figure 9.3 Suggested method of vial reconstitution to avoid environmental exposure. (a) When reconstituting vial, insert a second needle to allow air to escape when adding diluent for injection. (b) When shaking the vial to dissolve the powder, push in second needle up to Luer connection and cover with a sterile swab. (c) To remove reconstituted solution, insert syringe needle and then invert vial. Ensuring that tip of second needle is above fluid, withdraw the solution. (d) Remove air from syringe without spraying into the atmosphere by injecting air back into vial.

*Procedure guidelines: **Administration of injections** (cont'd)*

Multidose vial: powder

Action	Rationale
1 Clean the rubber cap with the chosen antiseptic and let it dry.	To prevent bacterial contamination of the drug.
2 Insert a 21 G needle into the cap to vent the bottle (Fig. 9.3a).	To prevent pressure differentials, which can cause separation of needle and syringe.
3 Inject the correct diluent slowly into the powder within the ampoule.	To ensure that the powder is thoroughly wet before it is shaken and is not released into the atmosphere.
4 Remove the needle and the syringe.	
5 Place a sterile topical swab over the venting needle (Fig. 9.3b) and shake to dissolve the powder.	To prevent contamination of the drug or the atmosphere. To mix the diluent with the powder and dissolve the drug.

Note: the nurse may encounter other presentations of drugs for injection, e.g. vials with a transfer needle, and should follow the manufacturer's instructions in these instances.

6 Inspect the solution for cloudiness or particulate matter. If this is present, discard. Follow hospital guidelines on what action to take, e.g. return drug to pharmacy.	To prevent patient from receiving an unstable or contaminated drug.
7 Clean the rubber cap with an appropriate antiseptic and let it dry.	To prevent bacterial contamination of the drug.
8 Withdraw the prescribed amount of solution, and inspect for pieces of rubber which may have 'cored out' of the cap (Fig. 9.3c). *Note*: coring can be minimized by inserting the needle into the cap, bevel up, at an angle of 45° to 60°. Before complete insertion of the needle tip, lift the needle to 90° and proceed (Fig. 9.4).	To prevent the injection of foreign matter into the patient.

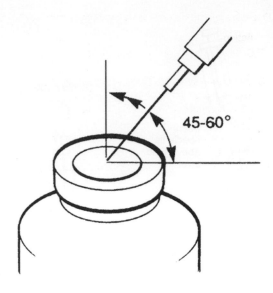

Figure 9.4 Method to minimize coring.

*Procedure guidelines: **Administration of injections** (cont'd)*

Action	Rationale
9 Remove air from syringe without spraying into the atmosphere by injecting air back into the vial (see Fig. 9.3d) or replace the sheath on the needle and tap the syringe to dislodge any air bubbles. Expel air.	To reduce risk of contamination of practitioner. To prevent aerosol formation. To ensure that the correct amount of drug is in the syringe.
10 Change the needle.	To reduce the risk of infection. To avoid possible trauma to the patient if the needle has barbed. To avoid tracking medications through superficial tissues. To ensure that the correct size of needle is used for the injection.

Subcutaneous injections

Action	Rationale
1 Explain and discuss the procedure with the patient.	To ensure that the patient understands the procedure and gives his/her valid consent.
2 Consult the patient's prescription chart, and ascertain the following: (a) Drug (b) Dose (c) Date and time of administration (d) Route and method of administration (e) Diluent as appropriate (f) Validity of prescription (g) Signature of doctor.	To ensure that the patient is given the correct drug in the prescribed dose using the appropriate diluent and by the correct route.
3 Assist the patient into the required position.	To allow access to the chosen site.
4 Remove appropriate garments to expose the chosen site.	To gain access for injection.
5 Choose the correct needle size.	To minimize the risk of missing the subcutaneous tissue and any ensuing pain.
6 Clean the chosen site with a swab saturated with isopropyl alcohol 70%.	To reduce the number of pathogens introduced into the skin by the needle at the time of insertion. (For further information on this action see 'Skin preparation', p. 196.)

*Procedure guidelines: **Administration of injections** (cont'd)*

Action	Rationale
7 Gently pinch the skin up into a fold.	To elevate the subcutaneous tissue, and lift the adipose tissue away from the underlying muscle (Workman 1999).
8 Insert the needle into the skin at angle of 45° and release the grasped skin (unless administering insulin when an angle of 90° should be used). Inject the drug slowly.	Injecting medication into compressed tissue irritates nerve fibres and causes the patient discomfort. The introduction of shorter insulin needles makes 90° the more appropriate angle (Trounce & Gould 2000).
9 Withdraw the needle rapidly. Apply pressure to any bleeding point.	To prevent haematoma formation.
10 Record the administration on appropriate sheets.	To maintain accurate records, provide a point of reference in the event of any queries and prevent any duplication of treatment.
11 Ensure that all sharps and non-sharp waste are disposed of safely and in accordance with locally approved procedures. For example, sharps into sharps bin and syringes into yellow clinical waste bag.	To ensure safe disposal and to avoid laceration or other injury to staff.

Intramuscular injections

Action	Rationale
1 Explain and discuss the procedure with the patient.	To ensure that the patient understands the procedure and gives his/her valid consent.
2 Consult the patient's prescription sheet, and ascertain the following: (a) Drug (b) Dose (c) Date and time of administration (d) Route and method of administration (e) Diluent as appropriate (f) Validity of prescription (g) Signature of doctor.	To ensure that the patient is given the correct drug in the prescribed dose using the appropriate diluent and by the correct route.
3 Assist the patient into the required position.	To allow access to the chosen site and to ensure the designated muscle group is flexed and therefore relaxed.
4 Remove the appropriate garment to expose the chosen site.	To gain access for injection.
5 Clean the chosen site with a swab saturated with isopropyl alcohol 70% for 30 seconds and allow to dry for 30 seconds (Workman 1999).	To reduce the number of pathogens introduced into the skin by the needle at the time of insertion, to prevent stinging sensation if alcohol is taken into the tissues upon needle entry. (For further information on this action see 'Skin preparation'.)
6 Stretch the skin around the chosen site.	To facilitate the insertion of the needle and to displace the underlying subcutaneous tissue.
7 Holding the needle at an angle of 90°, quickly plunge it into the skin.	To ensure that the needle penetrates the muscle.
8 Pull back the plunger. If no blood is aspirated, depress the plunger at approximately 1 ml every 10 seconds and inject the drug slowly. If blood appears, withdraw the needle completely, replace it and begin again. Explain to the patient what has occurred.	To confirm that the needle is in the correct position and not in a vein. This allows time for the muscle fibres to expand and absorb the solution (Workman 1999). To prevent pain and ensure even distribution of the drug.
9 Wait 10 seconds before withdrawing the needle.	To allow the medication to diffuse into the tissue.
10 Withdraw the needle rapidly. Apply pressure to any bleeding point.	To prevent haematoma formation.

*Procedure guidelines: **Administration of injections** (cont'd)*

Action	Rationale
11 Record the administration on appropriate charts.	To maintain accurate records, provide a point of reference in the event of any queries and prevent any duplication of treatment.
12 Ensure that all sharps and non-sharp waste are disposed of safely and in accordance with locally approved procedures, e.g. put sharps into sharps bin and syringes into yellow clinical waste bag.	To ensure safe disposal and to avoid laceration or other injury to staff.

Procedure guidelines: **Administration of rectal and vaginal preparations**

Equipment

1 Disposable gloves.
2 Topical swabs.

3 Lubricating jelly.
4 Prescription chart.

Procedure

Rectal preparations

For further information about the administration of rectal medication see the relevant sections in Ch. 13, Bowel care.

Vaginal pessaries

Action	Rationale
1 Explain and discuss the procedure with the patient.	To ensure that the patient understands the procedure and gives her valid consent.
2 Consult the patient's prescription sheet, and ascertain the following: (a) Drug (b) Dose (c) Date and time of administration (d) Route and method of administration (e) Validity of prescription (f) Signature of doctor.	To ensure that the patient is given the correct drug in the prescribed dose and by the correct route.
3 Select the appropriate pessary and check it with the prescription chart.	To ensure that the correct medication is given to the correct patient at the appropriate time.
4 Assist the patient into the appropriate position, either left lateral with buttocks to the edge of the bed or supine with the knees drawn up and legs parted.	To facilitate the correct insertion of the pessary.
5 Wash hands with bactericidal soap and water or bactericidal alcohol handrub, and put on gloves.	To minimize the risk of cross-infection.
6 Apply lubricating jelly to a topical swab and from the swab on to the pessary.	To facilitate insertion of the pessary and ensure the patient's comfort.
7 Insert the pessary along the posterior vaginal wall and into the top of the vagina. *Note*: This procedure is best performed late in the evening when the patient is unlikely to get out of bed.	To ensure that the pessary is retained and that the medication can reach its maximum efficiency.
8 Wipe away any excess lubricating jelly from the patient's vulval and/or perineal area with a topical swab.	To promote patient comfort.
9 Make the patient comfortable and apply a clean sanitary pad.	To absorb any excess discharge.

*Procedure guidelines: **Administration of rectal and vaginal preparations** (cont'd)*

Action	Rationale
10 Record the administration on appropriate charts.	To maintain accurate records, provide a point of reference in the event of any queries and prevent any duplication of treatment.

Procedure guidelines: **Topical applications of drugs**

Equipment

1 Clean non-sterile gloves.
2 Sterile topical swabs.

3 Applicators.

Procedure

Action	Rationale
1 Explain and discuss the procedure with the patient.	To ensure that the patient understands the procedure and gives his/her valid consent.
2 Check the patient's prescription chart.	To ensure that the patient is given the correct drug and dose.
3 Use aseptic technique if the skin is broken.	To prevent local or systemic infection.
4 Remove semisolid or stiff preparations from their containers with a gloved hand.	To minimize the risk of cross-infection from one part of the wound to another.
5 If the medication is to be rubbed into the skin, the preparation should be placed on a sterile topical swab. The wearing of gloves may be necessary.	To minimize the risk of cross-infection. To protect the nurse.
6 If the preparation causes staining, advise the patient of this.	To ensure that adequate precautions are taken beforehand and to prevent unwanted stains.
7 Record the administration on appropriate charts.	To maintain accurate records, provide a point of reference in the event of any queries and prevent any duplication of treatment.

Procedure guidelines: **Administration of drugs in other forms**

Procedure

Inhalations

Action	Rationale
1 Explain and discuss the procedure with the patient.	To ensure that the patient understands the procedure and gives his/her valid consent.
2 Seat the patient in an upright position if possible.	To permit full expansion of the diaphragm.
3 Consult the patient's prescription chart, and ascertain the following: (a) Drug (b) Dose (c) Date and time of administration (d) Route and method of administration (e) Diluent as appropriate (f) Validity of prescription (g) Signature of doctor.	To ensure that the patient is given the correct drug in the prescribed dose using the appropriate diluent and by the correct route.
4 Administer only one drug at a time unless specifically instructed to the contrary.	Several drugs used together may cause undesirable reactions or they may inactivate each other.

*Procedure guidelines: **Administration of drugs in other forms** (cont'd)*

Action	Rationale
5 Measure any liquid medication with a syringe.	To ensure the correct dose.
6 Clean any equipment used after use, and discard all disposable equipment in appropriate containers.	To minimize the risk of infection.
7 Correct use of inhalers is essential (see manufacturer's information leaflet) and will be achieved only if this is carefully explained and demonstrated to the patient. If further advice is required, contact the hospital pharmacist.	Incorrect use may result in most of the dose remaining in the mouth and/or being expelled almost immediately. This renders treatment ineffective.
8 Record the administration on appropriate charts.	To maintain accurate records, provide a point of reference in the event of any queries and prevent any duplication of treatment.

Gargles

Action	Rationale
1 Throat irrigations should not be warmer than body temperature.	Any liquid warmer may cause discomfort or damage tissue.

Nasal drops

Action	Rationale
1 Explain and discuss the procedure with the patient.	To ensure that the patient understands the procedure and gives his/her valid consent.
2 Consult the patient's prescription sheet, and ascertain the following: (a) Drug (b) Dose (c) Date and time of administration (d) Route and method of administration (e) Validity of prescription (f) Signature of doctor.	To ensure that the patient is given the correct drug in the prescribed dose and by the correct route.
3 Have paper tissues available.	To wipe away secretions and/or medication.
4 Clean the patient's nasal passages, with tissues or damp cotton bud.	To ensure maximum penetration for the medication.
5 Hyperextend the patient's neck (unless clinically contraindicated, e.g. cervical spondylosis).	To obtain a safe optimum position for insertion of the medication.
6 Avoid touching the external nares with the dropper.	To prevent the patient from sneezing.
7 Request the patient to maintain his/her position for 1 or 2 minutes.	To ensure full absorption of the medication.
8 Each patient should have his/her own medication and dropper.	To minimize the risk of cross-infection.
9 Record the administration on appropriate charts.	To maintain accurate records, provide a point of reference in the event of any queries and prevent any duplication of treatment.

Eye medications

For information on eye care see Ch. 31.

Ear drops

Action	Rationale
1 Explain and discuss the procedure with the patient.	To ensure that the patient understands the procedure and gives his/her valid consent.

*Procedure guidelines: **Administration of drugs in other forms** (cont'd)*

Action	Rationale
2 Consult the patient's prescription chart and ascertain the following: (a) Drug (b) Dose (c) Date and time of administration (d) Route and method of administration (e) Validity of prescription (f) Signature of doctor.	To ensure that the patient is given the correct drug in the prescribed dose using the appropriate diluent and by the correct route.
3 Ask the patient to lie on his/her side with the ear to be treated uppermost.	To ensure the best position for insertion of the drops.
4 Warm the drops to body temperature if allowed.	To prevent trauma to the patient.
5 Pull the cartilaginous part of the pinna backwards and upwards.	To prepare the auditory meatus for instillation of the drops.
6 Allow the drop(s) to fall in direction of the external canal.	To ensure that the medication reaches the area requiring therapy.
7 Request the patient to remain in this position for 1 or 2 minutes.	To allow the medication to reach the eardrum and be absorbed.
8 Record the administration on appropriate charts.	To maintain accurate records, provide a point of reference in the event of any queries and prevent any duplication of treatment.

Procedure guidelines: **Administration of intravenous drugs by continuous infusion**

This procedure may be carried out by the infusion of drugs from a bag, bottle or burette.

Equipment

1 Clinically clean receiver or tray containing the prepared drug to be administered.
2 Patient's prescription chart.
3 Recording chart or book as required by law or hospital policy.
4 Protective clothing as required by hospital policy for specific drugs.
5 Container of appropriate intravenous infusion fluid.
6 Swab saturated with isopropyl alcohol 70%.
7 Drug additive label.

Procedure

Action	Rationale
1 Explain and discuss the procedure with the patient.	To ensure that the patient understands the procedure and gives his/her valid consent.
2 Inspect the infusion in progress.	To check it is the correct infusion being administered at the correct rate and that the contents are due to be delivered on time in order for the next prepared infusion bag to be connected. To check whether the patient is experiencing any discomfort at the site of insertion, which might indicate the peripheral device needs to be resited.
3 Before administering any prescribed drug check that it is due and has not already been given.	To protect the patient from harm.
4 Before administering any prescribed drug, consult the patient's prescription chart and ascertain the following: (a) Drug (b) Dose (c) Date and time of administration (d) Route and method of administration	To ensure that the patient is given the correct drug in the prescribed dose using the appropriate diluent and by the correct route. To protect the patient from harm.

Procedure guidelines: **Administration of intravenous drugs by continuous infusion** *(cont'd)*

Action	Rationale
(e) Diluent as appropriate (f) Validity of prescription (g) Signature of doctor (h) The prescription is legible.	To comply with NMC (2002a) *Guidelines for the Administration of Medicines.*
5 Wash hands with bactericidal soap and water or bactericidal alcohol handrub, and assemble the necessary equipment.	
6 Prepare the drug for injection described in the Procedure guidelines: Administration of injections.	
7 Check the name, strength and volume of intravenous fluid against the prescription chart.	To ensure that the correct type and quantity of fluid are administered.
8 Check the expiry date of the fluid.	To prevent an ineffective or toxic compound being administered to the patient.
9 Check that the packaging is intact and inspect the container and contents in a good light for cracks, punctures, air bubbles.	To check that no contamination of the infusion container has occurred.
10 Inspect the fluid for discoloration, haziness and crystalline or particulate matter.	To prevent any toxic or foreign matter being infused into the patient.
11 Check the identity and amount of drug to be added. Consider: (a) Compatibility of fluid and additive (b) Stability of mixture over the prescription time (c) Any special directions for dilution, e.g. pH, optimum concentration (d) Sensitivity to external factors such as light (e) Any anticipated allergic reaction. If any doubts exist about the listed points, consult the pharmacist or appropriate reference works.	To minimize any risk of error. To ensure safe and effective administration of the drug. To enable anticipation of toxicities and the nursing implications of these.
12 Any additions must be made immediately before use.	To prevent any possible microbial growth or degradation.
13 Wash hands thoroughly using bactericidal soap and water or bactericidal alcohol handrub.	To minimize the risk of cross-infection.
14 Place infusion bag on flat surface.	To prevent puncturing the side of the infusion bag when making additions.
15 Remove any seal present.	To expose the injection site on the container.
16 Clean the site with the swab and allow it to dry.	To reduce the risk of contamination.
17 Inject the drug using a new sterile needle into the bag, bottle or burette. A 23 or 25 G needle should be used.	To minimize the risk of contamination. To enable resealing of the latex or rubber injection site.
18 If the addition is made into a burette at the bedside:	
(a) Avoid contamination of the needle and inlet port.	To minimize the risk of contamination.
(b) Check that the correct quantity of fluid is in the chamber.	To ensure the correct dilution.
(c) Switch the infusion off briefly.	To ensure a bolus injection is not given.
(d) Add the drug.	
19 Invert the container a number of times, especially if adding to a flexible infusion bag.	To ensure adequate mixing of the drug.
20 Check again for haziness, discoloration and particles. This can occur even if the mixture is theoretically compatible, thus making vigilance essential.	To detect any incompatibility or degradation.
21 Complete the drug additive label and fix it on the bag, bottle or burette.	To identify which drug has been added, when and by whom.

*Procedure guidelines: **Administration of intravenous drugs by continuous infusion** (cont'd)*

Action	Rationale
22 Place the container in a clean receptacle. Wash hands and proceed to the patient.	To minimize the risk of contamination.
23 Check the identity of the patient with the prescription chart and infusion bag.	To minimize the risk of error and ensure the correct infusion is administered to the correct patient.
24 Check that the contents of the previous container have been delivered.	To ensure that the preceding prescription has been administered.
25 Switch off the infusion. Place the new infusion bag on a flat surface and then disconnect empty infusion bag.	To ensure that the administration set spike will not puncture the side wall of the infusion bag.
26 Push the spike in fully without touching the spike and hang the new infusion bag on the infusion stand.	To reduce the risk of contamination.
27 Restart the infusion and adjust the rate of flow as prescribed.	To ensure that the infusion will be delivered at the correct rate over the correct period of time.
28 If the addition is made into a burette, the infusion can be restarted immediately following mixing and recording and the infusion rate adjusted accordingly.	
29 Ask the patient whether any abnormal sensations, etc., are experienced.	To ascertain whether there are any problems that may require nursing care and refer to medical staff where appropriate.
30 Discard waste, making sure that it is placed in the correct containers, e.g. sharps into a designated receptacle.	To ensure safe disposal and avoid injury to staff. To prevent reuse of equipment.
31 Complete the patient's recording chart and other hospital and/or legally required documents.	To maintain accurate records. To provide a point of reference in the event of any queries. To prevent any duplication of treatment.

Procedure guidelines: **Administration of drugs by intermittent infusion**

Equipment

Equipment for this procedure is as described for the previous procedure (i.e. items 1–7), together with the following:

8 Intravenous administration set.
9 Intravenous infusion stand.
10 Clean dressing trolley.
11 Clinically clean receiver or tray.
12 Sterile needles and syringes.
13 20 ml for injection of a compatible flush solution, e.g. 0.9% sodium chloride or 5% dextrose.

14 Heparin, in accordance with hospital policy, plus sterile injection cap.
15 Alcohol-based lotion for cleaning injection site, e.g. chlorhexidine in 70% alcohol.
16 Alcohol-based hand wash solution or rub.
17 Sterile dressing pack.
18 Hypoallergenic tape.

Procedure

Action	Rationale
1 Explain and discuss the procedure with the patient.	To ensure that the patient understands the procedure and gives his/her valid consent.
2 Before administering any prescribed drug, check that it is due and has not been given already. Check that the information contained in the prescription chart is complete, correct and legible.	To protect the patient from harm.

*Procedure guidelines: **Administration of drugs by intermittent infusion** (cont'd)*

Action	Rationale
3 Before administering any prescribed drug, consult the patient's prescription chart and ascertain the following: (a) Drug (b) Dose (c) Date and time of administration (d) Route and method of administration (e) Diluent as appropriate (f) Validity of prescription (g) Signature of doctor (h) The prescription is legible.	To ensure that the patient is given the correct drug in the prescribed dose using the appropriate diluent and by the correct route. To protect the patient from harm. To comply with NMC (2002a) *Guidelines for the Administration of Medicines.*
4 Prepare the intravenous infusion and additive as described for the previous procedure (i.e. items 2–13).	
5 Prime the intravenous administration set with infusion fluid mixture and hang it on the infusion stand.	To ensure removal of air from set and check that tubing is patent. To prepare for administration.
6 Draw up 10 ml of compatible flush solution for injection in two separate syringes, using an aseptic technique.	To ensure sufficient flushing solution is available.
7 Draw up solution (as per hospital policy) to be used for maintaining patency, e.g. 0.9% sodium chloride.	To prepare for administration.
8 Place the syringes in a clinically clean receiver or tray on the bottom shelf of the dressing trolley.	To ensure top shelf is used for sterile dressing pack in order to minimize the risk of contamination.
9 Collect the other equipment and place it on the bottom shelf of the dressing trolley.	To ensure all equipment is available to commence procedure.
10 Place a sterile dressing pack on top of the trolley.	To minimize risk of contamination.
11 Check that all necessary equipment is present.	To prevent delays and interruption of the procedure.
12 Wash hands thoroughly using bactericidal soap and water or bactericidal alcohol handrub before leaving the clinical room.	To minimize the risk of cross-infection.
13 Proceed to the patient. Check patient's identity with prescription chart and prepared drugs.	To minimize the risk of error and ensure the correct drug is given to the correct patient.
14 Open the sterile dressing pack.	To minimize the risk of cross-infection.
15 Add lotion for cleaning the injection cap to the gallipot in order to wet the low-linting swabs.	To ensure the swabs can be used for cleaning when sufficient alcohol-based lotion is applied.
16 Wash hands with bactericidal soap and water or with a bactericidal alcohol handrub.	To minimize the risk of cross-infection.
17 If peripheral device is in situ remove the patient's bandage and dressing.	To observe the insertion site.
18 Inspect the insertion site of the device.	To detect any signs of inflammation, infiltration, etc. If present, take appropriate action.
19 Wash hands as above (see item 16).	To minimize the risk of contamination.
20 Put on gloves, if appropriate.	To protect against contamination with hazardous substances, e.g. cytotoxic drugs.
21 Place a sterile towel under the patient's arm.	To create a sterile area on which to work.
22 (a) If using a needleless injection system, clean the cap with alcohol-soaked swabs.	To minimize the risk of contamination and maintain a closed system.
(b) If using an injectable cap, clean the connection between the cap and the device/	To minimize the risk of contamination and to prevent blood spillage.

*Procedure guidelines: **Administration of drugs by intermittent infusion** (cont'd)*

Action	Rationale
extension set then remove the cap while applying digital pressure at the point in the vein where the cannula tip rests.	
23 Inject gently 10 ml of 0.9% sodium chloride for injection.	To confirm the patency of the device.
24 Check that no resistance is met, no pain or discomfort is felt by the patient, no swelling is evident, no leakage occurs around the device and there is a good back-flow of blood on aspiration.	To ensure the device is patent.
25 Connect the infusion to the device.	To commence treatment.
26 Open the roller clamp.	To check the infusion is flowing freely.
27 Check the insertion site and ask the patient if he/she is comfortable.	To confirm that the vein can accommodate the extra fluid flow and that the patient experiences no pain, etc.
28 Adjust the flow rate as prescribed.	To ensure that the correct speed of administration is established.
29 Tape the administration set in a way that places no strain on the device, which could in turn damage the vein.	To reduce the risk of mechanical phlebitis or infiltration.
30 If peripheral device is in situ cover it with a sterile topical swab and tape it in place.	To maintain asepsis.
31 Remove gloves, if used.	
32 If the infusion is to be completed within 30 minutes, bandaging is unnecessary and the patient may be instructed to keep the arm resting on the sterile towel. Otherwise reapply bandage.	To reduce the risk of dislodging the device.
33 The equipment must be cleared away and new equipment only prepared when required at the end of the infusion.	To ensure that the equipment used is sterile prior to use.
34 Monitor flow rate and device site frequently.	To ensure the flow rate is correct and the patient is comfortable, and to check for signs of infiltration.
35 When the infusion is complete, wash hands using bactericidal soap and water or bactericidal alcohol handrub, and recheck that all the equipment required is present.	To maintain asepsis and ensure that the procedure runs smoothly.
36 Stop the infusion when all the fluid has been delivered.	To ensure that all of the prescribed mixture has been delivered and prevent air infusing into the patient.
37 Put on non-sterile gloves, if appropriate.	To protect against contamination with hazardous substances.
38 Disconnect the infusion set and flush the device with 10 ml of 0.9% sodium chloride or other compatible solution for injection. (A 'minibag' may be used to flush the drug through the tubing but the cost implications of this as well as the risk to patients on restricted intake should be considered before this is adopted routinely.)	To flush any remaining irritating solution away from the cannula.
39 Attach a new sterile injection cap if necessary.	To maintain a closed system.
40 Flushing must follow.	To maintain the patency of the device.
41 Clean the injection site of the cap with a swab saturated with chlorhexidine in 70% alcohol.	To minimize the risk of contamination.
42 Administer flushing solution (using a 23 or 25 G needle if necessary) using the push pause technique and ending with positive pressure.	To maintain the patency of the device and if needle used enable reseal of the injection site.

*Procedure guidelines: **Administration of drugs by intermittent infusion** (cont'd)*

Action	Rationale
43 If a peripheral device is in situ cover the insertion site and cannula with a new sterile low-linting swab. Tape it in place. Apply a bandage.	To minimize the risk of contamination of the insertion site. To reduce the risk of dislodging the cannula.
44 Remove gloves, if used.	
45 Ensure that the patient is comfortable.	
46 Record the administration on appropriate charts.	To maintain accurate records, provide a point of reference in the event of any queries and prevent any duplication of treatment.
47 Discard waste, placing it in the correct containers, e.g., sharps into a designated container.	To ensure safe disposal and avoid injury to staff. To prevent reuse of equipment.

Procedure guidelines: **Administration of drugs by direct injection, bolus or push**

This procedure may be carried out via any of the following:

1 The injection or Y site of an intravenous administration set.

2 An injection cap attached to any vascular access device.

3 An extension set, multiple adaptor or stopcock (one-, two- or three-way).

Equipment

1 Clinically clean receiver or tray containing the prepared drug(s) to be administered.

2 Patient's prescription chart.

3 Protective clothing as required by hospital policy or specific drugs.

4 Clean dressing trolley.

5 Clinically clean receiver or tray.

6 Sterile needles and syringes.

7 0.9% sodium chloride, 20 ml for injection or compatible solution.

8 Flushing solution, in accordance with hospital policy.

9 Alcohol-based solution for cleaning injection site, e.g. chlorhexidine in 70% alcohol.

10 Sterile dressing pack.

11 Hypoallergenic tape.

12 Sharps container.

Procedure

Action	Rationale
1 Explain and discuss the procedure with the patient.	To ensure that the patient understands the procedure and gives his/her valid consent.
2 Before administering any prescribed drug, check that it is due and has not been given already. Check that the information contained in the prescription chart is complete, correct and legible.	To protect the patient from harm.

3 Before administering any prescribed drug, consult the patient's prescription sheet and ascertain the following:
  (a) Drug
  (b) Dose
  (c) Date and time of administration
  (d) Route and method of administration
  (e) Diluent as appropriate
  (f) Validity of prescription
  (g) Signature of doctor
  (h) The prescription is legible.
	To ensure that the patient is given the correct drug in the prescribed dose using the appropriate diluent and by the correct route.
	To protect the patient from harm.
	To comply with NMC (2002a) *Guidelines for the Administration of Medicines.*

Procedure guidelines: **Administration of drugs by direct injection, bolus or push** *(cont'd)*

Action	Rationale
4 Select the required medication and check the expiry date.	Treatment with medication that is outside the expiry date is dangerous. Drugs deteriorate with storage. The expiry date indicates when a particular drug is no longer pharmacologically efficacious.
5 Wash hands with bactericidal soap and water or bactericidal alcohol handrub, and assemble necessary equipment.	To minimize the risk of infection.
6 Prepare the drug for injection as per procedure described earlier.	
7 Prepare a 20 ml syringe of 0.9% sodium chloride (or compatible solution) for injection, as described, using aseptic technique.	To use for flushing between each drug.
8 Draw up flushing solution, as required by hospital policy.	To prepare for administration.
9 Place syringes in a clinically clean receptacle on the bottom shelf of the dressing trolley, along with the receptacle containing any drug(s) to be administered.	To ensure top shelf is used for sterile dressing pack in order to minimize the risk of contamination.
10 Collect the other equipment and place it on the bottom of the trolley.	To ensure all equipment is available to commence procedure.
11 Place a sterile dressing pack on top of the trolley.	To minimize the risk of contamination.
12 Check that all necessary equipment is present.	To prevent delays and interruption of the procedure.
13 Wash hands thoroughly.	To minimize the risk of infection.
14 Proceed to the patient and check identity with prescription chart and prepared drug.	To minimize the risk of error and ensure the correct patient.
15 Open the sterile dressing pack. Add lotion to wet the low-linting swab.	
16 Wash hands with bactericidal soap and water or with bactericidal alcohol handrub.	To reduce the risk of infection.
17 If a peripheral device is in situ, remove the bandage and dressing (if appropriate).	To observe the insertion site.
18 Inspect the insertion site of the device.	To detect any signs of inflammation, infiltration, etc. If present, take appropriate action (Problem solving).
19 Observe the infusion, if in progress.	To confirm that it is infusing as desired.
20 Check whether the infusion fluid and the drugs are compatible. If not, change the infusion fluid to 0.9% sodium chloride to flush between the drugs.	To prevent drug interaction. Some manufacturers may recommend that the drug is given into the injection site of a rapidly running infusion.
21 Wash hands or clean them with an alcohol handrub.	To minimize the risk of infection.
22 Place a sterile towel under the patient's arm.	To create a sterile field.
23 Clean the injection site with a swab saturated with chlorhexidine in 70% alcohol and allow to dry.	To reduce the number of pathogens introduced by the needle at the time of the insertion. To ensure complete disinfection has occurred.
24 Switch off the infusion or close the fluid path of a tap or stopcock.	To prevent excessive pressure within the vein. To prevent contact with an incompatible infusion fluid. To allow the nurse to concentrate on the site of insertion and injection.
25 If a peripheral device is in situ use a sterile 23 or 25 G needle if the injection is made through a resealable site and gently inject 0.9% sodium chloride. This may not be necessary if the patient has a 0.9% sodium chloride infusion in progress.	To enable resealing of the site at the end of the injection. To confirm patency of the vein. To prevent contact with an incompatible infusion solution.
26 Open the roller clamp of the administration set fully. Inject the drug at a speed sufficient to slow but not	To prevent a back-flow of drug up the tubing. To prevent excessive pressure within the vein. To prevent speed shock.

*Procedure guidelines: **Administration of drugs by direct injection, bolus or push** (cont'd)*

Action	Rationale
stop the infusion and inject the drug smoothly in the direction of flow at the specified rate.	
27 Ensure used needles and syringes are disposed of immediately into appropriate sharps container (or are returned to tray). Do not leave any sharps on opened sterile pack.	To reduce the risk of needlestick injury and to prevent contamination of pack.
28 Observe the insertion site of the device throughout.	To detect any complications at an early stage, e.g. extravasation or local allergic reaction.
29 Blood return and/or 'flashback' must be checked frequently throughout the injection (i.e. every 3–5 ml; Weinstein 2000).	To confirm that the device is correctly placed and that the vein remains patent.
30 Consult the patient during the injection about any discomfort, etc.	To detect any complications at an early stage, and ensure patient comfort.
31 If more than one drug is to be administered, flush with 0.9% sodium chloride between administrations by restarting the infusion or changing syringes.	To prevent drug interactions.
32 At the end of the injection, flush with 0.9% sodium chloride by restarting the infusion or attaching a syringe containing 0.9% sodium chloride.	To flush any remaining irritant solution away from the device site.
33 Observe the insertion site of the cannula carefully.	To detect any complications at an early stage. Extra pressure within the vein caused by both fluid flow and injection of the drug may cause rupture.
34 After the final flush of 0.9% sodium chloride adjust the infusion rate as prescribed or open the fluid path of the tap/stopcock or use flushing solution.	To continue delivery of therapy. To maintain the patency of the cannula.
35 If a peripheral device is in situ cover the insertion site with new sterile low linting swab and tape it in place.	To minimize the risk of contamination of the insertion site.
36 Apply a bandage.	To reduce the risk of dislodging the cannula.
37 Make sure that the patient is comfortable.	
38 Record the administration on appropriate charts.	To maintain accurate records, provide a point of reference in the event of any queries and prevent any duplication of treatment.
39 Dispose of used syringes with needles, unsheathed, directly into a sharps container during procedure or place back on to plastic tray and then dispose of in a sharps container as soon as possible. *Do not* disconnect needle from syringe prior to disposal. Other waste should be placed into the appropriate plastic bags.	To avoid needlestick injury.

Problem solving

The problems associated with injection and infusion of intravenous fluids and drugs fall into two categories:

1 Local venous complications associated with the cannula insertion site.
2 Systemic problems which affect the whole patient, exerting effects on vital organs and their functions.

The nurse must regularly observe the insertion site, the infusion and the patient to detect any complications at the earliest possible moment and to prevent progression to more serious conditions. Early detection is aided by paying attention to the patient's comments of discomfort or pain. The patient's symptoms and physical signs both constitute reasons for resiting of the peripheral device or discontinuation of the infusion. Signs and symptoms are used as problem headings.

Problem solving (cont'd)

Problem	Possible causes	Preventive nursing measures	Suggested action
Infusion slows or stops.	Change in position of the following:		
	(a) Patient.	Check the height of the fluid container if the patient is active and receiving an infusion using gravity flow.	Adjust the height of the container accordingly. But the infusion should not hang higher than 1 m (above the patient) as the increased height will result in increased pressure and possible rupture of the vessel/device.
	(b) Limb.	Prevent by avoiding use of joints when inserting peripheral devices.	Move the arm or hand until infusion starts again.
		Instruct the patient on the amount of movement permitted. Continued movement could result in mechanical phlebitis.	Retape, bandage or splint the limb again carefully in the desired position. Take care not to cause damage to the limb.
	(c) Administration set.	Tape the administration set so that it cannot become kinked or occluded.	Check for kinks and/or compression if the patient is active or restless and correct accordingly.
	(d) Cannula.	Tape the cannula firmly to prevent movement. It may come into contact with the vein wall or a valve. Infusions sited in small veins are prone to this problem.	Remove the bandage and dressing and manoeuvre the peripheral device gently, without pulling it out of the vein, until the infusion starts again. Retape carefully.
	Technical problems:		
	(a) Negative pressure prevents flow of fluid.	Ensure that the container is vented using an air inlet.	Vent if necessary, using venting needle.
	(b) Empty container.	Check fluid levels regularly.	Replace the fluid container before it runs dry.
	(c) Venous spasm due to chemical irritation or cold fluids/drugs.	Dilute drugs as recommended. Remove solutions from the refrigerator a short time before use.	Apply a warm compress to soothe and dilate the vein, increase the blood flow and dilute the infusion mixture.
	(d) Injury to the vein.	Detect any injury early as it is likely to progress and cause more serious conditions (see below).	Stop the infusion and request resiting of the cannula.
	(e) Occlusion of the device due to fibrin formation.	Maintain a continuous, regular fluid flow or ensure that patency is maintained by flushing or by placement of a stylet. Instruct the patient to keep arm below the level of the heart if ambulant.	Remove extension set/injection cap and attempt to flush the cannula gently using a 10 ml syringe of 0.9% sodium chloride. If resistance is met, stop and request a resiting of the peripheral device (see Ch. 44, Vascular access devices).
	(f) The cannula has become displaced either completely or partially, i.e. fluid or drug has infiltrated into the surrounding tissues ('tissued'). If the drugs were vesicant in nature this would then be defined as extravasation.	Tape the cannula and the administration set so that no stress is placed on them. Instruct the patient on the amount of movement permitted.	Confirm that infiltration of drugs has/has not occurred by: (i) inspecting the site for leakage, swelling, etc.; (ii) testing the temperature of the skin – it will be cooler if infiltration has occurred; (iii) comparing the size of the limb with the opposite limb; (iv) lowering the infusion below the height of the limb. If the vein is patent, blood will flow back into the administration set.

Problem solving (cont'd)

Problem	Possible causes	Preventive nursing measures	Suggested action
			Once infiltration has been confirmed, stop the infusion and request a resiting of the device. If the infusion is allowed to progress, discomfort and tissue damage will result. Apply cold or warm compresses to provide symptomatic relief, whichever provides the most comfort for the patient. Reassure the patient by explaining what is happening.
			(v) If extravasation, follow hospital policy and procedure (see Ch. 10, Drug administration: cytotoxic drugs).
Erythema (inflammation) around the insertion site, and/or pain and swelling	Phlebitis due to:		Failure to detect and act when phlebitis is at an early stage, for whatever reason, will result in painful and incapacitating thrombophlebitis. Dislodgement of a thrombus could cause a pulmonary embolus (Lamb 1999; Weinstein 2000).
	(a) Sepsis.	Adhere to aseptic techniques when performing all intravenous procedures (RCN 2003)	Stop the infusion, remove the device and request the resiting of the cannula. Follow hospital policy about sending equipment for bacterial analysis. Clean the area and apply a sterile dressing. Check regularly.
	(b) Chemical irritation.	Dilute drugs according to instructions. Check compatibilities carefully to reduce the risk of particulate formation. Administer the drugs as an infusion instead of a bolus injection. Be aware of the factors involved, e.g. pH (Lamb 1999). Apply local heat above the cannula site (Lamb 1999). Apply a glycerol trinitrate (GTN) patch to aid vasodilatation (Wright *et al.* 1985; Hecker 1988).	Stop the infusion and request a resiting of the device. If the infusion is allowed to progress, tissue damage and severe pain will result. Apply cold or warm compresses to provide symptomatic relief. Encourage movement of the limb. Reassure the patient by explaining what is happening.
	(c) Mechanical irritation.	Tape, bandage or splint the limb if the infusion is sited at a point of flexion. Use an extension set to minimize manipulation of the device. Instruct the patient on the amount of movement permitted (Campbell 1996; Jackson 1998; Taylor 2000).	Stop the infusion and remove the device and request a resiting of the device. Although inflammation of this type progresses more slowly, it will cause discomfort. Provide symptomatic relief as above. Encourage movement and reassure the patient by explaining what is happening.
	Infection with or without discharge.	Adhere to aseptic techniques when performing all intravenous procedures. Observe all recommendations for equipment changes, etc.	Stop the infusion and request a resiting of the device. Follow hospital policy about sending equipment for bacterial analysis. Clean the area and apply a sterile dressing. Check regularly. Observe the patient for signs of systemic infection.
	Cellulitis due to: **(a)** Sepsis. **(b)** Non-specific sterile inflammation.	As above.	As above. Due to the nature of the connective tissue any infection or inflammation spreads quickly, especially if the limb is oedematous.

Problem solving (cont'd)

Problem	Possible causes	Preventive nursing measures	Suggested action
	Local allergic reaction, e.g. flare reaction which occurs with doxorubicin.	Ask whether the patient has any allergies before administration of any drugs or fluids, including sensitivities to topical solutions, which may cause erythema at the site. Check whether the particular medication is commonly associated with local or venous flushing.	Observe the patient for systemic reaction. Treat the local area symptomatically. Reassure the patient. Inform medical staff.
Local oedema.	During infusion or injection: (a) Infiltration. (b) Phlebitis. (c) Extravasation of medication (see Ch. 10, Drug administration: cytotoxic drugs).	Tape the device and administration set so that no stress is placed on the cannula. Use an extension set. Instruct the patient on the amount of movement permitted. Check regularly for swelling, e.g. tightness of bandages or around rings. Observe the patient carefully throughout drug administration.	Stop the infusion and request resiting of the cannula before proceeding. Apply warm compresses to provide symptomatic relief. Reassure the patient by explaining what is happening. Stop the injection immediately extravasation is suspected. Act in accordance with hospital policy. Some drugs may cause inflammation and supportive, symptomatic relief will be required. Others may have the potential to cause necrosis of tissue and further action may be necessary.
Oedema of the limb.	Infiltration.	Tape the device and administration set so that no stress is placed on the device, which in turn can lead to damage of the vein. Use an extension set. Instruct the patient on the amount of movement permitted. Check regularly for swelling, as above.	Stop the infusion and request resiting of the device. Provide symptomatic relief and support. Reassure the patient.
	Circulatory overload.	Administer infusion fluids at the prescribed rate and do not make sudden alterations of flow. Use infusion equipment wherever possible and administration set with anti free flow systems. Be aware of the patient's renal and cardiac status. Monitor intake and output routinely (Lamb 1999; Weinstein 2000).	Slow the infusion. Monitor vital signs for increase in blood pressure and respirations. Place the patient in an upright position and keep him/her warm to promote peripheral circulation and relieve stress on the central veins. Reassure the patient. Notify a doctor immediately.
Pain at the insertion site.	All of the previous listed conditions may be accompanied by soreness or pain.	As previously listed.	Provide local symptomatic relief, e.g. warmth, as required. Administer systemic analgesia, as prescribed, if necessary.
Pyrexia, rigors, tachycardia.	Septicaemia.	Adhere to aseptic techniques when performing all intravenous procedures. Inspect all equipment, infusion fluids, etc., before use. Observe recommendations for additives, equipment changes and general management. Avoid the use of equipment that can increase the risk of contamination, e.g. stopcocks (Lamb 1999).	Notify a doctor immediately. Follow hospital policy about sending equipment for bacterial analysis.

Problem solving (cont'd)

Problem	Possible causes	Preventive nursing measures	Suggested action
Decrease in blood pressure, tachycardia, cyanosis, unconsciousness.	Embolism: **(a)** Air.	Check the containers and change before they run through, especially bottles. Clear all air from tubing before commencing infusion. Check all connections regularly and make sure they are secure. Use infusion equipment with air in line detectors.	Turn the patient onto left side and lower the head of the bed to prevent air from entering the pulmonary artery. Notify a doctor immediately. Administer oxygen (Lamb 1999; Weinstein 2000; RCN 2003). Reassure the patient.
	(b) Particle.	Check all infusion fluids before and after any additions have been made. Check drug compatibility and stability. Observe the solution throughout the infusion for precipitate formation (Trissel 2003).	As above, but also change the container and administration set. Replace with new equipment and 0.9% sodium chloride infusion from a different batch. Follow hospital policy about sending contaminated fluid and equipment for bacterial analysis.
Itching, rash, shortness of breath.	Allergic reaction due to sensitivity to an intravenous fluid, additive or drug.	Ask the patient whether he/she has any allergies *before* administration of any drugs or fluids. Check whether the particular medication is commonly associated with any allergic reactions and observe the patient during treatment.	Stop drug infusion or injection and maintain the patency of the vascular access device using 0.9% sodium chloride. Notify a doctor immediately. Reassure the patient. Ensure that hydrocortisone and adrenaline are available.
Flushed face, headache, congestion of the chest, possibly progressing to loss of consciousness.	Speed shock due to too rapid administration of drugs. May be a small volume (Lamb 1999; Weinstein 2000).	Administer drugs and infusion at the correct rate. Check the flow rate frequently. Use infusion equipment with anti-free-flow administration sets if the delivery rate is crucial.	As above.

References and further reading

Allwood, M.C. (1984) Diamorphine mixed with antiemetic drugs in plastic syringes. *Br J Pharm Pract*, **6**, 88–90.

Arduino, M.J., Bland, L.A., Danzig, L.E. *et al.* (1997) Microbiological evaluation of needleless and needle access devices. *Am J Infect Control*, **25**(5), 377–80.

Arndt, M. (1994) Research and practice: how drug mistakes affect self-esteem. *Nurs Times*, **90**(15), 27–31.

Audit Commission (2001) *A Spoonful of Sugar: Medicines Management in NHS Hospitals*. Audit Commission, London.

Beyea, S.C. & Nicholl, L.sH. (1995) Administration of medications via the intramuscular route: an integrative review of the literature and research based protocol for the procedure. *Appl Nurs Res*, **5**(1), 23–33.

Bird, C. (1990) A prescription for self-care. *Nurs Times*, **86**(43), 52–5.

BMA & RPS (2003) British National Formulary. British Medical Association and Royal Pharmaceutical Association, London.

Brenneis, C. *et al.* (1987) Local toxicity during subcutaneous infusion of narcotics. *Cancer Nurs*, **10**(4), 172–6.

British Pharmacopoeia (2002) Volume 2. London, pp. 1860–909.

Brock, A.M. (1979) Self-administration of drugs in the elderly. *Nurs Forum*, **18**(4), 340–57.

Brown, J., Moss, H. & Elliot, T. (1997) The potential for catheter microbial contamination from a needleless connector. *J Hosp Infect*, **36**(3), 181–9.

Bruera, E., Legis, M.A. & Kuehn, N. (1990) Hypodermoclysis for the administration of fluids and narcotic analgesics in patients with advanced cancer. *J Pain Sympt Manage*, **5**(4), 218–20.

Burden, M. (1994) A practical guide to insulin injections. *Nurs Stand*, **8**(29), 25–9.

Campbell, J. (1996) Intravenous drug therapy. *Prof Nurse*, **11**(7), 437–42.

Central Health Services Council (1958) *Report of Joint Sub-Committee on the Control of Dangerous Drugs and Poisons in Hospitals* (Chairman J.K. Aitken). Stationery Office, London.

Cerchietti, L., Navigante, A., Sauri, A. & Palazzo, F. (2000) Hypodermoclysis for control of dehydration in terminal-stage cancer. *Int J Palliat Nurs*, **6**(8), 370–4.

Cole, D. (1999) Selection and management of central venous access devices in the home setting. *J Intravenous Nurs*, **22**(6), 315–19.

Constans, T. *et al.* (1991) Hypodermoclysis in dehydrated elderly patients – local effects with and without hyaluronidase. *J Palliat Care*, **7**(2), 10–12.

Cookson, S. *et al.* (1998) Increased blood stream infection rates in surgical patients associated with variation from recommended use and care following implementation of a needleless device. *Infect Control Hosp Epidemiol*, **19**(1), 23–7.

Cresswell, J. (1999) *Nurse Prescribing Handbook*. Association of Nurse Prescribing and Community Nurse, UK.

Daniels, L.E. (1995) The physical and psychosocial implications of central venous access devices in cancer patients: a review of the literature. *J Cancer Care*, **4**, 141–5.

Dann, T.C. (1969) Routine skin preparation before injection: an unnecessary procedure. *Lancet*, **ii**, 96–7.

Danzig, L.E. *et al.* (1995) Bloodstream infections associated with a needleless intravenous infusion system in patients receiving home infusion therapy. *JAMA*, **273**(23), 1862–4.

Dawkins, L., Britton, D., Johnson, I., Higgins, B. & Dean, T. (2000) A randomised trial of winged Vialon cannulae and metal butterfly needles. *Int J Palliat Nurs*, **6**(3), 110–16.

Deeks, P. & Byatt, K. (2000) Are patients who self-administer their medicines in hospital more satisfied with their care? *J Adv Nurs*, **31**(2), 395–400.

Department of Health (2001) *National Service Framework for Older People*. Stationery Office, London.

DHSS (1976) *Health Services Development, Addition of Drugs to Intravenous Fluids, HC(76)9 (Breckenridge Report)*. Stationery Office, London.

Dickman, A., Littlewood, C. & Varga, J. (2002) Compatibility data tables. In: *The Syringe Driver: Continuous Subcutaneous Infusions in Palliative Care*. Oxford University Press, Oxford, pp. 75–150.

DoH (1988) *Guidelines for the Safe and Secure Handling of Medicines (The Duthie Report)*. Stationery Office, London.

DoH (1989) *Report of the Advisory Group on Nurse Prescribing*. Crown One. Stationery Office, London.

DoH (1998) *Review of Prescribing, Supply and Administration of Medicines. A Report on the Supply and Administration of Medicines under Group Protocols*. Crown Two. Stationery Office, London.

DoH (1999) *Review of Prescribing, Supply and Administration of Medicines. Final Report*. Crown Three. Stationery Office, London.

DoH (2001) Guidelines for preventing infections associated with the insertion and maintenance of central venous catheters. *J Hosp Infect*, **47**(Suppl), S47–67.

DoH (2003a) *Supplementary Prescribing*. NHS, London. www.doh.gov.uk/supplementary prescribing.

DoH (2003b) *Supplementary Prescribing by Nurses and Pharmacists within the NHS in England*. NHS, London.

Donnelly, M. (1999) The benefits of hypodermoclysis. *Nurs Stand*, **13**(52), 44–5.

Dorr, T. & Von Hoff, D. (1993) *Cancer Chemotherapy Handbook*, 2nd edn. Appleton & Lange, Hemel Hempstead.

Dougherty, L. (1997) Reducing risks of complications in IV therapy. *Nurs Stand*, **12**(5), 40–2.

Dougherty, L. (2002) Delivery of intravenous therapy. *Nurs Stand*, **16**(16), 45–52.

Downie, G., MacKenzie, J. & Williams, A. (2000) Administration of medicines. In: *Pharmacology and Drugs Management for Nurses*, 2nd edn. Churchill Livingstone, London, pp. 495–557.

Ellershaw, J. *et al.* (1995) Dehydration and the dying patient. *J Pain Symptom Manage*, **10**(3), 192–7.

Epperson, E.L. (1984) Efficacy of 0.9% sodium chloride injection with and without heparin for maintaining indwelling intermittent injection sites. *Clin Pharm*, **3**, 626–9.

Fainsinger, R. & Bruera, E. (1997) When to treat dehydration in a terminally ill patients. *Support Care Cancer*, **5**, 205–11.

Fainsinger, R. *et al.* (1994) The use of hypodermoclysis for rehydration of terminally ill cancer patients. *J Pain Symptom Manage*, **9**, 298–302.

Ferrand, S. & Campbell, A. (1996) Safe, simple subcutaneous fluid administration. *Br J Hosp Med*, **55**(11), 690–2.

Field, P.A. (1981) A phenomenological look at giving an injection. *J Adv Nurs*, **6**(4), 291–6.

Gatford, J. & Anderson, R. (1998) *Nursing Calculations*, 5th edn. Churchill Livingstone, Edinburgh.

Gladstone, J. (1995) Drug administration errors: a study into the factors underlying the occurrence and reporting of drug errors in a district general hospital. *J Adv Nurs*, **22**(4), 628–37.

Glynn, A. *et al.* (1997) *Hospital Acquired Infection – Surveillance Policies and Practice*. Central Public Health Laboratory, London.

Hamilton, H. & Fermo, K. (1998) Assessment of patients requiring IV therapy via a central venous route. *Br J Nurs*, **7**(8), 451–60.

Hanchett, M. & Kung, L.Y. (1999) Do needleless intravenous systems increase the risk of infection? *J Intravenous Nurs*, **22**(6), 117–21.

Hirsch, C. & Faull, C. (2000) Standards for setting up and maintaining subcutaneous drug administration via a syringe driver. Poster, Palliative Care Congress, University of Warwick.

Hockley, J. *et al.* (1995) Audit to pinpoint IV drug administration pitfalls. *Nurs Times*, **91**(51), 33–4.

Hutton, M. (1998) Numeracy skills for IV calculations. *Nurs Stand*, **12**(43), 49–56.

Hyde, L. (2002) Legal and professional aspects of intravenous therapy. *Nurs Stand*, **16**(26), 39–42.

Hypodermoclysis Working Group (2000) *Hypodermoclysis – Guidelines on the Technique*. CP Pharmaceuticals, Wrexham.

Intravenous Nursing Society (1998) Revised intravenous nursing standards of practice. *J Intraven Nurs*, **21**(15), Suppl 1S.

Jackson, A. (1998) A battle in vein infusion phlebitis. *Nurs Times*, **94**(4), 68–71.

Jones, V.A. & Hanks, G.W. (1986) New portable infusion pump for prolonged administration of opioid analgesics in patients with advanced cancer. *Br Med J*, **292**, 1496.

Josephson, A. *et al.* (1985) The relationship between intravenous fluid contamination and the frequency of tubing replacement. *Infect Control*, **9**, 367–70.

Koivistov, V.A. & Felig, P. (1978) Is skin preparation necessary before insulin injection? *Lancet*, **i**, 1072–3.

Kuhn, M.M. (1989) *Pharmacotherapeutics. A Nursing Process Approach*, 2nd edn. F.A. Davis, Philadelphia.

Lamb, J. (1999) Local and systemic complications of intravenous therapy. In: *Intravenous Therapy in Nursing Practice* (eds L. Dougherty & J. Lamb). Churchill Livingstone, Edinburgh, pp. 163–93.

Laverty, D., Mallett, J. & Mulholland, J. (1997) Protocols and guidelines for managing wounds. *Prof Nurse*, **13**(2), 79–80.

Lenz, C.L. (1983) Make your needle selection right to the point. *Nursing (US)*, **13**(2), 50–1.

Lipschitz, S., Campbell, A.J., Roberts, M.S. *et al.* (1991) Subcutaneous fluid administration in elderly subjects: validation of an underused technique. *J Am Geriatr Soc*, **39**, 6–9.

Lonsway, R.A. (2001) IV therapy in the home. In: *Infusion Therapy in Clinical Practice*, 2nd edn. W.B. Saunders, Philadelphia, pp. 501–34.

Luebke, M.A. *et al.* (1998) Comparison of the microbial barrier properties of a needleless and conventional needle based intravenous access system. *Am J Infect Control*, **26**, 437–41.

Luker, K. & Wolfson, D. (eds) (1999) Introduction. In: *Medicines Management for Clinical Nurses*. Blackwell Science, Oxford.

Luker, K.A., Austin, L., Hogg, C. *et al.* (1998) Nurse–patient relationships: the context of nurse prescribing. *J Adv Nurs*, **28**, 235–42.

Maki, D.G. (1992) Infections due to infusion therapy. In: *Hospital Infections* (eds J.V. Bennett & P.S. Bradman), 3rd edn. Little, Brown & Co., Boston.

Maki, D.G. & Ringer, M. (1987) Evaluation of dressing regimens for prevention of infection with peripheral intravenous catheters. *J Am Med Assoc*, **256**(17), 2396–403.

Maki, D. *et al.* (1987) Prospective study replacing administration sets for intravenous therapy, at 48 to 72 hour intervals. *J Am Med Assoc*, **258**(13), 1777–81.

Mallett, J., Faithfull, S., Guerrero, D. *et al.* (1997) Nurse prescribing by protocol. *Nurs Times*, **93**(8), 50–2.

Martin, P.J. (1994) Professional updating through open learning as a method of reducing errors in the administration of medicines. *J Nurs Manage*, **2**(5), 209–12.

McClelland, B. (2001) *Handbook of Transfusion Medicine*, 2nd edn. HMSO, London.

McGraw, C. & Drennan, V. (2001) Self administration of medicine and older people. *Nurs Stand*, **15**(18), 33–6.

McHale, J. (2002) Extended prescribing: the legal implications. *Nurs Times*, **98**(32), 36–8.

Mendelson, M.H. *et al.* (1998) Study of a needleless intermittent intravenous access system for peripheral infusions: analysis of staff, patient and institutional outcomes. *Infect Control Hosp Epidemiol*, **19**(6), 401–6.

Mitten, T. (2001) Subcutaneous drug infusions: a review of problems and solutions. *Int J Palliat Nurs*, **7**(2), 75–85.

NHS Executive (2000) *Health Service Circular HSC 2000/26. Patient Group Directions (England Only)*. SI 2000, No. 1919. NHS Executive, Leeds.

NHSE (1998a) *Nurse Prescribing. A Guide for Implementation*. Stationery Office, London.

NHSE (1998b) *Nurse Prescribing. Implementing the Scheme Across England*. HSC 1998/232. Stationery Office, London.

Nicol, M. (1999) Safe administration of IV therapy. In: *Intravenous Therapy in Nursing Practice* (eds L. Dougherty & J. Lamb). Churchill Livingstone, Edinburgh.

Nicolson, H. (1986) The success of the syringe driver. *Nurs Times*, **82**, 49–51.

NMC (2001a) *Covert Administration of Medicines can be Justified*. Press statement, 5th September. Nursing and Midwifery Council, London.

NMC (2001b) *UKCC Position Statement on the Covert Administration of Medicines – Disguising Medicine in Food and Drink*. Nursing and Midwifery Council, London.

NMC (2001c) Circular 25/2002. Nursing and Midwifery Council, London.

NMC (2002a) *Guidelines for the Administration of Medicines*. Nursing and Midwifery Council, London.

NMC (2002b) *Code of Professional Conduct*. Nursing and Midwifery Council, London.

Noble-Adams, R. (1995) Dehydration: subcutaneous fluid administration. *Br J Nurs*, **4**(9), 488–94.

NPC (National Prescribing Centre) (2001) *Maintaining Competency in Prescribing: An Outline Framework to Help Nurse Prescribers*. NHS, London.

NPC (2003a) *Supplementary Prescribing. A Resource to Help Healthcare Professionals to Understand the Framework and Opportunities*. NHS, London.

NPC (2003b) *Maintaining Competency in Prescribing: An Outline Framework to Help Nurse Supplementary Prescribers*. NHS, London.

Nystrom, B. *et al.* (1983) Bacteraemia in surgical patients with intravenous devices: a European multicentre incidence study. *J Hosp Infect*, **4**, 338–49.

Osbourne, J., Blais, K. & Hayes, J.S. (1999) Nurses' perceptions: when is it a medication error? *J Nurs Admin*, **29**(4), 33–8.

Pelletier, G. (1995) Intravenous therapy calculations. In: *Intravenous Therapy: Clinical Principles and Practices* (eds J. Terry, L. Baranowski, R.A. Lonsway *et al.*), W.B. Saunders, Philadelphia, pp. 366–78.

Peragallo-Dittko, V. (1997) Rethinking subcutaneous injection technique. *Am J Nurs*, **97**(5), 71–2.

Perdue, L. (1995) Intravenous complications. In: *Intravenous Therapy: Clinical Principles and Practices* (eds J. Terry, L. Baranowski, R.A. Lonsway, *et al.*), pp. 419–46. W.B. Saunders Philadelphia.

Perucca, R. (1995) Obtaining vascular access. In: *Intravenous Therapy: Clinical Principles and Practices* (eds J. Terry, L. Baranowski, R.A. Lonsway *et al.*), pp. 377–91. W.B. Saunders, Philadelphia.

Pickstone, M. (1999) *A Pocketbook for Safer IV Therapy*. Medical Technology and Risk Series, Scitech.

RCN (2003) *Standards for Infusion Therapy*. Royal College of Nursing, London.

Regnard, C.F. & Davies, A. (1986) *A Guide to Symptom Relief in Advanced Cancer*. Haigh and Hochland, Manchester.

Rodger, M.A. & King, L. (2000) Drawing up and administering intra-muscular injection: a review of the literature. *J Adv Nurs*, **31**(3), 574–82.

Ross, J.R., Saunders, Y., Cochrane, M. & Zepetella, G. (2002) A prospective, within-patient comparison between metal butterfly needles and Teflon cannulae in subcutaneous infusion of drugs to terminally ill hospice patients. *Palliat Med*, **16**, 13–16.

Royal Pharmaceutical Society of Great Britain (1997) *From Compliance to Concordance*. Royal Pharmaceutical Society of Great Britain, London.

Sani, M. (1999) Pharmacological aspects of IV therapy. In: *Intravenous Therapy in Nursing Practice* (eds L. Dougherty & J. Lamb). Churchill Livingstone, Edinburgh.

Scales, K. (1996) Legal and professional aspects of intravenous therapy. *Nurs Stand*, **11**(3), 41–8.

Sexton, J. (1999) The nurse's role in medicines administration – legal and procedural framework. In: *Medicines Management for Clinical Nurses* (eds K. Luker & D. Wolfson). Blackwell Science, Oxford.

Shepherd, M. (2002a) Medicines 2. Administration of medicines. *Nurs Times*, **98**(16), 45–8.

Shepherd, M. (2002b) Medicines 3. Managing medicines. *Nurs Times*, **98**(17), 43–6.

Simmonds, B.P. (1983) CDC guidelines for the prevention and control of nosocomial infections: guidelines for prevention of intravascular infections. *Am J Infect Control*, **11**(5), 183–9.

Speechley, V. (1986) The nurse's role in intravenous management. *Nurs Times*, 2 May, 31–2.

Speechley, V. & Toovey, J. (1987) Factsheets: problems in IV therapy 1, 2, 3. *Prof Nurse*, **2**(8), 240–42; **2**(12), 413; **3**(3), 90–1.

Springhouse Corporation (1999) *Handbook of Infusion Therapy.* Springhouse, Pennsylvania.

Steiner, N. & Bruera, E. (1998) Methods of hydration in palliative care patients. *J Palliat Care*, **14**(2), 6–13.

Taxis, K. & Barber, N. (2003) Ethnographic study on the incidence and severity of intravenous drug errors. *Br Med J*, **326**, 684–7.

Taylor, N.J. (2000) Fascination with phlebitis. *Vasc Access Devices*, **5**(3), 24–8.

Torrence, C. (1989) Intramuscular injection, part 1 and 2. *Surg Nurses*, **2**(5), 6–10; **2**(6), 24–7.

Treloar, A., Beats, B. & Philpot, M. (2000) A pill in the sandwich: covert medication in food and drink. *J R Soc Med*, **93**, 408–11.

Trissel, L.A. (2003) *Handbook on Injectable Drugs*, 12th edn. American Society of Health System Pharmacists, Bethesda.

Trounce, J. & Gould, D. (2000) *Clinical Pharmacology for Nurses*, 16th edn. Churchill Livingstone, London.

Twycross, R., Willcock, A. & Thorp, S. (1998) Syringe drivers. In: *Palliative Care Formulary*. Radcliffe Medical Press, Oxford, pp. 183–202.

Weinstein, S.M. (2000) *Plumer's Principles and Practices of Intravenous Therapy*, 7th edn. Lippincott, Philadelphia.

Wilson-Barnett, J. & Batehup, L. (1992) *Patients' Problems: A Research Base for Nursing Care*, Chapter 3. Scutari Press, London.

Workman, B. (1999) Safe injection techniques. *Nurs Stand*, **13**(39), 47–52.

Wright, A. *et al.* (1985) Use of transdermal glyceryl trinitrate to reduce failure of intravenous infusion due to phlebitis and extravasation. *Lancet*, **ii**, 1148–50.

10

Drug administration: cytotoxic drugs

Chapter contents

Definition

The term cytotoxic literally translated means 'toxic to cells'. Hence these drugs are those which kill cells (malignant or non-malignant).

Reference material

Cytotoxic drug handling by nursing, pharmacy and other health care professionals has been acknowledged as an occupational hazard (Ferguson & Wright 2002). Cytotoxic drugs have been shown to be mutagenic, teratogenic and carcinogenic when given at therapeutic levels to animals and humans to destroy malignant cells (Dougherty 1999; Goodman 2000). Patients have been shown to develop secondary cancers as a result of treatment with cytotoxic drugs and such risks may be acceptable when patients have a life-threatening illness (Ferguson & Wright 2002). However, these effects are not acceptable to personnel involved in the reconstitution and administration of cytotoxic drugs and the handling of waste and spills. The risk to health associated with exposure is measured by the time, dose and routes of exposure. Cytotoxic drugs can be absorbed through the skin (although with the majority of the compounds there is little or no absorption through intact skin, the exceptions are those which are lipid soluble) (Weinstein 2000). Skin exposure can be by contact with contaminated equipment used in preparing or administering the drugs or during the handling and disposal of waste. In the latter instance this is because drugs and metabolites can be excreted in urine and stools up to 48 hours after administration (Valanis *et al.* 1993; Ferguson & Wright 2002). Drugs can also be ingested by contaminated food, or be inhaled as a result of aerosolization of powder or liquid during reconstitution. On the basis of the evidence available at present, risks to personnel involved in the reconstitution and administration of cytotoxic drugs fall into two categories – local effects and systemic effects:

- Local effects are usually caused by direct contact with the skin, eyes and mucous membranes, e.g. dermatitis, inflammation of mucous membranes, excessive lacrimation, pigmentation, blistering (associated with mustine) and other miscellaneous, allergic reactions (Goodman 2000; Weinstein 2000).
- Cytotoxic drugs may also have harmful short- or long-term systemic effects if inhaled or ingested during preparation. These effects include light-headedness, dizziness, nausea, headache, rashes and skin discoloration (Goodman 2000).

A number of experimental studies have suggested that serious long-term effects may result from exposure to cytotoxic drugs. Effects include chromosomal abnormalities (Waksvik et al. 1987) and reproductive function disorders including infertility (Selevan et al. 1985; Valanis et al. 1997). Mutagenic substances have been found in the urine and serum of cytotoxic drug handlers, including nurses (Ames et al. 1975; Falck et al. 1979; Vennit et al. 1984; Kaijser et al. 1990; Newman et al. 1994). It has been shown that although alterations in cell structure have been detected, they appear to be transient and of a low level. It has yet to be demonstrated whether these changes in cell structure are harmful and whether this level of mutagenesis can be equated with more serious consequences. There are also many limitations in testing blood and urine due to the range of agents which cannot be detected, low levels of drugs and metabolites and reduced sensitivity of the tests (Ferguson & Wright 2002). This has led to difficulties when offering staff monitoring and surveillance and it is less common to do extensive biological testing as there are no data to support a cause and effect.

The hazards of handling cytotoxic drugs are well recognized along with the requirement to adhere to safety measures recommended in order to protect all staff who prepare, administer and handle cytotoxic drugs or waste products. *Control of Substances Hazardous to Health (COSHH) Regulations* were introduced and updated in 2002. Under these regulations employers are obliged to identify substances which are a hazard to staff, as well as who may be exposed, how the drugs should be handled and what to do in the event of a spill or accident. They also ensure that staff have access to the ideal environment, protective clothing, policies and procedures, a system of monitoring and recording effects, and any necessary equipment such as spill kits (RCN 1998). This includes consideration of the following:

1 The environment: the most effective means of minimizing the hazard is to arrange for all cytotoxic drugs to be prepared on a named patient basis by trained pharmacy staff in a specially equipped area (RCN 1998;

Dougherty 1999). Chemotherapy should be reconstituted in a vertical class II or III biological safety cabinet with laminar flow or an isolator if drugs are prepared on the ward (RCN 1998; ONS 1999; Goodman 2000; Weinstein 2000; Ferguson & Wright 2002). Cabinets should be situated in a specified or dedicated area with access restricted to trained or supervised personnel.

2 Protective clothing: protective clothing should always be worn during all types of cytotoxic drug handling. There are minimum requirements for the type and degree of protective clothing which are based on possible exposure and type of environment.

(a) Gloves: gloves should be worn at all times and appear to be the only type of protective clothing which most practitioners consistently wear when handling cytotoxic drugs (Dougherty 1999). No type of glove is completely impermeable to every cytotoxic agent and there is no consensus as to which glove material offers the best protection (Dougherty 1999; Goodman 2000; Weinstein 2000). The key points to consider when selecting gloves are thickness and integrity as the main factors which affect permeation rates include glove thickness, lipophilicity, the nature of the solvent in which the cytotoxic drug is dissolved and glove material composition (Weinstein 2000; Ferguson & Wright 2002). Using poor-quality low-cost gloves is neither safe nor cost effective. The risk of allergic reactions in health care workers to latex and powdered medical gloves has been well documented in recent years. The NHSE issued a Health Service Circular (HSC 1999/186) which recommended that health care organizations limit their use of these types of gloves. Powder-free gloves should be used for handling cytotoxic drugs. If gloves are changed regularly during each work session, and immediately if contaminated with cytotoxic agent or punctured, then double gloving should be unnecessary (Ferguson & Wright 2002). It appears that most authors agree that double gloving is only required in the case of dealing with a spill.

(b) Gowns: the literature supports the use of a disposable gown for both reconstitution and administration. It has been suggested that a long-sleeved, non-absorbent gown made of a low-linting, low-permeability material such as Tyvek is used (Powell 1996; Cass et al. 1997; Weinstein 2000). Armlets and plastic aprons can be substituted for long-sleeved gowns during administration, and some experts recommend the use of Sarcrex laminated or Tyvek aprons to provide protection (Ferguson & Wright 2002).

(c) Goggles: goggles are used to protect the eyes from splashes and particles and should fully cover the eyes to protect the handler. Goggles should meet EN 166-168 requirements and be worn whenever reconstituting or dealing with a spill (Goodman 2000; Ferguson & Wright 2002).

(d) Masks: these should be worn whenever there is a possibility of inhalation or the drug is being prepared in an uncontrolled environment. Masks should conform to BSEN149: 1992 standard. The key factor with regard to requirements for respiratory protective equipment is that it fits well and is sealed properly to the wearer's face. A range of different sizes of disposable masks should be made available to health care workers (Ferguson & Wright 2002). A suitable dust mask or particulate respirator, such as the 3M 8810, affords the best protection.

There is no doubt that the existence of a formal hospital policy for handling has been shown to have a positive influence in the use of personal protective equipment yet it appears that there may be poor compliance among practitioners regarding guidelines and policies, and many health care workers underestimate the risk of exposure from cytotoxic drugs (ONS 1999; Goodman 2000; Ferguson & Wright 2002).

Risk assessment

A full risk assessment under the *COSHH Regulations* must be made by all departments and wards handling, preparing or administering cytotoxics. The assessment should identify all appropriate procedures for the safety of staff. A generic COSHH assessment form for the administration and reconstitution of chemotherapy out of hours should be kept in all ward COSHH assessment files. Ward sisters/charge nurses have a duty to ensure that all staff on the ward are made aware of the COSHH assessment procedures.

The questionnaire should include details of the individual performing the procedure, patient's details and the reason for which the reconstitution was performed. Information from the questionnaires can then be collated and passed to the safety committee, e.g. the Safe Handling of Hazardous Therapeutic Substances (SHOHTS) Committee which should include the consultant occupational health doctor and representatives from pharmacy, clinical divisions, wards and Health and Safety. All cases of reconstitution out of hours should be reviewed and procedures that did not comply with the Safe Handling Policy investigated. Recommendations can then be proposed to the Health and Safety Committee.

Occupational health offers staff protection by monitoring. Routine health surveillance should be carried out for staff directly involved in handling cytotoxics on a regular basis, e.g. certain staff working in the pharmacy. Routine health surveillance is not usually performed for individuals reconstituting on isolated occasions. However, in the unlikely event that some nursing staff are reconstituting on a regular basis they can be monitored by the Cytotoxic Health Surveillance Programme. This comprises regular general health screening and the use of specific tests to determine if an individual has been exposed to harmful levels of cytotoxic substances.

Health surveillance is carried out by:

1. Annual 'cytotoxic health questionnaires' which cover:
   - Detailed medical history of the individuals
   - Exposure record
   - Personal protective equipment used
   - Control measures in place
   - Symptoms which may be attributed to the effects of harmful levels of cytotoxic drugs, e.g. headache, dizziness, eye or skin irritation.
2. Six-monthly blood tests are taken which include full blood count, urea and electrolytes and liver function tests.
3. Six-monthly urinalysis is performed to detect raised protein, presence of glucose, blood and bilirubin and to detect any abnormal cytology.
4. In the event that any abnormalities are present, the individual is referred to the occupational health doctor.

The Health and Safety Executive (2003) have now produced a document on the safe handling of cytotoxic drugs. National evidence-based guidelines have been implemented in an attempt to reduce exposure, provide adequate protective equipment, ensure regular staff monitoring and provide effective written procedures for dealing with preparation, administration, disposal and dealing with spills and accidents (RCN 1998; Dougherty 1999). In order to limit exposure, cytotoxic drugs should only be prepared by skilled, knowledgeable and experienced health care professionals (ONS 1999; Goodman 2000; Langhorne & Barton-Burke 2001).

Procedure guidelines: **Protection of the environment**

The safest method of reconstituting cytotoxic drugs outside a pharmacy department is to use an isolator. There is a variety of systems and each will have specific instructions for its use. The following procedure is for the Envair 'Mini-Iso' isolator. The system creates a negative pressure in the isolator by drawing air out by a fan and passing it through a HEPA filter, which will trap any cytotoxic drug powder or aerosol which may escape from the drug vial during reconstitution.

*Procedure guidelines: **Protection of the environment** (cont'd)*

When used as instructed the isolator will minimize the risk to nurses when reconstituting any dose of cytotoxic drugs, but it will not protect the drug from the risk of microbial contamination so aseptic technique must always be used.

Nursing staff should not be involved in the routine reconstitution of cytotoxic drugs, as this is the function of the pharmacy department. However, there may be emergency situations when the nurse is requested to prepare chemotherapy and it is essential that this is performed safely. It should only be undertaken by competent, confident staff who have received appropriate training and have previous experience in the procedures required. The following procedure should be used for guidance.

Safe reconstitution using an isolator

Equipment

1 One pair of disposable non-sterile gloves.
2 Syringes, needles.

3 Drug to be reconstituted and appropriate diluent.
4 Appropriate cleaning solution.

Procedure

Action	Rationale
1 Prior to commencing reconstitution carefully check the gauntlets, especially the fingers and at the point of attachment to the isolator.	The gauntlets are designed for prolonged use, they need to be changed when torn or punctured.
2 Place hand through slot on right of the top cover of the isolator and press the green button.	To enable the isolator to be switched on.
3 Allow the isolator to run for 3–4 minutes and ensure that the gauge needle is reading over 50 pascals before use.	To ensure that the isolator is prepared to be operated safely.
4 Assemble all equipment required.	To avoid interruption of work.
5 Put on a pair of non-sterile gloves which should be worn under the isolator gloves and when passing equipment into or out of the isolator.	To provide extra operator protection in case of damage to the gauntlets while preparing the drug.
6 Open the door on the right side of the isolator by turning the handle anticlockwise through 180°.	To allow equipment to be placed inside the isolator.
7 Place equipment into the isolator and close and lock the door (by turning 180° clockwise).	To ensure doors are securely closed so that negative pressure can be achieved.
8 Place hands into gauntlets.	
9 Reconstitute the dose in the usual way (see Ch. 9, Drug administration) using aseptic technique.	To minimize the risk of contamination.
10 Move everything to the right prior to removing hands from gauntlets.	To enable easy removal of the prepared drug and waste.
11 Leave the isolator fan on.	To ensure any spills/aerosols are contained within the isolator.
12 Open the isolator door and remove all equipment.	
13 Dispose of waste in usual way.	To reduce the risk of contamination and needlestick injury.
14 Moisten a sheet of paper with cleaning spray provided and wipe inside of isolator.	To maintain equipment in good clean working order.
15 Turn off isolator by pushing green button.	
16 Complete cytotoxic reconstitution surveillance form and send to occupational health department.	To ensure follow-up and health surveillance check.

Management of spillage

Equipment

1 Two plastic overshoes.
2 Two disposable armlets.

3 Two clinical waste bags.
4 Two pairs of disposable non-sterile latex or nitrile gloves.

*Procedure guidelines: **Protection of the environment** (cont'd)*

5 Goggles (non-disposable) – EN 166-168.
6 Particulate respirator mask.
7 Plastic apron.
8 Gown.

9 Paper towels.
10 Plastic bucket.
11 Copy of spillage procedure.

Procedure

Action	Rationale
1 Act immediately.	Any spillage may become a health hazard.
2 Collect spillage kit.	It contains all necessary equipment.
3 Put on both pairs of gloves, goggles and a gown and then a disposable plastic apron over the gown.	To provide personal protection.
4 If there is visible powder spill, put on a good-quality particulate respirator mask.	To prevent inhalation of powder.
5 If spillage is on the floor, put on overshoes.	For protection and to minimize the spread of contamination.
6 Wipe up powder spillage quickly with well dampened paper towels, starting at the outer edge of the spill area and working in a circular motion towards the middle to contain spill (Cass *et al.* 1997), and dispose of them as 'high-risk' waste.	To prevent dispersal of powder. To prevent spread of contamination to a wider area. To protect others and ensure safe disposal by incineration.
7 Mop up liquids which have been spilled on a hard surface with paper towels, starting at the outer edge of the spill area and working in a circular motion towards the middle to contain spill (Cass *et al.* 1997), and dispose of them as 'high-risk' waste.	To prevent spread of contamination to a wider area. To protect others and ensure safe disposal by incineration.
8 Wash hard surfaces at least twice with copious amounts of cold, soapy water and dry with paper towels. The floor should then be given a routine clean as soon afterwards as possible. If spillage has occurred on a carpet it will require cleaning as soon as possible.	To remove residual contamination.
9 If spillage is on clothing, remove it as soon as possible and treat as 'soiled linen'.	To decontaminate clothing without hazard to laundry staff.
10 If spillage has penetrated clothing, wash contaminated skin liberally with soap and cold water.	To decontaminate skin and prevent drug absorption.
11 If spillage is on bed linen put on gloves and an apron, change it immediately and treat as 'soiled linen'.	To protect the patient. To protect the laundry staff.
12 If an accident or spillage involving direct skin contact occurs, the area should be washed thoroughly with soapy water as soon as possible. In the event of a cytotoxic splash to the eye, irrigate thoroughly with 0.9% sodium chloride or tap water for approximately 2 minutes.	To decontaminate the area and minimize the risk of drug absorption and damage.
13 Any accident or spillage by nursing staff involving direct skin contact with a cytotoxic drug must be reported to the occupational health department and manager as soon as possible after the first aid is performed and appropriate documentation completed (see Guidelines below).	To ensure that details of accidental contact are entered in the nurse's health record, and appropriate follow-up is initiated.

*Procedure guidelines: **Protection of the environment** (cont'd)*

Health surveillance for a spillage involving skin contact with cytotoxic drugs

Action

1 Complete cytotoxic incident investigation form:
  - Full details of the incident.
  - Details of the immediate first aid provided, e.g. washing and removal of contaminated clothing.
  - Details of personal protective equipment worn at the time.
  - The full name of the drug involved and the individual components of the constituent, including diluents.

2 A risk assessment is performed using the information provided. The risk assessment evaluates the health association with the exposure which itself is measured by the time, dose and routes of exposure.

3 Completion of the Cytotoxic Health Questionnaire which includes a detailed medical history of the individual and examination. Details of immediate effects are noted, e.g. skin effects, headaches, dizziness, and if changes are present the employee is referred to the occupational health doctor for further assessment, advice and treatment.

4 Blood tests are taken which include routine blood count and biochemistry and liver function tests.

5 Urinalysis is performed and details of protein, glucose, blood, bilirubin and bladder cytology are noted.

6 The occupational health nurse will contact the Health and Safety team to obtain details of risk assessments performed on the ward.

7 Repeat bloods should be taken on day 7 and day 28 following the incident and any health effects noted. If there are any changes, the employee should be referred to the occupational health doctor.

Disposal of waste

Action	Rationale
1 'Sharps' should be placed in the special container provided.	To ensure incineration and to prevent laceration and/or inoculation during transit and disposal.
2 Dry waste, intravenous administration sets and other contaminated material should be placed in 'high-risk' waste disposal bags.	To ensure careful handling and disposal by incineration.
3 Any part dose of a drug remaining should be placed in a special waste container.	
4 Reusable trays and other equipment should be washed with copious amounts of water followed by the usual procedure for disinfection.	To reduce the risk of cross-contamination and cross-infection.
5 Unused doses of cytotoxics should be returned, unopened, to the pharmacy.	To enable them to be relabelled and reissued, stability permitting, or to be destroyed safely.

Disposal of excreta from patients receiving cytotoxic drugs

Few cytotoxic agents are excreted as unchanged drug or active metabolites in urine or faeces. However, in order to comply with universal precautions, gloves should now always be worn, thus minimizing risks to all staff.

Procedure guidelines: **Protection of staff during accidental exposure to cytotoxic drugs**

Action	Rationale
1 Contamination of the skin, mucous membranes and eyes should be treated promptly. All areas should be washed with copious amounts of tap water or 0.9% sodium chloride for approximately 2 minutes. Eye wash may be available.	To minimize the risk of any local damage to tissue.

Procedure guidelines: **Protection of staff during accidental exposure to cytotoxic drugs** *(cont'd)*

Action	Rationale
2 Accidental infiltration of the skin with a vesicant drug should be treated as an extravasation and the appropriate procedure followed (see Management of extravasation of vesicant drugs, below).	To minimize the risk of any local damage to tissue.
3 If erythema and/or other local reaction occurs in any circumstances, contact the occupational health unit or a member of the medical staff so that appropriate treatment may be advised.	To prevent further damage and/or complications.
4 It is essential after any accident involving direct contact with a cytotoxic drug, or if any local or systemic symptoms occur after handling such a drug, that the occupational health unit should be contacted.	To assist with recording and monitoring of staff exposure.
5 If pregnancy is suspected or intended, the occupational health unit should be contacted.	To discuss future work patterns and any anxiety that may be felt.

Routes of administration

Cytotoxic drugs can be administered via a variety of routes (see Ch. 9, Drug administration). However, regardless of the route used there are certain preadministration principles which the nurse should apply. The nurse should remember that the administration of medicines is a collaborative process which involves the nurse, doctor and pharmacist. The nurse must identify and remedy any knowledge or practice deficit (NMC 2002).

1 *Provision of information*: the patient should be fully informed of all the possible side-effects of chemotherapy, how to cope with any effects at home and the types of supportive therapy they may receive, as well as where and how they are to receive the drugs. They should then receive written information, which should be used to reinforce verbal explanation and will enable patients to spend time reading and formulating any questions about treatments (Goodman 2000).

2 *Gaining the patient's consent*: consent must be obtained before chemotherapy is commenced and every time the patient is changed from one protocol/regimen to another. The standard NHS consent form dictates the amount of information necessary in order to obtain valid consent. For example, if there is a possibility that the patient may require a blood transfusion then the patient and the doctor must sign to state that this has been discussed with the patient. One copy of the consent form is kept in the medical notes whilst the other is given to the patient (DOH 2002).

3 *Ascertaining whether the patient is fit for treatment*, e.g. full blood count, renal function: certain blood results are required in order to:

(a) Calculate the dose of drug, e.g. in the case of platinum-based drugs ethylenediaminetetra-acetic acid (EDTA) or 24-hour urine collection for creatinine is required

(b) Ensure that the patient is fit enough to receive the treatment and if any of the blood results are too low, then supportive therapy may be prescribed.

4 *Calculating body surface area*: this is done by using the patient's height and weight and should be performed at each visit. The surface area is then determined using a nomogram, and this will then be used to calculate the dose of drug. The patient's height and weight should be recorded on the prescription chart.

Familiarization with the chemotherapy regimen

The nurse should ensure that the prescription states:

- The date
- The chemotherapy regimen (many chemotherapy prescriptions are computer generated to reduce the risk of error)
- The correct dose
- The route of administration.

The prescription should be signed by the medical practitioner and verified by a pharmacist.

Intravenous administration

Definition

This is the administration of cytotoxic drugs via a peripheral or central vein and is the most commonly used route for the administration of cytotoxic drugs.

Table 10.1 Arguments for using either a large- or small-gauge peripheral vascular access device

Larger	Smaller
1 Enables irritant drugs to reach general circulation quickly, without irritating peripheral veins. 2 Administration time is decreased and therefore patient does not need to spend as much time in a stressful environment.	1 Less chance of puncturing the posterior vein wall. 2 Less likely to cause trauma and result in scar formation. 3 Less pain on needle insertion. 4 Increased blood flow around small needle increases dilution of drug and reduces risk of chemical phlebitis.

Indications

Intravenous administration enables:

- Rapid and reliable delivery of a cytotoxic drug to the tumour site
- Rapid dilution of a drug which reduces local irritation and the risk of tissue damage.

Reference material

Choosing the appropriate device

Cytotoxic drugs may be administered via a winged infusion device (CVAD), a peripheral cannula or a central venous access device. A winged infusion device is used mainly for bolus injections of non-vesicant drugs, due to the potential risk of infiltration associated with steel needles (Dougherty 1999). A peripheral cannula is used for bolus injections and short or intermittent infusions of both vesicant and non-vesicant drugs (see Table 10.1). This device is associated with phlebitis and requires repeated resiting (Dougherty 1999). A central venous catheter is useful for patients with poor venous access, those at high risk of extravasation and for those undergoing long-term, high dose or continuous infusional chemotherapy (Dougherty 1999; Weinstein 2000). These devices are associated with infection and thrombosis (Gabriel 1999).

When the peripheral route is used a winged infusion device or cannula may be used. The insertion site of choice should be the large veins of the forearm (cephalic or basilic) as these are easier to access, reduce the risk of chemical phlebitis and result in fewer problems if extravasation should occur (Weinstein 2000). The next area of choice would be the dorsum of the hand, then the wrist. The antecubital fossa should only be used as the last resort as it can limit movement and is associated with problems if extravasation occurs in this area (Dougherty 1999; Weinstein 2000). The general rule is to start distally and proceed proximally where possible and also to alternate the arms (Weinstein 2000) to ensure that the same veins are not being used and damaged by chemical and mechanical irritation.

When using the peripheral intravenous route the following should be adhered to

- Patency should be checked at the start of administration by achieving a blood return and then flushing with 10 ml of 0.9% sodium chloride to ensure there is no resistance, swelling or pain. Blood return should then be checked after every 2–4 ml of drug is administered (Dougherty 1999; Weinstein 2000).
- The site should be assessed for signs of phlebitis.
- The site should be observed when a bolus injection is administered, particularly if a vesicant drug, for signs of infiltration or extravasation.
- Certain vesicants must not be administered as infusions into a peripheral vein as the risk of extravasation and damage is greater than via the central venous route (Weinstein 2000).

In addition, where possible a new site should be used for vesicants, to ensure the vein is healthy and patent, although this may not always be possible. There are some controversial issues related to peripheral intravenous cytotoxic drug administration (see Table 10.2).

CVADs have the advantage of providing a more reliable form of vascular access. This is because the problems associated with peripheral devices such as phlebitis, venous irritation and pain are eliminated as central venous access enables rapid dilution and circulation of the drug. However, extravasation can still occur as a result of a damaged catheter, port needle dislodgement or fibrin sheath formation along the length of the catheter (Mayo 1998).

Methods

Cytotoxic drugs may be administered as a direct bolus injection, a bolus via the side arm of a rapid infusion of 0.9% sodium chloride or a continuous infusion. The

Table 10.2   Controversial issues: use of antecubital fossa

For	Against
1 Larger veins permit rapid infusion of drug.	1 Mobility is restricted.
2 Larger veins allow irritant drugs to reach general circulation more quickly and with less irritation than small veins.	2 Risk of extravasation is increased if patient tends to be mobile.
3 Easier to palpate and therefore increases successful insertion of device.	3 Early recognition of extravasation is difficult due to the deep veins. This means there is less chance of observing swelling which could go undetected. The patient may also have a delayed reaction to pain.
	4 Damage can result in loss of structure and function, ulceration and fibrosis.

choice is dependent on:

- The type of cytotoxic drug, e.g. etoposide is only given as an infusion
- Pharmacological considerations, e.g. stability, need for dilution
- Degree of venous irritation, e.g. vinorelbine is a highly irritant drug
- Whether the drug is a vesicant
- The type of device in situ (Dougherty 1999).

The advantage of the bolus injection is that the integrity of the vein and any early signs of extravasation can be observed more easily than during an infusion. However, bolus injection can increase the risk of venous irritation due to the constant contact of the drug with the intima of the vein, resulting in venospasm and pain (Dougherty 1999). It could also lead to inappropriate rapid administration of the drug (Weinstein 2000).

Bolus injections administered via the side arm of a rapid infusion of solution ensure greater dilution of potentially irritating drugs and enable rapid removal of the drug from the insertion site and smaller vessels. The disadvantages are that a small vein may not allow rapid flow of the infusate and this may result in the drug backing up the tubing. The practitioner also has to interrupt the flow in order to check blood return (Dougherty 1999).

Adding the drug to an infusion bag allows for greater dilution, thus reducing the possibility of chemical irritation. Some drugs may only be administered as infusions owing to the type of side-effects associated with them (e.g. hypotension with etoposide) and long-term continuous infusions, e.g. 5-fluorouracil (5-FU), may also be necessary to reduce the risk of side-effects such as diarrhoea. Patency and device position cannot be easily assessed and the longer the infusion, the greater the possibility of device dislodgement, extravasation or infiltration and general complications associated with the device (Weinstein 2000).

Procedure guidelines: **Intravenous administration of cytotoxic drugs**

The aim of the procedure for administration of chemotherapy intravenously is to protect both nurse and patient from contamination and also to prevent extravasation of drugs which could result in local tissue damage. The large majority of cytotoxic agents will be delivered to the ward/unit individually packaged for delivery to a named patient, by injection or infusion. If this is not so, specific guidelines should be followed (see Procedure guidelines: Protection of the environment).

Procedure

Action	Rationale
1 Explain and discuss the procedure with the patient. Evaluate the patient's knowledge of cytotoxic therapy. If this knowledge appears to be inadequate, offer an explanation of the use, action, dose and potential side-effects of the drug or drugs involved.	To ensure that the patient understands the procedure and gives his/her valid consent. The patient has a right to information.
2 Put on gloves and an apron before commencing the procedure.	To protect the nurse from local contamination of skin or clothing. *Note*: with careful handling technique, this risk is minimal but splashes can occur when changing syringes or infusion containers.

*Procedure guidelines: **Intravenous administration of cytotoxic drugs** (cont'd)*

Action	Rationale
3 Prepare necessary equipment for an aseptic administration procedure, and ensure that this is followed carefully (see Ch. 9, Drug administration).	To minimize the risk of local and/or systemic infection. Patients are frequently immunosuppressed and at greater risk of hospital-acquired infection.
4 Check that all details on the syringe or infusion container are correct when compared with the patient's prescription, before opening the sterile packaging.	To ensure the patient is given the correct drug which has been dispensed for him/her. To prevent wastage.
5 Be aware of the immediate effects of the drug.	To observe the patient during administration. To be prepared to manage any side-effects that occur.
6 Take the medication and the prescription chart to the patient. Check the patient's identity and the dose to be given.	To prevent error.
7 Inspect the device site, and consult the patient about sensation around the device insertion site.	To detect any problems, e.g. phlebitis, which would render the device unusable.
8 Check the patency of the vein for blood return and then flush using 0.9% sodium chloride.	To determine whether the vein will accommodate the extra fluid flow and irritant drugs and remain patent.
9 Protect the patient from contact with the drugs by:	
(a) Ensuring the needle (if used) is inserted or a syringe (if using a needleless injection system) is attached carefully into the injection site of the administration set, extension set or cannula injection cap.	To prevent exiting on the other side of the intravenous equipment and contaminating or inoculating the patient.
(b) Taking care when removing the blind hub, changing needles/syringes, and inserting the administration set into the infusion container or changing bags (which must be done with the bag lying flat on a hard surface).	To avoid leakage or splashes and contamination of the nurse or patient. To prevent mis-spiking the bag and puncturing it.
(c) Securing a good connection between needle and syringe by always using Luer–Lok syringes.	To prevent leakage or separation, which may occur due to pressure during administration, resulting in spray and contamination.
(d) Checking the injection site or injection cap at the end of the procedure.	To ensure that there is no leakage.
(e) Acting promptly if any contamination is noted and washing the area with cold water or 0.9% sodium chloride.	To prevent any local reaction and absorption on skin, mucous membranes, etc.
10 Administer drugs in the correct order, antiemetics then cytotoxic drugs, i.e. vesicants first.	To ensure that those agents likely to cause tissue damage are given when venous integrity is greatest, i.e. at the beginning of the administration process.
11 Ensure the correct administration rate.	To prevent 'speed shock'. To prevent extra pressure and irritation within the vein.
12 Observe the vein throughout for signs of infiltration or extravasation, e.g. swelling or leakage at the site of injection. Note the patient's comments about sensation at the site, e.g. pain.	To detect any problems at the earliest moment. To prevent any damage to soft tissue, and to enable the remainder of the drug(s) to be given correctly at another site. To enable prompt treatment to be given, thus minimizing local damage, and possibly preserving venous access for future treatment. (For further information see Management of extravasation of vesicant drugs.)
13 Flush the device with 0.9% sodium chloride between drugs and after administration.	To prevent drug interaction. To prevent leakage of drug from the puncture site, on removal of the device.
14 Be aware of the patient's comfort throughout the procedure.	To minimize trauma to the patient. To involve the patient in treatment and detect any side-effects and/or problems that may then be avoided at the next treatment.
15 Record details of the administration in the appropriate documents.	To prevent any duplication of treatment and to provide a point of reference in the event of queries.

Extravasation of vesicant drugs

Definition

Extravasation is the inadvertent administration of vesicant solution or medication into surrounding tissues which can lead to tissue necrosis, while infiltration is the inadvertent administration of non-vesicant solutions/medications into the surrounding tissues (Goodman 2000; INS 2000; Perdue 2001; RCN 2003). A vesicant is any solution or medication that causes the formation of blisters with subsequent sloughing of tissues resulting from tissue necrosis (Goodman 2000; Perdue 2001). Irritants are drugs capable of causing inflammation and irritation but if these drugs infiltrate they rarely cause any tissue breakdown (ONS 1999; Stanley 2002).

Reference material

Prevention of extravasation

Extravasation is a condition that is often under-diagnosed, undertreated and under-reported (Stanley 2002). The incidence of extravasation is estimated to be between 0.1 and 7% of cytotoxic drug administration (Gault & Challands 1997; CP Pharmaceuticals 1999). Even when practitioners have many years of experience, extravasation of vesicant agents can occur and is an extremely stressful event, but is not in itself an act of negligence (Goodman 2000; Weinstein 2001). Early detection and treatment are crucial if the consequences of an untreated or poorly managed extravasation are to be avoided. These may include:

- Pain from necrotic areas
- Physical defect
- The cost of hospitalization and plastic surgery
- Delay in the treatment of disease
- Psychological distress
- Litigation – nurses are now being named in malpractice allegations and extravasation injuries are an area for concern (Gault & Challands 1997; Camp Sorrell 1998; Schulmeister 1998; CP Pharmaceuticals 1999; Weinstein 2000; Dougherty 2003).

The nurse's focus should be on safe intravenous technique and implementing strategies to minimize the risk (Weinstein 2000). This includes the following strategies.

Monitoring the site

Confirming venous patency by flushing with 0.9% sodium chloride solution prior to administration of vesicants and frequent monitoring thereafter. Checking blood return after every 2–4 ml when giving a bolus injection and assessing for any swelling (Goodman 2000; Weinstein 2000; Vandergrift 2001; Stanley 2002).

Location of the device

The most appropriate site for the location of a peripheral cannula is considered to be the forearm (Gault & Challands 1997; Weinstein 2000; Stanley 2002). However, a large straight vein over the dorsum of the hand is preferable to a smaller vein in the forearm (Weinstein 2001). Siting over joints should be avoided as tissue damage in this area may limit joint movement in the future. It is also recommended that the antecubital fossa should never be used for the administration of vesicants because of the risk of damage to local structures such as nerves and tendons (McCaffrey Boyle & Engelking 1995; Shulman et al. 1998; Dougherty 1999; Weinstein 2000; Stanley 2002).

Patients at risk

Extra caution and observation should be carried out in patients who are at increased risk of extravasation (See Box 10.1).

Sequence of drugs

Vesicants should be given first (see Table 10.3).

Types of devices

The use of steel needles is associated with a greater risk of extravasation and should be discouraged and a plastic cannula should be used instead (Gault & Challands 1997; How & Brown 1998; Stanley 2002). Vesicants should be given via a newly established cannula wherever possible and consideration should be given to changing the cannula site after 24 hours. However, if the fluid runs freely, there is good blood return and there are no signs of erythema, pain or swelling at the site, there is no reason to inflict a second cannulation on the patient (Weinstein 2000). Consideration should be given to a CVAD if peripheral access is difficult.

Method of administration

Many vesicants must be given as a slow bolus injection, often via the side arm of a fast-running intravenous infusion of a compatible solution, e.g. doxorubicin or

---

Box 10.1 Patients at risk of extravasation (Shulman et al. 1998; CP Pharmaceuticals 1999; Goodman 2000)

- Infants and young children
- Elderly patients
- Those who are unable to communicate, e.g. sedated, unconscious, confused, language issues
- Those with chronic diseases, e.g. cancer, peripheral vascular disease, SVC syndrome, lymphoedema
- Those on medications – anticoagulants, steroids
- Those who have undergone repeated intravenous cannulation/venepuncture
- Those with fragile veins or who are thrombocytopenic

Table 10.3 Drug sequencing – rationale for administering vesicant drugs first or last (Weinstein 2000; Stanley 2002)

Vesicants first	Vesicants last
1 Vascular integrity decreases over time.	1 Vesicants are irritating and increase vein fragility.
2 Vein is most stable and least irritated at start of treatment.	2 Venous spasm may occur and mask signs of extravasation.
3 Initial assessment of vein patency is most accurate.	
4 Patient's awareness of changes more acute.	

epirubicin via an infusion of 0.9% sodium chloride. If repeated infusions are to be given then a CVAD may be more appropriate (Weinstein 2000; Stanley 2002).

Skill of the practitioner

Correct choice of device and location, the ability to use the most appropriate vasodilatation techniques, early recognition of extravasation and prompt action come from ensuring only skilled and knowledgeable practitioners administer vesicant drugs and/or insert the vascular access device (McCaffrey Boyle & Engelking 1995; Gault & Challands 1997; Stanley 2002). Successful cannulation at the first attempt is ideal, as vesicants have been known to seep into tissues at a vein entry site of a previous cannulation (Gault & Challands 1997; Perdue 2001).

Patient information

Adequate information given to patients will ensure early recognition and co-operation as patients are the first to notice pain. Patients should be informed of the potential problems of administering vesicants and the possible consequences of extravasation (Goodman 2000; Weinstein 2000; Perdue 2001; Stanley 2002).

Drugs capable of causing tissue necrosis

Before administration of vesicant cytotoxic drugs the nurse should know which agents are capable of producing tissue necrosis. The following is a list of those in common use:

Group A drugs	*Group B drugs*
Vinca alkaloids	Amsacrine
Vinblastine	Carmustine (concentrated solution)
Vindesine	Dacarbazine (concentrated solution)
Vinorelbine	Dactinomycin
Vincristine	Daunorubicin
Vinflunine	Doxorubicin
Paclitaxel	Epirubicin
	Idarubicin
	Mithramycin
	Mitomycin C
	Mustine
	Streptozocin

If in any doubt, the drug data sheet should be consulted or reference made to a research trial protocol. Drugs should not be reconstituted to give solutions which are higher than the manufacturer's recommended concentration, and the method of administration should be checked, e.g. infusion, injection.

A variety of vesicant non-cytotoxic agents in frequent use are also capable of causing severe tissue damage if extravasated. They include:

Group A drugs	*Group B drugs*
Calcium chloride	Aciclovir
Calcium gluconate	Amphotericin
Phenytoin	Cefotaxime
Hypertonic solutions	Diazepam
of sodium bicarbonate	Digoxin
(greater than 5%)	Ganciclovir
Therapeutic radiopharmaceuticals,	Potassium chloride
e.g. MIBG	(>40 mmol/l)
	Mannitol

This potential hazard should always be remembered. The actions listed in this procedure may not be appropriate in all these instances. Drug data sheets should always be checked and the pharmacy departments should be consulted if the information is insufficient, regarding action to take if a vesicant drug extravasates.

Signs and symptoms of extravasation

Extravasation should be suspected if:

1 The patient complains of burning, stinging pain or any other acute change at the injection site. This should be distinguished from a feeling of cold, which may occur with some drugs, or venous spasm which can be caused by irritation usually accompanied by pain described as an achiness or tightness (Goodman 2000). Any change of sensation warrants further investigation (Goodman 2000).

2 Induration, swelling or leakage occurs at the injection site.

3 Blanching of the skin occurs (Springhouse 2002). Erythema can occur around the injection site but this is not usually present immediately. It is important that this is distinguished from a 'flare' reaction which is a red streak, flush or even 'blistering' often associated with doxorubicin (Vandergrift 2001). This occurs in 3–6% of patients (How & Brown 1998) and does not cause any pain, although the area may feel itchy. It is caused by a venous inflammatory response to histamine release, is characterized by redness and blotchiness and may result in the formation of small weals, having a similar appearance to a nettle rash. It usually subsides in 30–60 minutes, with 86% resolving within 45 minutes (How & Brown 1998; ONS 1999; Goodman 2000), but it responds well within a few minutes to the application of a topical steroid (CP Pharmaceuticals 1999; Weinstein 2000; Vandergrift 2001).

4 Blood return is one of the most misleading of all signs. If blood return is sluggish or absent this may indicate lack of patency and incorrect position of the device. If no other signs are apparent this should not be regarded as an indication of a non-patent vein, as a vein may not bleed back for a number of reasons and extravasation may occur even in the event of good blood return. Any change in blood flow should be investigated (Goodman 2000; Weinstein 2000; Stanley 2002; Springhouse 2002) (see Ch. 44, Vascular access devices).

5 A resistance is felt on the plunger of the syringe if drugs are given by bolus (Vandergrift 2001; Stanley 2002).

6 There is absence of free flow when administration is by infusion, once other reasons have been excluded, e.g. position (Vandergrift 2001; Stanley 2002).

Note: one or more of the above may be present. If extravasation is suspected or confirmed, action must be taken immediately (Weinstein 2000).

Management of extravasation

The management of extravasation of chemotherapy agents is controversial and there is little documented evidence of efficacy. No antidote has received clear validation in controlled clinical trials and no randomized trials managing cytotoxic extravasation in humans have been completed (Bertolli 1995). Some studies performed on animals have demonstrated both effective and ineffective treatments but extrapolation from animals to humans is limited (ONS 1999). Other studies have been small with low numbers of patients. Another problem is that it is often difficult to ascertain whether any extravasation has actually occurred (Weinstein 2000). Therefore recommendations are based on more consistent experimental evidence, cumulative clinical experience from available case reports and uncontrolled studies and empirical guidelines (Bertolli 1995). Drugs where there is evidence of effective management include: anthracyclines (Rudolph & Larson 1987), vinca alkaloids (Bertolli 1995; CP Pharmaceuticals 1998), CT contrast media (Federle *et al.* 1998) and paclitaxel (Bertolli *et al.* 1997).

The management of extravasation involves several stages including:

Stage 1: stopping infusion and withdrawing (aspirating) drug

It appears that most authors are agreed that withdrawing as much of the drug as possible, as soon as extravasation is suspected, is beneficial (Rudolph & Larson 1987; Cox *et al.* 1988; ONS 1999; Weinstein 2000; Vandergrift 2001). However, withdrawal is only possible during bolus injections. Aspiration may be successful if extravasation presents itself as a raised blister, but may be unsuccessful if tissue is soft and soggy (CP Pharmaceuticals 1999; Stanley 2002). It may help to reduce the size of the lesion (Vandergrift 2001). In practice it may achieve little and often distresses the patient (Gault & Challands 1997). The likelihood of withdrawing blood (as suggested by Ignoffo & Friedman 1980) is small and the practitioner may waste valuable time attempting this (Dougherty 1999) which could lead to delay in the rest of the management procedure.

Stage 2: removing device

Some clinicians advocate that the peripheral vascular access device be left in situ in order to instil the antidote via the device and into the affected tissues (Ignoffo & Friedman 1980; Cox *et al.* 1988; Weinstein 2000; Stanley 2002). However, others recommend that the peripheral device should be removed to prevent any injected solution increasing the size of the affected area (Rudolph & Larson 1987; CP Pharmaceuticals 1999; Vandergrift 2001). There appears to be no research evidence to support either practice.

Stage 3: applying hot or cold packs

Cooling appears to be a better choice, with the exception of the vinca alkaloids, than warming (Bertolli 1995; CP Pharmaceuticals 1999). Cold causes vasoconstriction, localizing the extravasation and perhaps allowing time for local vascular and lymphatic systems to contain the drug. It should be applied for 15–20 minutes, 3–4 times a day for up to 3 days (Gault & Challands 1997; CP Pharmaceuticals 1999; ONS 1999). Heat promotes healing after the first 24 hours by increasing the blood supply

(ONS 1999; Weinstein 2000). It also decreases local drug concentration, increasing the blood flow which results in enhanced resolution of pain and reabsorption of local swelling.

Stage 4: use of antidotes

A number of antidotes are available, but again there is a lack of scientific evidence to demonstrate their value. There appear to be two main methods: (1) localize and neutralize (using hyaluronidase) (CP Pharmaceuticals 1999) and (2) spread and dilute (using an antidote) (Stanley 2002). Administration of antidotes if not via the cannula is by the pincushion technique; that is, instilling small volumes around and over the areas affected using a small gauge (25) needle towards the centre of a clock face. The procedure causes considerable discomfort to patients and if large areas are to be tackled analgesia should be considered (Stanley 2002). Hyaluronidase is an enzyme which destroys tissue cement and helps to reduce or prevent tissue damage by allowing rapid diffusion of the extravasated fluid and promoting drug absorption. The usual dose is 1500 IU (Bertolli 1995; CP Pharmaceuticals 1998; Vandergrift 2001). It should be injected within 1 hour of extravasation and ideally through the intravenous device delivering the enzyme to the same tissue (Gault & Challands 1997; CP Pharmaceuticals 1998; Weinstein 2000; Vandergrift 2001; Stanley 2002). Corticosteroids have long been advocated as a treatment for anthracycline extravasation in reducing inflammatory components, although inflammation is not a prominent feature of tissue necrosis (Camp Sorrell 1998; CP Pharmaceuticals 1999) and they appear to have little benefit. Data now discourage the use of locally injected steroids, as there is little evidence to support their use (Bertolli 1995; Gault & Challands 1997). However, given as a cream they can help to reduce local trauma and irritation (Stanley 2002). Reports on the clinical use of topical dimethyl sulfoxide (DMSO) show it is effective and well tolerated in extravasation (Bertolli 1995). However, this is based on a high dose (95%) and only 50% is easily available in the UK (Stanley 2002).

Stage 5: elevation of limb

This is recommended as it minimizes swelling (Rudolph & Larson 1987; Powell 1996) and movement should be encouraged to prevent adhesion of damaged areas to underlying tissue (Dougherty 1999).

Stage 6: surgical techniques

Some centres suggest that a plastic surgery consultation be performed as part of the management procedure in order to remove the tissue containing the drug. Surgical

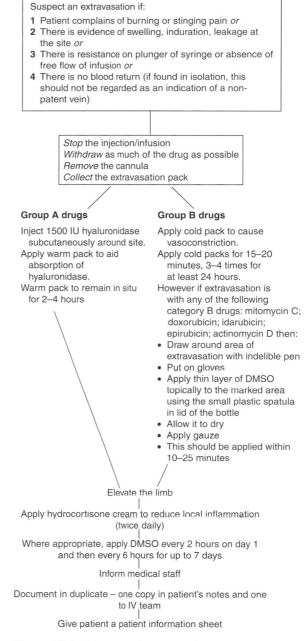

Figure 10.1 Treatment of extravasation.

intervention with doxorubicin is recommended, especially if the lesion is greater than 2 cm, there is significant residual pain 1–2 weeks after extravasation or there is minimal healing 2–3 weeks after injury (ONS 1999; Vandergrift 2001). Liposuction or a flush-out technique can remove extravasated drug without resorting to excision and skin grafting. A liposuction cannula can be used to aspirate extravasated material and subcutaneous fat. If there is little subcutaneous fat, e.g. preterm infants, then the saline flush-out technique is recommended, particularly if done within the first 24 hours. It has been suggested as a less traumatic and cheaper procedure than surgery. Four small stab incisions are made and large volumes of 0.9% sodium chloride are administered which flush out the extravasated drug (Gault & Challands 1997).

Extravasation kits

The use of extravasation kits has been recommended (CP Pharmaceuticals 1999; Goodman 2000; Stanley 2002). Kits should be assembled according to the particular needs of individual institutions. They should be kept in all areas where staff are regularly administering vesicant drugs, so staff have immediate access to equipment (Dougherty 1999). The kit should be simple to avoid confusion, but comprehensive enough to meet all reasonable needs (Stanley 2002). (See guidelines for minimal content.) Instructions should be clear and easy to follow and the use of a flow chart enables staff to follow the management procedure in easy steps (see Fig. 10.1).

Mixed vesicant extravasation

Consideration should be given to the management of mixed vesicant drug extravasation in terms of which drug to treat with which antidote. It has been recommended to act in accordance with the drug which possesses the most deleterious properties (How & Brown 1998). In the case of VAMP this would be doxorubicin.

Informing the patient

Patients should always be informed when an extravasation has occurred and be given an explanation of what has happened and what management has been carried out (McCaffrey Boyle & Engelking1995). An information sheet should be given to patients with instructions of what symptoms to look out for and when to contact the hospital during the follow-up period (Dougherty 1999).

Extravasation from CVAD

CVADs have decreased the incidence of extravasation. However, whilst the incidence is lower the severity of the injuries is far greater as detection tends to occur later (Stanley 2002). Extravasation can occur as a result of a leaking or damaged catheter, fibrin sheath formation (Mayo 1998) or a port needle dislodgement (Schulmeister 1998; ONS 1999). The consequences of an extravasation of a CVAD are more serious and require immediate consultation. Management is usually by surgical intervention and washout of affected tissues.

Wound management

Should the injury not heal, assessment of the wound is important to ensure the best dressing product is chosen (Irving 2001).

Documentation

An extravasation must be reported and fully documented as it is an accident and the patient may require follow-up care (NMC 2002). Information may also be used for statistical purposes, for example collation and analysis using the green card scheme devised by St Chad's Hospital, Birmingham (Stanley 2002). Finally it may be required in case of litigation, which is now on the increase (CP Pharmaceuticals 1999; Weinstein 2000; Irving 2001).

The procedure detailed here represents the policy of The Royal Marsden Hospital for the management by nursing staff of extravasation injury, drawn up with the assistance of pharmacist and medical colleagues. It relates specifically to the management of extravasation of a drug from a peripheral cannula.

Procedure guidelines:
Management of extravasation when using a peripheral cannula

Equipment

To assist the nurse, an extravasation kit should be assembled and should be readily available in each ward/unit. It contains:

1 Instant cold pack × 1/instant hot pack × 1 (or reusable packs which can be frozen or heated as required).
2 Hyaluronidase 1500 IU/2 ml sterile water.
3 Hydrocortisone cream 1% 15 g tube × 1.
4 2 ml syringes × 1.

5 25 G needles × 2.
6 Alcohol swabs.
7 Documentation forms.
8 Copy of extravasation management procedure.
9 Patient information leaflet.

*Procedure guidelines: **Management of extravasation when using a peripheral cannula** (cont'd)*

Procedure

Action	Rationale
1 Explain and discuss the procedure with the patient.	To ensure that the patient understands the procedure and gives his/her valid consent.
2 Stop injection or infusion *immediately*, leaving the cannula in place.	To minimize local injury. To allow aspiration of the drug to be attempted.
3 Aspirate any residual drug from the device and suspected extravasation site.	To minimize local injury by removing as much drug as possible and only attempt if appropriate. Subsequent damage is related to the volume of the extravasation, in addition to other factors.
4 Remove the cannula.	To prevent the device from being used for antidote administration.
5 Collect the extravasation pack and take it to the patient.	It contains all the equipment necessary for managing extravasation.
6 Group A drugs: Draw up hyaluronidase 1500 IU in 1 ml water for injection and inject volumes of 0.1–0.2 ml subcutaneously at points of the compass around the circumference of the area of extravasation. Apply warm pack.	This is the recommended agent for group A drugs. The warm pack speeds up absorption of the drug by the tissues.
Group B drugs: Apply cold pack or ice instantly.	To localize the area of extravasation, slow cell metabolism and decrease the area of tissue destruction. To reduce local pain.
However, if extravasation is with any of the following category B drugs: mitomycin C; doxorubicin; idarubicin; epirubicin; actinomycin D then: • Draw around area of extravasation with indelible pen • Put on gloves • Apply thin layer of DMSO topically to the marked area using the small plastic spatula in lid of the bottle • Allow it to dry • Apply gauze • This should be applied within 10–25 minutes.	This is the recommended agent for these anthracyclines and helps to reduce local tissue damage.
7 Where possible elevate the extremity and/or encourage movement.	To minimize swelling and to prevent adhesion of damaged area to underlying tissue, which could result in restriction of movement.
8 Inform a member of the medical staff at the earliest opportunity.	To enable actions differing from agreed policy to be taken if considered in the best interests of the patient. To notify the doctor of the need to prescribe any other drugs.
9 Apply hydrocortisone cream 1% twice daily, and instruct the patient how to do this. Continue as long as erythema persists.	To reduce local inflammation and promote patient comfort.
10 Where appropriate, apply DMSO every 2 hours on day 1 and then every 6 hours for up to 7 days (patients will need to have this prescribed as a TTO and continue treatment at home where necessary).	To help reduce local tissue damage.
11 Heat pack (group A drugs) should be reapplied after initial management for 2–4 hours. Cold packs (group B drugs) should be applied for 15–20 minutes, 3–4 times a day for up to 3 days.	To localize the steroid effect in the area of extravasation. To reduce local pain and promote patient comfort.

*Procedure guidelines: **Management of extravasation when using a peripheral cannula** (cont'd)*

Action	Rationale
12 Provide analgesia as required.	To promote patient comfort. To encourage movement of the limb as advised.
13 Document the following details, in duplicate, on the form provided: (a) Patient's name/number (b) Ward/unit (c) Date, time (d) Signs and symptoms. (e) Venepuncture site (on diagram). (f) Drug sequence. (g) Drug administration technique, i.e. 'bolus' or infusion. (h) Approximate amount of the drug extravasated. (i) Diameter, length and width of extravasation area. (j) Appearance of the area. (k) Step-by-step management with date and time of each step performed and medical officer notification. (l) Patient's complaints, comments, statements. (m) Indication that patient's information sheet given to patient. (n) Follow-up section. (o) Whether photograph was taken. (p) If required, when patient referred to plastic surgeon. (q) Signature of the nurse.	To provide an immediate full record of all details of the incident, which may be referred to if necessary. To provide a baseline for future observation and monitoring of patient's condition. To comply with NMC guidelines.
14 Explain to the patient that the site may remain sore for several days.	To reduce anxiety and ensure continued co-operation.
15 Observe the area regularly for erythema, induration, blistering or necrosis. *Inpatients*: monitor daily. Where appropriate, take photograph.	To detect any changes at the earliest possible moment.
16 All patients should receive written information explaining what has occurred, what management has been carried out, what they need to look for at the site and when to report any changes. For example, increased discomfort, peeling or blistering of the skin should be reported immediately.	To detect any changes as early as possible, and allow for a review of future management. This may include referral to a plastic surgeon.
17 If blistering or tissue breakdown occurs, begin sterile dressing techniques and seek advice regarding wound management.	To minimize the risk of a superimposed infection and increase healing.
18 Depending on size of lesion, degree of pain, type of drug – refer to plastic surgeon.	To prevent further pain or other complications as chemically induced ulcers rarely heal spontaneously.

Oral administration

Definition

The administration of cytotoxic drugs via the oral route.

Indications

The oral route is convenient, economical, non-invasive and sometimes less toxic than the other routes (Goodman 2000). Most oral drugs are absorbed well if the gastrointestinal tract is functioning normally. However the oral route can be unreliable for a number of reasons, including:

- Patients may not comply with therapy (although this is uncommon with chemotherapy), may forget or may feel the side-effects associated are too unpleasant, e.g. nausea and vomiting, hot flushes (Goodman 2000). However, the use of antiemetics as well as rescheduling the timing of the dose administered may prove beneficial.

- Patients may not take medications as instructed. However, it is imperative that the nurse ensures that the patient understands the importance of timing and schedule of the medication prescribed. The use of medication cards can assist the patient to record the doses of medication that have been taken.
- Some patients may experience difficulty taking tablets or capsules, and therefore attempt to crush them which could result in changes to the tablets' disposition and effectiveness.

Reference material

Nurses administering tablets or capsules should use a non-touch technique to avoid damage and contamination of the tablets or capsules and contamination of themselves. If tablets have to be counted, this should be done using a triangle, which should be washed and dried after use. Many tablets are coated and this protects the drug in its inner core. There is no risk of contamination if these coatings are not broken. A small number of tablets are compressed powders, but there appears to be no risk of contamination where there is no free powder visible. It is important that these tablets are not crushed because they will then release powder which could be inhaled. Capsules are also not a risk if they have not been opened or broken or have not leaked. They should not be crushed or opened and the powder tipped out. Any visible spillage should be dealt with as previously directed (see Procedure guidelines: Protection of the environment).

Intramuscular and subcutaneous injection

Definition

The administration of cytotoxic drugs by injection into the muscle or subcutaneous tissues.

Indications

Intramuscular and subcutaneous injections are a useful route:

- When administering therapy in the community
- For patient convenience
- When regular administration is required and journeys to the hospital are impractical, e.g. younger or elderly patients on maintenance therapy.

It is also useful if venous access is limited although only small volumes (up to 3 ml) are recommended using this route (Goodman 2000; Sewell *et al.* 2002).

Reference material

Only a few cytotoxic drugs can be administered via these routes due to a number of factors:

- The irritant nature of the drugs and/or tissue damage
- Incomplete absorption may occur
- Bleeding as a result of thrombocytopenia
- Discomfort of regular injections.

Cytotoxic and biological agents administered in this way are:

- Methotrexate
- Bleomycin
- Cytosine arabinoside
- L-Asparaginase
- Ifosfamide
- Interferon
- Colony stimulating factor (Sansivero & Barton-Burke 2001; Stanley 2002).

Although the volume of drug and diluent handled is less than for the intravenous route, preparation and reconstitution of the agents should be commensurate with the information listed under Procedure guidelines: Protection of staff during accidental exposure to cytotoxic drugs, above. The nurse should continue to wear gloves during administration. Spillage and disposal of equipment should be dealt with as previously directed (see Procedure guidelines: Protection of the environment, above) and systems of work modified to ensure these guidelines are followed. Where community nurses are to be responsible for administration, they must be supplied with adequate information when the patient is discharged.

Recommendations about administration should be followed carefully, e.g. deep intramuscular injection using a Z-track technique to prevent leakage onto the skin (Goodman 2000) and rotation of sites to prevent local irritation developing. The skin should be cleaned with antiseptic prior to injection (Sansivero & Barton-Burke 2001) and the smallest needle used, the gauge of which will allow passage of the solution to minimize discomfort and scarring.

Topical application

Definition

Topical application is the application of cream or ointments containing cytotoxic agents.

Indications

Topical application is only suitable for superficial lesions and has been found to be useful in the treatment of cutaneous malignant lesions, e.g. cutaneous T-cell lymphomas, basal cell carcinoma, squamous cell carcinoma and Kaposi's sarcoma (Goodman 2000).

Reference material

Topical agents include mustine and 5-FU (Goodman 2000). The most widely used is 5% 5-FU cream, which is usually applied once or twice daily until significant penetration of the damaged or diseased skin can be achieved, and a typical response pattern has been observed. This can take up to 4 weeks when local erythema, blistering and ulceration occur. Once the affected skin starts sloughing, regranulization of normal tissue will begin to occur (Sewell *et al.* 2002).

Considerations include safe handling when applying the cream by wearing gloves and using low-linting swabs or non-metal applicators. It is important to protect the normal skin and avoid the eyes and other mucous membranes. The affected area should not be washed vigorously during the treatment (Goodman 2000). The area should be observed for any adverse reactions such as pain, pruritus and hyperpigmentation, which may result in discontinuation and subsequent dose reduction.

Intrathecal administration

Definition

Intrathecal administration is the administration of cytotoxic drugs into the central nervous system (CNS) via the cerebrospinal fluid. This is usually achieved using a lumbar puncture (Goodman 2000; Stanley 2002).

Indications

Intrathecal administration has proved to be of benefit in prophylactic treatment in cases of leukaemias and some lymphomas, where the CNS may provide a sanctuary site for tumour cells not reached during systemic chemotherapy (Goodman 2000). It has no place in the treatment of CNS metastases of solid tumours (Stanley 2002).

Reference material

Intrathecal administration is only appropriate for a limited number of drugs:

- Thiotepa
- Cytarabine
- Methotrexate.

Chemotherapy administered using this route has the potential to cause great harm (Sewell *et al.* 2002) and has been associated with the deaths of at least 13 patients since 1985. The risks of intrathecal chemotherapy have been well documented in *An Organization with a Memory* and the government set a target to eliminate the incidents of patients dying or being paralysed by maladministered intrathecal injections by the end of 2001 (DOH 2000). Two reports on injection errors (Toft 2001) gave rise to the publication of the national guidance for the safe administration of intrathecal chemotherapy. All trusts which administer intrathecal chemotherapy have been required to comply with the guidance since the end of 2001.

The key requirements of the guidance are noted in Box 10.2.

The advantage of this route is that it allows the direct access to the CNS of drugs which do not normally cross the blood–brain barrier in sufficient amounts and thus ensures constant levels of the drug in this area. The main disadvantage is that it requires a standard lumbar puncture before the drug can be injected, and this may need to be performed on a daily to weekly basis (Goodman 2000; Stanley 2002). Although this can be quick and easy to perform it can be distressing for the patient, and could even result in CNS trauma and infection. It may also only reach the epidural or subdural spaces and therefore the concentrations in the ventricles may not be therapeutic (Goodman 2000). However, central instillation of the drug into the ventricle can be achieved via an Ommaya reservoir which is surgically implanted through the cranium (Goodman 2000; Sewell *et al.* 2002). It carries more risks but provides permanent access and can be inserted under local or general anaesthetic (Goodman 2000; Sansivero & Barton-Burke 2001).

The preparation of the drug must be performed using aseptic technique to reduce the risk of infection and the drug should be free from preservatives to reduce neurotoxicity. Cerebrospinal fluid removal and medications should not be more than 2 ml/min. Expected side-effects of neurotoxicity related to the drugs include headache, nausea and vomiting, drowsiness, fever, stiff neck, ataxia and blurred vision (Sansivero & Barton-Burke 2001). Neurological and vital signs checks should be obtained at least every 1–2 hours initially, and then on a scheduled frequency. Observations should include signs of infection, headache and signs of increasing intracranial pressure, and monitoring the function of the pump or reservoir (Goodman 2000).

Box 10.2 Key requirements of the safe administration of intrathecal chemotherapy (DoH HSC 2003/10)

- The Chief Executive, who has overall responsibility for ensuring compliance with the guidance, should identify a 'designated lead' to oversee compliance within the Trust.
- A register must be established and maintained which lists designated personnel who have been trained and authorized to prescribe, dispense, issue, check or administer intrathecal chemotherapy.
- A formal induction programme must be provided for all new staff including training that is appropriate to their role in prescribing, dispensing, checking, issuing or administering of chemotherapy.
- Annual reviews of competence are required for all professional staff (nurses, doctors, pharmacy) who remain on the register.
- All staff involved with chemotherapy must be provided with a written protocol, which reflects both the national guidance and additional local information.
- Intrathecal chemotherapy must only be prescribed by a Medical Consultant, Associate Specialist or Specialist Register whose name is on the register. SHOs must never prescribe.
- A purpose-designed intrathecal chemotherapy chart must be used.
- Intrathecal chemotherapy drugs must only be dispensed and issued by pharmacy staff on the register. These drugs must only be transported from the pharmacy by the administering doctor or pharmacy staff on the register.
- Intrathecal chemotherapy drugs must be administered after intravenous chemotherapy drugs and should only be issued following written confirmation that any intravenous chemotherapy drugs have already been administered. The only exception is where intrathecal chemotherapy is being given to a child under general anaesthesia.
- Intrathecal chemotherapy must be administered in a designated, separate area and under normal circumstances only within normal working hours.
- The administering doctor must use a formal checking procedure to ensure that the right drug is given to the right patient. These checks must be completed with a chemotherapy-trained nurse (or a nurse trained and deemed competent to carry out this check if a chemotherapy-trained nurse is not available) the patient and, if appropriate, a relative or guardian. The nurse checking must be on the designated register. The checks made by the administering doctor and nurse must be recorded on the prescription chart prior to administration.

Intrapleural instillation

Definition

Introduction of cytotoxic drugs, or other substances, into the pleural cavity.

Indications

Pleural effusion is a common complication of malignant disease and may pose a considerable management problem. Installation should occur following drainage of an effusion to prevent or delay a recurrence caused by malignant cells, as after aspiration alone 60% will recur (Goodman 2000).

The most common neoplasms associated with the development of malignant pleural effusions are those of the:

- Breast
- Lung
- Gastrointestinal tract
- Prostate
- Ovary (Goodman 2000).

Such effusions can be very distressing to the patient, causing progressive discomfort, dyspnoea and death from respiratory insufficiency.

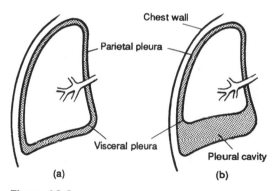

Figure 10.2 Lung anatomy. (a) Normal lung anatomy showing pleura. (b) Lung demonstrating presence of pleural effusion.

The alteration in normal anatomy due to the pressure of an effusion is illustrated in Fig. 10.2. In health less than 5 ml of transudate fluid is present between the visceral and parietal pleurae. This fluid acts as a lubricant and hydraulic seal (see Ch. 20, Intrapleural drainage). Infections and malignancies disrupt this mechanism, often repeatedly. Patients may survive for months or years, therefore effective palliation is important in maintaining or improving their quality of life. Administering chemotherapy via this route may alleviate symptoms and also has the potential for delivering the drugs to a site of poor systemic penetration (Sewell *et al.* 2002).

Reference material

Several methods have been used to treat pleural effusions, including:

- Surgical techniques, such as ablation of the pleural space
- Radiotherapy
- Systemic chemotherapy
- The insertion of a small-bore catheter placement and the installation of a pleural shunt (Sewell *et al.* 2002) to deliver cytotoxic agents.

In addition, instillation of sclerosing agents into the pleural space has been used and been reported to have highly variable success rates of 20–88% (Sewell *et al.* 2002). These agents have included talc, radioactive phosphorus, BCG, tetracycline and, more recently, cytotoxic drugs. The drug most frequently instilled is bleomycin, but others include mitozantrone, doxorubicin, mustine and thiotepa (Goodman 2000; Sewell *et al.* 2002).

Cytology may show the presence of tumour cells in effusion fluid, but even when these are absent, instillation of drugs may be effective in preventing recurrence due to the inflammatory reaction which obliterates the pleural space.

Improvements in equipment used, for example flexible cannulae or catheters, and lengthening of both the initial drainage period and that following instillation of the drug have contributed to increased patient comfort and greater effectiveness. The insertion of small-bore percutaneously placed catheters or ports, as well as pleuroperitoneal shunts (Goodman 2000), has been found to be useful for recurrent effusions.

The literature recommends that the patient should be turned regularly following instillation of the drug to facilitate its complete distribution over the pleural surfaces. It has been recommended that the timing for turning should be every 15 minutes for between 2 and 6 hours (Quan 1999). The rationale for such turning is based on clinical observation and there is a lack of work comparing patients who are turned with those who are not.

Local pleural pain and inflammation can last for 24–48 hours after instillation. Good symptom management should focus upon emesis control, adequate analgesia and emotional support and chest tube security to ensure patient comfort (Goodman 2000).

Procedure guidelines: **Administration of intrapleural drugs**

The procedure and problem solving related to intrapleural drainage (see Ch. 20) should be consulted for all aspects of thoracic drainage. The following information covers specific points regarding drug instillation.

Procedure

Instillation of drug

Action	Rationale
1 Explain and discuss the procedure with the patient.	To ensure that the patient understands the procedure and gives his/her valid consent.
2 Administer premedication to patients if prescribed.	To relax the patient.
3 Prepare the required equipment (see Ch. 9, Procedure guidelines: Administration of injections) and cytotoxic drug with protective wear as necessary.	To ensure the procedure goes smoothly without interruption.
4 Assist the doctor with the installation and provide support for the patient.	To increase the efficiency of the procedure and reduce discomfort for the patient.
5 At the end of the procedure clamp the drainage tube and leave for the desired period.	To prevent back-flow of the drug.

Rotation of patient

Action	Rationale
1 Assess the clinical status of the patient and ability to tolerate the desired rotation.	To prevent discomfort the patient may feel and to ensure that the doctor is informed of the patient's inability to comply.

*Procedure guidelines: **Administration of intrapleural drugs** (cont'd)*

Action	Rationale
2 Turn the patient in the following rotation: (a) Left side (b) Supine (c) Right side (d) Prone	To ensure that the drug coats and washes the pleural cavity completely.
3 Carry out the rotations as instructed. Examples are as follows: (a) 5 minutes in each position, repeated once, equals 20 minutes. (b) 30 minutes in each position, repeated once, equals 2 hours. (c) 1 hour in each position equals 4 hours.	As above.
4 Observe regularly for patient comfort. Administer analgesic as required.	To keep the patient comfortable and free from pain.
5 Record the patient's respirations and colour at least every 15 minutes for 1 hour, then every hour until stable, then 4-hourly, or as frequently as the patient's condition dictates. Record temperature at least 4-hourly.	To ensure there is no change in respiratory function following the procedure. To observe for pyrexia, a common side-effect that may indicate a developing infection or a reaction to chemotherapy.

Drainage of thoracotomy tube

Action	Rationale
1 Ensure the patient is in a comfortable position, and is aware of any limitations about movement.	To prevent discomfort or dislodgement of the drainage tube.
2 Unclamp the chest tube.	To allow drainage of the drug instilled.
3 Maintain the underwater seal until a volume of less than 50 ml is drained during 24 h for 2 consecutive days or for a maximum of 7 days, or in consultation with medical staff.	To allow complete drainage of the drug instilled, and any additional fluid.
4 Record the colour and amount of fluid drained on the appropriate documents.	To monitor the immediate effectiveness of therapy.

Problem solving

Problem	Cause	Suggested action
Local or systemic effects associated with specific cytotoxic drugs, e.g. rigors due to bleomycin.	Absorption of the drug into circulation in sufficient quantities to cause toxicity.	Be aware that this can occur. Initiate preventive action, e.g. obtain a prescription for corticosteroid cover to prevent rigors, or observe for a reaction and treat symptomatically.

Intravesical instillation

Definition

Intravesical instillation is the instillation of cytotoxic drugs directly into the bladder, via a urinary catheter.

Indications

Intravesical instillation has been shown to be effective in the treatment of small, multiple, superficial, well differentiated, non-invasive papillomatous carcinomas. It also minimizes recurrence in patients with a history of multiple tumours known readily to seed locally (Stanley 2002).

Reference material

Instillation of cytotoxic agents, and now immunotherapy, into the bladder via a urinary catheter has been used for many years in selected cases and has proven to be an effective and simple method of controlling and treating superficial bladder cancer (Reymann 1993). In measurable disease, average response rates are 60%. Approximately 30% of patients experience a complete response. Cytotoxic drugs found to be effective include:

- Thiotepa
- Mitomycin C
- Doxorubicin
- Epirubicin
- Mitoxantrone
- BCG.

Intravesical installation allows a high concentration of drug to bathe the endothelium, which enables localized treatment to the tumour and limits the systemic absorption so toxicity is reduced. Systemic toxicity is a problem with thiotepa, but otherwise the main problems are local inflammation, pain, burning on urination,

frequency and occasional haematuria. There is also the inconvenience for the patients. In addition a urinary tract infection may develop so the procedure should be performed using an aseptic technique.

Treatment protocols vary. Instillation involves the insertion of a urinary catheter and drainage of the bladder. Instillation of the drug usually takes about 50–60 minutes; it is retained for 1–2 hours with frequent movement to disperse the drug through the bladder (Goodman 2000; Sewell *et al.* 2002). Therapy may be repeated on alternating days for three doses or weekly for varying lengths of time (4–12 weeks).

Patients should be instructed in good personal hygiene such as washing hands and genitalia thoroughly after voiding and the toilet should be flushed at least twice after voiding. Increased intake during dwell time will increase the dilution of medication required and may reduce side-effects (Goodman 2000).

Procedure guidelines: **Intravesical instillation of cytotoxic drugs**

Other relevant procedures are urinary catheterization (see Ch. 16) and bladder lavage and irrigation (see Ch. 12). Details of required procedure and problems which may be encountered are given in these chapters. The following guidelines and problem solving deal with specific aspects of chemotherapy administration.

Equipment

1 Urotainer containing prescribed drug in clinically clean tray (delivered from pharmacy reconstitution unit).
2 Sterile gloves.
3 Disposable apron and eye protection.
4 Gate clip or equivalent clamp for catheter.
5 Catheter drainage bag, if catheter is to remain in position.
6 10 or 20 ml sterile syringe.
7 Small dressing pack, containing sterile field.

Procedure

Action	Rationale
1 Explain and discuss the procedure with the patient.	To ensure that the patient understands the procedure and gives his/her valid consent.
2 Check the patient's full blood count, as instructed by the medical staff, and inform them of any deficit before administration.	Absorption of the drug through the bladder wall may cause some myelosuppression. However, there are differing opinions as to whether regular checks are necessary.
3 Check all the details on the container of cytotoxic drug against the patient's prescription chart.	To minimize the risk of error and comply with legal requirements.
4 Assemble all necessary equipment, including the cytotoxic drug container, and proceed to the patient.	To ensure that the instillation proceeds smoothly and without interruption.
5 Screen the patient's bed/couch.	To ensure privacy during the procedure.
6 Check that the patient's identity matches the patient's details on the prescription chart.	To ensure that the correct patient has been identified. To reduce the risk of error.
7 If patient does not have a catheter in situ, then pass a catheter (see Ch. 12, Bladder lavage and irrigation).	
8 Ensure the bladder is empty of urine.	To prevent dilution of the drug.
9 Put on an apron/eye protection.	To protect the nurse from contact with the cytotoxic drugs. With correct technique the risk of contamination is minimal, but splashes can occur.

Procedure guidelines: **Intravesical instillation of cytotoxic drugs** *(cont'd)*

Action	Rationale
10 Using aseptic technique and sterile gloves, proceed to place a receiver under the end of the catheter to catch any urine and disconnect the drainage bag.	To protect the patient from infection. To protect the nurse from drug spillage. To gain access to the catheter. To prevent urine from soiling the bed.
11 Remove the cover from the urotainer, connect to the catheter and release the clamp.	To facilitate drug instillation.
12 Allow gravity to instil the cytotoxic drug into the bladder. Gentle squeezing may be needed to assist this process.	Rapid instillation would be uncomfortable for the patient, especially if the bladder is small or scarred from previous treatment or disease.
13 When the correct volume has been instilled, slide urotainer clamp over filling port.	To prevent drainage of drug from the bladder.
14 If the catheter is to be removed, withdraw the water from the catheter balloon (if appropriate – some catheters do not have a balloon: see Ch. 16) using the sterile syringe and remove the catheter using gentle traction. Dispose of equipment into yellow clinical waste bag and seal.	The catheter may not be required for continued urinary drainage, and may have been inserted to facilitate drug administration, particularly in the outpatient department. The risk of infection is greater if the catheter remains in situ.
15 Make the patient comfortable.	
16 Provide outpatients with information about the amount of movement required.	Following outpatient instillation, the journey home is usually sufficient to coat the bladder mucosa.
17 When the drug has been in the bladder for 1 hour, request the patient to micturate or slide clamp across filling port and place receiver under connectors. Disconnect urotainer and connect new drainage bag.	One hour is the usual time specified for intravesical drugs to ensure the maximum therapeutic effect with minimum toxicity. To prevent contamination of bed linen.
18 Advise the patient on fluid intake, suggesting ways in which he or she may increase it in the following 24-hour period. Patients should be aware that their urine may be cloudy.	To provide a good fluid output, washing out the bladder and reducing the likelihood of local irritation or difficulty in urination due to debris from the tumour. To make patients aware of this side-effect.
19 Instruct the patient to report any discomfort or inability to pass urine immediately to ward staff or general practitioner/district nurse, or to telephone the hospital if anxious.	To detect and resolve any problems at the earliest moment. To reduce anxiety experienced by the patient.

Problem solving

Problem	Cause	Suggested action
No drainage of urine when the catheter is inserted.	Bladder is empty or the catheter is in the wrong place, e.g. in the urethra or in a false track. False tracks may develop after repeated cystoscopy or bladder surgery.	Do not inflate the balloon but tape the catheter to the skin to keep it in position. Check when the patient last micturated. Encourage the patient to drink a few glasses of fluid. Do not give the drug until urine flow is seen or correct positioning of the catheter is established. Inform a doctor if no urine has drained during the next 30 minutes.
Haematuria.	Trauma of catheterization or loosening of blood clots following cystoscopy by fluid injected into the bladder.	Inform a doctor. Observe the patient for signs of clot retention, shock, haemorrhage or fluid retention. Encourage the patient to drink fluids.
Leakage from around the catheter following administration of the drug.	Catheter slipping out of the bladder or bladder spasm caused by the drug.	Check the position of the catheter. Inform a doctor if leakage persists. Protect the patient's skin by wrapping sterile topical swabs around the catheter. Estimate the volume lost by leakage. Wash contaminated skin thoroughly.

Problem solving

Problem	Cause	Suggested action
Abdominal pain or discomfort.	Peritoneal irritation following placement of catheter.	Knowledge of these side-effects. Observe for a reaction and treat symptomatically.
	Incomplete drainage of the dialysate solution.	
	Failure to warm dialysate solution to body temperature.	
	Chemical peritonitis resulting from chemotherapeutic agent.	
	Bacterial peritonitis.	
Leakage from around the catheter following administration of the drug.	Peritoneum is not intact or catheter is not entirely within peritoneal cavity.	Strict aseptic technique required. Dressings to be changed frequently. When skin around the catheter has healed, there should be no further leakage.

Intra-arterial administration

Definition

Intra-arterial administration is the delivery of a cytotoxic drug to the tumour site by catheterization of the artery providing the blood supply to the affected organ. This allows a high concentration of drug to be delivered.

Indications

Intra-arterial chemotherapy has been used to treat a variety of malignancies at a number of different sites. These include:

- Head and neck lesions
- Liver metastases from colorectal cancer
- Sarcomas/melanomas of upper and lower limb (including isolated limb perfusion)
- Carcinoma of the stomach
- Carcinoma of the breast
- Carcinoma of the cervix (Weinstein 2000).

The tumour site determines which artery will be used to deliver the chemotherapy since it is the artery supplying the tumour which is cannulated. The commonest route is the hepatic artery (Goodman 2000).

Reference material

The advantage of the route is that it facilitates the delivery of high concentrations of drug to the primary or secondary tumour mass (Sewell *et al.* 2002). A reduction in systemic circulating levels of drugs has been shown to occur in many circumstances resulting in a corresponding reduction in side-effects to the patient (Goodman 2000). The cytotoxic drugs used vary with the histology and site of the tumour. All of the following have been administered via the intra-arterial route:

- Actinomycin D
- BCNU (carmustine)
- Bleomycin
- Cisplatin
- Doxorubicin
- 5-FU (5-fluorouracil)
- 5-FUDR (fluorodeoxyuridine)
- Methotrexate
- Melphalan
- Mitomycin C
- Vincristine.

The main disadvantage of this route is that very high levels of drug in a perfused organ may result in excessive tissue damage (Sewell *et al.* 2002). It also requires the insertion of an arterial device. Two main methods are used for infusional chemotherapy; these are termed external and internal arterial infusions.

The external method involves radiographic placement of an arterial catheter and attachment to an external infusion pump (Goodman 2000). Temporary catheter placement is used for short-term therapies, i.e. from hours up to 5 days. Therapy can be given intermittently for several courses. This method is unsuitable for long-term use

(6 months or longer) as it is uncomfortable, inconvenient and expensive, although a subcutaneous implanted port increases the patient's comfort and freedom (Goodman 2000).

Once the catheter is in place and secured, cytotoxic drugs may be administered by:

- Injection – using a syringe
- Small volume infusion – using a syringe pump
- Large volume infusion – using a volumetric pump.

Internal or implantable methods involve the surgical placement of a totally implantable pump and appear to have a lower complication rate than the external method. The catheter is inserted into an appropriate artery and attached to the pump, which is filled with chemotherapy. This approach is more frequently used for colorectal cancer metastases to the liver.

Confirmation that the artery supplies the desired area can be achieved by instillation of yellow fluorescent dye if the tumour site is visible, or contrast medium if an internal organ such as the liver is the target area.

All delivery systems must provide adequate pressure to combat arterial pressure, i.e. 300 mmHg (Goodman 2000). The majority of infusion pumps meet this requirement. Patient education is very important as the patient may have to maintain the implantable pump and be able to recognize any complications or malfunctions.

Principles of nursing care

Insertion is an operative procedure and consent must be obtained. Adequate explanation to the patient is essential, especially what to expect on return to the ward.

The area of insertion should be shaved or otherwise prepared and the period of fasting should be checked with the anaesthetist.

The catheter is inserted in theatre or in the X-ray department and its position checked at that time. The catheter is then secured and an occlusive dressing applied. This should *not* be touched as it is essential that the catheter is *not* displaced.

A three- or one-way tap is connected to the catheter and it is at this point that all manipulations take place. An extension set should be connected to this at the time of insertion or on return to the ward to prevent unnecessary handling near the skin exit site.

The system will consist of: catheter/tap/extension set/administration set and infusion device.

Certain general rules apply:

1 The dressing must not be touched but should be observed regularly for signs of bleeding. This should be reported immediately to the medical staff, including the radiologist.

2 All procedures or manipulations must be performed using aseptic technique.

3 All connections must be Luer locking to prevent exsanguination, air embolism or disconnection under pressure.

4 The catheter must be clamped securely or switched off using the tap in situ before any equipment changes.

5 A positive pressure greater than arterial pressure must be maintained at all times.

6 When chemotherapy is not being infused, the flushing solution must be used to maintain patency. This should be via a syringe or syringe pump during transfer between wards or departments, or via a syringe pump or infusion pump in the ward. A nurse escort may be necessary for transfers. It should be delivered at the minimum rate sufficient to combat arterial pressure and maintain patency, approximately 3–5 ml per hour or 10 drops per minute, dependent on the device used. If a specialist delivery system is used, then manufacturers' instructions should be followed.

7 The patient must be instructed on the amount of mobility allowed. This may vary depending on the site of the catheter. Assistance may be needed to maintain personal hygiene and relieve pressure in order to prevent the development of pressure ulcers on all points of contact.

8 The position of the catheter may be checked daily by X-ray, which will be performed on the ward. Fluoroscopy and instillation of dye are other methods of confirming position.

9 At the end of treatment, the patency of the arterial catheter should be maintained using an appropriate flushing solution until a decision has been made about removal. Instructions for this and the amount of heparin to be used should be prescribed in advance to enable the nurse to initiate the procedure when appropriate.

10 Before removal, the tap may be switched off and the catheter allowed to clot. The catheter should be removed by a doctor and firm pressure applied for at least 5 minutes or until all bleeding has ceased. A dressing should be applied to the site. Pressure dressings are not indicated if bleeding has ceased as they can obscure the formation of a haematoma.

Complications associated with intra-arterial chemotherapy

1 Arterial occlusion and thrombosis: the literature indicates that thrombosis occurs in over 40% of arteries catheterized for over 48 hours. However,

this is dependent on the vessel used. Most catheters used for chemotherapy delivery pose no problem and will remain patent for the treatment period. However, a thrombus may embolize causing vascular insufficiency, distal or central embolism (Weinstein 2000). When occlusion occurs due to thrombus formation or spasm, blood flow is usually maintained by the collateral circulation until the vessel recovers. Presence of a pulse and the colour of the area should be checked daily or a Doppler flow meter may be used. Any abnormality should be reported to the medical staff and radiologist. The catheter should be removed by the doctor using firm, steady traction, in an attempt to prevent dislodging any thrombus present. The condition of the patient and the limb/area should be observed carefully at the time that vital signs are measured.

2 Damage to the artery, arteriovenous fistula, aneurysm formation: the incidence of these is low and the likelihood of problems occurring can be minimized by gentle handling of the catheter and immobilization of the limb/area as soon as appropriate.

3 Chemical hepatitis and biliary sclerosis: the occurrence of these will be evident from elevated liver enzymes. Therefore, monitoring of liver function tests is important. Any elevation is usually transient.

4 Exsanguination/air embolism: the seriousness of an air embolus depends on the siting of the arterial catheter and whether it is a direct route to the carotid artery and so to the brain. Luer–Lok connections must be used throughout the pathway. These should be checked at regular intervals, and continuous flow maintained. Care must be taken when changing equipment to prevent blood loss occurring or air entering the catheter, e.g. shut off the tap, firm clamping, if necessary.

Problem solving

Problem	Cause	Action
Haemorrhage.	Excessive movement.	Observe the dressing at regular intervals. Monitor pulse and blood pressure at least 4 hourly.
		Instruct the patient on the amount of movement permitted and to report any feeling of faintness, or oozing noted on dressing.
	Insufficient pressure on site following removal of catheter.	After removal of the catheter, vital signs and the dressing should be observed at least every 15 minutes for 2 hours.
		Whether the patient should remain on bedrest for 24 hours is dependent on the site where the patient has been catheterized.
		If bleeding occurs, pressure should be applied immediately and a member of the medical staff contacted.
Displacement of the catheter.	Dressing disturbed.	Do not disturb the dressing.
	Excessive movement by patient.	Instruct the patient on amount of movement permitted. Check position daily.
Infection.	Poor aseptic technique.	Strict asepsis must be maintained for all procedures and manipulations of the arterial catheter. Temperature must be taken at least every 4 hours and any pyrexia investigated.
Extravasation of drugs/failure of drug to reach target area (both rare).	Incorrect placement of catheter.	If there is any doubt concerning the placement of the catheter the doctor and radiologist should be notified, as extravasation of the drug may lead to ulceration and necrosis.

References and further reading

Ames, B.N. *et al.* (1975) Methods for detecting carcinogens and mutagens with the salmonella/mammalian microsome mutagenicity test. *Mutat Res*, **31**, 347–64.

Bertolli, G. (1995) Prevention and management of extravasation of cytotoxic drugs. *Drug Saf*, **12**(4), 245–55.

Bertolli, G., Cafferata, M. & Ardizzoni, A. (1997) Skin ulceration potential of paclitaxel in a mouse skin model in vivo. *Cancer*, **79**, 2266–9.

Bingham, E. (1985) Hazards to health care professionals from antineoplastic drugs. *N Engl J Med*, **313**, 1120–22.

Camp Sorrell, D. (1998) Developing extravasation protocols and monitoring outcomes. *J Intraven Nurs*, **21**(4), 232–9.

Cass, Y. *et al.* (1997) Health and safety aspects of cytotoxic services. In: *The Cytotoxic Handbook*, 3rd edn (eds M. Allwood, A. Stanley & P. Wright). Radcliffe Medical Press, Oxford, pp. 35–54.

Colls, B.M. (1985) Safety of handling cytotoxic agents: a cause for concern by pharmaceutical companies. *Br Med J*, **291**, 318–19.

Cooke, J. *et al.* (1987) Environmental monitoring of personnel who handle cytotoxic drugs. *Pharm J*, **239** (6452, Suppl R2).

Cox, K., Stuart-Harris, R.A., Addini, G. *et al.* (1988) The management of cytotoxic drug extravasation: guidelines drawn up by a working party for the Clinical Oncological Society of Australia. *Med J Aust*, **148**, 185–9.

CP Pharmaceuticals (1999) *How Quickly Could You Act?* CP Pharmaceuticals, Wrexham.

DoH (2000) *An Organisation with a Memory*. Stationery Office, London.

DoH (2002) *Reference Guide to Consent for Examination or Treatment*. Stationery Office, London.

DoH (2003) HSC 2003/10. *Updated National Guidance on the Safe Administration of Intrathecal Chemotherapy*. DoH, London.

Dougherty, L. (1999) Obtaining peripheral venous access. In: *Intravenous Therapy in Nursing Practice* (eds L. Dougherty & J. Lamb). Churchill Livingstone, Edinburgh.

Dougherty, L. (1999) Safe administration of intravenous cytotoxic drugs. In: *Intravenous Therapy in Nursing Practice* (eds L. Dougherty & J. Lamb). Churchill Livingstone, Edinburgh.

Dougherty, L. (2003) An expert witness working within the legal system in the United Kingdom. *J Vas Ass Net* **8**(2), 29–37.

Elliot, T.S.J. & Tebbs, S.E. (1998) Prevention of central venous catheter related infection. *J Hosp Infect*, **40**, 193–201.

Falck, K. *et al.* (1979) Mutagenicity in urine of nurses handling cytotoxic agents. *Lancet*, **i**, 1250.

Federle, M., Chang, P.J. & Confer, S. (1998) Frequency and effects of extravasation of non isotonic CT contrast media during rapid bolus injection. *Radiology*, **206**, 637–40.

Ferguson, L. & Wright, P. (2002) Administration of chemotherapy. In: *The Cytotoxic Handbook*, 4th edn (eds M. Alwood *et al.*). Radcliffe Medical Press, Oxford.

Gabriel, J. (1999) Long-term central venous access. In: *Intravenous Therapy in Nursing Practice* (eds L. Dougherty & J. Lamb). Churchill Livingstone, Edinburgh.

Gault, D.T. (1993) Extravasation injuries. *Br J Plast Surg*, **46**(2), 91–6.

Gault, D. & Challands, J. (1997) Extravasation of drugs. *Anaesth Rev*, **13**, 223–41.

Goodman, I. (1998) Development of national evidence based clinical guidelines for the administration of cytotoxic chemotherapy. *Eur J Oncol Nurs*, **2**(1), 43–50.

Goodman, M. (2000) Chemotherapy: principles of administration. In: *Cancer Nursing – Principles and Practice* (eds C. Henke Yarbro *et al.*). Jones and Bartlett, Massachusetts.

Health and Safety Executive (1983) *Precautions for the Safe Handling of Cytotoxic Drugs. Medical Series*. Stationery Office, London.

Health and Safety Executive (2002) *The Control of Substances Hazardous to Health Regulations*. Stationery Office, London.

Health and Safety Executive (2003) *Safe Handling of Cytotoxic Drugs*. HSE, London (in press).

Heckler, F.R. (1989) Current thoughts on extravasation injuries. *Clin Plast Surg*, **16**(3), 557–63.

How, C. & Brown, J. (1998) Extravasation of cytotoxic chemotherapy from peripheral veins. *Eur J Oncol Nurs*, **2**(1), 51–8.

Ignoffo, R.J. & Friedman, M.A. (1980) Therapy of local toxicities caused by extravasation of cancer chemotherapeutic drugs. *Cancer Treat Rev*, **7**, 17–27.

Intravenous Nursing Society (INS) (2000) *Standards*. INS, Massachusetts.

Irving, V. (2001) Managing extravasation injuries in preterm infants. *NT Plus*, **97**(35), 40–6.

Kaijser, G.P. *et al.* (1990) The risks of handling cytotoxic drugs, 1. Methods of testing exposure. *Pharm Weekbi*, **12**(6), 217–27.

Kotilainen, H.R. (1989) Latex and vinyl examination gloves – quality control procedures and implications for health care workers. *Arch Intern Med*, **149**, 2749–53.

Labuhn, K. *et al.* (1998) Nurses' and pharmacists' exposure to antineoplastic drugs: findings from industrial hygiene scans and urine mutagenicity tests. *Cancer Nurs*, **21**(2), 79–89.

Langhorne, M. & Barton-Burke, M. (2001) Chemotherapy administration: general principles for nursing practice:. In: *Cancer: A Nuring Process Approach*, 3rd edn (eds M. Barton-Burke, G. Wilkes & K. Ingwerson). Jones and Bartlett, Massachusetts.

Mayo, D.J. (1998) Fibrin sheath formation and chemotherapy extravasation: a case report. *Supp Care Cancer*, **6**, 51–6.

McCaffrey Boyle, D. & Engelking, C. (1995) Vesicant extravasation: myths and realities. *Oncol Nurs Forum*, **22**(1), 57–65.

Newman, M.A. *et al.* (1994) Urinary biological monitoring markers of anticancer drug exposure in oncology nurses. *Am J Public Health*, **84**(5), 852–5.

Nguyen, T.V. *et al.* (1982) Exposure of pharmacy personnel to mutagenic antineoplastic drugs. *Cancer Res*, **42**, 4792–6.

NMC (2002) *Code of Professional Conduct*. NMC, London.

Oncology Nursing Society (ONS) (1999) *Cancer Chemotherapy Guidelines and Recommendations for Practice*, 2nd edn. Oncology Nursing Press, Pittsburgh.

Otto, S.E. (1995) Advanced concepts in chemotherapy drug delivery. *Reg Ther I Intraven Nurs*, **18**(4), 170–6.

Parker, L.A. *et al.* (1989) Small bore catheter drainage and sclerotherapy for malignant pleural effusions. *Cancer*, **64**, 1218–21.

Perdue, M.B. (2001) Intravenous complications. In: *Infusion Therapy in Clinical Practice*, 2nd edn (eds J. Hankin *et al*). W.B. Saunders, Philadelphia.

Priestman, T.J. (1989) *Cancer Chemotherapy: An Introduction*, 3rd edn. Springer, Berlin.

Quan, W. (1999) Malignant, pleural, peritoneal and pericardial effusions and meningeal infiltrates. In: *Handbook of Chemotherapy*, 5th edn (ed. R.T. Skeet). Lippincott, Williams & Wilkins, Philadelphia.

RCN (1998) *Clinical Practice Guidelines – The Administration of Cytotoxic Chemotherapy*. Royal College of Nursing, Oxford.

RCN (2003) *Standards for Infusion Therapy*. Royal College of Nursing, London.

Reymann, P.E. (1993) *Chemotherapy Principles of Administration* in *Cancer Nursing Principles and Practice*, 3rd edn (eds S.L. Groenwald, M. Goodman, M.H. Frogge & C.H. Yarbro). Jones & Bartlett Publishers, Boston, Chap. 15.

Rittenberg, C.N., Gralla, R.J. & Rehmeyer, T.A. (1995) Assessing and managing venous irritation with vinorelbine tartrate. *Oncol Nurs Forum*, **22**(4), 707–10.

Rudolph, R. & Larson, D.L. (1987) Etiology and treatment of chemotherapeutic agent extravasation injuries: a review. *J Clin Oncol*, **5**(7), 1116–26.

Sansivero, G. & Barton-Burke, M. (2001) Chemotherapy administration: general principles for vascular access. In: *Cancer: A Nursing Process Approach*, 3rd edn (eds M. Barton-Burke, G. Wilkes & K. Ingwerson). Jones and Bartlett, Massachusetts.

Schulmeister, L. (1989) Needle dislodgement from implanted venous access devices – inpatients and outpatient experiences. *J Intraven Nurs*, **12**, 90–2.

Schulmeister, L. (1998) A complication of vascular access device insertion. *J Intraven Nurs*, **21**(4), 197–202.

Selevan, S.G. *et al.* (1985) A study of occupational exposure to antineoplastic drugs and fetal loss in nurses. *N Engl J Med*, **19**, 1173–8.

Sewell, G., Summerhayes M. & Stanley, A. (2002) Administration of chemotherapy. In: *The Cytotoxics Handbook*, 4th edn (eds M. Allwood *et al.*). Radcliffe Medical Press, Oxford.

Shulman, R., Drayan, S. & Harries, M. (1998) Management of extravasation of IV drugs. In: *UCL Injectable Drug Administration*. Blackwell Science, Oxford.

Springhouse Corporation (2002) Chemotherapy infusions. In: *Intravenous Therapy Made Incredibly Easy*. Springhouse Corporation, Philadelphia.

Stanley, A. (2002) Managing complications of chemotherapy administration. In: *The Cytotoxic Handbook*, 4th edn (eds M. Allwood *et al.*). Radcliffe Medical Press, Oxford.

Stokes, M. *et al.* (1987) Permeability of latex and polyvinyl chloride gloves to fluorouracil and methotrexate. *Am J Hosp Pharm*, **44**, 1341–6.

Taskinen, H.K. (1990) Effects of parental occupational exposures on spontaneous abortion and congenital malformation. *Scand J Work Environ Health*, **16**, 297–314.

Taylor, L. (1962) A catheter technique for intrapleural adminstration of alkylating agents: a report of ten cases. *Am J Med Sci*, **244**(6), 706–16.

Thomas, P.H. & Fenton May, V. (1987) Protection offered by gloves to carmustine exposure. *Pharm J*, **238**, 775–7.

Toft, B. (2001) *External Inquiry into the Adverse Incident that Occurred at the Queen's Medical Centre, Nottingham, on 4th January 2001*. Department of Health, London.

Tsang, V. *et al.* (1990) Pleuroperitoneal shunt for recurrent malignant pleural effusion. *Thorax*, **45**, 369–72.

Tully, J.L., Friedland, G.H., Baldrini, L.M. *et al.* (1981) Complications of intravenous therapy with steel needles and teflon catheters: a comparative study. *Am J Med*, **70**, March, 702–6.

Valanis, B. *et al.* (1997) Occupational exposure to antineoplastic agents and self reported infertility among nurses and pharmacists. *J Occup Environ Med*, **39**(6), 574–80.

Valanis, B.G., Vollmer, W.M. Labuhn, K.T. *et al.* (1993) Acute symptoms associated with antineoplastic drug handling among nurses. *Cancer Nurs*, **16**(4), 288–95.

Vandergrift, K.V. (2001) Oncologic therapy. In: *Infusion Therapy in Clinical Practice*, 2nd edn (eds J. Hankin *et al.*). W.B. Saunders, Philadelphia.

Vennit, S. *et al.* (1984) Monitoring exposure of nursing and pharmacy personnel to cytotoxic drugs: urinary mutation assays and urinary platinum as markers of absorption. *Lancet*, **i**, 74–6.

Waksvik, H. *et al.* (1987) Chromosome analysis of nurses handling cytostatic agents. *Cancer Treat Rep*, **65**, 607–10.

Weinstein, S. (2000) Antineoplastic therapy. In: *Plumer's Principles and Practices of Intravenous Therapy*, 7th edn. Lippincott, Philadelphia, pp. 474–548.

11

Drug administration: delivery (infusion devices)

Chapter contents

Definition

An infusion device is designed to deliver measured amounts of drug or fluid via a number of routes (e.g. intravenous, subcutaneous or epidural) over a period of time. This is set at an appropriate rate to achieve the desired therapeutic response and prevent complications.

Indications

The nurse has a responsibility to determine the correct rate in individual circumstances and to maintain that rate throughout the infusion. The nurse can achieve this by mechanical means such as gravity flow or by the use of an electronic infusion device. The following factors should be considered when selecting an appropriate infusion delivery system:

1 Risk to the patient of:
  (a) Overinfusion
  (b) Underinfusion
  (c) Uneven flow
  (d) High delivery pressure
  (e) Inadvertent bolus
  (f) Extravascular infusion
2 Delivery parameters:
  (a) Infusion rate and volume required
  (b) Accuracy required (over a long or short period of time)
  (c) Alarms required
  (d) Ability to infuse into site chosen (venous, arterial, subcutaneous)
  (e) Suitability of device for infusing drug (e.g. ability to infuse viscous drugs)
3 Environmental features:
  (a) Ease of operation
  (b) Frequency of observation and adjustment

Box 11.1 Complications of inadequate flow control

Complications associated with overinfusion:
1 Fluid overload with accompanying electrolyte imbalance.
2 Metabolic disturbances during parenteral nutrition, mainly related to serum glucose levels.
3 Toxic concentrations of medications, which may result in a shock-like syndrome ('speed shock').
4 Air embolism, due to containers running dry before expected.
5 An increase in venous complications, e.g. chemical phlebitis, caused by reduced dilution of irritant substances (Weinstein 2000).

Complications associated with underinfusion:
1 Dehydration.
2 Metabolic disturbances.
3 A delayed response to medications or below therapeutic dose.
4 Occlusion of a cannula/catheter due to slow flow or cessation of flow.

Box 11.2 Groups at risk of complications associated with flow control

---

1 Infants and young children.
2 The elderly.
3 Patients with compromised cardiovascular status.
4 Patients with impairment or failure of organs, e.g. kidneys.
5 Patients with major sepsis.
6 Patients suffering from shock, whatever the cause.
7 Postoperative or post-trauma patients.
8 Stressed patients, whose endocrine homeostatic controls may be affected.
9 Patients receiving multiple medications, whose clinical status may change rapidly (Springhouse 2002).

(c) Type of patient (neonate, child, very sick)
(d) Mobility of patient (Medical Devices Agency 1995).

Reference material

Infusion devices are commonly used to manage intravenous administration (Quinn 2000) and the aim is to ensure the delivery of a drug or fluid to a patient at a constant rate over a set period of time with no adjustment to 'catch up'. This is not only to ensure a therapeutic response but also to avoid complications of over- and underinfusion (Box 11.1).

The nurse must have knowledge of the solutions, their effects, rate of administration, factors which affect flow of infusion, as well as the complications which could occur when flow is not controlled (Weinstein 2000). The nurse should have an understanding of which groups require accurate flow control in order to prevent complications (Box 11.2) and how to select the most appropriate device for accuracy of delivery to best meet the patient's flow control needs (according to age, condition, setting and prescribed therapy) (Weinstein 2000).

The use of infusion devices, both mechanical and electronic, has increased the level of safety in intravenous therapy. However, it is recommended that a clearly defined structure for management of infusion systems must exist within a trust (Medical Devices Agency 2003).

Criteria for selection of an infusion device include rationalization of devices, clinical requirement, education, compatibility with other equipment, disposables, product support, costs, service and maintenance and regulatory issues, e.g. compliance with European Community directives (Medical Devices Agency 2000; Quinn 2000; DoH 2001). Strategies need to be developed for replacement of old, obsolete or inappropriate devices (Medical Devices Agency 2000; Quinn 2000; DoH 2001), planned service maintenance programmes and acceptance testing (Medical Devices Agency 1998). A useful checklist has been produced by the Medical Devices Agency for staff to follow prior to using a medical device to ensure safe practice (Medical Devices Agency 2000).

Many thousands of infusion devices are now being used within hospitals and in the community. Between 1990 and 2000 there were 1485 incidents reported to the Medical Devices Agency which involved infusion pumps (Medical Devices Agency 2003). In 50% of incidents no cause was established. However, of the remaining incidents, 27% were attributed to user error (misloading administration set or syringe, setting wrong rate, confusing pump type, etc.) and 20% to device-related issues (poor maintenance, cleaning, etc.) (Williams & Lefever 2000; Medical Devices Agency 2003). In any 100 reports involving pumps, over 50% are overinfusions (Medical Devices Agency 2000). In theory any infusion system can be misused; in practice, syringe pumps have given rise to the most significant problems in terms of patient mortality and morbidity (Fox 2000; Medical Devices Agency 2003; NPSA 2003). The high frequency of human error has highlighted the need for more formalized, validated, competency-based training and assessment (Pickstone 2000; Quinn 2000; Medical Devices Agency 2003). As the main users of infusion devices in direct patient care, nurses must be competent with both simple and complex devices (McConnell *et al.* 1996). Health care professionals are personally accountable for their use of infusion devices and therefore must ensure they have the appropriate training (Medical Devices Agency 2001). They must be familiar with the device they are using and not attempt to operate any device that they have not been fully trained to use (Murray & Glenister 2001). Education can be problematic, often inadequate, and its nature and quality vary greatly (McConnell 1995). The most frequently identified methods of training for staff are reading the user/instruction manual, trial and error (self taught) and consulting policy and procedure manuals (McConnell 1995; McConnell *et al.* 1996). 'Hands on' training is a major constituent of learning to use the equipment and teaching may be carried out by another member of staff or as part of in-service training. As a minimum, the training should cover the device, drugs and solutions, and the practical procedures related to setting up the device and problem solving (Medical Devices Agency 2001, 2002). Staff should also be made aware of the mechanisms for reporting faults with devices and procedures for adverse incident reporting within their trust and to the Medical Devices Agency and National Patient Safety Agency (Medical Devices Agency 2001).

Factors influencing flow rates

The following factors may increase or decrease intravenous flow rates, particularly with mechanical devices using gravity flow, so the nurse should recheck the infusion rate regularly to ensure the prescribed flow rate is maintained.

Type of fluid and container

The composition, viscosity and concentration of the fluid affect flow (Weinstein 2000; Quinn 2000; Springhouse 2002). For example, an infusion of cold blood (which is viscous when cold, Macklin 1999) or irritants will result in venospasm and impede the flow rate. This can be resolved by use of a warm pack over the cannula site and the limb (Weinstein 2000; Springhouse 2002). Intravenous fluids run by gravity and so any changes in the height of the container will alter the flow rate. The optimum height of the container above the patient is 1 m (Springhouse 2002; Medical Devices Agency 2003) and it will usually provide 70 mmHg of pressure, which is adequate to overcome venous pressure (normal range in an adult is 25–80 mmHg) (Macklin 1999; Pickstone 1999; Springhouse Corporation 1999). Therefore any alterations in the patient's position may alter the flow rate and necessitate a change in the speed of the infusion to maintain the appropriate rate of flow (Weinstein 2000; Perucca 2001).

Type of administration set

The flow rate of the infusion may be affected in several ways:

1 Roller clamps or screw clamps, used to adjust and maintain rates of flow on gravity infusions, vary considerably in their efficiency and accuracy which is often dependent on a number of variables such as patient movement and height of infusion container (Weinstein 2000; Perucca 2001). Roller clamps should be positioned on the upper third of the tubing near the fluid container, making access convenient for staff and out of the way of the patient (Perucca 2001). The clamp should be repositioned or the tubing will develop a memory (cold creep). This is when the tubing tries to retain its round shape and pushes the clamp open, while pinched tubing does not reopen (Perucca 2001; Medical Devices Agency 2003). The roller clamp should be used as the primary means of occluding the tubing even if there is an anti-free-flow device (Medical Devices Agency 2003).

2 The diameter/inner lumen size and the length of tubing will also affect flow (Quinn 2000). Microbore sets have a narrow lumen and flow is restricted to some degree. However, these sets may be used as a safeguard against 'runaway' or bolus infusions by either an integrated anti-siphon valve or anti-free flow device (Weinstein 2000; Quinn 2000; Perucca 2001).

3 Inclusion of other in-line devices, e.g. filters, may also affect the flow rate (Perucca 2001; Medical Devices Agency 2003).

Type of vascular access device

The flow rate may be affected by any of the following:

- The condition and size of the vein, e.g. phlebitis can reduce the lumen size and decrease flow (Weinstein 2000).

- The gauge of the cannula/catheter (Weinstein 2000; Springhouse 2002; Medical Devices Agency 2003).

- The position of the device within the vein, i.e. whether it is up against the vein wall.

- The site of the vascular access device, e.g. the flow may be affected by the change in position of a limb – such as a decrease in flow when a patient bends their arm if a cannula is sited over the elbow joint (Springhouse 2002).

- Kinking, pinching or compression of the cannula/catheter or tubing of the administration set may cause variation in the set rate (Springhouse 2002; Medical Devices Agency 2003).

- Occlusion of the device due to clot formation, which may result from a BP cuff on the infusion arm, with the patient lying on the side of the infusion (Quinn 2000).

The patient

Patients occasionally adjust the control clamp or other parts of the delivery system, for example changing the height of the infusion container, thereby making flow unreliable. Some pumps now have tamper-proof features. Positioning of the patient will affect flow and patients should be instructed to keep the arm lower than the infusion if the infusion is reliant on gravity (Dolan 1999).

Complications associated with lack of flow control

Fluid/electrolyte imbalance

Circulatory overload (isotonic fluid expansion)

A critical and common complication of intravenous therapy is circulatory overload, which is *isotonic fluid expansion*. It is caused by infusion of fluids of the same tonicity as plasma into the vascular circulation, for example 0.9% sodium chloride. As isotonic solutions do not affect osmolarity, water does not flow from the extracellular to the intracellular compartment. The result is that the extracellular compartment expands in proportion to the fluid infused (Weinstein 2000). Because of the electrolyte concentration, no extra water is available to enable the kidneys selectively to excrete and restore the balance. Patients at risk include older people, those with impaired renal and cardiac function and children (Dougherty 2002).

Early manifestations include:

- Weight gain
- A relative increase in fluid intake compared to output
- A high bounding pulse pressure, indicating a high cardiac output
- Raised central venous pressure measurements
- Peripheral hand vein emptying time longer than normal. (Peripheral veins will usually empty in 3–5 seconds when the hand is elevated and will fill in the same length of time when the hand is lowered to a dependent position; Weinstein 2000.)
- Peripheral oedema.

Progression of circulatory overload will lead to dyspnoea and cyanosis due to pulmonary oedema and neck vein engorgement (Weinstein 2000). If fluid administration is allowed to continue unchecked, it can result in left-sided heart failure, circulatory collapse and cardiac arrest (Edwards 2001; Dougherty 2002). Early detection results in simple treatment and consists of withholding all fluids until excess water and electrolytes have been eliminated by the body and/or administration of diuretics to promote rapid diuresis (Weinstein 2000). However, careful monitoring should continue to prevent isotonic contraction occurring (where there is loss of fluid and electrolytes isotonic to the extracellular fluid such as blood and large volumes of fluid from diarrhoea and vomiting; Weinstein 2000).

If a patient is receiving large quantities of electrolyte-free water, such as glucose 5% in water to replace losses from gastric suction, vomiting, diarrhoea, diuresis or insensible loss, *hypotonic expansion* may develop. This involves both extracellular and intracellular compartments (Weinstein 2000).

Hypertonic expansion occurs when the volume of body water is increased by infusion of hypertonic saline (Weinstein 2000).

Dehydration (hypertonic contraction)

This occurs when water is lost without corresponding loss of salts (Weinstein 2000) and occurs in patients unable to take sufficient fluids (elderly, unconscious or incontinent patients) or who have excess insensible water loss via skin and lungs or as a result of certain drugs in excess. Manifestations include:

- Thirst (although this may be absent in the elderly)
- Weight loss
- Negative fluid balance
- Irritability and restlessness
- Diminishes skin turgor
- Dry mouth and furrowed tongue.

Hypotonic contraction occurs when fluids containing more salt than water are lost and this results in a decrease in osmolarity of the extracellular compartment. Infants are at greatest risk, especially if they have diarrhoea (Weinstein 2000). It may also result from the loss of salt from various sources – excess diuresis, fistula drainage, burns, vomiting or sweating. Manifestations include:

- Weight loss
- Negative fluid balance
- Weak, thready, rapid pulse rate
- Increased 'hand filling time'
- Increased skin turgor.

Treatment of dehydration is replacement of fluids and electrolytes.

Speed shock

Speed shock is a systemic reaction that occurs when a substance foreign to the body is rapidly introduced into the circulation (Dougherty 2002). This complication can manifest following administration of intravenous bolus injections or when large volumes of fluid are given too rapidly. This should not be confused with pulmonary oedema, which relates to the volume of fluid infused into the patient. Rapid, uncontrolled administration of drugs will result in toxic concentrations reaching vital organs. Toxicity may be manifested by an exaggeration of the usual pharmacological actions of the drug or by signs and symptoms specific for that drug or class of drugs. The most extreme toxic response which can occur if a drug is given at a dose or rate exceeding that recommended is termed the lethal response.

Signs of speed shock may include:

- Flushed face
- Headache and dizziness
- Congestion of the chest
- Tachycardia and fall in blood pressure
- Syncope
- Shock
- Cardiovascular collapse (Weinstein 2000).

Prevention of speed shock is achieved by reducing the drop size, for example by the use of paediatric burette sets or infusion devices. When commencing an infusion using gravity flow, check that the solution is flowing freely before adjusting the rate. Movement of the patient or the device within the vessel can cause the infusion to flow more or less freely after a few minutes of setting the rate (Weinstein 2000). Always close the roller clamp prior to removing the set from the pump. Although most pumps have an anti-free-flow mechanism, it is still recommended to switch off the clamp (Pickstone 1999). Administration must be slowed down or discontinued and the medical staff notified. If speed shock occurs it may be necessary to administer antidotes and diuretics (see Problem solving).

Siphonage

Uncontrolled flow from a syringe is called siphonage; this is a result of gravity or leakage of air into the syringe and administration set. Siphonage can occur whether or not the syringe is fixed into an infusion device (Pickstone 1999; Quinn 2000).

The height of the syringe and air leaking into the syringe barrel can be equally catastrophic. To minimize the risk of siphonage the following steps need to be taken:

- Intravenous administration extension sets should always be micro/narrow bore in diameter.
- Wide-bore extension sets should be avoided.
- Position of the syringe pump should always be as close to the heart as is practically possible.

- High-risk infusions warrant the use of extension sets with an integral anti-siphonage valve (Quinn 2000).

Paediatric considerations

Infusion therapy within the paediatric setting requires very specific skills (Sundquist 2001). Competency in calculation of paediatric dosages, maintaining a stringent fluid balance, use of paediatric-specific devices and management of complications are paramount.

Principles of equipment selection and application

The Medicines and Healthcare Products Regulatory Agency (MHRA), formerly the Medical Devices Agency, has made recommendations on the safety and performance of infusion devices in order to enable users to make the appropriate choice of equipment to suit most applications (Medical Devices Agency 2003). The new classification system has been divided into three major categories according to the potential risks involved. These are shown in Table 11.1. A pump suited to the most risky category of therapy (A) can be safely used for the other categories (B and C). A pump suited to category B can be used for B and C, whereas a pump with the lowest specification (C) is suited only to category C therapies (Medical Devices Agency 2003) (see Fig. 11.1). Hospitals will be required to label each infusion pump with its category and it will be necessary to know the category of the proposed therapy and match it with a pump of the same or better category. A locally produced list of drugs/fluids by their categories will need to be provided to all device users (Medical Devices Agency 2003).

Requirements of devices

Accuracy of delivery

In order to meet requirements for high-risk and neonatal infusions, pumps must be accurate to within $\pm 5\%$ of the set rate when measured over a 60-minute period (Perucca 2001; Springhouse 2002). They also have to satisfy short-term, minute to minute accuracy requirements which determine smoothness and consistency of output (Pickstone *et al.* 1994).

Occlusion response and pressure

Flow will occur if the pressure at the tip of an intravascular device is just fractionally above the pressure in the vein; the pressure does not need to be excessive. In an adult peripheral vein pressure is approximately 25 mmHg, while in a neonate it measures 5 mmHg

Table 11.1 Therapy categories and performance parameters

Therapy category	Therapy description	Patient group	Critical performance parameters
A	Drugs with narrow therapeutic margin	Any	Good long-term accuracy Good short-term accuracy
	Drugs with short half-life	Any	Rapid alarm after occlusion Small occlusion bolus
	Any infusion given to neonates	Neonates	Able to detect very small air embolus (volumetric pumps only) Small flow rate increments Good bolus accuracy Rapid start-up time (syringe pumps only)
B	Drugs, other than those with a short half-life	Any except neonates	Good long-term accuracy Alarm after occlusion
	Total parenteral nutrition (TPN) Fluid maintenance Transfusions	Volume sensitive except neonates	Small occlusion bolus Able to detect small air embolus (volumetric pumps only) Small flow rate increments
	Diamorphine	Any except neonates	Bolus accuracy
C	TPN Fluid maintenance Transfusions	Any except volume sensitive or neonates	Long-term accuracy Alarm after occlusion Small occlusion bolus Able to detect air embolus (volumetric pumps only) Incremental flow rates

Crown copyright material is reproduced with the permission of the Controller of HMSO and Queen's Printer for Scotland. Medical Devices Agency (2003).

(Auty 1995). Most pumps have a variable pressure setting which allows the user to use their own judgement about the pressure needed to deliver therapy safely. It can be set as low as 100–250 mmHg (2–5 psi) for infusions of vesicants or routine infusions via healthy veins (Perucca 2001) or a maximum of 10 psi in positional central venous catheters. The common setting is 200–400 mmHg (4–8 psi); (Macklin 1999). Flow is dependent upon pressure divided by resistance. If very long extension sets of small internal bore are used the resistance to flow can increase dramatically (Auty 1995). If any set is occluded this increases resistance and infusate will not flow into the vein. The longer the occlusion occurs, the greater the pressure and the pump will continue to pump until an occlusion alarm is activated. There are two types of occlusions defined – upstream, between the pump and the container, and downstream, which is between the pump and the patient. An upstream occlusion alarms when a vacuum is created in the upstream tubing or full reservoir, due to collapsed or empty plastic fluid container or clamped/kinking tubing. A downstream occlusion is

when the pressure required by the pump exceeds a certain psi limit (Perucca 2001). Devices have 2–3 levels of differential pressure settings (psi ratings) and can sense a change in pressure usually 5 psi over baseline (Weinstein 2000).

Pumps alarm at a pressure termed 'occlusion alarm pressure' and many pumps allow the user to set the pressure within a range (Auty 1995). Therefore the time it takes to alarm depends on the rate of flow – high rates alarm more quickly. When the alarm is activated, a certain amount of stored bolus will be present and it is important that a large bolus is not released into the vein as this could lead to rupture of the vein or constitute overinfusion (Auty 1995).

Air-in-line detectors are designed to detect only visible or microscopic 'champagne' bubbles. They should not create anxiety over small particles of air but alert the nurse to the integrity of the system. Most air bubbles detected are too small to have a harmful effect (Perucca 2001).

The Medical Devices Agency (2003) has set performance criteria for infusion pumps; see Table 11.1.

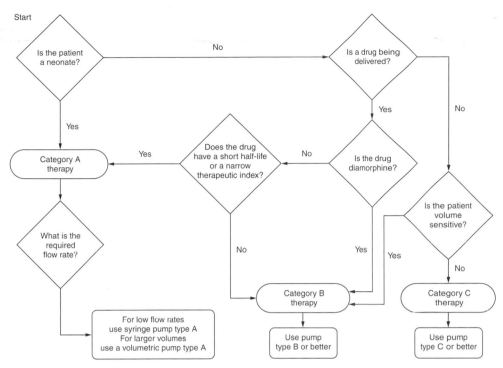

Figure 11.1 Decision tree for selection of infusion device. Crown copyright material is reproduced with the permission of the Controller of HMSO and Queen's Printer for Scotland. Medical Devices Agency (2003).

Infusion devices

Gravity infusion devices

Gravity flow

Gravity infusion devices depend entirely on gravity to drive the infusion. The system consists of an administration set containing a drip chamber and utilizing a roller clamp to control the flow, which is usually measured by counting drops (Pickstone 1999). The indications for use are:

- Delivery of fluids without drug additives
- Administration of drugs or fluids where adverse effects are not anticipated if the infusion rate varies slightly
- Where the patient's condition does not give cause for concern and no complication is predicted.

Gravity infusions are ideal for infusing fluids which do not need to be infused with absolute precision. The pressure is dependent on the height of the container above the infusion site as well as the other factors mentioned previously. Roller clamps used to adjust and to maintain rates of flow on gravity infusions vary considerably in their efficiency and accuracy (Clarkson 1995). Flow rate is calculated using a formula which requires the following

information: the volume to be infused, the number of hours the infusion is running over and the drop rate of the administration set (which will differ depending on type of set). The number of drops per millilitre is dependent on the type of administration set used and the viscosity of the infusion fluid. Increased viscosity causes the size of the drop to increase. For example, crystalloid fluid administered via a solution set is delivered at the rate of 20 drops/ml; the rate of packed red cells given via a blood set will be calculated at 15 drops/ml.

The rate of administration of a continuous or intermittent infusion may be calculated from the following equation (Pickstone 1999):

$$\frac{\text{Volume to be infused}}{\text{Time in hours}} \times \frac{\text{Drop rate}}{60 \text{ minutes}} = \text{Drops per minute}$$

In this equation, 60 is a factor for the conversion of the number of hours to the number of minutes.

Advantages and disadvantages
The advantages of the gravity flow system are that it is usually familiar to most staff and is simple to set up. It is low cost and the infusion of air is less likely than with electronic devices (Pickstone 1999). However, the

system does require frequent observation and adjustment due to:

- The tubing changing shape over time
- Creep or distortion of tubing made of PVC
- Fluctuations of venous pressure which can affect the flow of the solution
- The roller clamp can be unreliable, leading to inconsistent flow rates.

There can also be variability of drop size and if the roller clamp is inadvertently left open free flow will occur. Infusion rates with viscous fluids can be reduced (particularly if administered via small cannulae) and there is a limitation on the type of infusion as it is not suitable for arterial infusions – this is because viscosity and arterial flow offer a high resistance to flow which cannot be overcome by gravity flow (Dolan 1999; Pickstone 1999).

Gravity drip rate controllers

A controller is a mechanical device that operates by gravity. These devices use standard solution sets and although they look much like a pump, they have no pumping mechanism. The desired flow rate is set in drops per minute and controlled by battery or mains powered occlusion valves (Medical Devices Agency 2003).

Advantages and disadvantages
Although they can maintain a drip rate within 1%, volumetric accuracy is not guaranteed and many of the disadvantages associated with gravity flow still remain. The main advantages are they are relatively inexpensive and can usually use standard gravity sets. They also incorporate some audible and visual alarm systems (Medical Devices Agency 2003).

Infusion pumps

These devices pump fluid from an infusion bag or bottle via an administration set (Dolan 1999).

Volumetric pumps

A volumetric pump works by calculating the volume delivered. This is achieved when the pump measures the volume displaced in a 'reservoir'. The reservoir is an integral component of the administration set. The pump calculates that every fill and empty cycle of the reservoir delivers a given amount of solution (Perucca 2001). The mechanism of action may be piston generated or linear peristaltic – where fingers in the pump move in a wave-like manner pushing the fluid out of the chamber (Pickstone 1999). The indications

for use are all large volume infusions, both venous and arterial.

Most volumetric pumps have a linear peristaltic pumping mechanism, although some use cassettes. All are mains and battery powered, with the rate selected in millilitres per hour. The accuracy of flow is usually within 5% when measured over a period of time, which is more than adequate for most clinical applications (Pickstone 1999).

Advantages and disadvantages
These pumps are able to overcome resistance to flow by increased delivery pressure and do not rely on gravity. This generally makes the performance of pumps predictable and capable of accurate delivery over a wider range of flow rates (Medical Devices Agency 2003).

The pumps also incorporate a wide range of features including air-in-line detectors, variable pressure settings and comprehensive alarms such as end of infusion, KVO (keep vein open, where the pump switches to a low flow rate, e.g. 5 ml/hour, in order to continue flow to prevent occlusion of the device) and low battery. Many have a secondary infusion facility, which is to allow for intermittent therapy, e.g. antibiotics. The pump is programmed to switch to a secondary set and, when completed, it reverts back to the primary infusion at the previously set rate. The changing hospital environment has led to an increased demand on volumetric pumps, which in turn has resulted in the development of multichannel and dual-channel infusion pumps. These pumps may consist of two devices with an attached housing or of several infusion channels within a single device (Perucca 2001).

The disadvantages are that these are usually relatively expensive and often dedicated administration sets are required. The use of the wrong set could result in error even if the pump appears to work. Some are complicated to set up, which can also lead to errors (Medical Devices Agency 2003).

Syringe pumps

Syringe pumps are low-volume, high-accuracy devices designed to infuse at low flow rates. The plunger of a syringe containing the substance to be infused is driven forward by the syringe pump at a controlled rate to deliver it to the patient (Medical Devices Agency 2003).

Syringe pumps are useful in intensive care situations where small volumes of highly concentrated drugs need to be infused.

The volume for infusion is limited to the size of the syringe used in the device, which is usually a 60 ml syringe, but most pumps will accept different sizes and brands of syringe. These devices are calibrated for delivery in millilitres per hour.

Advantages and disadvantages

Syringe pumps are mains and/or battery powered, are usually easy to operate and tend to cost less than volumetric pumps. The alarm systems are becoming more comprehensive but include low battery, end of infusion and syringe clamp open alarm. Most of the problems associated with the older models, for example free flow, mechanical backlash (slackness which causes start-up and alarm delays) and incorrect fitting of the syringe, have been eliminated in the newer models (Pickstone 1999; Medical Devices Agency 2003).

Specialist pumps

Patient-controlled analgesia (PCA) pumps

PCA devices are typically syringe pumps (although some are based on volumetric designs) (Auty 1995; Medical Devices Agency 2003). The syringe pump forces down on the syringe piston, collapsing the syringe at a preset rate, but the distinguishing feature is the ability of the pump to deliver doses on demand, which occurs when the patient pushes a button (Perucca 2001). Whether or not the dose is delivered is determined by preset parameters in the pump. That is, if the maximum amount of drug over a given period of time has already been delivered, a further dose cannot be delivered.

PCA pumps are useful for patients who require analgesia. PCA pumps are used more in the acute setting, but are also useful in ambulatory situations.

Infusion options of a PCA pump are usually categorized into three types:

- Basal: a 'baseline' rate can be accompanied by intermittent doses requested by patients. This aims to achieve pain relief with minimal medication, but not necessarily to achieve a pain-free state (Perucca 2001).
- Continuous: designed for the patient who needs maximum pain relief without the option of demand dosing, e.g. epidural.
- Demand: drug delivered by intermittent infusion when button is pushed and can be used alone or supplemented by the basal rate. Doses can be limited by a designated maximum amount (Perucca 2001).

The PCA pump can dispense a bolus dose, with an initial bolus dose being called a loading dose. This may benefit patients as the one time dose is significantly higher than a demand dose in order to achieve immediate pain relief.

Advantages and disadvantages

These devices offer a 'lock-out' feature (when a key or a combination of numbers is necessary to gain access to pump controls) which is designed for patient safety. These pumps have an extensive memory capability which can be accessed through the display via a printer or computer. This facility is critical for the pump's effective use in pain relief (Perucca 2001), as it enables the clinician to determine when and how often demand is made by a patient and what total volume has been infused (Perucca 2001). It has also been shown that they increase patient satisfaction, patients require less sedation, anxiety is reduced and so are nursing time and time in hospital (Ripamonti & Bruera 1997).

Anaesthesia pumps

These are syringe pumps designed for delivery of anaesthesia or sedation and must only ever be used for that purpose. They should be restricted to operating theatres or critical care units and should be clearly labelled. They infuse at a very high flow rate and have a high-rate bolus facility in order to deliver the induction dose of anaesthesia quickly (Dolan 1999).

Ambulatory infusion devices

Ambulatory devices are small devices which were developed to allow patients more freedom and enable the patient to continue with normal activities or to move unencumbered by a large infusion device (Perucca 2001). They are used for small volumes of a variety of drugs and are mainly designed for patients to wear and use when ambulant.

Ambulatory devices range in size and weight from small enough to fit into a pocket to large enough to require a rucksack. The solution containers are often more cumbersome than the actual pump itself. Due to their size the available capacity may be low and alarms provided may be limited. Considerations for selection of an ambulatory device include the following:

- Type of therapy
- Patient's ability to understand
- Drug stability
- Frequency of doses
- Reservoir volumes required
- Control of flow/flow rates
- Type of access
- Cost effectiveness
- Portability
- Convenience.

Ambulatory pumps fall into two categories: mechanical and battery-operated infusion devices.

Mechanical infusion devices

These are simple and compact but may not necessarily be cost effective as they are usually disposable. The mechanism for delivery is by balloon or simple spring, or they may be gas-powered.

Elastomeric balloons

These are made of a soft rubberized material capable of being inflated to a predetermined volume and the drug is then administered over a very specific infusion time. The balloon is encapsulated inside a rigid transparent container which may be round or cylindrical. The rate of infusion is not controlled by the balloon but by the diameter of the restricting outlet located in the preattached tubing. It is designed for single use that supplies the patient's need for a single dose infusion of drugs, e.g. intermittent small volume parenteral therapies such as delivery of antibiotics. Its small size causes little disruption to the patient's daily activities and it tends to be well tolerated (Perucca 2001).

Spring mechanism

Spring coil piston syringes have a spring which powers the plunger of a syringe in the absence of manual pressure. The volume is restricted by the size of the syringe, which is usually prefilled. The spring coil container tends to be a multidose, small-volume administration device and is a combination of a spring coil in a collapsible flattened disk. Its shape can accommodate many therapies and volumes (Perucca 2001).

Epidural pumps

These pumps are a method of providing analgesia (most commonly a combination of opioids and anaesthetic agents) via a fine catheter inserted directly into the epidural space. As a form of analgesia delivery, the efficacy of the epidural route has been well highlighted (Wheatley *et al.* 2001).

Battery-operated infusion devices

Battery-operated pumps are small and light enough to be carried around by the patient without interfering with most everyday activities. They are operated using rechargeable or alkaline batteries but, owing to their size, the available battery capacity tends to be low. The length of time the battery lasts is often dependent on the rate the pump is set at. Most give an output in the form of a small bolus delivered every few minutes. Most devices have an integral case or pouch which allows the pump and the reservoir/syringe to be worn with discretion by the patient. There are two types: ambulatory volumetric infusion pumps and syringe drivers.

Ambulatory volumetric infusion pumps

An ambulatory volumetric infusion pump is an infusion device which pumps in the same way as a large volumetric pump, but by nature of its size it is portable and useful in the ambulatory setting.

This pump is suitable for patients who have been prescribed continuous infusional treatment for a period of time, for example from 4 days to 6 months, and enables the patients, where appropriate, to receive treatment at home, because it is small and portable.

The advantages of the ambulatory pump are that it:

- Is able to deliver drugs continuously or intermittently
- Delivers drugs accurately over a set period of time
- Improves potential outcomes of treatment by delivering treatment continuously
- Heightens patients' independence and control by allowing them to be at home and participate in their own care
- Is compact, light and easy to use
- Has audible alarm systems.

The disadvantages are that:

- It may require the insertion of a central venous access device, which has associated complications and problems.
- It could malfunction at home, which could be distressing and dangerous for the patient.
- In spite of its ease of use, some patients may not be able to cope with it at home.
- Patients may have to adapt their lifestyle to cope with living with a pump continuously.

Syringe drivers

A syringe driver is a portable battery-operated infusion device. It is used to deliver drugs at a predetermined rate via the appropriate parenteral route. Typical applications include its use in pain control, cytotoxic chemotherapy, coronary care and neonatal care. It may also be used for the administration of heparin and insulin, and treatment of thalassaemia. The syringe driver should be used for patients who are unable to tolerate oral medication for whatever reason, for example, in nausea and vomiting, dysphagia, intestinal obstruction, local disease or sometimes in intractable pain which is unrelieved by oral medications and where rapid dose titration is required. In addition, patients who are weak, agitated or unconscious may benefit from subcutaneous infusions. It is mainly used for administration of drugs via the subcutaneous route, but may be used intravenously too.

Subcutaneous drug infusions using a syringe driver are commonly used in palliative care. Drugs administered by subcutaneous infusion include opioid analgesics, antiemetics, anxiolitic sedatives, corticosteroids, non-steroidal anti-inflammatory drugs and anticholinergic drugs (Doyle *et al.* 1998).

The Sims (Graseby) Medical MS16A and MS26 syringe drivers are typical examples of the drivers in use;

however, other types are available and nurses should follow the manufacturer's instruction manual for details of their use. The MS16A allows drug administration on an hourly rate. This driver is clearly marked with a pink '1HR' in the bottom right hand corner of the driver. The MS26 delivers drugs on a 24-hourly rate. This driver is clearly marked with a yellow '24 h' in the bottom right hand corner of the driver (Fig. 11.2). It is important that users are aware that the MS16A syringe driver is calibrated in millimetres per hour, and the MS26 is calibrated in millimetres per day. The MS series of syringe drivers may be used with most sizes and brands of plastic syringes, although it is recommended to use those with Luer–Lok facility to avoid leakage or accidental disconnection.

The advantages of the syringe driver are:

- It avoids the necessity of intermittent injections.
- Mixtures of drugs may be administered.
- Infusion timing is accurate, which is particularly advantageous in the community where the ability to constantly monitor the rate is not feasible.
- The device is lightweight and compact, allowing mobility and independence (it usually weighs approximately 175 g including the battery and measures about 165 × 53 × 23 mm).
- Rate can be increased (see additional notes at end of chapter).
- Simple calculations of dosage are required over a 12- or 24-hour period.

- It allows patients to spend more time at home with their symptoms managed effectively.

The disadvantages are:

- The patient may become psychologically dependent on the device.
- Inflammation or infection may occur at the insertion site of the subcutaneous cannula.
- The rate calculation can be confusing for the novice because there are two different types of devices, particularly if the patient's dose requirements alter (see 'Additional notes' at end of Guidelines).
- The alarm system of some syringe drivers, e.g. the Sims (Graseby), operates only if the plunger is obstructed. It does not alert the nurse if the flow is too rapid or if the skin site has perished.

Summary

Careful calculation and control of flow rates are essential as delivery of fluids and medications may be critical owing to any of the factors mentioned above. There are many infusion control devices available to assist the nurse in this task, ranging from the simple to the complex. Nurses should have a sound knowledge of how the device works or seek assistance from a colleague. Many organizations now use only one type of device in each category. Standardization of equipment reduces confusion and therefore reduces the risk of user error (Murray & Glenister 2001).

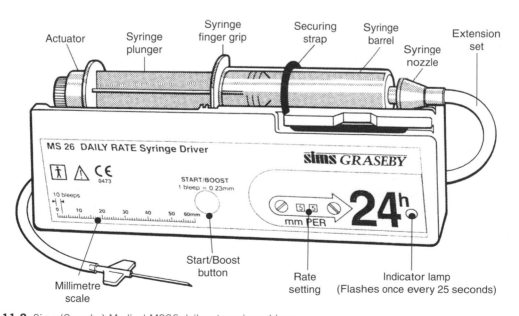

Figure 11.2 Sims (Graseby) Medical MS26 daily rate syringe driver.

Procedure guidelines: **Subcutaneous administration of drugs using a syringe driver (e.g. Sims (Graseby) Medical MS26)**

Equipment

1 Syringe driver MS26.
2 Battery (PP3 size, 9 volt alkaline).
3 Plastic peripheral cannulae (e.g. Insyte 24 G) and microbore driver set (100 cm) with needle-free Y connector injection site (or 100 cm winged infusion set).
4 Luer–Lok syringe of suitable size (e.g. 10 ml).
5 Swab saturated with isopropyl alcohol 70%.
6 Transparent adhesive dressing.
7 Drugs and diluent.
8 Needle (to draw up drug).
9 Drug additive label.
10 Patient's prescription.

Calculating the rate setting for administration of drugs using a syringe driver (e.g. Sims (Graseby) Medical MS26) over a 24-hour period (using a BD Plastipak Luer–Lok syringe)

1 Measure stroke length in mm. The stroke length is the *length* of fluid to be infused, i.e. the distance the plunger has to travel (irrespective of the number of ml) (Fig. 11.3).
2 Check the delivery time (previously prescribed) in days.
3 Calculate:

Example:
Stroke length = 48 mm
Delivery time = 1 day
Rate setting   = 48 mm
Set rate using screwdriver provided (see Fig. 11.4).
See instruction booklets provided with individual syringe driver.

$$\text{Rate} = \frac{\text{Fluid length}}{\text{Infusion period in days}}$$

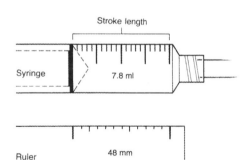

Figure 11.3 Measuring stroke length.

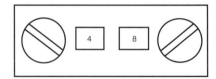

Figure 11.4 Setting the rate.

Procedure guidelines: **Preparation of the syringe for 24-hour drug administration using the Sims (Graseby) Medical MS26 syringe driver**

Action	Rationale
1 Calculate and check dosage of drugs required over a 24-hour period.	To establish correct dosages of drugs.
2 Using a 10 ml BD Plastipak Luer–Lok syringe, draw up drugs required with diluent to measure a total volume of 7.8 ml.	To ensure accuracy and avoid any infusion errors.
3 Establish the correct rate setting of the driver using the correct calculation.	To monitor rate and ensure drug is infused safely.

Procedure guidelines: **Priming the infusion set**

	Action	Rationale
1	Using previously prepared syringe, connect a 100 cm microbore driver set with needle-free Y connector injection site.	This length of tubing allows patient greater freedom of movement.
2	Gently depress the plunger until the infusion tubing is filled to the end.	This removes extraneous air from the system. Adding further diluent to the syringe reduces the potency and therefore the effect of drug to be infused.
3	Having previously calculated the rate setting, allow time for speedier first infusion rate.	Ensures patient receives drugs immediately and accurately. (Usually priming the set reduces delivery time by approximately half an hour.) Do not alter previously calculated rate setting despite volume reduction in barrel of syringe.

Procedure guidelines: **Inserting the winged infusion set or cannula**

	Action	Rationale
1	Explain and discuss the procedure with the patient.	To ensure that the patient understands the procedure and gives his/her valid consent.
2	Assist the patient into a comfortable position.	
3	Expose the chosen site for infusion (see subcutaneous infusion sites in Ch. 9, Drug administration).	
4	Clean the chosen site with a swab saturated with 70% isopropyl alcohol. Wait until the alcohol evaporates.	To reduce the risk of infection.
5	Grasp the skin firmly.	To elevate the subcutaneous tissue.
6	Insert the infusion needle into the skin at an angle of 45° and release the grasped skin. (If using a cannula, remove the stylet and connect the extension set.)	Positioning shallower than 45° may shorten the life of the infusion site.
7	Connect the syringe to the syringe driver (see instructions below).	To ensure the syringe is connected correctly to the syringe driver.
8	Record, in the appropriate documents, that the infusion has been commenced.	To comply with local drug administration policies and ensure the safe administration and monitoring of the infused drug.

Connecting syringe to syringe driver

	Action	Rationale
1	Place the syringe on the syringe driver along the grooved lines, with barrel clamp firmly in position.	To ensure the syringe is in the correct position.
2	Secure in place with rubber strap.	To ensure the syringe is securely clamped to the barrel.
3	Slide the actuator assembly along the lead screw by pressing white release button as shown in Fig. 11.5, until it rests against the end of the plunger.	To enable the pump mechanism to operate correctly.
4	Secure plunger with additional safety clamp (Fig. 11.6).	To ensure extra security and minimize the risk of errors in infusional rates.
5	Press start/test button to commence infusion. The indicator light should flash to indicate functioning syringe pump.	To check the infusion device is operating correctly.

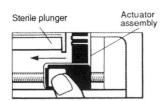

Figure 11.5 Connecting syringe to syringe driver.

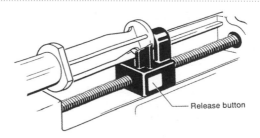

Figure 11.6 Securing the plunger.

*Procedure guidelines: **Inserting the winged infusion set or cannula** (cont'd)*

Additional notes

1   Different manufacturers of syringes have different barrel sizes, e.g. 7.8 ml in a 10 ml syringe made by one company may yield a different stroke length to 7.8 ml in a 10 ml syringe made by another.

2   If more than one drug is to be administered, for example analgesic and antiemetic, it is important not to increase the rate of the syringe driver to yield more pain relief, as this will increase the antiemetic dose.

3   If 'breakthrough' analgesia is required, it is preferable to administer the equivalent of a 4-hourly dose as an injection using the needle-free Y connector injection site or as a separate extra statim subcutaneous injection (when a winged infusion set is in use). Bolus pushes using the boost button are not recommended, for the following reasons:

   (a) Those outlined in point 2 above.

   (b) A 'boost' push yields only 0.23 mm of extra analgesia.

   (c) Pain assessment is more difficult and evaluation of pain control is hindered.

   (d) Inaccuracies of infusion time may occur as a result.

4   Accurate documentation of the site, rate, flow, start time and drugs used is imperative in order to avoid confusion and errors among staff.

5   Appropriate education/teaching material, e.g. syringe driver instruction manual and guidelines on problem solving, is required for both the patients and staff, as these are not easily available in the community.

Problem solving

Problem	Possible causes	Preventive nursing measures	Suggested action
Infusion pump alarming:			
(a) Air detected	Air bubbles in administration set.	Ensure all air is removed from all equipment prior to use.	Remove all air from the administration set and restart the infusion.
(b) Tube misload	Administration set has been improperly loaded.	Ensure set is loaded correctly.	Check that the set is loaded correctly and reload if necessary.
(c) Upstream occlusion	Closed clamp, obstruction or kink in the administration set is preventing fluid flow.	Ensure the container/fluid bag has been adequately pierced by the administration spike.	Inspect the administration set and restart the infusion.
		Ensure that the tubing is taped to prevent kinking.	If tubing is kinked, reposition, tape and restart infusion.
		Ensure the regulating (roller) clamp is open.	Check the administration set and open the clamp; restart the infusion.
(d) Downstream occlusion	Phlebitis/infiltration or extravasation.	Observe site regularly for signs of swelling, pain and erythema.	Remove peripheral device, provide symptomatic relief where appropriate. Initiate extravasation procedure Resite as appropriate.
	Closed distal clamp.	Ensure clamps are open.	Locate distal occlusion, restart infusion.
(e) KVO alert (keep vein open).	The volume infused is complete and the device is infusing at the KVO rate.	Programme in a new volume as appropriate.	Do not turn the device off. Allow KVO mode to run to maintain patency of device. Prepare new infusion or discontinue as appropriate.

Problem solving (cont'd)

Problem	Possible causes	Preventive nursing measures	Suggested action
Infusion devices malfunctioning (electrical/mechanical).	Not charging at mains.	Ensure that the device is kept plugged in where appropriate.	Change device and remove device from use until fully charged. Send to works department to check plug.
	Low battery.	Check lead is pushed in adequately.	
	Batteries keep requiring replacement.	Do not use small rechargeable batteries in ambulatory devices	
	Technical fault.	Ensure all infusion devices are serviced regularly	Remove infusion device from use and contact BME (biomedical engineering) department or relevant personnel.
	Device soiled inside mechanism.	Maintain equipment and keep clean and free from contamination.	Remove administration set, wipe pump, reload. Do not use alcohol-based solutions on internal mechanisms.
Unstable infusion device.	Mounted on old, poorly maintained stands.	Ensure that stands are maintained and kept clean. Replace old stands.	Remove device from stand. Remove stand and send to works department for repair.
	Mounted on incorrect stands.	Ensure the correct stands are used.	Check the stand and change to appropriate stand.
	Equipment not balanced on stand.	Ensure that all equipment is balanced around the stand.	Remove devices and attach to two stands if necessary. Balance equipment.
Under/overinfusion.	Technical fault with equipment.	Ensure regular servicing of devices.	Remove device from use immediately and label to prevent further use. Report incident to medical staff and nursing staff. Report to appropriate person, e.g. nurse specialist or an electro-biomedical engineer for checking. Complete an incident form. Inform head of risk management and MHRA as appropriate.
	Incorrect rate setting.	Ensure that the rate is calculated prior to commencing infusion. Check infusion rate regularly within the first hour and at start of each shift to ensure correct rate is set.	Check patient's condition. Inform medical staff and senior member of nursing staff.

References and further reading

DoH (2001) *Controls Assurance Standards.* Stationery Office, London.

Dolan, S. (1999) Intravenous flow control and infusion devices. In: *Intravenous Therapy in Nursing Practice* (eds L. Dougherty & J. Lamb), pp. 195–222. Churchill Livingstone, Edinburgh.

Dougherty, L. (2002) Delivery of intravenous therapy. *Nurs Stand*, **16**(16), 45–56.

Dougherty, L., Viner, C. & Young, J. (1998) Establishing ambulatory chemotherapy at home. *Prof Nurse*, **13**(6), 356–60.

Doyle, D., Hanks, G.W. & MacDonald, N. (1998) *Oxford Textbook of Palliative Medicine*, 2nd edn. Oxford University Press, Oxford.

Edwards, S. (2001) Regulation of water, sodium and potassium: implications for practice. *Nurs Stand*, **15**(22), 36–45.

Fox, N. (2000) Armed and dangerous. *Nurs Times*, **96**(44), 24–6.

Macklin, D. (1999) What's physics got to do with it? – A review of the physical principles of fluid administration. *J Vasc Access Networks*, Summer, 7–11.

McConnell, E.A. (1995) How and what staff nurses learn about the medical devices they use in direct patient care. *Res Nurs Health*, **18**, 165–72.

McConnell, E.A. *et al.* (1996) Australian registered nurse medical device education: a comparison of simple vs complex devices. *J Adv Nurs*, **23**, 322–8.

Medical Devices Agency (1997) Selection and use of infusion devices for ambulatory applications. *Device Bulletin, Medical Devices Agency DB 9703*, March.

Medical Devices Agency (1998) *Medical Device and Equipment Management for Hospital and Community Based Organisations.* Medical Devices Agency 9801. Medical Devices Agency, London.

Medical Devices Agency (2000) *Equipped to Care.* Medical Devices Agency, London.

Medical Devices Agency (2001) *Devices in Practice.* Medical Devices Agency, London.

Medical Devices Agency (2003) *Infusion Systems Device Bulletin.* DB 9503. Medical Devices Agency, London.

Morling, S. & Ford, L. (1997) IV therapy: selection, use and management of infusion pumps. *Br J Nurs*, **6**(19), 1094–1102.

Murray, W. & Glenister, H. (2001) How to use medical devices safely. *Nurs Times*, **97**(43), 36–8.

NPSA (2003) *Risk Analysis of Infusion Devices.* National Patient Safety Agency, London.

Perucca, R. (2001) Types of infusion therapy equipment. *Infusion Therapy in Clinical Practice* (eds J. Hankin *et al.*). W.B. Saunders, Philadelphia.

Pickstone, M. (1999) *A Pocketbook for Safer IV Therapy.* Medical Technology and Risk Series. Scitech, Kent.

Pickstone, M. (2000) Using the technology triangle to assess the safety of technology-controlled clinical procedures in critical care. *Int J Intens Care*, **7**(2), 90–6.

Quinn, C. (2000) Infusion devices: risks, functions and management. *Nurs Stand*, **14**(26), 35–41.

Springhouse Corporation (1999) *Handbook of Infusion Therapy.* Springhouse, Pennsylvania.

Springhouse Corporation (2002) *Intravenous Therapy Made Incredibly Easy.* Springhouse Corporation, Pennsylvania.

Sundquist, S.B. (2001) Didactic components of a comprehensive paediatric competency programme. *J Infus Nurs*, **24**(6), 367–74.

Weinstein, S. (2000) *Plumer's Principles and Practices of Intravenous Therapy*, 7th edn. Lippincott, Philadelphia.

Wheatley, R., Schug, S. & Watson, D. (2001) Safety and efficacy of postoperative epidural analgesia. *Br J Anaesth*, **87**(1), 47–61.

Williams, C. & Lefever, J. (2000) Reducing the risk of user error with infusion pumps. *Prof Nurse*, **15**(6), 382–4.

12

Elimination: bladder lavage and irrigation

Chapter contents

Definitions

Lavage

Bladder lavage is the washing out of the bladder with sterile fluid.

Irrigation

Bladder irrigation is the continuous washing out of the bladder with sterile fluid.

Indications

Bladder lavage or irrigation is indicated for the following reasons:

Lavage

- To clear an obstructed catheter.
- To remove the potential souces of obstruction, e.g. blood clots or sediment from infection.

Irrigation

- To prevent the formation and retention of blood clots, e.g. following prostatic surgery.
- On rare occasions to remove heavily contaminated material from a diseased urinary bladder.

Reference material

Solutions used for lavage and irrigation

A number of solutions are available for cleaning the bladder and the selection of a particular solution will depend on its therapeutic properties in relation to the patient's needs.

The agent most commonly recommended for lavage and irrigation is 0.9% sodium chloride. This should be used in every case unless an alternative solution is prescribed. It is isotonic so it does not affect the body's fluid or electrolyte levels, therefore large volumes may be used as necessary. Three-litre bags of 0.9% sodium chloride are available for irrigation purposes.

Careful monitoring of bladder irrigation is essential for, although not a common complication, absorption of irrigation fluid can occur. This leads to electrolyte imbalance and circulatory overload, producing a potentially critical situation. Absorption is most likely to occur in theatre where irrigation fluid, devoid of sodium or potassium, is forced under pressure into the prostatic veins (Forristal & Maxfield 1997), but the risk remains while irrigation continues. For this reason it is important that fluid balance should be monitored carefully during irrigation (Scholtes 2002). 0.9% sodium chloride is not used during surgery as the electrolytes it contains interfere with the diathermy; therefore glycine is used (Gilbert & Gobbi 1989).

Water should never be used to irrigate the bladder as it will be readily absorbed by the process of osmosis. Water may be used as a purely mechanical means to flush out catheters for patients at home (Addison 2000).

The use of bladder washouts is an area where there is considerable confusion and controversy (Getliffe 1996a; Rew 1999). Poor levels of knowledge have been found among nurses with regard to the type of washout fluid to use in specific circumstances and also the frequency of administration (Bailey 1991). Bladder lavage has been used in the management of catheter associated infections, catheter encrustation and blockage (Getliffe 1996a).

A number of prepacked sterile washout solutions or, as they are now commonly called, catheter maintenance solutions are available; these include the following:

- 0.9% sodium chloride is used for mechanical flushing to remove tissue debris and small blood clots.
- Chlorhexidine 0.02% is used to prevent or reduce bacterial growth, in particular *Escherichia coli* and *Klebsiella*.
- Mandelic acid (1%) is used to prevent the growth of urease-producing bacteria by acidifying the urine.
- 6% citric acid solution, 'solution R', is used to dissolve persistent crystallization in the catheter or bladder.
- 3.23% citric acid and magnesium oxide solution, 'Suby G', is used to prevent, and dissolve, crystallization in the catheter or bladder (Rew & Woodward 2001).

Catheter-associated infection

Catheter-associated urinary tract infections are a common complication occurring in over 90% of patients within 4 weeks of catheterization (Jewes *et al.* 1988). The risk of catheter-associated bacteriuria increases by 5–8% a day during catheterization (Mulhall *et al.* 1988) and is inevitable in long-term patients (Getliffe 1996b). Antibiotics will not prevent infection in long-term catheterized patients and their use is not recommended unless systemic symptoms are present (Simpson 2001). Bladder washouts using antibiotic or antiseptic solutions in order to prevent, reduce or treat urinary tract infections have been commonly used, but these have been found to be ineffective.

Chlorhexidine has been shown to be ineffective against a number of commonly occurring pathogens. It may, in fact, remove sensitive bacteria in the normal urethral flora, allowing subsequent colonization by resistant organisms (Davies *et al.* 1987; Stickler *et al.* 1987; King & Stickler 1992). Other solutions reviewed include noxythiolin, providone iodine, acetic acid and a range of antibiotics (Rao & Elliott 1988). These have also been shown not to be effective. Therefore their use in long-term catheterized patients is not advocated (Stickler & Chawla 1987; Stickler 1990).

Catheter-associated urinary infections are difficult to treat as bacteria adhere to the surface of the catheter in the form of a biofilm. Bacteria in this biofilm are generally less susceptible to antimicrobial agents than their free-living counterparts (Gristina *et al.* 1987). Three theories have been suggested to explain why this may happen:

- Microbial secretions 'bind' the biofilm to the surface, making it difficult to remove and for antibiotic and antiseptic agents to penetrate (Getliffe 1996b; Liedl 2001).
- Cells in the biofilm exist in a slow-growing or starved state and are therefore not very susceptible to many antimicrobial agents (Getliffe 1996b; Liedl 2001).
- The micro-organisms in the biofilm undergo cellular changes so they develop into a different phenotype that has different sensibility to antibiotic agents than their free-living counterparts (Liedl 2001).

Bacteria in the urine may be successfully killed but may persist in the biofilm and restart the cycle of infection (Stickler *et al.* 1987). As yet there is no catheter material that resists biofilm formation in the clinical setting (Getliffe 1996b; Morris *et al.* 1997).

Catheter encrustations and blockages

Recurrent catheter encrustation and blockage is a common problem with approximately 50% of catheterized patients being susceptible (Kohler-Ockmore 1992; Getliffe 1994a). Catheter blockage may occur as the result of detrusor spasm, twisted drainage tubing or constipation, but the most common reason is the formation of encrustation on the catheter surface and within its lumen (Getliffe 1996a).

Catheter encrustations commonly consist of magnesium, ammonium phosphate (struvite) and calcium phosphate (Getliffe 1996b) which precipitate from urine when it becomes alkaline during infection from urease-secreting micro-organisms (Mobley & Warren 1987; Getliffe 1996a). The urease producers implicated most commonly in catheter encrustations are of the *Proteus* species, in particular *Proteus mirabilis* (Getliffe 1996b; Stickler & Hughes 1999; Liedl 2001).

The development of catheter encrustations may lead to:

- Blockage of the catheter lumen
- Bypassing of urine
- Retention of urine
- Pain
- Recatheterization (Rew 1999).

Getliffe's (1994a) study attempted to identify characteristics of patients who were at greater risk of obstructing their catheters. Patients who 'blocked' their catheters were found to have high urinary pH and ammonia concentrations. High ammonia concentration and alkaline urine are found when urine is infected with urease producing micro-organisms, such as *P. mirabilis*. Significantly more females were classed as 'blockers'; this may be due to the greater risks females have of developing catheter associated urinary infections (Kennedy *et al.* 1983), as the shorter female urethra may allow more rapid colonization. 'Blockers' were also found to be significantly less mobile than 'non-blockers'. There was no significant relationship noted between non-blockers and high average daily fluid intake; this study therefore does not support the advice conventionally given to 'drink plenty' to reduce mineral precipitation.

There have been very few clinical studies about the use of bladder washouts. 0.9% sodium chloride has been shown to have no effect in dissolving encrustations but may, through the mechanical effect of flushing, dislodge debris (Flack 1993).

A study carried out by Kennedy *et al.* (1992) showed that citric acid solution with (Suby G) and without magnesium oxide (solution R) administered twice weekly for 3 weeks did not have a demonstrable effect in preventing crystal formation. However, 6% citric acid solution R has been shown to dissolve fragments of struvite renal calculi following lithotripsy (Holden & Rao 1991). Catheter encrustations may be dissolved using this solution but potential inflammatory tissue reactions of the urothelium limit its use (Getliffe 1996a). Getliffe (1996a) suggests it may be used prior to catheter removal to dissolve external encrustations, which cause pain and tissue trauma on withdrawal of the catheter. Getliffe's (1994b) *in vitro* study suggested that mandelic acid solution may be particularly effective in reducing encrustation.

Mandelic acid 1% has been shown to be effective in removing *Pseudomonas* species from the urine of catheterized patients, although it needs to be used twice a day for a long period (on average 19 days). It has also shown to be a biocidal agent against some biofilms of single or mixed bacterial species (Stickler & Hewitt 1991). This agent is thought to have a dual role, first in reducing urinary pH and second in dissolving struvite and calcium phosphate deposits. However, tissue reactions to mandelic acid 1% in clinical situations have yet to be demonstrated, as does its efficacy in the presence of urinary elements such as mucin and organic debris (Getliffe 1996a; Rew 1999).

Potential risks to the bladder urothelium associated with bladder lavage solutions have raised concerns. Dilute acid solutions have been shown to remove the surface layer of mucus in the bladder (Parsons *et al.* 1970) and an increased shedding of urethelial cells has been observed following washouts (Elliot *et al.* 1989). Reassessment of bladder irrigation methods and the indication for their use is therefore called for.

There has been little research to advise on the frequency with which washouts should be used or the volumes of solution needed. It has been suggested that 'mini' washouts regularly performed would be effective at reducing encrustations and minimizing irritant effects on the bladder (Getliffe 1994a; Getliffe & Dolman 1997). A catheter lumen holds 4–5 ml of fluid, therefore smaller volumes of 10–20 ml would still completely fill the catheter lumen and bathe the catheter tip. Therefore the bladder mucosa would not be exposed to large volumes of washout solution. Getliffe (1994a) suggests that washouts could then be performed more frequently without increasing the risk of tissue damage. This suggestion has been supported by an *in vitro* study by Getliffe *et al.* (2000). Two sequential washouts with 50 ml of Suby G retained for 15 minutes were found to be significantly better at removing encrustations than a single washout of 100 ml; this theory has yet to be tested in a clinical setting. It is recognized by researchers that further work is needed in the whole sphere of bladder lavage.

Patient assessment

There are a number of risks associated with bladder lavage and the procedure should not be undertaken lightly. Patients should be assessed and a catheter history should be noted before a decision to use bladder washouts is made. Assessment of all aspects of catheter care should be taken, including:

- Patient activity and mobility
- Diet and fluid intake

- Standards of patient hygiene
- Patients' and/or carers' ability to care for the catheter (Getliffe 1996a; Rew 1999).

Newly catheterized patients should be monitored to ascertain how long the catheter remains in situ before showing signs of blockage, without any interference with prophylactic washouts. A catheter history should be established, and documented, to enable future care to be planned (Rew 1999). In order to develop a distinct pattern of catheter history, Norberg *et al.* (1983) suggest that three to five consecutive catheters should be observed before treatment, if needed, is instigated.

An important aspect of management, for patients where a clear pattern of catheter history can be established, is the scheduling of catheter changes prior to likely blockages (Getliffe 1996b). In patients where no clear pattern emerges, or for whom frequent catheter changes are traumatic, acidic bladder lavages can be beneficial in reducing catheter encrustations (Getliffe 1996a; Rew 1999).

Cytotoxic agents given intravesically

For details on the administration of cytotoxic agents, see Ch. 10, Drug administration: Cytotoxic drugs, Procedure guidelines: Intravesical instillation of cytotoxic drugs.

Catheters used for irrigation

A three-way urinary catheter must be used for irrigation in order that fluid may simultaneously be run into, and drained out from, the bladder. A large-gauge catheter (16–24) is often used to accommodate any clot and debris which may be present. This catheter is commonly passed in theatre when irrigation is required, e.g. after

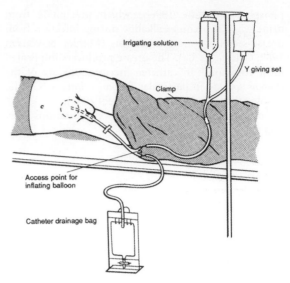

Figure 12.1 Closed urinary drainage system with provision for intermittent or continuous irrigation.

prostatectomy (Maxfield *et al.* 1994). Occasionally if a patient is admitted with a heavily contaminated bladder, e.g. blood clots, bladder irrigation may be started on the ward. If the patient has a two-way catheter, this must be replaced with a three-way type (Fig. 12.1).

It is recommended that a three-way catheter is passed if frequent intravesical instillations of drugs or antiseptic solutions are prescribed and the risk of catheter obstruction is not considered to be very great. In such cases the most important factor is minimizing the risk of introducing infection and maintaining a closed urinary drainage system, for which the three-way catheter allows.

Procedure guidelines: **Bladder lavage**

Equipment

1 Sterile dressing pack.
2 Sterile bladder syringe, 60 ml.
3 Sterile jug.
4 Antiseptic solution.
5 Bactericidal alcohol handrub.
6 Clamp.

7 New catheter bag (for balloon two-way catheter) or sterile spigot (for three-way catheter).
8 Sterile receiver.
9 Sterile solution for lavage.
10 Absorbent sheet.

Procedure

Action	Rationale
1 Explain and discuss the procedure with the patient.	To ensure that the patient understands the procedure and gives his/her valid consent.

*Procedure guidelines: **Bladder lavage** (cont'd)*

Action	Rationale
2 Screen the bed. Ensure that the patient is in a comfortable position allowing access to the catheter.	For the patient's privacy and to reduce the risk of cross-infection. Curtains are drawn at this stage so that dust and airborne organisms disturbed by the curtains do not settle on the sterile field.
3 Perform the procedure using an aseptic technique.	To minimize the risk of infection. (For further information on aseptic technique see Ch. 4.)
4 If necessary, draw up solutions using a 60 ml syringe, preferably with needle adapter. Cap the syringe and place it in a sterile receiver.	It is easier to draw up solutions from vials in the clinical area than at the bedside.
5 Take the trolley to the bedside, disturbing the screens as little as possible. Open the outer wrappings of packs and put them on the top shelf of the trolley.	To minimize airborne contamination. To begin to prepare equipment for procedure.
6 Prepare the sterile field. Pour the lavage solution into the sterile jug.	To prepare equipment for procedure.
7 Place absorbent sheet under the catheter junction and clamp the catheter. Wash hands with bactericidal alcohol handrub.	To prevent leakage when the catheter is disconnected. To reduce the risk of infection.
8 Put on sterile gloves, place sterile towel under the junction of the catheter and the tubing of the drainage bag and disconnect them.	To create a sterile field and reduce the risk of cross-infection. When the patient has a three-way catheter the drainage bag will not need disconnecting as the washout fluid is injected through the side-arm of the catheter. This should be spigotted off after use and the fluid remaining in the bladder will drain into the catheter bag.
9 Clean gloved hands with a bactericidal alcohol handrub. Clean around the end of the catheter with sterile low-linting gauze and an antiseptic solution.	To remove surface organisms from gloves and catheter and thus reduce the risk of introducing infection into the catheter.
10 Draw up the irrigating fluid into the bladder syringe and insert the nozzle into the end of the catheter.	To prepare syringe for lavage.
11 Release the clamp on the catheter and gently inject the contents of the syringe into the bladder, trying not to inject air.	Rapid injection of fluid could be uncomfortable for the patient. Large volumes of air in the bladder cause distension and discomfort.
12 Remove the syringe and allow the bladder contents to drain by gravity into a receiver placed on a sterile towel.	To allow catheter to drain gently. To reduce risk of cross-infection.
13 Repeat steps 11 and 12 of the procedure until the washout is complete or the returning fluid is clear.	To ensure the bladder is free of contaminants.
14 If the fluid does not return naturally, aspirate gently with the syringe.	Gentle suction is sometimes required to remove obstructive material from the catheter. If suction is applied too forcefully the urothelium may be sucked into the eyes of the catheter, preventing drainage and causing pain and trauma which may predispose to infection (Lowthian 1991; Macaulay 1994).
15 Connect a new catheter bag or sterile spigot if a three-way catheter is in place, and allow the remaining fluid to drain out.	A closed drainage system must be re-established as soon as possible to reduce the risk of bacterial invasion through the catheter.
16 If the solution is to remain in the bladder, the catheter should be clamped when all the fluid has been injected and the clamp released after the desired period.	To allow solution to act on bladder mucosa/catheter.
17 Measure the volume of washout fluid returned and compare it with the volume of fluid injected. Record any discrepancies of volume in the appropriate documents.	To keep an accurate record of urinary output and to observe for catheter obstruction.
18 Make the patient comfortable, remove equipment, clean the trolley, and wash hands.	To reduce the risk of cross-infection.

Procedure guidelines: **Administering a catheter maintenance solution**

Equipment

1 Sterile dressing pack.
2 Antiseptic solution.
3 Bactericidal alcohol handrub.

4 Absorbent sheet.
5 New catheter bag.
6 Catheter maintenance solution.

Procedure

Action	Rationale
1 Explain and discuss the procedure with the patient.	To ensure that the patient understands the procedure and gives his/her valid consent.
2 Screen the bed. Ensure that the patient is in a comfortable position, allowing the nurse access to the catheter.	For the patient's privacy and to reduce the risk of cross-infection. Curtains are drawn at this stage so that dust and airborne organisms disturbed by the curtains do not settle on the sterile field.
3 Perform the procedure using aseptic technique.	To minimize the risk of infection. (For further information on aseptic technique see Ch. 4.)
4 Take the trolley to the bedside, disturbing the screens as little as possible. Open the outer wrappings of packs and put them on the top shelf of the trolley.	To minimize airborne contamination. To begin to prepare the equipment for the procedure.
5 Remove outer packaging from catheter maintenance solution and place sterile solution container on to the sterile field.	To prepare equipment for the procedure.
6 Expose the whole length of the catheter and observe for any signs of discharge, meatal problems and length of catheter in patient. (If patient is using a leg bag, remove straps and place bag on the bed before exposing the catheter.) Place the absorbent pad under catheter drainage bag junction.	To prepare patient for procedure. To detect for signs of infection, skin excoriation or displacement of catheter. If any signs noted report to medical staff as appropriate.
7 Wash hands with bactericidal rub and put on sterile gloves. Place sterile towel under catheter junction.	To reduce the risk of infection.
8 Slide clamp on solution container tubing to closed, remove the security ring on the solution container connection port and loosen cover from the connection port.	To prevent fluid loss when connection port is opened. To prepare equipment.
9 Squeeze the end of the catheter together just above the connection to the drainage bag. Disconnect the drainage bag, keeping the catheter squeezed. Remove the cover from the connecting port on the solution container and insert it into the catheter. Release the catheter.	To prevent urine leaking from the catheter.
10 Slide the clamp open on the solution container, raise the bag slightly above the level of the bladder and allow the required amount of the solution to flow into the bladder. Gentle pressure may be needed initially to start the flow.	Rapid instillation of fluid could be uncomfortable for the patient.
11 If the fluid is to be retained for a period of time close the clamp and place the bag on the bed. Reposition the covers and ensure the patient is comfortable for the required time.	To allow the solutions time to act on the bladder/mucosa/catheter. For the patient's privacy and comfort.
12 When the solution is to be removed, ensure the bag is below the level of the bladder, open the clip and allow the solution to drain back.	For gravity to help facilitate drainage.
13 When all the solution has drained back out of the bladder, close the clamp, disconnect the solution container and connect a new drainage bag. Note the amount of fluid returned.	To prevent spillage of solution. To re-establish closed drainage system.

*Procedure guidelines: **Administering a catheter maintenance solution** (cont'd)*

Action	Rationale
14 Make the patient comfortable, remove and dispose of equipment, clean the trolley and wash hands.	To reduce risk of cross-infection.
15 Sign prescription chart. Document that catheter maintenance solution has been administered and note any complication or problems encountered with the procedure.	To maintain accurate records. Provide a point of reference in the event of any queries and prevent duplication of treatment.

Procedure guidelines: **Continuous bladder irrigation**

Equipment

1 Sterile dressing pack.
2 Antiseptic solution.
3 Bactericidal alcohol handrub.
4 Clamp.
5 Sterile irrigation fluid.

6 Disposable irrigation set.
7 Infusion stand.
8 Sterile jug.
9 Absorbent sheet.

Procedure

Commencing bladder irrigation

Action	Rationale
1 Explain and discuss the procedure with the patient.	To ensure that the patient understands the procedure and gives his/her valid consent.
2 Screen the patient and ensure that he or she is in a comfortable position allowing access to the catheter.	For the patient's privacy and to reduce the risk of cross-infection. Curtains are drawn at this stage so that dust and airborne organisms disturbed by the curtains do not settle on the sterile trolley.
3 Perform the procedure using an aseptic technique.	To minimize the risk of infection. (For further information on aseptic technique, see Ch. 4.)
4 Open the outer wrappings of the pack and put it on the top shelf of the trolley.	To prepare equipment.
5 Insert the end of the irrigation giving set into the fluid bag and hang the bag on the infusion stand. Allow fluid to run through the tubing so that air is expelled.	To prime the irrigation set so that it is ready for use. Air is expelled in order to prevent discomfort from air in the patient's bladder.
6 Clamp the catheter and place absorbent sheet under the catheter junction.	To prevent leakage of urine through the irrigation arm when the spigot is removed. To contain any spillages.
7 Clean hands with a bactericidal alcohol handrub. Put on gloves.	To minimize the risk of cross-infection.
8 Place a sterile paper towel under the irrigation inlet of the catheter and remove the spigot.	To create a sterile field. To prepare catheter for connection to irrigation set.
9 Discard the spigot and gloves.	To prevent reuse and reduce risk of cross-infection.
10 Put on sterile gloves. Clean around the end of the irrigation arm with sterile low-linting gauze and an antiseptic solution.	To remove surface organisms from gloves and catheter and to reduce the risk of introducing infection into the catheter.
11 Attach the irrigation giving set to the irrigation arm of the catheter. Keep the clamp of the irrigation giving set closed.	To prevent overdistension of the bladder, which can occur if fluid is run into the bladder before the drainage tube has been unclamped.
12 Release the clamp on the catheter tube and allow any accumulated urine to drain into the catheter bag. Empty the urine from the catheter bag into a sterile jug.	Urine drainage should be measured before commencing irrigation so that the fluid balance may be monitored more accurately.
13 Discard the gloves.	These will be contaminated, having handled the catheter bag.

Procedure guidelines: Continuous bladder irrigation (cont'd)

Action	Rationale
14 Set irrigation at the required rate and ensure that fluid is draining into the catheter bag.	To check that the drainage system is patent and to prevent fluid accumulating in the bladder.
15 Make the patient comfortable, remove unnecessary equipment and clean the trolley.	To reduce the risk of cross-infection.
16 Wash hands.	To reduce the risk of cross-infection.

Care of the patient during irrigation

Action	Rationale
1 Adjust the rate of infusion according to the degree of haematuria. This will be greatest in the first 12 hours following surgery (average fluid input is 6–9 litres during the first 12 hours, falling to 3–6 litres during the next 12 hours). The aim is to obtain a drainage fluid which is rosé in colour.	To remove blood from the bladder before it clots and to minimize the risk of catheter obstruction and clot retention.
2 Check the volume in the drainage bag frequently when infusion is in progress, e.g. half-hourly or hourly, or more frequently as required.	To ensure that fluid is draining from the bladder and to detect blockages as soon as possible, also to prevent overdistension of the bladder and patient discomfort. To empty catheter drainage bags before they reach capacity.
3 Using rubber-tipped 'milking' tongs, 'milk' the catheter and drainage tube, as required.	To remove clots from within the drainage system and to maintain an efficient outlet.
4 Record the fluid balance chart accurately. The fluid balance of all patients having bladder irrigation must be monitored.	So that urine output is known and any related problems, e.g. renal dysfunction, may be detected quickly and easily.

Bladder irrigation recording chart

The bladder irrigation recording chart (Fig. 12.2) is designed to provide an accurate record of the patient's urinary output during the period of irrigation.

Procedure for use of chart

Record the time (column A) and the fluid volume in each bag of irrigating solution (column B) as it is put up.

When the irrigating fluid has all run from the first bag into the bladder, record the original volume in the bag in column C. Record the corresponding time in column A. Do not attempt to estimate the fluid volume run-in while a bag is in progress as this will be inaccurate. If, however, a bag is discontinued, the volume run-in can be calculated by measuring the volume left in the bag and deducting this from the original volume. This should be recorded in column C.

The catheter bag should be emptied as often as is necessary, the volume being recorded in column D and the corresponding time in column A. The catheter bag must also be emptied whenever the bag of irrigating fluid is empty, and the volume recorded in column D.

When each bag of fluid has run through, add up the total volume drained by the catheter in column D, and write this in red. Subtract from this the total volume run-in (column C) to find the urine output (D − C = E). Write this in column E. Draw a line across the page to indicate that this calculation is complete and continue underneath for the next bag.

Patient name: Hospital no:

(A) Date and time	(B) Volume put up	(C) Volume run in	(D) Total volume out	(E) Urine	(F) Urine running total
10/7/96					
10.00	2000				
10.30			700		
11.10			850		
11.40		2000	600		
			2150	150	150
11.45	2000				
12.30			500		
13.15			700		
14.20		2000	800		
			2400	400	550
14.25	2000				
15.30			850		
17.00	Irrigation stopped	1200	800		
			1650	450	1000

Figure 12.2 Bladder irrigation recording chart.

Problem solving

Problem	Cause	Suggested action
Fluid retained in the bladder when the catheter is in position.	Fault in drainage apparatus, e.g.	
	Blocked catheter	'Milk' the tubing. Wash out the bladder with 0.9% sodium chloride.
	Kinked tubing	Straighten the tubing.
	Overfull drainage bag	Empty the drainage bag.
	Catheter clamped off	Unclamp the catheter.
Distended abdomen related to an overfull bladder during the irrigation procedure.	Irrigation fluid is infused at too rapid a rate.	Slow down the infusion rate.
	Fault in drainage apparatus.	Check the patency of the drainage apparatus.
Leakage of fluid from around the catheter.	Catheter slipping out of the bladder.	Insert the catheter further in. Decompress balloon fully to assess the amount of water necessary. Refill balloon until it remains in situ, taking care not to overfill beyond safe level (see manufacturer's instructions).
	Catheter too large or unsuitable for the patient's anatomy.	If leakage is profuse or catheter is uncomfortable for the patient, replace the catheter with one of smaller size.
Patient experiences pain during the lavage or irrigation procedure.	Volume of fluid in the bladder is too great for comfort.	Reduce the fluid volume within the bladder.
	Solution is painful to raw areas in the bladder.	Inform the doctor. Administer analgesia as prescribed.
Retention of fluid with or without distended abdomen, with or without pain.	Perforated bladder.	Stop irrigation. Maintain in recovery position. Call medical assistance. Monitor vital signs. Monitor patient for pain, tense abdomen.

For further details, see Ch. 16, Elimination: urinary catheterization, Problem-solving with catheter in place.

References and further reading

Addison, R. (2000) *Bladder Washout/Irrigation/Instillations. A Guide for Nurses.* B. Braun Medical, Sheffield.

Bailey, S. (1991) Using bladder washouts. *Nurs Times*, **87**(24), 75–6.

Cox, A.J., Harries, J.E., Hukins, D.W.L. *et al.* (1987) Calcium phosphate in catheter encrustation. *Br J Urol*, **59**, 159 63.

Davies, A.J. *et al.* (1987) Does instillation of chlorhexidine into the bladder of catheterised geriatric patients help reduce bacteriuria? *J Hosp Infect*, **9**, 72–5.

Dudley, M.N. & Barriere, S.L. (1981) Antimicrobial irrigations in the prevention and treatment of catheter-related urinary tract infections. *Am J Hosp Pharm*, **38**, 59–65.

Elliott, T. (1990) Disadvantages of bladder irrigation (in catheterized patients. Brief research report). *Nurs Times*, **86**, 52.

Elliott, T.S. *et al.* (1989) Bladder irrigation or irritation? *Br J Urol*, **64**, 391–4.

Ferrie, B.G., Glen, E.S. & Hunter, B. (1979) Long-term urethral catheter drainage. *Br Med J*, **2**(6197), 1046–7.

Fillingham, S. & Douglas, J. (1997) *Urological Nursing.* Baillière Tindall, London.

Flack, S. (1993) Finding the best solution. *Nurs Times*, **11**, 68–74.

Forristal, H. & Maxfield, J. (1997) Prostatic problems. In: *Urological Nursing*, 2nd edn (eds S. Fillingham & J. Douglas). Baillière Tindall, London.

Getliffe, K.A. (1994a) The characteristics and management of patients with recurrent blockage of long-term urinary catheters. *J Adv Nurs*, **20**, 140–49.

Getliffe, K.A. (1994b) The use of bladder wash-outs to reduce urinary catheter encrustation. *Br J Urol*, **73**, 696–700.

Getliffe, K.A. (1996a) Bladder instillations and bladder washouts in the management of catheterized patients. *J Adv Nurs*, **23**, 548–54.

Getliffe, K. (1996b) Care of urinary catheters. *Nurs Stand*, **11**(11), 47–54.

Getliffe, K.A. & Dolman, M. (1997) *Promoting Continence: A Clinical and Research Resource*. Baillière Tindall, London.

Getliffe, K., Hughes, S.C. & Le Claire, M. (2000) The dissolution of urinary catheter encrustation. *Br J Urol*, **85**(1), 60–4.

Gilbert, V. & Gobbi, M. (1989) Bladder irrigation (principles and methods). *Nurs Times Nurs Mirror*, **85**, 40–2.

Griffith, D.P. & Musher, O.N. (1976) Urease: the primary cause of infection induced urinary stones. *Invest Urol*, **13**(5), 346–82.

Gristina, A.G., Hobgood, C.D., Webb, L.X. & Myrvik, Q.N. (1987) Adhesive colonisation of biomaterials and antibiotic resistance. *Biomaterials*, **8**, 423–6.

Hedelin, H., Eddeland, A., Larsson, L. *et al.* (1984) The composition of catheter encrustations, including the effects of allopurinol treatment. *Br J Urol*, **56**, 250–4.

Holden, D. & Rao, P.N. (1991) Management of staghorn stones using a combination of lithotripsy, percutaneous nephrolithotomy and solution R irrigation. *Br J Urol*, **67**, 13–17.

Jewes, L.A., Gillespie, W.A., Leadbetter, A. *et al.* (1988) Bacteriuria and bacteraemia in patients with long-term indwelling catheters: a domiciliary study. *J Med Microbiol*, **26**, 61–5.

Kennedy, A.P. *et al.* (1983) Factors relating to the problems of long-term catheterization. *J Adv Nurs*, **8**, 207–12.

Kennedy, A.P. *et al.* (1992) Assessment of the use of bladder washouts/instillations in patients with long term indwelling catheters. *Br J Urol*, **70**, 610–15.

King, J.B. & Stickler, D.J. (1992) The effects of repeated instillations of antiseptics on catheter-associated urinary tract infections. *Urol Res*, **20**, 403–7.

Kohler-Ockmore, J. (1992) Urinary catheter complications. *J District Nurs*, **10**(8), 18–20.

Liedl, B. (2001) Catheter-associated urinary tract infections. *Curr Opin Urol*, **11**(1), 75–9.

Lowthian, P. (1991) Using bladder syringes sparingly. *Nurs Times*, **87**(10), 61–4.

Macaulay, D. (1994) Urinary drainage systems. In: *Urological Nursing* (ed. C. Laker). Scutari Press, Harrow.

Maxfield, J. *et al.* (1994) Prostatic problems. In: *Urological Nursing* (ed. C. Laker). Scutari Press, Harrow.

Mobley, H.L.T. & Warren, J.W. (1987) Urease positive bacteriuria and obstruction of long-term urinary catheters. *J Clin Microbiol*, **25**, 2216–17.

Morris, N.S., Stickler, D.J. & Winters, C. (1997) Which indwelling urethral catheters resist encrustations by *Proteus mirabilis* biofilms? *Br J Urol*, **80**, 58–63.

Mulhall, A.B., Chapman, R.G. & Crow, R.A. (1988) Bacteriuria during indwelling urethral catheterisation. *J Hosp Infect*, **11**(3), 253–62.

Norberg, B., Norberg, A. & Parkhede, U. (1983) The spontaneous variation in catheter life in long-stay geriatric patients with in-dwelling catheters. *Gerontology*, **29**, 332–5.

Parsons, C.L., Mulholland, S.G. & Anwar, H. (1970) Antibacterial activity of bladder surface mucin duplicated by exogenous glycosaminoglycan (heparin). *Infect Immun*, **25**, 552–4.

Rao, G.G. & Elliott, T.S.J. (1988) Bladder irrigation. *Age Ageing*, **17**(6), 373–8.

Rew, M. (1999) Use of catheter maintenance solutions for long-term catheters. *Br J Nurs*, **8**(11), 708–15.

Rew, M. & Woodward, S. (2001) Troubleshooting common problems associated with long-term catheters. *Br J Nurs*, **10**(12), 764–74.

Roe, B.H. (1989) Use of bladder washouts: a study of nurses' recommendations. *J Adv Nurs*, **14**(6), 494–500.

Roe, B. (1990) The basis for sound practice. *Nurs Stand*, **4**, 25–7.

Scholtes, S. (2002) Management of clot retention following urological surgery. *Nurs Times*, **98**(28), 48–50.

Simpson, L. (2001) Indwelling urethral catheters. *Nurs Stand*, **15**(46), 47–54.

Stickler, D.J. (1990) The role of antiseptics in the management of patients undergoing short term indwelling bladder catheterisation. *J Hosp Infect*, **16**, 89–108.

Stickler, D.J. & Chawla, J.C. (1987) The role of antiseptics in the management of patients with long term indwelling bladder catheters. *J Hosp Infect*, **10**, 219–28.

Stickler, D.J. & Hewitt, P. (1991) Activity of antiseptic against biofilms of mixed bacterial species growing on silicone surfaces. *Eur J Microbiol Infect*, **10**, 416–21.

Stickler, D. & Hughes, G. (1999) Ability of *Proteus mirabilis* to swarm over urethral catheters. *Eur J Clin Microbiol Infect Dis*, **18**(3), 206–8.

Stickler, D.J., Clayton, C.L. & Chawla, J.C. (1987) The resistance of urinary tract pathogens to chlorhexidine bladder washouts. *J Hosp Infect*, **10**, 28–39.

Stickler, D.J. *et al.* (1981) Some observations on the activity of three antiseptics used as bladder irrigants in the treatment of UTI in patients with indwelling catheters. *Paraplegia*, **19**, 325–33.

Elimination: bowel care

Chapter contents

Definitions

Diarrhoea

Diarrhoea results when the balance among absorption, secretion and intestinal motility is disturbed (Hogan 1998). It has been defined as an 'abnormal increase in the quantity, frequency and fluid content of stool and associated with urgency, perianal discomfort and incontinence' (Basch 1987).

Constipation

Constipation results when there is a delayed movement of intestinal content through the bowel (Walsh 1997). It is characterized by infrequent, hard, dry stools, which may be difficult to pass (Norton 1996a; Winney 1998).

Reference material

Bowel elimination is a sensitive issue and providing effective care and management for problems associated with it can be problematic. Many patients are too embarrassed to discuss bowel function and will often delay reporting problems, despite the sometimes severe impact these symptoms have on their quality of life (Cadd *et al.* 2000). Generally complaints will be either that the patient has diarrhoea or is constipated. These should be seen as symptoms of some underlying disease or malfunction and managed accordingly.

The nurse's priority is to effectively assess the nature and cause of the problem, to help find resolutions and to inform and support the patient. This requires sensitive communication skills to dispel embarrassment and ensure a shared understanding of the meanings of the terms used by the patient (Smith 2001).

Anatomy and physiology

The main events of digestion and absorption occur in the small intestine. The small intestine begins at the pyloric sphincter of the stomach, coils through the abdomen and opens into the large intestine at the ileocaecal junction. It is approximately 6.4 m in length and is divided into three segments: the duodenum, jejunum and ileum. The mucosal surface of the small intestine is covered with finger-like processes called villi, which increase the surface area available for absorption and digestion. A number of digestive enzymes are also secreted by the small intestine (Tortora & Grabowski 2002).

Movement through the small bowel is divided into two types, segmentation and peristalsis. Segmentation refers to the localized contraction of the intestine, which mixes the intestinal contents and brings particles of food into contact with the mucosa for absorption. Intestinal content usually remains in the small bowel for 3–5 hours and it is moved along by peristaltic action. These actions are controlled by the autonomic nervous system (Tortora & Grabowski 2002).

Absorption of nutrients, electrolytes and water occurs by diffusion, facilitated diffusion, osmosis and active transport. Water can move across the intestinal mucosa in both directions (Tortora & Grabowski 2002). There are differences in the water and sodium absorption between the jejunum, ileum and colon. The sodium concentration in the intraluminal contents of the jejunum is kept at approximately 90 mmol/l by the ready absorption and secretion of sodium through the loose intracellular junctions of the jejunal mucosa. Water absorption is controlled by the osmolarity of the intraluminal fluid. Sodium absorption, in the ileum, takes place against a concentration gradient and the absorption of water results in only about a litre of effluent passing through into the colon (Woods 1996).

From the ileocaecal sphincter to the anus the colon is approximately 1.5 m in length. Its main function is to eliminate the waste products of digestion by the propulsion of faeces towards the anus. In addition, it produces mucus to lubricate the faecal mass, thus aiding its expulsion. Other functions include the absorption of fluid and electrolytes, the storage of faeces and the synthesis of vitamins B and K by bacterial flora (Tortora & Grabowski 2002).

Faeces consist of the unabsorbed end products of digestion, bile pigments, cellulose, bacteria, epithelial cells, mucus and some inorganic material. They are normally semi-solid in consistency and contain about 70% water (Tortora & Grabowski 2002).

The movement of faeces through the colon towards the anus is by peristaltic action. Three to four times a day there is a strong peristaltic wave. This wave begins at the middle of the transverse colon and quickly drives the colonic contents into the rectum. This is known as the *gastrocolic reflex*, and it is initiated by food in the stomach (Tortora & Grabowski 2002). The colon absorbs about 2 litres of water in 24 hours. If faeces are not expelled they will, therefore, gradually become hard due to dehydration and will be difficult to expel. If there is insufficient roughage (fibre) in the faeces, colonic stasis occurs. This leads to continued water absorption and the faeces will harden still further.

Faeces normally remain in the sigmoid colon until the stimulus to defecate occurs. This stimulus varies in individuals according to habit. The stimulus can be controlled by conscious effort. After a few minutes the stimulus disappears and does not return for several hours. If these natural reflexes are inhibited on a regular basis they are eventually suppressed and reflex defecation is inhibited. The result is that the individual becomes severely constipated. In response to the stimulus faeces move into the rectum (Norton 1996b; Taylor 1997; Tortora & Grabowski 2002).

The rectum is very sensitive to rises in pressure, even of 2–3 mmHg, and distension will cause a perineal sensation with a consequent desire to defecate. A co-ordinated reflex empties the bowel from mid-transverse colon to the anus. During this phase the diaphragm, abdominal and levator ani muscles contract and the glottis closes. Waves of peristalsis occur in the distal colon and the anal sphincter relaxes, allowing the evacuation of faeces (Tortora & Grabowski 2002).

Diarrhoea

Diarrhoea can be characterized according to its onset and duration (acute or chronic) or by type (secretory, osmotic or mixed). Sudden onset acute diarrhoea is very common, it is usually self-limiting and lasts less than 2 weeks. It often requires no investigation or treatment (Shepherd 2000). The causes of acute diarrhoea include:

- Dietary indiscretion (eating too much fruit, alcohol abuse)
- Allergy to food constituents
- Infective:
  (a) Traveller's diarrhoea
  (b) Viral gastroenteritis
  (c) Food poisoning
- Contrast media for screening purposes (Taylor 1997; Campbell & Lunn 1999).

Chronic diarrhoea generally lasts longer than 2 weeks and may have more complex origins (Hogan 1998). Chronic causes include:

- Inflammatory bowel disease, e.g. ulcerative colitis, Crohn's disease

- Malabsorption, e.g. coeliac disease, tropical sprue
- Organic disease, e.g. neoplasms, diverticulitis
- Endocrine disorders, e.g. thyrotoxicosis, diabetes, VIPoma, carcinoid tumours
- Intestinal obstruction including faecal obstruction
- Miscellaneous colitis including pseudomembranous colitis, blind loop syndrome, radiation enteritis, gut reaction and drug therapy, e.g. laxatives, antibiotics, chemotherapy (Fallon & O'Neill 1997; Taylor 1997).

Diarrhoea can have profound physiological and psychosocial consequences on a patient. Severe or extended episodes of diarrhoea may result in dehydration, electrolyte imbalance and malnutrition. Patients not only have to cope with increased frequency of bowel movement but may have abdominal pain, cramping, proctitis and anal or perianal skin breakdown. Food aversions may develop or patients may stop eating altogether as they anticipate subsequent diarrhoea following intake. Consequently this may lead to weight loss and malnutrition. Fatigue, sleep disturbances, feelings of isolation and depression are all common consequences for those experiencing diarrhoea (Hogan 1998). Patients with a stoma may also need to change their appliances more frequently and skin excoriation may occur which can exacerbate distress (Campbell & Lunn 1999). The impact of severe diarrhoea should not be underestimated. It is highly debilitating, may cause patients on long-term therapy to be non-compliant and can be a life-threatening problem (Kornblau *et al.* 2000).

Assessment

The cause of diarrhoea needs to be identified before effective treatment can be instigated. This may include clinical investigations such as stool cultures for bacterial, fungal and viral pathogens or a more formal medical evaluation of the gastrointestinal tract (Kornblau *et al.* 2000).

Ongoing nursing assessment is essential for ensuring individualized management and care. The lack of a systematic approach to assessment and poor documentation, however, cause problems in effective management of diarrhoea (Cadd *et al.* 2000; Smith 2001). Nurses need to be aware of contributing factors and be sensitive to patients' beliefs and values in order to provide holistic care. A comprehensive assessment is therefore essential and should include:

1. History of onset, frequency and duration of diarrhoea
2. Consistency and colour of stool: presence of blood, fat, mucus
3. Symptoms associated with diarrhoea, e.g. pain, nausea, vomiting, fatigue, weight loss, fever
4. Recent lifestyle changes, emotional disturbances, or travel abroad
5. Fluid intake and dietary history including any cause and effect relationships between food consumption and bowel action
6. Normal medication including recent antibiotics, laxatives or chemotherapy
7. Effectiveness of antidiarrhoeal medication (dose and frequency)
8. Significant past medical history, e.g. bowel resection, pancreatitis, pelvic radiotherapy
9. Hydration status (e.g. evaluation of mucous membranes and skin turgor)
10. Perianal or peristomal skin integrity
11. Stool cultures for bacterial, fungal and viral pathogens
12. Patient's preferences and own coping strategies including non-pharmacological interventions and their effectiveness (Taylor 1997; Hogan 1998; Cadd *et al.* 2000).

Management

Once the cause of diarrhoea has been established management should be focused on resolving the cause of the diarrhoea and providing physical and psychological support for the patient. Most cases of chronic diarrhoea will resolve once the underlying condition is treated, e.g. drug therapy for Crohn's disease, or with dietary management, e.g. for coeliac disease. Episodes of acute diarrhoea, usually caused by bacteria or viruses, generally resolve spontaneously and are managed by symptom control and the prevention of complications (Shepherd 2000).

All episodes of acute diarrhoea must be considered potentially infectious until proved otherwise. The risk of spreading the infection to others can be reduced by adopting universal precautions such as wearing of gloves, aprons and gowns, disposing of all excreta immediately and, ideally, nursing the patient in a side room with access to their own toilet. Advice should be sought from infection control teams.

The prevention and/or correction of dehydration is the first step in managing an episode of diarrhoea. Simple steps to encourage patients to drink include:

- Providing drinks to suit individual taste preferences
- Adding ice to drinks
- Ice-lollies
- Using china cups or glass instead of plastic or polystyrene cups.

Dehydration can be corrected by using oral rehydration solutions, for example WHO oral rehydration salts, or by intravenous fluids and electrolytes.

Antimotility drugs such as loperamide, codeine phosphate and co-phenotrope may be useful in some cases, for example in blind loop syndrome and radiation enteritis. These drugs reduce gastrointestinal motility to relieve the symptoms of abdominal cramps and reduce the frequency of diarrhoea (Shepherd 2000). It is important to rule out any infective agent as the cause of diarrhoea before using any of these drugs as they may make the situation worse by slowing the clearance of the infective agent (Taylor 1997). Occasionally intractable diarrhoea may be reduced by a subcutaneous infusion of octreotide, but this is more commonly indicated in patients with a high output of diarrhoea from a stoma (Fallon & O'Neill 1997).

Preserving the patient's privacy and dignity is essential during episodes of diarrhoea. The nurse has an important role in minimizing the patient's distress by adjusting language and using terms that are appropriate to the individual to reduce embarrassment (Smith 2001) and by listening to the patient's preference for care (Cadd et al. 2000).

It is important that the patient has easy access to clean toilet and washing facilities and that requests for assistance are answered promptly. Skin care is also essential to prevent bacteria present in faecal matter from destroying the skin's cellular defence and causing skin damage. This is particularly important with diarrhoea since it has high levels of faecal enzymes that come easily into contact with the perianal skin (Le Lievre 2002). The anal area should be gently cleaned with warm water immediately after every episode of diarrhoea (Taylor 1997). Soap should be avoided, unless it is an emollient, to avoid excessive drying of the skin. Gentle patting of the skin is preferred for drying to avoid friction damage. Talcum powder should not be used and barrier creams should be applied sparingly, gently layered on in the direction of the hair growth rather than rubbed into the skin (Le Lievre 2002).

Constipation

Constipation occurs when there is a failure of colonic propulsion (slow transit), or a failure to evacuate the rectum or a combination of these problems (Norton 1996a). It has been estimated that 2–20% of people eating a Western diet experience constipation (Cook et al. 1999). Its management is dependent on its cause. There are many possible causes and many patients may be affected by more than one causative factor (see Fig. 13.1).

There is no one universally accepted definition of constipation; it is open to individual interpretation, which can lead to confusion. There are a range of symptoms which are commonly characterized as constipation.

These include:

• Reduced or infrequent defecation
• Difficulty in defecation
• Hard stools
• Bulky stools
• Pellet-sized stools
• A feeling of incomplete emptying of rectal contents (Norton 1996a; Maestri-Banks 1998; Winney 1998).

Constipation is associated with abdominal pain or cramps, feelings of general malaise or fatigue and feelings of bloatedness. Nausea, anorexia, headaches, confusion, restlessness, retention of urine, faecal incontinence and halitosis may also be present in some cases (Norton 1996b; Maestri-Banks 1998).

Chronic constipation is defined by the Rome Criteria as demonstrating at least two of the following symptoms which should be present for at least 3 months:

• Straining for at least 25% of the time
• Lumpy/hard stool for at least 25% of the time
• A sensation of incomplete evacuation for at least 25% of the time
• Two or fewer bowel movements a week (Merec Bulletin 1999).

While constipation is not life-threatening it does cause a great deal of distress and discomfort.

The myth of daily bowel evacuation being essential to healthy living has persisted through the centuries. It is thought that less than 10% of the population has a bowel evacuation daily (Edwards 1997). This myth has resulted in laxative abuse becoming one of the commonest types of drug abuse in the Western world. The cost to the NHS of prescribing medications to treat constipation has been estimated as £47 million (Petticrew 1997). An individual's bowel habit is dictated by their diet, lifestyle and environment. The notion of what is a 'normal' bowel habit varies considerably. Studies reveal that in the USA and UK 95% of people pass three stools per week (Bartolo & Wexner 1995). Normal bowel movement has been defined as ranging between three times a day and three times a week (Nazarko 1996). Given that there is such a wide normal range it is important to establish the patient's usual bowel habit and the changes that have occurred.

Assessment

Assessment and the identification of the underlying cause and/or identification of any contributory cause are instrumental to the successful management of constipation. There are many factors which may affect normal

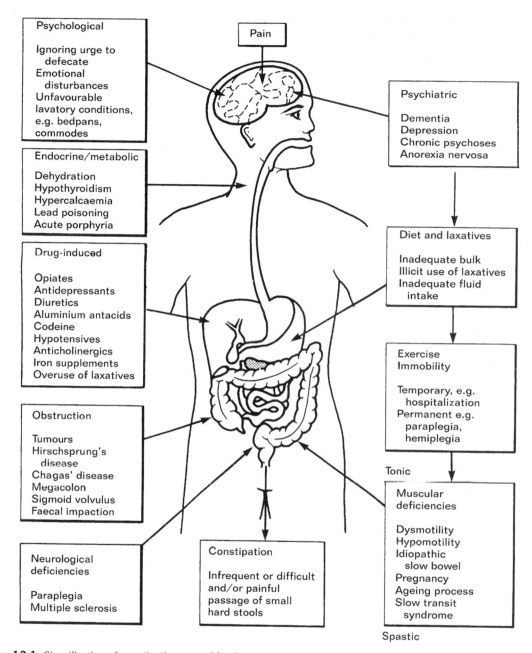

Figure 13.1 Classification of constipation – combined sources.

bowel functioning. These include:

- Change in diet
- Change in fluid intake
- Lack of exercise
- The use of drugs, e.g. analgesics, antacids, iron preparations, antidepressants

- Lack of privacy, e.g. having to use shared toilet facilities, commodes or bedpans
- Change in patient's normal routine
- Disease process or symptoms, e.g. neoplasm, vomiting
- X-ray investigation of the bowel involving the use of barium.

A careful history of a patient's bowel habits should be taken, with particular note taken of the following:

1 Any changes in the patient's usual bowel activity. How long have these changes been present and have they occurred before?
2 Frequency of bowel action
3 Volume, consistency and colour of the stool
4 Presence of mucus, blood, undigested food or offensive odour
5 Presence of pain or discomfort on defecation
6 Use of oral or rectal medication to stimulate defecation and its effectiveness.

The assessment should also include a dietary history (including fluid intake), significant medical history and present medical situation, current medication, recent lifestyle changes such as decrease in mobility/physical activity or change in home circumstances, and psychological status, e.g. depression. A digital rectal examination should also be performed to assess the contents of the rectum and to identify conditions which may cause discomfort such as haemorrhoids or anal fissure (Winney 1998; Hinriches & Huseboe 2001).

Management

The effective treatment of constipation relies on the cause being identified. Constipation can be categorized as either primary or secondary. Factors that lead to the development of primary constipation include:

• An inadequate diet (low fibre)
• Poor fluid intake
• A lifestyle change
• Ignoring the urge to defecate.

Constipation that is attributed to a disease process or surgical and/or medical conditions such as anal fissures, colonic tumours or hypercalcaemia is classified as secondary constipation. Constipation of unknown cause must be investigated before treatment is instigated (Taylor 1997; Teahon 1999).

Dietary manipulations may help to resolve mild constipation, although it is much more likely to help prevent constipation from recurring. Increasing dietary fibre increases stool bulk, which in turn improves peristalsis and stool transit time. This results in a softer stool being delivered to the rectum (Norton 1996b). The UK average daily fibre intake of 12–13 g could be usefully doubled to help improve bowel health. However, care should be taken to increase dietary bran intake gradually as bloating and abdominal discomfort can result from a sudden increase (Cummings 1994; Norton 1996b). Other sources of dietary laxatives

should be encouraged, for example prunes contain diphenylisatin and onions contain indigestible sugars (Norton 1996b).

Dietary changes need to be taken in combination with other lifestyle changes. Daily fluid intake should be between 2 and 2.5 litres (Taylor 1997; Day 2001). Fruit juices such as orange and prune juice can help stimulate bowel activity (Winney 1998) and coffee has been shown to stimulate colonic motor and bowel activity (Brown *et al.* 1990; Addison 1999a). The motor response takes place within minutes of drinking coffee and can last for up to 90 minutes (Addison 2000a). There is a need for further studies to examine the role of dietary manipulations in the management of constipation, particularly the function of dietary fibre and fluid intake (Addison 2000b).

Patients should be advised not to ignore the urge to defecate and to allow sufficient time for defecation (Norton 1996b). It is important that the correct posture for defecation is adopted. Crouching or a 'crouch like' posture is considered anatomically correct (Taylor 1997). The use of a foot stool by the toilet may enable patients to adopt a better defecation posture (Norton 1996b). The use of the bedpan should always be avoided if possible. The poor posture adopted while using a bedpan has been shown to cause extreme straining during defecation (Lewin 1976; Taylor 1997). Patients should be supported with pillows to enable them to achieve an upright position if the use of a bedpan is unavoidable.

Where possible patients should be encouraged to increase their level of exercise. Therapies such as homeopathy and reflexology may be utilized (Emly *et al.* 1997; Rankin-Box 2000).

Laxatives are the most commonly used treatment for constipation (Table 13.1). In general they should be used as a short-term measure to help relieve an episode of constipation as long-term use can perpetuate constipation and a dependence on laxatives can develop (Butler 1998).

Laxatives

Weller (1989) defines laxatives as medicines that loosen bowel contents and encourage evacuation. A laxative with a mild or gentle effect is also known as an aperient and one with a strong effect is referred to as a cathartic or a purgative. Purgatives should be used only in exceptional circumstances, i.e. where all other interventions have failed, or when they are prescribed for a specific purpose. Wherever possible the most natural means of bowel evacuation should be employed.

The many different types of laxatives available may be grouped into four types according to the action they have (Table 13.1).

Table 13.1 Types of laxative

Type of laxative	Example	Brand names and sources
Stool softeners	Synthetic surface active agents, liquid paraffin	Agarol, Dioctyl, Petrolager, Milpar
Osmotic agents	Sodium, potassium and magnesium salts	Magnesium sulphate, milk of magnesia, lactulose
Stimulant laxatives	Sodium picosulphate, glycerin	Senna, Senokot, bisacodyl, Dulcolax, co-danthrusate, Picolax, glycerol
Bulk producers	Dietary fibre Mucilaginous polysaccharides Methylcellulose	Bran, wholemeal bread, Fybogel (ispaghula), Normacol (sterculia)

Stool softeners

These act by lowering the surface tension of faeces which allows water to penetrate and soften the stool. They may also have a weak stimulatory effect (Barrett 1992), but drugs of this type are often given in combination with a chemical stimulant. Softening agents take 24–48 hours to work (Martindale 1993).

Liquid paraffin acts as a lubricant as well as a stool softener by coating the faeces and allowing easier passage. However, its use should be avoided as there are a number of problems associated with this preparation. The use of liquid paraffin interferes with the absorption of fat-soluble vitamins. Accidental inhalation of droplets of liquid paraffin may result in lipoid pneumonia (Barrett 1992; Taylor 1997).

Osmotic agents

These may be divided into two subgroups: lactulose and magnesium preparations. Lactulose is a synthetic disaccharide which exerts an osmotic effect in the small bowel. Distension of the small bowel induces propulsion which in turn reduces transit time. Colonic bacteria metabolize lactulose into a short chain organic salt which is then absorbed; therefore the osmotic effect does not continue throughout the colon (Barrett 1992). This process of metabolism also produces gas which in turn stimulates colonic movements and increases bacterial growth. This results in increased stool weight and thus colonic transit time is shortened (Spiller 1994). Bowel action may occur 3 hours after administration or up to 48 hours later (Taylor 1997). Flatulence, cramps and abdominal discomfort are associated with high dosages. Magnesium preparations also exert an osmotic effect on the gut and additionally they stimulate the release of cholecystokinin. This encourages intestinal mobility and fluid secretion (Nathan 1996). They have a rapid effect, working within 2–6 hours. Fluid intake is important with these preparations as patients may easily become dehydrated (Martindale 1993). These

preparations should be avoided in patients with renal or hepatic impairment (Taylor 1997).

Stimulant laxatives

These stimulate the nerve plexuses in the gut wall causing irritation and increased peristalsis in the small and large bowel (Barrett 1992; Nathan 1996). Abdominal cramping may be increased if the stool is hard and a stool softener may be used in combination with this group of drugs (Taylor 1997; ABPI 1999). Long-term use of these laxatives should be avoided, except for patients on long-term opiates, as they may lead to impaired bowel function such as atonic non-functioning colon (Taylor 1997; ABPI 1999).

Preparations containing Danthron are restricted to certain groups of patients, i.e. the elderly, the terminally ill and some cardiac patients, as some rodent studies have indicated a potential carcinogenic risk (Taylor 1997; ABPI 1999). Danthron preparations should not be used for incontinent patients especially those with limited mobility as prolonged skin contact will colour the skin pink or red and superficial sloughing of the discoloured skin will occur (Taylor 1997; ABPI 1999).

Bulking agents

These work by retaining water and promoting microbial growth in the colon. This increases faecal mass production which stimulates peristalsis. Ispaghula husk (Isogel, Regulan) and sterculia (Normacol) both trap water in the intestine by the formation of a highly viscous gel which softens faeces, increases weight and reduces transit time (Butler 1998). These agents need plenty of fluid in order to work (2–3 litres per day) (Taylor 1997). They take a few days to exert their effect so are not suitable to relieve acute constipation. They are not suitable for use in patients who have bowel obstruction or reduced muscle tone. Increasing the bulk may worsen impaction, lead to increased colonic faecal loading or even intestinal obstruction (Norton 1996b), and may also increase the risk of faecal incontinence (Ardron & Main 1990). Other potentially harmful effects include malabsorption of minerals, calcium, iron and fat-soluble vitamins, and reduced bioavailability of some drugs (Taylor 1997). Another problem initially is that bulk laxatives tend to distend the abdomen, often making the patient feel full and uncomfortable. Sometimes this leads to temporary anorexia (Taylor 1997).

Studies have now shown that there are a number of types and components of 'dietary fibre', which makes this too imprecise a term for health care professionals to use: its closest, more exact description is now 'non-starch polysaccharides'. A more detailed discussion of this area can be found in *Dietary Reference Values for Food Energy and Nutrients for the United Kingdom* (DoH 1991).

Enemas

Definition

An enema is the introduction into the rectum or lower colon of a stream of fluid for the purpose of producing a bowel action or instilling medication (Clarke 1988).

Indications

Enemas may be prescribed for the following reasons:

- To clean the lower bowel before surgery; X-ray examination of the bowel using contrast medium; before endoscopy examination or in cases of severe constipation
- To introduce medication into the system
- To soothe and treat irritated bowel mucosa
- To decrease body temperature (due to contact with the proximal vascular system)
- To stop local haemorrhage
- To reduce hyperkalaemia (calcium resonium)
- To reduce portal systemic encephalopathy (phosphate enema).

Contraindications

Enemas are contraindicated under the following circumstances:

- In paralytic ileus
- In colonic obstruction
- Where the administration of tap water or soap and water enemas may cause circulatory overload, water intoxication, mucosal damage and necrosis, hyperkalaemia and cardiac arrhythmias

- Where the administration of large amounts of fluid high into the colon may cause perforation and haemorrhage
- Following gastrointestinal or gynaecological surgery, where suture lines may be ruptured (unless medical consent has been given)
- The use of micro-enemas and hypertonic saline enemas in patients with inflammatory or ulcerative conditions of the large colon
- Recent radiotherapy to the lower pelvis unless medical consent has been given (Addison 2000a).

Reference material

Types of enemas

Evacuant enemas

An evacuant enema is a solution introduced into the rectum or lower colon with the intention of its being expelled, along with faecal matter and flatus, within a few minutes. The following solutions are used:

- Phosphate enemas with standard or long rectal tubes in single-dose disposable packs
- Dioctyl sodium sulphosuccinate 0.1%, sorbitol 25% in single-dose disposable packs
- Sodium citrate 450 mg, sodium alkysulphoacetate 45 mg, sorbic acid 5 mg in single-dose disposable packs.

Enemas containing dioctyl sodium sulphosuccinate lubricate and soften impacted faeces. Phosphate enemas are useful in bowel clearance before X-ray examination and surgery.

Retention enemas

A retention enema is a solution introduced into the rectum or lower colon with the intention of being retained for a specified period of time. Three types of retention enema are in common use:

- Arachis oil (may be obtained in a single-dose disposable pack)
- Olive oil
- Prednisolone.

Enemas containing olive oil or arachis oil will soften and lubricate impacted faeces. These work by penetrating faeces, increasing the bulk and softness of stools. They work most effectively when warmed to body temperature and retained for as long as possible (Clarke 1988). Retention enemas given to administer medications will be prescribed by the doctor. The product must be checked with the prescription before its administration.

Procedure guidelines: **Administration of enemas**

Equipment

1 Disposable incontinence pad.
2 Disposable gloves.
3 Topical swabs.
4 Lubricating jelly.

5 Rectal tube and funnel (if not using a commercially prepared pack).
6 Solution required or commercially prepared enema.
7 Bath thermometer.

Procedure

Action	Rationale
1 Explain and discuss the procedure with the patient.	To ensure that the patient understands the procedure and gives his/her valid consent.
2 Ensure privacy.	To avoid unnecessary embarrassment to the patient.
3 Allow patient to empty bladder first if necessary.	A full bladder may cause discomfort during the procedure.
4 Ensure that a bedpan, commode or toilet is readily available	In case the patient feels the need to expel the enema before the procedure is completed.
5 Warm the enema to the required temperature by immersing in a jug of hot water, testing with a bath thermometer. A temperature of 40.5–43.3°C is recommended for adults. Oil retention enemas should be warmed to 37.8°C.	Heat is an effective stimulant of the nerve plexi in the intestinal mucosa. An enema temperature of body temperature or just above will not damage the intestinal mucosa. The temperature of the environment, the rate of fluid administration and the length of the tubing will all have an effect on the temperature of the fluid in the rectum.
6 Assist the patient to lie in the required position, i.e. on the left side, with knees well flexed, the upper higher than the lower one, and with the buttocks near the edge of the bed.	This allows ease of passage into the rectum by following the natural anatomy of the colon. In this position gravity will aid the flow of the solution into the colon. Flexing the knees ensures a more comfortable passage of the enema nozzle or rectal tube.
7 Place a disposable incontinence pad beneath the patient's hips and buttocks.	To reduce potential infection caused by soiled linen. To avoid embarrassing the patient if the fluid is ejected prematurely following administration.
8 Wash hands with bactericidal soap and water or bactericidal alcohol handrub, and put on disposable gloves.	To minimize the risk of cross-infection.
9 Place some lubricating jelly on a topical swab and lubricate the nozzle of the enema or the rectal tube.	To prevent trauma to the anal and rectal mucosa by reducing surface friction.
10 Expel excessive air and introduce the nozzle or tube slowly into the anal canal while separating the buttocks.	The introduction of air into the colon causes distention of its walls, resulting in unnecessary discomfort to the patient, and increases peristalsis. The slow introduction of the lubricated tube will minimize spasm of the intestinal wall.
(A small amount of air may be introduced if bowel evacuation is desired.)	(Evacuation will be more effectively induced due to the increased peristalsis.)
11 Slowly introduce the tube or nozzle to a depth of 10–12.5 cm.	This will bypass the anal canal (2.5–4 cm in length) and ensure that the tube or nozzle is in the rectum.
12 If a retention enema is used, introduce the fluid slowly and leave the patient in bed with the foot of the bed elevated by 45° for as long as prescribed.	To avoid increasing peristalsis. The slower the rate at which the fluid is introduced the less pressure is exerted on the intestinal wall. Elevating the foot of the bed aids in retention of the enema by force of gravity.
13 If an evacuant enema is used, introduce the fluid slowly by rolling the pack from the bottom to the top to prevent backflow, until the pack is empty or the solution is completely finished.	The faster the rate of flow of the fluid the greater the pressure on the rectal walls. Distention and irritation of the bowel wall will produce strong peristalsis which is sufficient to empty the lower bowel.

*Procedure guidelines: **Administration of enemas** (cont'd)*

Action	Rationale
14 If using a funnel and rectal tube, adjust the height of the funnel according to the rate of flow desired.	The forces of gravity will cause the solution to flow from the funnel into the rectum. The greater the elevation of the funnel, the faster the flow of fluid.
15 Clamp the tubing before all the fluid has run in.	To avoid air entering the rectum and causing further discomfort.
16 Slowly withdraw the tube or nozzle.	To avoid reflex emptying of the rectum.
17 Dry the patient's perineal area with a gauze swab.	To promote patient comfort and avoid excoriation.
18 Ask the patient to retain the enema for 10–15 minutes before evacuating the bowel.	To enhance the evacuant effect.
19 Ensure that the patient has access to the nurse call system, is near to the bedpan, commode or toilet, and has adequate toilet paper.	To enhance patient comfort and safety. To minimize the patient's embarrassment.
20 Remove and dispose of equipment.	To minimize risk of cross-infection.
21 Wash hands.	To minimize risk of cross-infection.
22 Record in the appropriate documents that the enema has been given, its effects on the patient and its results (colour, consistency, content and amount of faeces produced, using the Bristol Stool Chart (Gill 1999)).	To monitor the patient's bowel function.

Problem solving

Problem	Cause	Suggested action
Unable to insert the nozzle of enema pack or rectal tube into the anal canal.	Tube not adequately lubricated.	Apply more lubricating jelly.
	Patient in an incorrect position.	Ask the patient to draw knees up further towards the chest.
	Patient apprehensive and embarrassed about the situation. Patient unable to relax anal sphincter.	Ensure adequate privacy and give frequent explanations to the patient about the procedure. Ask the patient to take deep breaths and 'bear down' as if defecating.
Unable to advance the tube or nozzle into the anal canal.	Spasm of the canal walls.	Wait until spasm has passed before inserting the tube or nozzle more slowly, thus minimizing spasm. Ask patient to take slow deep breaths to help to relax.
Unable to advance the tube or nozzle into the rectum.	Blockage by faeces.	Withdraw tubing slightly and allow a little solution to flow and then insert the tube further.
	Blockage by tumour.	If resistance is still met, stop the procedure and inform a doctor.
Patient complains of cramping or the desire to evacuate the enema before the end of the procedure.	Distension and irritation of the intestinal wall produce strong peristalsis sufficient to empty the lower bowel.	Temporarily stop the infusion of fluid by clamping the tubing or lowering the funnel until the patient says the feeling has subsided. If the feeling does not subside, stop procedure and allow patient to evacuate bowel.
Patient unable to open bowels after an evacuant enema and the fluid has not returned.	Reduced neuromuscular response in the bowel wall.	Insert a rectal tube and try to siphon the fluid off. Measure and record the amount. If this is not successful, perform rectal lavage. (For further information, see Rectal lavage, p. 300.) Measure and record the amount returned.

Suppositories

Definition

A suppository is a medicament in a base that melts at body temperature when inserted into the rectum (Churchill Livingstone 1996).

Indications

The use of suppositories is indicated under the following circumstances:

- To empty the bowel before certain types of surgery
- To empty the bowel to relieve acute constipation or when other treatments for constipation have failed
- To empty the bowel before endoscopic examination
- To introduce medication into the system
- To soothe and treat haemorrhoids or anal pruritus.

Contraindications

The use of suppositories is contraindicated when one or more of the following pertain:

- Chronic constipation, which would require repetitive use
- Paralytic ileus
- Colonic obstruction
- Following gastrointestinal or gynaecological operations, unless on the specific instructions of the doctor.

Reference material

Administration of suppositories

The use of suppositories dates back to about 460 BC. Hippocrates recommended the use of cylindrical suppositories of honey smeared with ox gall (Hurst 1970). The torpedo-shaped suppositories commonly used today came into being in 1893, when it was recommended that they were inserted apex first (Moppett 2000). This practice has been questioned by Abd-el Maeboud *et al.* (1991) who suggest that suppositories should be inserted blunt end first. This advice is based on anorectal physiology for if a suppository is inserted apex first the circular base distends the anus and the lower edge of the anal sphincter fails to close tightly. The normal squeezing motion (reverse vermicular contraction) of the anal sphincter fails to drive the suppository into the rectum. These factors can lead to anal irritation and expulsion of the suppository (Moppett 2000). A clinical study based on this evidence demonstrated that patients found insertion and retention of suppositories much easier using the base-first method.

There are several different types of suppository available. Retention suppositories are designed to deliver drug therapy, e.g. analgesia, antibiotic, NSAID. Those designed to stimulate bowel evacuation include glycerine, bisacodyl and sodium bicarbonate. Lubricant suppositories, e.g. glycerine, should be inserted directly into the faeces and allowed to dissolve to enable softening of the faecal mass. However, stimulant types, such as bisacodyl, must come into contact with the mucous membrane of the rectum if they are to be effective. Other types, such as sodium bicarbonate and anhydrous sodium acid phosphate, exert their influence by releasing carbon dioxide, causing rectal distension when they contact water or mucous membrane.

Procedure guidelines: **Administration of suppositories**

Equipment

1 Disposable incontinence pad.
2 Disposable gloves.
3 Topical swabs or tissues.
4 Lubricating jelly.
5 Suppository(ies) as required (check prescription before administering a medicinal suppository, e.g. aminophylline).

Procedure

Action	Rationale
1 Explain and discuss the procedure with the patient. If you are administering a medicated suppository, it is best to do so after the patient has emptied his/her bowels.	To ensure that the patient understands the procedure and gives his/her valid consent. To ensure that the active ingredients are not impeded from being absorbed by the rectal mucosa or that the suppository is not expelled before its active ingredients have been released.
2 Ensure privacy.	To avoid unnecessary embarrassment to the patient.

*Procedure guidelines: **Administration of suppositories** (cont'd)*

Action	Rationale
3 Ensure that a bedpan, commode or toilet is readily available.	In case of premature ejection of the suppositories or rapid bowel evacuation following their administration.
4 Assist the patient to lie in the required position, i.e. on the left side, with the knees flexed, the upper higher than the lower one, with the buttocks near the edge of the bed.	This allows ease of passage of the suppository into the rectum by following the natural anatomy of the colon. Flexing the knees will reduce discomfort as the suppository is passed through the anal sphincter.
5 Place a disposable incontinence pad beneath the patient's hips and buttocks.	To avoid unnecessary soiling of linen, leading to potential infection and embarrassment to the patient if the suppositories are ejected prematurely or there is rapid bowel evacuation following their administration.
6 Wash hands with bactericidal soap and water or bactericidal alcohol handrub, and put on gloves.	To reduce the risk of cross-infection.
7 Place some lubricating jelly on the topical swab and lubricate the blunt end of the suppository if it is being used to obtain systemic action. Separate the patient's buttocks and insert the suppository blunt end first, advancing it for about 2–4 cm. Repeat this procedure if a second suppository is to be inserted.	Lubricating reduces surface friction and thus eases insertion of the suppository and avoids anal mucosal trauma. Research has shown that the suppository is more readily retained if inserted blunt end first (Abd-el-Maeboud *et al.* 1991). (For further information, see Suppositories, above.) The anal canal is approximately 2–4 cm long. Inserting the suppository beyond this ensures that it will be retained.
8 Once suppository(ies) has been inserted, clean any excess lubricating jelly from the patient's perineal area.	To ensure the patient's comfort and avoid anal excoriation.
9 Ask the patient to retain the suppository(ies) for 20 minutes, or until he or she is no longer able to do so. If medicated suppository given remind patient that its aim is not to stimulate evacuation and to retain suppository for at least 20 minutes or as long as possible.	This will allow the suppository to melt and release the active ingredients.
10 Remove and dispose of equipment. Wash hands.	To reduce risk of infection.
11 Record that the suppository(ies) have been given, the effect on the patient and the result (amount, colour, consistency and content, using the Bristol Stool Chart (Gill 1999)) in the appropriate documents.	To monitor the patient's bowel function.

Digital rectal examination

A digital rectal examination (DRE) is carried out by inserting a lubricated gloved finger into the rectum. The reasons for performing this test include:

- To establish whether faecal matter is present in the rectum and if so, to assess the amount and consistency
- To assess the need for rectal medication and to evaluate its efficacy in certain circumstances, e.g. in patients who have diminished anal/rectal sensation
- For digital stimulation to trigger defecation by stimulating the recto-anal reflex
- To assess anal sphincter function and tone
- To assess anal/rectal sensation.

This examination should not be a primary investigation for constipation but should only be performed after a full assessment. Discussion with medical staff should occur to confirm diagnosis and jointly plan appropriate interventions to treat the constipation (RCN 2003).

Before carrying out a DRE the perineal and perianal area should be checked for signs of rectal prolapse, haemorrhoids, anal skin tags or lesions, foreign bodies or infestations. The condition of the skin should be noted, as should the type and amount of any discharge or leakage. If any of these abnormalities are seen DRE should not be carried out until advice is taken from a specialist nurse or medical practitioner (RCN 2003).

Precautions

Special care should be used in performing DRE in patients when disease processes or treatments in particular affect the anus or the bowel mucosa. These conditions include:

- Active inflammation of the bowel, e.g. ulcerative colitis
- Recent radiotherapy to the pelvic area
- Rectal/anal pain

- Rectal surgery or trauma to the anal/rectal area
- Obvious rectal bleeding
- Spinal injury patients with autonomic dysreflexia
- Patients with known allergies, e.g. latex
- Patients with a history of abuse.

Procedure guidelines: **Digital rectal examination**

Equipment

1 Disposable incontinence pad.
2 Disposable gloves (check if patient allergic to latex).
3 Lubricating gel.
4 Tissues or topical swabs.

Procedure

Action	Rationale
1 Explain and discuss procedure with the patient.	To ensure that the patient understands the procedure and gives his/her valid consent.
2 Ensure privacy.	To avoid unnecessary embarrassment to the patient.
3 Ensure that a bedpan, commode or toilet is readily available.	DRE can stimulate the need for bowel movement.
4 Assist the patient to lie in the left lateral position with knees flexed, the upper knee higher than the lower knee, with the buttocks towards the edge of the bed.	This allows ease of digital examination into the rectum, by following the natural anatomy of the colon. Flexing the knees reduces discomfort as the examining finger passes the anal sphincter.
5 Place a disposable incontinence pad beneath the patient's hips and buttocks.	To reduce potential infection caused by soiled linen. To avoid embarrassing the patient if faecal staining occurs during or after the procedure.
6 Wash hands with bactericidal soap and water or bactericidal alcohol handrub and put on disposable gloves.	To minimize the risk of cross-infection.
7 Place some lubricating gel on a swab and gloved index finger.	To minimize discomfort as lubrication reduces friction and to ease insertion of the finger into the anus/rectum. Lubrication also helps minimize anal mucosal trauma.
Inform patient you are about to proceed and explain same.	Assists with patient co-operation with the procedure.
8 Observe anal area prior to the insertion of the finger into the anus for evidence of skin soreness, excoriation, swelling, haemorrhoids, rectal prolapse and infestation.	May indicate incontinence or pruritus. Swelling may be indicative of possible mass or abscess. Abnormalities such as bleeding, discharge or prolapse should be reported to medical staff before any examination is undertaken (RCN 2000).
Proceed to insert finger into the anus/rectum.	
9 On insertion of finger assess anal sphincter control; resistance should be felt.	Digital insertion with resistance indicates good internal sphincter tone, poor resistance may indicate the opposite (Addison 1999b).
10 Digital examination may feel faecal matter within the rectum; note consistency of any faecal matter.	May establish loaded rectum and indicate constipation and the need for rectal medication.
11 Clean anal area after the procedure.	To prevent irritation and soreness occurring. Preserves patient dignity and personal hygiene.
12 Remove gloves and dispose of equipment in appropriate clinical waste bin. Wash hands with bactericidal soap and water.	To minimize the risk of cross-infection.
13 Assist patient into a comfortable position and offer toilet facilities as appropriate.	To promote comfort.

*Procedure guidelines: **Digital rectal examination** (cont'd)*

Action	Rationale
14 Document findings and report to medical team.	To ensure continuity of care and assist in nursing diagnosis so appropriate corrective action may be initiated.

Manual evacuation

Manual evacuation of the rectum is an invasive procedure which should only be performed when necessary and after individual assessment. Advances in oral and rectal treatments have reduced the need for manual evacuations to be performed. For certain patients, such as those with spinal injuries, this procedure may be the only suitable bowel-emptying technique.

Nurses who have received appropriate training may perform manual evacuation. They should ensure that their employer has defined policies and procedure for undertaking this role (RCN 2003; Withell 2000). If appropriate, the patient and their personal carer may wish for the carer to maintain their established programme of bowel management (Harrison 2000).

Indications for assisted evacuation of bowels (manual evacuation or digital stimulation) include:

- Faecal impaction
- Incomplete defecation
- Inability to defecate
- If other bowel-emptying techniques have failed
- Neurogenic bowel dysfunction
- In patients with spinal injury (RCN 2003).

Patients are at risk of rectal trauma if these procedures are not performed with care or knowledge. The nurse should be aware of any conditions which may contraindicate performance of these procedures (see precautions listed above for DRE). Manual evacuation of faeces can be distressing, it may be painful and can be a dangerous procedure. In particular, stimulation of the vagus nerve in the rectal wall can slow the patient's heart, in addition to the risk of bowel perforation and bleeding (Powell & Rigby 2000).

If this procedure is used as an acute intervention the patient's pulse rate should be recorded before and during the process. Patients with a spinal injury should also have their blood pressure measured before, during and at the end of the procedure. A baseline blood pressure measurement should be available for comparison (RCN 2003). Every time the procedure is performed the consistency of the stool should be noted before continuing. If the stool is hard and dry lubricant suppositories should be inserted and left for 30 minutes before commencing. If the stool is too soft to remove effectively, consider delaying the procedure for 24 hours to allow further water

reabsorption to occur. During the procedure the nurse should observe the patients for signs of:

- Distress, pain or discomfort
- Bleeding
- Autonomic dysreflexia – hypertension, bradycardia, headache, flushing above the level of the spinal injury, sweating, pallor below the level of spinal injury, nasal congestion (Harrison 2000)
- Collapse (RCN 2003).

Autonomic dysreflexia is unique to patients with spinal cord injury. It is an abnormal response from the autonomic nervous system to a painful (noxious) stimulus perceived below the level of spinal cord injury (Powell & Rigby 2000; Harrison 2000). Distended bowel caused by constipation or impaction can lead to autonomic dysreflexia and therefore it is important that an effective programme of bowel management is established and followed (Harrison 2000).

Managing bowel problems such as constipation and prolonged bowel evacuation in patients following spinal cord injury requires a multimodality approach. This includes dietary fibre, digital stimulation, enemas, suppositories, stool softeners and abdominal massage (Amir *et al.* 1998; Addison & White 2002). Digital stimulation is a method of initiating the defecation reflex by dilating the anus, by either a finger or an anal dilator (Norton 1996a). This approach is only useful if the rectum is full.

Rectal lavage

Definition

Rectal lavage is the washing out of the rectum using large volumes of non-sterile fluid.

Indications

Rectal lavage is performed for the following purposes:

- To clear the lower bowel before investigation by barium enema and thus enable good images to be obtained
- To assist in clearing the lower bowel before major abdominal surgery and thus decrease the risk of infection and aid satisfactory healing
- To clear the lower bowel of residual faecal matter following previous surgery, e.g. formation of colostomy.

Contraindications

Rectal lavage is contraindicated in patients who have a history of any one of the following:

- Severe or prolapsed haemorrhoids
- Anal fissure
- Inflammatory bowel disease
- Large tumour in the rectum or sigmoid colon
- Post-radiation proctitis
- Internal fistulae
- Pelvic radiotherapy
- Recent bowel surgery
- Congestive cardiac failure
- Impaired renal function.

In the first eight of the contraindications listed above, the reason for employing caution is because of the damage that could be inflicted by the mechanical aspects of rectal lavage. When the bowel has already been traumatized there is a greater potential risk of causing irritation or, in extreme cases, perforation while inserting the catheter and running large volumes of fluid in and out of the rectum.

With the last two contraindications the potential risk lies with the possibility of large amounts of fluid and/or electrolytes becoming absorbed through the bowel. (Generally speaking, with the amounts and type of fluid used and the relatively short time that it stays in the bowel, this should not present a major problem.)

Caution should be exercised when giving tap water lavage to infants or patients with altered kidneys or cardiac reserve, but otherwise tap water is the solution of choice.

Reference material

Choice of fluid

Several solutions can be used to clear the bowel.

Hypertonic solutions

Hypertonic solutions, e.g. sodium phosphate and sodium acid phosphate in solution, act by drawing water from the intestinal cells by osmosis. This increases the fluid in the faecal mass, causing first distension then contraction and defecation.

For patients who have a large amount of faecal matter to evacuate, small volumes of these solutions are very effective. Hypertonic solutions should not be given to patients whose capacity to utilize sodium is affected, as some sodium may be absorbed. These solutions are available as commercially prepared enemas but are not suitable for administration in large volumes.

Tap water

Rectal lavage is a procedure that is normally used in combination with other methods of clearing the bowel, e.g. oral aperients and dietary restrictions. In this situation, it can be anticipated that there will be very little residue remaining in the lower bowel. What is needed, therefore, is a simple, non-sterile solution that can be used with relative safety in large volumes to wash out the residual faecal matter. The solution which fulfils these criteria ideally is tap water.

Rectal lavage using tap water is not without risk as large volumes of this hypotonic solution can upset the patient's electrolyte balance. Water is drawn by osmosis into the intestinal cells and water intoxication can result, with symptoms of weakness, sweating, pallor, vomiting, coughing and dizziness. However, this is a relatively rare complication and generally tap water is very well tolerated.

The other advantages of tap water are as follows:

- It is cheap and easily available.
- It can be easily warmed to the correct temperature (37°C).
- It is non-irritant to the bowel mucosa.
- It does not cause excessive peristalsis with resulting cramps and colic.

Isotonic saline

An isotonic saline solution can be substituted for patients with compromised electrolyte status. This is prepared by adding 2 level teaspoons of salt to 1 litre of plain water. Its effect on the bowel is similar to that of water in that it stimulates peristaltic action by distending the intestinal walls. With isotonic saline, however, there is less danger of electrolyte imbalance.

Choice of catheter

Several manufacturers produce rectal catheters. The criteria for selection should be as follows:

- The catheter should be of an adequate length. Most are approximately 30 cm long.
- The lumen should be large enough to allow the free drainage of particulate matter, i.e. a minimum Charrière gauge of 24.
- The tip of the catheter should be open ended or have large opposed eyelets to minimize the possibility of blockage.
- The catheter should be made from a soft flexible material; rubber or plastic is suitable.

Procedure guidelines: **Administration of rectal lavage**

Equipment

1 Rectal lavage pack containing a large funnel, rubber tubing, straight connector, 1 litre jug and rectal catheter (Charrière gauge 24). (Commercial packs are also available.)
2 Non-sterile topical swabs.
3 Lubricating jelly.
4 Disposable gloves.
5 Disposable incontinence pad.
6 Plastic sheet and draw sheet.
7 Large non-sterile jug.
8 Bucket.
9 Gate clip or clamp.
10 Toilet paper or tissues.
11 Disposable plastic apron.
12 Large disposable bag.
13 Measured volume of warm tap water (37–40°C).

Procedure

Action	Rationale
1 Explain and discuss the procedure with the patient.	To ensure that the patient understands the procedure and gives his/her valid consent.
2 Prepare the area, i.e. the patient's bed or a couch. Protect the bed or couch with plastic sheet and draw sheet. Place a disposable incontinence pad on the floor.	To prevent non-disposable equipment becoming contaminated with faecal matter, thus minimizing the risk of cross-infection.
3 Wash hands with bactericidal soap and water or bactericidal alcohol handrub, and dry hands, clean the trolley and prepare the equipment for the procedure by opening the pack and laying out the contents on the top of the shelf.	Although this is not an aseptic procedure, care must be taken to avoid unnecessary contamination.
4 Attach a large disposable bag to the trolley.	To provide a suitable receptacle for safe disposal of potentially large amounts of contaminated waste.
5 Fill a large non-sterile jug with a measured volume of warm (37–40°C) tap water. Check the temperature with a lotion thermometer. Place the filled jug on the lower shelf of the trolley. Put a bucket for receiving effluent by the side of the bed or couch.	As the bowel is not sterile, there is no need to use sterile fluid. A large volume needs to be available for use, up to a maximum of six litres, although the total amount used will vary with each patient and may be much less. If the solution is too warm, the intestinal mucosa may be damaged; if too cold, unnecessary cramping may occur.
6 Assist the patient to lie in the required position, i.e. on the left side, with the knees well flexed, the upper knee higher than the lower one, and with the buttocks near the edge of the bed. Tilt the foot of the bed slightly upwards if possible.	This position allows ease of access for insertion of the catheter into the rectum, follows the natural anatomy of the colon and aids gravity in promoting the flow of fluid into the sigmoid and descending colon. Tilting the bed also aids the flow.
7 Check that the patient's clothing is tucked out of the way and that both the patient and the bed are adequately protected. Ensure that the patient is as comfortable as possible before continuing with the procedure.	As the procedure can be lengthy and is potentially messy, the patient needs to be as relaxed and well protected as possible.
8 Wash hands with bactericidal soap and water or bactericidal alcohol handrub, and put on disposable gloves and a disposable plastic apron.	To reduce the risk of cross-infection.
9 Connect up the funnel, tubing and rectal catheter, using a straight connector between the latter two items. Fix a gate clamp or clip in position approximately 15 cm from the end of the rectal catheter.	To allow the tubing and the catheter to be primed and filled with fluid, thus preventing the entry of air into the rectum and discomfort to the patient.
10 Using a non-sterile topical swab lubricate the last 15 cm of the rectal catheter with a generous amount of lubricating jelly.	To aid insertion and minimize patient discomfort and trauma to the rectal mucosa.
11 Fill a small jug with 1 litre from the measured volume of warm tap water.	A small jug is more manageable and allows measurement of the amount of fluid used each time.

Procedure guidelines: **Administration of rectal lavage** *(cont'd)*

Action	Rationale
12 Prime the catheter and the tubing.	To prepare equipment.
13 Gently insert 7.5–10 cm of the catheter into the rectum.	The rectum is approximately 12.5 cm long and the anal canal 2.5 cm. Inserting the catheter 7.5–10 cm ensures that the rectum will be adequately filled with the minimum trauma to the patient.
14 Encourage the patient to take deep breaths.	Deep breathing relaxes the anal sphincter.
15 Check that the patient is comfortable.	
16 Fill the funnel with approximately 400 ml of fluid from the jug.	The rectum will hold 200–400 ml without causing trauma.
17 Hold the funnel about 30 cm above the rectum, release the clamp and allow the fluid to run into the rectum, holding the catheter in position.	Aqueous solution exerts pressure of 0.225 kg for every 30 cm of elevation. The pressure should not exceed 0.45 kg as this may cause cramping or even rupture of the intestinal wall.
18 Ask the patient to rock gently from side to side.	To ensure efficient lavage of the bowel lumen.
19 Before the funnel is completely empty, invert it over the bucket to allow the lavage fluid and faecal matter to drain out.	To prevent unnecessary amounts of air entering the rectum and causing the patient discomfort.
20 Refill the funnel with another measure of fluid, keeping the tubing pinched or clamped and the funnel at patient level until it is filled.	To prevent entry of air into rectum and discomfort to the patient.
21 Repeat the last two procedures until:	
(a) The effluent runs clear	If the bowel is not clear after this volume, other methods need to be employed.
(b) A maximum volume of 6 litres has been used.	
22 Note how much fluid was used during the procedure.	To ensure that not more than 6 litres are used to reduce the risk of circulatory fluid overload.
23 At the end of the procedure:	
(a) Measure the amount of effluent obtained and compare it with the volume run in.	To ensure that the patient has not absorbed fluid in such a quantity that will carry the risk of fluid overload.
(b) Clear away and dispose of equipment.	To minimize risk of cross-infection.
(c) Ensure that the patient is clean and tidy.	
24 Settle the patient into bed, on an incontinence pad and with a bedpan or commode at hand.	To minimize risk of infection caused by soiled linen.

Problem solving

Problem	Cause	Suggested action
Fluid will not run in freely.	Catheter is pressed against the bowel wall.	Gently manoeuvre the catheter around in the rectum.
	Catheter is blocked with faecal material	Remove the catheter and unblock. Reinsert and recommence procedure.
	Insufficient gravity flow.	Raise the funnel slightly but not above a height of 50 cm.
Leakage of fluid around the catheter.	Poor positioning of the catheter or displacement following insertion. Poor tone of the anal sphincter muscles.	Check that the catheter is 7–10 cm into the rectum. Hold it gently in position. Ask the patient to try and tighten muscles as fluid is run in. Elevate the foot of the bed to aid flow.
Discomfort and/or cramping when the fluid is run in.	Fluid is too cold.	Check the temperature of the fluid and warm to a temperature of 37–40°C.

Problem solving (cont'd)

Problem	Cause	Suggested action
	Pressure of the fluid entering the rectum is too high.	Lower the funnel to stop fluid from running until the spasm passes, but leave the catheter in to relieve distension.
	Extreme tension and anxiety.	When the spasm has passed, gradually raise the funnel and allow fluid to enter very slowly. Encourage deep breathing through the mouth to relax the abdominal muscles and decrease colonic pressures.
	Perforation of the rectum.	Stop the procedure immediately. Check the patient's vital signs. Inform a doctor.
Severe pain accompanied by perspiration, pallor and tachycardia.	Perforation of the gut around the site of a large tumour due to increased peristalsis.	Check the patient's vital signs. Inform a doctor. Do not allow the patient to eat or drink until seen by a doctor as patient may require emergency surgery.
Blood is returned in the effluent.	Insertion of the catheter has caused internal haemorrhoids to bleed.	Stop the procedure and inform a doctor. Record the appropriate amount of blood that has been passed and observe further bowel motions.
	Trauma to rectal mucosa.	
Large discrepancy between amount of fluid run in and the effluent obtained.	Excessive leakage on to pads during the procedure.	Try to estimate the amount of fluid on pads, etc.
	Patient has retained a certain amount of fluid that may be passed later.	Measure carefully all subsequent bowel actions.
	Patient has absorbed the excess fluid.	Check the patient's vital signs. Record further intake and output carefully. Inform a doctor.
Sudden onset of pallor, perspiration, vomiting, coughing and dizziness.	Water intoxication due to absorption of water from the rectum.	Stop the procedure immediately. Inform a doctor. Check the patient's vital signs.

References and further reading

Abd-el-Maeboud, K.H., El-Naggar, T. & El-Hawi, E.M.M. (1991) Rectal suppositories: commonsense mode of insertion. *Lancet*, **338**, 798–800.

ABPI (1999) *ABPI Compendium of Data Sheets and Summaries of Product Characteristics 1999–2000*. Datapharm Publications.

Addison, R. (1999a) Practical procedures for nurses. Fluid intake and continence care. *Nurs Times*, **95**(49), insert.

Addison, R. (1999b) Practical procedures for nurses. Digital rectal examination 1. *Nurs Times*, **33**(1), 95.

Addison, R. (2000a) Fluid intake: how coffee and caffeine affect continence. *Nurs Times*, **96**(40) (Suppl), 7–8.

Addison, R. (2000b) Fluids, fibre and constipation. *Nurs Times*, **96**(31) (Suppl), 11–12.

Addison, R. & White, M. (2002) Spinal injury and bowel management. *NT Plus*, **98**(4), 61–2.

Amir, I., Sharma, R., Bauman, W.A. *et al.* (1998) Bowel care for the individual with spinal cord injury: comparison of four approaches. *Spinal Med*, **21**(1), 21–4.

Ardron, M.E. & Main, A.N.H. (1990) Management of constipation. *Br Med J*, **300**, 1400.

Barrett, J.A. (1992) Faecal incontinence. In: *Clinial Nursing Practice. The Promotion and Management of Continence* (ed. B. Roe). Prentice Hall, New York.

Bartolo, D.G.C. & Wexner, S.D. (1995) *Constipation, its Etiology, Evaluation and Management*. Butterworth Heinemann, Philadelphia.

Basch, A. (1987) Symptom distress changes in elimination. *Semin Oncol Nurs*, **3**(4), 287–92.

Brown, S.R., Cann, P.A. & Read, N. (1990) Effect of coffee on distal colon function. *Gut*, **31**, 450–53.

Butler, M. (1998) Laxatives and rectal preparations. *Nurs Times*, **94**(3), 56–8.

Cadd, A., Keatinge, D., Henssen, M. *et al.* (2000) Assessment and documentation of bowel care management in palliative care: incorporating patient preferences into the care regimen. *J Clin Nurs*, **9**, 228–35.

Campbell, T. & Lunn, D. (1999) Colorectal cancer. Part 3 patient care. *Prof Nurse*, **15**(2), 117–21.

Churchill Livingstone (1996) *Dictionary of Nursing*, 17th edn. Churchill Livingstone, London.

Clarke, B. (1988) Making sense of enemas. *Nurs Times*, **84**(30), 40–4.

Cook, T., Frall, S., Gough, A. & Lennard, F. (1999). The conservative management of constipation in adults. *J Assoc Chart Physiother Women's Health*, **85**, 24–8.

Cummings, J.H. (1994) Non-starch polysaccharides (dietary fibre) including bulk laxatives in constipation. In: *Constipation* (eds M.A. Kamm & J.E. Lennard-Jones). Wrightson Biomedical, Petersfield.

Day, A. (2001) The nurse's role in managing constipation. *Nurs Stand* **16**(8), 41–4.

DoH (1991) *Report on Health and Social Subjects 41, Dietary Reference Values for Food Energy and Nutrients for the United Kingdom*, pp. 61–71. Stationery Office, London.

Edwards, C. & Dolman, E. (1997) Down, down and away! An overview of adult constipation and faecal incontinence. In: *Promoting Continence. A Clinical and Research Resource* (eds K. Getliffe & E. Dolman). Baillière Tindall, London.

Emly, M., Wilson, L. & Darby, J. (1997) Abdominal massage for adults with learning disabilities. *Nurs Times*, **97**(30) (Suppl), 61–2.

Fallon, M. & O'Neill, B. (1997) Clinical review. ABC of palliative care: constipation and diarrhoea. *Br Med J*, **315**, 1293–6.

Gill, D. (1999) Practical procedures for nurses. Stool specimen assessment. *Nurs Times*, **95**, 26.

Harrison, P. (2000) *HDU/ICU Managing Spinal Injury: Critical Care*. Spinal Injuries Association, London.

Hinriches, M.D. & Huseboe, J. (2001) Research based protocol: management of constipation. *J Gerontol Nurs*, **27**(2), 17–28.

Hogan, C.M. (1998) The nurse's role in diarrhoea management. *Oncol Nurs Forum*, **25**(5), 879–86.

Hurst, Sir A. (1970) *Selected Writings of Sir Arthur Hurst* (1989–1944). Spottiswode, Ballantyne.

Kornblau, A., Benson, R., Catalano, S. *et al.* (2000) Management of cancer treatment-related diarrhea: issues and therapeutic strategies. *J Pain Symptom Manage*, **19**(2), 118–29.

Le Lievre, S. (2002) An overview of skin care and faecal incontinence. *Nurs Times (NT Plus)*, **98**(4), 58–9.

Lewin, D. (1976) Care of the constipated patient. *Nurs Times*, **72**, 444–6.

Maestri-Banks, A. (1998) An overview of constipation – causes and treatment. *Int J Palliat Nurs*, **4**(6), 271–5.

Martindale, W. (1993) *The Extra Pharmacopea*, 30th edn. (ed. J.E.F. Reynolds). Pharmaceutical Press, London.

Merec Bulletin (1999) The management of constipation. *Merec Bull*, **10**(a), 33–7.

Moppett, S. (2000) Which way is up for a suppository? *Nurs Times*, **96**(19) (Suppl), 12–13.

Nathan, A. (1996) Laxatives. *Pharm J*, **257**, 52–5.

Nazarko, L. (1996) Preventing constipation in older people. *Prof Nurse*, **11**(12), 816–18.

Norton, C. (1996a) *Nursing for Continence*, 2nd edn. Beaconsfield, Beaconsfield.

Norton, C. (1996b) The causes and nursing management of constipation. *Br J Nurs*, **5**(20), 1252–8.

Petticrew, W. (1997) Treatment of constipation in older people. *Nurs Times*, **93**(48), 55–6.

Powell, M. & Rigby, D. (2000) Management of bowel dysfunction: evacuation difficulties. *Nurs Stand*, **14**(47), 47–54.

Rankin-Box, D. (2000) An alternative approach to bowel disorders. *Nurs Times*, **96**(19) (Suppl), 24–5.

RCN (2003) *Digital Rectal Examination and Manual Removal of Faeces: Guidance for Nurses*. RCN, London.

Shepherd, M. (2000) Treating diarrhoea and constipation. *Nurs Times (NT Plus)*, **96**(6), 15–16.

Smith, S. (2001) Evidence-based management of constipation in the oncology patient. *Eur J Oncol Nurs*, **5**(1), 18–25.

Spiller, R.C. (1994) *Diarrhoea and Constipation*. Libra Pharm, Petroc Press.

Taylor, C. (1997) Constipation and diarrhoea. In: *Gastroenterology* (eds L. Bruce & T.M.D. Finlay). Churchill Livingstone, Oxford.

Teahon, E. (1999) Constipation. In: *Essential Coloproctology for Nurses* (eds T. Porret & N. Daniel). Whurr, London.

Tortora, G.A. & Grabowski, S.R. (2002) *Principles of Anatomy and Physiology*. John Wiley and Sons, New York.

Walsh, M. (1997) *Watson's Clinical Nursing and Related Sciences*, 5th edn. Baillière Tindall, London.

Weller, B. (1989) *Encyclopaedic Dictionary of Nursing and Health Care*. Baillière Tindall, Eastbourne.

Winney, J. (1998) Constipation. *Nurs Stand*, **13**(11), 49–56.

Withell, B. (2000) A protocol for treating acute constipation in the community setting. *Br J Commun Nurs*, **5**(3), 110–17.

Woods, S. (1996) Nutrition and the short bowel syndrome. In: *Stoma Care Nursing: A Patient-Centred Approach* (ed. C. Myres). Edward Arnold, London.

Elimination: continent urinary diversions

Chapter contents

Definition

A urinary diversion is a surgically created system for removing urine from the body when either the bladder or urethra is either non-existent or no longer viable. There are two main types: a urostomy (see Ch. 15, Elimination: stoma care) and continent urinary diversions. Continent urinary diversions differ in that a system is created to collect and store urine before it is removed from the body.

Indications for formation of a continent urinary diversion

A continent urinary diversion may be formed to:

- Store and expel urine from the body if the lower urinary tract is defective or absent
- Offer patients a choice of urinary diversion
- Improve or maintain the individual's body image, psychological and social well-being by removing the necessity of wearing external devices, e.g. urostomy pouch or incontinence pads (Randles 1990; Leaver 1997).

Continent urinary diversions are increasingly available as an alternative to the conventional ileal conduit (see Ch. 15, Elimination: stoma care).

Reference material

Principles of a continent urinary diversion

A continent urinary diversion is surgically constructed to replace a defective or non-existent lower urinary tract. It consists of three components:

- A reservoir to store urine
- A continence mechanism to retain urine in the reservoir
- A channel or tunnel to let the urine out (Leaver 1996, 1997).

> **Box 14.1** Types of continent urinary diversion with catheterizable stomas
>
> 1 Mitrofanoff pouch   4 Mainz pouch
> 2 Kock pouch   5 Indiana pouch
> 3 Benchekroun pouch   6 Le bag

The reservoir can be the bladder itself, an augmented bladder or made completely of ileum, colon or a combination of the two. The continence mechanism may be constructed during the operation using the same tissues used to construct the reservoir or an existing valve or sphincter may be utilised (Leaver 1997). Five types of continence system have been identified:

- The flutter valve, created by the intussusception of a segment of bowel, usually ileum, e.g. Kock nipple
- The flap valve, created by tunnelling a narrow tube between the muscle and mucosal layers of the reservoir, e.g. Mitrofanoff valve
- The ileocaecal valve
- The urethral sphincter
- The anal sphincter.

The channel or tunnel component can be formed by utilizing other tube/tunnel-like structures such as the appendix, ureter or fallopian tube. Alternatively, a segment of ileum or colon can be used (Leaver 1996).

There are a number of different types of continent diversions performed today; these include those with catheterizable stomas, rectal bladders and orthotopic neobladders. The aim of these diversions is to mimic, as far as possible, the normal bladder function. The goals are:

- To create a pouch with the ability to hold an adequate volume of urine at low pressure
- To preserve and protect the upper tract by preventing reflux
- To prevent or minimize the absorption of urine, thus avoiding metabolic disturbances
- To control urine voiding by sphincter control or self-catheterization (Razor 1993; Leaver 1996).

Indications for surgical formation of a continent urinary diversion

The indications for the formation of a continent urinary diversion and an ileal conduit are similar (see Ch. 15, Elimination: stoma care). These include:

- Congenital abnormalities, e.g. bladder extrophy
- Pelvic cancers, e.g. bladder, cervical

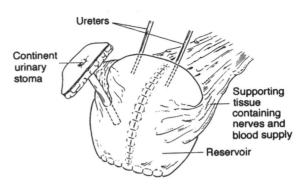

Figure 14.1 Continent urinary diversion.

- Neuropathic bladder – a condition where the nerve impulses do not reach the bladder as the result of an underlying disease or injury, e.g. myelomeningocoele
- Trauma
- Incontinence
- Interstitial cystitis
- Radiation fibrosis
- Irreparable fistula
- An existing diversion, e.g. ileal conduit (Woodhouse 1991; Leaver 1994; Dixon *et al.* 2001).

Continent urinary diversions with catheterizable stomas

There are a number of different types of continent urinary diversions with catheterizable stomas performed today (Box 14.1). These procedures differ in construction, using different structures to form the reservoir and tunnel and different techniques to create the continence mechanism. The outcomes for patients and the nursing care involved are essentially similar in most cases. The most commonly performed procedure of this type in the UK is arguably the Mitrofanoff (Leaver 1996) (Fig. 14.1).

This type of diversion involves the patient having two admissions into hospital. The first is to form the continent urinary diversion. Following the operation, a sterile fine-bore tube is left in the continent urinary stoma to keep it patent and allow the urine to drain into a catheter bag. After recovering from the operation, patients are taught how to take care of the tubing, leg bags and night drainage systems. Patients are then discharged home to be readmitted 6 weeks after the operation to be taught self-catheterization. This admission lasts between 24 and 48 hours. During this time, patients are taught self-catheterization and encouraged to practise the technique. Nursing staff are available to detect and rectify any problems. This allows patients time to gain confidence in self-catheterization before they return home.

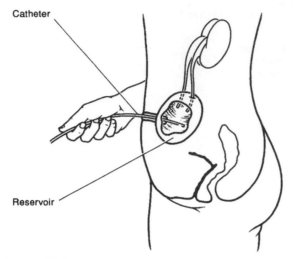

Figure 14.2 Self-catheterization into the continent urinary stoma.

In a continent urinary diversion the urine drains into the urinary reservoir or bladder through the ureters. Patients can self-catheterize into the continent urinary stoma every 4–6 hours to empty the urine reservoir (Fig. 14.2). This is achieved by the patient adjusting any restrictive clothing and inserting a special tube into the continent urinary stoma, pointing the other end into the toilet. When urine has drained out the tube is removed, washed with water and replaced in its container (usually a plastic bag, spectacle case or cosmetic bag).

Before each discharge, patients are given verbal and written advice (Horn 1990), and can contact the hospital 24 hours a day.

The Mitrofanoff pouch was devised in the late 1970s/early 1980s by Paul Mitrofanoff (1980) in France. Initially, it was devised for patients with bladder neck obstruction or incompetence. The bladder was preserved and the appendix was used as the continent urinary stoma. One end of the appendix is buried in a submuscular tunnel in the bladder, forming an obstructing flap valve. The other end is brought to the surface of the abdominal wall to form a continent stoma. As the bladder fills with urine more pressure is put on the valve, causing it to become even more obstructed. A catheter is passed into the stoma along the channel, through the valve and into the bladder when the patient wants to empty their bladder (Leaver 1996).

Mitrofanoff's principle can be adapted to suit each individual patient taking into account their underlying condition and the available body tissues (Duckett & Snyder 1985; Leaver 1994). For example, patients with urinary incontinence may have their bladder preserved and urethra oversewn; a tunnel may then be fashioned using their appendix. Other patients with bladder cancer following cystectomy may have a new 'bladder' constructed from a segment of ileum and, in the absence of an appendix, another segment of ileum may be used to construct the tunnel.

Rectal bladder

A type of rectal bladder, the ureterosigmoidostomy, is the oldest known continent urinary diversion (Fisch & Hohenfellner 1992). In this procedure the ureters are directly implanted into the sigmoid colon, where the urine and faeces mix and are evacuated via the anus. This procedure became unpopular because of continual complications of infection, electrolyte imbalance, loss of renal function, renal calculi, the high rate of incontinence, especially at night, and its poor reputation for morbidity and mortality (Leaver 2002).

Improved understanding of how some complications arise, development in surgical techniques and greater ability to manage electrolyte imbalances have all led to renewed interest in the rectal bladder (Woodhouse & Christofides 1998; Leaver 2002). High-pressure peristalsis in the bowel has been shown to cause the reflux of faeces into the kidneys (Coffey 1911). If the bowel is detubularized this high pressure can be overcome. To detubularize the rectum, it is opened longitudinally and closed transversely to form a pouch, which remains continuous with the sigmoid colon (Fig. 14.3a). The ureters are implanted into this pouch. This pouch is called the sigma-rectum pouch or Mainz Sigma II. This modified pouch acts as a reservoir for urine until the patient is ready to void. The patient can, in time, distinguish between needing to void urine and opening their bowels even though both events take place via the rectum (Leaver 2002).

Orthotopic neobladder

In this type of diversion the neobladder is constructed by using the ileum or a section of the large colon and then it is anastomosed to the urethra to allow voiding in the conventional way (Pontieri-Lewis & Vates 1993) (Fig. 14.3b). Therefore this procedure is only suitable for patients where the urethra is left intact. As a radical cystectomy for female patients typically involves a total urethrectomy, the orthotopic neobladder is more commonly indicated for men (Pontieri-Lewis & Vates 1993) although this procedure is beginning to be offered more frequently to women (Dixon *et al.* 2001).

The ability to pass urine naturally via the urethra and maintaining a normal anatomical appearance are the major advantages of this procedure. Patients need to use the Valsalva manoeuvre to empty the neobladder and some may find this difficult and may need to perform clean intermittent self-catheterization to achieve this. Pelvic floor exercises should be taught preoperatively and performed on a daily basis. Continence can be

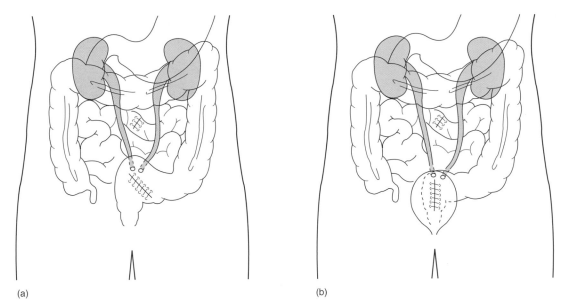

(a)   (b)

Figure 14.3 (a) Mainz Sigma II or rectal bladder. (b) Orthotopic neobladder.

problematic; most patients (83–96%) achieve continence during the day (Arai *et al.* 1999), but may experience night-time incontinence.

Patient selection

Patients are selected carefully for this type of surgery. They must be physically and psychologically able to undergo a lengthy major procedure. Patients need to have an adequate renal function and a healthy bowel, particularly if the bladder is to be replaced with a reservoir constructed from a segment of bowel (Horn 1990; Razor 1993; Leaver 1996).

It is important to ensure that patients undergoing the formation of a rectal bladder have good anal sphincter control. This can be established with the porridge test. A sloppy porridge enema is instilled into the patient's rectum and the patient needs to hold 300 ml for 3–4 hours without leaking. It is important that during this time the patient performs as many usual activities as possible, i.e. walking, climbing stairs, etc. The porridge imitates the contents of the rectum postoperatively (Leaver 1997).

Patients undergoing catheterizable continent diversions must be motivated towards self-catheterization and be dextrous enough to manipulate a nelaton catheter.

Specific preoperative preparation

Patients undergo the usual preparation for anaesthesia (see Ch. 30, Perioperative care). Only the specific preparation is discussed here although physical preparation may vary according to the individual surgeon's preference.

Preoperative counselling

Once patients have been selected as suitable candidates, psychological preparation should begin as soon as possible. Boore (1978), Hayward (1978), Zeimer (1983), Morris *et al.* (1989), Raleigh *et al.* (1990) and Roberts (1991) have illustrated the importance of preoperative information and explanation in reducing postoperative physical and psychological stress to the individual following the formation of a stoma (ileal conduit or colostomy). Their research is also applicable to patients receiving continent urinary diversion stomas. This is discussed in Ch. 15, Elimination: stoma care.

Patients should receive a full explanation of their operation and the type or types of urinary diversion which are available for them, including all the advantages and disadvantages of each diversion. The amount and type of information should be adapted to the individual's requirements. The stoma nurse or specialist is valuable in the preoperative stage. Many patients focus on the lack of appliance wearing in these types of surgery and are blind to the complications of the surgery itself (Leaver 2002). They should be shown pictures of the appropriate urinary diversion and encouraged to familiarize themselves with the equipment: pouches, wafers, catheterization tubes and bladder syringes.

Useful aids

Useful aids for teaching patients and helping them to understand the procedure and the implications it may have on their lives include the following:

- Information booklets
- Videos
- Diagrams/photographs
- Samples of equipment
- Contact with others who have the same type(s) of continent diversion, ideally of a similar age, sex and background to the patient.

Bowel preparation

Patients need to commence a regimen to evacuate all faecal matter from the intestine 2–3 days before surgery. Patients may be admitted for all of this preparation or they may start the regimen at home. The regimen used depends on the surgeon's preference. It is necessary to clear the bowel to:

- Prevent hard faecal masses from impacting proximal to an anastomosis
- Prevent faeces spilling from the cut ends of the bowel during the operation
- Reduce bacterial contamination when the bowel is opened (Alexander-Williams 1980).

Patients undergoing this procedure are at risk of developing hypovolaemia and electrolyte imbalance. Therefore, it is important that the fluid loss is replaced orally or intravenously (Skinner & Lieskovsky 1988; Woodhouse 1989).

Sexual dysfunction

Following the formation of a continent urinary diversion possible sexual impairment for both men and women may occur. This is the same as for other stoma patients and is discussed in Ch. 15, Elimination: stoma care.

Pre- and postoperative counselling is given to each patient and partner. Each person's potential sexual dysfunction should be discussed and treated individually.

Specific postoperative care

Reconstruction of the lower urinary tract is a lengthy procedure and has a significant complication rate (Leaver 1996). Patients may require a short stay in a high dependency unit after surgery. Postoperative care is similar to that for major abdominal surgery, with special attention to urinary output and the patency of the many drainage tubes (Fig. 14.4). Extensive experience has shown that to allow healing of the continent diversion and to reduce the risk of urine leaking into the peritoneum it is important that the reservoir is kept

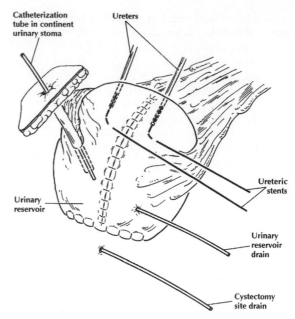

Figure 14.4 Siting of wound drains to reduce risk of haematoma and abscess formation.

empty for 4–8 weeks depending on the type of diversion that has been performed.

The drains and catheters used are unique to the type of diversion and determined by the surgeon's preference. They can often be overwhelming for the patient so each tube should be explained and an anticipated date for its removal should be given to reduce anxiety (Dixon *et al.* 2001). There will often be one or two fine-bore catheters placed in the ureters (ureteric stents) which will initially drain most of the urine. One or two catheters may be present in the new reservoir to keep it drained; these can become blocked with debris or mucus (which is produced by the bowel) so they should be flushed with sterile 0.9% sodium chloride twice daily starting from day 1 postoperatively. Initially only 20 ml should be used but this should increase to 100 ml on day 4 postoperatively.

Patients who have undergone a catheterizable continent diversion or orthotopic neobladder should be taught how to perform this procedure, as it will have to be maintained following their discharge home.

The ureteric stents, if present, are gently pulled on day 7 after the operation to remove them. If resistance is felt the stents should be left in and the procedure repeated on a daily basis, until the stents slide out. Generally the stents are totally removed by day 10. By this time wound drains, the nasogastric tube or gastrostomy tube and all intravenous catheters should also have been removed. After this time the patient may have a cystogram or 'pouchogram' performed to check that the reservoir is intact. If there are no leaks detected on this examination the pouch catheter is removed. Patients with a catheterizable continent diversion or neobladder are left with one catheter, which is on free drainage. They are discharged home for 4–6 weeks with this catheter in place on free drainage and with instructions to carry out at least twice daily washouts. This is to ensure that the urine drains and the reservoirs are not stretched at any time. Some patients prefer to be discharged with both the stoma catheter and pouch catheter in place, although only one is usually on free drainage.

Patients with a rectal bladder will now start voiding via the anus. The new bladder will start to stretch and its volume capacity will increase. Voiding will eventually be every 2–4 hours, often emptying once at night (Leaver 2002).

Patient education before discharge

All patients who have undergone continent urinary diversion have similar discharge needs. They are taught how to recognize a urinary tract infection and advised to drink at least 2–3 litres of fluid daily to reduce the risk of this happening. All patients undergoing continent diversion are advised to wear a medical alert bracelet, so that if they are found unconscious at any time a doctor or nurse will be aware of the surgery that has been performed.

Patients with an orthotopic neobladder are advised to undertake pelvic floor muscle exercises 4–6 times a day to promote continence (Razor 1993).

Patients who have a diversion with a catheterizable stoma are taught how to flush their catheters and wash out their reservoirs to prevent blockages and mucus build-up. These patients are then readmitted in 3–4 weeks to have their catheters removed and reservoirs activated and to be taught self-catheterization.

Patients should be seen by the nurse specialist before discharge and a request for community nurses to continue support at home should be made. An explanatory letter and the relevant literature are supplied. Patients are encouraged to seek advice from the ward staff at any time.

Second admission

Patients with catheterizable stomas are readmitted 6 weeks after the operation to expand the pouch and to be taught intermittent self-catheterization. The stoma catheter is clamped and patients are encouraged to drink fluids. This allows the pouch to fill up with urine and helps the patient establish what sensation is experienced as this happens. Patients have described this sensation as a feeling of fullness, bloated feeling, discomfort or an ache. However, some patients experience no sensations at all when the pouch is full and have to establish a voiding programme to avoid overfilling of the pouch. The stoma catheter is released after 2–3 hours, depending on how the patient tolerates the sensation and on the amount of fluid drunk. This process is repeated 1–2 times more, during the day, to continue expanding the pouch. Experience has shown that at this stage the average pouch capacity is 250–300 ml. The pouches are generally constructed to hold 500 ml and it may take several weeks to reach this target. Patients continue to expand their pouch at their own pace once they are discharged.

Once the pouch has been initially stretched, the catheter is removed and the catheterization procedure is explained and demonstrated. See 'Teaching intermittent self-catheterization', below. Patients should be supervised during the catheterization process until they are competent and confident with the procedure. Generally, patients remain in hospital for 1–2 days.

Discharge advice

Once proficient with the new continent diversion patients are discharged home with a 2–4 week outpatient clinic appointment to see the surgeon and nurse specialist. Before patients are discharged they should be informed about the following:

- To empty pouch every 4–6 hours to prevent overdistension and to always empty pouch before participating in strenuous activities to minimize the pressure put on the pouch. If the pouch becomes too full there is a risk of trauma to, or rupture of, the pouch, leakage of urine via the tunnel or, because of increased pressure on the valve, it may make catheterization difficult or impossible (Leaver 1997).
- To ensure an undisturbed sleep by reducing the amount of fluid the patient drinks 3 hours before going to sleep. The patient should catheterize or void before going to sleep and on waking.
- To keep a catheter available at all times (in suit, car, handbag, at work and at home), in case the patient needs to empty the urine.
- A small amount of mucus may leak from the continent urinary stoma and a piece of gauze can be worn to protect clothing.

Patients should be informed that it could take time to become accustomed to and gain confidence in their new continent urinary diversion. They should be given contact details of appropriate nursing staff who may be called for advice and reassurance.

Long- and short-term problems

A number of complications have been identified; these may be short-term 'teething' problems while the pouch settles down and the patient becomes familiar with it. However, some patients require further surgery or treatment to rectify problems to ensure their pouch function is acceptable. The most common complications are:

* Infection
* Stenosis of the stoma
* Leakage via the stoma
* Inability to empty pouch
* Loss of tunnel
* High-pressure bladder system
* Stone formation
* Metabolic acidosis
* Renal damage
* Pouch rupture
* Incontinence
* Skin irritation with Mainz II if anal sphincter leaks
* Secondary malignancy following Mainz II due to the high risk posed by the mixture of urine and faeces in the bowel. Neoplasms usually are seen 20–30 years after surgery (Stewart 1986). Yearly endoscopic follow-up should be carried out from the 12th post-operative year in order to detect any tumours early (Woodhouse & Christofides 1998; Wagstaff et al. 1991; McCahill et al. 1992; Woodhouse 1994). As the formation of a continent urinary diversion is a relatively new surgical technique the long-term complications (other than those listed above) are unknown. Therefore patients remain on long-term follow-up at those centres where these procedures are performed.

Psychological effects

Several surveys have been undertaken to compare ileal conduits with Mitrofanoff/Kock's continent urinary diversions in terms of social and sexual effects, and to assess the effect on the patient of converting an ileal conduit to a continent urinary diversion (Boyd et al. 1987; Mansson et al. 1988, 1991; Oishi et al. 1993). Each examined the effect of cystectomy and investigated issues such as depression, adjustment to the new skills required for self-catheterization or use of stoma appliances, and changes in social, sports and sexual activity. The evidence suggests that patients are able to learn the manual skills required of them, but that all experience some degree of depression and altered body image. Patients with ileal conduits reported a more negative body image and a higher incidence of depression compared with the other two groups. Patients with a primary continent urinary diversion also exhibited depression and altered body image. Patients whose ileal conduit was converted to a continent urinary diversion experienced less depression and fewer negative changes in body image. It is conjectured that this is because these patients perceive a definite improvement in their situation when the conversion is carried out (Boyd et al. 1987; Mansson et al. 1988, 1991; Oishi et al. 1993).

These studies did not investigate altered body image or psychological morbidity in patients whose ileal conduits or continent urinary diversions were performed for non-malignant disease. Kennedy et al. (1993), however, describe the experiences of four women who had successful pregnancies following continent urinary diversions for non-malignant disease.

The importance of the role of stoma therapists and nursing staff in providing information tailored for the individual and in teaching new skills is recognized by patients, and it is suggested that these functions play a part in adjustment to changes brought about by surgery (Boyd et al. 1987; Mansson et al. 1988, 1991; Oishi et al. 1993).

Teaching intermittent self-catheterization of a continent urinary diversion stoma

Definition

Intermittent self-catheterization is when patients insert a self-catheterization catheter into the urinary reservoir via the continent urinary stoma using a clean technique. It is performed to evacuate or instil fluids, after which the tube is removed.

Indications

Intermittent self-catheterization may be carried out for the following reasons:

* To empty the contents of the urinary reservoir every 4–6 hours. If the reservoir is left too long between emptying it can become overstretched and lose its elasticity.
* To allow irrigation of the urinary reservoir for the removal of mucus which may occlude the continent urinary stoma.

Reference material

The following research has been gathered from urethral self-catheterization. However, the same principles would apply to a continent urinary stoma.

Intermittent self-catheterization is intended to make life easier and not more complicated. It is associated with a lower incidence of urinary tract infection than long-term indwelling catheters (Lapides 1971; Lapides *et al.* 1974; Diokno *et al.* 1983; Lindenhall *et al.* 1994).

Types of tubing used for intermittent self-catheterization

Catheters used for intermittent self-catheterization should be smooth surfaced and flexible. The nelaton-type of catheter, which is made of soft plastic and has two drainage eyes at one end and a funnel at the other, is most commonly used for patients with continent diversions. The smallest size of catheter which will drain the reservoir at an acceptable speed should be used (Busuttil-Leaver 1997). If the continent stoma and tunnel has been constructed from a fine tube-like structure, such as a ureter or fallopian tube, a small gauge catheter (6–10 ch) may be needed. Fine-bore feeding tubes have been used

in some instances (Horn 1990; see Ch. 16 Elimination: urinary catheterization).

Teaching self-catheterization

Intermittent self-catheterization should be taught in a place that offers privacy, with a good clear light and a mirror (bathroom, toilet or at the patient's bedside) (Horn 1990). It is a clean and not a sterile procedure. Patients can learn self-catheterization with the aid of a mirror or by touch, and are observed and assisted by a nurse until they are proficient (see Procedure guidelines: Self-catheterization, below).

During the day patients are encouraged to drink 2–3 litres of fluid to reduce the risk of any urinary tract infection and to catheterize every 4–6 hours to prevent the reservoir becoming distended and losing its elasticity. However, patients can reduce their fluid intake during the evening so that they need catheterize only before they go to sleep and again when they get up in the morning.

Procedure guidelines: **Self-catheterization of a continent urinary diversion stoma**

Equipment

1 Catheters for catheterization depending upon the size of the stoma.
2 Tissues.
3 Clean jug or bowl.
4 Low-linting gauze and non-allergenic skin protective tape to cover stoma if it oozes mucus.

Procedure

Action	Rationale
1 Explain and discuss the procedure with the patient.	To ensure that the patient understands the procedure and gives his/her valid consent.
2 Collect all equipment necessary for the procedure.	To ensure all the equipment required is easily available.
3 Take the equipment to the toilet, bathroom or screened bed area. Ensure there is a good light and a full-length mirror.	To ensure the patient's privacy. To ensure the patient can see the stoma clearly.
4 The equipment should be arranged on a clean surface and within easy reach for the procedure.	To reduce the risk of contamination by surface bacteria. So that equipment is easily available.
5 The patient needs to remove any inhibiting clothing.	To ensure the patient can examine the stoma.
6 The patient should wash their hands with soap and water, then dry them.	To ensure the hands are clean.
7 The patient should look at the stoma, if necessary with the aid of a hand or full-length mirror.	To look for mucus and swelling around the stoma.
8 The patient should wipe away any mucus with a tissue soaked in warm water and gently pat dry.	To ensure the opening of the stoma is clear and mucus does not block the catheter during insertion into stoma.
9 If catheter is self-lubricating, open catheter container and fill with tap water. If it is not, lubricate tip of catheter with water-soluble lubricant.	To act as a lubricant to allow the tube to enter the urinary reservoir without causing internal trauma.
10 Ensure the untipped end of the tube is in a receiver, i.e. jug, bowl or toilet.	To ensure the urine goes into a bowl and not onto the patient.

no fear of leakage or odour and the appliance should be comfortable, unobtrusive, easy to handle and disposable. The ostomate should be allowed a choice from the management systems available. It is also important to identify and manage problems with the stoma or peristomal skin early. When choosing the appropriate management system for the new ostomate, factors which need to be considered include:

- Type of stoma
- Type of effluent
- Patient's mental capacity
- Manual dexterity
- Lifestyle
- Condition of peristomal skin
- Siting of stoma
- Patient preference (Black 2000a).

Management systems available: pouches, plugs and irrigation

Pouches

Although some people whose stomas were created several years ago are wearing non-disposable rubber bags, most appliances used today are made from an odour-proof plastic film. These pouches adhere to the body by a hydrocolloid wafer or flange (Taylor 2000). Pouches may be opaque or clear and often have a soft backing to absorb perspiration. They usually have a built-in integral filter containing charcoal to neutralize any odour.

Choosing the right size

It is important that the flange of the appliance fits snugly around the stoma within 0.5 cm of the stoma edge. This narrow edge is left exposed so that the appliance does not rub on the stoma. Ileostomies may need a closer fit to protect the peristomal skin from exposure to enzymes in the effluent. Stoma appliances usually come with measuring guides to allow for choice of size. During the first weeks the oedematous stoma will reduce in size and the appliances will have to be changed accordingly.

Fear of malodour

Pouches usually have a built-in integral filter containing charcoal to neutralize any odour when flatus is released. There are also various deodorizers available. The individual should be reassured that any problems with odour or leakage will be investigated and that in most circumstances the problem will be solved with alternative appliances or accessories (Bryant 1993; Black 1997).

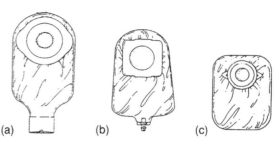

Figure 15.6 Stoma equipment. (a) Drainable bowel stoma pouch; (b) urostomy pouch; (c) closed bag.

Types of pouch

The type of pouch used will depend on the type of stoma and effluent expected.

Closed pouches are mainly used when formed stool is expected, e.g. sigmoid colostomy (Fig. 15.6c). These pouches have a flatus filter and need to be changed once or twice a day.

Drainable pouches are used when the effluent is fluid or semi-formed, i.e. ileostomy or transverse colostomy (Fig. 15.6a). These pouches have specially designed filters, which are less likely to become blocked or leak faecal fluid. These pouches need to be emptied regularly and the outlet rinsed carefully and then closed with a clip or 'roll-up' method. They may be left on for up to 3 days.

Urostomy pouches have a drainage tap for urine and should be emptied regularly (Fig. 15.6b). They can be attached to a large bag and tubing for night drainage. These pouches can remain on for up to 3 days.

One- or two-piece systems

All types of pouch (closed, drainable or with a tap) as described above fall into one of two broad categories: one-piece or two-piece systems.

- One-piece. This comprises a pouch attached to an adhesive wafer that is removed completely when the pouch is changed. This is an easy system for an ostomate with arthritis to handle.
- Two-piece. This comprises a wafer onto which a pouch is clipped. It can be used with sore and sensitive skin because when the pouches are removed the flange is left intact and so the skin is left undisturbed. The patient must, however, have dexterity to clip the bag securely on to the flange (Willis 1995; Heenan 1996).

Plug system

Patients with colostomies may be able to stop the effluent by inserting a plug into the stoma lumen. This plug swells in the moist environment and behaves as a seal. This system should only be introduced by a stoma nurse specialist (Taylor 2000).

Accessories

The specific products in this section have been mentioned as examples of what aids are available and reference to them is not necessarily intended as a recommendation.

Solutions for skin and stoma cleaning

Mild soap and water, or water only, are sufficient for skin and stoma cleaning. It is important that all soap residues are removed as they may interfere with pouch adhesion. Detergents, disinfectants and antiseptics cause dryness and irritation and should not be used. The stoma is not a wound or a lesion and should be regarded as a resited urethra or anus.

Skin barriers

1 Creams.

Unless made specifically for use on peristomal skin, creams should not be used, as the residual surface film of grease prevents adherence of the appliance. Creams usually have a soothing and moisturizing effect.

Use: for sensitive skin, as a protective measure.

Method: use sparingly; massage gently into the skin until completely absorbed; excess grease may be wiped off with a soft tissue.

Example: Chiron barrier cream (aluminium chlorohydrate 2% in an emulsified base) (*ABPI Compendium* 1999–2000).

Precaution: not to be used on broken or sore skin.

2 Skin gels/sealants.

Use: act as a film on the skin, first to prevent irritation and, second, to give protection as it is removed with the adhesive of the bag, thus preventing removal of the stratum corneum of the skin.

Method: pat onto the skin gently; dries quickly.

Examples: Skin Gel, Skin Prep.

Precaution: should not be used on broken skin as they contain alcohol and cause stinging (*ABPI Compendium* 1999–2000).

3 Protective wafers.

Use: these are hypoallergenic and are designed to cover and protect skin, and allow healing if the skin is sore or broken. May be useful in cases of skin reaction or allergy to the adhesive or an appliance.

Method: the wafers may be cut with the aid of a template (pattern) to the required shape and fitted on to the skin. The appliances are then attached to the wafer. The rim of the wafer should not press against the stoma but should fit to 0.5 cm around it.

Examples: Stomahesive or Comfeel type of wafers. Stomahesive is composed of gelatin, pectin, sodium carboxymethycellulose and polyisobutylene (Martindale 1993); it adheres painlessly to normal, erythematous, moist or broken skin; it is available in three sizes.

Precautions: allergy may occur, but rarely.

4 Protective rings.

Use: protective rings are used to provide skin protection around the stoma; they will protect a smaller area than the wafers mentioned above. They are also useful to fill in 'dips' or 'gulleys' in the skin.

Method: like the wafers, they have an adhesive side and may be applied directly to the skin. They form an integral part of some of the appliances.

Example: Salts Cohesive seals.

Precautions: as for protective wafers above.

5 Pastes.

Use: useful to fill in crevices and 'gulleys' in the skin to provide a smooth surface for an appliance.

Method: Stomahesive – a syringe may be used to apply paste. Either leave for 60 seconds after applying to the skin, when the surface will be dry, making the paste easier to mould into the skin contour, or apply with a spatula, or wet the finger first to prevent the paste sticking and mould the paste immediately. Will sting on raw areas as it contains alcohol. Apply a little Orahesive powder to these areas first.

Examples: Stomahesive paste, Soft paste.

6 Protective paste

Use: to protect raw areas. Does not contain alcohol so will not cause irritation (useful for fistula problems).

Method: Orabase, similar to Stomahesive paste in composition but with the addition of liquid paraffin. Liquid paraffin will inhibit adhesives sticking so care must be taken to ensure Orabase paste is not applied under appliances.

Examples: Orabase paste.

7 Powders.

Use: for protection of sore or raw areas without impeding adhesion of the appliance.

Method: sprinkle on affected areas.

Example: Orahesive powder.

Adhesive preparations

1 Lotions.

Use: only required when appliance does not adhere well to the skin, e.g. because of leakage, uneven site, or if abdominal fistulae present.

Method: the individual products differ considerably in their method of application and it is recommended that the user consults the manufacturer's instructions.

Example: Saltair solution.

Convex devices

Use: these devices are designed to be used with retracted stomas. The convex shape allows a greater seal round the stoma by filling in any crevices caused by retraction, scars or skin creases.

Method: convexity may be achieved by fitting specially designed plastic inserts into the baseplate of a two piece appliance or by using appliances with built in convexity.

Examples: Convex inserts, Impression range of appliances.

Deodorants

1 Aerosols.

Use: to absorb odour.

Method: one or two puffs into the air before emptying or removal of appliance.

Examples: Atmacol, Limone, Naturcare.

2 Drops and powders.

Use: for deodorizing bag contents.

Method: before fitting pouch or after emptying and cleaning drainable pouch, squeeze tube two or three times.

Examples: Ostobon deodorant powder, Chironair odour control liquid.

3 Flatus filters (charcoal filled) usually incorporated into the bag.

Use: to allow gradual release of flatus from the bag while allowing absorption of odour by the charcoal. The charcoal may only be effective for between 6 and 12 hours, depending on brand of filter.

Procedure guidelines: **Stoma care**

These procedural guidelines contain the basic information needed for changing a stoma appliance. Modifications may be made according to the following factors:

1 The place of change, i.e. bathroom, bedside, availability of sink, etc.
2 The person changing the appliance, i.e. nurse, patient or carer.
3 Type of appliance used, e.g. one- or two-piece, closed or drainable.
4 Any accessories used, e.g. flatus filters, hypoallergenic tape, barrier creams.

Equipment

1 Clean tray holding:
   (a) Tissues
   (b) New appliances
   (c) Disposal bags for used appliances and tissues
   (d) Relevant accessories, e.g. flatus filters, tape.
2 Bowl of warm water.
3 Soap (if desired).
4 Jug for contents of appliance.
5 Gloves. (It is now common practice and, in many cases, hospital policy, to wear gloves when dealing with blood and body fluids due to risk of infections. Thus they should be worn for cleaning stomas. It is recognized that it could be difficult to attach an appliance with gloves in situ (due to adhesive), but once the stoma has been cleaned of excreta and blood, gloves may be removed to apply bag.) This practice should be explained to patients so that they do not feel it is just because they have a stoma that gloves are worn.

Procedure

Action	Rationale
1 Explain and discuss the procedure with the patient.	To ensure that the patient understands the procedure and gives his/her valid consent.
2 Explain the procedure.	To familiarize the patient with the procedure.
3 Ensure that the patient is in a suitable and comfortable position where the patient will be able to watch the procedure, if well enough. A mirror may be used to aid visualization.	To allow good access to the stoma for cleaning and for secure application of the stoma bag. The patient will become familiar with the stoma and will also learn much about the care of the stoma by observation of the nurse (Bryant 1993).
4 Use a small protective pad to protect the patient's clothing from drips if the effluent is fluid and apply gloves for nurse's protection.	Avoids the necessity for renewing clothing or bedclothes and demoralization of the patient as a result of soiling.
5 If the bag is of the drainable type, empty the contents into a jug before removing the bag.	For ease of handling the appliance and prevention of spillage.

*Procedure guidelines: **Stoma care** (cont'd)*

Action	Rationale
6 Remove the appliance. Peel the adhesive off the skin with one hand while exerting gentle pressure on the skin with the other.	To reduce trauma to the skin. Erythema as a result of removing the appliance is normal and quickly settles (Broadwell 1987).
7 Remove excess faeces or mucus from the stoma with a damp tissue.	So that the stoma and surrounding skin are clearly visible.
8 Examine the skin and stoma for soreness, ulceration or other unusual phenomena. If the skin is unblemished and the stoma is a healthy red colour, proceed.	For the prevention of complications or the treatment of existing problems.
9 Wash the skin and stoma gently until they are clean.	To promote cleanliness and prevent skin excoriation.
10 Dry the skin and stoma gently but thoroughly.	The appliance will attach more securely to dry skin.
11 Apply a clean appliance.	
12 Dispose of soiled tissues and the used bag. Rinse the bag through in the sluice with water, wrap it in a disposable bag and place it in an appropriate plastic bin. At home the bag should be emptied into the toilet; a closed bag may be cut at the lower end using scissors especially reserved for this purpose, then rinsed using a jug or by holding it under the flushing water. Wrap the bag in newspaper, tie it in a plastic bag and dispose of it in a rubbish bag.	Faecal material in waste bags is a potential source of infection. Excreta should be disposed of down the sluice or toilet.
13 Wash hands thoroughly using bactericidal soap and water or bactericidal alcohol handrub.	To prevent spread of infection by contaminated hands.

Procedure guidelines: **Collection of a specimen of urine from an ileal conduit or urostomy**

Equipment

1 Sterile dressing pack.
2 Soft catheter – Nelaton type, not larger than 12 or 14 Fr.
3 Disposable plastic apron.
4 Universal specimen container.
5 Skin cleaning solution.
6 Bactericidal alcohol handrub.
7 Clean stoma appliance.

Procedure

Action	Rationale
1 Explain and discuss the procedure with the patient.	To ensure that the patient understands the procedure and gives his/her valid consent.
2 Ensure that the patient is in a comfortable position, e.g. sitting up, supported by pillows, and that the stoma is easily accessible.	For patient comfort and to allow access to the stoma.
3 Screen the bed, then wash hands using bactericidal soap and water or bactericidal alcohol handrub and dry them.	For the patient's privacy and to reduce the risk of cross-infection (see Ch. 4, Aseptic technique). Curtains are drawn at this stage so that dust and airborne organisms disturbed by the curtains do not settle on the sterile trolley.
4 Prepare the trolley and take it to the patient's bedside.	To ensure equipment is easily available.
5 Put on a disposable plastic apron.	To reduce risk of cross-infection.
6 Remove the sterile dressing pack, catheter and receiver from their outer wrappings. Place them on the top shelf of the trolley.	To prepare equipment.
7 Remove the appliance from the stoma and cover the stoma with a clean topical swab.	To absorb any spillage from the stoma.

Procedure guidelines: Collection of a specimen of urine from an ileal conduit or urostomy (cont'd)

Action	Rationale
8 Clean hands with a bactericidal alcohol handrub, and put on clean disposable gloves before opening the sterile field on the trolley.	To reduce the risk of introducing infection into the stoma during the procedure.
9 Remove the non-linting gauze with forceps, check and discard it. Arrange a towel to absorb spillage from the stoma.	To keep the areas as clean as possible and to protect the patient and the bedclothes from spilled urine.
10 Clean around the stoma with water or saline, from the centre outwards.	Good cleaning of the area reduces the risk of introduction of surface pathogens into the ileal loop.
11 Apply gentle skin traction to allow stomal opening to be more visible. Insert the catheter tip gently to a depth of 2.5–5 cm only and wait for urine to drain through. Collect the sample in the specimen container. The recommended volume is 3–5 ml.	To avoid catheter coming into contact with external surfaces of stoma. Gentle handling reduces the risk of ileal perforation and is more comfortable for the patient. To ensure adequate sample of urine for bacteriological assessment.
12 Remove the catheter and seal in the specimen container. Remove gloves and attend to stoma care and apply a pouch as usual. Make the patient comfortable.	To prevent spillage of sample. To ensure patient comfort.
13 Dispose of equipment.	
14 Wash hands with bactericidal soap and water and dry.	To reduce risk of cross-infection.
15 Check that the specimen is labelled correctly and dispatch it to the laboratory with the appropriate forms.	

Procedure guidelines: **Removal of stoma bridge or rod**

Equipment

1 Clean tray holding:
  (a) Tissues
  (b) New appliances
  (c) Disposal bags for used appliances and tissues
  (d) Relevant accessories, e.g. belt.

2 Bowl of warm water.
3 Soap if desired.
4 Jug for contents of appliance.
5 Gloves.

Procedure

Action	Rationale
1 Explain and discuss the procedure with the patient.	To ensure that the patient understands the procedure and gives his/her valid consent.
2 Ensure the patient is in a suitable and comfortable position.	To allow good access to the stoma for cleaning and for secure application of stoma bag.
3 Apply gloves.	To reduce risk of cross-infection.
4 If the bag is of the drainable type, empty the contents into a jug before removing the bag.	For ease of handling the appliance and prevention of spillage.
5 Remove the appliance. Peel the adhesive off the skin with one hand while exerting gentle pressure on the skin with the other.	To reduce trauma to the skin. Erythema as a result of removing the appliance is normal and quickly settles (Broadwell 1987).
6 Remove excess faeces or mucus from the stoma with a damp tissue.	So that the stoma and surrounding skin are clearly visible.
7 (a) Slide the bridge gently to one side to ensure the mobile wing of the bridge is away from the stoma. Turn this wing so that it becomes flush with the bridge. Gently slide the bridge through the stoma loop (see Fig. 15.7).	To prepare bridge for removal.

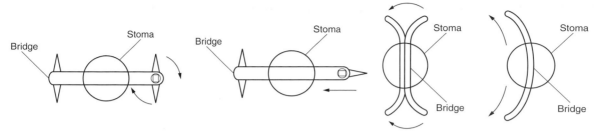

Figure 15.7 Removal of stoma bridge or rod.

Procedure guidelines: ***Removal of stoma bridge or rod*** *(cont'd)*

Action	Rationale
(b) Fold the bridge in half so that the bridge appears in a 'C' shape. Gently slide the bridge through the stomal loop (see Fig. 15.7).	
8 Examine the skin and stoma for soreness, ulceration or other unusual phenomena. If the skin is unblemished and the stoma is a healthy red colour, proceed. If the skin is red and/or broken, treat as outlined in Problem solving, below. If the stoma is not a healthy red colour inform medical and/or stoma care nurse.	For the prevention of complications or the treatment of existing problems (see Problem solving)
9 Wash the skin and stoma gently until they are clean.	To promote cleanliness and prevent skin excoriation.
10 Dry the skin and stoma gently but thoroughly.	The appliance will attach more securely to dry skin.
11 Apply a clean appliance.	To contain effluent from the stoma.
12 Dispose of soiled tissues, the bridge and the used bag.	To prevent environmental contamination.
13 Wash hands with bactericidal soap and water or bactericidal alcohol handrub.	To reduce risk of cross-infection.

Problem solving

Stoma

Problem	Cause	Suggested action
Leakage of urine or faeces.	Ill-fitting appliance.	Remeasure stoma and ensure a snug-fitting appliance. Prepare template for future use.
	Skin creases or 'gulleys' preventing correct application of adhesive.	Build up indented areas and fill in gulleys to create a smooth surface, e.g. using paste.
	Infrequent emptying of drainable bag leading to stress on adhesion.	Drainable bags should be emptied frequently, e.g. 2–3-hourly if necessary.
Sore skin.	Leakage.	As above.
	Skin reaction to adhesive.	Change to an appliance from another manufacturer or apply a protective square between skin and adhesive. Anti-inflammatory agents may be required for very severe reactions.
	Poor hygiene.	Improve the technique of nurses, patient or carers.
Odour.	Ill-fitting appliance; lack of seal between skin and adhesive.	Fit the appliance with care. Consider a change of the type of appliance.
	Poor hygiene.	Improve the technique of nurses, patient or carers.
	Poor technique, e.g. when emptying drainable bag.	Empty the bag, then rinse the end with water to ensure that it is clean before closing.

Problem solving (cont'd)

Urostomy specimen

Problem	Cause	Suggested action
Stoma specimen of urine contaminated.	Contaminants introduced during specimen collection.	Take a repeat specimen, observing aseptic procedure and cleaning the stoma well.
Ileum perforated during specimen collection.	Catheter too hard or inserted too roughly.	Report to a doctor immediately.
Difficulty passing catheter into conduit.	Small degree of retraction of ileum.	Apply gentle pressure to the area around the stoma to make it protrude.
	Unpredictable direction of ileum.	Gently insert your little (gloved) finger into the stoma to determine the direction of the conduit. Insert the catheter tip along this line.

Useful addresses

1 Association for Spina Bifida and Hydrocephalus (ASBAH), 42 Park Road, Peterborough PE1 2UQ (Tel: 01733 555988)

2 British Colostomy Association, 13–15 Station Road, Reading, Berkshire RG1 1LG (Tel: 0118 9391537 or 0800 3284257)

3 IA (Ileostomy and Internal Pouch Support Group), PO Box 132, Scunthorpe, DN15 9YW (Tel: 01724 720150 or 0800 0184724)

4 Urostomy Association, 'Buckland', Beaumont Park, Danbury, Essex CM3 4DE (Tel: 0124 5224294)

References and further reading

ABPI Compendium of Data Sheets and Summaries of Product Characteristics 1999–2000. Datapharm Publications, London.

Ashford, L. (1998) Erectile dysfunction. *Prof Nurse*, **13**(9), 603–608.

Bass, E.M., Del Pino, A., Tan, A., Pearl, R.K., Orsay, C.P. & Abcarian, H. (1997) Does preoperative stoma marking and education by the enterostomal therapist affect outcome? *Dis Colon Rectum*, **40**(4), 440–2.

Beddows, J. (1997) Alleviating pre-operative anxiety in patients: a study. *Nurs Stand*, **11**(37), 35–8.

Black, P. (2000a) Practical stoma care. *Nurs Stand*, **14**(41), 47–55.

Black, P. (2000b) *Holistic Stoma Care*. Baillière Tindall, London.

Black, P.K. (1994a) Stoma care: a practical approach. *Nurs Stand*, **8**(34), *RCN Nurs Update*, Learning Unit 045.

Black, P.K. (1994b) Choosing the correct stoma appliance. *Br J Nurs*, **3**(11), 545–6, 548, 550.

Black, P.K. (1997) Practical stoma care. *Nurs Stand*, **11**(47), 49–55.

Black, P.K. (1998) Update. Colostomy. *Prof Nurse*, **13**(12), 851–7.

Blackley, P. (1998) *Practical Stoma, Wound and Continence Management*. Research Publications, Australia.

Boore, J.R.P. (1978) *A Prescription for Recovery: The Effect of Preoperative Preparation of Surgical Patients on Postoperative Stress, Recovery and Infection*. RCN, London.

Borwell, B. (1994) Colostomies and their management. *Nurs Stand*, **8**(45), CE article 332.

Borwell, B. (1997a) Ileo-anal pouch surgery and its after-care. *Commun Nurse*, August.

Borwell, B. (1997b) The psychosexual needs of a stoma patient. *Prof Nurse*, **12**(4), 250–55.

Borwell, B. (1997c) Psychological considerations of stoma care nursing. *Nurs Stand*, **11**(48), 49–55.

Borwell, B. (1999) Sexuality and stoma care. In: *Stoma Care in the Community* (ed. P. Taylor). Nursing Times Books, London.

Bridgewater, S.E. (1999) Dietary considerations. In: *Stoma Care in the Community. A Clinical Resource for Practitioners* (ed. P. Taylor). Nursing Times Books, London, pp. 187–202.

Broadwell, D.C. (1987) Peristomal skin integrity. *Nurs Clin North Am*, **22**(2), 321–32.

Bryant, R.A. (1993) Ostomy patient management: care that engenders adaptation. *Cancer Invest*, **11**(5), 565–77.

Cottam, J. (1999) Recovering after stoma surgery (Know How series). *Commun Nurse*, **5**(9), 24–5.

Crooks, S. (1994) Foresight that leads to improved outcome: stoma care nurses' role in siting stomas. *Prof Nurse*, **10**(2), 89–92.

Davis, K. (1996) Irrigation technique. In: *Stoma Care Nursing – A Patient-Centred Approach* (ed. C. Myers). Arnold, London.

Gelister, J.F. & Woodhouse, C.R. (1991) Role of continent suprapubic diversion in pelvic cancer. *Br J Urol*, **68**, 376–9.

Hayward, J. (1978) *Information – A Prescription Against Pain*. RCN, London.

Heath, H. & White, I. (2001) *The Challenge of Sexuality in Health Care*. Blackwell Science, London.

Heenan, A.L.J. (1996) Two piece stoma systems. *Prof Nurse*, **11**(5), 313–14.

Heywood Jones, I. (1994) Skills update. Stoma care. *Commun Outlook*, December.

Horn, S. (1991) Nursing patients with a continent urinary diversion. *Nurs Stand*, **4**(21), 24–6.

Huish, M., Kumar, D. & Stones, C. (1998) Stoma surgery and sex problems in ostomates. *Sex Marital Ther*, **13**(3), 311–28.

Hulten, L. & Palselius, I. (1996) Are dietary restrictions necessary for ileostomy surgery? *Eurostoma*, **13**, 20.

Ivimy, A. (1997) Postoperative recovery is influenced by preoperative care. *Eurostoma*, **17**, 8–9.

Kelly, L. (1995) Patients becoming people. *J Community Nurs*, August, 12–16.

Kelly, M.P. & Henry, T. (1992) A thirst for practical knowledge: stoma patients' opinions of the services they receive. *Prof Nurse*, **7**(6), 350–6.

Kirby, R., Carson, C. & Goldstein, I. (1999) *Erectile Dysfunction: A Clinical Guide*. Isis Medical Media, Oxford.

Leaver, R. (1996) Continent urinary diversions: the Mitrafanoff principle. In: *Stoma Care Nursing – A Patient-Centred Approach* (ed. C. Myers). Arnold, London.

Martindale (1993) *The Extra Pharmacopoeia*, 13th edn (ed. J.E.F. Reynolds). Pharmaceutical Press, London.

Mowdy, S. (1998) The role of the WOC nurse in an ostomy support group. *J Wound Ostomy Continence Nurses*, **25**, 51–4.

Myers, C. (1996) *Stoma Care Nursing – A Patient-Centred Approach*. Arnold, London.

Newey, J. (1998) Causes and treatment of erectile dysfunction. *Nurs Stand*, **12**(47), 39–40.

Nicholls, R.J. & Williams, J. (1998) *Ulcerative Colitis*. Convatec, Uxbridge.

Ortiz, H. *et al.* (1993) Does the frequency of colostomy hernia depend on the colostomy location in the abdominal wall? *World Council Enterost Ther J*, **13**(2), 13–14.

Price, B. (1990) *Body Image Nursing: Concepts and Care*. Prentice Hall, New York.

Price, B. (1993) Profiling the high risk altered body image patient. *Sen Nurse*, **13**(4), 17–21.

Pullen, M. (1998) Support role. *Nurs Times*, **94**(47).

Rheaume, A. & Gooding, B.A. (1991) Social support, coping strategies, and long term adaptation to ostomy among self-help group members. *J Enterost Ther*, **18**, 11–15.

Salter, M. (1992) Body image: the person with a stoma, Part 1. *Wound Manage*, **2**(2), 8–9.

Salter, M. (1995) Guest editorial: some observations on body image. *World Council Enterost Ther*, **15**(3), 4–7.

Salter, M. (1996) Sexuality and the stoma patient. In: *Stoma Care Nursing – A Patient-Centred Approach* (ed. C. Myers). Arnold, London.

Salter, M. (1997) *Altered Body Image: The Nurse's Role*. Baillière Tindall, London.

Schover, L.R. (1986) Sexual rehabilitation of the ostomy patient. In: *Ostomy Care and the Cancer Patient* (eds D.B. Smith & D.E. Johnson). Grune & Stratton, Orlando.

Taylor, P. (2000) Choosing the right stoma appliance for a colostomy. *Nurse Prescrib Commun Nurse*, **6**(9), 35–8.

Topping, A. (1990) Sexual activity and the stoma patient. *Nurs Stand*, **4**(41), 24–6.

Wade, B. (1989) Nursing care of the stoma patient. *Surg Nurse*, **2**(5), Suppl, ix–xii.

Wells, D. (2000) *Caring for Sexuality in Health and Illness*. Churchill Livingstone, London.

Willis, J. (1995) Stoma care principles and product type. *Nurs Times*, **91**(2), 43–5.

Winkley, M. (1998) Pre-operative fasting. *Nurs Times*, **94**(40).

Wood, S. (1998) Nutrition and stoma patients. *Nurs Times*, **94**(48).

16

Elimination: urinary catheterization

Chapter contents

Definition

Urinary catheterization is the insertion of a special tube into the bladder, using aseptic technique, for the purpose of evacuating or instilling fluids.

Indications

Male

In the male, urinary catheterization may be carried out for the following reasons:

- To empty the contents of the bladder, e.g. before or after abdominal, pelvic or rectal surgery and before certain investigations
- To determine residual urine
- To allow irrigation of the bladder
- To bypass an obstruction
- To relieve retention of urine
- To introduce cytotoxic drugs in the treatment of papillary bladder carcinomas
- To enable bladder function tests to be performed
- To measure urinary output accurately, e.g. when a patient is in shock, undergoing bone marrow transplantation or receiving high-dose chemotherapy
- To relieve incontinence when no other means is practicable.

Female

In the female, urinary catheterization may be carried out for the nine reasons listed above and for two further reasons:

- To empty the bladder before childbirth, if thought necessary
- To avoid complications during intracavitary insertion of radioactive caesium.

Table 16.1 Types of catheter

Catheter type	Material	Uses
Balloon (Foley) two-way catheter: two channels, one for urine drainage; second, smaller channel for balloon inflation	Latex, PTFE coated latex, silicone elastomer coated, 100% silicone, hydrogel coated	Most commonly used for patients who require bladder drainage (short-, medium- or long-term)
Balloon (Foley) three-way irrigation catheter: three channels, one for urine; one for irrigation fluid; one for balloon inflation	Latex, PTFE coated latex, silicone, plastic	To provide continuous irrigation (e.g. after prostatectomy). Potential for infection is reduced by minimizing need to break the closed drainage system (Gilbert & Gobbi 1989; Mulhall *et al.* 1993)
Non-balloon (Nelaton) or Scotts, or intermittent catheter (one channel only)	PVC and other plastics	To empty bladder or continent urinary reservoir intermittently; to instil solutions into bladder

Reference material

Catheter selection

A wide range of urinary catheters are available, made from a variety of materials and with different design features. Careful assessment of the most appropriate material, size and balloon capacity will ensure that the catheter selected is as effective as possible, that complications are minimized and that patient comfort and quality of life are promoted (Pomfret 1996; Robinson 2001). Types of catheter are listed in Table 16.1, together with their suggested use. Catheters should be used in line with the manufacturer's recommendations, in order to avoid product liability (RCN 1994).

Balloon size

In the 1920s, Fredrick Foley designed a catheter with an inflatable balloon to keep it positioned inside the bladder. Balloon sizes vary from 2.5 ml for children to 30 ml. The latter is used to aid haemostasis after prostatic surgery. Large balloon catheters (30 ml) weigh approximately 48 g, causing pressure on the bladder neck and pelvic floor and potential damage to these structures (Kristiansen *et al.* 1983; Pomfret 2000; Robinson 2001). These catheters are associated with leakage of urine, pain and bladder spasm as they can cause irritation to the bladder mucosa and trigone (Stewart 1998; Robinson 2001). Large balloons are inclined to sit higher in the bladder, allowing a residual pool of urine to collect below the balloon, providing a reservoir for infection (Getliffe 1996; Pomfret 2000).

Consequently, a 5–10 ml balloon is recommended for adults, and a 3–5 ml balloon for children. Care should be taken to use the correct amount of water to fill the balloon because too much or too little may cause distortion of the catheter tip. This may result in irritation and trauma to the bladder wall consequently causing pain, spasm, bypassing and haematuria. If underinflated, one

or more of the drainage eyes may become occluded or the catheter may become dislodged. Overinflation risks rupturing the balloon and leaving fragments of balloon inside the bladder (Pomfret 2000; Robinson 2001).

Catheter balloons ought to be only filled with sterile water. Tap water and 0.9% sodium chloride should not be used as salt crystals and debris may block the inflation channel, causing difficulties with deflation. Any microorganisms which may be present in tap water can pass through the balloon into the bladder (Falkiner 1993; Stewart 1998).

Catheter size

Urethral catheters are measured in charrières (ch). The charrière is the outer circumference of the catheter in millimetres and is equivalent to three times the diameter. Thus a 12 ch catheter has a diameter of 4 mm.

Potential side-effects of large-gauge catheters include:

- Pain and discomfort
- Pressure ulcers, which may lead to stricture formation.
- Blockage of paraurethral ducts
- Abscess formation (Edwards *et al.* 1983; Crow *et al.* 1986; Roe & Brocklehurst 1987; Blandy & Moors 1989; Winn 1998).

The most important guiding principle is to choose the smallest size of catheter necessary to maintain adequate drainage (McGill 1982). If the urine to be drained is likely to be clear, a 12 ch catheter should be considered. Larger gauge catheters may be necessary if debris or clots are present in the urine (Pomfret 1996; Winn 1998).

Length of catheter

There are three lengths of catheter currently available:

- Female length: 23–26 cm
- Paediatric: 30 cm
- Standard length: 40–44 cm.

The shorter female length catheter is often more discreet and less likely to cause trauma or infections because movement in and out of the urethra is reduced. Infection may also be caused by the longer catheter looping or kinking (Pomfret 2000; Robinson 2001). In obese women or those in wheelchairs, however, the inflation valve of the shorter catheter may cause soreness by rubbing against the inside of the thigh, and the catheter is more likely to pull on the bladder neck; therefore, the standard length catheter should be used (Pomfret 2000; Godfrey & Evans 2000; Evans *et al.* 2001).

Tip design

Several different types of catheter tip are available in addition to the standard round tip. Each tip is designed to overcome a particular problem:

- The *Tieman-tipped catheter* has a curved tip with one to three drainage eyes to allow greater drainage. This catheter has been designed to negotiate the membranous and prostatic urethra in patients with prostatic hypertrophy.
- The *Whistle-tipped catheter* has a lateral eye in the tip and eyes above the balloon to provide a large drainage area. This design is intended to facilitate drainage of debris, e.g. blood clots.
- The *Roberts catheter* has an eye above and below the balloon to facilitate the drainage of residual urine.

Catheter material

A wide variety of materials are used to make catheters. The key criterion in selecting the appropriate material is the length of time the catheter is expected to remain in place. Three broad time scales have been identified:

- Short-term (1–14 days)
- Short- to medium-term (2–6 weeks)
- Medium- to long-term (6 weeks–3 months).

Patients should be assessed individually as to the ideal time to change their catheters. The use of a catheter diary will help to ascertain a pattern of catheter blockages so changes can be planned accordingly.

The principal catheter materials are as follows.

1 *Polyvinylchloride (PVC).* Catheters made from PVC or plastic are quite rigid. They have a wide lumen, which allows a rapid flow rate; however, their rigidity may cause some patients discomfort. They are mainly used for intermittent catheterization or postoperatively. They are recommended for short-term use only (Pomfret 1996).

2 *Latex.* Latex is a purified form of rubber and is the softest of the catheter materials. It has a smooth surface, with a tendency to allow crust formation. Latex absorbs water and consequently the catheter may swell, reducing the diameter of the internal lumen and increasing its external diameter (Pomfret 2000; Robinson 2001). It has been shown to cause urethral irritation (Wilksch *et al.* 1983) and therefore should only be considered when catheterization is likely to be short-term. Hypersensitivity to latex has been increasing in recent years (Woodward 1997) and latex catheters have been the cause of some cases of anaphylaxis (Young *et al.* 1994). Woodward (1997) suggests that patients should be asked whether they have ever had an adverse reaction to rubber products before catheters containing latex are utilized.

3 *Teflon (polytetrafluoroethylene; PTFE) or silicone elastomer coatings.* A Teflon or silicone elastomer coating is applied to a latex catheter to render the latex inert and reduce urethral irritation (Slade & Gillespie 1985). Teflon or silicone elastomer coated catheters are recommended for short- or medium-term catheterization.

4 *All silicone.* Silicone is an inert material which is less likely to cause urethral irritation. Silicone catheters are not coated, and therefore have a wider lumen. The lumen of these catheters, in cross-section, is crescent or D-shaped, which may induce formation of encrustation (Pomfret 1996). Because silicone permits gas diffusion, balloons may deflate and allow the catheter to fall out prematurely (Studer 1983; Barnes & Malone-Lee 1986). These catheters may be more uncomfortable as they are more rigid than the latex-cored types (Pomfret 2000). All silicone catheters are suitable for patients with latex allergies. Silicone catheters are recommended for long-term use.

5 *Hydrogel coatings.* These catheters are made of an inner core of latex encapsulated in a hydrophilic polymer coating have recently been developed. The polymer coating is well tolerated by the urethral mucosa, causing little irritation. Hydrogel coated catheters become smoother when rehydrated, reducing friction with the urethra. They are inert (Nacey & Delahunt 1991), and are reported to be resistant to bacterial colonization and encrustation (Roberts *et al.* 1990; Woollons 1996). Hydrogel coated catheters are recommended for long-term use.

6 The *conformable catheter* is designed to conform to the shape of the female urethra, and allows partial filling of the bladder. The natural movement of the urethra on the catheter, which is collapsible, is intended to prevent obstructions (Brocklehurst *et al.* 1988). They are made of latex and have a silicone elastomer coating. Conformable catheters are approximately 3 cm longer than conventional catheters for women.

Research into new types of catheter materials is ongoing, particularly examining materials that resist the formation of biofilms and reduce instances of urinary tract infections. Catheters coated with a silver alloy have been shown to prevent urinary tract infections (Saint *et al.* 1998). However, the studies which demonstrated this benefit were all small scale and a number of questions about the long-term effects of using such catheters, such as silver toxicity and argyria, need to be addressed. As these catheters are much more expensive a cost-effectiveness analysis should also be carried out before they are used more widely (Best Practice 2000; Centre for Reviews and Dissemination Reviewers 2002).

Anaesthetic lubricating gel

The use of anaesthetic lubricating gels is well recognized for male catheterization, but there is some controversy in their use for female catheterization. In males the gel is instilled directly into the urethra and then external massage is used to move the gel down its length. In female patients the anaesthetic lubricating gel or plain lubricating gel is applied to the tip of the catheter only, if it is used at all. It has been suggested that most of the lubricant is wiped off the catheter at the urethral introitus so therefore it fails to reach the urethral tissue (Muctar 1991).

These differences in practice imply that catheterization is a painful procedure for men but is not so for women. This assumption is not based on any empirical evidence or on any biological evidence. Other than the differences in length and route, the male and female urethra are very similar except for the presence of lubricating glands in the male urethra (Tortora & Grabowski 2002). The absence of these lubricating glands in the female urethra suggests that there is perhaps a greater need for the introduction of a lubricant. Women have complained of pain and discomfort during catheterization procedures (Mackenzie & Webb 1995), suggesting that the use of anaesthetic lubricating gels must be reconsidered. Trauma can occur during catheterization, which in turn can increase the risk of infection. Using sterile lubrication gels can reduce these risks (Pratt *et al.* 2001). Since there is a lack of research to clarify the efficacy of lubricating gels, practice must be based on the research evidence that is available and the physiology and anatomy of the urethra.

Infections

Catheter-associated infections are the most common hospital-acquired infection, possibly accounting for up to 45% of all hospital infection (Winn 1996). The maintenance of a closed drainage system is central in reducing the risk of catheter-associated infection. It is thought that micro-organisms reach the bladder by two possible routes: from the urine in the drainage bag or via the space between the catheter and the urethral mucosa (Gould

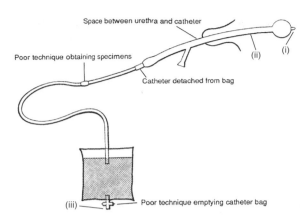

Figure 16.1 Common sites of cross-infection in a catheterized patient. (i) On catheter tip during insertion. (ii) Migration on the inside of the catheter via biofilm. (iii) Connection points of linked systems.

1994; Getliffe 1995). The most common sites where bacteria may enter the system are illustrated in Fig. 16.1. To reduce the risk of infection it is important to keep manipulations of the closed system to a minimum; this includes unnecessary emptying, changing the drainage bags or taking samples. Before handling catheter drainage systems hands must be decontaminated and a pair of clean non-sterile gloves should be worn (Pratt *et al.* 2001). All urine samples should only be obtained via the specially designed sampling ports using an aseptic technique.

Urine drainage bags should only be changed according to clinical need, i.e. when that catheter is changed or if the bag is leaking, or at times dictated by the manufacturer's instructions, for example every 5–7 days (Wilson 1998; Pratt *et al.* 2001). Urine drainage bags positioned above the level of the bladder and full bags cause urine to reflux which is associated with infection. Therefore bags should always be positioned below the level of the bladder to maintain an unobstructed flow and emptied appropriately. Urine drainage bags should be hung on suitable stands to avoid contact with the floor. In situations when dependent drainage is not possible, the system should be clamped until dependent drainage can be resumed (Kunin 1997). When emptying drainage bags, clean separate containers should be used for each patient and care should be taken to avoid contact between the drainage tap and the container (Pratt *et al.* 2001).

Meatal cleaning

Cleaning the urethral meatus, where the catheter enters the body, is a nursing procedure intended to minimize infection of the urinary tract. Studies examining the use of a variety of antiseptic, antimicrobial agents or soap and water found that there was no reduction in bacteriuria when using any of these preparations for meatal cleaning compared to routine bathing or showering (Pratt *et al.* 2001). Further studies support the view that vigorous meatal cleaning is unnecessary and may increase the risk of infection (Saint & Lipsky 1999). Therefore it is recommended that routine personal hygiene is all that is needed to maintain meatal hygiene (Pratt *et al.* 2001).

Drainage bags

A wide variety of drainage systems are available. Selecting a system involves consideration of the reasons for catheterization, the intended duration, the wishes of the patient and infection control issues (Wilson & Coates 1996).

Urine drainage bags are available in a wide selection of sizes ranging from the large 2 litre capacity bag, which is used more commonly in non-ambulatory patients and overnight, to 350–750 ml leg bags. There are also large drainage bags that incorporate urine-measuring devices, which are used when very close monitoring of urine output is required.

There are a number of different styles of body-worn or leg bags. They allow patients greater mobility, they can be worn under the patient's own clothes and therefore are much more discreet, helping to preserve the patient's privacy and dignity. Shapes vary from oblong to oval and some have cloth backing for greater comfort in contact with the skin. Others are ridged to encourage an even distribution of urine through the bag, resulting in better conformity to the leg. The length of the inlet tube also varies (direct, short, long and adjustable length) and the intended position on the leg, i.e. thigh, knee or lower leg, determines which length is used. The patient should be asked to identify the most comfortable position. Several different tap designs exist and patients must have the manual dexterity to operate the mechanism. Most leg bags allow for larger 1–2 litre bags to be connected via the outlet tap, to increase capacity for night-time use.

Leg drainage bags

A variety of supports are available for use with these bags, including sporran waist belts, leg holsters, knickers/pants and leg straps (Roe 1992).

Catheter valves

Catheter valves, which eliminate the need for drainage bags, are also available. The valve allows the bladder to fill and empty intermittently, and is particularly appropriate for patients who require long-term catheterization, as they do not require a drainage bag.

Catheter valves are only suitable for patients who have good cognitive function, sufficient manual dexterity to manipulate the valve and an adequate bladder capacity. It is important that catheter valves are released at regular intervals to ensure that the bladder does not become overdistended. As catheter valves preclude free drainage they are unlikely to be appropriate for patients with uncontrolled detrusor overactivity, ureteric reflux or renal impairment (Fader *et al.* 1997). Catheter valves are designed to fit with linked systems so it is possible for patients to connect to a drainage bag. This may be necessary when access to toilets may be limited, for example overnight or on long journeys.

Catheter valves are licensed by the Department of Health to remain in situ for 5–7 days and this corresponds with most manufacturers' recommendations (Pomfret 1996). Little research into the advantages and disadvantages of catheter valves has been completed.

Suprapubic catheterization

Suprapubic catheterization is the insertion of a catheter through the anterior abdominal wall into the dome of the bladder. The procedure is performed under general or local anaesthesia, using a percutaneous system (Kirkwood 1999). A number of different suprapubic catheters are available. A trocar is used with all types of catheters in order to make the tract through which the catheter is threaded. Specifically designed catheters incorporate a fixing plate, which requires sutures to secure the catheter to the skin of the abdomen. For long-term use a Foley catheter is adequate. Large charrière size (18–22 ch) hydrogel coated or 100% silicone catheters are recommended (Winder 1994).

Suprapubic catheterization does offer some advantages over urethral catheterization. There is a reduction in the risk of patients developing urinary tract infection, as the bacterial count on the abdominal skin is less than around the perineal and perianal areas, although bacteriuria and encrustation still occur in susceptible patients (Winn 1998; Simpson 2001). Urethral integrity is retained and it allows for the resumption of normal voiding after surgery. Clamping the suprapubic catheter allows urethral voiding to occur, and the clamp can be released if voiding is incomplete. Pain and catheter-associated discomfort are reduced. Patient satisfaction is increased as, for some, their level of independence is increased and sexual intercourse can occur with less impediment (Hammarsten & Lindquist 1992; Barnes *et al.* 1993; Fillingham & Douglas 1997; Wilson 1998).

There are a number of risks and disadvantages associated with suprapubic catheterization:

- Bowel perforation and haemorrhage at the time of insertion

- Infection, swelling, encrustation and granulation at insertion site
- Pain, discomfort or irritation for some patients
- Bladder stone formation and possible long-term risk of squamous cell carcinoma
- Urethral leakage (Addison & Mould 2000).

Caring for a suprapubic catheter is the same as for a urethral catheter. Immediately following insertion of a suprapubic catheter, aseptic technique should be employed to clean the insertion site. Dressings may be required if secretions soil clothing, but they are not essential. Once the insertion site has healed (7–10 days), the site and catheter can be cleaned during bathing using soap, water and a clean cloth (Fillingham & Douglas 1997).

Intermittent self-catheterization (ISC)

This is not a new technique, although it has become noticeably more popular in recent years.

The procedure involves the episodic introduction of a catheter into the bladder to remove urine. After this the catheter is removed, leaving the patient catheter-free between catheterizations. In hospital this should be a sterile procedure because of the risks of hospital-acquired infection. However, in the patient's home a clean technique may be used (Wilson 1998; Lapides *et al.* 2002). Catheterization should be carried out as often as necessary to stop the bladder becoming overdistended and to prevent incontinence (Bennett 2002). How frequent this is depends on the individual but may vary from once a week, to once a day to four to six times a day.

The advantages of intermittent catheterization over indwelling urethral catheterizations include improved quality of life, as patients are free from bulky pads or indwelling catheters and drainage bags, greater patient satisfaction and greater freedom to express sexuality. In addition, urinary tract complications are minimized and normal bladder function is maintained (Webb *et al.* 1990;

Bakke & Malt 1993; Chai *et al.* 1995; Bakke *et al.* 1997; Getliffe 1997).

Patients suitable for intermittent self-catheterization include:

- Those with a bladder capable of storing urine without leakage between catheterizations
- Those who can comprehend the technique
- Those with a reasonable degree of dexterity and mobility to position themselves for the procedure and manipulate the catheter
- Those who are highly motivated and committed to carry out the procedure (Colley 1998)
- Those who have a willing partner to perform the technique (i.e. if agreeable to both).

Nelaton catheters are generally used to carry out intermittent self-catheterizations. These catheters are available in standard, female and paediatric lengths and in charrière sizes 6–24. They are normally manufactured from plastic but there is also a non-PVC, chlorine-free catheter obtainable. Some Nelaton catheters are coated with a lubricant which is activated by soaking the catheter in water for a short while; others are packaged with a lubricant gel which coats the catheter as it slides out of the packaging. These catheters are for single use only. Uncoated catheters, which require separate lubrication, may be reused by a single patient for up to a week, but the catheter must be rinsed in running water and properly dried after use; between uses it should be kept in a clean bag or container (Barton 2000).

In 1970, Lasides, in the USA, found that patients using a clean rather than a sterile technique did not encounter problematic urinary tract infection. The catheters used for intermittent self-catheterization are technically described as semi-disposable, i.e. they are designed to be washed and reused for a limited period only, usually 1 week.

They should always be rinsed in running water and properly dried after use; between uses they should be kept in a container such as a plastic envelope (Simcare 1989).

Procedure guidelines: **Urinary catheterization**

Equipment

1 Sterile catheterization pack containing gallipots, receiver, low-linting swabs, disposable towels.
2 Disposable pad.
3 Sterile gloves.
4 Selection of appropriate catheters.
5 Sterile anaesthetic lubricating jelly.
6 Universal specimen container.
7 0.9% sodium chloride or antiseptic solution.
8 Bactericidal alcohol handrub.
9 Gate clip.
10 Hypoallergenic tape.
11 Scissors.
12 Sterile water.
13 Syringe and needle.
14 Disposable plastic apron.
15 Drainage bag and stand or holder.

Procedure guidelines: **Urinary catheterization** *(cont'd)*

Procedure

Male

Action	Rationale
1 Explain and discuss the procedure with the patient.	To ensure that the patient understands the procedure and gives his valid consent.
2 (a) Screen the bed.	To ensure patient's privacy. To allow dust and airborne organisms to settle before the field is exposed.
(b) Assist the patient to get into the supine position with the legs extended.	To ensure the appropriate area is easily accessible.
(c) Do not expose the patient at this stage of the procedure.	To maintain patient's dignity and comfort.
3 Wash hands using bactericidal soap and water or bactericidal alcohol handrub.	To reduce risk of infection.
4 Put on a disposable plastic apron.	To reduce risk of cross-infection from micro-organisms on uniform.
5 Prepare the trolley, placing all equipment required on the bottom shelf.	The top shelf acts as a clean working surface.
6 Take the trolley to the patient's bedside, disturbing screens as little as possible.	To minimize airborne contamination.
7 Open the outer cover of the catheterization pack and slide the pack onto the top shelf of the trolley.	To prepare equipment.
8 Using an aseptic technique, open the supplementary packs.	To reduce the risk of introducing infection into the bladder.
9 Remove cover that is maintaining the patient's privacy and position a disposable pad under the patient's buttocks and thighs.	To ensure urine does not leak onto bedclothes.
10 Clean hands with a bactericidal alcohol handrub.	Hands may have become contaminated by handling the outer packs.
11 Put on sterile gloves.	To reduce risk of cross-infection.
12 Place sterile towels across the patient's thighs and under buttocks.	To create a sterile field.
13 Wrap a sterile topical swab around the penis. Retract the foreskin, if necessary, and clean the glans penis with 0.9% sodium chloride or an antiseptic solution.	To reduce the risk of introducing infection to the urinary tract during catheterization.
14 Insert the nozzle of the lubricating jelly into the urethra. Squeeze the gel into the urethra, remove the nozzle and discard the tube. Massage the gel along the urethra.	Adequate lubrication helps to prevent urethral trauma. Use of a local anaesthetic minimizes the discomfort experienced by the patient.
15 Squeeze the penis and wait approximately 5 minutes.	To prevent anaesthetic gel from escaping. To allow the anaesthetic gel to take effect.
16 Grasp the penis behind the glans, raising it until it is almost totally extended. Maintain grasp of penis until the procedure is finished.	This manoeuvre straightens the penile urethra and facilitates catheterization (Stoller 1995). Maintaining a grasp of the penis prevents contamination and retraction of the penis.
17 Place the receiver containing the catheter between the patient's legs. Insert the catheter for 15–25 cm until urine flows.	The male urethra is approximately 18 cm long.
18 If resistance is felt at the external sphincter, increase the traction on the penis slightly and apply steady, gentle pressure on the catheter. Ask the patient to strain gently as if passing urine.	Some resistance may be due to spasm of the external sphincter. Straining gently helps to relax the external sphincter.

Procedure guidelines: **Urinary catheterization** *(cont'd)*

	Action	Rationale
19	Either remove the catheter gently when urinary flow ceases, or:	
(a)	When urine begins to flow, advance the catheter almost to its bifurcation.	Advancing the catheter ensures that it is correctly positioned in the bladder.
(b)	Gently inflate the balloon according to the manufacturer's direction, having ensured that the catheter is draining properly beforehand.	Inadvertent inflation of the balloon in the urethra causes pain and urethral trauma.
(c)	Withdraw the catheter slightly and attach it to the drainage system.	
(d)	Support the catheter, if the patient desires, either by using a specially designed support, e.g. Simpla G-Strap, or by taping the catheter to the patient's leg. Ensure that the catheter does not become taut when patient is mobilizing or when the penis becomes erect. Ensure that the catheter lumen is not occluded by the fixation device or tape.	To maintain patient comfort and to reduce the risk of urethral and bladder neck trauma. Care must be taken in using adhesive tapes as they may interact with the catheter material (Pomfret 1996).
20	Ensure that the glans penis is clean and then reduce or reposition the foreskin.	Retraction and constriction of the foreskin behind the glans penis (paraphimosis) may occur if this is not done.
21	Make the patient comfortable. Ensure that the area is dry.	If the area is left wet or moist, secondary infection and skin irritation may occur.
22	Measure the amount of urine.	To be aware of bladder capacity for patients who have presented with urinary retention. To monitor renal function and fluid balance. It is not necessary to measure the amount of urine if the patient is having the urinary catheter routinely changed.
23	Take a urine specimen for laboratory examination, if required (see Ch. 39, Specimen collection).	For further information, see the procedure on collection of a catheter specimen of urine, below.
24	Dispose of equipment in a yellow plastic clinical waste bag and seal the bag before moving the trolley.	To prevent environmental contamination. Yellow is the recognized colour for clinical waste.
25	Draw back the curtains.	
26	Record information in relevant documents; this should include reasons for catheterization, date and time of catheterization, catheter type, length and size, amount of water instilled into the balloon, batch number, manufacturer, any problems negotiated during the procedure, and a review date to assess the need for continued catheterization or date of change of catheter.	To provide a point of reference or comparison in the event of later queries.

Female

	Action	Rationale
1	Explain and discuss the procedure with the patient.	To ensure that the patient understands the procedure and gives her valid consent.
2 (a)	Screen the bed.	To ensure patient's privacy. To allow dust and airborne organisms to settle before the sterile field is exposed.
(b)	Assist the patient to get into the supine position with knees bent, hips flexed and feet resting about 60 cm apart.	To enable genital area to be seen.
(c)	Do not expose the patient at this stage of the procedure.	To maintain the patient's dignity and comfort.
3	Ensure that a good light source is available.	To enable genital area to be seen clearly.
4	Wash hands using bactericidal soap and water or bactericidal alcohol handrub.	To reduce risk of cross-infection.

*Procedure guidelines: **Urinary catheterization** (cont'd)*

Action	Rationale
5 Put on a disposable apron.	To reduce risk of cross-infection from micro-organisms on uniform.
6 Prepare the trolley, placing all equipment required on the bottom shelf. (Also, see section on catheter selection.)	To reserve top shelf for clean working surface.
7 Take the trolley to the patient's bedside, disturbing screens as little as possible.	To minimize airborne contamination.
8 Open the outer cover of the catheterization pack and slide the pack on the top shelf of the trolley.	To prepare equipment.
9 Using an aseptic technique, open supplementary packs.	To reduce risk of introducing infection into the urinary tract.
10 Remove cover that is maintaining the patient's privacy and position a disposable pad under the patient's buttocks.	To ensure urine does not leak onto bedclothes.
11 Clean hands with a bactericidal alcohol handrub.	Hands may have become contaminated by handling of outer packs, etc.
12 Put on sterile gloves.	To reduce risk of cross-infection.
13 Place sterile towels across the patient's thighs.	To create a sterile field.
14 Using low-linting swabs, separate the labia minora so that the urethral meatus is seen. One hand should be used to maintain labial separation until catheterization is completed.	This manoeuvre provides better access to the urethral orifice and helps to prevent labial contamination of the catheter.
15 Clean around the urethral orifice with 0.9% sodium chloride or an antiseptic solution, using single downward strokes.	Inadequate preparation of the urethral orifice is a major cause of infection following catheterization. To reduce the risk of cross-infection.
16 Insert the nozzle of the lubricating jelly into the urethra. Squeeze the gel into the urethra, remove the nozzle and discard the tube.	Adequate lubrication helps to prevent urethral trauma. Use of a local anaesthetic minimizes the patient's discomfort.
17 Place the catheter, in the receiver, between the patient's legs.	To provide a temporary container for urine as it drains.
18 Introduce the tip of the catheter into the urethral orifice in an upward and backward direction. If there is any difficulty in visualizing the urethral orifice due to vaginal atrophy and retraction of the urethral orifice, the index finger of the 'dirty' hand may be inserted in the vagina, and the urethral orifice can be palpated on the anterior wall of the vagina. The index finger is then positioned just behind the urethral orifice. This then acts as a guide, so the catheter can be correctly positioned (Jenkins 1998). Advance the catheter until 5–6 cm has been inserted.	The direction of insertion and the length of catheter inserted should bear relation to the anatomical structure of the area.
19 Either remove the catheter gently when urinary flow ceases, or:	
(a) Advance the catheter 6–8 cm.	This prevents the balloon from becoming trapped in the urethra.
(b) Inflate the balloon according to the manufacturer's directions, having ensured that the catheter is draining adequately.	Inadvertent inflation of the balloon within the urethra is painful and causes urethral trauma.
(c) Withdraw the catheter slightly and connect it to the drainage system.	
(d) Support the catheter, if the patient desires, either by using a specially designed	To maintain patient comfort and to reduce the risk of urethral and bladder neck trauma. Care must

*Procedure guidelines: **Urinary catheterization** (cont'd)*

Action	Rationale
support, e.g. Simpla G-Strap, or by taping the catheter to the patient's leg. Ensure that the catheter does not become taut when patient is mobilizing. Ensure that the catheter lumen is not occluded by the fixation device or tape.	be taken in using adhesive tapes as they may interact with the catheter material (Pomfret 1996).
20 Make the patient comfortable and ensure that the area is dry.	If the area is left wet or moist, secondary infection and skin irritation may occur.
21 Measure the amount of urine.	To be aware of bladder capacity for patients who have presented with urinary retention. To monitor renal function and fluid balance. It is not necessary to measure the amount of urine if the patient is having the urinary catheter routinely changed.
22 Take a urine specimen for laboratory examination if required.	For further information, see the procedure on collection of a catheter specimen of urine, below.
23 Dispose of equipment in a yellow plastic clinical waste bag and seal the bag before moving the trolley.	To prevent environmental contamination. Yellow is the recognized colour for clinical waste.
24 Draw back the curtains.	
25 Record information in relevant documents; this should include reasons for catheterization, date and time of catheterization, catheter type, length and size, amount of water instilled into the balloon, batch number, manufacturer, any problems negotiated during the procedure and a review date to assess the need for continued catheterization or date of change of catheter. *Note*: beware of patient having a vasovagal attack. This is caused by the vagal nerve being stimulated so that the heart slows down, leading to a syncope faint. If it happens, lie the patient down in the recovery position. Inform doctors.	To provide a point of reference or comparison in the event of later queries.

Procedure guidelines for patients: **Intermittent self-catheterization**

Equipment

1 Mirror (for female patients).
2 Appropriately sized catheters for male/female patients.
3 Lubricating gel.
4 Clean container (e.g. plastic envelope) for catheter.

Procedure

Female

Action	Rationale
1 Wash hands using bactericidal soap and water or bactericidal alcohol handrub.	To reduce risk of cross-infection.
2 Take up a comfortable position, depending on mobility (e.g. sitting on toilet; standing with one foot placed on toilet seat).	To facilitate insertion of intermittent catheter.
3 Spread the labia (the lips at the entrance to the vagina) and wash genitalia, from front to back, with soap and water, then dry.	To reduce the risk of introducing infection.
4 Open catheter packaging or container. If using an uncoated catheter a water-soluble lubricating gel may be applied to the surface of the catheter. If using a coated catheter pre-soak it in water to activate the slippery coating (Barton 2000).	To prepare catheter and to ease insertion.

Procedure guidelines for patients: Intermittent self-catheterization (cont'd)

Action	Rationale
5 Find the urethral opening above the vagina. A mirror can be used to help identify the urethral opening. Gently insert the catheter into the urethra, taking care not to touch the part of the catheter entering the body.	To reduce risk of introducing an infection.
6 Drain the urine into the toilet or suitable container. When the urine stops flowing slowly remove the catheter, halting if more urine starts to flow.	To ensure that the bladder is completely emptied.
7 Before removing the catheter from the urethra put a finger over the funnel end of the catheter and then remove the catheter from the urethra.	To trap urine in the catheter and prevent spillage on to clothing or the floor.
8 Hold the catheter over the toilet or suitable container and remove finger from the funnel end to release the trapped urine.	To prevent spillage on to clothing or the floor.
9 If using a coated catheter dispose of the catheter in a suitable receptacle.	To prevent environmental contamination.
If the catheter is uncoated and is to be reused wash through with tap water.	To remove urine.
Allow to drain then dry the outside of the catheter. Store in a dry container (as per manufacturer's instructions).	To reduce risk of infection.
These catheters may be used for 5–7 days.	
NB: If carrying out this procedure in hospital a new catheter must be used every time.	To reduce the risk of hospital-acquired infections.
10 Wash hands with soap and water.	To reduce the risk of infection.

Male

Action	Rationale
1 Wash hands using bactericidal soap and water or bactericidal alcohol handrub.	To prevent infection.
2 Stand in front of a toilet or a low bench with a suitable container if it is easier.	To catch urine.
3 Clean glans penis with plain water. If the foreskin covers the penis it will need to be held back during the procedure.	To reduce risk of infection.
4 Open catheter packaging or container. If using an uncoated catheter a water-soluble lubricating gel may be applied to the surface of the catheter. If using a coated catheter pre-soak it in water to activate the slippery coating.	To prepare catheter and to ease insertion.
5 Hold penis with the non-dominant hand upwards towards your stomach.	To prevent trauma to the penoscrotal junction.
6 Hold the catheter with the dominant hand, being careful not to touch the part of the catheter entering the body, and gently insert it into the opening of the urethra. Advance the catheter into the bladder.	To reduce the risk of introducing an infection.
There will be a change of feeling as the catheter passes through the prostate gland and into the bladder.	The prostate gland surrounds the urethra just below the neck of the bladder and consists of much firmer tissue.
It may be a little sore on the first few occasions only. If there is any resistance, do not continue. Withdraw the catheter and contact a nurse or doctor.	This can enlarge and cause an obstruction, especially in older men.
7 Drain the urine into the toilet or suitable container. When the urine stops flowing slowly remove the catheter, halting if more urine starts to flow.	To ensure that the bladder is completely emptied.

*Procedure guidelines for patients: **Intermittent self-catheterization** (cont'd)*

Action	Rationale
8 Before removing the catheter from the urethra put a finger over the funnel end of the catheter and then remove the catheter from the urethra.	To trap urine in the catheter and prevent spillage on to clothing or the floor.
9 Hold the catheter over the toilet or suitable container and remove finger from the funnel end to release the trapped urine.	Hold the catheter over the toilet or suitable container and remove finger from the funnel end to release the trapped urine.
10 If using a coated catheter dispose of the catheter in a suitable receptacle.	To prevent environmental contamination.
If the catheter is uncoated and is to be reused wash through with tap water.	To remove urine.
Allow to drain then dry the outside of the catheter. Store in a dry container (as per manufacturer's instructions). These catheters may be used for 5–7 days.	To reduce risk of infection.
NB: If carrying out this procedure in hospital a new catheter must be used every time.	To reduce the risk of hospital-acquired infections.
11 Wash hands with soap and water.	To reduce the risk of infection.
12 Standing in front of a mirror is helpful for patients with a large abdomen.	For ease of observation.

Procedure guidelines: **Collection of a catheter specimen of urine**

Equipment

1 Swab saturated with isopropyl alcohol 70%.
2 Gate clip.
3 Sterile syringe and needle.
4 Universal specimen container.

Procedure

Action	Rationale
1 Explain and discuss the procedure with the patient.	To ensure that the patient understands the procedure and gives his/her valid consent.
2 Screen the bed.	To ensure the patient's privacy.
3 Only if there is no urine in the tubing, clamp the tubing below the rubber cuff until sufficient urine collects. (An access point is now available on catheter bags.)	To obtain an adequate urine sample.
4 Wash hands using bactericidal soap and water or bactericidal alcohol handrub.	To reduce risk of infection.
5 Clean the access point with a swab saturated with 70% isopropyl alchohol.	To reduce risk of cross-infection.
6 Using a sterile syringe and needle (if necessary), aspirate the required amount of urine from the access point (Fig. 16.2).	If the catheter bag or tubing is punctured it causes leakage carrying organisms with it. Specimens collected from the catheter bag may give false results due to organisms proliferating there.
Needle sampling port: insert the needle into the port at an angle of 45° and aspirate the required amount of urine, withdraw the needle.	To reduce the risk of the needle going straight through the tubing.
Needleless sampling port: insert the syringe firmly into the centre of the sampling port (following manufacturer's instructions). Aspirate the required amount of urine and disconnect the syringe.	To reduce the risk of needlestick injury.

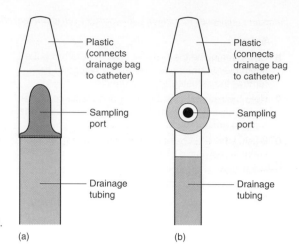

Figure 16.2   Taking a specimen. (a) Needle sampling port. (b) Needleless sampling port.

(a)   (b)

*Procedure guidelines: **Collection of a catheter specimen of urine** (cont'd)*

Action	Rationale
7 Reclean access point with a swab saturated with 70% isopropyl alchohol.	To reduce contamination of access point and to reduce risk of cross-infection.
8 Place the specimen in a sterile container.	To ensure that only organisms for investigation are preserved.
9 Wash and dry hands with bactericidal soap and water.	To reduce risk of cross-infection.
10 Unclamp if necessary.	To allow drainage to continue.
11 Make the patient comfortable.	
12 Label the container and dispatch it (with the completed request form) to the laboratory as soon as possible after sample is taken to allow more accurate results from culture.	To ensure the best possible conditions for laboratory tests.

Procedure guidelines: **Emptying a catheter bag**

Equipment

1 Swabs saturated with 70% isopropyl alcohol.
2 Clean jug.
3 Disposable gloves.
4 Sterile jug.

Procedure

Action	Rationale
1 Explain and discuss the procedure with the patient.	To ensure that the patient understands the procedure and gives his/her valid consent.
2 Wash hands using bactericidal soap and water or bactericidal alcohol handrub, and put on disposable gloves.	To reduce risk of cross-infection.
3 Clean the outlet valve with a swab saturated with 70% isopropyl alcohol.	To reduce risk of infection.
4 Allow the urine to drain into the appropriate jug.	To empty drainage bag and accurately measure volume of contents.
5 Close the outlet valve and clean it again with a new alcohol-saturated swab.	To reduce risk of cross-infection.

Procedure guidelines: Emptying a catheter bag (cont'd)

Action	Rationale
6 Cover the jug and dispose of contents in the sluice, having noted the amount of urine if this is requested for fluid balance records.	To reduce risk of environmental contamination.
7 Wash hands with bactericidal soap and water.	To reduce risk of infection.

Procedure guidelines: **Removing a catheter**

Equipment

1 Dressing pack containing sterile towel, gallipot, foam swab or non-linting gauze.
2 Disposable gloves.
3 Needle and syringe for urine specimen, specimen container.
4 Syringe for deflating balloon.

Procedure

Action	Rationale
1 Catheters are usually removed early in the morning.	So that any retention problems can be dealt with during the day.
2 Explain procedure to patient and inform him or her of potential postcatheter symptoms, i.e. urgency, frequency and discomfort which are often caused by irritation of the urethra by the catheter.	So that patient knows what to expect, and can plan daily activity.
	For adequate flushing of bladder, especially to dilute and expel debris and infected urine, if present.
3 Clamp below the sampling port until sufficient urine collects. Take a catheter specimen of urine using the sampling port.	To obtain an adequate urine sample and to assess whether postcatheter antibiotic therapy is needed.
4 Wearing gloves, use saline to clean the meatus and catheter, always swabbing away from the urethral opening.	To reduce risk of infection.
In women, never clear from the perineum/vagina towards the urethra.	To help reduce the risk of bacteria from the vagina and perineum contaminating the urethra.
5 Release leg support.	For easier removal of catheter.
6 Having checked volume of water in balloon (see patient documentation), use syringe to deflate balloon.	To confirm how much water is in the balloon. To ensure balloon is completely deflated before removing catheter.
7 Ask patient to breathe in and then out; as patient exhales, gently – but quickly – remove catheter. Male patients should be warned of discomfort as the deflated balloon passes through the prostate gland.	To relax pelvic floor muscles.
8 Clean meatus, tidy away equipment, and make the patient comfortable. Symptoms should resolve over the following 24–48 hours. If not, further investigation may be needed. Encourage patient to exercise and to drink 2–3 litres of fluid per day.	

Problem solving

With catheter in place

Problem	Cause	Suggested action
Urinary tract infection introduced during catheterization.	Faulty aseptic technique. Inadequate urethral cleaning. Contamination of catheter tip.	Inform a doctor. Obtain a catheter specimen of urine.

Problem solving (cont'd)

Problem	Cause	Suggested action
Urinary tract infection introduced via the drainage system.	Faulty handling of equipment. Breaking the closed system. Raising the drainage bag above bladder level.	Inform a doctor. Obtain a catheter specimen of urine.
No drainage of urine.	Incorrect identification of external urinary meatus (female patients).	Check that catheter has been sited correctly.
	Blockage of catheter.	In the female if catheter has been wrongly inserted in the vagina, leave the catheter in position to act as a guide, re-identify the urethra and catheterize the patient. Remove the inappropriately sited catheter.
	Empty bladder.	When changing the catheter, clamp the catheter 30 min before the procedure. On insertion of the new catheter, urine will drain.
Urethral mucosal trauma.	Incorrect size of catheter. Procedure not carried out correctly or skilfully. Movement of the catheter in the urethra.	Recatheterize the patient using the correct size of catheter. Check the catheter support and apply or reapply as necessary.
	Creation of false passage as a result of too rapid insertion of catheter.	Nurse may need to remove the catheter and wait for the urethral mucosa to heal.
Inability to tolerate indwelling catheter.	Urethral mucosal irritation.	Nurse may need to remove the catheter and seek an alternative means of urine drainage.
	Psychological trauma. Unstable bladder. Radiation cystitis.	Explain the need for and functioning of the catheter.
Inadequate drainage of urine.	Incorrect placement of a catheter.	Resite the catheter.
	Kinked drainage tubing.	Inspect the system and straighten any kinks.
	Blocked tubing, e.g. pus, urates, phosphates, blood clots.	If a three-way catheter, such as Foley, is in place, irrigate it. If an ordinary catheter is in use, milk the tubing in an attempt to dislodge the debris; then replace it with a three-way catheter.
Fistula formation.	Pressure on the penoscrotal angle.	Ensure that correct strapping is used.
Penile pain on erection.	Not allowing enough length of catheter to accommodate penile erection.	Ensure that an adequate length is available to accommodate penile erection.
Paraphimosis.	Failure to retract foreskin after catheterization or catheter toilet.	Always retract the foreskin.
Formation of crusts around the urethral meatus.	Increased urethral secretions collect at the meatus and form crusts, due to irritation of urothelium by the catheter (Fillingham & Douglas 1997).	Correct catheter toilet.

Problem solving (cont'd)

Problem	Cause	Suggested action
Leakage of urine around catheter.	Incorrect size of catheter.	Replace with the correct size, usually 2 ch smaller.
	Incorrect balloon size.	Select catheter with 10 ml balloon.
	Bladder hyperirritability.	Use Roberts tipped catheter. As a last resort, bladder hyperirritability can be reduced by giving diazepam or anticholinergic drugs.
Unable to deflate balloon.	Valve expansion. Valve displacement.	1 Check the non-return valve on the inflation/deflation channel. If jammed, use a syringe and needle to aspirate by means of the inflation arm above the valve.
	Channel obstruction.	2 Obstruction by a foreign body can sometimes be relieved by the introduction of a guidewire through the inflation channel.
		3 Inject 3.5 ml of dilute ether solution (diluted 50/50 with sterile water or 0.9% sodium chloride) into the inflation arm.
		4 Alternatively, the balloon can be punctured suprapubically using a needle under ultrasound visualization.
		5 Following catheter removal the balloon should be inspected to ensure it has not disintegrated, leaving fragments in the bladder.
		Note: steps 2 to 4 should be attempted by or under the directions of a urologist. The patient may require cystoscopy following balloon deflation to remove any balloon fragments and to wash the bladder out.

After removal of the catheter

Problem	Cause	Suggested action
Dysuria.	Inflammation of the urethral mucosa.	Ensure a fluid intake of 2–3 litres per day. Advise the patient that dysuria is common but will usually be resolved once micturition has occurred at least three times. Inform medical staff if the problem persists.
Retention of urine.	May be psychological.	Encourage the patient to increase fluid intake. Offer the patient a warm bath. Inform medical staff if the problem persists.
Urinary tract infection.		Encourage a fluid intake of 2–3 litres a day. Collect a specimen of urine. Inform medical staff if the problem persists. Administer prescribed antibiotics.

References and further reading

Addison, R. (2001) Intermittent self-catheterisation. *Nurs Times*, **97**(20), 67 9.

Addison, R. & Mould, C. (2000) Risk assessment in suprapubic catheterization. *Nurs Stand*, **14**(36), 43–6.

Bakke, A. & Malt, U.F. (1993) Social functioning and general well being in patients treated with clean intermittent catheterisation. *J Psychosom Res*, **37**(4), 371–80.

Bakke, A., Digranes, A. & Hoisaeter, P.A. (1997) Physical predictors of infection in patients treated with clean intermittent catheterisation: a prospective 7-year study. *Br J Urol*, **79**(1), 85–90.

Barnes, D.G., Shaw, P.J.R., Timoney, A.G. & Tsokos, N. (1993) Management of the neuropathic bladder by supra-pubic catheterisation. *Br J Urol*, **72**, 169–72.

Barnes, K.E. & Malone-Lee, J. (1986) Long-term catheter management: minimising the problem of premature replacement due to balloon deflation. *J Adv Nurs*, **11**, 303–7.

Barton, R. (2000) Intermittent self-catheterisation. *Nurs Stand* **15**(9), 1–9.

Bennett, E. (2002) Intermittent self-catheterisation and the female patient. *Nurs Stand*, **30**(17), 37–42.

Best Practice (2000) Management of short term indwelling urethral catheters to prevent urinary tract infections. *Best Practice* **4**(1), 1–6.

Blandy, J.P. & Moors, J. (1989) *Urology for Nurses*. Blackwell Science, Oxford.

Brocklehurst, J.C. *et al.* (1988) A new urethral catheter. *Br J Med*, **296**, 1691–3.

Centre for Reviews and Dissemination Reviewers (2002) Management of short term indwelling urethral catheters to prevent urinary tract infections: a systematic review. Database of Abstracts of Reviews of Effectiveness, York.

Chai, T., Chung, A.K., Belville, W.D. & Faerber, G.J. (1995) Compliance and complications of clean intermittent catheterisation in the spinal-cord injured patient. *Paraplegia*, **33**(3), 161–3.

Colley, W. (1998) Catheter care 1. *Nurs Times*, **94**(23), insert.

Crow, R.A. *et al.* (1986) *A Study of Patients with an Indwelling Catheter and Related Nursing Practice*. Nursing Practice Unit, University of Surrey.

Cruickshank, J.P. & Woodward, S. (2001) *Management of Continence and Urinary Catheter Care*. Mark Allen, London.

Doherty, W. (2000) Intermittent self-catheterisation: draining the bladder. *Nurs Times*, **96**(31), 13.

Edwards, L.E. *et al.* (1983) Post-catheterisation urethral strictures: a clinical and experimental study. *Br J Urol*, **55**, 53–6.

Evans, A., Painter, D. & Feneley, R. (2001) Blocked urinary catheters: nurses' preventive role. *Nurs Times*, **97**(1), 37–8.

Fader, M., Pettersson Brooks, R. & Dean, G. *et al.* (1997) A multi-centre comparative evaluation of catheter valves. *Br J Nurs*, **6**(7), 359–67.

Falkiner, F.R. (1993) The insertion and management of indwelling urethral catheters – minimising the risk of infection. *J Hosp Infect*, **25**, 79–90.

Fillingham, S. & Douglas, J. (1997) *Urological Nursing*, 2nd edn. Baillière Tindall, London.

German, K., Rowley, P., Stone, P., Kumar, U. & Blackford, H.N. (1997) A randomized cross-over study comparing the use of a catheter valve and a leg-bag in urethrally catheterised male patients. *Br J Urol*, **79**(1), 96–8.

Getliffe, K. (1995) Care of urinary catheters. *Nurs Stand*, **10**(1), 25–31.

Getliffe, K. (1996) Care of urinary catheters. *Nurs Stand*, **11**(11), 47–54.

Getliffe, K. (1997) Catheters and catheterisation. In: *Promoting Continence: A Clinical and Research Resource* (eds K. Getliffe & M. Dolman). Baillière Tindall, London.

Gilbert, A. & Gobbi, M. (1989) Making sense of bladder irrigation. *Nurs Times*, **85**(16), 40–2.

Godfrey, H. & Evans, A. (2000) Management of long-term catheters: minimising complications. *Br J Nurs*, **9**(2), 74–81.

Gould, D. (1994) Keeping on tract. *Nurs Times* **90**(40), 58–64.

Hammarsten, J. & Lindquist, K. (1992) Supra-pubic catheter following transurethral resection of the prostate: a way to decrease the number of urethral strictures and improve the outcome of operation. *J Urol*, **147**, 648–52.

Jenkins, S.C. (1998) Digital guidance of female urethral catheterization. *Br J Urol*, **82**, 589–90.

Kirkwood, L. (1999) Taking charge. *Nurs Times*, **95**(6), 63–4.

Kristiansen, P. *et al.* (1983) Long-term urethral catheter drainage and bladder capacity. *Neurol Urodyn*, **2**, 135–43.

Kunin, C.M. (1997) *Urinary Tract Infections: Detection, Prevention and Management*, 5th edn. Williams and Wilkins, Baltimore.

Lapides, J., Diokno, A.C., Silber, S.M. & Lowe, B.S. (2002) Clean, intermittent self-catheterization in the treatment of urinary tract disease. *J Urol*, **167**(4), 1584–6.

Leaver, R. & Pressland, D. (2001) Intermittent self-catheterisation in urinary tract reconstruction. *Br J Commun Nurs*, **6**(5), 253–8.

Mackenzie, J. & Webb, C. (1995) Gynopia in nursing practice: the case of urethral catheterization. *J Clin Nurs*, **4**, 221–6.

McGill, S. (1982) Catheter management: it's size that's important. *Nurs Mirror*, **154**, 48–9.

Milligan, F. (1999) Male sexuality and urethral catheterisations: a review of the literature. *Nurs Stand*, **13**(38), 43–7.

Moore, K. (1995) Intermittent self-catheterisation: research based practice. *Br J Nurs*, **4**(18), 1057–63.

Muctar, S. (1991) The importance of a lubricant in transurethral interventions. *Urologue (B)*, **31**, 153–5 [translation].

Mulhall, A.B., King, S., Lee, K. & Wiggington, E. (1993) Maintenance of closed urinary drainage systems: are practitioners aware of the dangers? *J Clin Nurs*, **2**, 135–40.

Nacey, J.N. & Delahunt, B. (1991) Toxicity study of first and second generation hydrogel-coated latex catheters. *Br J Urol*, **67**, 314–16.

Pomfret, I. (2000) Catheter care in the community. *Nurs Stand*, **22**(14), 46–51.

Pomfret, I.J. (1996) Catheters: design, selection and management. *Br J Nurs*, **5**(4), 245–51.

Pratt, R.J., Pellowe, C., Loveday, H.P. & Robinson, N. (2001) Guidelines for preventing infections associated with the insertion and maintenance of short-term indwelling urethral catheters in acute care. *J Hosp Infect*, **47**(Suppl), S39–46.

RCN (1994) *Guidelines on Male Catheterisation: The Role of the Nurse*. Royal College of Nursing, London.

Roberts, J.A. *et al.* (1990) Bacterial adherence to urethral catheters. *J Urol*, **144**, 264–9.

Robinson, J. (2001) Urethral catheter selection. *Nurs Stand,* **25**(15), 39–42.

Roe, B.H. (1992) Use of indwelling catheters. In: *Clinical Nursing Practice: The Promotion and Management of Continence* (ed. B.H. Roe). Prentice Hall, Hemel Hempstead.

Roe, B.H. & Brocklehurst, J.C. (1987) Study of patients with indwelling catheters. *J Adv Nurs,* **12**, 713–18.

Ryan-Woolley, B. (1987) *Urinary Catheters: Aids for the Management of Incontinence.* King's Fund Project Paper No. 65. King's Fund, London.

Saint, S. & Lipsky, B.A. (1999) Preventing catheter-associated bacteriuria. Should we? Can we? How? *Arch Intern Med,* **159**, 800–8.

Saint, S., Elmore, J.G., Sullivan, S.D., Emerson, S.S. & Koepsell, T.D. (1998) The efficacy of silver alloy-coated urinary catheters in preventing urinary tract infection: a meta-analysis. *Am J Med,* **105**(3), 236–41.

Simcare (1989) *Intermittent Self-Catheterization – A Guide for Patients' Families.* Simcare, Lancing.

Simpson, L. (2001) Indwelling urethral catheters. *Nurs Stand,* **15**(46), 47–54, 56.

Slade, N. & Gillespie, W.A. (1985) *The Urinary Tract and the Catheter: Infection and Other Problems.* John Wiley, Chichester.

Stewart, E. (1998) Urinary catheters: selection, maintenance and nursing care. *Br J Nurs,* **7**(19), 1152–61.

Studer, U.E. (1983) How to fill silicone catheter balloons. *Urology,* **22**, 300–2.

Thakar, R. & Stanton, S. (2000) Management of urinary incontinence in women. *Br Med J,* **323**(7272), 1326–31.

Tortora, G.A. & Grabowski, S.R. (2002) *Principles of Anatomy and Physiology.* John Wiley and Sons, New York.

Webb, R.J., Lawson, A.L. & Neal, D.E. (1990) Clean intermittent self-catheterisation in 172 adults. *Br J Urol,* **65**(1), 20–3.

Wilksch, J. *et al.* (1983) The role of catheter surface morphology and extractable cytotoxic material in tissue reactions to urethral catheters. *Br J Urol,* **55**, 48–52.

Wilson, M. (1998) Infection control. *Prof Nurse Study Suppl,* **13**(5), S10–13.

Wilson, M. & Coates, D. (1996) Infection control and urine drainage bag design. *Prof Nurse,* **11**(4), 245–52.

Winder, A. (1994) Suprapubic catheterisation. *Commun Outlook,* **4**(12), 25–6.

Winn, C. (1996) Catheterisation: extending the scope of practice. *Nurs Stand,* **10**(52), 49–56.

Winn, C. (1998) Complications with urinary catheters. *Prof Nurse Study Suppl,* **13**(5), S7–10.

Woodward, S. (1997) Complications of allergies to latex urinary catheters. *Br J Nurs,* **6**(4), 786–93.

Woollons, S. (1996) Urinary catheters for long-term use. *Prof Nurse,* **11**(12), 825–32.

Young, A.E., Macnaughton, P.D., Gaylard, D.G. & Weatherly, C. (1994) A case of latex anaphylaxis. *Br J Hosp Med,* **52**(11), 599–600.

17

External compression and support in the management of lymphoedema

Chapter contents

Definitions

The terms 'compression' and 'support' refer to the application of different pressures to a limb.

- Compression is achieved by the direct application of external pressure (Eagle 2001) as the forces of an elastic garment or bandage pull in and exert pressure on the tissues below.
- The application of a semi-rigid support to a swollen limb results in a massaging effect on the tissues below and pressure arises from the body tissues and muscles as they push outwards against the firm encasement provided by the garment or bandage (Thomas & Nelson 1998).

The type of material from which garments or bandages are made can therefore determine whether support or compression is applied, with elastic garments providing compression and inelastic garments or low-stretch bandages providing support.

Under support, a relatively low resting pressure is experienced when the muscle is inactive during rest. This contrasts with a high working pressure during exercise of the muscle as it contracts within the inelastic garment or bandage, resulting in a massaging effect on the tissues below and the stimulation of lymph drainage (Todd 2000). There is a less pronounced effect achieved with compression where the resting and working pressures are higher. The elastic garment or bandage pulls in along the length of the limb, stretching as the muscle expands and providing a high resting pressure when it is at rest (Todd 2000).

The circumference of the limb determines the pressure exerted by the garment or bandage, with the highest pressure achieved where the limb is narrowest. When a garment or bandage is applied to a limb of normal proportions, therefore, the highest pressure will be achieved at the ankle or wrist, with graduated, reducing pressure along the length of the limb as the circumference increases (Thomas & Nelson 1998).

Indications

External graduated pressure in the form of support or compression is the mainstay of conservative management for lymphoedema. It is important for several reasons:

- It ensures that fluid in the limb travels towards the root of the limb.
- It limits the formation of fluid in the tissues.
- It contains the tissues of the swollen limb and helps to maintain a normal shape to the limb.
- It helps to maximize the effect of the muscle pump.

Elastic compression is primarily indicated when the lymphoedema is mild and uncomplicated (Todd 2000). It is also used to maintain the reduced size of a swollen limb after the use of bandaging. Support, provided by low stretch bandages or the more rigid types of hosiery, is indicated when the lymphoedema is moderate to severe and the limb has swollen out of shape. It is also effective when fibrosis of the subcutaneous tissues is present, due to the massaging effect on the tissues of the low resting pressures and high working pressures.

Contraindications for external graduated pressure

- Arterial disease in the arm or leg
- Acute stages of deep vein thrombosis in the leg
- Acute infections of the limb, e.g. cellulitis
- Cardiac oedema (Callam *et al.* 1997).

Reference material

There are many reasons why a limb may swell and the appearance of oedema represents an increase in extracellular fluid volume (Stanton 2000). Dependency or gravitational oedema is commonly seen in the immobile patient when the immobility results in minimal lymph drainage. Swelling can also occur in chronic venous disease of the lower limbs as a result of lymph drainage failure and increased capillary filtration (Stanton 2000).

Lymphoedema occurs because the lymphatics are reduced in number, obstructed, obliterated or simply fail to function. Tissue swelling then appears due to the failure of lymph drainage (Stanton 2000). Lymphoedema

is most commonly seen in cancer patients as a result of damage to lymph nodes following surgery and/or radiotherapy, but it can also occur as a result of local tumour obstruction in lymph node areas. A survey of 1200 breast cancer patients reported the prevalence of chronic arm oedema as 28%. The prevalence increased with time following treatment in patients who had received postoperative radiotherapy (Mortimer *et al.* 1996). There is no research to indicate the incidence of leg oedema following treatment for abdominal and pelvic tumours, soft tissue sarcomas and melanomas, although lymphoedema is known to occur following treatment for these tumours (Keeley 2000).

Lymphoedema can affect any part of the body including the face and head, but it most commonly affects a limb. The swelling can have physical, psychological and psychosocial implications for the patient and is associated with a number of complications arising from its development (Woods 2000a). Limb heaviness may lead to impaired function, reduced mobility and musculoskeletal problems (Tobin *et al.* 1993). Skin and tissue changes develop with increased lymph stasis in the oedematous limb and give rise to the characteristic deepened skin folds, distorted limb shape and hyperkeratosis associated with long-standing lymphoedema. There is an increased risk of local and systemic infection as a result of poor lymph drainage and recurrent acute inflammatory episodes are common (Mortimer 2000).

The experience of living with lymphoedema as a long-term chronic condition is a unique experience for each patient and can have an impact on many areas of the individual's life. Studies of breast cancer patients with arm swelling have highlighted the degree of psychological and psychosocial distress that can be experienced when lymphoedema develops (Tobin *et al.* 1993; Woods 1993; Woods *et al.* 1995). The physical and psychological effects of lymphoedema are not short-lived and enormous motivation and perseverance coupled with adaptation are demanded in order to achieve control or reduction of the swelling (Mason 2000).

Assessment of the patient with lymphoedema

Definition

Assessment has been defined as an expert activity (Benner 1984) which can have a dramatic effect on outcome for the individual patient (Derdiarian 1990). As lymphoedema is a unique experience for each patient, accurate assessment is essential if an individualized approach is to be achieved and the most appropriate treatment chosen.

Indications

When the use of external compression and support is being considered, a full and careful assessment will highlight the patient's main problems and any co-existing complications. This information is then used to set realistic treatment goals and to determine the approach to treatment. A number of treatments are used in combination during the management of lymphoedema and their choice and usefulness can be determined by the therapist and patient at the time of assessment.

A full assessment should include the following elements:

- *Details of the patient's medical history*: to determine whether external graduated pressure can be used safely on a lower limb where appropriate. Arterial insufficiency of the lower limb must be excluded prior to the use of external graduated pressure and patients with a history of diabetes or cardiac failure should undergo a medical assessment prior to the commencement of treatment and close supervision during its progress (Eagle 2001).
- *Physical assessment*: to determine the cause of the swelling and any symptoms or complicating factors, i.e. the cause and extent of the oedema, assessment of skin condition and limb shape, disease status.
- *Psychological assessment*: to determine the effect of the swelling on the patient, i.e. effect on relationships, personal concerns and fears.
- *Psychosocial assessment*: to determine the influence of the swelling upon the patient's life, i.e. influence upon limb function and mobility, employment, hobbies, activities, personal roles.

In order to evaluate the outcome of a plan of treatment, suitable outcome indicators are required (Jenns 2000). No standardized method of evaluating the outcome of a plan of treatment has been adopted but the measurement of limb volume using surface measurement is the most frequently used means of assessing response to treatment in lymphoedema management (Jenns 2000). The effect of treatment on the patient's psychological and psychosocial well-being should, however, also be monitored and this is frequently achieved in a more subjective manner where the patient's views are sought.

Measurement of limb volume

Definition

The measurement of limb volume is calculated from a series of circumference measurements taken along the length of the limb and applied to the formula for the volume of a cylinder (Sitzia 1995).

Indications

As part of the initial assessment of the patient, limb volume measurements can be calculated in order to:

- Determine the total excess volume of the swollen limb compared to the patient's contralateral normal limb
- Establish the distribution of the swelling along the limb
- Provide information to assist in the choice of external pressure.

Measurements can also be used to provide an objective method of determining response to treatment by indicating:

- Changes in the size and shape of the limb over time
- Changes in the excess volume
- The distribution of any volume loss or gain in the limb.

Reference material

A reliable method of assessing response to treatment is the measurement of limb volume. A variety of methods to measure volume have been used, including:

- Volume measured by water displacement (Kettle *et al.* 1958; Engler & Sweat 1962)
- Volume measured using an optoelectronic device (Stanton *et al.* 1997)
- Volume calculated from surface measurements (Sitzia 1995).

Each of these methods has advantages and disadvantages. The calculation of limb volume from surface measurements, however, is uncomplicated and inexpensive. Reproducibility is accurate if care is taken with the procedure and a standard format for the recording of the measurements is used (Woods 1994; Badger 1997).

The following points should be considered when using surface measurements in order to calculate limb volume:

1 Ensure that the same position is used for the same patient each time the limb is measured. The position of the limb will affect the measurements taken because the degree to which muscles are flexed or relaxed will influence the shape and size of the limb.

2 The limb should be marked afresh on each measuring occasion with a washable ink, even when measuring on consecutive days. Any increase or decrease in limb volume will influence the position of the marks on the limb.

3 Tension should not be exerted on the tape measure during measuring. If tension is applied it will vary between measurers and recordings will not be consistent.

4 The tape measure should be positioned so that it is horizontal around the limb, taking care to ensure that it is not pulled tightly.

5 The same number of measurements should be taken on both limbs each time measurements are taken. The normal limb would not be expected to change significantly in volume except following vigorous exercise or where there has been weight loss or gain; therefore the normal limb acts as a control in patients with unilateral swelling.

6 The starting point for the taking of measurements should be clearly identified by measuring and clearly recording the distance from the tip of the middle finger to the wrist. This starting point on the wrist should be used each time.

7 A standard format for the recording of measurements should be adopted to ensure that key points can be referred to.

Once measurement of the limb has been completed, a number of formulae may be used to calculate the limb

The formula for calculating the volume of a cylinder is $\dfrac{\text{circumference}^2}{\pi}$. The formula must be applied to each circumference measurement ($circ_1$, $circ_2$, ... $circ_n$) in order to calculate the volume of each segment; the volumes are totalled to give the total limb volume.

So $\left(\dfrac{circ_1 \times circ_1}{3.1415}\right) + \left(\dfrac{circ_2 \times circ_2}{3.1415}\right) + \left(\dfrac{circ_3 \times circ_3}{3.1415}\right)$
$+ \ldots$ etc.

Use of a programmable calculator will speed up the process of calculation.

Figure 17.1 Procedure for calculating volume from circumferences.

volume (Sitzia 1995; Badger 1997). The formula for the volume of a cylinder (Fig. 17.1) considers the limb as a series of cylinders, each with a height of 4 cm, and limb volume is calculated by totalling the volume of each section.

Procedure guidelines: **Calculation of limb volume**

Equipment

1 Ruler, preferably 30 cm or longer.
2 Tape measure; avoid those made from fabric which tends to stretch.

3 Felt-tip pen for marking the limb.
4 Record chart and pen.

Procedure for measuring lower limbs

Action	Rationale
1 Place the patient in a sitting position with the legs outstretched horizontally, preferably on a firm couch with adjustable height.	The lower limbs are relaxed and supported and the adjustable height means that the measurer can work without straining their back.
2 Standing on the outside of the leg, ask the patient to flex the foot to a right angle. Measure the distance from the base of the heel to the ankle, along the inside of the leg; mark the ankle, allowing at least 2 cm of leg to lie below the mark, and record the distance on the chart.	This establishes a reproducible fixed starting point for all subsequent measurements. *Note*: the marks represent a point midway through each cylinder segment, they do not represent the base of the cylinder, therefore at least half the segment (i.e. 2 cm) must lie below the mark.
3 Ask the patient to relax the foot. From the starting point mark the inside of the leg at 4 cm intervals along the length of the leg up to the groin; use the ruler for this.	Reducing the limb to 4 cm segments improves the accuracy of measurement since these segments resemble a cylinder more closely than does the whole limb. The formula used here assumes that the measurements are 4 cm apart.
4 Place the tape measure around the limb and measure the circumference at each marked point, recording each measurement on the chart. Make sure that the tape lies smoothly around the relaxed limb and that it does not lie at an angle. Decide at the outset whether the tape is to be placed above, below or on the mark and keep to the same position every time.	Ensuring that there are no gaps between the limb and the tape and ensuring that the procedure is the same each time reduces error.

*Procedure guidelines: **Calculation of limb volume** (cont'd)*

Action	Rationale
5 Repeat the process on the other leg, whether or not it is swollen.	If only one limb is affected the normal limb acts as the patient's own control.
6 If desired, a circumference measurement may be taken of the foot but this is *not* included in the calculation of volume.	The foot cannot be considered to be a cylinder and it is therefore inappropriate to include it in the calculation of volume.

Procedure for measuring upper limbs

Action	Rationale
1 Sit the patient in a chair with the arms extended in front and resting on the back of a chair. The arms should be as close to an angle of 90° to the body as possible.	The arms are supported and accessible at a standard height. Changing the angle of the arms to the body will result in changes in the measurements.
2 Measure the distance from the tip of the middle finger to the wrist. Mark the wrist, allowing at least 2 cm from where the hand joins the arm, and note down the distance.	This establishes a reproducible fixed starting point for all subsequent measurements. *Note*: The marks represent a point midway through each cylinder segment, they do not represent the base of the cylinder, therefore at least half the segment (i.e. 2 cm) must lie below the mark.
3 From the starting point mark along the inside length of the arm at 4 cm intervals up to the axilla; use the ruler for this.	Reducing the limb to 4 cm segments improves the accuracy of measurement since these segments resemble a cylinder more closely than does the whole limb.
4 Place the tape measure around the limb and measure the circumference at each marked point, recording each measurement on the chart. Make sure that the tape lies smoothly around the relaxed limb and that it does not lie at an angle. Decide at the outset whether the tape is to be placed above, below or on the mark and keep to the same position every time.	Ensuring that there are no gaps between the limb and the tape and ensuring that the procedure is the same each time reduces error.
5 Repeat the process on the other arm whether or not it is swollen.	If only one limb is affected the normal limb acts as the patient's own control.
6 If desired, a circumference measurement may be taken of the hand but this is *not* included in the calculation of volume.	The hand cannot be considered to be a cylinder and it is therefore inappropriate to include it in the calculation.

Phases of treatment

Treatment of lymphoedema can be approached in two phases: the maintenance phase and the intensive phase (Jenns 2000).

During the maintenance phase, the concept of self-care is promoted to encourage the patient to become independent in the long-term management and control of their swelling. Elastic compression garments are used and the therapist evaluates progress at regular intervals to ensure that they remain appropriate and that any problems can be identified at an early stage.

The intensive phase of treatment is a short, planned period of therapist-led treatment in which specific aims are identified and agreed between the patient and the therapist. Low-stretch bandages provide support to the swollen limb and are usually reapplied daily during a specified period of time.

Not all patients will follow both phases of treatment and many may only need to follow the maintenance phase.

Maintenance phase of treatment

Indications

Elastic compression garments are used during the maintenance phase of lymphoedema management in order to control limb swelling or to maintain a reduction in limb size following bandaging. They are usually combined with other elements of treatment including:

- A skin-care regimen to minimize the risks of infection
- Exercise to promote lymph drainage
- Massage to stimulate lymph drainage.

Elastic compression garments are most effective when patients have mild, uncomplicated swelling. They can also be used to control swelling and to provide support in the palliative treatment of oedema.

Contraindications

Elastic compression garments should not be used where there is:

- Arterial disease; blood supply may be further compromised.
- Distortion of limb shape; the garment will not fit.
- Skin folds; the garment will cause ridges and a tourniquet effect to the limb.
- Open wounds; the garment will become soiled and pose an infection risk.
- Fragile skin; application and removal of the garment may cause further damage to the skin.
- Lymphorrhoea; the garment will become wet and may cause skin excoriation.
- An acute infective episode (cellulitis); application and removal of the garment may be painful and cause damage to the friable skin.

Choosing elastic compression garments

The choice and fitting of an elastic compression garment should follow a detailed assessment of the patient (Eagle 2001) and should only be attempted by a health care professional with knowledge and appropriate skills to ensure patient safety.

A wide range of garments are available in different styles, materials and compression classes. Garments are manufactured as either round knit or flat knit. Round-knit garments, produced in one piece, are readily available in a variety of sizes 'off the shelf' and accommodate the needs of most patients. Flat-knit or 'made to measure' garments are suited to patients with specific needs and require accurate measurements to be taken to ensure a good fit. Consideration of the patient's ability must be taken into account when choosing a garment as a high degree of dexterity and strength may be required during its application and removal and this may be impractical for the patient.

Elastic compression garments are made in a number of compression classes and in lymphoedema management are usually provided in a compression class of an International Standard. These strong compression class garments are only available through a hospital or specialist orthotic supplier. Some compression stockings of a lower compression, made to British Standard specification, are available on prescription (FP10) but are generally of a lower compression than that required to treat

Table 17.1 British and continental standard compression class (in mmHg) measured at the ankle

Compression class	British standard	Continental standard
1	14–17	18.4–21.1
2	18–24	25.2–32.3
3	25–35	36.5–46.6

lymphoedema (Table 17.1). The highest compression provided by a garment when fitted can be found at the wrist or the ankle. The compression is then graduated along the length of the limb to encourage movement of the fluid out of the limb.

All areas influenced by swelling must be contained within the compression garment or further swelling will develop. Once fitted, the garment should feel comfortable and supportive, not tight and restrictive. The patient should be instructed concerning the application, removal and care of the garment to ensure that maximum effectiveness is achieved through its use.

Intensive phase of treatment

The intensive or reduction phase of treatment should always be carried out by a skilled therapist with the necessary skills and experience to apply bandages to the swollen limb, ensuring that pressure is graduated towards the root of the limb and evenly applied (Hampton 1998). Damage to the skin and tissues can occur if the bandages are incorrectly or inappropriately applied (Thomas & Nelson 1998).

Indications

The intensive phase of treatment is usually carried out for a short specified period of 2–3 weeks, necessitating daily bandaging of the swollen limb. Indications for this phase of treatment include:

- Large limbs: containment hosiery used on large swollen limbs may be ineffective due to the difficulties of applying sufficient tension to compress the limb (Stillwell 1973).
- Misshapen limbs: containment hosiery will promote the development of deep skin folds when the limb is awkwardly shaped. Foam or soft padding under bandages will smooth out the folds and restore normal shape to the limb.
- Severe lymphoedema: large limbs with long-standing oedema require high pressures to break down tissue fibrosis. Bandages provide a low resting and high active pressure which enables hardened tissues to soften.

- Lymphorrhoea: the leakage of lymph fluid from the skin responds readily to external pressure provided by bandages.
- Damaged or fragile skin: containment hosiery can cause damage to fragile skin. Bandages should be used until the skin condition improves.

Palliative care

Bandaging can be versatile and extremely useful in the palliative care setting when volume reduction may be unrealistic or not indicated. Support and comfort can be provided to a limb using a low level of pressure with a modified technique of bandaging designed around the patient's needs. The bandages can be left in place for 2–3 days and should not prevent the patient from maintaining full movement in their bandaged limb (Woods 2000b).

Preparation of the patient

The bandaging materials used on a swollen limb can be bulky and patients will therefore require appropriate information and advice concerning suitable clothing and footwear, which will accommodate the bulk of the bandages during the course of treatment. As the bandages are worn for 24 hours a day, advice will also be required concerning personal hygiene. The timing of appointments for the bandages to be replaced may need to consider opportunities to attend to personal hygiene and accommodate family and work commitments. The therapist should also discuss and outline with the patient an appropriate exercise regimen to be followed during the course of treatment, to ensure that maximum effectiveness is gained from the course of bandaging.

Verbal information given should be supported by written information and include details of what the patient should do if problems develop with the bandages and who to contact.

Principles to be followed in multilayer bandaging

Low-stretch bandages should always be used. These provide a low resting pressure to the swollen limb when the muscle is inactive and a high working pressure during activity when the muscle is pumping against the resistance created by the bandage (Todd 2000).

For bandaging to be effective the following principles must be considered.

- *An even pressure should be provided around the circumference of the limb*. Where the limb shape is irregular or distorted by swelling, an even profile can be achieved with the use of padding or foam to add bulk to an area where shape requires correcting.
- *The pressure from the bandages must be graduated along the length of the limb to ensure that the most pressure is achieved distally and the least proximally*. Graduated pressure will be achieved naturally in a regularly shaped limb where the circumference of the wrist or ankle is smaller than the circumference of the root of the limb. Graduated pressure can also be achieved by selecting the correct bandage width for the size of the limb and controlling the amount of bandage tension and overlap used. Moderate tension only should be used and the bandages should never be stretched to their maximum length.
- *The pressure applied to the limb should be adequate to counter the limb circumference*. Greater pressure is required when the circumference of the limb is large. This can be achieved by using more than one layer of bandages and selecting the correct width of bandage for the circumference of the limb.

The bandages should be left in place day and night and removed once every 24 hours. This enables skin hygiene to be attended to and the condition of the skin to be checked. Reapplication of the bandages then ensures that effective compression is maintained on the changing limb shape (Todd 2000).

The bandages should be comfortable for the patient and removed at any time if they cause any pain, numbness or discoloration (blueness) in the fingers or toes. This may indicate a variety of causes including too great a compression on the limb. A satisfactory outcome of treatment should be achieved within 2–3 weeks. The patient may then begin the maintenance phase of treatment where containment hosiery is fitted.

Evaluation of the bandaging procedure

Evaluation of each stage of the bandaging procedure is essential to ensure that the bandage and padding have been used appropriately and correctly.

The process of evaluation must be thorough and exhaustive and should include:

1 Continuous attention to the colour of the digits. Too much pressure will result in compromised circulation.
2 Continuous attention to the sensations experienced in the bandaged limb. The bandages should not cause pain, numbness or tingling.
3 The shape of the limb. A cylindrical contour should be achieved with the use of soft foam and padding.

4 The overlap of the bandages. This should be even and consistent with no gaps in the bandages.

5 The pressure achieved. This should feel even to the patient and there should be no creases in the bandages. Layers should be used appropriately.

Patient evaluation

The patient should feel comfortable and able to move their limb. Information should be given concerning when and how to remove the bandages if necessary.

Procedure guidelines: **The application of elastic compression garments**

The application of elastic garments can be greatly eased by the wearing of household rubber gloves during application which facilitate control of the garment and prevent damage to the fabric of the garment. Application aids are also available commercially and may assist some patients who experience difficulties. Any moisturizing cream should be applied at night-time rather than in the morning before putting the garment on. A very fine layer of talcum powder applied to hot sticky skin can ease application. If this is the first time that the patient has worn elastic compression garments, the therapist should explain to the patient that the feeling of pressure may feel strange for the first few hours, but that it should not cause pain in the limb or numbness in the digits or toes.

Procedure for applying elastic compression garments to the leg

Action	Rationale
1 Explain and discuss the procedure with the patient.	To ensure that the patient understands the procedure and gives his/her valid consent.
2 If possible, position the patient seated upright on a bed or couch and raise the height to a comfortable level.	To ensure the comfort of both the patient and nurse.
3 Turn the stocking inside-out to the heel.	This makes it easier to ease the stocking up.
4 Pull the foot of the stocking over the patient's foot.	
5 Turn the rest of the stocking back over the foot and up the leg.	
6 Ask the patient to keep the leg straight and if possible to push against the nurse.	
7 Starting at the foot, gradually ease the stocking into place over the heel and up the leg a bit at a time, until it is in its final position.	Since it is the material of the stocking that provides the pressure, it must be distributed evenly to ensure an even distribution of pressure.
8 Do not pull from the top.	This will cause the stocking top to become overstretched and will lead to an uneven distribution of the stocking material.
9 Once the stocking is in place, check that there are no creases or wrinkles, particularly around the joints.	Wrinkles cause chafing of the skin and constricting bands of pressure.
10 Check that the patient finds the stocking comfortable and ask that any feelings of pain, tingling or numbness be reported.	Pain, tingling or numbness indicates that the stocking has been either inappropriately applied or fitted.
11 To remove the stocking, peel the stocking off the limb from the top downwards. Do not roll it down.	Rolling the stocking can result in tight bands of material forming, which are difficult to move.

Procedure for applying elastic compression garments to the arm

Action	Rationale
1 Explain and discuss the procedure with the patient.	To ensure that the patient understands the procedure and gives his/her valid consent.
2 The patient may be seated or standing.	
3 Turn the sleeve inside-out to the wrist. Pull over the patient's hand. *Note*: if a glove or separate handpiece is worn, always put the sleeve on *after* the glove or handpiece.	To avoid increasing swelling in the hand.

Procedure guidelines: **The application of elastic compression garments** *(cont'd)*

Action	Rationale
4 Turn the rest of the sleeve back over the hand and up the arm.	
5 Ask the patient to grip something stable, such as a towel rail or the back of a chair.	This steadies the arm and gives the patient something to pull against.
6 Working from the hand or wrist, gradually ease the sleeve up the arm.	Since it is the material that provides the pressure, it must be evenly distributed to ensure an even distribution of pressure.
7 Do not pull up from the top.	This will cause the top to become overstretched and will result in an uneven distribution of pressure.
8 Once the sleeve is in place, check that there are no creases or wrinkles, particularly around the joints.	Wrinkles and creases cause chafing of the skin and constricting bands of pressure.
9 Check that the patient finds the sleeve comfortable and ask that any signs of pain, tingling or numbness be reported.	Pain, tingling or numbness indicate that the sleeve has been either inappropriately applied or fitted.
10 To remove the sleeve, peel the sleeve off the limb from the top. Do not roll it down.	Rolling the sleeve down can lead to tight bands of material forming which are difficult to move.

Procedure guidelines: **Standard multilayer compression bandaging**

This procedure should not be attempted by anyone who has not had specialist education in this area. The swollen limb should be clean and well moisturized with a bland cream (e.g. E45) before being bandaged. Pressure must be applied in a graduated profile, i.e. highest over the hand or foot, and gradually reducing as the limb is bandaged upwards, to ensure that fluid is encouraged to drain towards the root of the limb.

Thus, on a normally shaped limb, maintaining the same amount of bandage tension and the same amount of bandage overlap all the way up the limb will result in a natural graduation of pressure due to the gradual increase in the size of the limb from ankle to groin, or wrist to axilla. In cases where swelling has distorted the shape of the limb, additional padding is used to create a suitable profile on which to bandage, and adjustments may be needed in bandage tension and bandage overlap. Very large limbs may also require extra layers of bandage to be used in order to ensure that sufficient pressure is applied.

Equipment for bandaging an arm

1 Tubular stockinette.
2 Light retention bandages, 6 and 10 cm to bandage digits and to hold foam padding in place.
3 Padding, 6 cm roll.
4 Sheet of low-density foam.
5 Low-stretch bandages, 6 and 8 cm.
6 Tape.
7 Scissors.

Procedure

Action	Rationale
1 Explain and discuss the procedure with the patient.	To ensure that the patient understands the procedure and gives his/her valid consent.
2 If possible, the patient should be seated in a chair. The nurse should be positioned in front of the patient.	To ensure the comfort of both the patient and nurse.
3 Cut a length of tubular stockinette long enough to fit the patient's arm. Cut a small hole for the thumb and slip over the patient's arm.	To protect the skin from chafing.
4 The fingers must be bandaged (Fig. 17.2). Using a narrow light retention bandage anchor the bandage loosely at the wrist and bring across the back of the hand to the thumb. Bandage around the thumb from the tip downwards (start at the level of the nail bed). Do not pull the bandage tight but go gently and firmly.	To reduce or prevent swelling.

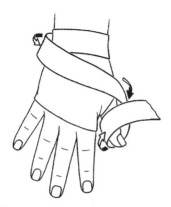

Figure 17.2 Bandaging swollen fingers.

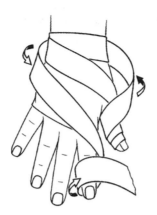

Figure 17.3 Bandage is taken under wrist, back over hand, to index finger.

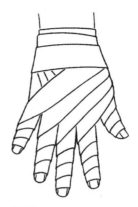

Figure 17.4 Finished bandage.

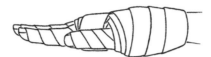

Figure 17.5 Palm and back of hand are padded out.

*Procedure guidelines: **Standard multilayer compression bandaging** (cont'd)*

Action	Rationale
Take the bandage under the wrist and back over the back of the hand to the index finger (Fig. 17.3). Again, bandage from the nail bed down to the webs of the finger. Repeat the same procedure for all fingers. Finish by tucking in the end of the bandage (Fig. 17.4).	
5 Check the colour and temperature of the tips of the fingers.	To ensure that the blood supply is not compromised.
6 Check that the patient can move the fingers and make a fist.	To check that the bandage is not too tight.
7 Using the roll of padding, cover the hand in a figure of eight, padding out the palm and back of the hand (Fig. 17.5).	Padding out the hand ensures even pressure distribution and protects the bony areas of the hand.
8 Using foam and padding, even out any exaggerated contours of the limb.	To create a smooth profile on which to apply the bandage.
9 Cut foam to fit the length of the arm from the wrist to axilla. Ensure that the width is sufficient to encircle the arm with a small overlap.	To protect the elbow joint and provide a smooth, even profile on which to bandage.
10 Wrap the foam around the arm, securing with a light retention bandage. Finish by tucking in the end of the bandage (Fig. 17.6).	
11 Take a 6 cm compression bandage and start by anchoring it loosely at the wrist. Advise the patient to hold their fingers apart whilst the hand is bandaged and take the bandage across the dorsum of the hand to wrap it twice around the hand close to the base of the fingers. Continue bandaging the hand firmly in a figure of eight until all of the hand is covered (Fig. 17.7).	To avoid constriction at the wrist.

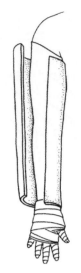

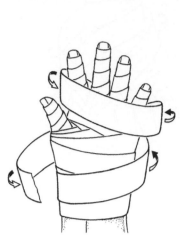

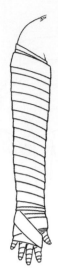

Figure 17.6 Foam is wrapped around arm, secured with a light retention bandage.

Figure 17.7 Hand is bandaged firmly in a figure of eight using a 6 cm compression bandage.

Figure 17.8 Starting at wrist, an 8 or 10 cm bandage is used to cover to top of arm, in a spiral fashion.

*Procedure guidelines: **Standard multilayer compression bandaging** (cont'd)*

Action	Rationale
Continue the rest of the bandage up the forearm in a spiral, covering half of the bandage with each turn. Keep the bandage as smooth as possible.	
12 Take an 8 or 10 cm bandage and, starting at the wrist, bandage in a spiral, still covering half of the bandage with each turn, up to the top of the arm (Fig. 17.8).	Two layers are used on the forearm to ensure that pressure is highest distally.
13 Secure the end of the bandage with tape.	
14 Once again, check the colour and sensations of the finger tips and check that the patient can move all joints.	To check that the blood flow is not compromised.
15 Remind the patient to use the limb as normally as possible, to exercise as advised and to remove the bandages if any pain, tingling or numbness is experienced.	To ensure good lymph flow and to prevent complications developing.

Equipment for bandaging a leg

1 Tubular stockinette.
2 Light retention bandages, 6 and 10 or 12 cm.
3 Padding, 10 and 20 cm.
4 Sheet of low-density foam.

5 Low-stretch compression bandages, 8, 10 and 12 cm.
6 Tape.
7 Scissors.

Procedure for bandaging a leg and the toes

Action	Rationale
1 Explain and discuss the procedure with the patient.	To ensure that the patient understands the procedure and gives his/her valid consent.
2 If possible, the patient should be seated upright on a bed or treatment couch. Raise the bed or couch to a comfortable height.	To ensure the comfort of both the patient and nurse.

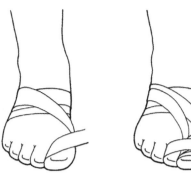

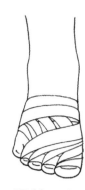

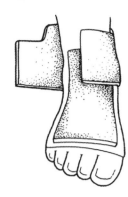

Figure 17.9   **Figure 17.10**   **Figure 17.11**   **Figure 17.12** Foam is used to cover dorsum of foot and around ankle.

*Procedure guidelines: **Standard multilayer compression bandaging** (cont'd)*

Action	Rationale
3 Cut a length of tubular stockinette long enough to fit the patient's leg. Slip over the leg.	To protect the skin from chafing.
4 If the toes are swollen or have a tendency to swell they must be bandaged. The little toe can be omitted. Using a narrow light retention bandage anchor the bandage around the foot and bring across the top of the foot to the big toe (Fig. 17.9). Bandage around the toe from the tip downwards (start at the level of the nail bed). Do not pull the bandage tight, but gently and firmly. Take the bandage under the foot and back over the top of the foot to the next toe (Fig. 17.10). Repeat the same procedure for each toe that needs to be bandaged. Finish by tucking in the end of the bandage (Fig. 17.11).	To reduce or prevent swelling. To prevent friction to and around the little toe.
5 Cut the foam into pads to fit over the dorsum of the foot, around the ankle (Fig. 17.12) and behind the knee (Fig. 17.13).	To protect bony prominences and joint flexures.
6 Secure the pads firmly in place with light retention bandages.	
7 Using foam and padding even out any exaggerated contours of the limb.	To create a smooth profile on which to apply the bandages.
8 Using a 10 cm roll of padding, apply firmly in a spiral up the leg, starting around the foot. Use the 20 cm padding over the thigh (Fig. 17.14).	To protect the skin and create a smooth profile on which to bandage.
9 Take an 8 cm compression bandage and start by anchoring it loosely at the ankle. Advise the patient to hold their foot at a 90° angle whilst it is bandaged and take the bandage across the dorsum of the foot to wrap it around the foot close to the base of the toes (Fig. 17.15). Continue bandaging the foot firmly, forming a figure of eight to cover the heel and ankle without leaving any gaps. Any surplus bandage should be taken up the leg in a spiral.	To avoid constriction at the ankle. Fluid will accumulate in any unbandaged areas.

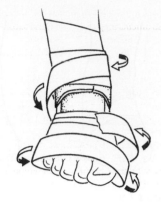

Figure 17.15 Bandaging foot using an 8 cm compression bandage and starting close to toes.

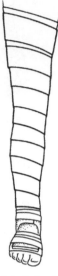

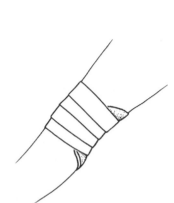

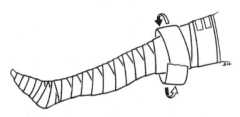

Figure 17.13 A foam pad is bandaged into position behind knee.

Figure 17.14 Rolls of padding are applied firmly in a spiral up leg, starting around foot.

Figure 17.16 Applying a second layer of bandage, from ankle to thigh.

Procedure guidelines: **Standard multilayer compression bandaging** *(cont'd)*

Action	Rationale
10 Using a 10 cm bandage, continue from where the first bandage finished, using a spiral up the leg and covering half of the bandage with each turn. Remember to bandage firmly. Use the widest bandage over the thigh. Secure the end of the last bandage with tape.	
11 Apply a second layer of bandage, from ankle to thigh, using a figure of eight. Secure the end with tape (Fig. 17.16).	To keep the bandages in place and provide additional pressure along the length of the leg.
12 Check the colour and temperature of the patient's toes. It may be difficult for the patient to flex the knee at first but this should get easier as the bandages loosen slightly.	To check that the blood flow is not compromised.
13 Remind the patient to use the limb as normally as possible, to exercise as advised and to remove the bandages if any pain, tingling or numbness is experienced.	To ensure good lymph flow and to prevent complications developing.

References and further reading

Badger, C. (1997) A study of the efficacy of multi-layer bandaging and elastic hosiery in the treatment of lymphoedema and their effects on the swollen limb. PhD thesis, Institute of Cancer Research.

Benner, P. (1984) *From Novice to Expert*. Addison-Wesley, California.

Callam, M.J., Ruckley, C.V., Dale, J.J. *et al.* (1997) Hazards of compression treatment of the leg: an estimate from Scottish surgeons. *Br Med J*, **295**, 1382.

Derdiarian, A. (1990) Effects of using systematic assessment instruments on patient and nurse satisfaction with nursing care. *Oncol Nurs Forum*, **17**(1), 95–101.

Eagle, M. (2001) Compression bandaging. *Nurs Stand*, **15**(38), 47–52.

Engler, H. & Sweat, R. (1962) Volumetric arm measurements: techniques and results. *Am Surg*, **28**, 465–8.

Hampton, S. (1998) Bandage application. In: *Compression Therapy: A Complete Guide*. Journal of Wound Care/EMAP Publishers, London, pp. 5–8.

Jenns, K. (2000) Management strategies. In: *Lymphoedema* (eds R. Twycross, K. Jenns & J. Todd). Radcliffe Medical Press, Oxford.

Keeley, V. (2000) Classification of lymphoedema. In: *Lymphoedema* (eds R. Twycross, K. Jenns & J. Todd). Radcliffe Medical Press, Oxford.

Kettle, J., Rundle, F. & Oddie, T. (1958) Measurement of upper limb volumes: a clinical method. *Aust N Z J Surg*, **27**, 263–70.

Mason, W. (2000) Exploring rehabilitation within lymphoedema management. *Int J Palliat Nurs* **6**(6), 265–73.

Mortimer, P. (2000) Acute inflammatory episodes. In: *Lymphoedema* (eds R. Twycross, K. Jenns & J. Todd). Radcliffe Medical Press, Oxford.

Mortimer, P., Bates, D., Brassington, H. *et al.* (1996) The prevalence of arm oedema following treatment for breast cancer. *Q J Med*, **89**, 377–80.

Sitzia, J. (1995) Volume measurement in lymphoedema treatment: examination of the formulae. *Eur J Cancer Care*, **4**, 11–16.

Stanton, A. (2000) How does tissue swelling occur? The physiology and pathophysiology of interstitial fluid formation. In: *Lymphoedema* (eds R. Twycross, K. Jenns & J. Todd). Radcliffe Medical Press, Oxford.

Stanton, A., Northfield, J., Holroyd, B. *et al.* (1997) Validation of an optoelectronic limb volumeter (Perometer). *Lymphology*, **30**, 77–97.

Stillwell, G. (1973) The Law of Laplace: some clinical applications. *Mayo Clin Proc*, **48**, 863–9.

Thomas, S. & Nelson, A. (1998) Graduated external compression in the treatment of venous disease. In: *Compression Therapy: A Complete Guide*. Journal of Wound Care/EMAP Publishers, London, pp. 1–4.

Tobin, M., Mortimer, P., Meyer, L. *et al.* (1993) The psychological morbidity of breast cancer related arm swelling. *Cancer*, **72**(11), 3348–52.

Todd, J. (2000) Containment in the management of lymphoedema. In: *Lymphoedema* (eds R. Twycross, K. Jenns & J. Todd). Radcliffe Medical Press, Oxford.

Twycross, R., Jenns, K. & Todd, J. (eds) (2000) *Lymphoedema*. Radcliffe Medical Press, Oxford.

Woods, M. (1993) Patients' perceptions of breast-cancer related lymphoedema. *Eur J Cancer Care*, **2**, 125–8.

Woods, M. (1994) An audit of swollen limb measurements. *Nurs Stand*, **9**(5), 24–6.

Woods, M. (2000a) Psychosocial aspects of lymphoedema. In: *Lymphoedema* (eds R. Twycross, K. Jenns & J. Todd). Radcliffe Medical Press, Oxford.

Woods, M. (2000b) Lymphoedema. In: *Stepping into Palliative Care: A Handbook for Community Professionals* (ed. J. Cooper). Radcliffe Medical Press, Oxford.

Woods, M., Tobin, M. & Mortimer, P. (1995) The psychological morbidity of breast cancer patients with lymphoedema. *Cancer Nurs*, **18**(6), 467–71.

18

Gene therapy for the management of cancer

Chapter contents

Definition

Gene therapy is the insertion, augmentation or substitution of a functioning gene into a cell to provide the cell with a new function, which will correct a genetic disorder, e.g. cystic fibrosis (Greisenbach *et al.* 2002) or correct a malformation to achieve a therapeutic effect (Palu *et al.* 1999; Barzon *et al.* 2000). In the case of cancer, the aim of gene therapy is to eliminate the malignant cell (Searle *et al.* 2002).

Reference material

Normal cells contain the mechanisms to repair damage to the genetic material. Cancer can occur when such mechanisms are absent or fail to protect against genetic error through cell division. This failure allows multiplication of abnormal cells, invasion of local tissue and ultimately distant metastases (Trahan Rieger 1997). The overall goal of gene therapy is to improve health by correcting the gene alteration in affected cells (Lea 1997).

The process by which genes are inserted, augmented or substituted into a cell is termed genetic modification. Genetic modification in relation to an organism means the altering of the genetic material by a method which does not occur naturally. Essentially, this means that in order for genetic modification to have occurred, there must be a change to an organism's genetic material using a method not based on mating or natural recombination (HSE 2000a). Genetic modification as part of human gene therapy activities takes the form of *ex vivo* (outside body) or *in vivo* (inside body) therapy. *Ex vivo* gene therapy is achieved by introducing the gene into the patient's cells in the laboratory and reinfusing them into the patient. *In vivo* describes the direct administration of the genetic material into the patient using an appropriate delivery system such as a virus, by methods such as injections or infusion (Sandhu *et al.* 1997).

Genetic modification involves the manipulation of nucleic acid and, in particular, DNA. Molecules of DNA contain information for cellular structure and function. Every cell in an organism contains a complete set of genes, 'the genome', which are found on chromosomes. Gene therapy involves ascertaining which gene controls which inherited feature, and then introducing, deleting or enhancing a particular trait in an organism, by altering its genetic composition. In most cases this involves extracting DNA from one organism, manipulating or restructuring it and then transferring it into another organism. Transfer usually takes place by attaching the gene of interest to another DNA carrier (vector). The most commonly used vectors are plasmids and genetically modified viruses (Galanis *et al.* 2001; Cemazar *et al.* 2002).

For example, one of the best viruses in terms of its potential ability to deliver therapeutic genes to cancer cells is the adenovirus (Vorburger & Hunt 2002). Other vectors that have been developed are retroviruses, parvoviruses and herpesviruses (Searle *et al.* 2002). The adenovirus contains DNA and can, therefore, be manipulated to transport a genetically modified gene into any cell it invades. The virus will do no harm as long as genes conferring virulence are removed when the new genes are inserted (Hull & Chester 2002). Genetic modification of the virus means its virulence is reduced and it can no longer replicate, which ensures viral infection cannot occur. The manipulated virus is called an 'attenuated' adenovirus (Kim *et al.* 2002). Viruses are useful as vectors as they are capable of invading living cells and replicating themselves only within the target cell. For example, an adenovirus can be genetically altered in such a way that it assumes command of tumour cells but not healthy ones. The virus replicates in the tumour causing cell death, however healthy non-tumour cells remain unaffected (Trahan Rieger 1997).

There are four potential uses for gene therapy:

1 Enhancement gene transfer, which involves transferring a gene that would enhance or improve a specific desirable trait.
2 Eugenics, which is genetic engineering of society to favour certain desirable human traits (Launis 2002).
3 Somatic cell gene transfer, which places a gene in a body cell other than an egg or sperm cell. Somatic cells are all of the body's non-reproductive cells. They are targets for gene therapy, as they cannot pass on the new trait to the patient's offspring (Nippert 2002).
4 Germline gene transfer, which makes inheritable alterations to egg or sperm cells, which can be passed on to future humans (Lea 1997).

Gene therapy has the potential to be used to treat disorders caused by a defect in a single gene. This may be inherited diseases such as cystic fibrosis, or diseases such as cancer (Bank 1996). Gene therapy is experimental and much is unknown about the immediate and future safety and toxicity effects. The only form of gene therapy currently being used is somatic cell therapy for human clinical trials in patients with incurable diseases.

Gene therapy has the potential to enhance useful properties or reduce unwanted properties of the genes being used. There are many different approaches to the choice of the genes. Examples include:

- Tumour suppressor genes: if the tumour suppressor genes that prevent or control abnormal cell growth become mutated, the cells may grow uncontrollably and become malignant (Lipinski *et al.* 2001).
- Tumour susceptibility genes: the tumour susceptibility genes are a class of genes which include oncogenes, tumour suppressor genes and DNA repair genes, that predispose an organism to the development of tumours (Loud *et al.* 2002).

The goal of traditional cancer treatments is to eliminate cancer cells, however during this process many normal cells may also be eliminated. Gene therapy is a novel therapeutic approach that targets disease directly at the molecular and cellular levels and is expected to be less toxic than traditional treatments such as chemotherapy and radiotherapy. Gene therapy allows for the modification of cancer cells using gene transfer, either to enhance host immunity or to act directly on cancer cells (Descamp *et al.* 1996). Gene therapy should therefore improve the quality of life for the patient with cancer. However, gene therapy research is still in its infancy and it is, therefore, too early to identify benefits (Marchisone *et al.* 2000).

Regulatory controls for gene therapy

All work with genetically modified organisms (GMO), including gene therapy, is controlled by the following regulations, the majority of which focus on safety. For example:

1 *The Genetically Modified Organisms (Contained Use) Regulations* (HSE 2000). These regulations implement the requirements of the EC Directive 8/81/EC on the contained use of genetically modified organisms. The regulations have been made under the powers of the Health and Safety at Work etc. Act (1974) and European Directive 98/81/EC (1998). The regulations are concerned with protecting both human health and the environment and are designed to ensure the safe use and handling of genetically

modified organisms under containment. 'Contained use' means any operation in which organisms are genetically modified or in which such genetically modified organisms are cultured, stored, used, transported, destroyed or disposed of and for which physical barriers, or a combination of physical barriers with chemical or biological barriers or both, are used to limit their contact with the general population and the environment (HSE 2000).

2 *The Control of Substances Hazardous to Health Regulations* (HSE 1999). These regulations require formal risk assessments and appropriate control measures to be provided in order to reduce potential health risks to those working with the genetically modified organisms. Information on the classification of genetically modified biological agents is provided within the Health and Safety Commission Advisory Committee on Genetic Modification (ACGM) Compendium of Guidance (HSC/ACGM 2000).

3 *The Management of Health and Safety at Work Regulations (1999)* requires a suitable and sufficient assessment of the risk to the health and safety of employees to which they are exposed at work, and of the risk to others arising out of their work activities.

4 *The Genetically Modified Organisms (Deliberate Release and Risk Assessment – Amendment) Regulations* (HSE 1997) deal with the deliberate release into the environment of genetically modified organisms to ensure adverse effects to the environment do not occur.

5 The use of viral vectors for gene therapy requires rigorous control of production and safety testing methods. Approval from the Medicines Control Agency and the Gene Therapy Advisory Committee (GTAC) should be obtained before any gene therapy research is attempted on humans (HSE 2000).

6 Other legislation that has a bearing on work with genetically modified organisms includes the Medicine Acts 1971 and 1968; European Council Regulations No. (EEC) 2309/93, The Personal Protection Equipment Regulations 1992 and part I of the Environmental Protection Act (EPA) 1990.

Regulation requirements

The main requirement of the Genetically Modified Organisms (Contained Use) Regulations (HSE 2000) is to ensure that exposure and harm to humans and the environment by GMO are reduced to the lowest level reasonably possible.

In order to do so, the regulations require organizations undertaking gene therapy to:

1 Establish a local Genetic Modification Safety Committee. All risk assessments for work with genetically

modified organisms must to be formally discussed and approved by the local Genetic Modification Safety Committee. It should be noted that research treatments such as gene therapy also need to be formally agreed by the health care organization's own local research ethics committee and by the Department of Health's Gene Therapy Advisory Committee (GTAC). The Gene Modification Safety Committee should have representation from all staff groups involved in GMO work within the organization. For health care activities this is likely to include medical, nursing, laboratory, facilities and ancillary staff representatives.

2 Appoint a Biological Safety Officer (BSO) or other suitably qualified competent person to offer specialist advice on gene modification risk assessment and containment.

3 Carry out risk assessments to assess the risks to human health and to the environment.

4 Record the risk assessment and identify appropriate containment measures required.

5 Submit advanced notification to the Health and Safety Executive (HSE) of an intention to use premises for genetic modification purposes and in certain circumstances receive HSE consent before work can start. Consideration of the recipient, the nature, activity and function of the vector, the inserted sequence, and the overall combination of host, vector and insert will need to be made before categorization can be decided. Establish the appropriate classification for the activity.

6 Notify the HSE of an intention to use premises for the first time for genetic modification activity. Subsequent notifications will then be dependent on the classification of activities undertaken.

7 Implement standards of occupational and environmental safety and levels of containment appropriate to the level of risk.

8 Identify emergency plans for dealing with adverse events involving GMO, e.g. spillage procedures.

9 Establish and implement procedures for the notification of adverse incidents associated with genetic modification activities.

The Genetically Modified Organisms (Contained Use) Regulations (2000) and the Control of Substances Hazardous to Health Regulations (1999) are enforced by the HSE. Failure to comply can lead to enforcement action and/or prosecution.

Classification

The Genetically Modified Organisms (Contained Use) Regulations (HSE 2000) require all activities involving genetically modified organisms to be classified into one of four classes, referred to as class 1, 2, 3 or 4. Classification depends on:

- Risk assessment factors such as the potential harmful effects of the genetically modified organisms to humans and/or the environment
- The characteristics of the proposed activity and the severity of any potential harmful effects
- The likelihood of harmful effects occurring and the level of containment required (HSE 2000).

To assist in the determination of the appropriate classification, reference should be made to guidance contained in Schedules 3, 4, 7 and 8 of the Genetically Modified (Contained Use) Regulations (HSE 2000). Further advice is available from the Health and Safety Commission Advisory Committee on Genetic Modification (ACGM) *Compendium of Guidance* 2000.

Risk assessments

One of the most important features of the Genetically Modified Organisms (Contained Use) Regulations (2000) is that a risk assessment must be made before any genetic modification work is undertaken. The risk assessment process must involve the classification of the genetically modified organism involved and identify the safety measures required to reduce the risk of exposure of humans and the environment to a genetically modified organism, to the lowest level reasonably practicable (HSE 2000).

Each individual risk assessment will, therefore, vary. However, each risk assessment should identify:

- The hazards of the activity
- The likelihood that the activity will give rise to harm (i.e. an accident, injury, ill-health or infection)
- The appropriate containment levels required and associated safety control measures
- The procedures for the inactivation of any waste materials produced as a result of the genetic modification activity
- The emergency plans in place to ensure safety in the event of a foreseeable accident occurring during the activity
- The appropriate level of training required for all personnel involved in the identified GMO activity
- Decontamination procedures
- Storage procedures for GMO materials.

The assessment should consider any hazards associated with the vector's pathogenicity, the inserted gene product, the area of use and the survivability of the organism in the environment. In addition, with respect to gene therapy, the risk assessment should consider possible risks to the patients receiving the treatment, other patients and visitors in the treatment area and to health care workers and others likely to come in contact with the genetically modified organism and/or the gene therapy patient.

Once the written risk assessment has been completed (usually by the principal investigator for the study) a copy must be reviewed and approved by the local Genetic Modification Safety Committee.

Standard operating procedures

Safety operating procedures must be prepared for all areas and staff involved in the gene therapy study. This would include areas involved in preparing and administering the therapy, those involved in diagnostic investigation following the administration of the therapy and those involved in the general care of the patient. Safety procedures for staff involved in ancillary tasks such as cleaning and waste disposal tasks should also be completed under the requirements of the Genetically Modified Organisms (Contained Use) Regulations (HSE 2000). The safety procedure documentation must reflect the safe practices necessary for the specified gene therapy protocol and identify responsibilities for compliance in each of the work areas identified.

The structure of the safety documentation should essentially include:

- A preamble, which describes the protocol and the genetically modified organism involved and the level of risk to those potentially affected by the work activity
- Storage and preparation procedures
- Administration precautions for pharmacy staff
- Safety procedures for staff involved in the care of the patient requiring gene therapy
- Safety procedures for transportation, analysis, packaging, storage and disposal of all biological samples and specimens taken during the gene therapy treatment period
- Waste disposal procedures
- Action to be taken for decontamination of spills of the genetically modified organisms
- Action to be followed for accidental exposure of staff, visitors and other patients to genetically modified organisms
- Arrangements for staff training (HSE 2000).

Nursing care

Potential safety issues include the immediate and long-term complications of gene therapy to the health care worker, patient, visitors and other patients. There is no current information related to the risk of health care workers to genetically modified organisms and no severe toxicity has been seen related to gene therapy (Lea 1997). However, studies are limited at this stage and, therefore, strict safety precautions must be observed at all times.

Current standards of safe practice are as follows:

1 The patient receiving gene therapy must be admitted into a single room with en-suite facilities. This room will have previously been agreed by the local Genetic Modification Safety Committee as suitable, when the protocol and risk assessment documentation was undertaken. Consideration may need to be given to the appropriateness of the ward to be used depending on the patient population and potential health issues associated with the vector used.

2 Negative pressure air conditioning is an advantage in eliminating any airborne contamination, but is not essential.

3 Only those persons who are providing direct patient care should enter the room during the treatment period.

4 Nursing staff should observe barrier nursing principles and ensure appropriate protective clothing is worn, i.e. water-repellent gown, gloves, respiratory face mask, safety goggles or spectacles, plus overshoes if contamination has occurred (see Ch. 5, Barrier nursing).

5 Hand washing procedures should be observed before entering and when leaving the patient's room (see Ch. 4, Aseptic technique).

6 In some cases the gene therapy can be administered to patients in the outpatient setting. The therapy should be administered in a room in outpatients or the day care department which has been approved previously as suitable. Although these patients are receiving their therapy on an outpatient basis, the restrictions and segregation that are adopted for inpatients are employed in the outpatient setting. The patient should be instructed to go directly to the designated room upon arriving at the hospital. In some cases a respiratory face mask may need to be worn by the patient on entering the hospital and removed on leaving the site. This requirement highlights the need to protect vulnerable patients within the hospital setting.

7 While genetic modification of the vector ensures that the virulence of the vector is reduced, microbiological monitoring of blood and body fluids is required to ensure that the patient is no longer excreting the vector, before barrier nursing restrictions can be reduced (Young 1997).

Gene therapy is still in its early stages of development (Wivel & Wilson 1998). However, there is a need for nurses to appreciate the importance that gene therapy may play in cancer prevention and control in the future (Peters 1997). Nurses must have a fundamental understanding of immunology, the administration (Loud *et al.* 2002) and the risks and potential benefits of gene therapy (Evans & Lahoti 2000). They must also be familiar with the gene therapy protocol to be able to provide help, support, education and advice to the patients and their families and at the same time good clinical care (Lea 1997). Anxiety and fatigue may result from being included in a treatment trial. Patients may also experience reduced levels of concentration and therefore the nurse may need to repeat instructions and provide encouragement during the treatment period (Jenkins *et al.* 1994). Continual observations are essential to identify toxicities as soon as possible.

In a survey carried out by Jenkins *et al.* (1994), which investigated the public's perception of gene therapy, it was found that the potential benefits were thought to be cure, prevention of genetic disease, disease control, medical advance and overall benefit to humanity worldwide. However, this survey group also expressed concerns related to the risk of genetic manipulation, including the danger of error or unethical use.

One concern about the use of viral vectors is that changes in the virus's genetic material could occur which would cause them to revert back to replication competent viruses, which could multiply after administration to the patient and cause a viral infection. Alternatively, retroviruses could insert themselves into the DNA of the patient to cause inactivation of a tumour suppressor gene, or activation of an oncogene, resulting in a malignancy. In addition, an immunological reaction to the viral vector protein may occur. For instance, the immune system may attack and neutralize the virus before it reaches its target (Wilson 1996).

To date, no serious adverse effects have been reported. Strict health and safety and infection control principles must be maintained at all times to reduce the risk of any adverse effect to a level as low as practically possible.

Consent

Currently, patients in the UK enrolled in gene therapy cancer clinical trials have had advanced cancers. The Gene Therapy Advisory Committee (GTAC), which gives approval for gene therapy research conducted on human subjects, carry out a case-by-case assessment with regard to patient group suitability. This assessment includes a review of the possible risks against the possible benefits. The GTAC needs to be convinced that the clinical management of the patient will not be impaired by the requirements of the trial (GTAC 2000).

Patients must be fully informed of the experimental nature of gene therapy treatments (Robinson *et al.* 1996). As much information as is available should be given to the patient in order for them to make an informed decision as to whether they wish to be included in the study or not (Hull & Chester 2002). The patient must sign a consent form (Young 1997) (see Ch. 1, Context of care).

Gene therapy options in the future

Ardern-Jones (1999) discusses how cancer due to inherited genetic factors represents 5–10% of the total cases of cancer. The identification of inherited cancer susceptibility genes and advances in gene therapy technology may, in the future, lead to modification of these genes by gene therapy (Flygenring 1999) to treat or prevent cancer (Vorburger & Hunt 2002). Knowledge gained from the Human Genome Project and related genetic research is already impacting on clinical practice. Oncology nurses are in an ideal situation to incorporate these emerging paradigms into their day-to-day care (Middelton *et al.* 2002).

Procedure guidelines: **Care of patients receiving gene therapy**

Preparation of patient

Action	Rationale
1 Evaluate patient's suitability for treatment.	To ensure patient's physical and psychological status is suitable for treatment and restrictions imposed by treatment.
2 Explain and discuss the procedure with the patient.	To ensure that the patient understands the procedure, which will enable the patient to make an informed decision regarding whether or not to participate in the study, and gives his/her valid consent.
3 Ensure the patient is aware of the barrier nursing restrictions, and the need to remain in the room during the treatment period.	Patients who understand the need for restrictions are more likely to comply and be satisfied with their care.
4 Ensure the relatives and visitors are aware of the reasons why barrier nursing restrictions are required.	In order for relatives to be able to encourage and support the patient during the barrier nursing care.
5 Encourage patients to bring books and entertainment items into the room.	To prevent a feeling of loneliness and boredom.
6 Ensure that all personal items are washable.	In the event of contamination with genetically modified material personal items will need to be cleaned before removal from the room.

Preparation of room

Action	Rationale
1 Room should include a television and video.	To prevent the patient being bored and leaving the single room.
2 Room should be stocked with all necessary equipment. This will include observation equipment.	Equipment used regularly by the patient should be left within the barrier nursing area to prevent possible spread of infection.
3 Place a clinical waste bag on a bag holder in the room.	To contain all waste, including used protective clothing.
4 Place a special waste bin with a biohazard label and a sharps disposal bin in the room.	To ensure immediate and safe disposal of special waste and sharps.
5 Place a specimen carrying box in room.	To store and transport specimens.
6 Put water-repellent gowns, disposable gloves, respiratory face mask with filtering face piece protection level 3 (FFP3), safety goggles or spectacles and overshoes outside the room. Masks and goggles are only required for class 2 GMO activity or when there is the risk of airborne contamination, for example if a patient has a productive cough or a tracheostomy.	To reduce the risk of contamination to clothing, skin, eyes, nose and mouth, and to reduce the risk of inhalation or ingestion of GMO. Staff and visitors are more likely to use the protective clothing if it is readily available.

Procedure guidelines: **Care of patients receiving gene therapy** *(cont'd)*

Action	Rationale
7 Ensure hand wash basin is stocked with bactericidal detergent, paper towels and bactericidal alcoholic handrub.	To ensure hand cleaning is undertaken before and after patient contact.

Entering the room

Action	Rationale
1 Ensure staff and visitors are aware of restrictions related to entering the room.	To ensure compliance with restrictions and ensure non-essential persons do not enter the patient's room.
2 Visitors and staff should be restricted to essential persons only.	To restrict entry to the room to those who are aware of the need to comply to the restrictions.
3 Pregnant staff should seek advice from occupational health staff before they enter the room.	There is no information to suggest there is a risk to the foetus, but as research is limited occupational health should undertake a risk assessment.
4 Young children and babies must not enter the room.	Young persons are unlikely to understand or be able to comply with restrictions.
5 Clean hands with bactericidal alcoholic handrub.	To reduce the risk of cross-infection.
6 Assess the condition of the patient and the room, so that appropriate clothing can be used before entering the room. This will include: (a) Water-repellent gown (b) Disposable gloves (c) Respiratory face mask (FFP3) if airborne contamination is likely to occur (d) Safety goggles or spectacles if airborne contamination is likely to occur (e) Overshoes if contamination of the floor has occurred.	
7 Enter the room and close the door.	To reduce the risk of airborne contamination leaving the room.

Attending to patient

Action	Rationale
1 Serve meals using normal crockery and cutlery.	Nicely prepared and served food will encourage the patient to eat their food.
2 Dispose of any uneaten food in the clinical waste bag in the room.	Food may be contaminated by saliva.
3 Wash used crockery and cutlery immediately in the ward's dishwasher.	Mechanical washing and heat will remove or kill all micro-organisms.
4 Place waste in yellow clinical waste bag. When half full, seal the bag with an identification tie and send for incineration.	Yellow is the recognized colour for clinical waste and this must be incinerated. To prevent contamination of the environment. To prevent overfilling of bag and potential spillage.
5 Label specimens and specimen request cards with a biohazard warning label, double bag in biohazard specimen carrying bag (also labelled by a biohazard warning label) and take to the appropriate laboratory in a washable, sealable box.	To warn laboratory workers of the possible risk. The box and double bag will contain spillages, if the specimen container becomes damaged.

Administration of gene therapy

Action	Rationale
1 Ensure only identified 'designated' staff should be involved in the administration of the gene therapy treatment.	To minimize the number of persons who could become contaminated if an accident occurs during administration of the gene therapy vaccine.

Procedure guidelines: **Care of patients receiving gene therapy** *(cont'd)*

Action	Rationale
2 Staff who directly administer the gene therapy vaccine should attend the occupational health department and, if appropriate, provide a sample of blood which will be stored in a freezer for 40 years.	Occupational health will ensure staff are fit to undertake this task and maintain appropriate health surveillance as required by the COSHH Regulations (1999).
3 Administer the treatment using an aseptic technique. For example, intravenously, subcutaneously, directly into the tumour or via an intraperitoneal catheter (see Ch. 9, Drug administration).	To minimize risk of cross-infection. As far as possible the administration procedures should minimize the potential risk of airborne exposure and/or inoculation.
4 Identify all equipment used to administer gene therapy as clinical waste and autoclave before incineration.	To comply with statutory waste disposal procedures, as there may be small amounts of gene therapy left in the administration equipment.

Accidental inoculation or spillage of gene therapy

Action	Rationale
1 In the event of an inoculation accident or contamination of the health care worker occurring during the administration of gene therapy, immediate action should be: (a) Make the inoculation area bleed. (b) Wash the area thoroughly. (c) Inform the occupational health department. (d) Inform the infection control officer. (e) Complete an accident/incident report form.	To ensure appropriate care is provided. An accident occurring at the time of treatment has increased significance due to the concentrated nature of the gene therapy.
2 Implement the follow-up care for inoculation and contamination accidents at the time of administration, which will be included in the risk assessment documentation.	To ensure that staff are aware of appropriate emergency procedures.
3 In the event of a sharps accident occurring after administration of gene therapy, handle as for routine sharps accidents.	Sharps accidents that occur which are not involved with the administration of gene therapy are not as significant as those that occur when gene therapy is involved, due to the diluted nature of the gene therapy following administration.
4 Clear up spillages using a standard spillage kit containing chlorine releasing tablets.	To contain and remove the contamination.

Readmission following gene therapy

Action	Rationale
1 Barrier nursing restrictions to be reinstated, if patient is readmitted within one week of discharge, until the clinician can reassess the condition of the patient.	The time during which excretion of the gene therapy occurs is unknown, therefore precautions are necessary until a risk assessment shows that barrier nursing is not necessary, i.e. the patient is no longer shedding the gene therapy vector.

Domestic staff

Action	Rationale
1 Thoroughly prepare and clean patient's room prior to the start of the gene therapy treatment.	To provide a pleasant and safe environment for the patient.
2 The room is only cleaned following the administration of the gene therapy, if stated in the risk assessment document.	If contamination of the environment is likely, the domestic staff should not enter the room.
3 The risk assessment will include information concerning the frequency with which the room is to be cleaned.	The domestic manager or supervisor needs to be informed so that the ward domestic is provided with the correct instructions.

*Procedure guidelines: **Care of patients receiving gene therapy** (cont'd)*

Action	Rationale
4 In the event that the risk assessment states the domestic staff may enter the room, cleaning should be undertaken as for guidelines for barrier nursing (see Ch. 5).	Employing barrier nursing principles will reduce risk of contamination of staff and the environment.
5 In the event that the risk assessment states the domestic may not enter the room, the patient should be informed of this before admission and asked to undertake minor cleaning tasks. This may include flushing the toilet with disinfectant after use.	Patients expect their hospital accommodation to be kept clean by the domestic department. Prior warning that this will not occur may help prevent patient dissatisfaction and complaint. To ensure disinfection of the toilet.
6 Following discharge of the patient the room and bathroom should be thoroughly cleaned using a detergent/bleach solution.	To ensure any contamination is removed. Bleach is particularly useful in destroying viruses.
7 Once cleaning is completed, the room can be used as normal.	Cleaning will remove any contamination, making it safe for other patients to be admitted into this area.

Linen

Action	Rationale
1 Place used linen in a red alginate bag, then in an outer red bag.	Red is the recognized colour for foul or infected linen. The laundry will process this type of laundry in a hot barrier wash.

Leaving the room

Action	Rationale
1 If wearing gloves, remove and discard them in the yellow clinical waste bag. Clean hands with bactericidal alcoholic handrub.	To remove pathogenic organisms acquired on the gloves during contact with patient. Hands inside gloves may become contaminated following contact with the patient.
2 Remove apron, overshoes, goggles and mask, taking care not to contaminate skin or clothing. Discard in yellow clinical waste bag. Clean hands with bactericidal alcoholic handrub.	To prevent contamination of pathogenic organisms acquired during contact with patient. Hands may have become contaminated when removing protective clothing.
3 Leave room and shut the door.	To reduce the risk of airborne spread of infection.
4 Clean hands with bactericidal alcoholic handrub.	Hands may have become contaminated from such items as the door handle.

Discontinuing restrictions

Action	Rationale
1 The risk assessment documentation for the trial will state when restrictions can be discontinued. Restrictions are generally discontinued when microbiological sampling shows that the patient is no longer excreting the micro-organism.	For some gene therapy trials it is possible to test the patient to see if they are infected. Early notification can result in a reduction in stringent barrier nursing procedures.

Discharge home

Action	Rationale
1 The patient will be discharged home when the clinician is satisfied that it is safe to do so.	Generally, restrictions are less once the patient is discharged into the community.
2 The patient should be asked to phone the clinician if problems occur following discharge from hospital.	It is essential that the person responsible for the research trial is available for help and advice when problems occur in the community.

Further advice

Health Service Executive (HSE) (2000) *A Guide to the Genetically Modified Organisms (Contained Use) Regulations.* Stationery Office, London.

For advice on general policy or interpretation relating to the Contained Use Regulations 2000 refer to:
Health and Safety Executive (HSE) Health Directorate Division B, Rose Court, 2 Southwalk Bridge, London SE1 9HS.

For advice on writing information leaflets for patients participating in gene therapy research, contact:
Gene Therapy Advisory Committee, Health and Safety Executive.

Latest UK gene therapy research details available from: www.open.gov.uk/doh/genetics/gtac.htm

References and further reading

Ardern-Jones, A. (1999) Developing roles of nursing in cancer prevention: the clinical nurse specialist in cancer genetics. *Oncol Nurs Today*, **4**(2), 11–13.

Bank, A. (1996) Human somatic cell gene therapy. *Bioassays*, **18**(12), 999–1007.

Barzon, L., Bonaguro, R., Palu, G. & Boscaro, M. (2000) New perspectives for gene therapy in endocrinology. *Eur J Endocrinol*, **143**(4), 447–66.

Cemazar, M., Sersa, G., Wilson, J. *et al.* (2002) Effective gene transfer to solid tumors using different nonviral gene delivery techniques: electroporation, liposomes, and integrin-targeted vector. *Cancer Gene Ther*, **9**(4), 399–406.

Descamp, V., Duffour, M.T., Mathieu, M.C. *et al.* (1996) Strategies for cancer gene therapy using adenoviral vectors. *J Mol Med*, **74**(4) 183–9.

Environmental Protection Act (1990). Stationery Office, London.

European Council Regulations No. (EEC) 2309/93. Stationery Office, London.

European Directive (1998) *The Contained Use of Genetically Modified Microorganisms.* 89(81)EC (Amending Directive 90(219)EEC). EC, Brussels.

Evans, D. & Lahoti, S. (2000) Adenovirus in cancer therapy: a gastrointestinal case study. *Gastroenterol Nurs*, **23**(1), 16–18.

Flygenring, B.G. (1999) Comments from Iceland. *Oncol Nurs Today*, **4**(2), 13–14.

Galanis, E., Vile, R. & Russell, S.J. (2001) Delivery systems intended for in vivo gene therapy of cancer: targeting and replication of competent viral vectors. *Crit Rev Oncol Hematol*, **38**(3), 177–92.

Griesenbach, U., Ferrari, S., Geddes, D.M. & Alton, E.W. (2002) Gene therapy progress and prospects: cystic fibrosis. *Gene Ther*, **9**(20), 1344–50.

GTAC (2000) *Report of the Adenoviral Working Party.* DOH, London.

Health Service Executive (HSE) (1997) *Genetically Modified Organisms (Deliberate Release and Risk Assessment – Amendment) Regulations.* Stationery Office, London.

Health Service Executive (HSE) (1999) *The Control of Substances Hazardous to Health (COSHH) Regulations.* Stationery Office, London.

Health Service Executive (HSE) (2000) *The Genetically Modified Organisms (Contained Use) Regulations.* Stationery Office, London.

Hull, D. & Chester, M. (2002) Gene therapy trials: a patient pathway. *Nurs Stand*, **17**(3), 39–42.

Jenkins J., Wheeler, V. & Albright, L. (1994) Gene therapy for cancer. *Cancer Nurs*, **17**(6), 447–56.

Kim, J., Cho, J.Y., Kim, J.H. *et al.* (2002) Evaluation of E1B gene-attenuated replicating adenoviruses for cancer gene therapy. *Cancer Gene Ther*, **9**(9), 725–36.

Launis, V. (2002) Human gene therapy and the slippery slope argument. *Med Health Care Philos*, **5**(2), 169–79.

Lea, D.H. (1997) Gene therapy: current and future implications for oncology nursing practice. *Semin Oncol Nurs*, **13**(2), 115–22.

Lipinski, K.S., Djeha, A.H. & Krausz, E. *et al.* (2001) Tumour-specific therapeutic adenovirus vectors: repression of transgene expression in healthy cells by endogenous p53. *Gene Ther*, **8**(4), 274–81.

Loud, J.T., Peters, J.A., Fraser, M. & Jenkins, J. (2002) Applications of advances in molecular biology and genomics to clinical cancer care. *Cancer Nurs*, **25**(2), 110–22.

Marchisone, C., Pfeffer, U., Del Grosso, F. *et al.* (2000) Progress towards gene therapy for cancer. *J Exp Clin Cancer Res*, **19**(3), 261–70.

Medicine Act (1971). Stationery Office, London.

Middelton, L., Dimond, E., Calzone, K. *et al.* (2002) The role of the nurse in cancer genetics. *Cancer Nurs*, **25**(3), 196–206.

Nippert, I. (2002) The pros and cons of human therapeutic cloning in the public debate. *J Biotechnol*, **98**(1), 53–60.

Palu, G., Bonaguro, R. & Marcello, A. (1999) In pursuit of new developments for gene therapy of human diseases. *J Biotechnol*, **68**(1), 1–13.

Peters, J.A. (1997) Applications of genetic technologies to cancer screening, prevention, diagnosis, prognosis and treatment. *Semin Oncol Nurs*, **13**(2), 74–81.

Robinson, K.D., Abernathy, E. & Conrad, K.J. (1996) Gene therapy of cancer. *Semin Oncol Nurs*, **12**(2), 142–51.

Sandhu, J.S., Keating, A. & Hozumi, N. (1997) Human gene therapy. *Crit Rev Biotechnol*, **17**(4), 307–26.

Searle, P.F., Spiers, I., Simpson, J. & James, N.D. (2002) Cancer gene therapy: from science to clinical trials. *Drug Delivery Syst Sci*, **2**(1), 5–13.

The Personal Protection Equipment Regulations (1992). Stationery Office, London.

The Health and Safety at Work Act etc. (1974) Stationery Office, London.

Trahan Rieger, P. (1997) Emerging strategies in the management of cancer. *Oncol Nurs Forum*, **24**(4), 728–37.

Vorburger, S.A. & Hunt, K.K. (2002) Adenoviral gene therapy. *Oncologist*, **7**(1), 46–59.

Wilson, T.M. (1996) Adenoviruses as gene-delivery vehicles. *N Engl J Med*, **334**(18), 1185–93.

Wivel, N.A. & Wilson, J.M. (1998) Methods of gene therapy. *Hematol Oncol Clin North Am*, **12**(3), 483–501.

Young, A. (1997) Gene therapy for oncology patients. *Nurs Times*, **93**(37), 50–2.

19

Haematological procedures: specialist, diagnostic and therapeutic

Chapter contents

Definition

Haematological procedures include bone marrow procedures and apheresis procedures (donor and therapeutic).

Bone marrow procedures

Bone marrow procedures involve the removal of haemopoietic tissue, usually from the iliac crest or sternum, using a special needle. In children aged less than 1 year the upper end of the tibia may be used (Beutler *et al.* 2001). Bone marrow procedures include the following:

- *Aspiration*: a needle is inserted into the marrow and a liquid sample of marrow is aspirated into a syringe. This is then spread onto a slide for microscopy and stained. A large amount of morphological information can be obtained by examining the slide of the aspirated marrow. An aspirate sample may also be used for a number of specialized investigations (Table 19.1) (Hoffbrand *et al.* 2001).
- *Trephine*: a trephine biopsy provides a solid core of bone including marrow and is examined as a histo logical specimen after fixation in formalin, decalcification and sectioning. The indications for undertaking trephine are shown in Table 19.1. Immunophenotyping may also be undertaken with a trephine biopsy (Hoffbrand *et al.* 2001).
- *Harvest*: at any given time, 90% of haemopoietic progenitor stem cells may be found in the bone marrow (Grundy 2000). One method of harvesting these stem cells is to collect them from the marrow with a needle and syringe.

Indications

Examination of the bone marrow, together with the prior examination of the blood, remains the gold standard required for the diagnosis of many haematological diseases (Ryan 2001). Bone marrow is harvested for

Table 19.1 Comparison of bone marrow aspiration and trephine biopsy (reproduced with kind permission from Hoffbrand *et al.* 2001)

	Aspiration	**Trephine**
Site	Posterior iliac crest or sternum (tibia in infants)	Posterior iliac crest
Stains	Romanowsky; Perls reaction (for iron)	Haematoxylin and eosin; reticulin (silver stain)
Result available	1–2 hours	1–7 days (according to decalcification method)
Main indications	Investigation of anaemia, pancytopenia, suspected leukaemia or myeloma, neutropenia, thrombocytopenia, etc.	Indications for trephine in addition to aspirate: suspicion of polycythaemia vera, myelofibrosis and other myeloproliferative disorders, aplastic anaemia, malignant lymphoma, secondary carcinoma, cases of splenomegaly or pyrexia of undetermined cause. Any case where aspiration gives a 'dry tap'
Special tests	Cytogenetics, microbiological culture, biochemical analysis, immunological and cytochemical markers, immunoglobulin or T-cell receptor gene analysis, DNA or RNA analysis for gene abnormalities, progenitor cell culture	Immunophenotyping

autologous or allogeneic transplantation or cryopreservation for both malignant and non-malignant conditions (Cottler-Fox 1999).

Apheresis procedures (donor or therapeutic)

Apheresis is the separation and collection of one or more blood components. It may be performed using either a single arm or two arm technique via a peripheral cannula. It can be performed using continuous or intermittent flow depending on the apheresis machine used (Burgstaler & Pineda 1994). The procedure for performing apheresis is complex and beyond the scope of this chapter and should only be performed by specially trained operators. Further information can be gained from the individual apheresis operator's manual. Apheresis procedures include the following:

- *Platelet depletion*: removal of circulating platelets, either from a donor or in order to reduce dangerously high levels such as in essential thrombocythaemia to prevent thrombosis.
- *Therapeutic plasma exchange*: removal of part of the plasma pool and replacing it with disease-free plasma. Used in diseases such as multiple myeloma, autoimmune disorders and idiopathic thrombotic thrombocytopenic purpura.
- *Red cell exchange*: used on patients with haematological disorders such as sickle cell anaemia, thalassaemia, polycythaemia and haemochromatosis. In sickle cell anaemia exchange transfusion may be needed if there is neurological damage, visceral sequestration or repeated painful crisis (Hoffbrand *et al.* 2001).

- *Rapid red cell transfusion*: for outpatient transfusion (to minimize length of time in hospital) and prevention of fluid overload in volume sensitive patients (McLeod *et al.* 1994).
- *White blood cell (mononuclear cell or polymorphonuclear cell) procedures*: used to remove excess white blood cells in patients with leukaemia, collecting donor T lymphocytes for immunotherapy or collecting donor granulocytes for treatment of acute sepsis (Hoffbrand *et al.* 2001).
- *Peripheral blood stem cell procedures*: used to harvest haemopoietic stem cells for autologous or allogeneic transplantation or cryopreservation for both malignant and non-malignant conditions (Proven *et al.* 1998).

Reference material

Anatomy and physiology

The yolk sac is the primary source of haemopoiesis from day 8 of gestation until birth. After birth, the marrow, located in the medullary cavity of the bone, then becomes the sole site of effective haemopoiesis (Abboud & Litchmann 2001). The marrow is one of the largest organs in the body, representing 3.4–4.6% of the total body weight (Monteil 1996).

Haemopoietic stem cells give rise to all haemopoietic cell lines. Stromal cells, fat cells and a microvascular network provide a suitable network for stem cell growth and development (Hoffbrand *et al.* 2001). There are two

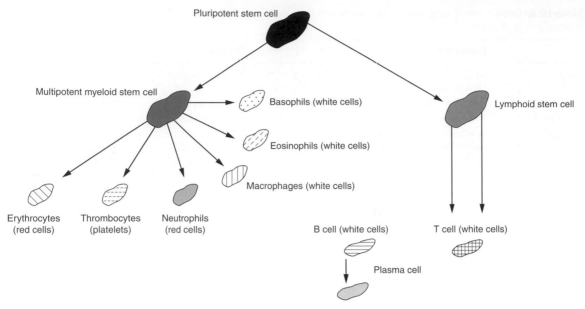

Figure 19.1 Diagrammatic representation of the bone marrow pluripotent stem cell and the cell lines that arise from it.

types of bone marrow:

- *Red marrow*: which is haemopoietically active and is found in the lower skull, vertebrae, shoulder and pelvic girdles, ribs and sternum.
- *Yellow marrow*: which is primarily made up of fat cells replacing haemopoietic cells in the bones of the hands, feet, legs and arms. This marrow has the ability to revert to haemopoietic tissue in certain circumstances such as haemolytic anaemia (Abboud & Litchmann 2001).

Blood cells

Blood cell growth and development is regulated by haemopoietic growth factors. Some growth factors are found naturally in the plasma but others are only detectable following an inflammatory or other stimulus (Hoffbrand *et al.* 2001). Growth factors include GM-CSF (granulocyte macrophage colony stimulating factor), G-CSF (granulocyte colony stimulating factor) and IL-6 (interleukin 6). All mature blood cells are derived from a common pluripotent haemopoietic stem cell. These cells mature and differentiate to provide the three types of blood cells (see Fig. 19.1).

- Red blood cells (erythrocytes): the main function is to carry oxygen to the tissues and to return carbon dioxide to the lungs. This gaseous exchange is facilitated by the protein haemoglobin contained in the erythrocyte (Hoffbrand *et al.* 2001). The normal

Table 19.2 Normal values (Hoffbrand *et al.* 2001)

	Males	Females	Males and females
Haemoglobin (g/dl)	13.5–17.5	11.5–15.5	
Erythrocytes ($\times 10^{12}$/l)	4.5–6.5	3.9–5.6	
Leucocytes ($\times 10^{9}$/l)			4.0–11.0
Platelets ($\times 10^{9}$/l)			150–400

values of haemoglobin and erythrocytes vary according to gender (see Table 19.2).
- White blood cells (leucocytes): the main function is to protect the body from infection. Leucocytes are divided into neutrophils, eosinophils and basophils (granulocytes); monocytes; and lymphocytes (T and B) (Turgeon 1999).
- Platelets: the main function is the formation of mechanical plugs during the normal haemostatic response to vascular injury (Hoffbrand *et al.* 2001).

Although 90% of haemopoietic stem cells live in the bone marrow, they can migrate to the peripheral blood following treatment with cytotoxic chemotherapy or the administration of haemopoietic growth factors. Exact protocols vary according to underlying disease, treatment regimens and local practice but involve one of three techniques.

- *Mobilization after standard chemotherapy alone* where no specific stimulus is given. Yields are variable and timing of harvesting may be difficult as individual

▒ Ideal location

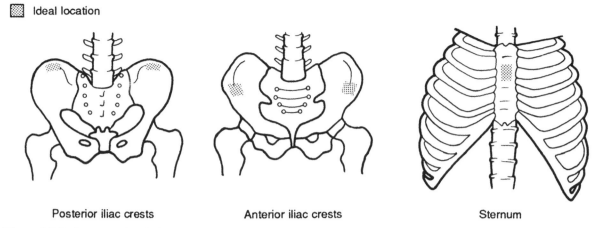

| Posterior iliac crests | Anterior iliac crests | Sternum |

Figure 19.2 Common sites for bone marrow examination, arranged in order of preference. Normally, only aspirations and not biopsies are done on the sternum because of its small size and proximity to vital organs.

marrow recovery varies and so the optimum time may be difficult to predict.

- *Mobilization following chemotherapy and with haemopoietic growth factor.* This regimen is the best evaluated (Proven *et al.* 1998), is most commonly used and enables more accurate prediction of optimum harvest time.
- *Mobilization with haemopoietic growth factor alone* is suitable for sibling or volunteer donors as well as patients in remission.

Haemopoietic stem cells can also be harvested from foetal tissue and umbilical cord blood (Cottler-Fox 1999).

Aspiration and trephine biopsy

Patients may be anxious about the procedure and a mild sedative may be indicated. The procedure is performed under local anaesthetic, although owing to the nature of the pain (often described as a dragging sensation) the actual aspiration procedure may still remain painful even when the site is numb. The posterior iliac crest is the preferred site for both aspiration and biopsy as there are no vital organs nearby that may be punctured. The position also means that the procedure can be performed outside the patient's line of vision (Fig. 19.2). In adults, the sternum and anterior iliac crest can also be used. In infants under 1 year old, the anteromedial surface of the tibia is an option, but the posterior iliac crest is preferred (Ryan 2001).

Contraindications

Bone marrow aspirate and trephine biopsy are contraindicated in those patients who are unable to co-operate or have a coagulation defect such as increased clotting time, unless this is correctable, as excessive bleeding or bruising may occur. Patients in extreme pain may not be able to adopt the lateral position for posterior iliac crest sampling. In this case the anterior iliac crest or, if biopsy is not needed, the sternum can be used (Beutler *et al.* 2001).

Bone marrow harvest

Bone marrow harvests are performed under a general anaesthetic. This is done because:

- The procedure may last for approximately 1 hour compared with the 15–30 minutes for an aspiration and biopsy.
- Multiple puncture sites are used and the patient may be approached from both sides (i.e. from both the pelvis and the sternum).
- The procedure can be very painful.

A volume of 1 litre or more (dependent on the harvest cell count in relation to the recipient's body weight) is aspirated from multiple puncture sites. If large volumes of marrow are harvested the patient may require a blood transfusion, or, following processing of the bone marrow, the donor's own red cells may be returned to them following the procedure. The marrow may be harvested for immediate use or may be cryopreserved for the future.

Complications of bone marrow procedures

Complications of bone marrow procedures are extremely rare but include the following:

- Cardiac tamponade: this is compression of the heart produced by the accumulation of blood or fluid in the

Haemopneumothorax

This is defined as blood and air in the pleural space, as a combination of factors already mentioned (Yeam & Sassoon 1997).

Empyema

This is defined as pus in the pleural space. Its main causes include rupture of an abscess of the lung, following pneumonia, pulmonary TB, or an infection following thoracic surgery (Kumar & Clarke 2002).

Collective signs and symptoms

The following signs and symptoms can occur in the conditions previously mentioned, individually or together depending on the patient's condition:

- Pallor
- Cyanosis
- Dyspnoea
- Increasing respiratory rate
- Reduced breath sounds on affected side
- Dullness of air entry, on listening to the chest with stethoscope
- Reduced chest movement on affected side
- Decrease in peripheral tissue oxygen saturations
- Pleuritic chest pain
- Cardiovascular change, i.e. increasing heart rate, decreasing blood pressure due to compression of the mediastinum and in turn the heart and surrounding vessels (Kumar & Clarke 2002).

Drain insertion site

Before insertion of an intrapleural drain the patient should have a chest X-ray reviewed by the doctor. The chest X-ray will confirm the site of the pneumothorax or effusion to be drained. Patients who are receiving anticoagulation therapy or who have platelet abnormalities should have appropriate haematological investigations – international normalized ratio (INR) or activated partial thromboplastin ratio (APTR) – to ascertain whether correction is required prior to insertion of the drain (Tang et al. 2002). If the INR or APTR is too high, bleeding could occur if left untreated.

Intrapleural drains are usually inserted in the chest, in an area which is known as the 'triangle of safety'. The mid-axillary line borders this area posteriorly, the level of the nipple inferiorly and the lateral border of the pectoralis major interiorly (Hyde et al. 1997; Peek et al. 2000; Tang et al. 2002). Once the drain has been placed in any position within the 'triangle of safety', re-expansion of the lung occurs. However, in cases of intrapleural adhesions or localized collection of pus or fluids, the

Table 20.1 Drain sizes

Reason for drainage	Size of catheter
Air	16–24 Fr
Blood	28–32 Fr
Pus	32–36 Fr
Debris associated with empyema	32–36 Fr

doctor will need to position the tip of the drain to assist drainage (Hyde et al. 1997; Tang et al. 2002).

Drain size

The size of tube used is dependent on the reason for drainage: see Table 20.1.

Stripping/milking of intrapleural drains

Milking and stripping are harmful and can result in lung damage. If the tubing becomes occluded, it should be replaced. Using the correct size of catheter should prevent tubes becoming occluded, therefore reducing the necessity of changing the drain (Tang et al. 2002).

Clamping of intrapleural drains

The British Thoracic Society Guidelines (Miller & Harvey 1993) discourage clamping of intrapleural drains as this can prevent air leaving the pleural space. This in turn can cause a pneumothorax which could progress to a life-threatening tension pneumothorax. There is also no need to clamp tubing when mobilizing or transporting patients to other departments as this may also cause a tension pneumothorax (Hyde et al. 1997). When changing the bottle system, it may be necessary to clamp the drain and during this process the patient should be under close observation for any signs of deterioration in breathing.

Drainage systems

Prepacked drainage systems are now available for drainage of pneumothoraces, haemothoraces or pleural effusions. The bottle has a screw top with two ports. One port has the underwater length of tubing attached. The second port has a shorter length of tubing attached which acts as the venting end and is exposed to air or could be attached to a suction unit. Venting prevents the build-up of pressure in the chest drainage system which could prevent evacuation of air or fluid (Fig. 20.2).

The underwater seal occurs when there is adequate water in the bottle, usually 500 ml of water. The distal end of the intrapleural drain is then attached to the underwater seal port of the chest drain bottle and immersed 2.5 cm below the level of the water. Incoming air bubbles through the water which acts as a one-way valve and prevents the backflow of air into the intrapleural space (McMahon-Parkes 1997).

For more complicated pneumothoraces or haemothoraces a plastic multichamber system incorporates the above one-bottle system into one unit. There are three chambers: the first is for drainage, the second chamber is the underwater seal and the third chamber is the vacuum or suction control. When this system is set up, water is placed in the water seal chamber to the indicated mark, and also placed in the suction control chamber to the required level. This system is a great improvement on the previous systems and enables patient mobility (Fig. 20.3).

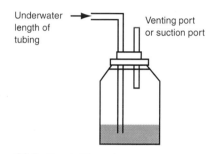

Figure 20.2 One-bottle system.

Maintenance of drainage systems during and after insertion

When the drain is attached to the drainage bottle bubbling or swinging should be observed; this indicates that air is being evacuated from the pleural space. As the lung re-inflates, the bubbling should decrease. If bubbling continues, a leak may be present in the patient's lung. Causes of air leaks may include:

- Blocked drain
- Inadequate drain size
- Poor tube connections
- Poor seal around the entry site to the lung.

The presence of an air leak should be assessed. Bubbling can occur in the underwater seal compartment. If bubbling occurs when the patient coughs, this would usually indicate the leak is only minor. However, continuous bubbling would indicate a serious air leak in the system. The drain and tube should be inspected thoroughly down to the level of the underwater seal to eliminate any external problems such as loose tubing connections or poor seal around the drain at the insertion site. A chest X-ray should also be ordered by the doctor to establish the position of the drain. Air leaks should be treated with caution. Prompt action is required such as referral to a specialist respiratory physician.

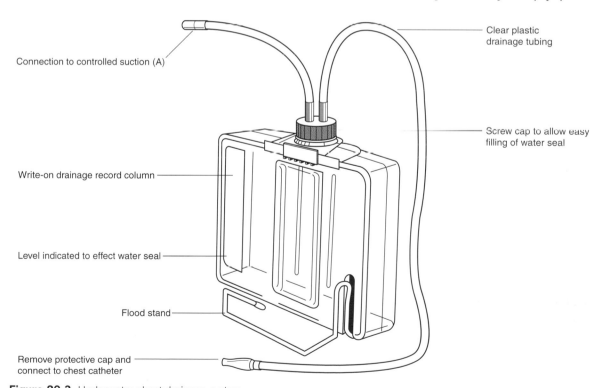

Figure 20.3 Underwater chest drainage system.

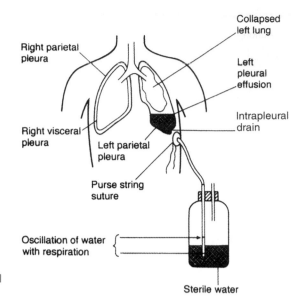

Figure 20.4 An intrapleural drain and underwater seal bottle are used to drain a left pleural effusion.

*Procedure guidelines: **Chest drain insertion** (cont'd)*

Action	Rationale
14 Check the drain is well secured.	To prevent movement of drain or loss of drain.
15 Ensure that there is bubbling/swinging of water in the bottle/tubing or drainage fluid and check there are no leaks around the site or that any loose connections exist within the drainage system.	To ensure there is no occlusion or leak which will prevent re-expansion of the lung or drainage of the fluid.
16 Ensure patient comfort following the procedure. Return the patient to an elevated position sitting in bed, well supported by pillows, and give further analgesia if required.	To ensure patient comfort in order to aid recovery and breathing.
17 Dispose of waste appropriately.	To reduce risk of cross-infection and sharps injury.

Suction for intrapleural drainage

Action	Rationale
1 Communicate with the patient during the application of suction and explain what is happening at each stage.	To keep the patient fully informed. To enable the patient to feel reassured.
2 Discuss analgesia management with the patient. Give analgesia to the patient as prescribed.	To ensure patient comfort.
3 Prepare the suction unit.	To maintain safety, ensuring the suction is set at low pressure.
4 Connect tube A (Fig. 20.3) to the suction unit, as directed by the medical team. Adjust the suction to required level prescribed, usually $-5\,cmH_2O$ to $-20\,cmH_2O$, and to a level which is tolerable for the patient.	To ensure patient comfort and to ensure suction is applied.
5 Position patient to aid comfort, ensuring the patient is pain free and relaxed.	To aid breathing for lung expansion. To aid patient comfort.
6 Monitor intrapleural drainage and record amount.	To maintain patient safety by observing level of suction and amount of fluid drained.
7 Check suction unit is working and suction pressure is maintained according to doctor's orders.	To maintain patient safety.

*Procedure guidelines: **Chest drain insertion** (cont'd)*

Postdrain procedure

Action	Rationale
1 Observe patient for any change in respiratory status: (a) Colour (b) Respiratory rate and pattern (c) Unequal chest movement (d) Peripheral tissue oxygen saturations (e) Blood gases.	These symptoms may indicate a change of chest drain position, occlusion of the drain or recurrence of pneumothorax or collection of fluid.
Observe patient for any change in cardiovascular status: (a) Heart rate (b) Blood pressure.	May indicate pressure on the cardiovascular system.
2 Ensure the drain remains well secured with suture and dressing.	To prevent movement of drain and ensure safety of patient.
3 Ensure the drain is well positioned with no loops or kinks.	To prevent occlusion of drain.
4 Ensure drain tubing is well supported at the side of the bed using tape and clamps.	To prevent drain pulling and dragging, causing trauma to the patient or movement of or the risk of the drain falling out.
5 Ensure drain tubing and connections are secure and attached to the drainage unit.	To ensure a sealed unit exists to prevent air entry into the pleura which could lead to further lung collapse.
6 Ensure a pair of clamps is available beside the patient in case of accidental disconnection.	To clamp drain and prevent further lung collapse.
7 Do not clamp drains other than in the case of accidental disconnection.	To prevent a high positive pressure which can be created when the drain is clamped and which can result in a tension pneumothorax.
8 Ensure chest drain remains at a level below the chest at all times.	This prevents backflow of fluid into the pleural space.
9 Do not milk or strip tubing other than in an emergency such as removal of an obstruction after discussion with doctor.	Milking or stripping can cause an increase in negative pressure which could result in damage to lung tissue.
10 Observe volume and type of drainage; is it clear/bloodstained, etc? Record on a fluid chart and in the nursing notes.	To ensure monitoring of type and volume of fluid loss.
11 Position patient comfortably in bed, sitting upright, well supported by pillows.	To aid patient comfort. To aid breathing and allow for full expansion of the lungs.
12 Change the position of the patient while in bed.	To reduce risk of breakdown in skin integrity.
13 Encourage mobilization of the patient, e.g. to sit in chair and also to walk aided by physiotherapist or nurse.	To encourage patient independence and prevent complications, e.g. pulmonary embolus, deep vein thrombosis, breakdown in skin integrity.
14 Ensure patient maintains mobility of arm on side of drain.	To prevent complications and reduce risk of immobility of arm.
15 Ensure patient remains pain free.	To relieve pain and aid recovery.
16 Maintain patient hygiene and mouth care. Assist patient in washing/mouth care because of restriction of movement due to drain.	To aid patient comfort and reduce the risk of infection.
17 Maintain normal oral and dietary intake.	To aid healing process. To reduce risk of dehydration and malnutrition. To reduce risk of infection.
18 Maintain a normal sleep pattern.	To allow patient to rest and aid recovery.
19 Ensure patient is kept occupied, e.g. reading, watching TV, listening to the radio.	To relieve boredom and aid recovery.

Procedure guidelines: **Removal of a chest drain**

Equipment

1 Sterile dressing pack containing gallipot, gauze, sterile towel.
2 Cleaning solution, e.g. 0.9% sodium chloride.
3 Sterile gloves.
4 Stitch cutter.
5 Sterile dressing.
6 Tape.
7 Chest drain clamps × 2.

Two nurses/assistants are required to facilitate safe removal of a chest drain. One is required to tie the suture and seal the site, and the other to remove the drain.

Procedure

Action	Rationale
1 Prepare patient for removal of the drain. Explain and discuss each step of the procedure with the patient.	To ensure the patient is well prepared, and to ensure their co-operation and consent.
2 Encourage patient to practise breathing exercises, as these are required to help with the procedure. The patient should be instructed to take three deep breaths in and out and on the fourth breath to hold the breath in. It is on this breath that the drain will be removed.	To prepare the patient and encourage co-operation. To allow the patient to practise the breathing exercises. To prevent the entry of air which can occur due to a negative intrathoracic pressure (Tomlinson & Treasure 1997).
3 Administer analgesia prior to procedure after discussion with doctor about the type and route of administration. The analgesia should be given at least half an hour before the procedure.	To minimize any pain during the procedure and to ensure the patient is pain free and able to co-operate.
4 Administer sedation on doctor's instruction, if considered appropriate, e.g. for an anxious patient.	To relieve anxiety and allow the patient to relax and co-operate and to enable the procedure to go ahead.
5 Discontinue suction if in use.	To prevent a tension pneumothorax.
6 Prepare trolley for procedure.	To aid the procedure.
7 Assist or set up the sterile procedure pack.	To minimize risk of infection and to have equipment ready.
8 Position patient comfortably.	To aid patient comfort.
9 Place protective pad underneath the patient and drain.	To absorb any ooze from the drain. To reduce risk of contamination of the patient and bed clothing.
10 Wash hands with bactericidal soap and water before touching the drain or dressing.	To reduce risk of infection.
11 Remove dressing from around drain site, examine sutures present: (a) tube retaining suture (anchor suture) and (b) purse-string suture; expose the ends of these sutures.	To prepare for drain removal and check what type of suture is present so that the suture can be used to form an airtight seal when the drain is removed.
12 Both assistants for the procedure must wash their hands and apply sterile gloves.	To reduce risk of infection.
13 First nurse/assistant prepares purse-string suture and loosens ends ready to tie the suture when the drain is removed.	To prepare for drain removal.
14 Second nurse/assistant prepares and cuts the anchor suture and ensures the drain is mobile and ready to remove.	To prepare for drain removal.
15 Second nurse/assistant asks the patient to start deep breathing exercises: to take three deep breaths then hold his/her breath on the fourth one while the drain is pulled out steadily and smoothly.	To aid in drain removal. Deep breathing exercises can help to prevent a tension pneumothorax. If a drain is removed too quickly or without due care a pneumothorax can occur due to rupture of the pleura.
16 First nurse/assistant will tie the purse-string suture securely to the skin.	To form an airtight seal and prevent air entry and formation of a pneumothorax.
17 Clean around site with 0.9% sodium chloride and apply an occlusive dressing.	To clean site, form an airtight seal and prevent air entry.

*Procedure guidelines: **Removal of a chest drain** (cont'd)*

Action	Rationale
18 Ensure that the patient is comfortable on completion of procedure by sitting the patient upright, and support with pillows.	To ensure patient comfort.
19 Dispose of waste appropriately.	To ensure safety and reduce risk of infection.
20 Observe and measure amount of drainage. Document on fluid chart and in nursing notes.	To maintain an accurate record of a legal document and to provide a point of reference for any queries.

Problem solving

Problem	Cause	Suggested action
Patient shows signs of respiratory distress, increased respiratory rate, uneven chest movement, decreasing peripheral tissue oxygen saturations.	Pneumothorax or tension pneumothorax.	Observe patient continually for change in vital signs. Inform doctor and administer oxygen. Prepare for re-insertion of chest drain.
Lack of drainage.	Kinking, looping or pressure on the tubing may cause reflux of fluid into the intrapleural space or may impede drainage, causing blocking of the intrapleural drain.	Check the system and straighten tubing as required. Secure the tubing to prevent a recurrence of the problem.
Fluid in drain not swinging.	Drain occluded due to position or occlusion.	Check no loops or kinks present in tubing. Lift drain, not higher than the patient's chest, to see if the obstruction will clear. Seek medical advice as the drain may need replacing.
Fluid in drain not bubbling.	Drain occluded or not correctly positioned.	Check no loops or kinks in the tubing. Lift tubing to see if it will clear.
Continual bubbling in chest drain bottle.	Air leak in system.	Check system for loose connections in tubing or around drainage unit. If no leak present in the drainage tubing the leak may be present in the lung. Inform doctor. Prepare chest drain insertion pack.
Leakage from drain site.	Bleeding or infection.	Remove the dressing and observe the site. Inform doctor, take swab. Clean and redress site. Discuss with medical team regarding prescription of antibiotic therapy.
Drainage from around drain site.	As a result of the insertion procedure. Incomplete closure with sutures. Infected insertion site.	Observe drain site, amount and type of drainage. Inform doctor. Take swab from site. Prepare suture pack to be available if required. Discuss with medical team regarding prescription of antibiotic therapy.
Accidental disconnection of the drainage tubing from the intrapleural drain.	Connections not secure.	Apply a clamp to the drain immediately in order to avoid air entering the pleural space. Re-establish the connection as soon as possible in order to re-establish drainage. If necessary, use a clean, sterile drainage tube; tubing may have been contaminated when it became disconnected. Report to the doctor, who may wish to X-ray. Record the incident in the relevant records. The patient may have been upset by the incident and will need reassurance.

Problem solving (cont'd)

Problem	Cause	Suggested action
Intrapleural drain falls out.	Drain not secure.	Pull the purse-string suture immediately to close the wound. Cover the wound with an occlusive sterile dressing. Check the patient's vital signs. Inform a doctor. The objective is to minimize the amount of air entering the pleural space. The drain will probably need reinserting. Prepare chest drain insertion pack. Reassure the patient with appropriate explanations.
Poor arm movement.	Restriction of arm movement due to position of drain.	Encourage movement of limb to keep mobile. Adjust analgesia as required.
Pain.	Drain pulling at site.	Try repositioning tubing, so that it is not dragging or irritating skin. Give analgesia as prescribed.
Restricted mobility of patient.	Due to position of drain and attachment to the drainage unit.	Explore with the patient the movement that is possible and aid them where help is required. Encourage mobility, aid patient to sit in chair. Work in liaison with physiotherapist. Encourage patient to move in bed and change position.

References and further reading

Adam, S.K. & Osborne, S. (1997) Respiratory problems. In: *Critical Care Nursing*. Oxford Medical Publications, Oxford, pp. 72–5.

Avery, S. (2000) Insertion and management of chest drains. *NT Plus*, **96**, 3–6.

Baumann, M.H. & Strange, C. (1997) The clinician's perspective on pneumothorax management. *Chest*, **112**(3), 822–8.

Berne, R.M. & Levy, M.N. (1998) Structure and function of the respiratory system. In: *Physiology*, 4th edn. Mosby, London, Chap. 32.

Calhorn Thomson, S., Wells, S. & Maxwell, M. (1997) Chest tube removal after cardiac surgery. *Crit Care Nurse*, **17**(1), 34–8.

Campbell, J. (1993) Making sense of underwater sealed drainage. *Nurs Times*, **89**(9), 34–6.

Carson, M. (1995) Minimizing pain when removing a chest tube. *Reg Nurse*, **58**(2), 19.

Carson, M.M., Barton, D.M., Morrison, C.G. *et al.* (1994) Managing pain during mediastinal chest tube removal. *Heart Lung*, **23**(6), 500–5.

Chernecky, C. & Shelton, B. (2001) Pulmonary complications in patients with cancer: diagnostic and treatment information for the noncritical care nurse. *Am J Nurs*, **101**(5), 24A–24H.

Couzza, C. (1995) Dislodged chest tube. *Nursing*, **25**(9), 33.

Ekstrowicz, N. (1997) Managing pain during chest tube insertion. *Nursing*, **27**(11), 28

Gallon, A. (1998) Pneumothorax. *Nurs Stand*, **39**(10), 35–9.

Godden, J. (1998) Managing the patient with a chest drain: a review. *Nurs Stand*, **12**(32), 35–9.

Gorden, P.A., Norton, J.M. & Guerra, J.M. (1997) Positioning of chest drain tubes: effects on pressure and drainage. *Am J Crit Care*, **6**, 33–8.

Gray, E. (2000) Pain management for patients with chest drains. *Nurs Stand*, **14**(23), 40–4.

Grodzin, C.J. & Baik, R.A. (1997) Indwelling small pleural catheter needle thoracentesis in the management of large pleural effusions. *Chest*, **111**(4), 981–8.

Guyton, A. (2000) Pulmonary ventilation. In: *A Textbook of Medical Physiology*, 10th edn. W.B. Saunders, Philadelphia, Chap. 37.

Hyde, J., Skyes, T. & Graham, T. (1997) Reducing morbidity from chest drains. *Br Med J*, **314** (7085), 914–15.

Kumar, P. & Clarke, C. (2002) *Clinical Medicine*. Mosby, St Louis.

Lazzara, D. (1996) Why is the Hemlich chest drain valve making a comeback? *Nursing*, **26**(12), 50–3.

Marieb, E.N. (2001) The respiratory system. In: *Human Anatomy and Physiology*, 5th edn. John Wiley, New York, Chap. 23.

McConnell, E. (1995) Clinical do's and don'ts. *Nursing*, **25**(8), 18.

McMahon-Parkes, K. (1997) Management of pleural drains. *Nurs Times*, **93**(52), 48–52.

Miller, A.C. & Harvey, J.E. (1993) Guidelines for the management of spontaneous pneumothorax. *Br Med J*, **307**, 114–16.

Patz, E.F. (1998) Malignant pleural effusions: recent advances and ambulatory sclerotherapy. *Chest*, **113**(1), Suppl 1, 74–7S.

Peek, G., Morcos, S. & Cooper, G. (2000) The pleural cavity. *Br Med J*, **320**, 1318–21.

Pettinicchi, T.A. (1998) Trouble shooting chest tubes. *Nursing*, **28**(3), 58–9

Pierce, L.N.B. (1995) *Guide to Mechanical Ventilation and Intensive Respiratory Care*. W.B. Saunders, London, Appendix 111, pp. 356–63.

Smith, R.D., Fallentine, J. & Kessel, S. (1995) Underwater chest drainage bringing the facts to the surface. *Nursing*, **25**(2), 60–3

Tang, A., Hooper, T. & Hassan, R. (1999) A regional survey of chest drains: evidence based practice? *Postgrad Med J*, **75**(886), 471–4.

Tang, A., Vellissaris, T. & Weeden, D. (2002) An evidence based approach to drainage of pleural cavity: evaluation of best practice. *J Eval Clin Pract*, **8**(3), 333–40.

Tooley, C. (2002) The management and care of chest drains. *Nurs Times*, **98**(26), 48–50.

Tortora, G. & Grabowski, S.R. (2000) The respiratory system. In: *Principles of Anatomy and Physiology*, 9th edn. John Wiley, New York, Chap. 23.

Yeam, I. & Sassoon, C. (1997) Haemothorax and chylothorax. *Curr Opin Pulmon Med*, **3**(4), 310–14.

Last offices

Chapter contents

Definition

Last offices is the care given to a deceased patient which demonstrates our respect for the dead and is focused on fulfilling religious and cultural beliefs as well as health and safety and legal requirements.

Reference material

Last offices has been carried out by nurses at least since the nineteenth century (Wolfe 1988) and is in many ways a traditional and ritualized nursing procedure which has not been based on research (Cooke 2000; Berry & Griffie 2001). This has resulted in some hospitals taking this procedure away from nurses and leaving the initial care of the body instead to the undertaker (Speck 1992). Administering last offices, however, often has symbolic significance for nurses and can be a fulfilling experience as it is the final demonstration of respectful, sensitive care given to a patient (Nearney 1998). Undertaking last offices also gives the message to the family and other patients that caring continues after death (Speck 1992). In administering last offices, nurses need to know the legal requirements for care of the dead and so it is essential that the correct procedures be followed. Every effort should also be made to accommodate the wishes of the patient's relatives (Neuberger 1994).

It is impossible to understand the laws and prohibitions about handling human bodies after death without having some idea of what that particular person's religion or philosophy has to say about the nature of human life and its value (Neuberger 1999). As the UK today is a multicultural and multifaith society, this offers a great challenge to nurses who need to be aware of the different religious and cultural rituals that may accompany the death of a patient. There are considerable cultural variations within and between people of different faiths, ethnic backgrounds and national origins in their approach to death and dying (Neuberger 1999). Whilst those who have settled in a society where there is a dominant faith or culture other than their own appear to increasingly adopt that dominant culture, in many ways they retain, almost deliberately to emphasize differences, their different practices at times of birth, marriage or death (Neuberger 1999). Approaches to death and dying also reveal as much of the attitude of society as a whole as they do about individuals within that society (Field *et al.* 1997).

Practices relating to last offices will vary depending on the patient's cultural background and religious practices (Nearney 1998). The following sections provide a guide to cultural and religious variations in attitudes to death and how individuals may wish to be treated. Given the current controversy over the use of 'factfiles' and the presentation of information on culture and religion in this way (Gunaratnam 1997; Smaje & Field 1997; Gilliat-Ray 2001), two key issues should be considered when applying this information to practice:

1 Few of us are whole hearted in our acceptance of the ways of our own religious or cultural group (Neuberger 1999).
2 Our motivation to categorize individuals into groups with clearly defined norms can lead to a lack of understanding of the complexities of religious and cultural practice and the processes of change and depersonalizes individuals and their families (Sampson 1982; Smaje & Field 1997; Neuberger 1999).

It is imperative that health care professionals establish the individual preferences of patients and encourage them to talk about the different patterns of observance within their own religious/cultural group.

The bibliography at the end of this chapter is by no means exhaustive, but may be used by nurses to deepen their understanding of issues surrounding death, and broaden their knowledge of and respect for other cultures and faiths.

Procedure guidelines: **Last offices**

Equipment

1 Bowl, soap, towel, two face cloths.
2 Razor (electric or disposable), comb, equipment for nail care.
3 Equipment for mouth care including equipment for cleaning dentures.
4 Identification labels ×2.
5 Documents required by law or hospital policy, e.g. notification of death cards.
6 Shroud or patient's personal clothing: night-dress, pyjamas, clothes previously requested by patient, or clothes which comply with family/cultural wishes.

7 Body bag if required (i.e. in event of actual or potential leakage of bodily fluids and/or infectious disease), and labels for the body defining the nature of the infection/disease.
8 Tape.
9 Gauze, tape, dressings and bandages if wounds present.
10 Valuables/property book.
11 Plastic bags for clinical and household waste.

Procedure

Action	Rationale
1 Inform the nurse in charge on the ward. Inform medical staff. Confirmation of death must be given. This is usually done by medical staff. If an expected death occurs during the night, the senior nurse on duty sometimes confirms death if an agreed policy has been implemented. An unexpected death must be confirmed by the attending medical officer. Confirmation of death must be recorded in a patient's medical and nursing notes.	A registered medical practitioner who has attended the deceased person during the last illness is required to give a medical certificate of the cause of death. The certificate requires the doctor to state the last date on which he/she saw the deceased alive and whether or not he/she has seen the body after death.
2 Inform and offer support to relatives and/or next of kin. Offer support of the Hospital Chaplain or other religious leader or other appropriate person, e.g. bereavement support officer.	To ensure relevant individuals are aware of patient's death. To provide sensitive care.

*Procedure guidelines: **Last offices** (cont'd)*

Action	Rationale
3 Inform other patients and discuss issues as appropriate.	Other patients are often aware that a death is expected or has occurred. It is important to inform them when someone dies so that they can be offered support and reassurance, and to answer any questions sensitively, so as to allay misconceptions and fears.
4 Put on gloves and apron.	To reduce risk of contamination with body fluids, and to reduce risk of cross-infection. Protective clothing, for example gloves and an apron, must be worn for carrying out last offices.
5 Lay the patient on his/her back with the assistance of two nurses (adhering to the manual handling policy). Remove all but one pillow. Support the jaw by placing a pillow or rolled-up towel on the chest underneath the jaw. Remove any mechanical aids such as syringe drivers, heel pads, etc. Apply gauze and tape to syringe driver sites and document actions in nursing documentation. Straighten the limbs.	To maintain the patient's dignity and for future management of the body, as rigor mortis occurs 2–6 hours after death, with full intensity within 48 hours and then disappearing within another 48 hours (Robbins 1995).
6 Close the patient's eyes by applying light pressure to the eyelids for 30 seconds.	To maintain the patient's dignity and for aesthetic reasons. Closure of eyes will also provide tissue protection in case of corneal donation (Green & Green 1992).
7 Drain the bladder by pressing on the lower abdomen.	Because the body can continue to excrete fluids after death.
8 Pack orifices with gauze if fluid secretion continues or is anticipated. If excessive leaking of bodily fluids occurs, consider suctioning.	Leaking orifices pose a health hazard to staff coming into contact with the body.
9 Exuding wounds should be covered with a clean absorbent dressing and secured with an occlusive dressing (e.g. Tegaderm).	The dressing will absorb any leakage from the wound site. Open wounds pose a health hazard to staff coming into contact with the body. If a post mortem is required, existing dressings should be left in situ and covered.
10 Remove drainage tubes, etc., unless otherwise stated, and document actions and any tubes remaining, e.g. Hickman lines. Open drainage sites may need to be sealed with an occlusive dressing (e.g. Tegaderm).	Open drainage sites pose a health hazard to staff coming into contact with the body. If a post mortem is required drainage tubes, etc., should be left in situ.
11 Wash the patient, unless requested not to do so for religious/cultural reasons (please refer to section on individual faiths in this chapter). If necessary, shave a male patient.	For hygienic and aesthetic reasons. As a mark of respect and a point of closure in the relationship between nurse and patient (Cooke 2000).
It may be important to family and carers to assist with washing, thereby continuing to provide the care given in the period before death.	It is an expression of respect and affection, part of the process of adjusting to loss and expressing grief.
12 Clean the patient's mouth using a foam stick to remove any debris and secretions. Clean dentures and replace them in the mouth if possible.	For hygienic and aesthetic reasons.
13 Remove all jewellery (in the presence of another nurse) unless requested by the patient's family to do otherwise. Jewellery remaining on the patient should be documented on the 'notification of death' form. Record the jewellery and other valuables in the patient's property book and store the items according to local policy.	To meet with legal requirements and relatives' wishes.
14 Dress the patient in personal clothing or shroud, depending on hospital policy or relatives' wishes.	For religious or cultural reasons and to meet family's or carers' wishes.

*Procedure guidelines: **Last offices** (cont'd)*

	Action	Rationale
15	Label one wrist and one ankle with an identification label. Complete any documents such as notification of death cards. Copies of such cards are usually required (refer to hospital policy for details). Tape one securely to clothing or shroud.	To ensure correct and easy identification of the body in the mortuary.
16	Wrap the body in a mortuary sheet, ensuring that the face and feet are covered and that all limbs are held securely in position.	To avoid possible damage to the body during transfer and to prevent distress to colleagues, e.g. portering staff.
17	Secure the sheet with tape.	Pins must not be used as they are a health and safety hazard to staff.
18	Place the body in a sheet and then a body bag if leakage of body fluids is a problem or is anticipated, or if the patient has certain infectious diseases (refer to Ch. 5, Barrier nursing).	Actual or potential leakage of fluid, whether infection is present or not, poses a health hazard to all those who come into contact with the deceased patient. The sheet will absorb excess fluid.
19	Tape the second notification of death card to the outside of the sheet (or body bag).	For ease of identification of the body in the mortuary.
20	Request the portering staff to remove the body from the ward and transport to the mortuary.	Decomposition occurs rapidly, particularly in hot weather and in overheated rooms. Many pathogenic organisms survive for some time after death and so decomposition of the body may pose a health and safety hazard for those handling the body (Cooke 2000). Autolysis and growth of bacteria are delayed if the body is cooled.
21	Screen off area where removal of the body will occur.	To avoid causing unnecessary distress to other patients, relatives and staff.
22	Remove gloves and apron. Dispose of equipment according to local policy and wash hands.	To minimize risk of cross-infection and contamination.
23	Record all details and actions within the nursing documentation.	To record the time of death, names of those present, and names of those informed.
24	Transfer property, patient records, etc., to the appropriate administrative department.	The administrative department cannot begin to process the formalities such as the death certificate or the collection of property by the next-of-kin until the required documents are in its possession.

Problem solving

Problem	Suggested action
Relatives not present at the time of the patient's death.	Inform the relatives as soon as possible of the death. Consider also that they may want to view the body before last offices are completed.
Relatives or next-of-kin not contactable by telephone or by the general practitioner.	If within the UK, local police will go to next-of-kin's house. If abroad, the British Embassy will assist.
Death occurring within 24 hours of an operation.	All tubes and/or drains must be left in position. Spigot any cannulae or catheters. Treat stomas as open wounds. Leave any endotracheal or tracheostomy tubes in place. Post-mortem examination will be required to establish the cause of death. Any tubes, drains, etc., may have been a major contributing factor to the death.
Unexpected death.	As above. Post-mortem examination of the body will be required to establish the cause of death.

Problem solving (cont'd)

Problem	Suggested action
Unknown cause of death.	As above.
Patient brought into hospital who is already deceased.	As above, unless patient seen by a medical practitioner within 14 days before death. In this instance the attending medical officer may complete the death certificate if he/she is clear as to the cause of death.
Patient with leaking wounds/orifices with or without infection present. Patient with hepatitis B or who is HIV positive.	For further information refer to Ch. 5, Barrier nursing: the infectious or immunosuppressed patient.
Patient who dies after receiving systemic radioactive iodine.	For further information refer to Ch. 35, Radioactive therapy: unsealed sources.
Patient who dies after insertion of gold grains, colloidal radioactive solution, caesium needles, caesium applicators, iridium wires or iridium hair pins.	Inform the physics department as well as appropriate medical staff. Once a doctor has verified death, the sources are removed and placed in a lead container. A Geiger counter is used to check that all sources have been removed. This reduces the radiation risk when completing the last offices procedures. Record the time and date of removal of the sources.
Patient and/or relative wishes to donate organs/ tissues for transplantation.	As stated in the Human Tissue Act 1961, patients with malignancies can only donate corneas and heart valves (and more recently tracheas). Contact local transplant co-ordinator as soon as decision is made to donate organs/tissue and before last offices is attempted. Obtain verbal and written consent from the next-of-kin, as per local policy. Prepare body as per transplant co-ordinator's instructions (Travis 2002).
Patient to be moved straight from ward to undertakers.	Contact senior nurse for hospital. Contact local Registry Office as release of Certificate for Burial or Cremation ('green' document) needs to be obtained. Liaise with chosen funeral directors and the deceased's family. Perform last offices as per religious/cultural/family wishes. Obtain written authority for removal of body by the funeral directors, from the next-of-kin. Document all actions and proceedings (Travis 2002).
Relatives want to see the body after removal from the ward.	Inform the mortuary staff in order to allow time for them to prepare the body. The body will normally be placed in the hospital viewing room. Ask relatives if they wish for a chaplain or other religious leader or appropriate person to accompany them. As required, religious artefacts should be removed from or added to the viewing room. The nurse should check that the body and environment are presentable before accompanying the relatives into the viewing room. The relatives may want to be alone with the deceased but the nurse should wait outside the viewing room in order that support may be provided should the relatives become distressed. After the relatives have left, the nurse should contact the portering service who will return the body to the mortuary.

Procedure guidelines: **Requirements for people of different religious faiths**

The following are only guidelines: individual requirements may vary even among members of the same faith. Varying degrees of adherence and orthodoxy exist within all the world's faiths. The given religion of a patient may occasionally be offered to indicate an association with particular cultural and national roots, rather than to indicate a significant degree of adherence to the tenets of a particular faith. If in doubt, consult the family members concerned.

Bahai

1 The body of the deceased should be treated with respect. Bahai relatives may wish to say prayers for the deceased person, but normal last offices performed by nursing staff are quite acceptable.
2 Bahai adherents may not be cremated or embalmed, nor may they be buried more than an hour's journey from the place of death. A special ring will be placed on the finger of the patient and should not be removed.
3 Bahais have no objection to post-mortem examination and may leave their bodies to scientific research or donate organs if they wish.

4 Further information can be obtained from the nearest Assembly of the Bahais (see telephone directory). Alternatively, contact:
  National Spiritual Assembly of the Bahais of the United Kingdom
  27 Rutland Gate, London SW7 1PD.
  Tel: 020 7590 8792.

Buddhism

1 There is no prescribed ritual for the handling of the corpse of a Buddhist person, so customary laying out is appropriate. However, a request may be made for a Buddhist monk or nun to be present.
2 As there are a number of different schools of Buddhism, relatives should be contacted for advice as some sects have strong views on how the body should be treated.
3 When the patient dies, inform the monk or nun if required (the patient's relatives often take this step). The body should not be moved for at least one hour if prayers are to be said.

4 There are unlikely to be objections to post-mortem examination and organ donation, although some Far Eastern Buddhists may object to this.
5 The patient's body should be wrapped in an unmarked sheet.
6 Cremation is preferred.
7 For further information contact:
  The Buddhist Hospice Trust,
  PO Box 123, Ashford, Kent TN24 9TF.

Christianity

1 There are many denominations and degrees of adherence within the Christian faith. In most cases customary last offices are acceptable.
2 Relatives may wish staff to call the hospital chaplain, or minister or priest from their own church to either perform last rites or say prayers.
3 Some Roman Catholic families may wish to place a rosary in the deceased patient's hands and/or a crucifix at the patient's head.
4 Some orthodox families may wish to place an icon (holy picture) at either side of the patient's head.

5 For further information consult the hospital chaplain or consult the telephone directory for the local denominational minister or priest. Alternatively, contact:
  Hospital Chaplaincies Council,
  Church House,
  Great Smith Street,
  London SW1 3NZ.
  Tel: 020 7898 1894.
  Useful website: www.nhs-chaplaincy-spiritualcare.org.uk

Hinduism

1 If required by relatives, inform the family priest or one from the local temple. If unavailable, relatives may wish to read from the *Bhagavad Gita* or make a request that staff read extracts during the last offices.
2 The family may wish to carry out or assist in last offices and may request that the patient is dressed in his or her own clothes. If possible, the eldest son should be present. A Hindu may like to have leaves of the sacred Tulsi plant and Ganges water placed in his/her mouth by relatives

before death. It is therefore imperative that relatives are warned that the patient's death is imminent. Relatives of the same sex as the patient may wish to wash his or her body, preferably in water mixed with water from the River Ganges. If no relatives are present, nursing staff of the same sex as the patient should wear gloves and apron and then straighten the body, close the eyes and support the jaw before wrapping in a sheet. The body should not be washed. Do not remove sacred threads or jewellery.

Procedure guidelines: **Requirements for people of different religious faiths** *(cont'd)*

3 The patient's family may request that the patient be placed on the floor and they may wish to burn incense.

4 The patient is usually cremated as soon as possible after death. Post-mortems are viewed as disrespectful to the deceased person, so are only carried out when strictly necessary. Consult the wishes of the family before touching the body.

5 For further information contact the nearest Hindu temple (see telephone directory) or:
   National Council of Hindu Temples (UK),
   40 Stoke Row, Coventry CV2 4JP.
   Tel: 0121 622 6946.

Jainism

1 The relatives of a Jainist patient may wish to contact their priest to recite prayers with the patient and family.

2 The family may wish to be present during the last offices and also to assist with washing. Not all families will want to perform this task, however.

3 The family may ask for the patient to be clothed in a plain white gown or shroud with no pattern or ornament and then wrapped in a plain white sheet. They may provide the gown themselves.

4 Post-mortems may be seen as disrespectful, depending on the degree of orthodoxy of the patient. Organ donation is acceptable.

5 Cremation is arranged whenever possible within 24 hours of death.

6 Orthodox Jains may have chosen the path of *Sallekhana*, that is, death by ritual fasting. Sallekhana is rarely practised today although it may still have an influence on the Jain attitude to death.

7 For further information contact:
   The Institute of Jainology,
   Unit 18, Silicon Business Centre,
   26 Wandsworth Road, Greenford,
   Middx UB6 7JZ.
   Tel: 020 8997 2300.

   The Jain Centre,
   32 Oxford Street,
   Leicester LE1 5XU.
   Tel: 0116 254 3091.

Jehovah's Witness

1 Routine last offices are appropriate. Relatives may wish to be present during last offices, either to pray or to read from the Bible. The family will inform staff should there be any special requirements, which may vary according to the patient's country of origin.

2 Jehovah's Witnesses usually refuse post-mortem unless absolutely necessary. Organ donation may be acceptable.

3 Further information can be obtained from the nearest Kingdom Hall (see telephone directory) or:
   The Medical Desk,
   The Watch Tower Bible and Tract Society,
   Watch Tower House, The Ridgeway,
   London NW7 1RN.
   Tel: 020 8906 2211.

Judaism

1 The family will contact their own Rabbi if they have one. If not, the hospital chaplaincy will advise. Prayers are recited by those present.

2 Traditionally the body is left for about 8 minutes before being moved while a feather is placed across the lips and nose to detect any signs of breath.

3 Usually close relatives will straighten the body, but nursing staff are permitted to perform any procedure for preserving dignity and honour. Wearing gloves, the body should be handled as little as possible but nurses may:
   (a) Close the eyes.
   (b) Tie up the jaw.
   (c) Put the arms parallel and close to the sides of the body leaving the hands open. Straighten the patient's legs.
   (d) Remove tubes unless contraindicated.
   Patients must not be washed and should remain in the clothes in which they died. The body will be washed by a nominated group, the Holy Assembly, which performs a ritual purification.

4 Watchers stay with the body until burial (normally completed within 24 hours of death). In the period before burial a separate non-denominational room is appreciated, where the body can be placed with its feet towards the door.

5 It is not possible for funerals to take place on the Sabbath (between sunset on Friday and sunset on Saturday). If death occurs during the Sabbath, the body will remain with the watchers until the end of the Sabbath. Advice should be sought from the relatives. In some areas, the Registrar's office will arrange to open on Sundays and Bank Holidays to allow for the registration of death where speedy burial is required for religious reasons. The Jewish Burial Society will know whether this service is offered in the local area.

6 Post-mortems are permitted only if required by law. Organ donation is sometimes permitted.

7 Cremation is unlikely but some non-orthodox Jews are now accepting this in preference to burial.

*Procedure guidelines: **Requirements for people of different religious faiths** (cont'd)*

8 For further information, contact:
  The Burial Society of the United Synagogue
  Tel: 020 8343 3456.

  The Office of the Chief Rabbi (Orthodox),
  735 High Road, North Finchley, London WC1N 9HN.
  Tel: 020 8343 6301.

Reform Synagogues of Great Britain,
The Sternberg Centre for Judaism,
80 East End Road, Finchley, London N3 2SY.
Tel: 020 8349 4731.

Union of Liberal and Progressive Synagogues,
Montagu Centre, 21 Maple Street,
London W1T 4BE.

Mormon (Church of Jesus Christ of the Latter Day Saints)

1 There are no special requirements, but relatives may wish to be present during the last offices. Relatives will advise staff if the patient wears a one or two piece sacred undergarment. If this is the case, relatives will dress the patient in these items.

2 For further information contact the nearest Church of Jesus Christ of Latter Day Saints (see telephone directory) or
  The Church of Jesus Christ of Latter Day Saints,
  751 Warwick Road, Solihull, West Midlands B91 3DQ.
  Tel: 0121 712 1145.

Muslim (Islam)

1 Where possible, the patient's bed should be turned so that their body (head first) is facing Mecca. If the patient's bed cannot be moved, then the patient can be turned on to their right side so that the deceased's face is facing towards Mecca.

2 Many Muslims object to the body being touched by someone of a different faith or opposite sex. If no family members are present, wear gloves and close the patient's eyes, support the jaw and straighten the body. The head should be turned to the right shoulder and the body covered with a plain white sheet. The body should not be washed nor the nails cut.

3 The patient's body is normally either taken home or taken to a mosque as soon as possible to be washed by another Muslim of the same sex. Burial takes place

preferably within 24 hours of death. Cremation is forbidden. Post-mortems are permitted only if required by law. Organ donation is not always encouraged although in the UK, a Fatwa (religious verdict) was given by the UK Muslim Law Council which now encourages Muslims to donate organs.

4 Further information can be obtained from:
  Islamic Cultural Centre,
  The London Central Mosque Trust Ltd,
  The Islamic Centre, 146 Park Road,
  London NW8 7RG.
  Tel: 020 7724 3363.

  Islamic Foundation,
  Markfield Dawah Centre, Ratby Lane, Markfield,
  Leics LE67 9RN.
  Tel: 01530 244944.

Rastafarian

1 Customary last offices are appropriate, although the patient's family may wish to be present during the preparation of the body to say prayers.

2 Permission for organ donation is unlikely and post-mortems will be refused unless absolutely necessary.

3 For further information contact:
  The Rastafarian Society
  290–296 Tottenham High Road, London N15 4AJ.
  Tel: 020 8808 2185.
  Useful website: www.rasta-man.co.uk/religion.htm

Sikhism

1 Family members (especially the eldest son) and friends will be present if they are able.

2 Usually the family takes responsibility for the last offices, but nursing staff may be asked to close the patient's eyes, support the jaw, straighten the body and wrap it in a plain white sheet.

3 Do not remove the '5 ks', which are personal objects sacred to the Sikhs:
  Kesh: do not cut hair or beard or remove turban.
  Kanga: do not remove the semi-circular comb, which fixes the uncut hair.

  Kara: do not remove bracelet worn on the wrist.
  Kaccha: do not remove the special shorts worn as underwear.
  Kirpan: do not remove the sword: usually a miniature sword is worn.

4 The family will wash and dress the deceased person's body.

5 Post-mortems are only permitted if required by law. Sikhs are always cremated.

6 Organ donation is permitted but some Sikhs refuse this as they do not wish the body to be mutilated.

*Procedure guidelines: **Requirements for people of different religious faiths** (cont'd)*

7 For further information contact the nearest Sikh temple or Gurdwara (see telephone directory). Alternatively, contact:
Sikh Missionary Society UK,
10 Featherstone Road, Southall, Middlesex UB2 5AA.
Tel: 020 8574 1902.

Sikh Educational and Cultural Association (UK),
Sat Nam Kutia, 18 Farncroft, Gravesend,
Kent DA11 7LT.
Tel: 01474 332356.

Zoroastrian (Parsee)

1 Customary last offices are often acceptable to Zoroastrian patients.
2 The family may wish to be present during, or participate in, the preparation of the body.
3 Orthodox Parsees require a priest to be present, if possible.
4 After washing, the body is dressed in the *Sadra* (white cotton or muslin shirt symbolizing purity) and *Kusti* (girdle woven of 72 strands of lambs' wool symbolizing the 72 chapters of the *Yasna* (Liturgy)).
5 Relatives may cover the patient's head with a white cap or scarf.
6 It is important that the funeral takes place as soon as possible after death.
7 Burial and cremation are acceptable. Post-mortems are forbidden unless required by law.

8 Organ donation is forbidden by religious law.
9 For further information contact:
The Zoroastrian Information Centre,
88 Compayne Gardens, London NW6 3RU.
Tel: 020 7328 6018.

In addition to the addresses given above, further information is available from:

The Shap Working Party on World Religions in Education
The National Society's RE Centre,
36 Causton Street, London SW1P 4AU.
Tel: 020 7932 1194.
Useful website: www.multifaithnet.org/mfnopenaccess/resource/zoroastrianism/descr-zo.htm

References and further reading

Ainsworth-Smith, I. & Speck, P. (1982) *Letting Go: Caring for the Dying and The Bereaved*. SPCK, London.

Albery, N. & Weinrich, S. (eds) (2000) *The New Natural Death Handbook*. Rider, London.

Barber, J., Campbell, A. & Morgan, L. (2000) Last Offices for a child/young person. In: *Clinical Care Manual for Children's Nursing*. Mark Allen, Dinton, Wiltshire, pp. 59–60.

Berry, P. & Griffie, J. (2001) Planning for the actual death. In: *Textbook of Palliative Care Nursing* (eds B. Ferrell & N. Coyle). Oxford University Press, Oxford, pp. 382–94.

Bradbury, M. (1999) *Representations of Death: A Sociological Perspective*. Routledge, London.

Braun, K.L., Pietsch, J.H. & Blanchett, P.L. (eds) (2000) *Cultural Issues in End of Life Decision Making*. Sage Publications, California.

Clark, D. & Seymour, J. (1999) *Reflections on Palliative Care*. Open University Press, Buckingham.

Cobb, M. (2001) *The Dying Soul. Spiritual Care at the End of Life*. Open University Press, Buckingham.

Commission for Racial Equality (1999) *CRE Factsheet: Ethnic Minorities in Britain*. CRE, London.

Cooke, H. (2000) *A Practical Guide to Holistic Care at the End of Life*. Butterworth-Heinemann, Oxford.

Davies, D.J. (1997) *Death, Ritual and Belief: The Rhetoric of Funerary Rites*. Cassell, London.

Department for Work & Pensions (2002) *What to do after a Death in England & Wales*. Stationery Office, London.

Dickenson, D., Johnson, M. & Katz, J.S. (eds) (2000) *Death, Dying and Bereavement*, 2nd edn. Sage Publications, London.

Docherty, B. (2000) Care of the dying patient. *Prof Nurse*, **12**, 752.

Eliade, M. & Couliano, I.P. (2000) *The Harper Collins Concise Guide to World Religions*. Harper, San Francisco.

Field, D., Hockey, J. & Small, N. (1997) *Death, Gender and Ethnicity*. Routledge, London.

Field, D., Hockey, J. & Small, N. (1997) Making sense of difference: death, gender and ethnicity in modern Britain. In: *Death, Gender and Ethnicity*. Routledge, London, pp. 1–28.

Firth, S. (1993) Cultural issues in terminal care. In: *The Future for Palliative Care: Issues of Policy and Practice* (ed. D. Clark). Open University Press, Buckingham, pp. 98–110.

Firth, S. (2001) *Wider Horizons: Care of the Dying in a Multi-cultural Society*. National Council for Hospice and Specialist Palliative Care Services, London.

Gilliat-Ray, S. (2001) Sociological perspectives on the pastoral care of minority faiths in hospital. In: *Spirituality in Health Care Contexts* (ed. H. Orchard). Jessica Kingsley Publishers, London, pp. 135–46.

Goldman, A. (ed.) (1999) *Care of the Dying Child*. Oxford University Press, Oxford.

Green, J. & Green. M. (1992) *Dealing with Death: Practices and Procedures*. Chapman and Hall, London.

Gunaratnam, Y. (1997) Culture is not enough: a critique of multi-culturalism in palliative care. In: *Death, Gender and Ethnicity* (eds D. Field, J. Hockey & N. Small). Routledge, London, pp. 166–86.

Hallam, E., Hockey, J. & Howard, G. (1999) *Beyond the Body. Death and Social Identity*. Routledge, London.

Harris, P. (2000) *What to Do When Someone Dies*. Which? London.

Helman, C.J. (2000) *Culture, Health and Illness*, 4th edn. Butterworth-Heinemann, London.

Henley, A. & Scott, J. (1999) *Culture, Religion and Patient Care*. Age Concern, London.

Hockey, J., Katz, J. & Small, N. (2001) *Grief, Mourning and Death Ritual*. Open University Press, Buckingham.

Howarth, G. & Jupp. P.C. (eds) (1996) *Contemporary Issues in the Sociology of Death, Dying and Disposal*. Macmillan, Basingstoke.

Hughes, S. & Henley, A. (1990) *Dealing with Death in Hospitals: Procedures for Managers and Staff*. King's Fund, London.

Jamieson, E.M., McCall, J.M. & Whyte, L.A. (2002) Care of the deceased person. In: *Clinical Nursing Practices*. Churchill Livingstone, Edinburgh, pp. 89–93.

Jewett, C.L. (1994) *Helping Children Cope with Separation and Loss*. Batsford, London.

Jupp, P.C. & Gittings, C. (1999) *Death in England. An Illustrated History*. Manchester University Press, Manchester.

Karmi, G. (1996) *The Ethnic Health Handbook. A Factfile for Health Care Professionals*. Blackwell Science, Oxford.

Keene, M. (2002) *World Religions*. Lion Publishing, Oxford.

Kowalak, J.P., Selena, A., Hughes & Mills, J.E. (2003) Postmortem care. In: *Best Practices. A Guide to Excellence in Nursing Care*. Lippincott Williams & Wilkins, Philadelphia, pp. 52–4.

Kubler-Ross, E. (1990) *Living with Dying and Death*. Souvenir, London.

Lawton, J. (2000) *The Dying Process. Patients' Experiences of Palliative Care*. Routledge, London.

National Council for Hospice and Specialist Palliative Care Services (1995) *Opening Doors: Improving Access to Hospital and Specialist Care Services by People in Black and Ethnic Communities*. National Council for Hospice and Palliative Care Services, London.

Nearney, L. (1998) Practical procedures for nurses. Last Offices, Part 1. *Nurs Times*, **94**(26), insert.

Nearney, L. (1998) Practical procedures for nurses. Last Offices, Part 2. *Nurs Times*, **94**(27), insert.

Nearney, L. (1998) Practical procedures for nurses. Last Offices, Part 3. *Nurs Times*, **94**(28), insert.

Neuberger, J. (1994) *Caring for Dying People of Different Faiths*. Lisa Sainsbury Foundation, London, pp. 775–801.

Neuberger, J. (1999) Cultural issues in palliative care. In: *Oxford Textbook of Palliative Medicine* (eds D. Doyle, G. Hanks & N. MacDonald). Oxford University Press, Oxford.

North Kent Council for Interfaith Relations (2002) *The Spiritual and Pastoral Care of Patients in Hospital and Their Relatives*. North Kent Council for Interfaith Relations, Kent.

Nursing Standard (2000) Last offices: patient hygiene. *Nurs Stand*, **15**(12), insert.

Nyatanga, B. (1997) International perspectives. Cultural issues in palliative care. *Int J Palliat Nurs*, **3**(4), 203–8.

O'Hagan, K. (2001) *Cultural Competence in the Caring Professions*. Jessica Kingsley, London.

Orchard, H. (ed.) (2001) *Spirituality in Health Care Contexts*. Jessica Kingsley, London.

Parkes, C.M., Laungani, P. & Young, B. (1997) *Death and Bereavement Across Cultures*. Routledge, London.

Philpin, S. (2002) Rituals and nursing: a critical commentary. *J Adv Nurs*, **38**(2) 144–51.

Rankin, J., Brown, A. & Gateshill, P. (1992) *Ethics and Religions*. Longman, London.

Rinpoche, S. (2002) *The Tibetan Book of Living and Dying*. Rider, London.

Robbins, J. (ed.) (1995) *Caring for the Dying Patient and the Family*, 3rd edn. Chapman and Hall, London.

Sambi, S.P. & Cole, W.O. (1990) Caring for Sikh patients. *Palliat Med*, **4**, 229–33.

Sampson, C. (1982) *The Neglected Ethic: Religious and Cultural Factors in the Care of Patients*. McGraw-Hill, Maidenhead.

Seale, C. (1998) *Constructing Death. The Sociology of Dying and Bereavement*. Cambridge University Press, Cambridge.

Sharma, D.L. (1990) Hindu attitudes towards suffering, dying and death. *Palliat Med*, **4**, 235–8.

Smaje, C. & Field, D. (1997) Absent minorities? Ethnicity and the use of palliative care services. In: *Death, Gender and Ethnicity* (eds D. Field, J. Hockey & N. Small). Routledge, London, pp. 142–65.

Speck, P. (1992) Care after death. *Nurs Times*, **88**(6), 20.

Spector, R. (1996) *Cultural Diversity in Health and Illness*, 4th edn. Appleton and Lange, Stanford.

Travis, S. (2002) *Procedure for the Care of Patients Who Die in Hospital*. Royal Marsden NHS Trust, London.

Weller, P. (ed.) (1997) *Religions in the UK: A Multi-Faith Directory*. University of Derby, Derby.

Wolfe, Z. (1988) *Nurses' Work: The Sacred and the Profane*. University of Pennsylvania Press, Philadelphia.

Bahai faith

Smith, P. (1998) *The Bahai Religion: A Short Introduction to Its History and Teachings*. George Ronald, Oxford.

Smith, P. (2000) *A Concise Encyclopaedia of the Bahai Faith*. Oneworld Publications, Oxford.

Buddhism

Gyatso, G.K. (2001) *Introduction to Buddhism: An Explanation of the Buddhist Way of Life*. Tharpa Publications, Ulverston, Cumbria.

Hagan, S. (1997) *Buddhism: Plain and Simple*. Penguin, London.

Maguire, J. (2001) *Essential Buddhism: A Guide to Beliefs and Practices*. Pocket Books, New York.

Northcott, N. (2002) Nursing with dignity. Part 2: Buddhism. *Nurs Times*, **98**(10), 36–8.

Sibley, D. (1997) Caring for dying Buddhists. *Int J Palliat Nurs*, **3**(1), 26–30.

Snelling, J. (1998) *The Buddhist Handbook: A Complete Guide to Buddhist Teaching and Practice*. Rider, London.

Stokes, G. (2000) *Buddha: A Beginner's Guide*. Hodder & Stoughton, London.

Williams, P. (1989) *Mahayana Buddhism*. Routledge, London.

Christianity

Christmas, M. (2002) Nursing with dignity, part 3. Christianity I. *Nurs Times*, **98**(11), 37–9.

Cross, F.L. & Livingstone, E.L. (1997) *The Oxford Dictionary of the Christian Church*. Oxford University Press, Oxford.

Edwards, D.L. (1999) *What Anglicans Believe*. Mowbray, London.

Grenz, S.J. (1998) *What Christians Believe and Why*. Paternoster Press, Carlisle.

Littleton, M. (2001) *Jesus.* John Knox Press, Westminster.

McManners, J. (ed.) (2002) *The Oxford History of Christianity.* Oxford Paperbacks, Oxford.

Papadopoulos, I. (2002) Nursing with dignity, part 4. Christianity II. *Nurs Times,* **98**(12), 36–7.

Stott, J. (2002) *Basic Christianity.* Intervarsity Press, London.

Ware, T. (1997) *The Orthodox Church.* Penguin, London.

Hinduism

Cross, S. (2002) *Way of Hinduism.* Thorsons, London.

Flood, G. (2001) *An Introduction to Hinduism.* Cambridge University Press, Cambridge.

Henley, A. (1983) *Caring for Hindus and Their Families: Religious Aspects of Care.* National Extension College, Cambridge.

Jootun, D. (2002) Nursing with dignity, part 7. Hinduism. *Nurs Times,* **98**(15), 38–40.

Klostermaier, K.K. (2000) *Hinduism: A Short History.* Oneworld Publications, Oxford.

Laungani, P. (1997) Death in a Hindu family. In: *Death and Bereavement Across Cultures* (eds C. Parkes, P. Laungani & B. Young). Routledge, London, pp. 52–72.

Wordsworth Classics (1997) *The Bhagavad Gita.* Wordsworth, Hertfordshire.

Jainism

Dundas, P. (2002) *The Jains.* Routledge, London.

Jehovah's Witnesses

Cumberland, W.H. (1986) The Jehovah's Witness tradition. In: *Caring and Curing: Health and Medicine in the Western Religious Traditions* (eds R. Numbers & D. Amundsen). Macmillan, New York, pp. 468–85.

Simpson, J. (2002) Nursing with dignity, part 9. Jehovah's Witnesses. *Nurs Times,* **98**(17), 36–7.

Watchtower (1996) *Jehovah's Witnesses: Religious and Ethical Position on Medical Therapy, Child Care and Related Matters.* Hospital Information Service, Britain.

Judaism

Collins, A. (2002) Nursing with dignity, part 1. Judaism. *Nurs Times,* **98**(9), 33–5.

Katz, J.S. (1996) Caring for dying Jewish people in a multi-cultural/religious society. *Int J Palliat Nurs,* **2**(1), 43–7.

Lancaster, B. (1997) *The Elements of Judaism.* Element, London.

Neuberger, J. (1999) Spiritual issues. Judaism and palliative care. *Eur J Palliat Care,* **6**(5), 166–8.

Neusner, J. (2002) *Judaism.* Penguin, London.

Wigoder, N., Skolnick, F. & Himelstein, S. (2002) *The New Encyclopaedia of Judaism.* New York University Press, New York.

Wood, C. (2002) *Living Judaism.* Heinemann Library, New York.

Mormonism

Bush, L.E. (1986) The Mormon tradition. In: *Caring and Curing: Health and Medicine in the Western Religious Traditions* (eds R. Numbers & D. Amundsen). Macmillan, New York, pp. 397–420.

Eliason, E.A. (ed.) (2001) *Mormons and Mormonism.* University of Illinois Press, Illinois.

Muslim faith

Akhtar, S. (2002) Nursing with dignity, part 8. Islam. *Nurs Times,* **98**(16), 40–2.

Gordon, M.S. (2002) *Islam.* Duncain Baird, London.

Henley, A. (1982) *Caring for Muslims and Their Families: Religious Aspects of Care.* National Extension College, Cambridge.

Horrie, C. & Chippindale, P. (2001) *What is Islam? A Comprehensive Introduction.* Virgin, London.

Lewis, P. (1994) *Islamic Britain.* I.B. Tauris, London.

Penguin Classics (1999) *The Koran.* Penguin, London.

Ruthven, M. (2000) *Islam: A Very Short Introduction.* Oxford University Press, Oxford.

Sarwas, G. (1998) *Islam: Beliefs and Teachings.* Muslim Educational Trust, London.

Sheikh, A. & Gatrad, A.R. (2000) *Caring for Muslim Patients.* Radcliffe Medical Press, Oxford.

Paganism

Prout, C. (1992) Paganism. *Nurs Times,* **88**(33), 42–3.

Rastafarianism

Barrett, L.E. (1997) *The Rastafarians.* Beacons Press, Boston.

Baxter, C. (2002) Nursing with dignity, part 5. Rastafarianism. *Nurs Times,* **98**(13), 42–3.

Sikhism

Cole, W.O. & Sambhi, P. (1995) *The Sikhs. Their Religious Beliefs and Practices.* Sussex Academic Press, London.

Gill, B.K. (2002) Nursing with dignity, part 6. Sikhism. *Nurs Times,* **98**(14), 39–41.

Henley, A. (1983) *Caring for Sikhs and Their Families: Religious Aspects of Care.* National Extension College, Cambridge.

Kalsi, S.S. (1999) *The Simple Guide to Sikhism.* Global Books, New Jersey.

Mayled, J. (2002) *Living Religions. Living Sikhism.* Heinemann Library, New York.

Shackle, C., Mandair, A. & Singh, G. (eds) (2000) *Sikh Religion: Culture and Ethnicity.* Routledge Curzon, New York.

Singh, D. & Smith, A. (2001) *Religions of the World.* Hodder Wayland, Hove.

Zoroastrianism

Boyce, M. (2001) *Zoroastrianism.* Routledge Curzon, New York.

Clark, P. (1998) *Zoroastranism.* Sussex Academic Press, London.

Hinnells, J.R. (1996) *Zoroastrians in Britain.* Clarendon Press, Oxford.

Kreyenbroek, P.G. (2001) *Living Zoroastrianism.* Routledge Curzon, New York.

Lumbar puncture

Chapter contents

Definition

Lumbar puncture is a medical procedure which involves withdrawing cerebrospinal fluid (CSF) by the insertion of a hollow spinal needle with a stylet into the lumbar subarachnoid space (Hickey 2002).

Indications

A lumbar puncture and withdrawal of CSF, with or without the introduction of therapeutic agents, is performed for the following purposes.

- *Diagnosis*: CSF is normally a crystal clear, colourless and sterile liquid which resembles water. Analysis of the CSF for cells not normally present may be made to determine the presence of a pathological process (Bassett 1997). In addition, CSF pressure can be measured but is contraindicated in patients where raised intracranial pressure (RIP) is suspected or present due to the risk of 'brain herniation'.
- *Introduction of therapeutic agents*: for example, antibiotics or cytotoxic intrathecal chemotherapy in the presence of malignant cytology (Hickey 2002). Since December 2001 all UK trusts that undertake to administer intrathecal cytotoxic chemotherapy must ensure safe practice guidelines have been introduced and that they are fully compliant with National Guidelines on the Safe Administration of Intrathecal Chemotherapy (HSC 2001/022: DoH 2001).
- *Introduction of spinal anaesthesia for surgery* (Hickey 2002).
- *Introduction of radiopaque contrast medium*: used to provide radiopaque pictures (myelograms) of the spinal cord (Blows 2002). Myelograms are useful in diagnosing spinal lesions and in helping to plan surgery by isolating the level of the lesion.

Contraindications

The procedure should not be undertaken in the following circumstances.

- In patients with papilloedema, bacterial meningitis or deteriorating neurological symptoms, where raised intracranial pressure or an intracranial mass is suspected. In this situation, neuroimaging (CT or MRI scan) should be undertaken prior to lumbar puncture in order to avoid resultant potentially fatal brainstem compression, herniation or coning. However, a normal CT scan does not always ensure that it is safe to perform a lumbar puncture. Until better non-invasive procedures to monitor intracranial pressure become available and are routinely used, the decision to proceed must be left to clinical expertise and judgement.
- Local skin infection may result in meningitis by passage of the bacteria from the skin to the CSF during the procedure (Richards 1992). Cutaneous or osseous infection at the site of the lumbar puncture may be considered an absolute contraindication (Hickey 2002).
- In patients who are unable to co-operate or who are too drowsy to give a history. Patient co-operation is essential to minimize the potential risk of trauma associated with this procedure.
- In patients who have severe degenerative spinal joint disease. In such cases difficulty will be experienced both in positioning the patient and in accessing between the vertebrae (Hickey 2002).
- In those patients undergoing anticoagulant therapy or who have coagulopathies or thrombocytopenia (less than 50×10^9/litre). These patients are at increased risk of bleeding and therefore coagulopathies and thrombocytopenia must be corrected prior to undertaking lumbar puncture.

Reference material

Anatomy and physiology

The spinal cord lies within the spinal column, beginning at the foramen magnum and terminating about the level of the first lumbar vertebra (Fig. 22.1). Like the brain, the spinal cord is enclosed and protected by the meninges, that is, the dura mater, arachnoid mater and pia mater. The dura and arachnoid mater are separated by a potential space known as the subdural space. The arachnoid and pia mater are separated by the subarachnoid space which contains the CSF. Below the first lumbar vertebra the subarachnoid space contains CSF, the filum terminale and the cauda equina (the anterior and posterior roots of

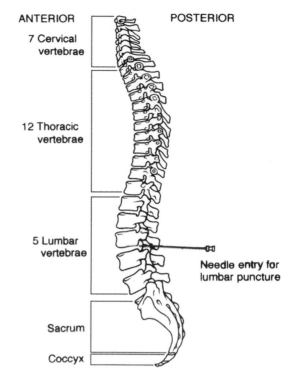

Figure 22.1 Lateral view of spinal column and vertebrae, showing needle entry site for lumbar puncture.

the lumbar and sacral nerves) (Weldon 1998). So as to avoid damage to the spinal cord, it is imperative that lumbar puncture is performed below the first lumbar vertebra where the cord terminates (Fig. 22.2).

The cord serves as the main pathway for the ascending and descending fibre tracts that connect the peripheral and spinal nerves with the brain (Weldon 1998). The peripheral nerves are attached to the spinal cord by 31 pairs of spinal nerves.

Cerebrospinal fluid (CSF)

CSF is formed primarily by filtration and secretion from networks of capillaries, called choroid plexuses, located in the ventricles of the brain. Eventually, absorption takes place through the arachnoid villi, which are finger-like projections of the arachnoid mater that push into the dural venous sinuses. CSF is clear, colourless and slightly alkaline, with a specific gravity of 1007 (Hickey 2002). In an adult, approximately 500 ml of CSF are produced and reabsorbed each day (Weldon 1998), with 120–150 ml present at one time. CSF constituents include:

- Water
- Mineral salts
- Glucose
- Protein (16–45 mg/dl) (Hickey 2002)
- Urea and creatinine.

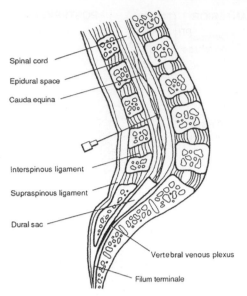

Figure 22.2 Lumbar puncture. Sagittal section through lumbosacral spine. The most common site for lumbar puncture is between L3 and L4 and between L4 and L5 as the spinal cord terminates at L1.

The functions of CSF include:

- To act as a shock absorber
- To carry nutrients to the brain
- To remove metabolites from the brain
- To support and protect the brain and spinal cord
- To keep the brain and spinal cord moist (Hickey 2002).

Sampling and CSF pressure

The amount of CSF withdrawn for sampling depends on the investigation required. In practice, approximately 5–10 ml of CSF are usually withdrawn, although investigations for cell count and Gram stain can be performed using 1 ml. The pressure of CSF can be measured at the time of lumbar puncture using a manometer. Normal CSF pressure falls within a range of 60–180 mmH$_2$O (Hickey 2002). Spinal pressure may be raised in the presence of cerbrovascular accident, a space-occupying lesion or bacterial meningitis.

Abnormalities of CSF

- A red discoloration of the CSF is indicative of the presence of blood, which is an abnormal finding. If the presence of blood is caused by a traumatic spinal tap, the blood will usually clot and the fluid clear as the procedure continues. If the presence of blood is due to subarachnoid haemorrhage, no clotting will occur (Lindsay *et al.* 1997).
- Turbidity, cloudy CSF, is indicative of the presence of a large number of white cells or protein and is an abnormal finding. The causes of such turbidity include infection or the secondary infiltration of the meninges with malignant disease, e.g. leukaemia or lymphoma.
- The presence of different types of blood cells in the CSF can be diagnostic of a variety of neurological disorders, e.g.
  (a) Erythrocytes are indicative of haemorrhage.
  (b) Polymorphonuclear leucocytes are indicative of meningitis or cerebral abcess.
  (c) Monocytes are indicative of a viral or tubercular meningitis or encephalitis.
  (d) Lymphocytes present in larger numbers are indicative of viral meningitis or infiltration of the meninges by malignant disease (Hickey 2002).
  (e) The presence of leukaemic blast cells is indicative of infiltration of the meninges by leukaemia.
  (f) Viral, bacterial or fungal cultures from the CSF sample are indicative of infection.

Investigations

A number of tests can be performed on CSF to aid diagnosis (Lindsay *et al.* 1997).

- *Culture and sensitivity.* Identifying the presence of micro-organisms would confirm the diagnosis of bacterial/fungal meningitis or a cerebral abscess. The isolation of the causative organism would enable the initiation of appropriate antibiotic or antifungal therapy.
- *Virology screening.* Isolation of a causative virus would enable appropriate therapy to be initiated promptly.
- *Serology for syphilis.* Tests include: Wasserman test (WR), venereal disease research laboratory (VDRL) and *Treponema pallidum* immobilization test (TPI).
- *Protein.* The total amount of protein in CSF should be 15.45 mg/dl (=154.5 μg/ml). Proteins are large molecules which do not readily cross the blood–brain barrier. There is normally more albumin (80%) than globulin in CSF as albumins are smaller molecules (Fischbach 1999). Raised globulin levels are indicative of multiple sclerosis, neurosyphilis, degenerative cord or brain disease. However, raised levels of total protein can be indicative of meningitis, encephalitis, myelitis or the presence of a tumour (Hickey 2002).

- *Cytology*. Central nervous system tumours or secondary meningeal disease tend to shed cells into the CSF, where they float freely. Examination of these cells morphologically after lumbar puncture will determine whether the tumour is malignant or benign (Fischbach 1999).

Instillation of chemotherapy

A number of drugs do not cross the blood–brain barrier so in the treatment and prophylaxis of some malignant diseases such as leukaemia and lymphoma, cytotoxic drugs, namely cytarabine, methotrexate and, rarely, thiopeta, may be administered intrathecally. Hydrocortisone may also be administered intrathecally. Care must be taken when administering intrathecal cytotoxic chemotherapy so as to ensure practice is safe and fully compliant with National Guidance on the Safe Administration of Intrathecal Chemotherapy (DoH HSC 2003/10). This guidance was issued as a result of the 13 patients who have died or been paralysed as a result of accidental intrathecal administration of vincristine intended for intravenous administration, between 1985 and 2001 (see Ch. 10, Drug administration: cytotoxic drugs).

Complications associated with lumbar puncture

- Infection (inadvertently introduced during procedure – there is a greater risk in the presence of neutropenia).

- Haemorrhage/localized bruising (may be caused by a traumatic procedure or in the presence of thrombocytopenia or a coagulopathy).
- Transtentorial or tonsillar herniation (if Queckenstedt's test is carried out in the presence of raised intracranial pressure).
- Headache. Frequency of post-lumbar puncture headache varies among studies and between diagnostic and therapeutic procedures. The following risk factors have been identified: young age; female gender; and the presence of headache before or at the time of the lumbar puncture. Less certain risk factors include low body mass index and previous experience of post-lumbar puncture headache (Evans *et al.* 2000). Research also suggests that the size of the needle used for the lumbar puncture may contribute to headache as a large gauge needle, such as an 18 gauge, may create a larger dural opening and the tip may tear dural fibres, delaying puncture closure. To minimize the risk of headache, a 25 gauge blunt-ended needle is recommended (Connolly 1999).
- Backache.
- Leakage from puncture site (Hickey 2002).
- The combination of intrathecal methotrexate with radiotherapy may cause arachnoiditis (irritation of the meninges), cerebral atrophy and necrosing encephalopathy (Steward *et al.* 1995). Arachnoiditis has also been reported when administering intrathecal methylprednisolone (Latham *et al.* 1997).

Procedure guidelines: **Lumbar puncture**

Equipment

1 Antiseptic skin-cleaning agents, e.g. chlorhexidine in 70% alcohol, isopropyl alcohol.
2 Selection of needles and syringes.
3 Local anaesthetic, e.g. lidocaine 1%.
4 Sterile gloves.
5 Sterile dressing pack.
6 Lumbar puncture needles of assorted sizes.
7 Disposable manometer.
8 Three sterile specimen bottles. (These should be labelled 1, 2 and 3. The first specimen, which may be bloodstained due to needle trauma, should go into bottle 1. This will assist the laboratory to differentiate between blood due to procedure trauma and that due to subarachnoid haemorrhage.)
9 Plaster dressing.

Procedure

Action	Rationale
1 Explain and discuss the procedure with the patient.	To ensure that the patient understands the procedure and gives his/her valid consent.
2 Assist patient into required position on a firm surface: (a) Lying (Fig. 22.3): • One pillow under the patient's head.	To ensure maximum widening of the intervertebral spaces and thus easier access to the subarachnoid space.

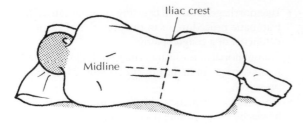

Figure 22.3 Position for lumbar puncture. Head is flexed onto chest and knees are drawn up.

*Procedure guidelines: **Lumbar puncture** (cont'd)*

Action	Rationale
• On side with knees drawn up to the abdomen and clasped by the hands.	
• Support patient in this position by holding him/her behind the knees and neck.	To avoid sudden movement by the patient which would produce trauma.
(b) Sitting:	
• Patient straddles a straight-backed chair so that his/her back is facing the doctor.	This position may be used for those patients unable to maintain the lying position. It allows more accurate identification of the spinous processes and thus the intervertebral spaces.
• Patient folds arms on the back of the chair and rests head on them.	
3 Continue to support, encourage and observe the patient throughout the procedure.	To facilitate psychological and physical well-being.
4 Assist doctor as required. Doctor will proceed to:	To monitor any physical or psychological changes.
(a) Clean the skin with the antiseptic cleaning agents	To ensure the removal of skin flora to minimize the risk of infection.
(b) Identify the area to be punctured and infiltrate the skin and subcutaneous layers with local anaesthetic	To minimize discomfort from the procedure.
(c) Introduce a spinal puncture needle between the second and third lumbar vertebrae and into the subarachnoid space	This is below the level of the spinal cord but still within the subarachnoid space.
(d) Ensure that the subarachnoid space has been entered and attach the manometer to the spinal needle, if required	To obtain a CSF pressure reading (normal pressure is 60–180 mmH$_2$O).
(e) Obtain the appropriate specimens of CSF (about 10 ml in total) for analysis. (Cell count and Gram stain can be performed using 1 ml of fluid.)	To establish diagnosis.
(f) Withdraw the spinal needle once specimens have been obtained, appropriate pressure measurements taken and intrathecal medication administered if required.	To minimize the risks of the procedure.
5 When the needle is withdrawn, apply pressure over the lumbar puncture site using a sterile topical swab.	To maintain asepsis and to stop blood and cerebrospinal fluid flow.
6 When all leakage from the puncture site has ceased, apply a plaster dressing.	To prevent secondary infection.
7 Make the patient comfortable. He/she should lie flat or the head should be tilted slightly downwards. Time to lie flat varies from hospital to hospital, but is usually around 4 hours if there is no headache.	To avoid headache and decrease the possibility of brainstem herniation (coning) due to a reduction in cerebrospinal fluid pressure.

*Procedure guidelines: **Lumbar puncture** (cont'd)*

Action	Rationale
8 Observe patient for the next 24 hours for the following:	
(a) Leakage from the puncture site	There may be a small amount of bloodstained oozing. The presence of clear fluid should be reported immediately to the doctor, especially if accompanied by fluctuation of other observations, as it may be a cerebrospinal fluid leak.
(b) Headache	Not unusual following lumbar puncture. Usually relieved by lying flat and, if ordered by the doctor, a mild analgesic.
(c) Backache	As above.
(d) Neurological observations/vital signs.	These may indicate signs of a change in intracranial pressure. (For further information on neurological observations and vital signs, see Ch. 26.)
9 Encourage a fluid intake of 2–3 litres in 24 hours.	To replace lost fluid and assist the patient to micturate, which may be difficult due to the supine position.
10 Remove equipment and dispose of as appropriate.	To prevent the spread of infection and reduce risk of needlestick injury.
11 Record the procedure in the appropriate documents.	To promote continuity of care and provide an accurate record for future reference.
12 Ensure that specimens are labelled appropriately and sent with the correct forms to the laboratory.	To ensure that the results are returned to the appropriate patient's notes.

Problem solving

Problem	Cause	Suggested action
Pain down one leg during the procedure.	A dorsal nerve root may have been touched by the spinal needle.	Inform doctor, who will probably move the needle. Reassure patient.
Headache following procedure (may persist for up to a week).	Removal of the sample of cerebrospinal fluid.	Reassure patient that it is a transient symptom. Ensure that he/she lies flat for specified period of time. Encourage a high fluid intake to replace fluid lost during procedure. Administer analgesics as ordered. If headache is severe and increasing, inform a a doctor – there is a possibility of rising intracranial pressure.
Backache following procedure.	(a) Removal of the sample of cerebrospinal fluid.	Reassure patient that it is usually a transient symptom. Ensure that he/she lies flat for appropriate period of time. Administer analgesic as ordered.
	(b) Position required for puncture.	
Fluctuation of neurological observations, i.e. level of consciousness, pulse, respirations, blood pressure or pupillary reaction.	Herniation (coning) of the brainstem due to the decrease of intracranial pressure. (Raised intracranial pressure is a contraindication to lumbar puncture.)	Observe patient constantly for signs of alteration in intracranial pressure. The frequency may be decreased as patient's condition allows. Report any fluctuations in these observations to a doctor immediately.
Leakage from the puncture site.	(a) Resolution of bleeding.	(a) No further action required.
	(b) Leakage of cerebrospinal fluid.	(b) Report immediately to a doctor, especially if accompanied by fluctuation in neurological observations (see Ch. 26).

References and further reading

Bassett, C. (1997) Medical investigations: principles and nursing management. Lumbar puncture. *Br J Nurs*, **6**(7), 405–6.

Blows, W. (2002) Diagnostic investigations, part 1: lumbar puncture. *Nurs Times*, **98**(36), 25–6.

Connolly, M.A. (1999) Clinical snapshot. Postdural puncture headache. *Am J Nurs*, **99**(11), 48–9.

Department of Health (2001) *National Guidance on the Safe Administration of Intrathecal Chemotherapy*. Department of Health, London.

Department of Health (2003) HSC 2003/10. *Updated National Guidance on the Safe Administration of Intrathecal Chemotherapy*. Department of Health, London.

Evans, R.W., Armon, C., Froham, E.M. & Goodin, D.S. (2000) Assessment: prevention of post-lumbar puncture headaches: report of the Therapeutics and Technology Assessment Subcommittee of the American Academy of Neurology. *Neurology*, **55**(7), 909–14.

Fischbach, F.T. (1999) *A Manual of Laboratory Diagnostic Tests*, 6th edn. Lippincott, Philadelphia.

Hickey, J. (2002) Cerebrospinal fluids and spinal procedures. In: *The Clinical Practice of Neurological and Neuroscience Nursing*, 5th edn. Lippincott, Philadelphia, pp. 89–91.

Latham, J.M., Fraser, R.D., Moore, R.J. *et al.* (1997) The pathological effects of intrathecal betamethasone. *Spine*, **22**(14), 1558–62.

Lindsay, K. *et al.* (1997) *Neurology and Neurosurgery Illustrated*, 3rd edn. Churchill Livingstone, Edinburgh.

Richards, P. (1992) Monitoring of cerebral function. *Br J Hosp Med*, **48**(7), 390–2.

Steward, W.P., Cassidy, J. & Kaye, S.B. (1995) Principles of chemotherapy. In: *Treatment of Cancer* (eds P. Price, K. Sikora & K. Halnan). Chapman and Hall Medical, London.

Weldon, K. (1998) Anatomy and physiology of the nervous system, pp. 1–28. In: *Neuro-Oncology for Nurses* (ed. D. Guerrero). Whurr, London.

Moving and handling
of patients

Definition

Manual handling operations are defined as:

> 'any transporting or supporting of a load (including the lifting, putting down, pushing, pulling, carrying or moving thereof) by hand or bodily force.' (HSAC 1998)

This chapter is primarily concerned with the manual handling of patients (commonly termed the moving and handling of patients).

Indications

When a patient cannot move independently nurses are involved in the moving and handling of patients (following individual patient assessment).

Reference material

Nurses are involved in the moving and handling of patients as well as inanimate loads such as medical equipment, and in many procedures with the potential to cause postural strain. This is due to the constraints of a poor environment as well as a lack of equipment. In such a demanding and stressful job, nurses are subject to cumulative strain and at risk of musculoskeletal problems – in particular back problems (Pheasant 1998).

For any manual handling operation to be considered successful it must meet two prime objectives. The handler needs to employ minimal effort, while the patient experiences minimal discomfort. These objectives can be achieved and the risk of injury reduced by undertaking a comprehensive assessment of the task's requirements. Risk assessments must be undertaken when manual handling cannot be avoided and there is a risk of injury. Where relevant, suitable equipment such as hoists, small handling aids and electronic profiling beds should be provided, as well as ongoing supervision in their use. The aim is to have fewer nurses injured and to increase comfort and safety for patients.

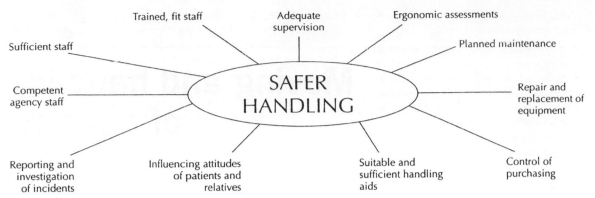

Figure 23.1 Factors that contribute to safer handling. (From *Manual Handling in the Health Services 1998*. Health and Safety Commission, 1998. Crown copyright material is reproduced with the permission of the Controller of Her Majesty's Stationery Office.)

The Royal College of Nursing Safer Patient Handling Campaign introduced in 1996 has changed the culture of manual handling within health care organizations. The implementation of a safer patient handling policy has prompted staff to question the practice of lifting patients manually (RCN 2000a, b, 2001).

A safer patient handling policy involves far more than simply training nurses in the latest handling techniques. Without management commitment to occupational health and safety, in consultation with employees, the risk to nurses will not be reduced (Fig. 23.1). The patient's perspective also needs to be taken into account – the experience of being moved physically by others can be unpleasant and frightening, especially if no prior explanation of the manoeuvre has been given. It can also be physically damaging to patients (Holmes 1998).

Epidemiology

It is well known that nursing is one of the occupational groups most likely to suffer from back pain. Stubbs and colleagues (Stubbs & Buckle 1994; Stubbs *et al.* 1983) provided a comprehensive account of this, and demonstrated that there is a significant incidence of back problems among nurses, which is a big factor in nurse wastage (Stubbs *et al.* 1986). It is many years since this seminal research, yet the picture has not greatly changed. Over 30% of nurses suffer back pain related to their work each year (Secombe & Smith 1996a, 1999) and therapists are no exception (Cromie *et al.* 2000). Therapists potentially put themselves at risk, as manual handling is an integral part of rehabilitation.

Research suggests that every year an estimated 80 000 nurses hurt their backs and 5% (3600) have to retire as a result (Secombe & Smith 1996b); 16% of nurses attribute

their back pain to handling of patients (NBPA/RCN 1998). In an RCN case a nurse was awarded £800 000 for back injury sustained at work (BBC Online 2000). This problem is not one that can be ignored; the price is too high for employers as well as employees. Training one nurse costs over £30 000, not to mention additional costs involved in litigation, covering sickness absence, recruiting new staff and possible effects on insurance premiums.

Musculoskeletal injuries are common amongst health care workers (HSE 1992, 1998; RCN 1995). In 2000/01 a total of 5084 manual handling accidents with over 3 days absence from work were reported to the Health and Safety Executive (HSE) under the Reporting of Injuries Diseases and Dangerous Occurrences 1995 (RIDDOR). This was 50% of the total accidents reported; 49% of the sites of injury were to the spine or back. The provision of equipment, appropriate training, risk assessments and protocols will help therapists, nurses and others involved with manual handling to undertake it as safely as possible. (Reportable incidents include those where an accident at work results in an absence from work of 3 days or more.)

Legal background, ergonomics and risk assessment

The Manual Handling Operations Regulations 1992 came into effect on 1 January 1993 under the terms of the *Health and Safety at Work Act 1974*, thereby implementing European Directive 90/269/EEC. The NHS has produced standards which are part of the control framework for risk management; these complement current and mandatory requirements. Criterion 13 of the Health and Safety Management relates to manual handling; it highlights the components needed to effectively control risk from manual handling.

- A manual handling policy understood by employees at all levels
- Access to competent advice from the backcare adviser/ manual handling co-ordinator/occupational health
- Availability of risk assessments for handling of both inanimate and animate loads
- Availability of training
- Equipment provision.

As a result, employers and employees acquired greater responsibilities for the design, development and maintenance of safe systems of practice. The regulations do not prohibit manual handling but state that all hazardous manual handling should be avoided (HSE 2001). If this is not possible then a 'suitable and sufficient' written assessment of the risk must be undertaken by the employer (or someone designated by the employer). Employers are required to provide suitable mechanical handling aids if the handling operation cannot be avoided, and training for employees in the use of equipment to maintain a safe working environment.

Employees must make use of safe systems of work implemented by their employers, and report to an appropriate person any hazards identified, as well as changes in their own ability to undertake manual handling tasks safely (e.g. pregnancy, back injury or deterioration in health status). In addition, employees are obliged:

> 'generally to make use of appropriate equipment provided for them in accordance with their training and the instructions, this would include machinery and other aids provided for the safe handling of loads.'
>
> (HSE 1998)

This law in relation to manual handling is based on the ergonomic approach. Ergonomics is a science concerned with the 'fit' between people and their work; it puts people first, taking into account their capabilities and limitations. Ergonomics makes sure that tasks, equipment, information and the environment suit each worker (HSE 2003). As with much health and safety law, the approach involves risk assessment by competent people. This involves looking at the task, individual, load and environment (TILE). This applies to both inanimate and animate loads.

Risk assessment is the first part of the risk management process. It involves identifying the problem, assessing the risk posed and using the information to decide ways of reducing the risk at source. Strategies and protocols should be considered in relation to manual handling; good risk assessment can be very effective as a risk reduction measure. Manual handling procedures involve both hazards and risks, factors which exist to a greater or lesser extent in any operation which involves the manual handling of a load. A hazard can be defined as something which has the potential to cause harm, while risk is an expression of probability of injury, in relation to the severity of the hazard. Hazards and risks are present for both nurses and patients involved in manual handling, particularly if an unsuitable system or method is employed.

There are many regulations in addition to The Manual Handling Operations Regulations (1992) that are relevant to manual handling, some of which are illustrated in Fig. 23.2.

In the context of legal requirements, the RCN, through the Advisory Panel on Back Pain in Nurses, has published a Code of Practice for the Handling of Patients (RCN

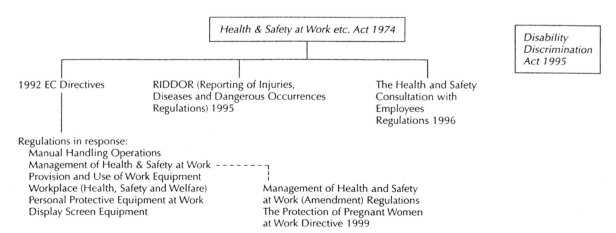

Figure 23.2 Nurses and manual handling: the legal context. In addition to criminal law, duties exist in civil law. These arise either from statutory provisions or from the common law, which is derived from the results of past cases.

2000b). The Code advocates that no nurse should be expected to move a patient where he/she bears most or all of the patient's weight and a hoist, sliding or other appropriate handling aid should always be used as appropriate, along with the required and associated education and training.

Manual handling assessments must be documented. Individual patient handling assessment should include:

- The patient's movement abilities
- The patient's physical and psychological circumstances and needs
- Instructions on handling aids and techniques
- The number of staff needed (NBPA/RCN 1998).

This must be documented in detail and should include, for example, the type of hoist to be used for a manoeuvre (such as a stretcher hoist) or, if a hoist sling is to be used, the size of the sling. Since risk assessment factors (for example a patient's condition) may change, reassessment is crucial and this too must be documented and communicated to all concerned (see Fig. 23.3 for a sample individual patient handling assessment form). More detailed advice on assessments of tasks and patients (including generic patient handling assessments) is given in the RCN's *Manual Handling Assessments in Hospital and the Community* (RCN 2001).

The risk of injury to both handler and patient can be reduced by fully assessing the task and identifying the best system for completing the procedure. However, assessment of the task and training are not sufficient on their own to minimize the risk or the incidence of back pain (Pheasant & Stubbs 1991). It is important that nurses understand how ergonomic principles contribute to providing and maintaining a safer environment for the handling of patients, and they must develop the ability to change their practices.

Ergonomic principles involve considering the 'fit' between a person and their work. To assess the fit, several aspects are taken into account, such as:

- The job being done and the demands on the worker
- The equipment being used (size, shape, etc.)
- The information used (how it is presented, accessed and changed)
- The physical environment (temperature, noise, lighting, etc.)
- The social environment (such as teamwork and supportive management)
- The physical aspects of a person (including body size and shape, fitness and strength) and psychological aspects (such as mental abilities and personality).

Biomechanics of load management

Biomechanics has been defined in the *Oxford Concise Dictionary* as 'the study of the mechanical laws relating to the movement or structure of living organisms' (Thompson 1995). Leggett (1998) explains in simple terms the biomechanics of human movement covering both mechanically and neurophysiologically based principles. She states that 'efficient movement of the human body involves the application of principles rather than the learning of techniques'.

When a person stands erect, most of the forces applied to the spine are the result of gravity acting upon the head and trunk. These forces are applied directly down through the spinal column, and very little muscular activity is required to maintain a stable upright position. However, when the trunk begins to move forward, away from the erect position, the nature and direction of the forces being applied to the spinal structure can change according to the lever principle. In the erect and near erect position the forces upon the spine are compressive, while in the stooped position forces can acquire harmful, shearing characteristics (Pheasant 1991). So the further a person moves away from an upright position, the more strain is put on the spine.

Owing to its gentle 'S' shape the spine is able to withstand considerable compressive forces being applied to it. This can be ten times more than it could withstand if it were a straight structure. Despite this, it can become easily damaged if those forces become torsional, twisting or shearing, affecting the surface of intervertebral discs.

Compression forces are caused by the greater effort exerted by the erector spinae muscles to maintain a counterbalance to the forward weight of the trunk and to the weight of any load being moved. They increase in direct proportion to the distance the load is held away from the operator's body (Pheasant 1991). Rotational or jerking movements can increase shearing forces by up to 400% (Nachemson 1981). It is always safer to move any load with the natural curves of the spine maintained and the object or patient as close to the body as possible with the weight of the load symmetrically spread through both arms. This makes use of the large, strong muscles of the hip and thigh to provide the momentum for the movement of the load, reducing the shearing forces produced in the back. This is not only safer but also more mechanically efficient. Mechanical efficiency is further improved by the use of low-friction devices and mechanical lifting aids.

It is also important to try to have a wide, stable base when manual handling so that the body is balanced with the line of gravity falling within that base.

Example

PATIENT HANDLING ASSESSMENT Patient Name: .... Hosp. No: ....

Body Build

Obese		Tall	
Above Average		Medium	
Average		Short	
Below Average			

Weight
(if known) .... (kgs)

Identify problems re: moving and handling and handling constraints
e.g. comprehension, language barrier, behaviour, co-operation, disability, weakness, pain, skin lesions, infusion, drains, equipment, space

History of Falls (if yes, describe)
No ☐ Yes ☐

1. If the patient is <u>totally independent for all tasks</u> and has no risk factors then tick ☐ and indicate low level of risk in the evaluation

2. Identify & document if patient will undergo a generic handling procedure during admission
    - Going to theatre/other department on trolley using patslide to transfer & 2 staff to assist ☐ tick

3. Complete patient capability, method and handling aids for each task then decide level of risk in the evaluation

Task	Patient's Capability	Specify Method/Handling Aids/Additional Information
Walking	Not Applicable ☐ Independent ☐ Supervision only ☐ Number of Staff	Walking aid (specify) Splint (specify)
Getting in /out of bed	Not Applicable ☐ Independent ☐ Supervision only ☐ Number of Staff	Hoist ☐ Sliding Sheet ☐ Sliding Board ☐
Transfers bed to chair/commode (vice versa)	Not Applicable ☐ Independent ☐ Number of Staff	Hoist ☐ Sliding Board ☐ Walking aid ☐
Transfers bed to trolley (vice versa)	Not Applicable ☐ Independent ☐ Number of Staff	Hoist ☐ Patslide ☐
Move up the bed	Not Applicable ☐ Independent ☐ Number of Staff	Indicate type of move - lying or sitting position Hoist ☐ Sliding Aid (fabric) ☐ Monkey Pole ☐
Toileting • Commode • Bed pan	Not Applicable ☐ Independent ☐ Number of Staff	Hoist ☐ Monkey Pole ☐
Bath or Shower	Not Applicable ☐ Independent ☐ Number of Staff	Ambulift ☐ Shower Chair ☐ Which Bath? Standard ☐ Parker ☐ Var height ☐

Other Tasks / Instructions:

Assessment Date: .... Review Date: .... Assessor's Signature: .... (Print Name)

Figure 23.3 Sample individual patient manual handling assessment form. It is important to constantly review and reassess the situation, completing a new, updated form as necessary.

Example

RISK ASSESSMENT CRITERIA			
Note any changes to the patient's condition, tasks, help required, method or equipment in the evaluation section			
LEVEL OF RISK	NUMBER OF STAFF	LIFTING AIDS OR EQUIPMENT	RISK FACTORS
High	3 or more	Required	The risk factors may alter the risk level and this is a professional judgement.
Medium	1 or 2	Required	
Low	0 or 1	NO equipment required	
DATE & TIME	DECIDE LEVEL OF RISK	PATIENT HANDLING CONTINUOUS EVALUATION	SIGNATURE

Figure 23.3 Sample individual patient manual handling assessment form. It is important to constantly review and reassess the situation, completing a new, updated form as necessary. (*continued*)

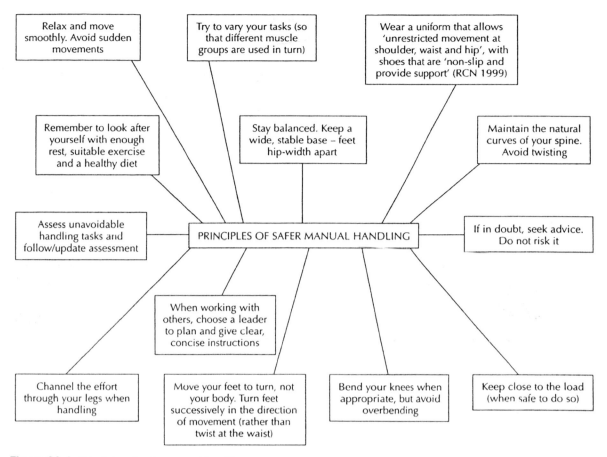

Figure 23.4 Principles of safer manual handling.

These basic principles of good manual handling are the cornerstone of back care training programmes. The aim is to encourage people to remember these principles and apply them (Fig. 23.4). Mechanical efficiency is further improved by using manual handling equipment, thus eliminating the need to lift patients physically.

Policy

Health care organizations must have a manual handling policy that is understood by employees at all levels. The policy should be produced following consultation with all concerned and agreed by a multidisciplinary team. Whether a 'no lifting' or minimal handling policy is appropriate has provoked extensive debate during the last few years. Using catchphrases in this way can lead to misinterpretation and can jeopardize the provision of safe and effective care. For example, 'no lifting' may mistakenly be taken to mean no lifting under any

circumstances. But there are clearly instances when lifting is appropriate, such as lifting or moving an object from the floor to avoid tripping over it or lifting a person's arm to wash it or dress a wound. On the other hand, minimal lifting policy is also open to a wide range of interpretations; what is minimal and how is it judged at the moment of providing care? A 'no lifting policy' means no lifting of all or most of a person's full body weight except in emergency or life-threatening situations, and must be clarified in the policy. A clear policy is unlikely to be the subject of misinterpretation (Backcare 1999).

Safety audits should be undertaken periodically and all the components of safety management systems should be included, i.e. policy, training, accident and incident reporting, risk assessments, equipment provision. Audits provide organizations with information, which enables them to develop and maintain their ability to manage risks and to determine areas for improvement (see Fig. 23.3).

The RCN recommend the introduction and implementation of a safer patient handling policy within all health care organizations. They suggest that such a policy might state:

'the manual handling of patients is eliminated in all but exceptional or life-threatening situations...patients are encouraged to assist in their own transfers and handling aids must be used whenever they can help to reduce risk, if this is not contrary to a patient's needs.'

(RCN 1996a)

The policy must be agreed, written down and communicated to all concerned. The roles, duties and responsibilities of managers, employees and occupational health and safety staff should be clear and guidance given on such aspects as assessment, reporting accidents and incidents, training content and requirements and equipment. A useful appendix to such a policy should include samples of assessment paperwork.

Equipment

Wherever patients requiring assisted mobility are cared for, appropriate equipment must be used. The range of equipment available includes:

- *Patient-handling slings*: cushioned material used by the assistant to help the patient to sit forward in bed, slide up in bed with a sliding sheet or lean forward in a chair
- *Handling belts*: used to give additional support when getting a patient to stand or when walking a patient and can ensure that the handler adopts a suitable posture
- *Sliding sheets*: made of slippery material and are used for moving dependant people
- *Transfer boards*: flat, rigid boards used to bridge the gap between two surfaces, for example wheelchair to bed, chair, commode or toilet
- *Turntables/turnplates*: circular discs positioned under the feet to help swivel/pivot transfers; useful for people with little or no lower limb function
- *Mobile hoists*: these are portable and versatile and are used for moving dependant patients from one area to another. They can be electric or hydraulic
- *Ceiling tracks*: eliminate the problem of moving round furniture and reduce the risk of injury to carers and nurses
- *Bath lifts*: hoists used to transfer patients into the bath.

More information on manual handling equipment is provided in *Handling People: Equipment, Advice and Information* (Disabled Living Foundation 2001).

It is useful for managers to keep an inventory of manual handling equipment used within their area. An inventory can help identify what equipment is missing. Staff should have the opportunity to learn about and try out equipment before using it to move or handle a person. This should be included as part of the pre-purchase evaluation.

A medical devices liaison officer or medical devices implementation group, where available within an organization, can provide information that has been published by the Medicines and Health care Products Regulatory Agency (MHRA) about the equipment.

The manager is responsible for ensuring that all assistive devices are adequately maintained in an efficient state and in good working order. Equipment must be suitable and safe for use, in line with the Provision and Use of Work Equipment Regulations (PUWER 1992/98) and the Lifting Operations and Lifting Equipment Regulations 1998 (LOLER 1998). All equipment should be CE marked in accordance with the Medical Devices Agency Regulations (MDA 1994).

Adverse incidents involving equipment must be reported to the Adverse Incidents Centre of the MHRA for investigation. The agency issues alerts in the form of hazard, safety or advice notices, hoping to prevent similar incidents happening again. In 2001 the MHRA (then the Medical Devices Agency) issued a safety notice concerning the risk of entrapment from electrically operated adjustable height beds and six notices in 2002 relating to patient hoists.

Hoists have now been designed which have the facility to lift patients from the ground on a stretcher, or with a hammock, sling attachment. Other hoists help physiotherapists when assisting patients to walk in rehabilitation. Sliding devices (for example Phil-E-Slide roller sheets) may be an effective way to help move someone up or down a bed. The traditional poles and canvas method of transferring a patient from bed to bed or bed to trolley can be replaced by more effective lateral transfer aids such as the Patslide. This information should be ascertained during the assessment. Patients may be able to use small aids such as 'monkey poles', rope ladders or patient hand blocks, which may allow them to be independent of the nurse while moving in bed. These are just a few examples of the hundreds of manual handling aids on the market.

The selection of use of an aid is based on individual patient assessment – one piece of equipment may be ideal for one patient but unhelpful to another. The key is taking account of the principles of safe handling, knowing what equipment is available and whom to contact for help or advice concerning other useful equipment which could be purchased or rented. An example of this is where a patient exceeds the safe working load of the hoist available on a ward – there should be a procedure already documented stating the action required in this situation. This may involve accessing equipment from elsewhere in the hospital or renting suitable heavy duty equipment. As with all manual handling issues the multidisciplinary approach is best.

Valuable sources of information outside the individual workplaces include the National Back Exchange (an association with a muldisciplinary membership which promotes the exchange and dissemination of information and ideas on back care) and the Disabled Living Foundation.

Emphasis on the avoidance of manual handling and the use of mechanical aids is prevalent in manual training today; however, a study by Dockrell *et al.* (1999) has shown that aids are underused. This study identified that the excuses nurses give for not using equipment include lack of time, lack of staff, equipment that is difficult to use, uncertainty about how to use equipment and patient discomfort. Increasing awareness through training programmes can help overcome these issues.

The more the manual handling techniques learnt are used, the more confident and skilled the user becomes. Overhead tracking hoists remove the strain of pushing and pulling a mobile hoist, although there is still some effort involved in positioning the sling. Nurses must recognize their own capabilities and seek advice as required. Even when using aids, prior assessment is essential to make the operation as safe as possible.

It must always be remembered that the use of any equipment must be commensurate with the manufacturer's guidelines and instructions, and that the use of equipment is kept under review for new information and developments in its use.

Training

Awareness training is only one aspect of a comprehensive manual handling programme (Fig. 23.1). No member of staff should undertake manual handling operations or use lifting aids until they have been trained and assessed as competent. Bank and agency staff should be given training in the policies and procedures of the organization (DoH 2001).

Training should include:

- The employer's manual handling policy
- Rudiments of spinal mechanics and the causes of back pain
- Principles of efficient body movement and posture
- Assessing risk and assessing the patient
- How to teach patients to move themselves
- Ergonomics – the environment and equipment
- Handling aids
- Back care, including awareness of good movement at work and at home

- Responsibilities for reporting risks and injuries (NBPA/RCN 1998).

Basic core training is to be followed up by refresher training:

'professional trainers have found that three to five days is needed to train health care staff who have had no previous relevant training or experience in manual handling. But training is an ongoing process and review or refresher courses need to be planned and implemented.'

(Health and Safety Commission 1998)

Refresher training frequency should be based on risk assessment. Signed training records must be kept by employers as well as details of the content of the training.

As well as a rolling programme of formal theoretical and practical classroom-based training there must be ongoing department-based training and supervision as part of a safe system of work. Managers must ensure that they and their staff understand, and are familiar with, the handling aids in their area and promote good manual handling practice. Training and supervision in the use of equipment are essential.

The RCN has produced guidelines on manual handling training, which include competencies for back care advisers, managers and staff (RCN 2000c). The aim of the guidance is to change attitudes and behaviour in managing manual handling risks in a variety of workplace settings. The core competencies outlined in the guidance would assist staff to develop their knowledge and skills in order to create a safe manual handling culture.

However, it should be noted that new equipment also brings new hazards (as shown by the Medical Devices Agency hazard and safety notices).

Summary

A team approach to manual handling policy, procedures, equipment selection and problem solving involves physiotherapists, occupational therapists and nurses sharing knowledge and working together for the benefit of the patient. Many patients may be able, with guidance and encouragement, to move themselves or assist nurses while being moved, and should be encouraged to help in ways that are compatible with their capabilities or health status. Manual handling assessments must be documented, implemented and updated. Nurses must be fully and regularly trained in manual handling by competent trainers and must always keep in mind the ergonomic principles of safer manual handling and back care.

Procedure guidelines: **Moving and handling of patients**

Procedure

Action	Rationale
1 Assess the needs of the patient, the environment and necessity for the procedure.	To ensure that action is in the patient's best interests. To ascertain whether there is sufficient space and appropriate equipment to perform procedure.
2 Inform all participating staff of the results of the assessment and confirm that details have been understood.	All staff participating in the procedure understand the plan of action in order to co-ordinate their actions correctly.
3 Prepare area by moving away any unwanted furnishings or equipment.	To provide an ergonomic workspace with sufficient space to manoeuvre and perform the required task.
4 Select appropriate equipment as specified in the hospital training programme and the assessments.	To ensure the patient is moved with the minimum of effort, safely, and experiences as little discomfort as is possible.
5 Assist the patient into the desired position, with one handler acting as leader and co-ordinator for the procedure.	To ensure that effort is exerted at the appropriate time by the handlers to prevent strain on the handlers.
6 Check that the patient is comfortable following the manoeuvre and store equipment correctly and in line with safe practice. Document any significant information.	To evaluate the methods used and maintain a safe working environment.

References and further reading

Backcare (1999) *Safer Handling of People in the Community*. Backcare, Teddington.

BBC News Online (2000) *Nurse wins £800 000 for back injury (15th February)*. BBC, London.

Cromie, J.E., Robertson, V.J. & Best, M.O. (2000) Musculoskeletal disorders in physical therapists: prevalence, severity, risks and responses. *Phys Ther*, **80**(4), 336–51.

Disabled Living Foundation (2001) Health and safety at work: legislation and guidance. In: *Handling People, Equipment, Advice and Information*. Disabled Living Foundation, London, pp. 1–9.

Dockrell, S., Duffy, A. & Burke, C. (1999) The use of lifting aids by hospital nurses. *Br J Rehabil Ther*, **6**(1), 20–5.

DoH (2001) *Controls Assurance Standards Health and Safety Management Criterion*. Department of Health, London.

Foster, L. (1996) Manual handling training and changes in work practices. *Occup Health*, **48**(11), 402–6, 417.

Health and Safety Commission (1998) New release 19th March. HSC, London.

Health Services Advisory Committee (1998) *Manual Handling in the Health Services*. HSE, Sudbury.

Holmes, D. (1998) Risk assessment: the practice. In: *Guide to the Handling of Patients*, revised 4th edn (ed. P. Lloyd). National Back Pain Association/RCN, London.

HSE (1992) *Successful Health and Safety Management*. HS(G) 65. Stationery Office, London.

HSE (1998) *Manual Handling Operations Regulations 1992. Guidance on the Regulations*, 2nd edn. HSE, Sudbury.

HSE (1998) *Manual Handling Operations Regulations*. Stationery Office, London.

HSE (1999) *Management of Health and Safety at Work Regulations, Approved Code of Practice and Guidance*. Stationery Office, London.

HSE (2001) *Handling Home Care: Achieving Safe, Efficient and Positive Outcomes for Care Workers and Clients*. Health and Safety Executive, London.

HSE (2003) *Understanding Ergonomics at Work*. HSE, Sudbury.

Leggett, P. (1998) The biomechanics of human movement. In: *Guide to the Handling of Patients*, revised 4th edn (ed. P. Lloyd). National Back Pain Association/RCN, London.

MDA (Medical Devices Agency) (1994) *The Medical Devices Regulation*. Medical Devices Agency, London.

Nachemson, A. (1981) Disc pressure measurement. *Spine*, **6**(1), 93–7.

National Back Exchange (2001) Manual handling training guidelines. *Column*, **13**(3), 12–13.

NBPA (National Back Pain Association)/RCN (1998) *Guide to the Handling of Patients*, 4th edn. NBPA/RCN, Teddington.

Pheasant, S. (1991) *Ergonomics: Work and Health*. Macmillan, Basingstoke.

Pheasant, S. (1998) Back injury in nurses – ergonomics and epidemiology. In: *Guide to the Handling of Patients*, revised 4th edn (ed. P. Lloyd). National Back Pain Association/RCN, London, pp. 30–8.

Pheasant, S. & Stubbs, D. (1991) *Lifting and Handling – An Ergonomic Approach*. National Back Pain Association/Thorn EMI UK Rental, London.

RCN (1995) *Hazards at Work. A Survey of 1600 Nurses Seeking Compensation for Back Injury*. Royal College of Nursing, London.

RCN (1996) *Introducing a Safer Patient Handling Policy*. Royal College of Nursing, London.

RCN (2000a) *Introducing Safer Patient Handling Policy*. Royal College of Nursing, London.

RCN (2000b) *Code of Practice for Patient Handling*. Royal College of Nursing, London.

RCN (2000c) *Manual Handling Training Guidance. Competencies for Manual Handling*. RCN, London.

RCN (2001) *Manual Handling Assessments in Hospitals and the Community*. Royal College of Nursing, London.

Secombe, I. & Smith, G. (1996a) *Manual Handling: Issues for Nurses*. Institute for Employment Studies, Brighton.

Secombe, I. & Smith, G. (1996b) *In the Balance: Registered Nurses Supply and Demand*. Institute for Employment Studies, Brighton.

Secombe, I. & Smith, G. (1999) *Report to the RCN on the Incidence of Back Injuries in Nurses*. Institute for Employment Studies, Brighton.

Stubbs, D. & Buckle, P. (1994) The epidemiology of back pain in nursing. *Nursing*, **2**(32), 935–7.

Stubbs, D. *et al.* (1983) Back pain in the nursing profession. Epidemiology and pilot methodology. *Ergonomics*, **26**(4), 755–65.

Stubbs, D. *et al.* (1986) Backing out: nurse wastage associated with back pain. *Int J Nurs Stud*, **23**(4), 325–36.

Thompson, D. (1995) *Oxford Concise Dictionary*, 9th edn. Clarendon Press, Oxford.

Tracy, M. (1998) Risk assessment: principles and preparation. In: *Guide to the Handling of Patients*, 4th edn. National Backpain Association/Royal College of Nursing, Teddington, pp. 90–4.

Tracy, M. & Tarling, C. (1998) The management responsibility. In: *Guide to the Handling of Patients*, 4th edn. National Backpain Association/Royal College of Nursing, Teddington, pp. 63–72.

Nutritional support

Chapter contents

Definition

Nutritional support refers to any method of giving nutrients which encourages an optimal nutritional status. It includes modifying the types of foods eaten, dietary supplementation, enteral tube feeding and parenteral nutrition.

Indications

Nutritional support should be considered for anybody unable to maintain their nutritional status by taking their usual diet.

- Patients unable to eat their usual diet (e.g. because of anorexia, mucositis, taste changes or dysphagia, see Problem solving) should be given advice on modifying their diet.
- Patients unable to meet their nutritional requirements, despite dietary modifications, should take dietary supplements.
- Patients unable to take sufficient food and dietary supplements to meet their nutritional requirements should be considered for an enteral tube feed.
- Patients unable to eat at all should have an enteral tube feed. Reasons for complete inability to eat include carcinoma of the head and neck area or oesophagus, surgery to the head or oesophagus, radiotherapy treatment to the head or neck, and fistulae of the oral cavity or oesophagus.
- Parenteral nutrition (PN) may be indicated in patients with a non-functioning or inaccessible gastrointestinal (GI) tract who are likely to be 'nil by mouth' for 5 days or longer. Reasons for a non-functioning or inaccessible GI tract include bowel obstruction, short bowel syndrome, gut toxicity following bone marrow transplantation or chemotherapy, major abdominal surgery, uncontrolled vomiting and enterocutaneous fistulae.

Patients in any group may have an increased requirement for nutrients due to an increased metabolic rate, as found in patients with burns, major sepsis, trauma or cancer cachexia (Bozzetti 2001; Thomas 2001).

Reference material

Assessment of nutritional status

Before the initiation of nutritional support the patient must be assessed. The purpose of assessment is to identify whether a patient is undernourished, the reasons why this may have occurred and to provide baseline data for planning and evaluating nutritional support (Nelson 2000). It is useful to use more than one method of assessing nutritional status. For example, a dietary history may be used to assess the adequacy of a person's diet but does not reflect actual nutritional status, whereas percentage weight loss does give an indication of nutritional status. However, percentage weight loss taken in isolation gives no idea of dietary intake and likelihood of improvement or deterioration in nutritional status (Sitges-Serra & Franch-Arcas 1995).

Nutrient intake

Nutrient intake can be assessed by a diet history (Thomas 2001). A 24-hour recall may be used to assess recent nutrient intake and a food chart may be used to monitor current dietary intake. A diet history may also be used to provide information on food frequency, food habits, preferences, meal pattern, portion sizes, the presence of any eating difficulty and changes in food intake (Reilly 1996). A food chart where all current food and fluid taken is recorded is a useful method for monitoring nutritional intake, especially in the hospital setting or when dietary recall is not reliable.

Body weight and weight loss

Body mass index or comparison of a patient's weight with a chart of ideal body weight gives a measure of whether the patient has a normal weight, is overweight or underweight, and may be calculated from weight and height using the following equation:

$$\text{Body mass index (BMI)} = \frac{\text{Weight (kg)}}{\text{Height (m)}^2}$$

These comparisons, however, are not a good indicator of whether the patient is at risk nutritionally, as an apparently normal weight can mask severe muscle wasting.

For children the amount and distribution of body fat are related to age and not health. A child's BMI should be plotted on age-related BMI centile charts (Thomas 2001; Shaw & Lawson 2001).

Of greater use is the comparison of current weight with the patient's usual weight. Percentage weight loss is a useful measure of the risk of malnutrition:

$$\text{\% Weight loss} = \frac{\text{Usual Weight} - \text{Actual Weight}}{\text{Usual Weight}} \times 100$$

An unintentional weight loss over 6 months of 10% represents malnutrition and a loss of 20%, severe malnutrition (Heymsfield & Matthews 1994; Wyszynski *et al.* 1998).

Sick children should have their weight and height measured frequently. Children over the age of 2 years in hospital should be weighed at least weekly (Shaw & Lawson 2001). These measurements must be plotted onto centile charts. A single weight or height cannot be interpreted as there is much variation of growth within each age group. It is only a matter of concern when a measurement falls above the 99.6th centile or below the 0.4th centile (Cole 1994). When there are a series of measurements and a child's weight or height deviates from a growth curve, this should be investigated.

Obesity and oedema may make interpretation of body weight difficult; both may mask loss of lean body mass and potential malnutrition (Pennington 1997). Accurate weighing scales are necessary for measurement of body weight. Patients who are unable to stand may require sitting scales for weight to be measured.

It is often not appropriate to weigh palliative care patients who may experience inevitable weight loss as disease progresses. Psychologically it may be difficult for patients to see that they are continuing to lose weight. Measures of nutritional status such as clinical examination and current food intake may still be used to assess patients without the need to weigh them.

Skinfold thickness

Skinfold thickness measurements can be used to assess stores of body fat. They are rarely used in routine nutritional assessment due to the insensitivity of the technique and the variation between measurements made by different observers. They are more appropriate for long-term assessments or research purposes. Calipers are used to measure the thickness of subcutaneous fat at four sites: the triceps, biceps, subscapular and supra-iliac. The measurements can be used to determine the percentage of body fat of a person (Durnin & Wolmersley 1974). Percentage charts for skinfold thickness measurements may be used to assess nutritional status (Thomas 2001, Appendix 6.4).

Bioelectrical impedance

Bioelectrical impedance analysis (BIA) is a simple technique which measures total body water and requires little patient co-operation (Walden & Klein 1992). The procedure involves the patient lying on a bed for a period of 5–10 minutes while electrodes are connected to the hand and foot. A small electrical current passes through the body which is undetectable by the patient. The principle of BIA relies on the difference in the electrical conductivity of the fat-free mass and fat mass of the body. Water is a good conductor of electricity and most water in the body is contained within fat-free mass. The small device with electrodes measures the impedance through the body of a small electrical current and calculates the body composition of the patient.

The equipment is easy to use but expensive. Results are compared with reference values for a healthy population. The measurements are of limited use in patients with grossly abnormal fluid balance, for example severe dehydration or ascites (Thomas 2001). It may be used for research studies or for monitoring nutritional status over a period of time (Heitman 1994).

Clinical examination

Observation of the patient may reveal signs and symptoms indicative of nutritional depletion.

- *Physical appearance*: emaciated, wasted appearance, loose clothing/jewellery.
- *Oedema*: will affect weight and may mask the appearance of muscle wastage. May indicate plasma protein deficiency and is often a reflection of the patient's overall condition.
- *Mobility*: weakness and impaired movement may result from loss of muscle mass.
- *Mood*: apathy, lethargy and poor concentration can be features of undernutrition.
- *Pressure sores and poor wound healing*: may reflect impaired immune function as a consequence of undernutrition and vitamin deficiencies (Thomas 2001).

Specific nutritional deficiencies may be identifiable in some patients. For example, thiamine deficiency characterized by dementia is associated with high alcohol consumption. Rickets is seen in children with vitamin D deficiency.

Subjective global assessment

Subjective global assessment is a clinical score, which can be obtained by a trained observer using a standardized questionnaire along with a physical examination, focused on nutritional status. The questionnaire includes questions about food intake, physical symptoms and weight loss and therefore encompasses a number of methods of assessing nutritional status (Naber *et al.* 1997).

Biochemical investigations

Biochemical tests carried out on blood may give information on the patient's nutritional status. The most commonly used are:

- *Plasma proteins.* Changes in plasma albumin may arise due to physical stress, changes in circulating volume, hepatic and renal function, shock conditions and septicaemia. Plasma albumin and changes in plasma albumin are not a direct reflection of nutritional intake and nutritional status as it has been shown that these may remain unchanged despite changes in body composition (Sitges-Serra & Franch-Arcas 1995). In addition, albumin has a long half-life of 21 days, so it cannot reflect recent changes in nutritional intake. It may be useful to review serum albumin concentrations in conjunction with C-reactive protein (CRP) which is an acute phase protein produced by the body in response to injury or trauma. CRP greater than 10 mg/litre and serum albumin less than 30 g/litre suggests 'illness'. CRP less than 10 mg/litre and serum albumin less than 30 g/litre suggests protein depletion (Elia 2001).
- *Haemoglobin.* This is often below haematological reference values in malnourished patients (men: 13.5–17.5 g/dl; women: 11.5–15.5 g/dl). This can be due to a number of reasons, such as loss of blood from circulation, increased destruction of red blood cells or reduced production of erythrocytes and haemoglobin, e.g. due to dietary deficiency of iron or folate.
- *Serum vitamin and mineral levels.* Clinical examination of the patient may suggest a vitamin or mineral deficiency. For example, gingivitis may be due to a deficiency of vitamin C, vitamin A, niacin or riboflavin. Goitre is associated with iodine deficiency, and tremors, convulsions and behavioural disturbances may be caused by magnesium deficiency (Shenkin 1995). Serum vitamin and mineral levels are rarely measured routinely, as they are expensive and often cannot be performed by hospital laboratories.
- *Immunological competence.* Total lymphocyte count may reflect nutritional status although levels may also be depleted with malignancy, chemotherapy, zinc deficiency, age and non-specific stress (Bodger & Heatley 2001).

If a patient is considered to be malnourished by one or more of the above methods of assessment then a referral to a dietitian should be made immediately (Burnham & Barton 2001).

Calculation of nutritional requirements

Energy requirements may be calculated using equations such as those derived by Schofield (1985), which take

Table 24.1 Guidelines for estimation of patient's daily protein and energy requirements (per kg body weight)

	Normal	Intermediate (moderate infection, postoperative patients, most cancer patients)	Severely hypermetabolic (multiple injuries, severe infection, severe burns)
Energy (kcal)	30	35–40	40–60
Nitrogen (g)	0.16	0.2–0.3	0.3–0.5
Protein (g)	1	1.3–1.9	1.9–3.1
Fluid (ml)	30–35	30–35	30–35 plus 500–700 ml additional fluid for every 1°C rise in temperature in pyrexial patients

into account weight, age, sex and injury. However, an easier method is to use body weight and allowances based on the patient's clinical condition (Table 24.1).

Fluid and nitrogen (or protein) requirements can be calculated in a similar way. If additional nitrogen is being given in situations where losses are increased, for example due to trauma, gastrointestinal losses or major sepsis, then additional energy intake is required to assist in promoting a positive nitrogen balance. Additional fluid of 500–750 ml is necessary for every 1°C rise in temperature in pyrexial patients (Thomas 2001).

Vitamin and mineral requirements calculated as detailed in the Committee on Medical Aspects of Food Policy (COMA) Report 41 on dietary reference values (DoH 1991) apply to groups of healthy people and are not necessarily appropriate for those who are ill. A patient deficient in a vitamin or mineral may benefit from additional supplements to improve a condition. For example, a malnourished patient with poor wound healing may benefit from an increase in vitamin C and zinc, although the evidence is controversial (ter Riet *et al.* 1995; Thomas 1997). Macronutrient and micronutrient requirements for children are also listed in the Committee on Medical Aspects of Food Policy (COMA) Report 41 on dietary reference values (DoH 1991). Calculations are usually done with the Reference Nutrient Intake (RNI). The child's actual body weight and not the expected body weight is used when calculating requirements. This is to avoid excessive feeding. For a very small child, the height age instead of the chronological age is the basis of calculation (Shaw & Lawson 2001).

Planning nutritional support

Many factors, including being in hospital, need to be taken into consideration when planning nutritional support. Within the *Essence of Care* framework (DoH 2001), food and nutrition were identified by patients as a fundamental area of care that is frequently unsatisfactory within the NHS.

Clinical benchmarking (DoH 2001) and the *Better Hospital Food* programme (NHS 2001) aim to address common problems that patients experience whilst in hospital. Box 24.1 outlines the benchmark for food and nutrition, identifying specific factors that need to be considered when reviewing service provision, in order to promote better practice.

Dietary supplements

These may be used to improve an inadequate diet or may be used as a sole source of nutrition if taken in sufficient quantity.

Sip feeds

These come in a range of flavours, both sweet and savoury, and are presented as a powder in a packet or ready prepared in a can or Tetrapak. Sip feeds contain whole protein, hydrolysed fat and carbohydrates. Most are called 'complete feeds' since they provide all protein, vitamins, minerals and trace elements to meet requirements if a prescribed volume is taken (Thomas 2001).

Energy supplements

Carbohydrates

Glucose polymers in powder or liquid form contain approximately 350 kcal per 100 g and 187–299 kcal per 100 ml respectively. Powdered glucose polymer is virtually tasteless and may be added to anything in which it will dissolve, e.g. milk and other drinks, soup, cereals and milk pudding; liquid glucose polymers may be fruit flavoured or neutral (Thomas 2001). Such supplements would be used to increase the energy content of the diet.

Fat

Fat may be in the form of long-chain triglycerides (LCT) or medium-chain triglycerides (MCT) and comes as a liquid which can be added to food and drinks. These oils provide 416–772 kcal per 100 ml – the oils with a lower energy value are presented in the form of an emulsion and those with a higher energy value are presented as pure oil (Thomas 2001).

Box 24.1 Food and nutrition benchmark (*food* includes drinks) (DoH 2001)

Agreed patient/client-focused outcome: patients/clients are enabled to consume food (orally) which meets their individual needs.

Indicators/information that highlight concerns which may trigger the need for benchmarking activity:

- Patient satisfaction surveys
- Complaints figures and analysis
- Audit results – including catering audit, nutritional risk assessments, documentation audit, environmental audit (including dining facilities)
- Contract monitoring, e.g. wastage of food, food handling and/or food hygiene training records

- Ordering of dietary supplements/special diets
- Audit of available equipment and utensils
- Educational audits/student placement feedback
- Litigation/Clinical Negligence Scheme for Trusts
- Professional concern
- Media reports
- Commission for Health Improvement reports

Factor	Benchmark of best practice
1 Screening/assessment to identify patients'/clients' nutritional needs	Nutritional screening progresses to **further assessment for all** patients/clients identified as '**at risk**'
2 Planning, implementation and evaluation of care for those patients who required a nutritional assessment	Plans of care based on **ongoing nutritional assessments** are devised, implemented and evaluated
3 A conducive environment (acceptable sights, smells and sounds)	The environment is **conducive to** enabling the **individual** patients/clients to eat
4 Assistance to eat and drink	Patients/clients **receive the care and assistance** they require with eating and drinking
5 Obtaining food	Patients/clients/carers, **whatever their communication needs**, have sufficient information to enable them to obtain their food
6 Food provided	Food that is provided by the service **meets the needs** of individual patients/clients
7 Food availability	Patients/clients have set meal times, are **offered a replacement meal** if a meal is missed and **can access snacks** at any time
8 Food presentation	Food is presented to patients/clients in a way that takes in to account what **appeals to them as individuals**
9 Monitoring	The amount of food patients actually eat is **monitored, recorded** and leads to **action** when cause for concern
10 Eating to promote health	**All opportunities** are used to encourage the patients/clients to eat to **promote their own health**

Other factors which may influence future food intake (e.g. surgery, chemotherapy or radiotherapy) also need to be taken into consideration when planning nutritional support, as clinical experience shows these may exert a deleterious effect on appetite and the ability to maintain an adequate nutritional intake (Newman *et al.* 1998).

Mixed fat and glucose polymer solutions and powders are available and provide 150 kcal per 100 ml or 486 kcal per 100 g, depending on the relative proportion of fat and carbohydrates in the product.

Products containing MCT are used in preference to those containing LCT where a patient suffers from gastrointestinal impairment causing malabsorption.

Always check with the manufacturer for the exact energy content of products.

Note: products containing a glucose polymer are unsuitable for patients with diabetes mellitus.

Protein supplements

These come in the form of a powder and provide 55–90 g protein per 100 g. Protein supplement powders may be added to any food or drink in which they will dissolve, e.g. milk, fruit juice, soup, milk pudding.

Energy and protein supplements are not used in isolation as these would not provide an adequate nutritional intake. They are used in conjunction with sip feeds and a modified diet. The detailed nutritional compositions of dietary supplements are available from the manufacturers.

Vitamin and mineral supplements

When dietary intake is poor a vitamin and mineral supplement may be required. This can often be given as a one-a-day tablet supplement that provides 100% of the dietary reference values.

Table 24.2 Suggestions for modification of diet

Eating difficulty	Dietary modification
Anorexia	Serve small meals and snacks
	Make food look attractive with garnish
	Fortify foods with butter, cream or cheese to increase energy content of meals
	Use alcohol, steroids, megestrol acetate or medroxyprogesterone as an appetite stimulant
	Encourage food that patient prefers
	Offer nourishing drinks between meals
Sore mouth	Offer foods that are soft and easy to eat
	Avoid dry foods that require chewing
	Avoid citrus fruits and drinks
	Avoid salt and spicy foods
	Allow hot food to cool before eating
Dysphagia	Offer foods that are soft and serve with additional sauce or gravy
	Some foods may need to be blended – make sure food is served attractively
	Supplement the diet with nourishing drinks between meals
Nausea and vomiting	Have cold foods in preference to hot as these emit less odour
	Keep away from cooking smells
	Sip fizzy, glucose-containing drinks
	Eat small frequent meals and snacks that are high in carbohydrate (e.g. biscuits and toast)
	Try ginger drinks and ginger biscuits
Early satiety	Eat small, frequent meals
	Avoid high-fat foods which delay gastric emptying
	Avoid drinking large quantities when eating
	Use prokinetics, e.g. metoclopramide, to encourage gastric emptying

Modification of diet

Practical information on modification of diet can be found in the Royal Marsden Hospital Patient Information Series *Eating Well When You Have Cancer – A Guide for Cancer Patients*. See also Table 24.2.

Enteral tube feeding

While the majority of patients will be able to meet their nutritional requirements orally, there is a group of individuals who will require enteral tube feeding either in the short term or on a more permanent basis. Several different feeding tubes are available.

Types of enteral feed tubes
Nasogastric/nasoduodenal
Nasogastric feeding is the most commonly used enteral tube feed and is suitable for short-term feeding for less than 4 weeks, for example postoperatively. Fine-bore feeding tubes should be used whenever possible as these are more comfortable for the patient than wide-bore tubes. They are less likely to cause complications such as rhinitis, oesophageal irritation and gastritis (Payne-James *et al.* 2001). Polyurethane or silicone tubes are preferable to polyvinyl chloride (PVC) as they withstand gastric acid and can stay in position longer than the 10–14 day lifespan of the PVC tube (Payne-James *et al.* 2001).

A wire introducer is provided with many of the tubes to aid intubation. The position of the nasogastric tube is checked with syringed aspirate of gastric content with a pH less than 3 and auscultation of the epigastrium. Both of these checks must be done. When one of these checks is unsuccessful tube position is confirmed with X-ray (Payne-James *et al.* 2001). Patients with oesophageal or head and neck tumours or reduced gag reflex or who are unconscious will have X-ray confirmation because they are at a higher risk for misplacement of the nasogastric tube.

Gastrostomy
A gastrostomy may be more appropriate than a nasogastric tube where feeding is for a period greater than 4 weeks. It avoids delays in feeding and discomfort associated with tube displacement. Suitable patients are those undergoing radical or hyperfractionated radiotherapy to the neck or children with solid tumours. They will require long-term enteral feeding because the treatment is intensive and prolonged. Percutaneous endoscopically guided gastrostomy (PEG) tubes are the gastrostomy tube of choice. They are made from polyurethane or silicone and are therefore suitable for short- or long-term feeding. A flange, flexible dome or inflated balloon holds the tube in position. The use of conventional balloon urinary catheters is now outdated, particularly as these are at risk of allowing gastric acid to leak at the tube entry site. However, gastrostomy tubes held in place with an inflatable balloon have the benefit over urinary catheters of being less likely to leak and are also made from polyurethane or silicone rather than from PVC. Clinical trials have shown that complications with PEG tubes, such as leakage, are rare (Riera *et al.* 2002).

For long-term feeding (i.e. longer than 1 month), a gastrostomy tube may be replaced with a button which is made from silicone. The entry site for feeding is flush with the skin, making it neat and less obvious than a gastrostomy tube. This is more cosmetically acceptable, especially for teenagers, but does require a certain amount of manual dexterity from the patient (Thomas 2001). The button is held in place by a balloon or dome inside the stomach (Griffiths 1996).

PEG tubes may be placed while the patient is sedated, thereby avoiding the risks associated with general anaesthesia.

When a patient cannot be endoscoped for insertion of a PEG tube then a radiologically inserted gastrostomy (RIG) can be used. RIGs are done in a few specialist centres. They are indicated for oesophageal patients with bulky tumours where it would be difficult to pass an endoscope. There is also documented risk of the endoscope seeding the tumour to the gastrostomy site (Pickhardt *et al.* 2002).

Jejunostomy

A jejunostomy is preferable to a gastrostomy if a patient has undergone upper gastrointestinal surgery or has severe delayed gastric emptying; in some cases it can be used to feed a patient with pyloric obstruction (Thomas 2001). Fine-bore feeding jejunostomy tubes may be inserted with the use of a jejunostomy kit, which consists of a needle-fine catheter. The use of needles and an introducer wire allows a fine-bore polyurethane catheter to be inserted into a loop of jejunum. Alternatively, some gastrostomy tubes allow the passage of a fine-bore tube into the jejunum.

Enteral feeding equipment

The administration of enteral feeds may be as a bolus, intermittent or continuous infusion, via gravity drip or pump-assisted (Table 24.3). There are many enteral feeding pumps available which vary in their range of flow rate from 1 ml to 300 ml per hour. The following systems may be used for feeding via a pump or gravity-drip:

- Feed is decanted into plastic bottles or PVC bags. The administration set may be an integral part of the bag. The feed is sterile until opened and decanting feed into reservoirs will increase the risk of contamination of the feed from handling (Payne-James *et al.* 2001). Malnourished and immunocompromised patients are particularly at risk from contamination and infection.
- The 'ready to hang system' has a glass bottle, plastic bottle or pack attached directly to the administration set. The bottles and packs are available in different types of feeds and sizes for flexibility. This is a closed sterile system. It has been shown to be successful in preventing exogenous bacterial contamination (Payne-James *et al.* 2001).

Enteral feeds

Commercially prepared feeds should be used for nasogastric, gastrostomy or jejunostomy feeding. Available in liquid or powder form, they have the advantage of being of known composition and are sterile when packaged.

1 Whole protein/polymeric feeds contain protein, hydrolysed fat and carbohydrate and so require digestion. These may provide 1 kcal/ml to 1.5 kcal/ml (see manufacturer's specifications). As the energy density of the feed increases so does the osmolarity. Hyperosmolar feeds tend to draw water into the lumen of the gut and can contribute to diarrhoea if given too rapidly. Fibre may be beneficial for maintaining gut ecology and function, rather than promoting bowel transit time (Thomas 2001).

2 Feeds containing MCT. In some whole protein feeds a proportion of the fat or LCT may be replaced with MCT. The feed often has a lower osmolarity, and is

Table 24.3 Methods of administering enteral feeds

Feeding regimen	Advantages	Disadvantages
Continuous feeding via a pump	Easily controlled rate Reduction of gastrointestinal complications	Patient connected to the feed for majority of the day May limit patient's mobility
Intermittent feeding via gravity or a pump	Periods of time free of feeding Flexible feeding routine May be easier than managing a pump for some patients	May have an increased risk of gastrointestinal symptoms, e.g. early satiety Difficult if outside carers are involved with the feed
Bolus feeding	May reduce time connected to feed Very easy Minimum equipment required	May have an increased risk of gastrointestinal symptoms Can be time consuming

therefore less likely to draw fluid from the plasma into the gut lumen. MCT is transported via the portal vein rather than the lymphatic system. These feeds are suitable for patients with fat malabsorption and maybe steatorrhoea (Cummings 2000).

3 Chemically defined/elemental feeds. These contain free amino acids, short-chain peptides or a combination of both as the nitrogen source. They are often low in fat or may contain some fat as MCT. Glucose polymers provide the main energy source. These feeds require little or no digestion and are suitable for those patients with impaired gastrointestinal function (Thomas 2001). They are hyperosmolar and low in residue.

4 Special application feeds. Low protein and mineral feeds may be used for patients with liver or renal failure.

High-fat, low-carbohydrate feeds may be used for ventilated patients because less carbon dioxide is produced per calorie intake compared with a low-fat, high-carbohydrate feed.

Very high energy and protein feeds may be used where nutritional requirements are exceptionally high, e.g. burns, severe sepsis. These feeds contain approximately double the amount of energy and protein compared to standard whole protein feeds.

5 Paediatric feeds are designed for children 1–6 years old and/or 8–20 kg in weight. The protein, vitamin and mineral profile is suitable for children. Generally they are lower in osmolarity than adult feeds. The whole protein/polymeric feeds are based on cow's milk but are lactose free. They may be with to without fibre. These feeds provide 1 kcal/ml to 1.5 kcal/ml for children who require additional energy and protein in a smaller volume. Protein hydrolysate feeds and elemental feeds are used in conditions such as food allergies or malabsorption. Some specialist centres use these feeds for enteral feeding during bone marrow transplants as children may have malabsorption caused by gut mucositis. The osmolarity of these feeds is higher than whole protein feeds. They need to be introduced carefully (Thomas 2001).

6 There is evidence to show that the addition of glutamine, arginine or omega-3 fatty acids to feeds may benefit postsurgical or septic patients (Thomas 2001).

Up-to-date information on the exact composition of dietary supplements and enteral feeds can be obtained from the manufacturers.

Monitoring enteral tube feeding

In order to avoid complications and ensure optimal nutritional status, it is important to monitor the following in patients on enteral tube feeds:

- Oral intake
- Body weight
- Urea and electrolytes
- Blood glucose
- Full blood count
- Fluid balance
- Tolerance to feed, e.g. nausea, fullness and bowel activity
- Quantity of feed taken
- Care of tube
- Care of stoma site.

Complications of enteral tube feeding

The type and frequency of complications related to tube feeding depend on the access route, underlying disease state, the feeding regimen and the patient's metabolic state (Payne-James *et al.* 2001) (Table 24.4).

Home enteral feeding

Patients who are unable to take sufficient food and fluids orally may be taught to manage enteral tube feeding at home. Home circumstances and the ability of the patient or carers to manage the feed must be considered before the patient is discharged. Adequate time should be allowed in the hospital setting for patients to become fully accustomed to the techniques of feed administration and care of the feeding tube, prior to discharge home.

Support in the form of the general practitioner, community nurse and community dietetic services should be established before discharge. If possible, a multidisciplinary discharge meeting may be of benefit to both the patient and the professionals involved. Many of the commercial feed companies organize for the patient's feed and equipment to be delivered to the patient's home, after consultation with the local community services (BAPEN 1994a). The hospital or community dietitian can arrange this. Early notification of discharge is essential as it usually takes a minimum of 7 days to set this up.

Termination of enteral tube feeding

It is important to ensure that an individual is able to meet their nutritional requirements orally prior to termination of the feed. Ideally, the feeds should be reduced gradually, according to the dietary intake (BAPEN 1999). It may be useful to maintain an overnight feed while the patient is establishing oral intake.

Parenteral nutrition

Parenteral nutrition (PN) is the direct infusion into a vein, of solutions containing the essential nutrients in

Table 24.4 Complications that may occur during enteral feeding

Complication	Cause	Solution
Aspiration	Regurgitation of feed due to poor gastric emptying Incorrect placement of tube	Medication to improve gastric emptying, e.g. metoclopramide Check tube placement Ensure patient has head at 45° during feeding
Nausea and vomiting	Related to disease/treatment Poor gastric emptying Rapid infusion of feed	Antiemetics Reduce infusion rate Change from bolus to intermittent feeding
Diarrhoea	Medication such as antibiotics, chemotherapy, laxatives Radiotherapy Disease-related, e.g. pancreatic insufficiency Gut infection	Antidiarrhoeal agent If possible discontinue antibiotics, avoid microbiological contamination of feed or equipment Send stool sample to check for gut infection
Constipation	Inadequate fluid intake Immobility Use of opiates or other medication causing gut stasis Bowel obstruction	Check fluid balance Administer laxatives/bulking agents If possible encourage mobility If in bowel obstruction, discontinue feed
Abdominal distension	Poor gastric emptying Rapid infusion of feed Constipation or diarrhoea	Reduce rate of infusion Gastric motility agents If possible encourage mobility Treat constipation or diarrhoea
Blocked tube	Inadequate flushing or failure to flush feeding tube Administration of medication via the tube	Prevent by flushing with 30–50 ml water before and after feeds or medication Use liquid or finely crushed medications If blocked, try warm water, soda water, sodium bicarbonate, fizzy soft drink, pancreatic enzymes

quantities to meet all the daily needs of the patient. While enteral feeding is the preferred route of nutritional support in terms of cost and mechanical, septic and metabolic complications (Mercadante 1998; Reilly 1998), parenteral nutrition may be indicated for patients with a prolonged ileus, uncontrolled vomiting or diarrhoea, severe radiation enteritis, short bowel syndrome or gastrointestinal obstruction.

Route of administration

The traditional method of access is a central venous catheter. The major hazard associated with the delivery of PN via a central venous catheter is infection. Therefore catheter insertion should take place using strict aseptic technique either within theatre or at the bedside (Hamilton *et al.* 1995; Fitzsimmons 1997; Weinstein 2000; Benton & Marsden 2002). A skin-tunnelled catheter is the catheter of choice for long-term nutrition. The number of lumens will depend on the patient's peripheral venous access and the number of additional therapies required. If veins are considered inadequate then a double or triple

lumen catheter should be inserted. Central venous access is required because PN solutions are hyperosmolar and there is a risk of thrombophlebitis associated with feeding into peripheral veins (Wilson & Jordan 2001; Springhouse 2002). However, it has been shown that with care and attention, peripheral veins can be used to provide short-term peripheral PN (Mercadante 1998). This would be via a midline or a peripherally inserted central catheter (PICC). (See Ch. 44, Vascular access devices.)

PN solution

The basic components of a PN regimen are provided by solutions of:

* *Amino acids* (nitrogen source). Commercially available solutions provide both essential amino acids, usually in proportions to meet requirements, and non-essential amino acids, such as alanine and glycine.
* *Glucose* (carbohydrate energy source). Glucose is the carbohydrate source of choice. It provides 3.75 kcal/g.

- *Fat emulsion* (fat energy source). Fat generates 9 kcal/g and its inclusion in PN is necessary to provide essential fatty acids. Fat usually provides 30–50% of non-nitrogen energy. Nitrogen : non-nitrogen energy is usually provided in the ratio of 1 : 150–200. An insufficient energy supply from carbohydrate and fat will encourage the use of nitrogen for energy.
- *Electrolytes*, e.g. sodium, potassium.
- *Vitamins*: both water-soluble and fat-soluble are required.
- *Trace elements*, e.g. zinc, copper, chromium, selenium (Thomas 2001).

Choice of a PN regimen

PN is usually administered from a single infusion container in which all the requirements for a 24-hour feed are premixed. Such infusions are either prepared by the hospital pharmacy or are purchased.

The regimen for a particular patient may be formulated according to the patient's needs for energy and nitrogen (see calculation of nutritional requirements, Table 24.1). The majority of commercial vitamin and mineral preparations aim to meet both short- and long-term requirements.

Standard PN regimens may be suitable for some patients who require short-term nutritional support or do not appear to have excessively altered nutritional requirements.

The choice of such regimens depends on the patient's body weight and nutritional requirements. To allow for the possible need to vary the constituents of the infusion in response to changes in the patient's electrolyte or nutritional requirements, PN solutions should be ordered daily. Once compounded, most PN preparations last up to 7 days (Weinstein 2000) and need to be stored in a refrigerator. However, some triple chamber PN bags can be stored at ambient temperatures and require mixing prior to administration.

Delivery of parenteral nutrition and recommendations for intravenous management

Administration sets should always be changed every 24 hours (Burnham 1999; DoH 2001; Wilson & Jordan 2001; Springhouse 2002), using an aseptic technique. Existing injection sites on the administration set should never be used for the giving of additional medications as PN is incompatible with numerous medications. If any additional medications, blood products or CVP readings are required then they should be given via a separate lumen or via a peripheral device.

A volumetric infusion pump must be used to ensure accurate delivery of PN. No bag should be used for longer

Table 24.5 Monitoring of PN (BAPEN 1996)

Parameter	Frequency of monitoring
TPR and blood pressure	Daily
Body weight	Daily
Fluid balance	Daily
Serum urea, creatinine and electrolytes	Initially and at least three times weekly
Blood glucose	Daily for the first week, if normal, twice weekly thereafter
Full blood count	Initially and at least three times weekly
Serum phosphate	48 hours after initiation of feeding, thereafter twice weekly
Serum magnesium	At least twice weekly (may be measured more often if the patient is on magnesium-depleting drugs, e.g. cyclosporin and cisplatin)
Alkaline phosphatase, alanine transaminase, bilirubin	Initially and at least twice weekly
Trace elements, e.g. selenium, copper, manganese, zinc	At least monthly

than 24 hours (Wilson & Jordan 2001; Springhouse 2002) and rates should never be adjusted more than ±10% (Weinstein 2000).

If the infusion must be discontinued the catheter should be flushed and patency maintained. Partly used PN bags should not be reused but must be discarded and a new one requested from the pharmacy.

Monitoring of PN

During intravenous feeding monitoring is necessary to detect and minimize complications (Table 24.5). Once feeding is established and the patient is biochemically stable then the frequency of monitoring may be reduced if the clinical condition of the patient permits. Additional patient monitoring such as 24-hour urine collection for urinary urea, nitrogen and serum zinc may be carried out where indicated, e.g. in severe malnutrition (Weinstein 2000).

Metabolic complications of PN

Metabolic complications should be detected by appropriate monitoring. Some more common complications are:

- *Fluid overload*. This may occur when other blood products and fluids are given concurrently. It may be possible to reduce the volume of a 24-hour bag of PN while maintaining the nutritional content. Pharmacy can advise on the feasibility of making such regimens.

- *Hyperglycaemia*. This may occur due to stress-induced insulin resistance or carbohydrate overload. A simultaneous sliding scale insulin infusion may be required. Failure to recognize hyperglycaemia may result in osmotic diuresis.
- *Hypoglycaemia*. Abrupt cessation of PN may result in a rebound hypoglycaemia. A reduction in infusion rate to half the rate prior to stopping the infusion may help prevent this occurring.
- *Azotaemia*. Raised plasma urea may indicate renal dysfunction or dehydration. Alterations in the nitrogen and non-protein energy content of the PN may be required, or an increase in fluid input (Payne-James *et al.* 2001).
- *Hypophosphataemia*. This is associated with excessive glucose infusion and the refeeding syndrome in malnourished patients (Thorell & Nordenström 2001). It is necessary to correct phosphate levels by providing additional phosphate prior to feeding. Phosphate levels should be monitored daily at the start of feeding. Introducing PN gradually in malnourished patients may help to prevent the refeeding syndrome.

Other complications such as metabolic acidosis, electrolyte disturbances, hyperammonaemia, hypernatraemia and hypokalaemia may require a review of the PN solution, rate of administration, additional fluids, blood products and drugs.

Termination of PN

Parenteral nutrition should not be terminated until oral or enteral tube feeding is well established (Weinstein 2000). The patient needs to be taking a minimum of 50% of their nutritional requirements via the enteral route. It is important that all members of the multidisciplinary team are involved in the decision to terminate PN.

Elective removal of catheter

See Ch. 44, Vascular access devices.

Home PN

There are few indications for home PN. It may be necessary in patients who have complete intestinal failure, e.g. short bowel syndrome due to Crohn's disease or radiation enteritis. The cost of home parenteral feeding is high and requires intensive training with an efficient and comprehensive back-up service. It is recommended that only hospitals which have the appropriate facilities to train patients and provide the necessary care in case of an emergency should be involved in home PN (BAPEN 1994a).

Multidisciplinary team

It is important that all members of the multidisciplinary team, including dietitian, nurse, doctor, pharmacist, catering department and community services, are involved in the patient's nutritional care to ensure a thorough and co-ordinated approach to nutritional management (BAPEN 1994b).

Procedure guidelines: **Nasogastric intubation with tubes using an introducer**

Equipment

1 Clinically clean tray.
2 Fine-bore nasogastric tube.
3 Introducer for tube.
4 Sterile receiver.
5 Sterile water.
6 10 ml syringe.
7 Hypoallergenic tape.
8 Adhesive patch if available.
9 Glass of water.
10 Lubricating jelly.
11 Indicator strips, e.g. pH Fix, 0–6, Fisher Scientific.

Prior to performing this procedure the patient's medical and nursing notes should be consulted to check for potential complications. For example, anatomical alterations due to surgery, such as a flap repair or the presence of a cancerous tumour, can prevent a clear passage for the nasogastric tube, resulting in pain and discomfort for the patient and further complications.

Procedure

Action	Rationale
1 Explain and discuss the procedure with the patient.	To ensure that the patient understands the procedure and gives his/her valid consent.

*Procedure guidelines: **Nasogastric intubation with tubes using an introducer** (cont'd)*

Action	Rationale
2 Arrange a signal by which the patient can communicate if he/she wants the nurse to stop, e.g. by raising his/her hand.	The patient is often less frightened if he/she feels able to have some control over the procedure.
3 Assist the patient to sit in a semi-upright position in the bed or chair. Support the patient's head with pillows. *Note*: The head should not be tilted backwards or forwards (Rollins 1997).	To allow for easy passage of the tube. This position enables easy swallowing and ensures that the epiglottis is not obstructing the oesophagus.
4 Select the appropriate distance mark on the tube by measuring the distance on the tube from the patient's ear lobe to the bridge of the nose plus the distance from the bridge of the nose to the bottom of the xiphisternum.	To ensure that the appropriate length of tube is passed into the stomach.
5 Wash hands with bactericidal soap and water or bactericidal alcohol handrub, and assemble the equipment required.	To minimize cross-infection.
6 Follow manufacturer's instructions to prepare the tube, e.g. injecting sterile water for injection down the tube and lubricating the proximal end of the tube with lubricating jelly.	Contact with water activates coating inside tube and on the tip. This lubricates the tube, assisting its passage through the nasopharynx and allowing easy withdrawal of the introducer.
7 Check that the nostrils are patent by asking the patient to sniff with one nostril closed. Repeat with the other nostril.	To identify any obstructions liable to prevent intubation.
8 Insert the rounded end of the tube into the clearer nostril and slide it backwards and inwards along the floor of the nose to the nasopharynx. If any obstruction is felt, withdraw the tube and try again in a slightly different direction or use the other nostril.	To facilitate the passage of the tube by following the natural anatomy of the nose.
9 As the tube passes down into the nasopharynx, unless swallowing is contraindicated, ask the patient to start swallowing and sipping water.	To focus the patient's attention on something other than the tube. A swallowing action closes the glottis, enabling the tube to pass into the oesophagus.
10 Advance the tube through the pharynx, as the patient swallows until the predetermined mark has been reached. If the patient shows signs of distress, e.g. gasping or cyanosis, remove the tube immediately.	The tube may have accidentally been passed down the trachea instead of the pharynx. Distress may indicate that the tube is in the bronchus.
11 Remove the introducer by using gentle traction. If it is difficult to remove, then remove the tube as well.	If the introducer sticks in the tube, it may be indicative that the tube is in the bronchus.
12 Secure the tape to the nostril with adherent dressing tape, e.g. Elastoplast (Burns *et al.* 1995). If this is contraindicated, a hypoallergenic tape should be used. An adhesive patch (if available) will secure the tube to the cheek.	To hold the tube in place. To ensure patient comfort.
13 Measure the part of the visible tube from tip of nose and record in care plan. Mark the tube at the exit site (nares) (Metheny & Titler 2001).	To provide a record to assist in detecting movement of the tube.
14 Check the position of the tube to confirm that it is in the stomach by using the following methods: **(a)** Taking an X-ray of chest and upper abdomen.	Feeding via the tube must not begin until the correct position of the tube has been confirmed. To confirm placement of radiopaque NG tube. X-ray of radiopaque tubes is the most accurate confirmation of position and is the method of choice in patients with altered anatomy, those who are aspirating or are unconscious with no gag reflex.
(b) Aspirating 2 ml of stomach contents and testing this with pH indicator strips (Rollins 1997). When	Indicator strips can distinguish between gastric acid (pH <3) and bronchial secretions (pH >6) (Rollins

*Procedure guidelines: **Nasogastric intubation with tubes using an introducer** (cont'd)*

Action	Rationale
aspirating fluid for pH testing, wait at least 1 hour after a feed or medication has been administered (either orally or via the tube). Before aspirating, flush the tube with 20 ml of air to clear other substances (Metheny *et al.* 1993). pH indicator strips should not be used on patients who are receiving acid-inhibiting agents (defined as H_2 receptor antagonists). With these patients the pH value of aspirate from the stomach will range from 0 to 6.0 (Metheny *et al.* 1993). Certain types of fine-bore feeding tubes cannot be aspirated, therefore it is necessary to take an X-ray of chest and upper abdomen.	1997; Colagiovanni 1999). To prove an accurate test result because the feed or medication may raise the pH of the stomach.
(c) Introducing 5 ml of air into the stomach via the tube and checking for a bubbling sound using a stethoscope placed over the epigastrium (Jones 1998). This should not be used as the sole or primary method of checking tube placement (Metheny & Titler 2001).	Air can be detected by a bubbling sound when entering the stomach. This test is not reliable as the only test of tube position as it has been shown to give false positive results (Metheny *et al.* 1990; Boyes & Kruse 1992; Arrowsmith 1993)

Procedure guidelines: **Nasogastric intubation with tubes without using an introducer, e.g. a Ryle's tube**

It is recommended that a nasogastric tube designed for feeding purposes be used wherever possible, e.g. fine-bore feeding tube, rather than a Ryle's tube which is used for drainage of gastric contents.

Equipment

1 Clinically clean tray.
2 Nasogastric tube that has been stored in a deep freeze for at least half an hour before the procedure is to begin, to ensure a rigid tube that will allow for easy passage.
3 Topical gauze.
4 Lubricating jelly.
5 Hypoallergenic tape.
6 20 ml syringe.
7 Indicator strips, e.g. pH Fix, 0–6, Fisher Scientific.
8 Receiver.
9 Spigot.
10 Glass of water.
11 Stethoscope.

Procedure

Action	Rationale
1 Explain and discuss the procedure with the patient.	To ensure that the patient understands the procedure and gives his/her valid consent.
2 Arrange a signal by which the patient can communicate if he/she wants the nurse to stop, e.g. by raising his/her hand.	The patient is often less frightened if he/she feels able to have some control over the procedure.
3 Assist the patient to sit in a semi-upright position in the bed or chair. Support the patient's head with pillows. Note: The head should not be tilted backwards or forwards (Rollins 1997).	To allow for easy passage of the tube. This position enables easy swallowing and ensures that the epiglottis is not obstructing the oesophagus.
4 Mark the distance which the tube is to be passed by measuring the distance on the tube from the patient's ear lobe to the bridge of the nose plus the distance from the bridge of the nose to the bottom of the xiphisternum.	To indicate the length of tube required for entry into the stomach.
5 Wash hands with bactericidal soap and water or bactericidal alcohol handrub, and assemble the equipment required.	To minimize cross-infection.

Procedure guidelines: Nasogastric intubation with tubes without using an introducer, e.g. a Ryle's tube (cont'd)

Action	Rationale
6 Check the patient's nostrils are patent by asking him/her to sniff with one nostril closed. Repeat with the other nostril.	To identify any obstructions liable to prevent intubation.
7 Lubricate about 15–20 cm of the tube with a thin coat of lubricating jelly that has been placed on a topical swab.	To reduce the friction between the mucous membranes and the tube.
8 Insert the proximal end of the tube into the clearer nostril and slide it backwards and inwards along the floor of the nose to the nasopharynx. If an obstruction is felt, withdraw the tube and try again in a slightly different direction or use the other nostril.	To facilitate the passage of the tube by following the natural anatomy of the nose.
9 As the tube passes down into the nasopharynx, ask the patient to start swallowing and sipping water.	To focus the patient's attention on something other than the tube. The swallowing action closes the glottis, enabling the tube to pass into the oesophagus.
10 Advance the tube through the pharynx as the patient swallows until the tape-marked tube reaches the point of entry into the external nares. If the patient shows signs of distress, e.g. gasping or cyanosis, remove the tube immediately.	Distress may indicate that the tube is in the bronchus.
11 Secure the tube to the nostril with adherent dressing tape, e.g. Elastoplast (Burns *et al.* 1995). If this is contraindicated, a hypoallergenic tape should be used. An adhesive patch (if available) will secure the tube to the cheek.	To hold the tube in place. To ensure patient comfort.
12 Check the position of the tube to confirm that it is in the stomach by using the following methods: (a) Taking an X-ray of chest and upper abdomen.	To confirm placement of radiopaque NG tube. X-ray of radiopaque tubes is the most accurate confirmation of position and is the method of choice in patients with altered anatomy, those who are aspirating or are unconscious with no gag reflex.
(b) Aspirating 2 ml of stomach contents and testing this with pH indicator strips (Rollins 1997). When aspirating fluid for pH testing, wait at least 1 hour after a feed or medication has been administered (either orally or via the tube). Before aspirating, flush the tube with 20 ml of air to clear other substances (Metheny *et al.* 1993). Feeding via the tube must not begin until the position of the tube has been confirmed.	Indicator strips can distinguish between gastric acid (pH <3) and bronchial secretions (pH >6) (Rollins 1997; Colagiovanni 1999). Wait at least 1 hour before aspirating to enable the feed or medication to be absorbed, otherwise an inaccurate test result will be obtained.
(c) Introducing 5 ml of air into the stomach via the tube and checking for a bubbling sound using a stethoscope placed over the epigastrium (Jones 1998). This should not be used as the sole or primary method of checking tube placement (Metheney & Titler 2001).	Air can be detected by a bubbling sound when entering the stomach. This method is not reliable as the only test of tube position as it has been shown to give false positive results (Metheny *et al.* 1990; Boyes & Kruse 1992; Arrowsmith 1993).

Procedure guidelines: **Care of a percutaneous endoscopically placed gastrostomy (PEG) tube**

This procedure should be performed daily and should begin approximately 36–48 hours following insertion. This will help maintain skin integrity and detect any problems early, e.g. infection, skin breakdown.

Equipment

1   Sterile procedure pack containing gallipot, low-linting gauze.

2   0.9% sodium chloride or antiseptic solution.

Procedure

Action	Rationale
1 Explain and discuss the procedure with the patient.	To ensure that the patient understands the procedure and gives his/her valid consent.
2 Perform procedure using aseptic technique. Self-caring patients should be taught socially clean technique.	To minimize the risk of cross-infection (for further information see procedure on aseptic technique, Ch. 4). Risk of cross-infection is greatly reduced if patients carry out self-care.
3 Remove postprocedural dressing if in place. Observe peristomal skin and stoma site for signs of infection, irritation or excoriation.	To gain access to stoma site. To detect complications early and instigate appropriate treatment.
4 Note the number of the measuring guide on the tube closest to the end of the external fixation device. Loosen the tube from the fixation device and ease fixation device away from the abdomen.	To ensure gastrostomy tube is reattached to the fixation device in the correct position. To ensure stoma site is thoroughly cleaned.
5 Clean the stoma site with a sterile solution such as 0.9% sodium chloride. Using low-linting gauze dry the area thoroughly.	To remove any exudate, to prevent infection and skin excoriation.
6 Rotate the gastrostomy tube 360°.	To prevent the tube adhering to the sides of the stoma tract.
7 Gently push the external fixation device against the abdomen.	To enable the gastrostomy tube to be reattached to the fixation device.
8 Gently but firmly pull the gastrostomy tube and attach to the fixation device.	To ensure that the tube is correctly secured.
9 Ensure the correct point on the measuring guide on the tube is placed closest to the end of the fixation device.	To ensure that the tube is correctly secured. If the patient gains weight the external fixation device should be released slightly to prevent pressure necrosis of the stoma site.
10 Do not cover the gastrostomy site with a new dressing unless there is a heavy discharge or leakage from the stoma site.	To encourage wound healing.
11 Do not use bulky dressings, particularly under the external fixation device.	This can increase the pressure on the internal retention disc or retention balloon and increase the risk of tissue necrosis and ulceration occurring in the stomach (Nutricia Clinical Care 1996).
12 Advise the patient not to use moisturizing creams or talcum powder around the stoma site.	To prevent infection and/or irritation to skin. The grease in creams can cause the external retention device to slip, allowing movement of the tube and increasing the risk of leakage and infection. Creams and talcs can affect the tube material, causing it to stretch or leak (Nutricia Clinical Care 1996).

Patients should be taught how to carry out this procedure themselves. Once the stoma site has healed (approximately 10 days postinsertion) it is no longer necessary to perform an aseptic technique. A socially clean procedure using soap and water to clean the stoma site should be adopted.

Procedure guidelines: **Care of a radiologically inserted gastrostomy (RIG) tube**

This procedure should be performed daily to maintain skin integrity and detect any problems early, e.g. infection, skin breakdown.

Equipment

1 Sterile procedure pack containing gallipot, low-linting gauze.

2 Sterile 0.9% sodium chloride.

Procedure

Action	Rationale
Follow points 1, 2, 3 and 5 of care of PEG tube (see above).	
6 Check that the T fasteners are intact. These will stay in place for 7–14 days after RIG insertion.	To enable the stomach to adhere to the abdominal wall.
7 Remove the T fasteners 7–14 days after insertion and secure fixation plate 1–2 cm away from the skin. Do not rotate the tube.	To prevent the RIG tube moving into the stomach.
8 Secure the tube to the skin with hypoallergenic tape. Do not secure near the stoma site.	To prevent the weight of the tube pulling on the exit site. Tape near the stoma site will make it difficult to clean.
9 Advise the patient not to use moisturizing creams or talcum powder.	To prevent infection and/or irritation to the skin.
10 Do not cover the gastrostomy site with a new dressing unless there is a heavy discharge or leakage from the stoma site.	To encourage wound healing.

Procedure guidelines: **Care of a jejunostomy feeding tube**

This procedure should be performed daily to maintain skin integrity and detect any problems early, e.g. infection, skin breakdown.

Equipment

1 Sterile procedure pack containing gallipot, low-linting gauze.

2 Sterile 0.9% sodium chloride.

Procedure

Action	Rationale
Follow points 1, 2, 3, 4 and 5 of care of PEG tube (see above).	
6 Check that the sutures on the retention device are intact. If not, advise medical staff and arrange for the retention device to be resutured.	To prevent accidental removal of the jejunostomy tube.
7 Secure the jejunostomy tube to the skin with hypoallergenic tape. The site may be covered with a dry dressing or left uncovered.	To prevent the weight of the tube pulling on the exit site.
8 Advise the patient not to use moisturizing creams or talcum powder.	To prevent infection and/or irritation to the skin.

Procedure guidelines: **Administration of drugs via enteral feeding tubes**

Equipment

1 50 ml enteral or catheter-tipped syringe.
2 Tap water or sterile water (for jejunostomy tubes or for patients who are immunosuppressed) (NICE 2003). Water should be fresh and kept covered.

3 Mortar and pestle or tablet crusher if tablets are being administered.

Procedure

Action	Rationale
1 Check whether patient can take medication orally, whether medication is necessary or if it can be temporarily suspended.	If patient can take medication orally this reduces the risk of tube blockage.
2 Consider whether an alternative route can be used, e.g. buccal, transdermal, topical, rectal or subcutaneous.	If patient can take medication via an alternative route this reduces the risk of tube blockage.
3 Check drug is absorbed from the site of delivery.	Some drugs may not be absorbed directly from the jejunum.
4 Clean hands with bactericidal soap and water or alcoholic handgel. Put on non-sterile gloves.	To minimize cross-infection and protect the practitioner from gastric/intestinal contents.
5 Stop the enteral feed and flush the tube with at least 30 ml of water (sterile water for jejunostomy administration), using an enteral or catheter-tipped syringe.	To clear the tube of enteral feed as this may cause a blockage or interact with medications. Sterile water should be used for jejunostomy tubes as water is bypassing the protective acidic environment of the stomach.
6 Where there is an absolute contraindication for medicine to be taken with feed: (a) Stop the feed 1–2 hours before and 2 hours after administration (this will depend on the drug), e.g. for phenytoin administration, stop feed 2 hours before and 2 hours after. (b) Consult with the dietitian to prescribe a suitable feeding regimen.	(a) To avoid interaction with enteral feed. (b) To ensure that the patient's nutritional requirements are met in the time available around medicine administration.
7 Prior to preparation, check with the pharmacist which medicines should never be crushed.	Some medications are not designed to be crushed. These include: (a) Modified-release tablets: absorption will be altered by crushing, possibly causing toxic side-effects (b) Enteric-coated tablets: the coating is designed to protect the drug against gastric acid (c) Cytotoxic medicines: this will risk exposing the practitioner to the drug.
8 Prepare each medication to be given separately. Volumes greater than 10 ml may be drawn up in a 50 ml syringe and administered via the tube. For small volumes (less than 10 ml) follow step 11. (a) Soluble tablets: dissolve in 10–15 ml water. (b) Liquids: shake well. For thick liquids mix with an equal volume of water. (c) Tablets: crush using a mortar and pestle or tablet crusher and mix with 10–15 ml water.	To avoid interaction between different medications and to ensure solubility.
9 Never add medication directly to the enteral feed.	To avoid interaction between medicines and feed.
10 Administer the medication through the tube via a 50 ml syringe. Rinse the tablet crusher or mortar with 10 ml water, draw up in a 50 ml syringe and flush this through the tube.	To ensure the whole dose is administered.

Procedure guidelines: **Administration of drugs via enteral feeding tubes** *(cont'd)*

Action	Rationale
11 If volumes of less than 10 ml are required the dose should be measured in a 10 ml oral syringe. The plunger of a 50 ml syringe should be removed and the 50 ml syringe connected with the enteral tube. The dose should then be administered into the barrel of the 50 ml syringe and the 10 ml syringe rinsed with water, which should also be administered via the barrel of the 50 ml syringe.	To ensure the whole dose is administered.
12 If more than one medicine is to be administered, flush between drugs with at least 10 ml of water to ensure that the drug is cleared from the tube.	To avoid interactions between medicines.
13 Flush the tube with at least 30 ml water following the administration of the last drug.	To avoid medicines blocking the enteral tube.
14 If the patient is on a fluid restriction or for a paediatric patient, consult the dietitian and pharmacist about the quantity of water to be given before and after medication.	To ensure that the patient does not exceed their fluid restriction or requirements.

Procedure guidelines: **Unblocking an enteral feeding tube**

Equipment

1 50 ml enteral or catheter-tipped syringe.
2 Tap water or sterile water (for jejunostomy tubes or for patients who are immunosuppressed) (NICE 2003). Water should be fresh and kept covered.

3 Fizzy water, e.g. soda water.

Procedure

Action	Rationale
1 Always flush the enteral tube before and after administration of feed and medication with at least 30 ml of water (sterile water for jejunostomy and for immunosuppressed patients).	To avoid the tube blocking. Sterile water should be used for jejunostomy tubes as water is bypassing the protective acidic environment of the stomach.
2 If the tube is blocked try to administer 50 ml warm water down the enteral tube and leave for 30 minutes. Boil the kettle, pour water into a clean cup and allow to cool until lukewarm.	To dissolve any medication or soften any feed plugs in the tube. To prevent hot water being administered via the feeding tube.
3 Flush tube with 50 ml water.	To remove blockage.
4 If unsuccessful try to administer 50 ml fizzy water, e.g. soda water, via the enteral tube and leave for 30 minutes.	To dislodge blockage.
5 Flush tube with 50 ml water.	To remove blockage.
6 If tube is still blocked consider use of a proprietary product designed to unblock tube. Follow manufacturer's instructions.	To break down plug. Such products contain digestive enzymes which may break down a protein plug but they may not unblock a tube blocked with medication.
7 Do not use a syringe smaller than 50 ml.	To avoid the tube being ruptured with the high pressure of a smaller syringe.
8 If all of the above are unsuccessful then the enteral tube will need replacing.	To ensure continued enteral access for the administration of feed, fluids and medication.

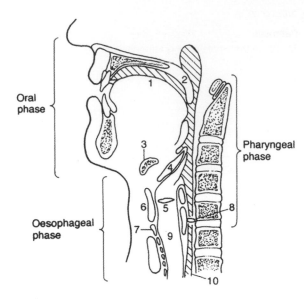

Figure 24.1   The normal swallow.
(1 tongue; 2 soft palate; 3 hyoid bone; 4 epiglottis;
5 vocal cords; 6 thyroid cartilage; 7 cricoid cartilage;
8 pharyngoesophageal sphincter; 9 trachea; 10 oesophagus.)
The oral, pharyngeal and oesophageal phases are separate
but highly co-ordinated (Groher 1997; Logemann 1998).

Problem solving

Supervision of patients with swallowing difficulties is important and in some cases patients may require support at meal
times, or when drinking, to carry out the recommended strategies. It is important for nurses to participate in educational
programmes for patients and carers in order to encourage awareness of the implications of dysphagia. Anxieties
associated with dysphagia should be allayed and confidence to undertake safe eating and drinking techniques built up.
Patients may experience one or a number of the following problems.

Problem	Cause	Prevention	Suggested action
Patient experiencing difficulties with drinking and/or eating (which may lead to dehydration, insufficient nutritional intake and compromised airway).	(a) Mechanical. Patients who have undergone surgery and/or radiotherapy to the oral cavity, pharynx, larynx, or trachea (including temporary or permanent tracheostomy) are likely to experience swallowing difficulties of a temporary or more persistent nature (Fig. 24.1). (b) Neurological. Patients who have tumours which affect the brainstem area and thus the cranial nerves will present with symptoms of dysphagia. These symptoms will continue as long as the disease and/or treatment effects are evident. (c) Oesophageal obstruction or dysfunction. Patients who have tumours of the upper gastrointestinal tract may well experience		Refer to specialist speech and language therapist for full assessment and management plan. Refer to dietitian for nutritional assessment and management plan.

Problem solving (cont'd)

Problem	Cause	Prevention	Suggested action
	discomfort and difficulty with the oesophageal phase of the swallow. The only way to alleviate oesophageal difficulties is through medical or surgical management. Swallowing therapy is not indicated in these circumstances, although the specialist speech and language therapist may be able to offer advice to minimize difficulties experienced by the patient.		
Dehydration and/or difficulty in maintaining adequate hydration.	Thin liquids (e.g. water) are difficult for the patient with dysphagia to manage. Watery liquids do not retain their cohesion in the mouth and therefore pass swiftly into the pharynx. Patients may avoid liquids of this consistency and become dehydrated.	Identify patients who are at risk.	Seek medical advice on the appropriateness of intravenous hydration.
Difficulty in maintaining a clear airway (may be severe enough to block airway in tracheostomy patients).	Inability to manage secretions, indicated by drooling and/or gurgly voice. Tracheostomy patients may feel breathing is laboured.	Monitor patient's progress carefully and regularly and liaise with the speech and language therapist about any changes noted.	Following assessment by specialist speech and language therapist, adjusting the patient's position may help (e.g. sitting posture and head position before and after swallowing). Oral suction may be required. See Ch. 41, Tracheostomy care.
Patient requires nutritional support and/or alternative feeding method.	Dysphagia and/or disease process leading to inadequate nutrition.	All patients with dysphagia should be fully assessed by a dietitian to ensure current nutritional requirements are met by nutritional support, alternative feeding method, normal diet, or a combination of these.	Nutritional support and/or alternative feeding method may be indicated following discussion with members of the multidisciplinary team. Following assessment by a specialist speech and language therapist recommendations may be made about sitting posture, head position, and consistency of food and drink. These will be individually tailored to the patient's needs. Nursing staff should monitor progress carefully, noting changes and reporting them to the appropriate professional.
Dysphagia in oral and/or pharyngeal stages of swallowing, related to head position and/or structural or neurological deficits.	Patients with tumours of the upper gastrointestinal tract may experience difficulty with the oesophageal phase of the swallow; patients with tumours affecting the brainstem/cranial nerves will experience dysphagia.		Proceed as advised by the specialist speech and language therapist: modified head positions, e.g. turned to the affected or unaffected side, tilted to the unaffected side, or chin flexed may be appropriate. Do *not* attempt these compensations without prior assessment and advice from a specialist speech and language therapist.

Problem solving (cont'd)

Problem	Cause	Prevention	Suggested action
Selecting suitable food and/or drink.	Not all members of the multidisciplinary team and/or catering and other staff may be aware of the extent of the patient's swallowing difficulties.	Liaise with specialist speech and language therapist, dietitian and catering.	Provide food and drink of a consistency which will not exacerbate the patient's problems. This might include soft foods, thickened liquids, or purées. Food and drink must be individually tailored to suit the patient.

References and further reading

Allison, S.P. (1999) *Hospital Food as Treatment*. British Association for Parenteral and Enteral Nutrition, Maidenhead.

Arrowsmith H. (1993) Nursing management of patients receiving a nasogastric feed. *Br J Nurs* **2**(21), 1053–8.

BAPEN (1994a) *Enteral and Parenteral Nutrition in the Community* (ed. M. Elia). British Association for Parenteral and Enteral Nutrition, Maidenhead.

BAPEN (1994b) *Organisation of Nutritional Support in Hospitals* (ed. D.B.A. Silk). British Association for Parenteral and Enteral Nutrition, Maidenhead.

BAPEN (1996) *Current Perspectives on Parenteral Nutrition in Adults* (ed. C.R. Pennington). British Association for Parenteral and Enteral Nutrition, Maidenhead.

BAPEN (1999) *Current Perspectives on Enteral Nutrition in Adults* (ed. C.A. McAtear). British Association for Parenteral and Enteral Nutrition, Maidenhead.

BAPEN (2003) *Tube Feeding and Your Medicines: A Guide for Patients and Carers*. www.bapen.org.uk

Benton, S. & Marsden, C. (2002) Training nurses to place tunnelled central venous catheters. *Prof Nurse*, **17**(9), 531–5.

Bodger, K. & Heatley, R.V. (2001) The immune system and nutrition support. In: *Artificial Nutritional Support in Clinical Practice*, 2nd edn (eds J. Payne-James, G. Grimble & D. Silk). Greenwich Medical Media, London.

Bond, S. (1997) *Eating Matters*. Centre for Health Services Research, University of Newcastle, Newcastle upon Tyne.

Boyes R.J. & Kruse J.A. (1992) Nasogastric and nasoenteric intubation. *Crit Care Clin* **8**(4), 865–78.

Bozzetti, F. (2001) Nutrition support in patients with cancer. In: *Artificial Nutritional Support in Clinical Practice*, 2nd edn (eds J. Payne-James, G. Grimble & D. Silk). Greenwich Medical Media, London.

Burke, A. (1997) *Hungry in Hospital*? Association of Community Health Councils for England and Wales, London.

Burnham, P. (1999) Parenteral nutrition. In: *Intravenous Therapy in Nursing Practice* (eds L. Dougherty & J. Lamb). Churchill Livingstone, Edinburgh, pp. 377–400.

Burnham, R. & Barton, S. (2001) The role of the nutrition support team. In: *Artificial Nutritional Support in Clinical Practice*, 2nd edn (eds J. Payne-James, G. Grimble & D. Silk). Greenwich Medical Media, London.

Burns, S.M., Martin, M., Robbins, V. *et al.* (1995) Comparison of nasogastric tube securing methods and tube types in medical intensive care patients. *Am J Crit Care*, **4**(3), 198–203.

Colagiovanni, L. (1999) Taking the tube. *Nurs Times*, **95**(21), 63, 64, 67, 71.

Cole, T.J. (1994) Do growth percentile charts need a face lift? *Br Med J*, **308**(6929), 641–2.

Cummings, J.H. (2000) Nutritional management of diseases of the gut. In: *Human Nutrition and Dietetics*, 10th edn (eds J.S. Garrow, W.P.T. James & A. Ralph). Churchill Livingstone, Edinburgh.

DoH (1991) *Dietary Reference Values for Food Energy and Nutrients for the United Kingdom*. COMA Report 41. Stationery Office, London.

DoH (1995) *Nutrition Guidelines for Hospital Catering*. Department of Health, London.

DoH (1996) *Hospital Catering: Delivering a Quality Service*. DoH/NHSE, London.

DoH (2001) *Essence of Care – Patient Focused Benchmarking for Health Care Professionals*. Department of Health, London.

DoH (2001) Guidelines for preventing infections associated with the insertion and maintenance of central venous catheters. *J Hosp Infect*, **47**(S), S47–67.

Durnin, J.B. & Wolmersley, J. (1974) Body fat assessed from total body density and its estimation from skinfold thickness: measurements on 481 men and women aged from 16 to 72 years. *Br J Nutr*, **32**, 77–9.

Elia, M. (2000) *Guidelines for Detection and Management of Malnutrition*. Malnutrition Advisory Group, British Association for Parenteral and Enteral Nutrition, Maidenhead.

Elia, M. (2001) Metabolic response to starvation, injury and sepsis. In: *Artificial Nutritional Support in Clinical Practice*, 2nd edn (eds J. Payne-James, G. Grimble & D. Silk). Greenwich Medical Media, London.

Fitzsimmons, C.L. (1997) Central venous catheter placement – extending the role of the nurse. *J R Coll Phys*, **31**(5), 533–5.

Griffiths, M. (1996) Single-stage percutaneous gastrostomy button insertion: a leap forward. *J Parent Enteral Nutr*, **20**(3), 237–9.

Groher, M. (1997) *Dysphagia: Diagnosis and Management*, 2nd edn. Butterworth Heinemann, Boston.

Hamilton, H., O'Byrne, M. & Nicholai, L. (1995) Central lines inserted by clinical nurse specialists. *Nurs Times*, **91**(17), 38–9.

Heitman, B. (1994) Impedance: a valid method in assessment of body composition? *Eur J Clin Nutr*, **48**, 228–40.

Heymsfield, S.B. & Matthews, D. (1994) Body composition: research and clinical advances – 1993 A.S.P.E.N. research workshop. *J Parent Enteral Nutr*, **18**(2), 91–103.

Jones, E. (1998) Surgical excision of a pharyngeal pouch. *Prof Nurse*, **13**(6), 378–81.

Logemann, J. (1998) *The Evaluation and Treatment of Swallowing Disorders*, 2nd edn. College Hill Press, San Diego.

Mercadante, S. (1998) Parenteral versus enteral nutrition in cancer patients: indications and practice. *Support Cancer Care*, **6**, 85–93.

Metheny, N.A. & Titler, M.G. (2001) Assessing placement of feeding tubes. *Am J Nurs*, **101**(5), 36–45.

Metheny N., Dettenmeier P., *et al.* (1990a) Detection of inadvertent respiratory placement of small bore feeding tubes: a report of 10 cases. *Heart Lung* **19**(6), 631–8.

Metheny N., McSweeney M. *et al.* (1990b) Effectiveness of the auscultatory method in predicting feeding tube location. *Nurs Res* **39**(5), 262–7.

Metheny, N., Reed, L., Wiersema, L. *et al.* (1993) Effectiveness of pH measurements in predicting tube placement: an update. *Nurs Res*, **42**(6), 324–31.

Naber, T.H.J., Schermer, T., de Bree, A. *et al.* (1997) Prevalence of malnutrition in nonsurgical hospitalised patients and its association with disease complications. *Am J Clin Nutr*, **66**, 1232–9.

Nelson, M. (2000) Methods and validity of dietary assessment. In: *Human Nutrition and Dietetics*, 10th edn (eds J.S. Garrow, W.P.T. James & A. Ralph). Churchill Livingstone, Edinburgh.

Newman, L.A., Vieira, F., Schwiezer, V. *et al.* (1998) Eating and weight changes following chemoradiation therapy for advanced head and neck cancer. *Arch Otolaryngol Head Neck Surg*, **124**, 589–92.

NHS (2001) *Better Hospital Food. The NHS Recipe Book Implementation Support Pack*. Stationery Office, London.

NICE (2003) *Care During Enteral Feeding. Infection Control – Prevention of Health Care Associated Infection in Primary and Community Care*. Clinical Guideline 2. NICE, London. Nutricia Clinical Care (1996) *The Flocare Gastrostomy Range: A Guide to Professional Care*. Nutricia Clinical Care, Cow & Gate Nutricia, Trowbridge.

Payne-James, J., Grimble, G. & Silk, D. (2001) Enteral nutrition: tubes and techniques of delivery. In: *Artificial Nutritional Support in Clinical Practice*, 2nd edn (eds J. Payne-James, G. Grimble & D. Silk). Greenwich Medical Media, London.

Pennington, C.R. (1997) Disease and malnutrition in British hospitals. *Proc Nutr Soc*, **56**, 393–407.

Pickhardt, P.J., Rohrmann, C.A. Jr & Cossentino, M.J. (2002) Stomal metastases complicating percutaneous endoscopic gastrostomy: CT findings and the argument for radiologic tube placement. *AJR Am J Roentgenol*, **179**(3), 735–9.

Reilly, H. (1996) Nutrition in clinical management: malnutrition in our midst. *Proc Nutr Soc*, **55**, 841–53.

Reilly, H. (1998) Parenteral nutrition: an overview of current practice. *Br J Nurs*, **7**(8), 461–7.

Riera, L., Sandiumenge, A., Calvo, C. *et al.* (2002) Percutaneous endoscopic gastrostomy in head and neck cancer patients. *J Otorhinolaryngol Relat Spec*, **64**(1), 32–4.

Rollins, H. (1997) A nose for trouble. *Nurs Times*, **93**(49), 66–7.

Royal Marsden NHS Trust (2002) *Eating Well When You Have Cancer – A Guide for Cancer Patients*. Royal Marsden NHS Trust, London.

Schofield, W.N. (1985) Predicting basal metabolic rate. New standards and review of previous work. *Human Nutr Clin Nutr*, **39C**, Suppl 15, 41.

Shaw, S. & Lawson, M. (2001) *Clinical Paediatric Dietetics*. Blackwell Science, Oxford.

Shenkin, A. (1995) Adult micronutrient requirements. In: *Artificial Nutrition Support in Clinical Practice* (eds J. Payne-James, G. Grimble & D. Silk). Edward Arnold, London, pp. 151–66.

Sitges-Serra, A. & Franch-Arcas, G. (1995) Nutrition assessment. In: *Artificial Nutrition Support in Clinical Practice* (eds J. Payne-James, G. Grimble & D. Silk). Edward Arnold, London, pp. 125–36.

Springhouse Corporation (2002) Parenteral nutrition. In: *IV Therapy Made Incredibly Easy*. Springhouse Corporation, Philadelphia, pp. 269–302.

ter Reit, G., Kessels, A.G. & Knipschild, P.G. (1995) Randomised clinical trial of ascorbic acid in the treatment of pressure ulcers. *J Clin Epidemiol*, **48**(12), 1453–60.

Thomas, B. (2001) *Manual of Dietetic Practice*. Blackwell Science, Oxford.

Thomas, D.R. (1997) Specific nutritional factors in wound healing. *Adv Wound Care*, **10**(4), 40–3.

Thorell, A. & Nordenström, J. (2001) Metabolic complications of parenteral nutrition. In: *Artificial Nutrition Support in Clinical Practice*, 2nd edn (eds J. Payne-James, G. Grimble & D. Silk). Greenwich Medical Media, London, pp. 445–59.

Walden, D. & Klein, S. (1992) Nutritional assessment. *Curr Opin Gastroenterol*, **8**, 286–9.

Weinstein, S.M. (2000) Parenteral nutrition. In: *Principles and Practice of Intravenous Therapy*, 7th edn. Lippincott, Philadelphia, pp. 353–410.

Wilson, J.M. & Jordan, N.L. (2001) Parenteral nutrition. In: *Infusion Therapy in Clinical Practice* (eds J. Hankin *et al.*). W.B. Saunders, Philadelphia.

Wyszynski, D.F., Crivelli, A., Ezquerro, S. *et al.* (1998) Assessment of nutritional status in a population of recently hospitalised patients. *Mecinina*, **58**, 51–7.

Observations

Chapter contents

Pulse

Definition

The pulse is a pressure wave that is transmitted through the arterial tree with each heart beat following the expansion and recoil of arteries during each cardiac cycle. A pulse can be palpated in any artery that lies close to the surface of the body (Fig. 25.1). The radial artery at the wrist is easily accessible and therefore often used but there are several other important areas for monitoring the pulse such as the carotid, femoral and brachial plexus (Marieb 2001).

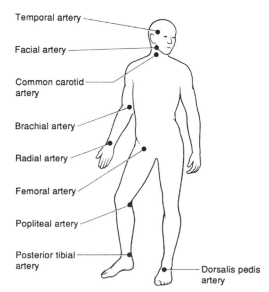

Temporal artery
Facial artery
Common carotid artery
Brachial artery
Radial artery
Femoral artery
Popliteal artery
Posterior tibial artery
Dorsalis pedis artery

Figure 25.1 Body sites where pulse is most easily palpated. The pulse can be felt in arteries lying close to the body surface.

Indications

The pulse is taken for the following reasons:

- To gather information on the heart rate, pattern of beats (rhythm) and amplitude (strength) of pulse
- To determine the individual's pulse on admission as a base for comparing future measurements
- To monitor changes in pulse.

Reference material

In health the arterial pulse is one of the measurements used to assess the effects of activity, postural changes and emotions on the heart rate. In ill health the pulse can be used to assess the effects of disease, treatments and response to therapy. Each time the heart beats it pushes blood through the arteries. The pumping action of the heart causes the walls of the arteries to expand and distend, causing a wave-like sensation which can then be felt as the pulse (Marieb 2001). The pulse is measured by lightly compressing the artery against firm tissue and by counting the number of beats in a minute.

The pulse is palpated to note the following:

- Rate
- Rhythm
- Amplitude.

Rate

The normal pulse rate varies in different client groups as age-related changes affect the pulse rate. The approximate range is illustrated in Table 25.1 (Timby 1989).

The pulse may vary depending on the posture of an individual. For example, the pulse of a healthy man may be around 66 beats per minute when he is lying down; this increases to 70 when sitting up, and 80 when he stands suddenly (Marieb 2001).

The rate of the pulse of an individual with a healthy heart tends to be relatively constant. However, when blood volume drops suddenly or when the heart has

Table 25.1 Normal pulse rates per minute at various ages

Age	Approximate range	Average
Newborn	120–160	140
1–12 months	80–140	120
12 months–2 years	80–130	110
2–6 years	75–120	100
6–12 years	75–110	95
Adolescent	60–100	80
Adult	60–100	80

been weakened by disease, the stroke volume declines and cardiac output is maintained only by increasing the rate of heart beat.

Cardiac output is the amount of blood pumped out by each heart ventricle in 1 minute, while the stroke volume is the amount of blood pumped out by a ventricle with each contraction. The relationship between these and the heart rate is expressed in the following equation:

$$\text{Cardiac output} = \text{Heart rate} \times \text{Stroke volume}$$

The heart rate and hence pulse rate are influenced by various factors acting through neural, chemical and physically induced homeostatic mechanisms (Fig. 25.2):

- Neural changes in heart rate are caused by the activation of the sympathetic nervous system which increases heart rate, while parasympathetic activation decreases heart rate (Ganong 1995).
- Chemical regulation of the heart is affected by hormones (adrenaline and thyroxine) and electrolytes (sodium, potassium and calcium) (Ganong 1995). High or low levels of electrolytes, particularly potassium, magnesium and calcium, can cause an alteration in the heart's rhythm and rate.
- Physical factors that influence heart rate are age, sex, exercise and body temperature (Marieb 2001).

Tachycardia is defined as an abnormally fast heart rate, over 100 beats per minute in adults, which may result from a raised body temperature, increased sympathetic response due to physical/emotional stress, certain drugs or heart disease (Marieb 2001).

Bradycardia is a heart rate slower than 60 beats per minute. It may be the result of a low body temperature, certain drugs or parasympathetic nervous system activation. It is also found in fit athletes when physical and cardiovascular conditioning occurs. This results in hypertrophy of the heart with an increase in its stroke volume. These heart changes result in a lower resting heart rate but with the same cardiac output (Marieb 2001). If persistent bradycardia occurs in an individual as a result of ill health, this may result in inadequate blood circulation to body tissues. A slowing of the heart rate accompanied by a rise in blood pressure is one of the indications of raised intracranial pressure.

Rhythm

The pulse rhythm is the sequence of beats. In health, these are regular. The co-ordinated action of the muscles of the heart in producing a regular heart rhythm is due to the ability of cardiac muscle to contract inherently without nervous control (Marieb 2001). The co-ordinated action of the muscles in the heart results from two

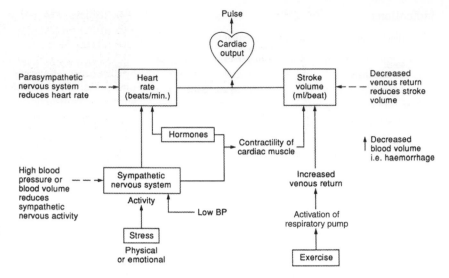

Figure 25.2 Influence of neural, chemical and physical factors on cardiac output and hence pulse.

physiological factors:

• Gap junctions in the cardiac muscles which form interconnections between adjacent cardiac muscles and allow transmission of nervous impulses from cell to cell (Marieb 2001).

• Specialized nerve-like cardiac cells that form the nodal system. These initiate and distribute impulses throughout the heart, so that the heart beats as one unit (Marieb 2001). These are the sinoatrial node, atrioventricular node, atrioventricular bundle and the Purkinje fibres.

The sinoatrial node is the pacemaker, initiating each wave of contraction. This sets the rhythm for the heart as a whole (Fig. 25.3). Its characteristic rhythm is called *sinus rhythm*.

Defects in the conduction system of the heart can cause irregular heart rhythms, or arrhythmias, resulting in uncoordinated contraction of the heart.

Fibrillation is a condition of rapid and irregular contractions. A fibrillating heart is ineffective as a pump (Marieb 2001). *Atrial fibrillation* is a disruption of rhythm in the atrial areas of the heart occurring at extremely rapid and uncoordinated intervals. The rapid impulses result in the ventricles not being able to respond to every atrial beat and, therefore, the ventricles contract irregularly. There are many causes of this condition, but the following are the most common: (1) ischaemic heart disease; (2) acute illness; (3) electrolyte abnormality; (4) thyrotoxicosis.

Ventricular fibrillation is an irregular heart rhythm characterized by chaotic contraction of the ventricles at very rapid rates. Ventricular fibrillation results in cardiac

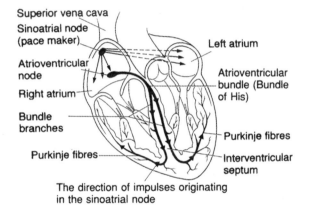

The direction of impulses originating in the sinoatrial node

Figure 25.3 Intrinsic conduction system of the heart.

arrest and death if not reversed with defibrillation and the injection of adrenaline (epinephrine). The cause of this condition is often myocardial infarction (MI), electrical shock, acidosis, electrolyte disturbances and hypovolaemia (Resuscitation Council UK 2000).

Body fluids are good conductors of electricity so it is possible through electrocardiography to observe how the currents generated are transmitted through the heart. The electrocardiograph provides a graphic representation and record (electrocardiogram) of electrical activity as the heart beats. The electrocardiogram (ECG) makes it possible to identify abnormalities in electrical conduction within the heart. The normal ECG consists of a series of three distinct areas called deflection waves. The first of these is the P wave, which results from an electrical impulse in the sinoatrial node. The large QRS complex results from ventricular depolarization, and

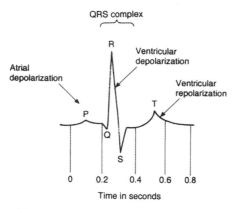

Figure 25.4 An ECG tracing illustrating normal deflection waves.

takes place prior to contraction of the heart muscles. The T wave is caused by ventricular repolarization. In a healthy heart, the size and rhythm of the deflection waves tend to remain constant (Fig. 25.4). Changes in the pattern or timing of the deflection in the ECG may indicate problems with the heart's conduction system, such as those caused by myocardial infarction (Marieb 2001). Examples of conduction abnormalities are shown in Figure 25.5.

Amplitude

Amplitude is a reflection of pulse strength and the elasticity of the arterial wall. The flexibility of the artery of the young adult feels different from the hard artery of the patient suffering from arteriosclerosis. It takes some clinical experience to appreciate the differences in amplitude. However, it is important to be able to recognize major changes such as the faint flickering pulse of the severely hypovolaemic patient or the irregular pulse in cardiac arrhythmias.

Assessing gross pulse irregularity

Paradoxical pulse is a pulse that markedly decreases in amplitude during inspiration. On inspiration, more blood is pooled in the lungs and so decreases the return to the left side of the heart; this affects the consequent stroke volume. A paradoxical pulse is usually regarded as normal, although in conjunction with such features as hypotension and dyspnoea, it may indicate cardiac tamponade.

When there is a gross pulse irregularity, it may be useful to use a stethoscope to assess the apical heart beat. This is done by placing the diaphragm of the stethoscope over the apex of the heart and counting the beats for 60 seconds. A second nurse should record the radial

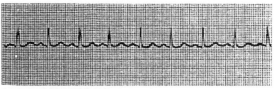

Normal sinus rhythm

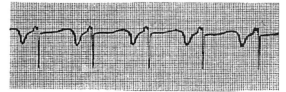

Junctional rhythm. Sinoatrial node is non-functional, P waves are absent and heart rate is paced by the AV node

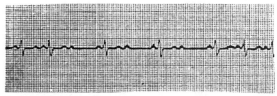

Second degree heart block. P waves are not conducted through the AV node

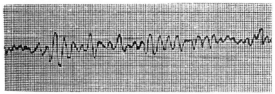

Ventricular fibrillation. Chaotic electrical conduction, grossly irregular. This is seen in an acute heart attack and electrical shock

Figure 25.5 Normal and abnormal ECG tracings.

pulse at the same time. The deficit between the two should be noted using, for example, different colours on the patient's chart to indicate the apex and radial rates (Docherty 2002).

Conditions where a patient's pulse may need careful monitoring are described below:

- Postoperative and critically ill patients require monitoring of the pulse to assess for cardiovascular stability. The patient's pulse should be recorded preoperatively in order to establish a baseline and to make comparisons. Hypovolaemic shock post surgery from the loss of plasma or whole blood results in a decrease in circulatory blood volume. The resulting acceleration in heart rate causes a tachycardia that can be felt in the pulse. The greater the loss in volume the more thready the pulse is likely to feel.

- Blood transfusions require the careful monitoring of the pulse as an incompatible blood transfusion may lead to a rise in pulse rate (BCSH 1999) (see Ch. 42, Transfusion of blood).
- Patients with local or systemic infections or inflammatory reactions require monitoring of their pulse to detect sepsis/severe sepsis. This is characterized by a decrease in the mean arterial pressure (MAP) and a rise in pulse rate (Bone 1997).

- Patients with cardiovascular conditions require regular assessment of the pulse to monitor their condition and the efficacy of medications.

Note: even where the patient has continuous ECG monitoring, such as in coronary care, A&E and ITU, it is still essential to manually feel a pulse to determine amplitude and volume and whether the pulse is irregular.

Procedure guidelines: **Pulse**

Procedure

	Action	Rationale
1	Explain and discuss the procedure with the patient.	To ensure that the patient understands the procedure and gives his/her valid consent.
2	Where possible, measure the pulse under the same conditions each time. Ensure that the patient is comfortable.	To ensure continuity and consistency in recording. To ensure that the patient is comfortable.
3	Place the second or third finger along the appropriate artery and press gently.	The fingertips are sensitive to touch. The thumb and forefinger have pulses of their own that may be mistaken for the patient's pulse.
4	Press gently against the peripheral artery being used to record the pulse.	The radial artery is usually used as it is often the most readily accessible.
5	The pulse should be counted for 60 seconds.	Sufficient time is required to detect irregularities or other defects.
6	Record the pulse rate.	To monitor differences and detect trends; any irregularities should be brought to the attention of the appropriate senior nursing and medical teams.

Note: in children under 2 years of age, the pulse should not be taken in this way; the rapid pulse rate and small area for palpation can lead to inaccurate data. The heart rate should be assessed by utilizing a stethoscope and listening to the apical heart beat.

---

12 Lead electrocardiogram (ECG)

Definition

A 12 lead ECG is a non-invasive procedure that is used to ascertain information about the electrophysiology of the heart. It is performed electively prior to various interventions such as surgery and anti-cancer chemotherapy. ECGs are also an important investigation during an acute situation, particularly in the presence of chest pain, haemodynamic disturbance or cardiac rhythm changes.

Procedure guidelines: **12 Lead ECG**

Equipment

1 ECG machine with chest and limb leads labelled respectively, e.g. LA to left arm, V1 to first chest lead.
2 Disposable electrodes.

3 Swabs saturated with 70% isopropyl alcohol.
4 Abrasive strips.

Procedure guidelines: **12 Lead ECG** *(cont'd)*

Procedure

Action	Rationale
1 Explain to the patient that the ECG is to be taken, that it is not a painful procedure and will be useful to aid diagnosis.	To ensure that the patient understands the procedure and gives his/her valid consent.
2 Ensure that the patient is comfortably positioned either lying or sitting.	To ensure optimal recording and comfort of the patient.
3 Clean limb and chest electrode sites (Fig. 25.6). If necessary, prepare skin by clipping hairs or use abrasive strip.	To ensure good grip and therefore good contact between skin and electrode which results in less electrical artefact.
4 Apply the ten electrodes as described in Fig. 25.6.	To obtain the ECG recording from vertical and horizontal planes.

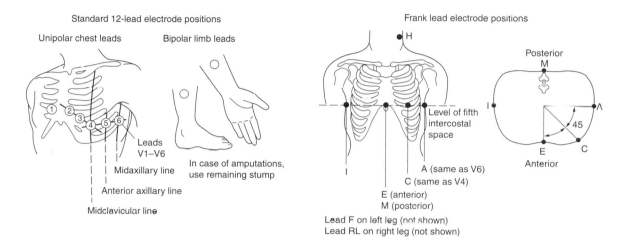

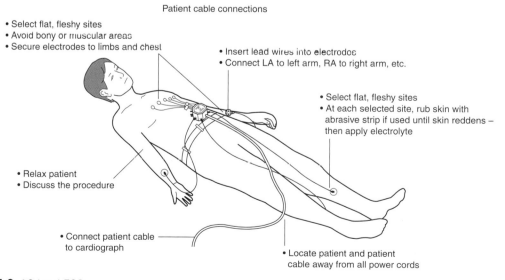

Figure 25.6 12 Lead ECG.

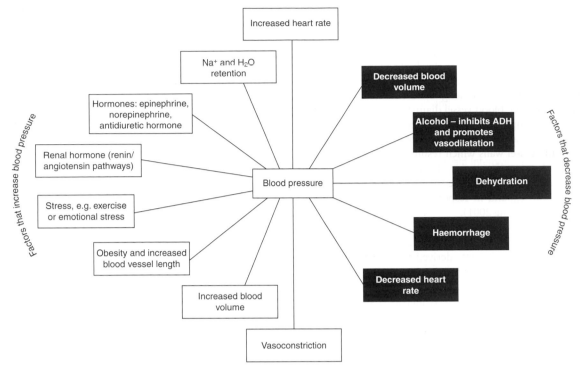

Figure 25.8 Factors that lead to a change in blood pressure.

or more blood pressure readings taken at rest, several days apart, exceeds the upper limits of what is considered normal for the patient.

Mean arterial pressure

The mean arterial pressure is the average pressure required to push blood through the circulatory system. This can be determined electronically or mathematically as well as by using an intra-arterial catheter and mercury manometer.

Mathematically, for example:

$$\text{Mean arterial pressure} = \frac{1}{3}\,\text{Systolic pressure} + \frac{2}{3}\,\text{Diastolic pressure}$$

A blood pressure of 130/85 mmHg gives a mean arterial pressure of 100 mmHg.

Methods of recording and equipment

There are two main methods for recording the blood pressure: direct and indirect. *Direct* methods are more accurate than indirect methods. The most accurate method of measuring blood pressure involves the insertion of a minute pressure transducer unit into an artery for transmission of a waveform or digital display on a monitor. The most commonly used techniques involve placing a cannula in an artery and attaching a pressure-sensitive device to the external end.

Patients who need to be constantly monitored, e.g. in theatres, high-dependency and intensive care units, may require such devices to be used. In such patients it is essential to have an early knowledge of any change in the blood pressure, as this may indicate a deterioration in condition and require prompt treatment.

The *indirect* method is the auscultatory method. This procedure is used to measure blood pressure in the brachial artery of the arm.

The sphygmomanometer

The sphygmomanometer (Fig. 25.9) consists of a compression bag enclosed in an unyielding cuff, and inflating bulb, pump or other device by which the pressure is increased, a manometer from which the applied pressure is read, and a control valve to deflate the system.

Manual sphygmomanometers

Mercury sphygmomanometers are generally reliable and accurate and have been the standard method for recording blood pressure. There are concerns

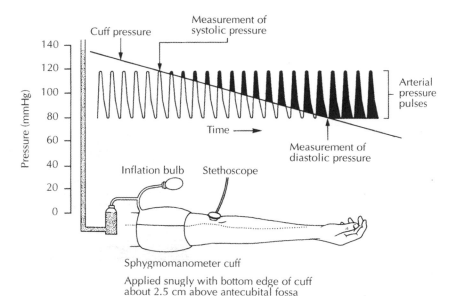

Figure 25.9 Using a sphygmomanometer, and the appearance and disappearance of Korotkoff's sounds.

regarding the safety and impact on the environment of medical devices containing mercury. There is no ban on the use of medical devices containing mercury in the UK but the Medical Devices Agency recommends 'the selection of mercury-free products when the opportunity arises' (MDA 2000). If mercury sphygmomanometers are used they should be in good repair and staff should be properly trained in their use. While in use, the measuring tube of the manometer should be kept in a vertical position, otherwise substantial errors can occur (Campbell *et al.* 1990). In the event of mercury spillage or disposal, proprietary kits are available to help contain the spillage and minimize the risk of mercury vapour forming. Local policies and the manufacturer's recommendations should be followed.

The most common types of error for mercury sphygmomanometers are:

- Rapid deflation of the cuff during measurement
- Improper placement (e.g. mercury column not vertical)
- Perished rubber tubing (McAlister & Straus 2001).

The other widely used type of manual sphygmomanometer is the aneroid sphygmomanometer. This is a mechanical device that measures the cuff pressure using a bellows connected to the cuff via rubber tubing. The pressure inside the bellows is transferred to a dial via a system of gears and levers (Beevers *et al.* 2001a). This type of sphygmomanometer can be calibrated properly, but is susceptible to inaccuracies or damage that would not be apparent to the user (O'Brien *et al.* 2001). The most common types of error for aneroid

sphygmomanometers are:

- Non-zeroed or bent indicators
- Cracked face plates
- Perished rubber tubing (McAlister & Straus 2001).

In addition, there are sources of error common to all methods of manual blood pressure measuring:

- Systematic error (e.g. lack of concentration, poor hearing, inattention to audible or visual cues)
- Failure to interpret the Korotkoff sounds correctly (discussed later in this section)
- Terminal digit preference (tendency to record blood pressures ending in '5' or '0')
- Bias (e.g. recording a blood pressure corresponding to what would be expected for the patient, not the actual reading) (Beevers *et al.* 2001b).

Non-invasive automated sphygmomanometers

Automated devices to measure blood pressure have been available for some time now. Devices are manufactured for a variety of different purposes, including home use. Generally, devices intended for home use are not found to be accurate or reliable enough for clinical use (O'Brien *et al.* 2001). The British Hypertension Society and the US Association for the Advancement of Medical Instrumentation (AAMI) regularly check blood pressure measuring devices and publish recommendations for their use.

Automatic blood pressure monitors are often oscillometric devices, where the measurement of blood pressure is based on the variations of pressure in the cuff caused by the pulsing of the artery directly underneath it (Berger 2001). For this reason, placement of the cuff over the artery is essential for accurate blood pressure reading.

As with all medical devices, use should be in accordance with the procedures recommended by the manufacturer. The principles of measuring an accurate blood pressure using an electronic device will be similar to manual recording of blood pressure with regard to patient factors such as positioning, choice and placement of the cuff. All medical devices should be properly serviced and maintained and may need calibration at intervals. Guidance should be sought from the manufacturer.

Users of electronic sphygmomanometers should also be aware that errors in measurement (for example, if there is a weak or thready pulse) may not be readily obvious to the operator and that manual blood pressure measurement may be indicated (Beevers *et al.* 2001a).

Parts of a sphygmomanometer

Cuff

The cuff is made of washable material that encircles the arm and encloses the inflatable rubber bladder. It is secured around the arm or leg by wrapping its tapering end to the encircling material, usually by Velcro.

Inflatable bladder

A bladder that is too short and/or too narrow will give falsely high pressures. The British Hypertension Society recommended in 1986 that the centre of the bladder should cover the brachial artery and that the bladder length should be 80% of the arm circumference and the width at least 40% (Gillespie & Curzio 1998).

Control valve, pump and rubber tubing

The control valve is a common source of error. It should allow the passage of air without excessive pressure needing to be applied on the pump. When the valve is closed it should hold the mercury at a constant level and, when released, it should allow a controlled fall in the level of mercury. The rubber tubing should be long (approximately 80 cm) and with airtight connections that can easily be separated to allow rapid deflation if required.

Campbell *et al.* (1990), in reviewing the methods for sphygmomanometer inaccuracies, found that errors in technique and equipment malfunction accounted for differences in readings of more than 15 mmHg. Problems with equipment malfunction were further supported in a study by Carney *et al.* (1995), who evaluated 463 sphygmomanometers and found that only 58% were in working order.

The stethoscope

Using the stethoscope it is possible to identify a series of five phases as blood pressure falls from the systolic to the diastolic. These phases are known as Korotkoff's sounds (Fig. 25.10).

When the cuff pressure has fallen to just below the systolic pressure, a clear but often faint tapping sound

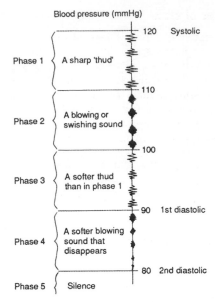

Figure 25.10 Korotkoff's sounds.

suddenly appears in phase with each cardiac contraction. The sound is produced by the transient and turbulent blood flowing through the brachial artery during the peak of each systole.

As the pressure in the cuff is reduced further, the sound becomes louder, but when the artery is no longer constricted and the blood flows freely, the sounds become muffled and then can no longer be heard. The diastolic pressure is usually defined as the cuff pressure at which the sounds disappear (Marieb 2001).

The stethoscope's diaphragm should be placed lightly over the point of maximal pulsation of the brachial artery (Petrie *et al.* 1997). The diaphragm is designed to amplify low-frequency sounds such as Korotkoff's sounds (Hill & Grim 1991). Excessive pressure on the stethoscope's diaphragm may partially occlude the brachial artery and delay the occurrence of Korotkoff's sounds. For this reason the diaphragm should not be tucked under the edge of the cuff.

Korotkoff's sounds form five phases:

1 The appearance of faint, clear tapping sounds which gradually increase in intensity.
2 The softening of sounds, which may become swishing.
3 The return of sharper sounds which become crisper but never fully regain the intensity of the phase 1 sounds.
4 The distinct muffling sound which becomes soft and blowing.
5 The point at which all sound ceases.

Sources of error

Much recent research has focused on the faulty techniques employed when blood pressures are taken (Campbell *et al.* 1990; Bogan *et al.* 1993; Kemp *et al.* 1994; Torrance & Serginson 1996; Gillespie & Curzio 1998). Blood pressure readings are altered by various factors that influence the patient, the techniques used and the accuracy of the sphygmomanometer. The variability of any readings can be reduced by an improved technique and by taking several readings (Campbell *et al.* 1990). In 1981 Thompson discussed the methodology of blood pressure recording and identified poor technique and observer bias as possible sources of error. He concluded that many nurses were inadequately trained in blood pressure measurement and that more attention needed to be paid to this area. In 1996 Beevers & Beevers found that observer error could be reduced if techniques for measuring blood pressure were taught repeatedly during medical and nursing training. Furthermore, the techniques should be reinforced regularly.

Similar conclusions were found in studies by Mancia *et al.* (1987), Feher & Harris St John (1992) and Torrance & Serginson (1996). Poor technique due to inadequate education can cause marked variation in the accuracy of measurements and can lead to inappropriate treatment decisions (Kemp *et al.* 1994).

Ambulatory blood pressure monitoring allows the measurement of trends in the patient's blood pressure over a longer period. For the assessment of hypertensive patients it is increasingly regarded as an important tool to assess blood pressure during normal daily activity (McAlister & Straus 2001). Ambulatory blood pressure is increasingly regarded as superior to individual blood pressure readings.

Variations in the procedure and frequency of taking blood pressure may be required in different patient groups with differing conditions. With a child it is important that the correctly sized cuff is used and that the average of repeated measurements is recorded. Low diastolic pressures are common in children and thus the pressure at muffling (Korotkoff phase 4) may be difficult to determine. Low diastolic pressures are common in elderly patients who may have atherosclerosis, and in patients with an increased cardiac output, i.e. as a result of pregnancy, exercise or hypothyroidism.

Patients with lines or shunts for dialysis in their arms or superior vena cava obstruction may be unsuitable for upper arm measurements of blood pressure; however, the blood pressure may be measured in the leg or forearm. For this procedure the patient lies prone and a thigh or large cuff is applied to the lower third of the thigh. The cuff is wrapped securely with its lower edge above the knee and its bladder centred over the posterior popliteal artery. The stethoscope diaphragm should be applied on the artery below the cuff. Systolic blood pressure is normally 20–30 mmHg higher in the leg than in the arm. The right sized cuff should be used for obtaining the blood pressure using the forearm, and the bladder should be centred over the radial artery below the elbow, and the cuff wrapped in a similar manner to the normal procedure. The stethoscope diaphragm should be positioned over the radial artery about 2.5 cm above the wrist. Forearm blood pressure measurements may vary significantly from an upper arm measurement, and therefore it is important to document cuff size and location (Hill & Grim 1991).

Patients who have had breast surgery with lymph node dissections and/or radiotherapy, or have lymphoedema should not have their blood pressure recorded on the affected side. This is due to the increased frailty of tissue in the area and the risk of developing lymphoedema. Patients should be told to only have their blood pressure taken on the unaffected arm or legs.

Conditions where a patient's blood pressure may need careful monitoring are described below.

- Hypertension is never diagnosed on a single blood pressure reading. Blood pressures are monitored to evaluate the condition of the patient and the effectiveness of medication (DoH 2000; Marieb 2001).
- Postoperative and critically ill patients require monitoring of blood pressure to assess for cardiovascular stability. The patient's blood pressure should be recorded preoperatively in order to establish a baseline for comparison.
- Patients receiving intravenous infusions require blood pressure monitoring to observe for circulatory overload. Certain chemotherapy protocols use protracted amounts of intravenous fluids. In this group of patients diuretics are frequently used to reduce the increase in blood volume which results in a rise in blood pressure. Careful monitoring of blood pressure, weight, kidney function and electrolytes is imperative to prevent fluid overload and electrolyte imbalance (Marini & Wheeler 1997).
- Patients with local or systemic infections or neutropenia require monitoring of their blood pressure in order to detect septicaemic shock. This is characterized by a change in the capillary epithelium and vasodilatation due to circulating cell mediation (Bone 1996), which permits loss of blood and plasma through capillary walls into surrounding tissues. The decrease in the circulating volume of blood results in impaired tissue perfusion, culminating in cellular hypoxia (Ganong 2001).

Procedure guidelines: **Manual blood pressure**

Equipment

1 Sphygmomanometer.

2 Stethoscope.

Procedure

Action	Rationale
1 Explain to the patient that blood pressure is to be taken and discuss the procedure.	To ensure that the patient understands the procedure and gives his/her consent.
2 Allow the patient to rest for 3 minutes if the patient is supine or seated and for 1 minutes if the patient is standing (Petrie *et al.* 1997).	To ensure an accurate reading is obtained. Normally blood pressure readings are measured with the patient in a sitting position (Ramsey *et al.* 1999).
3 Ensure that the upper arm is supported and positioned at heart level, with the palm of the hand facing upwards (Jevon *et al.* 2001).	To obtain an accurate reading. Measurements made with the arm dangling by the hip can be 11–12 mmHg higher than those made with the arm supported and the cuff at heart level. Measurements made with the arm raised can be falsely high (Beevers *et al.* 2001a).
4 Ensure that tight or restrictive clothing is removed from the arm (Petrie *et al.* 1997).	To obtain a correct reading.
5 Use a cuff that covers 80% of the circumference of the upper arm (Petrie *et al.* 1997).	To obtain a correct reading.
6 Apply the cuff of the sphygmomanometer snugly around the arm, ensuring that the centre of the bladder covers the brachial artery.	To obtain a correct reading.
7 Position the manometer within 1 m of the patient, and where it can be seen at eye level (Petrie *et al.* 1997).	To prevent the cuff tubing hanging down and causing a risk of being caught by objects or by the operator. The manometer should be at eye level to obtain an accurate recording.
8 Instruct the patient to stop eating, talking, etc., during blood pressure measurement.	Activity, including eating or talking, will cause an inaccurate high blood pressure to be recorded (McAlister & Straus 2001).
9 Inflate the cuff until the radial pulse can no longer be felt. This provides an estimation of the systolic pressure. Deflate the cuff completely and wait 15–30 seconds before continuing to measure (Hill & Grim 1991).	A low systolic pressure may be reported in patients who have an auscultatory gap. This is when Korotkoff's sounds disappear shortly after the systolic pressure is heard, and resume well above what corresponds to the diastolic pressure. About 5% of the population have an auscultatory gap and it is most common in those with hypertension (Hill & Grim 1991). This error can be avoided if the systolic pressure is first estimated by palpation.
10 The cuff is then inflated to a pressure 30 mmHg higher than the estimated systolic pressure.	Pressure exerted by the inflated cuff prevents the blood from flowing through the artery.
11 The diaphragm of the stethoscope should be placed over the pulse point of the brachial artery.	Apply just enough pressure on the stethoscope to keep it in its place over the brachial artery. Excessive pressure can distort sounds or make them persist for longer than normal (Londe & Klitzner 1984).
12 Do not tuck the diaphragm under the edge of the cuff (Petrie *et al.* 1997).	To prevent an inaccurate result due to the pressure exerted by the cuff on the brachial artery.
13 Deflate the cuff at 2 mmHg per second or per heart beat (Perloff *et al.* 1993).	At a slower rate of deflation venous congestion and arm pain can develop, resulting in a falsely low reading. At faster rates of deflation the mercury may fall too quickly, resulting in an imprecise reading (Perloff *et al.* 1993).

*Procedure guidelines: **Manual blood pressure** (cont'd)*

Action	Rationale
14 The measurement of systolic blood pressure is when a minimum of two clear repetitive tapping sounds can be heard. Diastolic pressure is measured at the point when the sound can no longer be heard.	To ensure that an accurate reading is obtained.
15 A record should be made of the systolic and diastolic pressures and comparisons made with previous readings. It should be recorded which arm was used to take the blood pressure. Any irregularities should be brought to the attention of the medical team.	The average of two or more blood pressure readings is often taken to represent a patient's normal blood pressure. Taking more than one measurement reduces the influence of anxiety and may provide a more accurate record (Hill & Grim 1991).
16 Remove the equipment and clean after use.	To reduce the risk of cross-infection.

Respiration

Definition

The function of the respiratory system is to supply the body with oxygen and remove carbon dioxide. This is achieved by the diffusion of gases between the air in the alveoli of the lungs and the blood in the alveolar capillaries (Marieb 2001).

Indications

The respiration rate is evaluated:

- To determine a baseline respiratory rate for comparisons
- To monitor changes in oxygenation or in respiration
- To evaluate the patient's response to medications or treatments that affect the respiratory system.

Reference material

The body cells require a continuous supply of oxygen to carry out their vital functions and this is provided by respiration (Marieb 2001). To accomplish respiration, four distinct events must occur:

1 Ventilation is where air is moved into and out of the lungs so that gas in the air sacs is replenished.
2 Gaseous exchange between the blood and the alveoli.
3 Oxygen and carbon dioxide are transported to and from the lungs by the cardiovascular system. This is called respiratory transportation.
4 Internal respiration is the cellular respiration that occurs in the cell where oxygen is utilized and carbon dioxide produced.

Control of respiration

Respiratory centre

The respiratory centre generates the basic pattern of breathing. It is located in the brain and is made up of

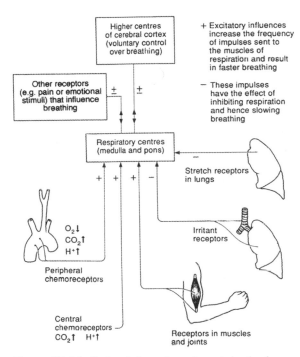

Figure 25.11 Factors influencing rate and depth of breathing.

groups of nerve cells in the reticular endothelial system of the medulla oblongata. Regular impulses are sent by these cells to the motor neurones in the anterior horn of the spinal cord which supply the intercostal muscles and the diaphragm (Ganong 2001). When the motor neurones are stimulated, the muscles contract and inspiration occurs. When the neurones are inhibited, the muscles relax and expiration follows.

Although the respiratory centre generates the basic rhythm, the depth and rate of breathing can be altered in response to the body's changing needs. The most important factors are those of nervous and chemical control (Fig. 25.11).

Nervous control

Lung tissue is stretched on inspiration and this stimulates afferent fibres in the vagus nerve. These impulses cause inspiration to cease and expiration occurs. Emotion, pain and anxiety also cause an increased respiratory rate (Marieb 2001).

Chemical control

An increase in the amount of carbon dioxide in the blood supplying the respiratory centre stimulates the respiratory centre and breathing becomes faster and deeper.

During exercise, carbon dioxide is produced in the muscles by the oxidation of carbohydrate. The amount of carbon dioxide in the blood increases and this stimulates the respiratory centre, producing an increase in depth and rate of respiration. More oxygen is made available in the alveoli for the blood to transport to the muscles, at the same time eliminating more carbon dioxide.

Any substance that, like carbon dioxide, lowers the pH of the blood will stimulate the respiratory centre. Figure 25.11 illustrates the factors influencing the rate and depth of breathing.

Patients with respiratory disease, e.g. emphysema and chronic bronchitis, who maintain high levels of carbon dioxide, will have arterial oxygen levels below 9 kPa (see Ch. 37, Respiratory therapy). This is termed the 'hypoxic drive'. This chronic elevation of the partial pressure of carbon dioxide results in the chemoreceptors becoming unresponsive to this chemical stimulus. The change in respiratory drive results in respiration being stimulated by decreases in oxygen levels rather than levels of carbon dioxide (Marieb 2001). This may be detrimental to the patient's respiration if oxygen is administered therapeutically at high levels.

Ventilation

Ventilation results from pressure changes transmitted from the thoracic cavity to the lungs (Fig. 25.12). Inspiration is initiated by contraction of the diaphragm and external intercostal muscles. This results in the rib cage rising up, and the thrusting forward of the sternum. The ribs also swing outwards, expanding the volume of the thorax (Marieb 2001). Because the lungs adhere tightly to the thoracic wall, attached by the layers of parietal and visceral pleura, this increases the intrapulmonary volume (Marieb 2001). Gases travel from an area of high pressure to areas of low pressure. The increased intrapulmonary volume results in a negative pressure of 1–3 mmHg less than the atmospheric pressure (Marieb 2001). The resulting pressure gradient causes air to rush into the lungs (Fig. 25.13).

Expiration is largely passive, occurring as the inspiratory muscles relax and the lungs recoil as a result of

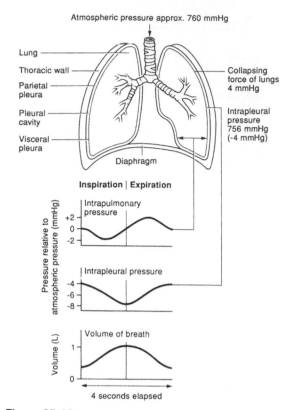

Figure 25.12 Intrapulmonary and intrapleural pressure relationships. Ventilation occurs due to pressure changes transmitted from the thoracic cavity to the lungs.

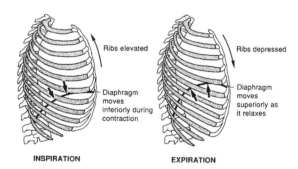

Figure 25.13 Changes in thoracic volume during breathing.

their elastic properties (Marieb 2001). When intrapulmonary pressure exceeds atmospheric pressure this compresses the microscopic air sacs (alveoli) and an expiration of gases occurs.

Disease that affects the pleura of the individual may influence ventilation. A chest wound or rupture of the visceral pleura may allow air to enter the pleural space

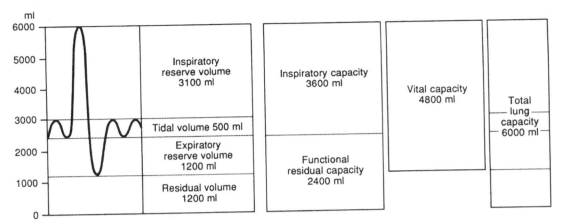

Figure 25.14 Respiratory volumes and capacities.

from the respiratory tract. The presence of air in the intrapleural space is referred to as a pneumothorax. Pleurisy, inflammation of the pleura where secretion of pleural fluid declines, causes a stabbing pain with each inspiration. Alternatively, an excessive increase in pleural secretions may hinder breathing (Marieb 2001). Air in the pleural space results in lung collapse (atelectasis). This affects the intrapulmonary pressure and hence ventilation.

The degree to which the lungs stretch and fill during inspiration and return to normal during expiration is due to the compliance and elasticity of lung tissue. Lung compliance depends on the elasticity of lung tissue and the flexibility of the thorax (Marieb 2001). When this is impaired, expiration becomes an active process, requiring the use of energy. The diseases that lower lung compliance are characterized by changes in the lung parenchyma. Examples include emphysema and fibrosing alveolitis, as a result of intrinsic or extrinsic means (Marieb 2001):

Intrinsic:	severe infection
	rheumatoid arthritis
	SLE (systemic lupus erythematosus)
Extrinsic:	pneumoconiosis
	psitticosis
	asbestosis
	oxygen fibrosis

In emphysema the lungs become progressively less elastic and more fibrous, which hinders both inspiration and expiration. The increased muscular activity results in greater energy required to breathe.

Compliance is diminished by any factor that:

- Reduces the natural resilience of the lungs
- Blocks the bronchi or respiratory passageways
- Impairs the flexibility of the thoracic cage.

Friction in the air passageways causes resistance and affects ventilation (Ganong 2001). Normally, airway resistance is reduced so that minimal opposition to airflow occurs. However, any factor that amplifies airway resistance such as the presence of mucus, tumour or infected material in the airways demands that breathing movements become more strenuous (Marieb 2001).

Respiratory volumes

The amount of air that is breathed varies depending on the condition of inspiration and expiration. Information about a patient's respiratory status can be gained by measuring various lung capacities, which consist of the sum of different respiratory volumes.

The respiratory volumes shown in Fig. 25.14 represent normal values for a healthy 20-year-old male weighing about 70 kg (Marieb 2001).

Tidal volume (TV)

The tidal volume is the amount of air inhaled or exhaled with each breath under resting conditions (about 500 ml).

Inspiratory reserve volume (IRV)

The inspiratory reserve volume is the amount of air that can be inhaled forcibly after a normal tidal volume inhalation (about 3100 ml).

Expiratory reserve volume (ERV)

The expiratory reserve volume is the maximum amount that can be exhaled forcibly after a normal tidal volume exhalation (about 1200 ml).

Residual volume (RV)

The residual volume is the amount of air remaining in the lungs after a forced expiration (about 1200 ml).

Respiratory capacities

Respiratory capacities are measured for diagnostic purposes. They consist of two or more respiratory lung volumes.

Total lung capacity (TLC)

The total lung capacity is the amount of air in the lungs at the end of a maximum inspiration.

$$TLC = TV + IRV + ERV + RV \ (6000 \ ml)$$

Vital capacity (VC)

The vital capacity is the maximum amount of air that can be expired after a maximum inspiration.

$$VC = TV + IRV + ERV \ (4800 \ ml)$$

Inspiratory capacity (IC)

The inspiratory capacity is the maximum amount of air that can be inspired after a normal expiration.

$$IC = TV + IRV \ (3600 \ ml)$$

Functional residual capacity (FRC)

The functional residual capacity is the amount of air remaining in the lungs after a normal tidal volume expiration.

$$FRC = ERC + RV \ (2400 \ ml)$$

Dead space

A percentage of the inspired air (about 120 ml) fills the respiratory passageways and does not contribute to gaseous exchange. This is termed the anatomical dead space.

Gaseous exchange

Oxygen in the inspired air enters while carbon dioxide leaves the blood in the lungs in the process of ventilation. These gases move in opposite directions in the alveoli by the mechanism of diffusion (Marieb 2001). Adjacent to the alveoli is a dense vascular network. Oxygen moves into the alveolar capillaries and carbon dioxide moves out (Fig. 25.15). This process is called gaseous exchange. Factors influencing this process include the partial pressure gradients, the width of the respiratory membrane and the surface area available.

The gaseous composition of the atmosphere and alveoli is demonstrated in Table 25.2. The atmosphere consists almost entirely of oxygen and nitrogen; the alveoli contain more carbon dioxide and water vapour and considerably less oxygen. These different figures reflect the following processes:

- Gaseous exchange in the lungs
- Humidification of air by the respiratory passageways
- The mixing of alveolar gas that occurs with each breath.

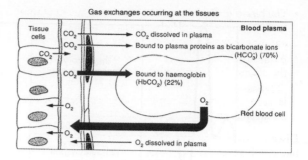

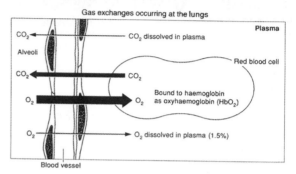

Figure 25.15 Transport and exchange of carbon dioxide and oxygen.

Table 25.2 Composition of gas in the atmosphere and alveoli

	Atmosphere inspired (%)	Alveoli (%)
Oxygen	20.9	13.7
Carbon dioxide	0.04	5.2
Nitrogen	78.6	74.9
Water	0.46	6.2

Respiratory transportation

Oxygen is carried in the blood in two ways, bound to the haemoglobin within the red blood cells and dissolved in plasma. Haemoglobin carries 98.5% of the oxygen from the lungs and the tissues. The amount of oxygen bound to haemoglobin depends on several factors:

- The partial pressure of oxygen (PaO_2) and the partial pressure of carbon dioxide ($PaCO_2$) in the blood. The gradient of partial pressure influences the rates of diffusion, the oxygen gradient being steeper than that of carbon dioxide. Carbon dioxide is transported from the tissue primarily as bicarbonate ions in the plasma (70%), whereas only small amounts are transported by haemoglobin in the red blood cells (22%).

- The blood pH influences the affinity of haemoglobin for oxygen: as the pH decreases, as in acidosis, the amount of oxygen unloaded in the tissues increases.
- As body temperature rises above normal levels, the affinity of haemoglobin for oxygen declines, and therefore oxygen unloading is enhanced. This effect is seen in localized temperature changes such as inflammation.

Diseases that reduce the oxygen-carrying ability of the blood, whatever the cause, are termed anaemia. This is characterized by oxygen blood levels that are inadequate to support normal metabolism (Marieb 2001). Common causes of anaemia include:

- Insufficient number of red cells, including destruction of red cells, haemorrhage and bone marrow failure
- Decreases in haemoglobin content, including iron deficiency anaemia and pernicious anaemia
- Abnormal haemoglobin, including thalassaemia and sickle cell anaemia (Marieb 2001).

Internal respiration

Internal respiration is the exchange of gases that occurs within the tissues between the capillaries and the cells. Carbon dioxide enters the blood and oxygen moves into the cells (Fig. 25.15).

Hypoxia is the result of an inadequate amount of oxygen delivered to body tissues. The blue coloration of tissues and mucosal membranes is termed cyanosis.

Lung defence mechanisms

The upper airway is designed to warm, humidify and filter inspired air. The nasal passages absorb noxious gases and trap inhaled particles. Smaller particles are removed by the cough reflex.

Observation of respiration

Respirations in an individual should be observed for rate, depth and pattern of breathing.

Rate

Rate and depth determine the type of respiration. The normal rate at rest is approximately 14–18 breaths per minute in adults and is faster in infants and children (Table 25.3). The ratio of pulse rate to respiration rate is approximately 5:1.

Changes in the rate of ventilation may be defined as follows. *Tachypnoea* is an increased respiratory rate, seen in fever, for example, as the body tries to rid itself of excess heat. Respirations increase by about 7 breaths per

Table 25.3 Respiratory rates (Timby 1989)

Age	Average range/minute
Newborn	30–80
Early childhood	20–40
Late childhood	15–25
Adulthood – male	14–18
Adulthood – female	16–20

minute for every 1°C rise in temperature above normal. They also increase with pneumonia, other obstructive airway diseases, respiratory insufficiency and lesions in the pons of the brainstem.

Bradypnoea is a decreased but regular respiratory rate, such as that caused by the depression of the respiratory centre in the medulla by opiate narcotics, or by a brain tumour.

Depth

The depth of respiration is the volume of air moving in and out with each respiration. This tidal volume is normally about 500 ml in an adult and should be constant with each breath. A spirometer is used to measure the precise amount (see Respiratory capacities). Normal, relaxed breathing is effortless, automatic, regular and almost silent.

Dyspnoea is undue breathlessness and an awareness of discomfort with breathing. There are several types of dyspnoea:

- Exertional dyspnoea is shortness of breath on exercise and is seen with heart failure.
- Orthopnoea is a shortness of breath on lying down which is relieved by the patient sitting upright. This is often caused by left ventricular failure of the heart.
- Paroxysmal nocturnal dyspnoea is a sudden breathlessness that occurs at night when the patient is lying down and is often caused by pulmonary oedema and left ventricular failure.

Pattern

Changes in the pattern of respiration are often found in disorders of the respiratory control centre. Examples of changes in respiratory pattern follow.

Hyperventilation is an increase in both the rate and depth of respiration. This follows extreme exertion, fear and anxiety, fever, hepatic coma, midbrain lesions of the brainstem, and acid–base imbalance such as diabetic ketoacidosis (Kussmaul's respiration) or salicylate overdose (in both of these situations the body compensates for the metabolic acidosis by increased respiration), as well as an alteration in blood gas concentration (either increased carbon dioxide or decreased oxygen). The breathing pattern is normally regular and consists of inspiration, pause, longer expiration and another pause. However, this may be altered by some defects and diseases. In adults, more than 20 breaths per minute is considered moderate, more than 30 is severe.

Apnoeustic respiration is a pattern of prolonged, gasping inspiration, followed by extremely short, inefficient expiration, seen in lesions of the pons in the mid-brain.

Cheyne–Stokes respiration is periodic breathing, characterized by a gradual increase in depth of respiration followed by a decrease in respiration, resulting in apnoea.

Biot's respiration is an interrupted breathing pattern, like Cheyne–Stokes respiration, except that each breath is of the same depth. It may be seen with spinal meningitis or other central nervous system conditions.

Conditions where a patient's respirations may need careful monitoring are described below.

- Patients with conditions that affect respiration, such as those described in the text, require monitoring of respiration to evaluate their condition and the effectiveness of medication.
- Postoperative and critically ill patients require monitoring of respiration. The patient's respiration should be recorded preoperatively in order to make significant comparisons. The breathing is observed to assess for the return to normal respiratory function.
- Patients receiving oxygen inhalation therapy or receiving artificial respiration require monitoring of breathing to assess respiratory function.

Oxygen saturation

Oxygen is transported to the body's tissues in the blood. The red blood cells contain haemoglobin molecules that bind with oxygen in the lungs and transport it to the tissues where it is released. When oxygen combines with haemoglobin it forms oxyhaemoglobin. Each haemoglobin molecule has the potential to bind with four oxygen molecules. When all the binding sites for oxygen are used then the haemoglobin is saturated with oxygen.

The oxygen saturation reading is a measure of the percentage of haemoglobin molecules saturated with oxygen. The normal arterial oxygen saturation is approximately 95–98% (Sims 1996).

Pulse oximetry

Pulse oximetry works on the principle that blood saturated with oxygen is a different colour from blood

Table 25.4 Respiratory assessment procedure

Observation	Rationale
Rate and regularity of respiration	Very slow or rapid breathing may be a sign of oxygenation or underlying change, for example due to sepsis
Observe for signs of respiratory effort: • Nasal flaring • Pursed lips • Use of accessory muscles such as the shoulder or neck muscles (sternomastoid or scalene)	These signs may show that the patient is making extra effort in breathing and may indicate changes in the respiratory status before other observations (e.g. oxygen saturation or rate)
Listen for cough or wheezing	Dry cough may be caused by viral infection, bronchial carcinoma or congestive cardiac failure Moist cough may be due to chronic bronchitis or asthma or bacterial infection Wheezing is caused by bronchospasm or bronchial obstruction
Assess respiratory history including smoking history, history of asthma, exertional shortness of breath or other respiratory symptoms	These factors will alert the nurse to potential patient problems or concurrent conditions
Assess sputum	White or opalescent sputum may be produced by asthmatics or patients with chronic bronchitis, but does not necessarily indicate infection Thick viscous sputum that is coloured indicates infection and should be sent for microbiology culture and sensitivity Frothy sputum indicates pulmonary oedema Haemoptysis can occur with infection, pulmonary embolism, malignant disease or trauma

depleted of oxygen. The probe for a pulse oximeter contains a red light source and a detector. These shine through the tissues of the body and work together to measure the colour difference between oxygenated and unoxygenated blood. The machine detects the pulse from an arterial blood source and is able to calculate the percentage of oxygen saturation by combining the detected colour changes of the blood combined with the detected pulse of the artery. Because of the way the pulse oximeter works, it is susceptible to error if it is not able to accurately measure the transmission of light through the tissues or detect the pulse of the artery.

Indications for pulse oximetry

- Monitoring effectiveness of oxygen therapy
- Sedation or anaesthesia
- Transport of patients who are unwell and require oxygenation assessment
- Haemodynamic instability (e.g. cardiac failure or MI) (Keenan 1995)
- Respiratory illness (e.g. asthma, chronic obstructive pulmonary disease (COPD)) (Place 2000)

- Monitoring during administration of respiratory depressant drugs, e.g. opiate epidural or patient-controlled analgesia.

Possible sources of error

Light transmission:
- Barriers or obstruction, e.g. nail varnish, dirt, foreign objects, bright or fluorescent room lighting, intravenous dyes used in imaging (Keenan 1995).

Pulse detection:
- Movement, rigors or shivering, poor circulation, atrial fibrillation (Woodrow 1999), vasoconstriction, arterial constriction or shock (Keenan 1995).

Limitations of pulse oximetry and oxygen saturation

Oxygen saturation is only one factor in oxygenation of the tissues. In anaemia it is possible to have high oxygen saturation readings, but inadequate amounts of oxygen reaching the tissues. Carbon monoxide (CO) exposure will lead to uptake of CO molecules in preference to O_2. As carboxyhaemoglobin is also bright red it can lead to significant overestimation of oxygen saturation when using pulse oximeters (Woodrow 1999).

Procedure guidelines: **Pulse oximetry**

Equipment

1 Pulse oximeter.

2 Alcohol swab.

Procedure

Action	Rationale
1 Explain to the patient that an oxygen saturation reading is needed and obtain consent to continue.	To ensure the patient understands the procedure and is able to provide valid consent.
2 Ensure that the patient is comfortable and warm enough, especially if continuous monitoring is needed.	To maintain patient comfort. Shivering will interfere with the pulse oximeter reading.
3 Wash your hands.	To minimize the risk of cross-infection.
4 Make sure the probe and equipment are clean and in good working order.	To minimize the risk of cross-infection and ensure that the equipment is suitable for use.
5 Select a suitable area for the probe (usually finger) and place the probe as directed by the manufacturer's instructions (see Fig. 25.16).	Proper function of the pulse oximeter will only be possible if the probe is placed as intended by the manufacturer.
6 Switch the pulse oximeter machine on.	
7 Make sure that the probe sensor is detecting the pulse and that it corresponds to the patient's pulse. This will usually be indicated by a beep in time with each detected pulse or a graphical indication of the pulse on a display panel.	To ensure that the probe is detecting the pulse.
8 Take the reading of the oxygenation saturation and document this in the patient's notes. Make a note of any oxygen administration.	To provide a written record of the patient's condition and therapy.
9 Ensure that any abnormal reading or observation is reported to the medical team.	To ensure that any patient problems are communicated.

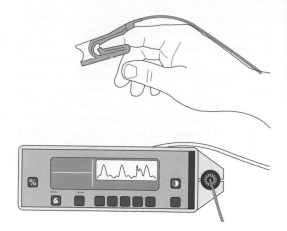

Figure 25.16 Pulse oximeter and finger probe.

Procedure guidelines: **Pulse oximetry** *(cont'd)*

Action	Rationale
10 If the reading is intermittent, remove the probe and ensure the patient is comfortable.	
11 If the oxygen saturation monitoring is continuous check the probe placement from time to time and reposition as necessary.	Leaving the probe on one digit for protracted periods of time may cause discomfort or lead to pressure damage.
12 Once oxygen saturation monitoring is completed, clean equipment and return to storage as appropriate.	Cleaning of the equipment, including the probe, will minimize the risk of cross-infection. Proper storage, including initiating battery recharging, will ensure that the equipment is ready for use when next required.

Peak flow

Definition

Peak expiratory flow rate (PEFR or peak flow) is a measurement of the highest rate at which air can be expelled from the lungs through an open mouth.

Reference material

Peak flow can be used as an indication of any restriction in the airway and is a useful assessment for asthma patients and others with respiratory symptoms. PEFR is one aspect of lung function assessment and is usually used in conjunction with assessment of the lung volume and other factors to give a more complete indication of lung function.

Timing of peak flow readings

For patients with asthma, the British Thoracic Society recommends measuring peak flows morning and evening before inhaled medication. In addition, a peak flow measurement should be taken 30 minutes after morning medications or nebulizers. Constriction of the airways will decrease the amount of air that can pass through and this will result in a lowered peak flow. Bronchodilators act to open the airways and allow a faster flow of air, resulting in an increase in peak flow (BTS 1997b).

Factors affecting peak flow

A patient's peak flow will vary due to age, sex and ethnic origin. Respiratory problems such as asthma, COPD or emphysema will also result in a reduction in peak flow. Assessment of any impairment should be against a recognized chart of normal values (see Fig. 25.17) or against the patient's best recorded measurements (BTS 1997b). In general, the result for a normal adult male would be 500–650 l/min and 400–500 l/min for a normal female.

In patients with asthma the peak flow reading will usually vary over time and in response to medication. Any significant deterioration in peak flow may signal the onset of acute severe asthma.

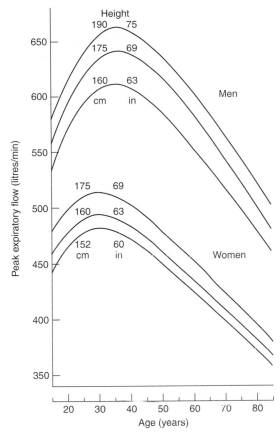

Figure 25.17 Chart of normal adult PF values. (*Source*: Gregg, I. & Nunn, A.J. (1989) *BMJ*, **298**, 1068–70, Reproduced with permission from BMJ.)

In the event of any life-threatening feature or pulse oximetry of less than 92%, arterial blood gases should be measured.

Blood gas markers for a severe life-threatening asthma attack:

- Normal or high $PaCO_2$ (5–6 kPa, 36–45 mmHg)
- Severe hypoxia, PaO_2 < (less than) 8 kPa/60 mmHg regardless of oxygen therapy
- Low pH or high H^+.

Box 25.1 Recognition and assessment of asthma

Features of acute severe asthma
- Peak flow ≤ (less than or equal to) 50% of the predicted value (Fig. 25.17) or best readings
- Unable to finish sentence in one breath
- Respirations ≥ (greater than or equal to) 25 breaths per minute
- Pulse over 110 beats per minute

Life-threatening features
- Peak flow < (less than) 33% of predicted or best readings
- Cyanosis, silent chest or feeble respiratory effort
- Bradycardia or hypotension
- Confusion, exhaustion or coma

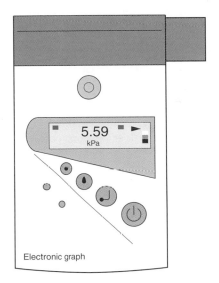

Electronic graph

Figure 25.18 Electronic peak flow meter.

Severe and life-threatening asthma attacks can occur without patient distress. Not all features above may be evident, but if one or more symptoms are noted and there is a deterioration, the medical team should be contacted urgently (BTS 1997b).

Procedure guidelines: **Peak flow reading using manual peak flow meter**

Equipment

1 Peak flow meter.

2 Observation chart.

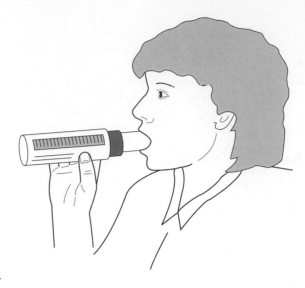

Figure 25.19 Manual peak flow meter in use.

Procedure guidelines: **Peak flow reading using manual peak flow meter** *(cont'd)*

Procedure

Action	Rationale
1 Explain the procedure to the patient and obtain consent.	To ensure the patient understands the procedure and gives valid consent.
2 Establish patient's current and best peak flow readings or predicted peak flow.	To allow for comparison and assessment of the patient's reading.
3 Wash and dry hands.	To minimize cross-infection.
4 Collect and assemble equipment. Attach mouthpiece to meter if required (see specific documentation).	
5 Move the indicator to the zero mark prior to reading.	To ensure the reading is accurate.
6 Place the patient in their usual position for readings.	To ensure consistency of readings, the British Thoracic Society recommends sitting.
7 Ask the patient to take a deep breath in and place their lips around the mouthpiece.	To ensure accuracy of reading.
8 Ask the patient to breathe out through the peak flow meter as hard as possible.	To ensure accuracy of reading.
9 Take a note of the reading and ask the patient to repeat the reading twice more.	
10 Return the patient to a comfortable position.	
11 Discard the used mouthpiece (if appropriate), wash your hands and store the peak flow meter ready for next use.	To minimize cross-infection.
12 Record the highest peak flow reading in the patient record, noting time of reading and any nebulized therapy. Inform medical staff of any abnormality in the reading.	To provide an accurate record of assessment.

Temperature

Definition

Body temperature represents the balance between heat gain and heat loss.

Indications

Monitoring the patient's temperature is an important aspect of nursing assessment. Temperature needs to be measured accurately and monitored effectively to enable temperature changes to be detected quickly and any necessary intervention commenced (Watson 1998). Measurement of body temperature is carried out for two reasons:

- To determine the patient's temperature on admission as a baseline for comparison with future measurements.
- To monitor fluctuations in temperature.

Reference material

All tissues produce heat as a result of cell metabolism, and this is increased by exercise and activity (Marieb 2001). Body temperature is usually maintained between 36 and 37.5°C regardless of the environmental temperature (Marini & Wheeler 1997). Humans are described as homoiothermic, that is, having a core temperature that remains constant in spite of environmental changes. The body core generally has the highest temperature while the skin is the coolest (Fig. 25.20). Core temperature reflects the heat of arterial blood and represents the balance between the heat generated by body tissues in metabolic activity and that lost through various mechanisms.

A relatively constant temperature is maintained by homeostasis, which is a constant process of heat gain and heat loss. The body requires stability of its temperature to produce an optimum environment for biochemical and enzymic reactions to maintain cellular function. A body temperature above or below this normal range affects total body function (Marieb 2001). A temperature above 41°C can cause convulsions and a temperature of 43°C renders life unsustainable.

The hypothalamus within the brain acts as the body's thermostat, controlling the body's temperature by various physiological mechanisms (Fig. 25.21). Heat is gained through metabolic activity of the body, especially of the muscles and liver. Heat loss is achieved through the skin by the processes of radiation, convection, conduction and evaporation.

Various factors cause fluctuations of temperature:

- The body's circadian rhythms cause daily fluctuations. The body temperature is higher in the evening than in the morning (Brown 1990). Minor & Waterhouse (1981) in a research study recorded a difference of 0.5–1.5°C between morning and evening measurements.
- Ovulation can elevate the body's temperature as it influences the basal metabolic rate (Tortora & Grabowski 2003).
- Exercise and eating cause an elevation in temperature (Marieb 2001).
- Extremes of age affect a person's response to environmental change. The young or elderly are unable to

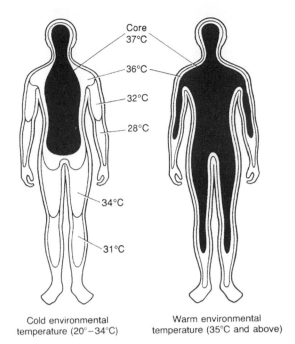

Figure 25.20 Body core and skin temperatures.

maintain an efficient equilibrium. Thermoregulation is inadequate in the newborn and especially in low-birth-weight babies. In older people there is an increased sensitivity to cold and the body temperature is generally lower (Nakamura *et al.* 1997).

Hypothermia is where body temperature drops and mechanisms to increase heat production are ineffective. This causes a decline in the metabolic rate and a resulting decrease in all bodily functions. Clinical hypothermia is when the core temperature falls below 35°C; if the temperature falls below 35°C the patient will start to shiver severely (Edwards 1997). However, it frequently escapes detection due to symptoms being non-specific and an oral thermometer's failure to record in the appropriate range (Marini & Wheeler 1997). Hypothermia is often multifactorial in origin and can arise as a result of:

- Environmental exposure
- Medications that can either alter the perception of cold, increase heat loss through vasodilatation or inhibit heat generation, e.g. alcohol, paracetamol
- Metabolic conditions, e.g. hypoglycaemia and adrenal insufficiency
- The exposure of the body and internal organs during surgery and the use of drugs which dampen the vasoconstrictor response (Marini & Wheeler 1997).

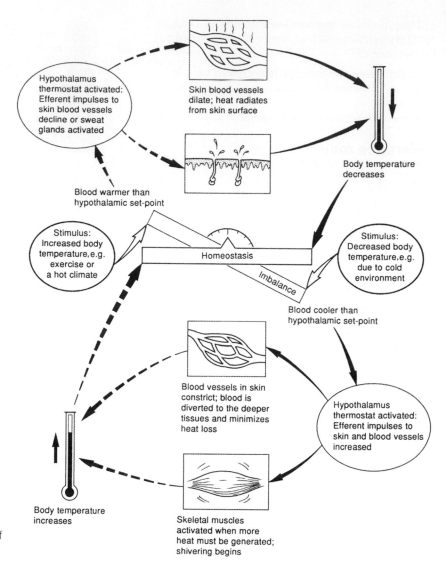

Figure 25.21 Mechanisms of body temperature regulation.

Pyrexia is defined as a significant rise in body temperature. Sudden temperature elevations usually indicate infection. However, other life-threatening non-infectious causes of fever are often overlooked (see Table 25.5).

Fever caused by pyrexia is the result of the internal thermostat resetting to higher levels. This resetting of the thermostat is the result of the action of pyrogens that are chemical substances now known to be cytokines. Cytokines are chemical mediators which are involved in cellular immunity. They enhance the immune response and are released from white blood cells, injured tissues and macrophages. This causes the hypothalamus to release prostaglandins which in turn

Table 25.5 Non-infectious causes of hyperthermia

Alcohol withdrawal	Malignant hyperthermia
Anticholinergic drugs	Neuroleptic malignant
Allergic drug or transfusion	syndrome
reaction	Pheochromocytoma
Autonomic insufficiency	Salicylate intoxication
Crystalline arthritis (gout)	Status epilepticus
Drug allergy	Stroke or CNS damage
Heat stroke	Vasculitis
Hyperthyroidism	Agonist drugs
Malignancy	

Table 25.6 Grades of pyrexia

Low-grade pyrexia	Normal to 38°C	Indicative of an inflammatory response due to a mild infection, allergy, disturbance of body tissue by trauma, surgery, malignancy or thrombosis
Moderate to high-grade pyrexia	38–40°C	May be caused by wound, respiratory or urinary tract infections
Hyperpyrexia	40°C and above	May arise because of bacteraemia, damage to the hypothalamus or high environmental temperatures

reset the hypothalamic thermostat. The body then promotes heat-producing mechanisms such as vasoconstriction. Heat loss is reduced, the skin becomes cool and the person 'shivers'. This is often called a rigor (Marieb 2001). A rigor is marked by shivering and the patient complains of feeling cold. The temperature quickly rises as a result of the normal physiological response to cold. This results in the following physiological changes.

- Thermoreceptors in the skin are stimulated, resulting in vasoconstriction. This decreases heat loss through conduction and convection.
- Sweat gland activity is reduced to minimize evaporation.
- Shivering occurs, muscles contract and relax out of sequence with each other, thus generating heat.
- The body increases catecholamine and thyroxine levels, elevating the metabolic rate in an attempt to increase temperature (Damanhouri & Tayeb 1992).

All of these changes contribute to a rise in metabolism with an increase in carbon dioxide excretion and the need for oxygen. This leads to an increased respiratory rate. When the body temperature reaches its new 'setpoint' the patient no longer complains of feeling cold, shivering ceases and sweating commences.

There are several grades of pyrexia, and these are described in Table 25.6.

There are different methods for lowering body temperature. As paracetemol can mask the function of the hypothalamus, it must be used with caution as it can slow down the automatic internal cooling functions of the body (Adam & Osborrne 1997). Antipyretic drugs can cause a marked fall in temperature (Connell 1997). It is thought that these drugs inhibit the inflammatory action of prostaglandins, affecting the hypothalamus by temporarily resetting the thermostat to normal levels. However, these drugs must be used with caution in patients with established liver disease or a history of gastric bleeding as they can cause gastric irritation and put an increased strain on a diseased liver to break down the drug.

Fanning is of benefit for moderate to high pyrexias. Fanning and tepid sponging are not recommended while the patient's temperature is still rising as this will only make the patient feel colder, cause distress (Sharber 1997) and cause the peripheral thermoreceptors to detect a decrease in temperature that leads the hypothalamus to initiate heat-gaining activities such as shivering and peripheral vasoconstriction (Krikler 1990).

Recordings of body temperature are an index of biological function and are a valuable indicator of a patient's health.

Temperature recording sites

Traditionally, the mouth, axillae or rectum have been the preferred sites for obtaining temperature readings. This is due to their accessibility. With the development of new technology the use of the tympanic membrane is increasingly becoming popular, as it is less invasive and provides rapid results (Burke 1996). The increasing use of tympanic membrane thermometers has also been influenced by the Health and Safety Executive directive for health care professionals to replace mercury devices where possible (Smith 2000).

Oral

To most accurately measure the temperature orally, the thermometer is placed in the posterior sublingual pocket of tissue at the base of the tongue (Torrance & Semple 1998). This area is in close proximity to the thermoreceptors which respond rapidly to changes in the core temperature, hence changes in core temperatures are reflected quickly here (Marini & Wheeler 1997).

Oral temperatures are affected by the temperatures of ingested foods and fluids and by the muscular activity of chewing. A respiratory rate that exceeds 18 breaths per minute, together with a patient who smokes, will also reduce the core temperature values (Marieb 2001).

It is important that the thermometer is placed in the sublingual pocket and not in the area under the front of the tongue as there may be a temperature difference of up to 1.7°C between these areas. This temperature difference is due to the sublingual pockets being more protected from the air currents which cool the frontal areas (Neff *et al.* 1989). Oxygen therapy has been shown not to affect the oral temperature reading (Hasler & Cohen 1982; Lim-Levy 1982).

Rectal

The rectal temperature is often higher than the oral temperature because this site is more sheltered from the external environment. Rectal thermometry has been demonstrated in clinical trials to be more accurate than oral thermometry. The researchers (Jensen *et al.* 1994) conclude that rectal thermometry is the more accurate route for daily measurements, but is more invasive, often unacceptable for the patient and time consuming. Although this method is more precise, fever can still be detected by oral screening. If greater accuracy is required the rectal method offers greater precision. The presence of soft stool may separate the thermometer from the bowel wall and give a false reading, especially if the central temperature is changing rapidly. In infants this method is not recommended as it carries a risk of rectal ulceration or perforation.

A rectal thermometer should be inserted at least 4 cm in an adult to obtain the most accurate reading.

Axillary

The axilla is considered less desirable than the other sites because of the difficulty to achieve accurate and reliable readings as it is not close to major vessels, and skin surface temperatures vary more with changes in temperature of the environment (Woollens 1996). It is usually only used for patients who are unsuitable for, or who cannot tolerate, oral thermometers, e.g. after general anaesthetic, or patients with mouth injuries (Edwards 1997).

To take an axillary temperature reading the thermometer should be placed in the centre of the armpit, with the patient's arm firmly against the side of the chest. It is important that the same arm is used for each measurement as there is often a variation in temperature between left and right (Heindenreich & Giuffe 1990).

Whichever route is used for temperature measurement, it is important that this is then used consistently, as switching between sites can produce a record that is misleading or difficult to interpret.

Time for recording temperatures

The average person experiences circadian rhythms which make their highest body temperature occur in the late afternoon or early evening, i.e. between 4 PM and 8 PM. The most sensitive time for detecting pyrexias appears to be between 7 PM and 8 PM (Angerami 1980). Samples *et al.* (1985) found the highest temperature between 5 PM and 7 PM. These studies suggest the most useful time to measure and detect an abnormal temperature would be approximately 6 PM. This should be considered when interpreting variations in 4- or 6-hourly observations, and when taking once-daily temperatures.

Types of thermometer

A variety of thermometers are now available, from clinical glass thermometers with oral or rectal bulbs to the electronic sensor thermometer to the tympanic thermometer. Mercury thermometers have been used extensively in the past, but it has been shown they are unable to detect temperatures lower than 34.5°C (94°F) or higher than 40.5°C (105°F). They are also slow to respond to temperature changes (Marini & Wheeler 1997). The use of electronic devices is therefore preferable where there are extremes of temperature or where there are temperature fluctuations. Other types of thermometer include those listed by Docherty (2000):

- Single-use plastic-coated strips with heat-sensitive recorders (dots) which change colour to indicate the temperature (record from 35.5°C to 40.4°C)
- Digital analogue probe thermometers with plastic disposable sheets (record from 32°C to 42°C)
- Invasive thermometers attached to a pulmonary artery catheter (record from 0°C to 50°C) (O'Toole 1997; Braun *et al.* 1998).

Tympanic membrane thermometer

The tympanic thermometer uses infra-red light to detect thermal radiation (Woodrow 2000). Temperature is measured by inserting the probe into the auditory canal; the probe then records the amount of infra-red energy given off by the tympanic membrane. The tympanic route has become popular because it is hygienic, non-invasive, simple to use, comfortable for the patient and quick to register (Bartlett 1996). However, inconsistent study results have highlighted problems with the accuracy and reliability of these devices (Fawcett 2001). A common problem with using tympanic thermometers is poor technique (Gilbert *et al.* 2002), leading to inaccurate temperature measurements. The placement of the probe to fit snugly within the ear canal (see Fig. 25.22) is crucial as differences between the opening of the ear canal and the tympanic membrane can be as much as 2.8°C (Hudek *et al.* 1998). Jevon & Jevon (2001) highlight other causes of false readings which include dirty or cracked probe lens, incorrect installation of the probe cover and short time intervals between measurements (less than 2–3 minutes).

Conditions where a patient's temperature requires careful monitoring

1 Patients with conditions that affect basal metabolic rate, such as disorders of the thyroid gland, require

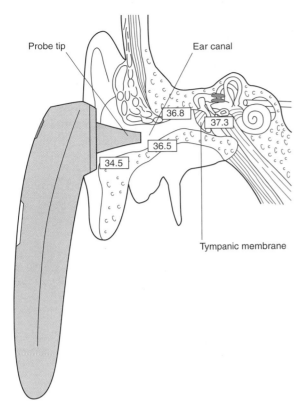

Probe tip

Ear canal

36.8

37.3

36.5

34.5

Tympanic membrane

Figure 25.22 Tympanic membrane thermometer.

monitoring of body temperature. Hypothyroidism is a condition where an inadequate secretion of hormones from the thyroid gland results in a slowing of physical and metabolic activity; thus the individual

has a decrease in body temperature. Hyperthyroidism is excessive activity of the thyroid gland; a hypermetabolic condition results, with an increase in all metabolic processes. The patient complains of a low heat tolerance. Thyrotoxic crisis is a sudden increase in thyroid hormones and can cause a hyperpyrexia (Mize *et al.* 1993).

2 Postoperative and critically ill patients require monitoring of temperature. The patient's temperature should be observed preoperatively in order to make any significant comparisons. In the postoperative period the nurse should observe the patient for hyperthermia or hypothermia as a reaction to the surgical procedures (Mize *et al.* 1993).

3 Patients with a susceptibility to infection, for example those with a low white blood cell count (less than 1000 cells/mm^3), or those undergoing radiotherapy, chemotherapy or steroid treatment, will require a more frequent observation of temperature. The fluctuation in temperature is influenced by the body's response to pyrogens. Immunocompromised patients are less able to respond to infection. Bacteraemia means a bacterial invasion of the bloodstream. Septic shock is a circulatory collapse as a result of severe infection. Pyrexia may be absent in those who are immunosuppressed or in the elderly.

4 Patients with a systemic or local infection require monitoring of temperature to assess development or regression of infection.

5 Pyrexia can occur when patients are receiving a blood transfusion but severe transfusion reactions usually occur within the first 15 minutes of starting (BSCH 1999).

Procedure guidelines: **Temperature**

Equipment

1 Tympanic membrane thermometer.

2 Disposable probe covers.

Procedure

Action	Rationale
1 Explain and discuss procedure with the patient.	To ensure that the patient understands the procedure and gives his/her valid consent.
2 Wash your hands.	To minimize the risks of cross-infection and contamination.
3 Document to ensure the same ear is used for consecutive readings.	Anatomical differences between the two ears can result in a difference of up to 1°C.
4 Remove thermometer from the base unit and ensure the lens is clean and not cracked. Use a dry wipe to clean if required.	Alcohol-based wipes should not be used as this can lead to a false low temperature measurement.

*Procedure guidelines: **Temperature** (cont'd)*

Action	Rationale
5 Place disposable probe cover on the probe tip, ensuring the manufacturer's instructions are followed.	The probe cover protects the tip of the probe and is necessary for the functioning of the instrument.
6 Gently place the probe tip in the ear canal to seal the opening, ensuring a snug fit.	To prevent air at the opening of the ear from entering it, causing a false low temperature measurement.
7 Press and release SCAN button.	To commence the instrument scanning.
8 Remove probe tip from the ear as soon as the thermometer display reads DONE, usually indicated by bleeps.	Measurement usually complete within 2 seconds.
9 Read the temperature display.	Document in the patient's records.
10 Press RELEASE/EJECT button to discard probe cover.	Probe covers are for single use only.
11 Replace thermometer in base unit.	

Urinalysis

Definition

Urinalysis is the testing of the physical characteristics and composition of freshly voided urine.

Indications

The composition of urine can change dramatically as a result of disease processes. It may contain red blood cells, glucose, proteins, white blood cells or bile (Marieb 2001). The presence of such abnormalities in urine is an important warning sign of illness and may be helpful in clinical assessment in the following ways:

- To determine the individual's urine status on admission as a baseline for comparisons with future assessments
- To monitor changes in urinary constituents as a response to medication
- To be used as a screening test to gather information about physical status.

Reference material

Urine is formed in the kidneys, which process approximately 180 litres of blood-derived fluid a day. Approximately 1.5% of this total actually leaves the body. Urine formation and the simultaneous adjustment of blood composition involves three processes (Marieb 2001) (Fig. 25.23):

- Glomerular filtration
- Tubular reabsorption
- Tubular secretion.

Glomerular filtration occurs in the glomeruli of the kidney, which act as non-selective filters. Filtration occurs as

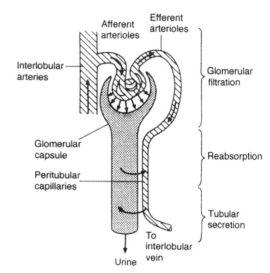

Figure 25.23 A nephron depicted diagrammatically to show the three major mechanisms by which urine is produced.

a result of increased glomerular blood pressure caused by the difference in diameter between afferent and efferent arterioles. The effect is a simple mechanical filter that permits substances smaller than plasma proteins to pass from the glomeruli to the glomerular capsule (Marieb 2001).

Tubular reabsorption then occurs, removing necessary substances from the filtrate and returning them to the peritubular capillaries. Tubular reabsorption is an active process that requires protein carriers and energy. Substances reabsorbed include nutrients and most ions. It is also a passive process, however, driven by electrochemical gradients. Substances reabsorbed in this way include sodium ions and water. Creatinine and the metabolites of drugs are not reabsorbed either because of their size, insolubility or a lack of carriers. Most of the nutrients, 80% of the water and sodium ions, and the majority of actively transported ions are reabsorbed in the proximal convoluted tubules (Marieb 2001).

Reabsorption is controlled by hormones. Aldosterone increases reabsorption of sodium (and hence also water), and antidiuretic hormone (ADH) enhances reabsorption of water in the collecting tubules (Marieb 2001).

Tubular secretion is both an active and a passive process in which the tubules excrete drugs, urea, excess ions and other substances into the filtrate. It plays an important part in maintaining the acid–base balance of blood (Marieb 2001).

Regulation of urine concentration and volume occurs in the loop of Henle, where the osmolarity of the filtrate is controlled. As the filtrate flows through the tubules the permeability of the walls controls how dilute or concentrated the resulting urine will be. In the absence of ADH dilute urine is formed because the filtrate is not reabsorbed as it passes through the kidneys. As levels of ADH increase, the collecting tubules become more permeable and water moves out of the filtrate back into the blood. Consequently, smaller amounts of more concentrated urine are produced (Marieb 2001).

Characteristics of urine

Urine is typically clear, pale to deep yellow in colour and slightly acidic (pH 6), though pH can change as a result of metabolic processes or diet. Vomiting and bacterial infection of the urinary tract can cause urine to become alkaline. Urinary specific gravity ranges from 1.001 to 1.035, according to how concentrated the urine is (Fillingham & Douglas 1997; Marieb 2001).

The colour of urine is due to a pigment called urochrome which is derived from the body's destruction of haemoglobin. The more concentrated urine is, the deeper yellow it becomes. Changes in colour may reflect diet (e.g. beetroot or rhubarb), or may be due to blood or bile in the urine. If fresh urine is turbid (cloudy), the cause may be an infection of the urinary tract. The urinary tract is the most common site of bacterial infection. There are many predisposing factors (Fig. 25.24), the most common of which is instrumentation, that is, cystoscopy and urinary catheterization (Bayer 1997).

Bacteriuria is defined as the presence of bacteria in the urine. Because urine specimens can become contaminated with periurethral flora during collection, infection is distinguished by counting the number of bacteria. Significant bacteriuria is defined as a presence of more than 10^5 organisms per ml of urine in the presence of

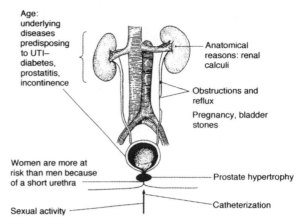

Figure 25.24 Urinary tract infections (UTI): predisposing factors.

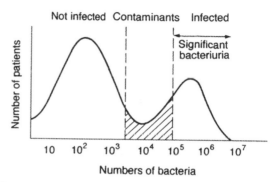

Figure 25.25 Significant bacteriuria. Specimens of urine are rarely sterile. A cut-off point is identified to distinguish true infection (significant bacteriuria) from effects of contamination from surrounding tissues.

clinical symptoms (Fig. 25.25). Covert bacteriuria is the presence of more than 10^5 organisms per ml of urine without clinical symptoms.

Fresh urine smells slightly aromatic. This can change as a result of disease processes such as diabetes mellitus, when acetone is present in the urine, giving it a fruity smell. The composition of urine can change dramatically as a result of disease, and abnormal substances may be present (see Table 25.7). Urinalysis can identify many of these substances, and should be part of every physical assessment (Cook 1996; Torrance & Elley 1998).

Renal clearance is the rate at which the kidneys clear a particular chemical from the plasma. Studies of renal clearance provide information about renal function or the course of renal disease. There is no single test of renal function.

Table 25.7 Changes to composition of urine and their possible causes

Abnormal constituent	Name of condition	Possible causes
Glucose	Glycosuria	Diabetes mellitus
Proteins	Proteinuria	May be seen in pregnancy and high-protein diets; heart failure; severe hypertension; infection; asymptomatic renal disease
Ketone bodies	Ketonuria	Starvation; untreated diabetes mellitus
Haemoglobin	Haemoglobinuria	Transfusion reaction; haemolytic anaemia; severe burns
Bile pigments	Bilirubinuria	Liver disease or obstruction of bile ducts
Erythrocytes	Haematuria	Bleeding in urinary tract: kidney stones, infection or trauma, or other urinary organs
Leucocytes	Pyuria	Urinary tract infection

Dipstick (reagent) tests

Strips that have been impregnated with chemicals are dipped quickly in urine and read as a means of testing urine. When dipped in urine, the chemicals react with abnormal substances and change colour. Although dipstick reagents have been primarily used as screening tools for protein or glucose in the urine, more sophisticated reagents are now available. These reagents test for nitrites and leucocyte esterase as indicators of bacterial infection. Leucocyte esterase is an enzyme from neutrophils not normally found in urine and is a marker of infection. Nitrites are produced in urine by the bacterial breakdown of dietary nitrates (Woodward & Griffiths 1993).

In the microbiology laboratory, urine samples constitute about 40% of the total workload; of these, 70–80% are not infected. This means that much time, energy and finances are wasted on unnecessary sample processing and investigation. Bayer (1997a, b) suggests an approach that gives the power to confidently avoid sending non-infected urine samples for microscopy and culture, enabling appropriate, timely and cost-effective patient management (see Fig. 25.26). However, there are still some concerns about the sensitivity of these sticks. Mills *et al.* (1992) concluded that dipstick reagents are a useful screening tool, but specimens still need to be examined in a microbiology laboratory to determine the nature and sensitivity of the infection for treatment. When interpreting the results of reagent sticks it is important to remember the limitations of the test as false negatives are possible.

Many drugs may influence urine tests (see Table 25.8). It is therefore important to assess the patient's medication when considering the results of dipstick urinalysis. The wide range of urine tests available and the ease with which they can be used have established the

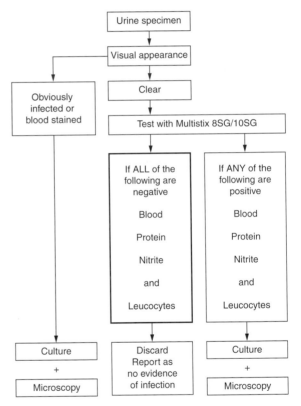

Figure 25.26 Testing strategy for UTI using Bayer reagent strips.

use of reagent sticks throughout clinical practice. It is important to be aware, however, that they do have limitations and that manufacturer's instructions should be followed carefully, as results, especially tests for glucose and protein, can influence treatment and care decisions.

Table 25.8 How drugs may influence the results of reagent sticks

Drug	Reagent test	Effect on the results
Ascorbic acid	Glucose, blood, nitrite	High concentrations may diminish colour
L-Dopa	Glucose	High concentrations may give a false negative reaction
	Ketones	Atypical colour
Nalidixic acid	Urobilinogen	Atypical colour
Probenacid		
Phenazopyridine (pyridium)	Protein	May give atypical colour
	Ketones	Coloured metabolites may mask a small reaction
	Urobilinogen, bilirubin	May mimic a positive reaction
	Nitrite	
Rifampicin	Bilirubin	Coloured metabolites may mask a small reaction
Salicylates (aspirin)	Glucose	High doses may give a false negative reaction

Procedure guidelines: **Reagent sticks**

Procedure

	Action	Rationale
1	Store reagent sticks in accordance with manufacturer's instructions. This often includes any dark place or in a refrigerator.	Tests may depend on enzymic reaction. To ensure reliable results.
2	Explain and discuss the procedure with the patient.	To ensure that the patient understands the procedure and gives his/her valid consent.
3	Obtain clean specimen of fresh urine from patient.	Urine that has been stored deteriorates rapidly and can give false results.
4	Dip the reagent strip into the urine. The strip should be completely immersed in the urine and then removed immediately and tapped against the side of the container.	To remove any excess urine.
5	Hold the stick at an angle.	Urine reagent strips should not be held upright when reading them because urine may run from square to square, mixing various reagents.
6	Wait the required time interval before reading the strip against the colour chart.	The strips must be read at exactly the time interval specified, or the reagents will not have time to react, or may be inaccurate.

Blood glucose

Definition

The body regulates the blood glucose levels by producing insulin. Insulin's main effect is to lower the blood glucose level, but it also influences protein and fat metabolism. If the pancreas fails to produce sufficient insulin, the level of glucose in the blood will remain high. Conversely, if too much insulin is made, or given, then the level of glucose in the blood remains low. In a healthy individual the body regulates the blood glucose to be maintained between 4 and 7 mmol/l (Cowan 1997).

Indications

Blood glucose monitoring is used to indicate when blood glucose is not within the normal range. Conditions where a patient's blood glucose may need careful monitoring are:

- To make a diagnosis of diabetes mellitus which is only confirmed following a glucose tolerance test (Burden 2001)
- In the acute management of unstable diabetic states: diabetic ketoacidosis, hyperosmolar non-ketotic coma and hypoglycaemia

- To make a diagnosis of hypoglycaemia
- To monitor and manage the treatment of both insulin-dependent diabetes mellitus (IDDM) and non-insulin-dependent diabetes mellitus (NIDDM).

Reference material

To maintain normal blood glucose levels, insulin and the counter-regulatory hormones, or stress hormones, must be in balance. These hormones, which include adrenaline, noradrenaline, cortisol, growth hormone and glucagon, are released in the event of stress (Sharp 1993).

During infection, major surgery or critical illness, people's regulatory hormone levels of cortisol, noradrenaline and glucagon will rise in response to the stressful event. This stimulates glycogen and fat breakdown, which causes the blood glucose levels to rise. In a healthy individual, insulin production would increase. In a person who is unable to raise his/her insulin levels, e.g. a diabetic, the result is hyperglycaemia (Curry & Weedon 1993). The majority of people who have diabetes will be known to be diabetic prior to this event but as many as one million people in the UK have the condition and do not know it (Diabetes UK 2000). However, there may be a proportion who have had no history of such a disorder, only becoming diabetic in response to their primary illness and treatment. An example of this is steroid-induced diabetes. This diagnosis does not mean that they will remain a diabetic, but that they may need careful monitoring after their recovery.

Hypoglycaemia

Hypoglycaemia is described as a blood glucose level that is unable to meet the metabolic demands of the body (Marini & Wheeler 1997). Often young and healthy individuals can be asymptomatic during this inadequate level of glucose in the blood. Early symptoms are sweating, tremor, weakness, nervousness, tachycardia and hypertension. Severe hypoglycaemia causes mental disorientation, convulsions, unconsciousness and shock (Tortora & Grabowski 2003). The most common cause is induced by insulin when combined with alcohol consumption, especially if alcohol is taken on an empty stomach (Marini & Wheeler 1997). In hospital, hypoglycaemia may occur when there is renal impairment, with insufficient clearing of insulin and with irregular or insufficient food intake (Marini & Wheeler 1997).

Other causes of hypoglycaemia are:

- Infection, which can result in hepatic failure, renal insufficiency, depletion of muscle glycogen and starvation

- Alcohol, which suppresses glyconeogenesis and nutritional intake. This induces a low insulin state, ketone production and fatty acid release
- Hepatic failure, which can be due to tumour infiltration, cirrhosis or hepatic necrosis
- Renal failure
- Salicylate poisoning
- Insulin-secreting tumours
- Surgery (Marini & Wheeler 1997).

Treatment should be by the administration of glucose. The route will depend on the conscious level of the individual and the treatment the patient has undergone, e.g. postoperatively it may be necessary to refrain from eating and drinking, as well as the recommendations of the medical staff.

Hyperglycaemia

When insulin is deficient or absent, blood glucose levels remain high after a meal. This is because insulin acts like a key, unlocking a door to allow glucose to enter the cell. If insulin is absent, the glucose is unable to enter most cells. When glucose levels become excessive (hyperglycaemia) the person will feel nauseated, and the body will precipitate the flight or fight response. The cells are starved of glucose and the body reacts inappropriately by producing reactions usually seen in states of fasting (hypoglycaemia). Processes such as glycogenolysis (the breakdown of glycogen to release glucose), lipolysis (the breakdown of stored fats into glycerol and fatty acids) and gluconeogenesis (the conversion of glycerol and amino acids into glucose) are instigated (Marieb 2001).

The blood glucose continues to rise and some of the glucose is excreted in the urine. As the level of glucose in the kidney increases, water reabsorption by the tubules becomes inhibited. This causes the body to excrete large amounts of urine (polyuria). The person will feel excessively thirsty (polydipsia) and will pass urine often and in large quantities. The person may also feel extremely hungry (polyphagia). The combination of polydipsia and polyuria will lead to dehydration, a fall in blood pressure and electrolyte imbalance. The acid–base imbalance caused by the loss of sodium and potassium (hypokalaemia) leads to the person complaining of abdominal pains, nausea and vomiting. As the patient's condition deteriorates, cardiac irregularities may occur with central nervous depression (Marini & Wheeler 1997) (Fig. 25.27).

Even though there is excessive glucose in the body, the body cannot utilize it, so an alternative source of energy has to be found. To compensate, the body starts to break down fats and protein. Fats are mobilized, which leads to

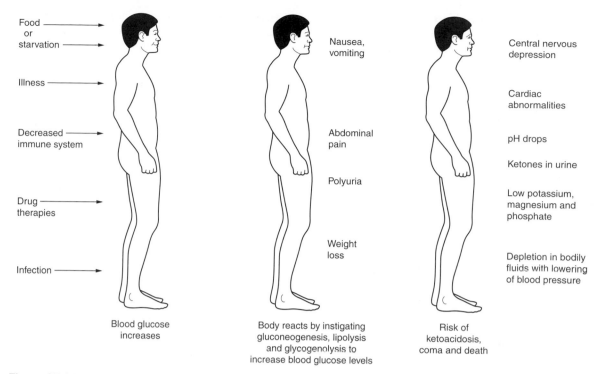

Blood glucose increases

Body reacts by instigating gluconeogenesis, lipolysis and glycogenolysis to increase blood glucose levels

Risk of ketoacidosis, coma and death

Figure 25.27 Effects of increasing glucose due to insufficient insulin production.

high levels of fatty acids in the blood (lipidaemia). This can also cause sudden and dramatic weight loss. The fatty acid metabolites, known as ketones, accumulate in the blood more rapidly than they can be excreted or used. The blood pH will fall, resulting in ketoacidosis and ketones being excreted into the urine. If ketoacidosis is allowed to continue it can become life-threatening as it disrupts all physiological processes, including oxygen transportation and heart activity. Depression of the nervous system leads to coma and death (Marieb 2001).

Diabetic ketoacidosis is a serious condition, which has a mortality rate of between 5 and 15% despite treatment (Marini & Wheeler 1997). It is a result of a deficiency of insulin and a high level of stress hormones. In the diabetic patient it is usually precipitated by a poor diet and inadequate medication and can be brought on by infection. The most prominent metabolic changes caused by ketoacidosis are metabolic acidosis and volume depletion.

Treatment involves fluid replacement, restoration of the acid–base imbalance and careful monitoring. If patients in a ketoacidotic state do not respond to fluid replacement and correction of the pH, then other conditions such as septic shock, bleeding, adrenal insufficiency, myocardial infarction and pancreatitis should be considered, and treated accordingly (Marini & Wheeler 1997).

The administration of intravenous insulin should be titrated by an infusion device, and measurements of blood glucose should be taken 1–2 hourly in order to guide the rate of delivery. If the blood glucose level does not fall within the first few hours it may indicate insulin resistance and the amount of insulin may need to be increased.

Note: care needs to be taken in the rapid reversal of fluid loss and electrolyte imbalance. Excessive fluids can cause sudden acid–base shifts and exacerbate hypokalaemia. Central nervous system acidosis and arrhythmias are preventable with constant monitoring. Once urine flow is re-established, potassium should be given. Magnesium and phosphate levels in the blood should also be monitored. A common complication after aggressive treatment is hypoglycaemia.

Blood glucose monitoring

Monitoring a patient's blood glucose provides an accurate indication of how the body is controlling glucose metabolism. In the short term, monitoring can prevent hypoglycaemia and ketoacidosis, and in the long term it can significantly reduce the risk of complications which affect the vascular and neural pathways by helping to maintain near-normal glucose levels (UKPDS 1998).

Blood testing is now known to be more accurate than urine testing as the result gives an indication of the current blood levels (Cowan 1997). The immediacy of results allows patients to receive appropriate care and advice. Blood samples can be taken from capillary, venous or arterial routes. The vessel used will depend on the accessibility of obtaining the blood sample, the frequency of testing and the condition of the patient. However, a recent meta-analysis questions the clinical efficiency and effectiveness of blood glucose self-monitoring (Coster et al. 2000).

It is essential that both the correct equipment is used and the operator is trained and proficient in its operation. Many different monitoring devices are currently available. Nursing and medical research has now been undertaken to identify the most accurate and practicable equipment (Trajanoski et al. 1996; Chan et al. 1997; Cowan 1997; Rumley 1997; Kirk & Rheney 1998; Batki et al. 1999).

Current methods for testing blood glucose rely on finger pricking but non-invasive blood glucose monitoring devices are being developed which would enable automatic detection of hypoglycaemia or hyperglycaemia (American Diabetes Association 2001). Non-invasive monitoring means checking blood glucose levels without puncturing the skin for a blood sample. One device approved is worn like a wristwatch and measures blood glucose via interstitial fluid (Pickup 2000).

Point-of-care testing (POCT), sometimes referred to as near-patient testing, is any test performed for a patient by a health care professional outside the laboratory setting (MDA 2002). There is a significant risk for errors to occur when using POCT. The Department of Health issued a hazard warning in 1987 and again in a 1996 safety notice. These warnings highlighted the need for formal training and strict quality control (DoH 1996). Quality assurance in relation to POCT is defined as the measures taken to ensure the test results are reliable (MDA 2002); this also aims to maintain the competency of all users. These hazard notices drew attention to the fact that a management or therapeutic decision based on an unreliable blood glucose result can prove fatal. Inaccurate results are often due to incorrect timing of the test, insufficient amount of blood taken and smearing of the sample (Heenan 1990). Staff undertaking POCT should be aware that certain patient conditions may lead to false and misleading results. The testing of blood glucose in the blood may be affected by the following.

- Hyperlipaemia (containing abnormal fat concentrations, for example cholesterol above 56.5 mmol/l). May elevate readings.

- Haematocrit values. If extremely high, i.e. above 55%, and blood glucose values are above 11 mmol/l, the value may be up to 15% too low. If the haematocrit level is low, i.e. less than 35%, the value may be up to 10% too high.
- Dialysis treatment. May elevate readings.
- Bilirubin values above 0.43 mmol/l, e.g. in jaundice. May elevate readings.
- Intravenous infusion of ascorbic acid (vitamin C). May depress readings.
- When there has been peripheral circulatory failure, e.g. following severe dehydration caused by hyperglycaemic–hyperosmolar state with or without ketoacidosis, hypotension, shock or peripheral vascular disease. In these cases the results of the blood sample taken from the peripheral blood, e.g. from a finger prick, may be much lower than laboratory measurements taken from venous or arterial sources. In these cases treatment should be based on laboratory measurements only (Sandler et al. 1990).

The Department of Health report (1996) highlights that there must be standardization in training, reliability and quality control. In order to achieve this, the following aspects need to be considered when selecting POCT blood glucose monitoring equipment.

1 Equipment is designed for use by non-laboratory staff and is suitable for use in the clinical environment.
2 All the equipment used is compatible and will give reliable results.
3 The biochemistry laboratory is involved in the purchase and maintenance of the equipment. This may involve the purchase of one type of device from one company for the whole hospital, to reduce costs and provide standardization (Lowes 1995).
4 The product should be easy to use and the staff should be involved in the choice of the device (Kirk & Rheney 1998).
5 The ongoing cost and maintenance of the device need to be considered; this should include buying strips, control solutions and the replacement of devices (Kirk & Rheney 1998).
6 There are written standard operating procedures available and kept with the device.
7 Training is given to the operators and records are kept of this. Following training the following learning outcomes should be demonstrated by the operator:
    (a) Knowledge of the basic principle of measurement and normal ranges
    (b) The proper use of the equipment as laid down by the operating instructions and specifications (Bayne 1997)

(c) The consequences of improper use

(d) Health and safety procedures for the collection of blood samples, i.e. to prevent spillage and needle-stick injuries

(e) The importance of complete documentation

(f) Use of appropriate calibration and quality control techniques

(g) An understanding that blood sugar analysis should only be used as a guide and a tool, with diagnosis and treatment decisions being based on confirmed laboratory results (DoH 1996).

There is a requirement to monitor the quality of the results of the device and the person operating it. This is both a hospital and a government directive. Independent quality control should be carried out with the collaboration of the biochemistry laboratory. External auditing of the quality control should be undertaken and this may be provided in the package offered by the company. Problems that can occur include compliance by both patient and staff, blood sampling problems, the quality of the solution, the external audit and the training needs of the individual (Lowes 1995).

Procedure guidelines: **Blood glucose monitoring**

Only nursing staff who have obtained a certificate of training for the equipment should undertake this task.

Equipment

1 Blood glucose monitor.
2 Test strips.
3 Control solution.
4 Finger-pricking device and lancets.

Procedure

Action	Rationale
1 Before taking the device to the patient the monitor needs to be checked for the following: (a) That one pack of test strips is open and has not been left exposed to the air and that they are in date. (b) That the monitor and the test strips have been calibrated together. (c) That if a new pack of strips is required, the monitor is recalibrated. (d) That a high and low internal quality control test is carried out prior to any patient sample being measured. (e) That the result of the internal quality control is recorded in the equipment log book and signed. (f) Ensure the needle from previous use has been ejected from the finger-pricking device.	To ensure accuracy of the result. The quality control and checks have been carried out in order to ensure the safety of the patient. To reduce the risk of needlestick injury.
2 Explain the procedure to the patient. Some patients may want to look away at the sight of a needle.	The patient should be aware of the procedure in order to allay some of his/her anxieties, and to be able to co-operate in the procedure.
3 Patients should be advised to wash their hands prior to blood sampling. The use of alcohol rub should be avoided. Encourage patients to keep their hands warm until sampling has been performed.	To ensure a non-contaminated result. To encourage good blood flow (Cowan 1997).
4 Ask the patient to sit or lie down.	To ensure the patient's safety as some patients may feel faint when blood is taken.
5 Wash your hands, and put on protective gloves.	To minimize the risk of cross-infection. To minimize the risk of contamination.
6 Use a disposable lancet (DoH 1990).	To minimize the risk of cross-infection. Disposable lancets are advised following an outbreak of hepatitis B in French and US hospitals.

*Procedure guidelines: **Blood glucose monitoring** (cont'd)*

Action	Rationale
7 Take a blood sample from the side of the finger using the lancet, ensuring that the site of piercing is rotated. Avoid frequent use of the index finger and thumb. The finger may bleed without assistance, or may need assistance by 'milking' to form a droplet of blood which is large enough to cover the test pad.	The side of the finger is used as it is less painful and easier to obtain a hanging droplet of blood. The site is rotated to reduce the risk of infection from multiple stabbing, the areas becoming toughened and to reduce pain.
8 Apply the blood to the testing strip. Some test strips are hydrophilic and are dosed/filled from the side and are not dropped directly onto the strip.	The window on the test strip allows verification of a correctly dosed strip.
9 Dispose of lancet in a container designed for sharps.	To reduce the risk of needlestick injury.
10 Depending on the type of monitor, the procedure will differ. See individual manuals and hospital policies.	To ensure the accuracy of the result.
11 Once the result is obtained, record immediately.	To ensure the accuracy of the result.
12 Dispose of waste appropriately. Remove gloves and dispose.	To reduce the risk of cross-infection.
13 Make the patient comfortable and observe site of test for bleeding.	To ensure the patient's comfort.
14 Wash hands.	To prevent cross-infection.

Central venous pressure

Central venous pressure (CVP) is the pressure of blood returning to or filling the right atrium. It indicates blood volume, vascular tone and cardiac function (Hudek *et al.* 1998). CVP is usually used to assess blood volume and to guide fluid management. It is important to remember that CVP is affected by:

- Intrathoracic pressure
- Vascular tone
- Obstruction (Woodrow 2002).

CVP measurement must be used as part of a wider clinical assessment, as the reading can be misleading if taken in isolation (Henderson 1997; Hatchett 2000). The CVP should be measured at the right atrial level, as it is a measure of the pressure of blood returning to the right atrium (Woodrow 2002). CVP is usually recorded at the mid-axilla (Fig. 25.28).

A variety of positions are suited to using the mid-axilla as a point of reference. Ideally, the patient should lie flat in a supine position to reflect the right atrial pressure. However, many breathless patients cannot tolerate lying supine, therefore the measurement can also be taken in a semi-recumbent or recumbent position (Hatchett 2000). It is vital that the same position is used on every measurement and it is therefore important to record and document the position.

If the patient is supine an alternative position is via the sternal angle (Fig. 25.29). It is important to use

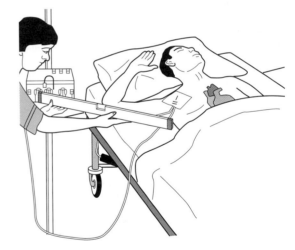

Figure 25.28 Measuring CVP from the mid-axilla.

just one method, to promote consistency, as readings from the sternal angle are about 5 cm lower than those taken from the mid-axilla (Hatchett 2000; Woodrow 2002). The site should be marked and recorded in the nursing notes as a reference. It is essential that the patient be fully informed before a CVP measurement is carried out.

Generally water manometers are used (Henderson 1997), but when patients are critically ill a more direct measurement is via an electronic transducer.

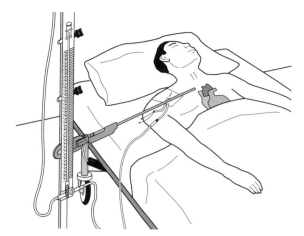

Figure 25.29 Measuring CVP from the sternal angle.

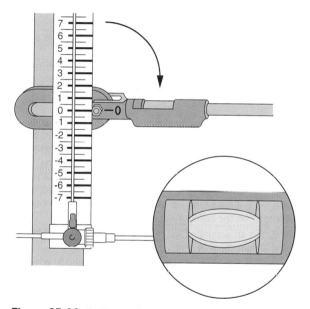

Figure 25.30 Setting and checking the baseline.

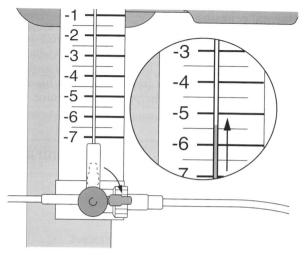

Figure 25.31 Turn off three-way tap to the patient.

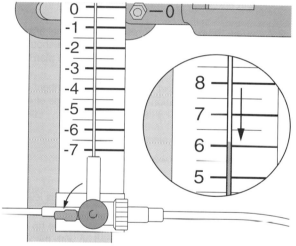

Figure 25.32 Turn off three-way tap to the intravenous fluid.

Zeroing a CVP

Zeroing a CVP is an essential part of measurement. The zero point will equal atmospheric (room) pressure. In critical care areas, monitors that can be set electronically usually measure CVPs. When measuring with water manometers the zero should align with the right atrial level (Fig. 25.30). This is usually checked by a spirit level.

Reading CVP

After zeroing, the chamber should be almost filled with fluid by turning the flow tap to allow fluid into the measure chamber, whilst closing the flow to the patient

(Fig. 25.31). Care should be taken not to get the air filter at the top wet, as a wet filter will resist air entry and give a false raised reading (Woodrow 2002). The tap should then be turned so the fluid flow is stopped and the chamber opened to the patient (Fig. 25.32). Gravity will cause the water level to fall until resistance from the patient's CVP matches the pressure of gravity. However, slight changes in pressure caused by the patient's respiration, usually 1 cm, will make the fluid fall in a swinging pattern, until it oscillates between two figures. The intrathoracic pressure represented by the fluid level in the chamber falls on inspiration so the higher figure should be recorded (Woodrow 2002). CVP can be measured in mmHg or cmH_2O.

Bartlett, E. (1996) Temperature measurement: why and how in intensive care. *Intens Crit Care Nurs*, **12**(1), 50–4.

Batki, A., Holder, R. & Thomason, H.L. *et al.* (1999) Selecting blood glucose monitoring systems. *Prof Nurse*, **14**(10), 715–23.

Bayer Diagnostics (1997a) *Urinary Tract Infection. Technical Information Bulletin No. 8.* Bayer Diagnostics, Newbury.

Bayer Diagnostics (1997b) *A Practical Guide to Urine Analysis.* Bayer Diagnostics, Newbury.

Bayne, C. (1997) How sweet it is: glucose monitoring equipment and interpretation. *Nurs Manage*, **28**(9), 52–4.

Beevers, M. & Beevers, G.B. (1996) Blood pressure measurement in the next century, a plea for stability. *Blood Press Monit*, **1**(2), 117–20.

Beevers, G., Lip, G.Y.H. & O'Brien, E. (2001a) Blood pressure measurement Part I. Sphygmomanometry: factors common to all techniques. *Br Med J*, **322**(7292), 981–5.

Beevers, G., Lip, G.Y.H. & O'Brien, E. (2001b) Blood pressure measurement Part II. Conventional sphygmomanometry: technique of auscultatory blood pressure measurement. *Br Med J*, **322**(7292), 1043–7.

Beevers, G., Lip, G.Y.H. & O'Brien, E. (2001c) Blood pressure measurement Part III. Automated sphygmomanometry: ambulatory blood pressure measurement. *Br Med J*, **322**, 1110–14.

Beevers, G., Lip, G.Y.H. & O'Brien, E. (2001d) Blood pressure measurement Part IV. Automated sphygmomanometry: self blood pressure measurement. *Br Med J*, **322**, 1167–70.

Berger, A. (2001) How does it work? Oscillatory blood pressure monitoring devices. *Br Med J*, **323**(7318), 9–19.

Bogan, B., Kritzer, S. & Deane, D. (1993) Nursing student compliance to standards for blood pressure measurement. *J Nurse Educ*, **32**(2), 90–2.

Bone, R.C. (1996) The pathogenesis of sepsis and rationale for new treatments. *Proceedings of the International Intensive Care Conference*, Barcelona.

Bone, R.C., Crodzin, C.J. & Balk, R.A. (1997) Sepsis: a new hypothesis for pathogenesis of the disease process. *Chest*, **112**(1), 235–43.

Braun, S.K., Preston, P. & Smith, R.N. (1998) Getting a better read on thermometry. *Reg Nurs*, **61**(3), 57–60.

British Committee for Standards in Haematology (BCSH) (1999) The administration of blood and blood components and the management of transfused patients. *Transfusion Med*, **9**, 227–38.

British Thoracic Society Standards of Care Committee (1997a) Current best practice for nebuliser treatment. *Thorax*, **52** (Suppl 2).

British Thoracic Society (1997b) Guidelines on asthma management: 1995 review and position statement. *Thorax*, **52** (Suppl).

Brown, S. (1990) Temperature taking – getting it right. *Nurs Stand*, **5**(12), 4–5.

Burden, M. (2001) Diabetes blood glucose monitoring. *Nurs Times*, **97**(8), 36–9.

Burke, K. (1996) The tympanic membrane thermometer in paediatrics: a review of the literature. *Accid Emergency Nurs*, **4**(4), 190–3.

Campbell, N.R. *et al.* (1990) Accurate, reproducible measurement of blood pressure. *Can Med Assoc J*, **143**(1), 19–24.

Carney, S.L., Gillies, A.H., Smith, A.J. & Smitham, S. (1995) Hospital sphygmomanometer use: an audit. *J Qual Clin Pract*, **15**(1), 17–22.

Casey, G. (2001) Oxygen transport and the use of pulse oximetry. *Nurs Stand*, **15**(47), 46–55.

Chan, J., Wong, R., Cheung, C. *et al.* (1997) Accuracy, precision and user-acceptability of self blood glucose monitoring machines. *Diabetes Res Clin Pract*, **36**(2), 91–104.

Connell, F. (1997) The causes and treatment of fever: a literature review. *Nurs Stand*, **12**(11), 40–3.

Cook, R. (1996) Urinalysis: ensuring accurate urine testing. *Nurs Stand*, **10**(46), 49–55.

Coster, S. *et al.* (2000) Self-monitoring in type 2 diabetes mellitus: a meta-analysis. *Diabetic Med*, **17**(11), 755–61.

Cowan, T. (1997) Blood glucose monitoring devices. *Prof Nurse*, **12**(8), 593–7.

Curry, M. & Weedon, L. (1993) Balancing act. *Nurs Times*, **89**(23), 50–2.

Damanhouri, Z. & Tayeb, O.S. (1992) Animal models for heat stroke studies. *J Pharmacol Toxicol Meth*, **28**, 119–27.

Diabetes UK (2000) *Diabetes in the UK – The Missing Millions.* Diabetes UK, London.

Docherty, B. (2000) Temperature recording. *Prof Nurse*, **16**(3), 943.

Docherty, B. (2002) Cardiorespiratory physical assessment for the acutely ill. *Br J Nurs*, **11**(12), 800–7.

DoH (1990) *Lancing Devices for Multi-Patient Capillary Sampling: Avoidance of Cross Infection by Correct Selection and Use.* DEF 42/00/10003. Medical Services Directorate, 14 Russell Square, London.

DoH (1996) *Extra-Laboratory Use of Blood Glucose Meters and Test Strips: Contraindications, Training and Advice to Users.* Medical Devices Agency Adverse Incident Centre Safety Notice 9616, June.

DoH (2000) *National Service Framework for Coronary Heart Disease – Modern Standards and Service Models.* Department of Health, London.

Edwards, S. (1997) Measuring temperature. *Prof Nurse*, **13**(2), 55–7.

Fawcett, J. (2001) The accuracy and reliability of the tympanic membrane thermometer – a literature review. *Emerg Nurse*, **8**(9), 13–17.

Feather, C. (2001) Blood pressure measurement. *Nurs Times*, **97**(4), 33–4.

Feher, M. & Harris St John, K. (1992) Blood pressure measurement by junior hospital doctors: a gap in medical education? *Health Trends*, **24**(2), 59–61.

Fillingham, S. & Douglas, J. (eds) (1997) *Urological Nursing.* Baillière Tindall, London.

Ganong, W.F. (1995) *Review of Medical Physiology*, 17th edn. Appelton & Lange, Norwalk, Connecticut.

Ganong, W.F. (2001) *Review of Medical Physiology*, 20th edn. McGraw Hill Education, New York.

Gilbert, M., Barton, A.J. & Counsell, C.M. (2002) Comparison of oral and tympanic temperatures in adult surgical patients. *Appl Nurs Res*, **15**(1), 42–7.

Gillespie, A. & Curzio, J. (1998) Blood pressure measurement: assessing staff knowledge. *Nurs Stand*, **12**(23), 35–7.

Hasler, M. & Cohen, J. (1982) The effect of oxygen administration on oral temperature assessment. *Nurs Res*, **31**, 265–8.

Hatchett, R. (2000) Central venous pressure measurement. *Nurs Times*, **96**(15), 49–50.

Heenan, A. (1990) Blood glucose measurement. *Nurs Times*, **86**(4), 65–8.

Heindenreich, T. & Giuffe, M. (1990) Post-operative temperature measurement. *Nurs Res*, **39**(3), 153–5.

Henderson, N. (1997) Central venous lines. *Nurs Stand*, **11**(42), 49–56.

Hill, M.N. & Grim, C.M. (1991) How to take a precise blood pressure. *Am J Nurs*, **91**(2), 38–42.

Hudek, C.M., Gallo, B.M. & Morton, P.G. (1998) *Critical Care Nursing: A Holistic Approach,* 7th edn. Lippincott, New York.

Hypertension Influence Team (2000) *Let's Do It Well – Nurse Learning Pack*. Hypertension Influence Team, London.

Jensen, B.N. *et al.* (1994) The superiority of rectal thermometry to oral thermometry with regard to accuracy. *J Adv Nurs*, **20**, 660–5.

Jevon, P. (2000a) Pulse oximetry – 1. *Nurs Times*, **96**(26), 43–4.

Jevon, P. (2000b) Pulse oximetry – 2. *Nurs Times*, **96**(27), 43–4.

Jevon, P. (2001a) Measuring lying and standing BP – 1. *Nurs Times*, **97**(1), 41–2.

Jevon, P. (2001b) Measuring lying and standing BP – 2. *Nurs Times*, **97**(3), 41–2.

Jevon, P. & Jevon, M. (2001) Using a tympanic thermometer. *Nurs Times*, **97**(9), 43–4.

Jevon, P., Ewens, B. & Manzie, J. (2000) Measuring peak expiratory flow. Practical procedures for nurses, part 45.1. *Nurs Times*, **96**(38), 49–50.

Keenan, J. (1995) Pulse oximetry (cardiology update). *Nurs Stand*, **9**, 35–55.

Kemp, F., Foster, C. & McKinlay, S. (1994) How effective is training for blood pressure measurement? *Prof Nurse*, **9**(8), 521–4.

Kirk, J. & Rheney, C. (1998) Important features of blood glucose meters. *J Am Pharm Assoc (Washington)*, **8**(2), 210–19.

Krikler, S. (1990) Pyrexia: what to do about temperatures. *Nurs Stand*, **4**(25), 37–8.

Lim-Levy, F. (1982) The effect of oxygen inhalation on oral temperature. *Nurs Res*, **31**, 150–2.

Londe, S. & Klitzner, T. (1984) Auscultatory blood pressure measurement: effect of blood pressure on the head-on stethoscope. *West J Med*, **141**(2), 193–5.

Lowes, L. (1995) Accuracy in ward-based blood glucose monitoring. *Nurs Times*, **91**(13), 44–5.

Magee, L.A., Ornstein, M.P. & Von Dadelszen, P. (1999) Management of hypertension in pregnancy. *Br Med J*, **318**, 1332–6.

Mancia, G. *et al.* (1987) Alerting reaction and rise in blood pressure during measurement by physician and nurse. *Hypertension*, **9**, 209–15.

Marieb, E.M. (2001) *Human Anatomy & Physiology*. Benjamin Cummings, San Francisco.

Marini, J. & Wheeler, A. (1997a) *Critical Care Medicine: The Essentials*, 2nd edn. Williams and Wilkins, Baltimore, pp. 19–43.

Marini, J. & Wheeler, A. (1997b) *Critical Care Medicine: The Essentials*, 2nd edn. Williams and Wilkins, Baltimore, pp. 498–510.

Marini, J. & Wheeler, A. (1997c) *Critical Care Medicine*, 2nd edn. Williams and Wilkins, London, pp. 456–64.

McAlister, F.A. & Straus, S.E. (2001) Evidence based treatment for hypertension – measurement of blood pressure: an evidence based review. *Br Med J*, **322**, 908–11.

MDA (2000) *Blood Pressure Measurement Devices – Mercury and Non-mercury*. Medical Devices Agency, London.

MDA (2002a) *Management and Use of IVD Point-of-Care Test Devices*. Medical Devices Agency, London.

MDA (2002b) Self-monitoring in type 2 diabetes mellitus: a meta-analysis. *Diabet Med*, **17**(11), 755–61.

Mills, S.J. *et al.* (1992) Screening for bacteriuria in urological patients using reagent strips. *Br J Urol*, **70**, 314–17.

Mims, C.A. *et al.* (1993) *Medical Microbiology*. C.V. Mosby, London.

Minor, D.G. & Waterhouse, J.M. (1981) *Circadian Rhythms and the Human*. Wright, Bristol.

Mize, J., Koziol-McLain, J. & Lowenstein, S.R. (1993) The forgotten vital sign: temperature patterns and associations in 642 trauma patients at an urban level 1 trauma centre. *J Emerg Nurs*, **19**(4), 303–5.

Nakamura, K., Tanaka, M., Motohashi, Y. & Maeda, A. (1997) Oral temperatures in the elderly in nursing homes in summer and winter in relation to activities of daily living. *Int J Biometeorol*, **40**(2), 103–6.

Neff, J. *et al.* (1989) Effect of respiratory rate, respiratory depth, and open versus closed mouth breathing on sublingual temperature. *Res Nurs Health*, **12**, 195–202.

O'Brien, E., Waeber, B., Parati, G., Staessen, J. & Myers, M G. (2001) Blood pressure measuring devices: recommendations of the European Society of Hypertension. *Br Med J*, **322**(7285), 531–6.

O'Toole, S. (1997) Alternatives to mercury thermometers. *Prof Nurse*, **12**(11), 783–6.

Petrie, J.C., O'Brian, E.T., Litler, W.A. & deSwiet, M. (1997) *British Hypertension Society: Recommendations on Blood Pressure Measurement*, 2nd edn. British Hypertension Society, London.

Pickup, J. (2000) Sensitive glucose sensing in diabetes. *Lancet*, **355**(9202), 426–7.

Ramsay, L.E., Williams, B., Johnston, G.D. *et al.* (1999) British Hypertension Society guidelines for hypertension management 1999: summary. *Br Med J*, **319**(63), 1–5.

Resuscitation Council UK (2000) Adult Advanced Life Support 1–7. In: *The Advanced Life Support Manual*, 4th edn. Resuscitation Council UK, London.

Rokosky, J.S. (1981) Assessment of the individual with altered respiratory function. *Nurs Clin North Am*, **16**(2), 195–9.

Rumley, A. (1997) Improving the quality of near patient blood glucose measurement. *Annu Clin Biochem*, **34**(Part 2), 281–6.

Samples, F. *et al.* (1985) Circadian rhythms: basis for screening for fever. *Nurs Res*, **34**(6), 377–9.

Sandler, M. *et al.* (1990) Misleading capillary glucose measurements. *Practical Diabetes*, **7**, 210.

Sharber, J. (1997) The efficacy of tepid sponge bathing to reduce fever in young children. *Am J Emerg Med*, **15**(2), 188–92.

Sharp, S. (1993) Blood glucose monitoring in the intensive care unit. *Br J Nurs*, **2**(4), 209–14.

Sims, J. (1996) Making sense of pulse oximetry and oxygen dissociation curve. *Nurs Times*, **92**(1), 34–5.

Smith, G.R. (2000) Devices for blood pressure measurement. *Prof Nurse*, **15**(5), 337–40.

Thompson, D.R. (1981) Recording patients' blood pressure: a review. *J Adv Nurs*, **6**(4), 283–90.

Timby, B. (1989) *Clinical Nursing Procedure*. J.B. Lippincott, Philadelphia.

Torrance, C. & Elley, K. (1997) Respiration technique and observation – 2. *Nurs Times*, **93**(44), insert.

Torrance, C. & Elley, K. (1998) Urine testing 2 – urinalysis. *Nurs Times*, **94**(5), (Suppl 2).

Torrance, C. & Semple, M. (1998) Recording temperature. *Nurs Times*, **94**(3).

Torrance, C. & Serginson, E. (1996) Student nurses' knowledge in relation to blood pressure measurement by sphygmomanometry and auscultation. *Nurse Educ Today*, **16**(6), 397–402.

Tortora, G.J. & Grabowski, S.R. (2003) *Principles of Anatomy & Physiology*. John Wiley, New York.

Trajanoski, Z., Brunner, G., Gfrerer, R., Wach, P. & Pieber, T. (1996) Accuracy of home blood glucose meters during hypoglycaemia. *Diabetes Care*, **19**(12), 1412–15.

UK Prospective Diabetes Study Group (UKPDS) (1998) Tight blood pressure control and risk of macrovascular and microvascular complications in type 2 diabetes. *Br Med J*, **317**(7160), 703–13.

Watson, R. (1998) Controlling body temperature in adults. *Nurs Stand*, **12**(20), 49–55.

Woodrow, P. (1999) Pulse oximetry. *Nurs Stand*, **13**(42), 42–6.

Woodrow, P. (2000) *Intensive Care Nursing. A Framework for Practice*. Routledge, London.

Woodrow, P. (2002) Central venous catheters and central venous pressure. *Nurs Stand*, **16**(26), 45–51.

Woodward, M.N. & Griffiths, D.M. (1993) Use of dipsticks for routine analysis of urine from children with acute abdominal pain. *Br Med J*, **306**, 1512.

Woollens, S. (1996) Temperature measurement devices. *Prof Nurse*, **11**(8), 541–7.

Observations: neurological

Definition

Neurological observation relates to the evaluation of the integrity of an individual's nervous system.

Indications

Neurological observations are required to monitor and evaluate changes in the nervous system by indicating trends, thus aiding diagnosis and treatment, which in turn may affect prognosis and rehabilitation (Abelson 1982; Jennett & Teasdale 1984).

Reference material

Changes in neurological status can be rapid and dramatic or subtle, developing over minutes, hours, days, weeks or even months depending on the insult (Aucken & Crawford 1998). Therefore the frequency of neurological observations will depend upon the patient's condition and the rapidity with which changes are occurring or expected to occur.

Neurological function is assessed by observing five critical areas:

- Level of consciousness
- Pupillary activity
- Motor function
- Sensory function
- Vital signs.

Consciousness

Consciousness depends on two components:

- Arousability
- Awareness.

Arousability

This depends on the integrity of the reticular activating system (RAS) (Fig. 26.1). This core of nuclei extends from the brainstem to the thalamic nuclei in the cerebral hemispheres. Thus cognitive ability depends on the ability of the cerebral cortex to permit reciprocal stimulation and conscious behaviour.

Awareness

This requires an intact cerebral cortex to interpret sensory input and respond accordingly. This is the content of the consciousness (Scherer 1986).

Levels of consciousness may vary and are dependent on the location and extent of any neurological damage (Aucken & Crawford 1998). Previous and/or co-existing problems should be heeded when noting levels of

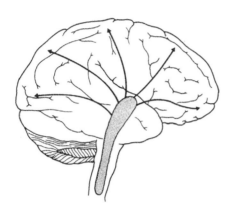

Figure 26.1 Reticular activating system.

consciousness, for example deafness, hemiparesis/hemiplegia.

Level of consciousness

Alterations in level of consciousness can vary from slight to severe changes, indicating the degree of brain dysfunction (Aucken & Crawford 1998). Consciousness ranges on a continuum from alert wakefulness to deep coma with no apparent responsiveness. Therefore, nurses must ensure that families and friends are involved at initial history taking and throughout care so as to chronicle accurately any change in neurological symptoms.

Terms such as 'fully conscious, semiconscious, lethargic or stuporous' to describe levels of consciousness are subjective and open to misinterpretation. Thus level of consciousness is often measured using the Glasgow Coma Scale (GCS) which was developed in 1974 at the University of Glasgow by Jennett and Teasdale (Table 26.1, Fig. 26.2). The GCS was designed to grade the severity of impaired consciousness in patients with traumatic head injuries or intracranial pressure (Aucken & Crawford 1998). The GCS is used worldwide, it is objective and provides a reliable and easy-to-use measure of conscious level. For example, a GCS score less than 8 is equated with a state of coma. When used consistently, the GCS provides a graphical representation that shows improvement or deterioration of the patient's conscious level at a glance (Fig. 26.2).

Table 26.1 Scoring activities of the Glasgow Coma Scale (from Aucken & Crawford 1998). Scores are added, with the highest score 15 indicating full consciousness

Eye opening		Scored 1–4
Spontaneously	4	Eyes open without need of stimulus
To speech	3	Eyes open to verbal stimulation (normal, raised or repeated)
To pain	2	Eyes open to central pain (tactile) only
None	1	No eye opening to verbal or painful stimuli
Verbal response		*Scored 1–5*
Orientated	5	Able to describe accurately details of time, person and place
Sentence	4	Can speak in sentences but does not answer orientation questions correctly
Words	3	Speaking incomprehensible, inappropriate words only
Sounds	2	Incomprehensible sounds following both verbal and painful stimuli
None	1	No verbal response following verbal and painful stimuli
Motor response		*Scored 1–6*
Obeys command	6	Follows and acts out commands, e.g. lifts up right arm
Localizes	5	Purposeful movement to remove noxious stimulus
Normal flexion	4	Flexes arm at elbow without wrist rotation in response to central painful stimulus
Abnormal flexion	3	Flexes arm at elbow with accompanying rotation of the wrist into spastic posturing in response to central pain
Extension	2	Extends arm at elbow with some inward rotation in response to central pain
None	1	No response to central painful stimulus

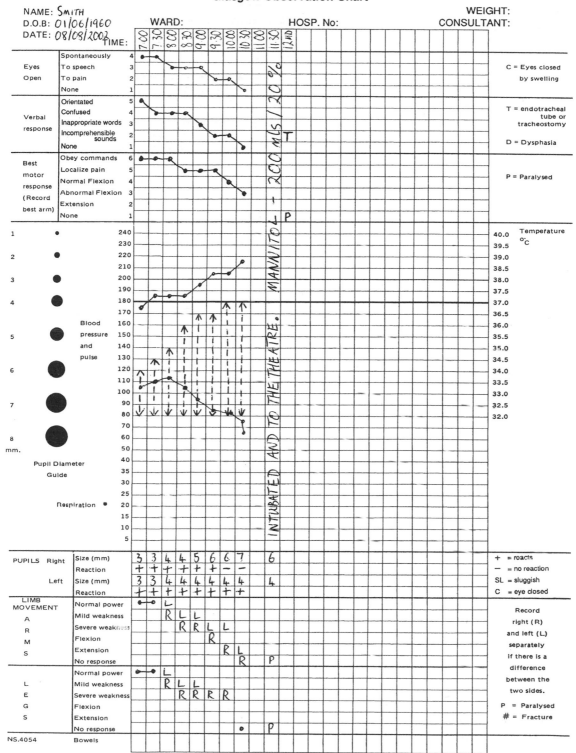

Figure 26.2 Glasgow Coma Scale.

Assessment of level of consciousness

Assessment involves three phases:

1 Eye opening
2 Evaluation of verbal response
3 Evaluation of motor response.

Evaluation of eye opening

Eye opening indicates that the arousal mechanism in the brain is active. Eye opening may be: spontaneous; to speech, e.g. spoken name; to painful stimulus; or not at all. Arousal (eye opening) is always the first measurement undertaken when performing the GCS, as without arousal, cognition cannot occur (Aucken & Crawford 1998). It must, however, be remembered that swollen or permanently closed eyes (e.g. after tarsorrhaphy surgery in which the upper and lower eyelids are partially or wholly joined to protect the cornea (Martin 1996)) will not open and do not necessarily indicate a falling conscious level.

Evaluation of verbal response

Verbal response may be:

- *Orientated*: the patient is aware of self and environment.
- *Confused*: the patient's responses to questions are incorrect and patient is unaware of self or environment.
- *Incomprehensible*: the patient may moan and groan without recognizable words.
- *Absent*: the patient does not speak or make sounds at all.

The absence of speech may not always indicate a falling level of consciousness. The patient may not speak English (though he/she can still speak), may have a tracheostomy or may be dysphasic. The patient may have a motor (expressive) dysphasia, and therefore be able to understand but unable to find the right word, or a sensory (receptive) dysphasia, being unable to comprehend what is being told to them. At times patients with expressive dysphasia may also have receptive problems; therefore it is important to make an early referral to a speech and language therapist. The nurse should also bear in mind that some patients may need a lot of stimulation to maintain their concentration to answer questions, even though they can answer them correctly. It is, therefore, important to note the amount of stimulation that the patient required as part of the baseline assessment (Aucken & Crawford 1998).

Evaluation of motor response

To obtain an accurate picture of brain function, motor response is tested by using the upper limbs because responses in the lower limbs reflect spinal function. (Aucken & Crawford 1998). The patient should be asked to obey commands; for example the patient should be asked to squeeze the examiner's hands (both sides) with the best motor response recorded. The nurse should note power in the hands and the patient's ability to release the grip. This is because some patients with cerebral dysfunction, for example those with diffuse brain disease, may show an involuntary grasp reflex where stimulation of the palm of their hand causes them to grip (Aucken & Crawford 1998). If movement is spontaneous, the nurse should note which limbs move, and how, for example whether the movement is purposeful.

Response to painful stimulus may be:

- *Localized*: the patient moves the other hand to the site of the stimulus.
- *Flexor*: the patient's limb flexes away from pain.
- *Extensor*: the patient's limb extends from pain.
- *Flaccid*: no motor response at all.

Evaluation of painful stimuli

Painful stimuli should be employed only if the patient does not respond to firm and clear commands. It is always important that the least amount of pressure to elicit a response is applied so as to avoid bruising the patient. As such, it should only be undertaken by experienced professionals (for suggested methods see below).

As the ability to localize pain is lost, various responses may be observed when painful stimuli are applied (Hudak *et al.* 1982). It is important to note, when applying a painful stimulus, that the brain responds to central stimulation and the spine responds first to peripheral stimulation (Aucken & Crawford 1998).

Central stimulation can be applied in the following ways (Lindsay *et al.* 1997; Aucken & Crawford 1998):

- *Trapezium squeeze*: using the thumb and two fingers, hold 5 cm of the trapezius muscle where the neck meets the shoulder and twist the muscle.
- *Supraorbital pressure*: running a finger along the supraorbital margin, a notch is felt. Applying pressure to the notch causes an ipsilateral (on that side) sinus headache. This method is not to be used if the facial bones are unstable, facial fractures are suspected or the assessor has sharp fingernails.
- *Sternal rub*: using the knuckles of a clenched fist to grind on the centre of the sternum. When applied adequately, marks are left on the skin as sternal tissue is tender and bruises easily. Please note that because of the danger of bruising, this method should not be used for repeated assessment but may be indicated if a decision as to whether to re-scan or alter management, e.g. proceed to surgery, is necessary.

Peripheral stimuli can be applied in the following way:

1 Place the patient's finger between assessor's thumb and a pencil or pen.
2 Pressure is gradually increased over a few seconds until the slightest response is seen.

Any finger can be used, although the third and fourth fingers are often most sensitive (Frawley 1990). Please note that because of the risk of bruising, pressure should not be applied to the nail bed. It must be remembered that nail bed pressure is a peripheral stimulus and should only be used to assess limbs that have not moved in response to a central stimulus (Aucken & Crawford 1998).

It cannot be overemphasized that the above methods of patient assessment should only be undertaken by appropriately qualified and trained nurses.

Table 26.2 Examination of pupils (from Fuller 1993)

What you find	Pupil size	Pupil reactiveness	Indication
Pupils equal	Pinpoint		Opiates or pontine lesion
	Small	Reactive	Metabolic encephalopathy
	Mid-sized	Fixed	Midbrain lesion
		Reactive	Metabolic lesion
Pupils unequal	Dilated	Unreactive	IIIrd nerve palsy
	Small	Reactive	Horner's syndrome

Evaluation of pupillary activity

Careful examination of the reactions of the pupils to light is an important part of neurological assessment (Table 26.2). The size, shape, equality, reaction to light (both direct and consensual responses, that is, the response from the eye that is not directly exposed to light) and position of the eyes should be noted. Are the eyes deviated upwards or downwards? Are both eyes conjugate (moving together) or dysconjugate (not moving together)? Impaired pupillary accommodation signifies that the midbrain itself may be suffering from pressure exerted by a swelling mass in the brain. Pupillary constriction and dilation are controlled by cranial nerve III (oculomotor) and any changes may indicate pressure on this nerve or brainstem damage (Fig. 26.3).

It should be noted that 'normal' visual function depends on a full and conjugate range of eye movements (cranial nerves III, IV, VI) in addition to normally functioning optic and oculomotor nerves and an intact visual centre in the occipital cortex (Aucken & Crawford 1998).

Evaluation of motor function

Damage to any part of the motor nervous system can affect the ability to move. Motor function assessment involves an evaluation of the following:

• Muscle strength
• Muscle tone
• Muscle co-ordination
• Reflexes
• Abnormal movements.

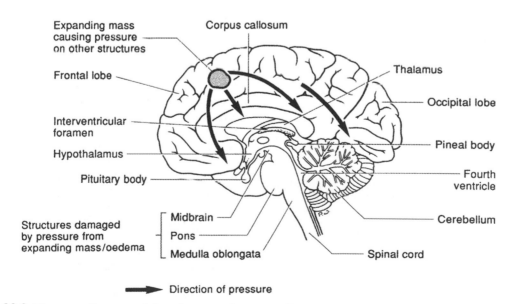

Figure 26.3 Diagrammatic representation of pressure from expanding mass and/or cerebral oedema.

Muscle strength

This involves testing the patient's muscle strength against one's own muscle resistance and then against the pull of gravity.

Muscle tone

This involves flexing and extending the patient's limbs on both sides and noting how well such movements are resisted. Increased resistance would denote increased muscle tone and vice versa.

Muscle co-ordination

Any disease or injury that involves the cerebellum or basal ganglia will affect co-ordination. Assessment of hand and leg co-ordination can be achieved by testing the rapidity and rhythm of alternating movements and of point-to-point movements.

Reflexes

Among the most important reflexes are: blink, gag and swallow, oculocephalic and plantar.

- *Blink*: this is a protective reflex and can be affected by damage to the Vth cranial nerve (trigeminal) and the VIIth cranial nerve (facial). Absence of the corneal reflex (Vth cranial nerve) may result in corneal damage. Facial weakness (VIIth cranial nerve) will affect eye closure.
- *Gag and swallow*: damage to the IXth cranial nerve (glossopharyngeal) and Xth cranial nerve (vagus) may impair protective reflexes. These two cranial nerves are always assessed together as their functions overlap. Muscle innervation of the palate is from the vagus, while sensation is supplied by the glossopharyngeal nerves (Aucken & Crawford 1998).
- *Oculocephalic*: this reflex is an eye movement that occurs only in patients with a severely decreased level of consciousness. In conscious patients this reflex is not present. When the reflex is present, the patient's eyes will move in the opposite direction from the side to which the head is turned. However, in patients with absent brainstem reflexes, the eyes will appear to remain stationary in the centre.
- *Plantar*: Abnormalities of plantar reflex will help to locate the anatomical site of the lesion. Upgoing plantar (extension) reflex is termed 'positive Babinski' and indicates an upper motor neurone lesion. It should be noted that in babies under 1 year of age upgoing plantar is normal (Aucken & Crawford 1998).

Abnormal movements

When carrying out neurological observations, any abnormal movements such as seizures, tics and tremors must be noted.

Sensory functions

Constant sensory input enables an individual to alter responses and behaviour to suit the environment. When disease or injury damages the sensory pathways, the sensory responses are always affected. Any assessment of sensory function should include an evaluation of the following:

- Central and peripheral vision
- Hearing and ability to understand verbal communication
- Superficial sensations (light touch, pain) and deep sensations (muscle and joint pain, muscle and joint position) (Hudak *et al.* 1982; Fuller 1993).

Vital signs

It is recommended that assessments of vital signs should be made in the following order:

1 Respirations
2 Temperature
3 Blood pressure
4 Pulse.

(See also Ch. 25, Observations.)

Respirations

Of these four vital signs, respiratory patterns give the clearest indication of how the brain is functioning because the complex process of respiration is controlled by more than one area of the brain. Any disease or injury that affects these areas may produce respiratory changes. The rate, character and pattern of a patient's respiration must be noted. Abnormal respiratory patterns are listed in Table 26.3.

Constant re-evaluation of the patient's ability to maintain and protect their airway is a concern when the GCS score is less than 8. At this stage, muscles often become flaccid and the use of the recovery position and airway adjuncts may need to be considered. Patients who have deteriorated may require artificial respiration in order to protect the airway from aspiration. Close working liaison with physiotherapists and speech and language therapists is important to minimize the danger of chest infections.

Temperature

Damage to the hypothalamus, the temperature-regulating centre, may result in grossly fluctuating temperatures (Nikas 1982).

Blood pressure, pulse and respirations

Observations of blood pressure, pulse and respirations will provide evidence of increased intracranial pressure.

Table 26.3 Abnormal respiratory patterns

Type	Pattern	Significance
Cheyne–Stokes	Rhythmic waxing and waning of both rate and depth of respirations, alternating regularly with briefer periods of apnoea. Greater than normal respiration, i.e. 16–24 breaths per minute.	May indicate deep cerebral or cerebellar lesions, usually bilateral; may occur with upper brainstem involvement
Central neurogenic hyperventilation	Sustained, regular, rapid respirations, with forced inspiration and expiration	May indicate a lesion of the low midbrain or upper pons areas of the brainstem
Apnoeustic	Prolonged inspiration with a pause at full inspiration; there may also be expiratory pauses	May indicate a lesion of the lower pons or upper medulla, hypoglycaemia or drug-induced respiratory depression
Cluster breathing	Clusters of irregular respirations alternating with longer periods of apnoea	May indicate a lesion of lower pons or upper medulla
Ataxic breathing	A completely irregular pattern with random deep and shallow respirations; irregular pauses may also appear	May indicate a lesion of the medulla

Table 26.4 Frequency of observations

Category	Frequency	Rationale
All patients diagnosed as suffering from neurological or neurosurgical conditions	At least 4-hourly, affected by the patient's condition	To monitor the condition of the patient so that any necessary action can be instigated
Unconscious patients (including ventilated and anaesthetized patients)	Frequency indicated by patient's condition	To monitor the condition closely and to detect trends so that appropriate action may be taken

When intracranial pressure is greater than 33 mmHg for even a short time, cerebral blood flow is significantly reduced. The resulting ischaemia stimulates the vasomotor centre, causing systemic blood pressure to rise. The patient becomes bradycardic and the respiratory rate falls. Abnormalities of blood pressure and pulse usually occur late, after the patient's level of consciousness has begun to deteriorate. This change in the blood pressure was first described by Cushing and is known as the Cushing reflex (Nikas 1982).

Frequency of observations

The frequency and type of neurological observation are matters of much debate (Price 2002). It is therefore not possible to be prescriptive, as the frequency will depend on the underlying pathology and possible consequences. For example, in a patient with a head injury and a skull fracture, there may be bruising to the brain (contusion), cerebral oedema and an extradural haemorrhage that will increase in size. The bruising and oedema may develop over a couple of days and gradually give rise to subtle neurological changes, whilst the extradural haemorrhage can develop very quickly and cause profound neurological changes over a matter of a few hours. Therefore such a patient may require frequent 30-minute GCS observations for the first 6 hours followed by 1–2-hourly observations for a further 48 hours. The nurse must be competent and take appropriate action if changes in the patient's neurological status occur, as well as reporting any subtle signs that may indicate deterioration, e.g. if the patient is incontinent, reluctant to eat, drink or initiate interaction. It should never be assumed that difficulty to rouse a patient is due to night-time sleep as even a deeply asleep patient with no focal deficit should respond to pain. Therefore if the patient requires an increased amount of stimulus to achieve the same GCS score, this may also be a pointer to subtle deterioration (see Table 26.4).

General points

The initial assessment of a patient should include a history (taken from relatives or friends if appropriate) including noting changes in: mood, intellect, memory and personality, since these may be indicators of a longstanding problem, e.g. brain tumour (Barker 1990).

Visual acuity

This may be tested using Snellen's chart or newspaper prints, with and without glasses if worn.

Visual fields

Lesions at different points in the visual pathways affect vision (Table 26.5). It should be noted that loss of vision is always described with reference to the visual fields rather than the retinal fields (Weldon 1998).

Table 26.5 Visual pathways (from Fuller 1993)

Defect	Implication
Monocular field defects	Lesion anterior to optic chiasm
Bitemporal field defects	Lesion at the optic chiasm
Homonymous field defects	Lesion behind the optic chiasm
Congruous homonymous field defects	Lesion behind lateral geniculate bodies

Procedure guidelines: **Neurological observations and assessment**

Note: the following describes a full neurological assessment. It may be inappropriate, unnecessary or impossible for the nurse to carry out all of the procedures every time the patient is observed.

Equipment

1 Pencil torch.
2 Thermometer.
3 Sphygmomanometer.
4 Tongue depressor.

5 Low-linting swabs.
6 Patella hammer.
7 Neurotips (refer to action 27).
8 Two test tubes (refer to action 28).

Procedure

Action	Rationale
1 Inform the patient, whether conscious or not, and explain and discuss the observations.	Sense of hearing is frequently unimpaired even in unconscious patients. It is important, as far as is possible, that the patient understands the procedure and gives his/her valid consent.
2 Talk to the patient. Note whether he/she is alert and is giving full attention or whether he/she is restless or lethargic and drowsy. Ask the patient who he/she is, the correct day, month and year, where he/she is, and to give details about family.	To establish whether the patient's level of consciousness is deteriorating. If the patient is becoming disorientated, changes will occur in this order: (a) Disorientation as to time (b) Disorientation as to place (c) Disorientation as to person.
3 Ask the patient to squeeze and release your fingers (include both sides of the body) and then to stick out the tongue.	To evaluate motor responses and to ensure that the response is not a reflex.
4 If the patient does not respond, apply painful stimuli. Suggested methods have been discussed earlier.	Responses grow less purposeful as the patient's level of consciousness deteriorates. As the condition worsens, the patient may no longer localize pain and respond to it in a purposeful way (Vernberg *et al.* 1983).
5 Record, precisely, the findings. Write exactly what stimulus was used, where it was applied, how much pressure was needed to elicit a response, and how the patient responded.	Vague terms can be easily misinterpreted. Record the patient's best response (Allen 1984).
6 Ask the patient to open their eyes. If the patient cannot do so, hold the eyelids open and note the size, shape and equality of the pupils.	To assess the size, shape and equality of the pupils as an indication of brain damage. Normal pupils are spherical, usually at mid-position and have a diameter ranging from 1.5 to 6 mm (Nikas 1982).
7 Darken the room, if necessary, or shield the patient's eyes with your hands.	To enable a better view of the eye.

Procedure guidelines: Neurological observations and assessment (cont'd)

Action	Rationale
8 Hold each eyelid open in turn. Move torch towards the patient from the side. Shine it directly into the eye. This should cause the pupil to constrict promptly.	To assess the reaction of the pupils to light. A normal reaction indicates no lesions in the area of the brainstem regulating pupil constriction.
9 Hold both eyelids open but shine the light into one eye only. The pupil into which the light is not shone should also constrict.	To assess consensual light reflex. Prompt constriction indicates intact connections between the brainstem areas regulating pupil constriction (Scherer 1986)
10 Record unusual eye movements.	To assess cranial nerve damage.
11 Extend your hands and ask the patient to squeeze your fingers as hard as possible. Compare grip and strength.	To test grip and ascertain strength. Record best arm in GCS chart to best reflect the potential outcome.
12 Note the rate, character and pattern of the patient's respirations.	Respirations are controlled by different areas of the brain. When disease or injury affects these areas, respiratory changes may occur.
13 Take and record the patient's temperature at specified intervals.	Damage to the hypothalamus, the temperature-regulating centre in the brain, will be reflected in grossly abnormal temperatures.
14 Take and record the patient's blood pressure and pulse at specified intervals.	To monitor signs of increased intracranial pressure. Hypertension and bradycardia usually occur late, after the patient's level of consciousness has begun to deteriorate. Call for medical assistance as soon as it is evident that there is a deterioration in the patient's level of consciousness (Scherer 1986; Tortora & Grabowski 1996).
15 Ask the patient to close the eyes and hold the arms straight out in front, with palms upwards, for 20–30 seconds. The weaker limb will 'fall away'.	To show weakness in limbs.
16 Stand in front of the patient and extend your hands. Ask the patient to push and pull against your hands. Ask the patient to lie on his/her back in bed. Place the patient's leg with knee flexed and foot resting on the bed. Instruct the patient to keep the foot down as you attempt to extend the leg. Flex the knee and place your hand in the flexion. Instruct the patient to straighten the leg while you offer resistance. *Note*: if a patient cannot follow the instruction due to a language barrier or unconsciousness, observe spontaneous movements and note how strong they appear. Then, if necessary, apply painful stimuli.	To test arm strength. If one arm drifts downwards or turns inwards, it may indicate hemiparesis. To test flexion and extension strength in the patient's extremities by having patient push and pull against your resistance.
17 Flex and extend all the patient's limbs. Note how well the movements are resisted.	To test muscle tone.
18 Ask the patient to pat the thigh as fast as possible. Note whether the movements seem slow or clumsy. Ask the patient to turn the hand over and back several times in succession. Evaluate co-ordination. Ask the patient to touch the back of the fingers with the thumb in sequence rapidly.	To assess hand and arm co-ordination. The dominant hand should perform better.
19 Extend one of your hands towards the patient. Ask the patient to touch your index finger, then his/her nose, several times in succession. Repeat the test with the patient's eyes closed.	To assess hand and arm co-ordination/cerebellar function.
20 Ask the patient to place a heel on the opposite knee and slide it down the shin to the foot. Check each leg separately.	To assess leg co-ordination.

Procedure guidelines: Neurological observations and assessment (cont'd)

Action	Rationale
21 Ask the patient to look up or hold the eyelid open. With your hand, approach the eye unexpectedly or touch the eyelashes.	To test the blink reflex.
22 Ask the patient to open the mouth, and hold down the tongue with a tongue depressor. Touch the back of the pharynx, on each side, with a low-linting swab.	To test the gag reflex.
23 Ask the patient to lie on his/her back in bed. Place your hand under the knee, raise and flex it. Tap the patellar tendon. Note whether the leg responds.	To assess the deep tendon reflex.
24 Stroke the lateral aspect of the sole of the patient's foot. If the response is abnormal (Babinski's response), the big toe will dorsiflex and the remaining toes will fan out.	To assess for upper motor neurone lesion.
25 Ask the patient to read something aloud. Check each eye separately. If vision is so poor that the patient is unable to read, ask the patient to count your upraised fingers or distinguish light from dark.	To test the visual acuity.
26 Occlude the ear with a low-linting swab. Stand a short way from the patient. Whisper numbers into the open ear. Ask for feedback. Repeat for both ears.	To test hearing and comprehension.
27 Ask the patient to close the eyes. Using the point of a Neurotip, stroke the skin. Use the blunt end occasionally. Ask patient to tell you what is felt. See if the patient can distinguish between sharp and dull sensations.	To test superficial sensations to pain.
28 Ask the patient to close the eyes. Fill two test tubes with water: one warm, one cold. Touch the patient's skin with each test tube and ask patient to distinguish between them.	To test superficial sensations to temperature.
29 Stroke a low-linting swab lightly over the patient's skin. Ask the patient to say what he/she feels.	To test superficial sensations to touch.
30 Ask the patient to close the eyes. Hold the tip of one of the patient's fingers between your thumb and index finger. Move it up and down and ask the patient to say in which direction it is moving. Repeat with the other hand. For the legs, hold the big toe.	To test proprioception (Netter 1975; Tortora & Grabowski 1996). *Definition of proprioception*: the receipt of information from muscles and tendons to the labyrinth that enables the brain to determine movements and the position of the body.

Emergency

31 Should seizures (epilepsy/fits) occur, maintain airway if possible by placing the patient in the recovery position. Do not insert artificial airway into patient's mouth during the tonic/clonic phase.	To maintain patient's safety and to assist in the diagnosis of any underlying pathology.
Record type of seizure, duration, any warning (aura) or incontinence the patient may have, as well as any postictal (after the fit) weakness (Todd's paralysis) or increase in drowsiness.	
Ensure the patient is closely observed until back to previous conscious level prior to ictus (fit).	
Anticonvulsants may be required as prescribed.	

References and further reading

Abelson, N.M. (1982) Observation of the neurosurgical patient. *Curiatonis*, **5**(3), 32–7.

Addison, C. & Crawford, B. (1999) Not bad, just misunderstood. *Nurs Times*, **95**, 52–3.

Allen, D. (1984) Glasgow Coma Scale. *Nurs Mirror*, **158**(2), 32.

Aucken & Crawford, (1998) Neurological observations. In: *Neuro-Oncology for Nurses* (ed. D. Guerrero). Whurr, London, pp. 29–65.

Barker, E. (1990) Brain tumour: frightening diagnosis, nursing challenge. *Registered Nurse*, **53**(9), 46–56.

Frawley, P. (1990) Neurological observations. *Nurs Times*, **86**(35), 29–34.

Fuller, G. (1993) *Neurological Examinations Made Easy*. Churchill Livingstone, Edinburgh.

Hudak, C.M. *et al.* (1982) Nervous system. In: *Critical Care Nursing*, 3rd edn (ed. B. Fuller). Lippincott, New Jersey, pp. 321–34.

Hudak, C.M. *et al.* (1982) Pathophysiology of CNS. In: *Critical care Nursing*, 3rd edn (ed. B. Fuller). Lippincott, New Jersey, pp. 335–48.

Hudak, C.M. *et al.* (1982) Management modalities. In: *Critical Care Nursing*, 3rd edn (ed. B. Fuller). Lippincott, New Jersey, pp. 349–78.

Hudak, C.M. *et al.* (1982) Assessment skills. In: *Critical Care Nursing*, 3rd edn (ed. B. Fuller). Lippincott, New Jersey, pp. 379–89.

Jennett, B. & Teasdale (1984) *An Introduction to Neurosurgery*, 4th edn. William Heinemann Medical Books, London, pp. 23–9.

Lindsay, K.W., Bone, I. & Callander, R. (1997) *Neurology and Neurosurgery Illustrated*, 3rd edn. Churchill Livingstone, Edinburgh.

Martin, E.A. (1996) *Oxford Concise Colour Medical Dictionary*. Oxford University Press, Oxford.

Netter, F.H. (1975) *IHL Printing of CIBA Collection of Medical Illustrations, Volume 1, Nervous System*. CIBA, Summit, New Jersey, pp. 58–9.

Nikas, D. (ed.) (1982) *The Critically Ill Neurosurgical Patient*. Churchill Livingstone, New York, pp. 1–27, 77–80, 100–103.

Price, T. (2002) Painful stimuli and the Glasgow Coma Scale. *Nurs Crit Care*, **7**(1), 17–23.

Scherer, P. (1986) The logic of coma. *Am J Nurs*, 542–9.

Shah, S. (1999) Neurological assessment. *Nurs Times*, **13**, 49–56.

Tortora, G.J. & Grabowski, S.R. (1996) *Principles of Anatomy and Physiology*, 8th edn. Harper Collins, London.

Vernberg, K. *et al.* (1983) The Glasgow Coma Scale: how do you rate? *Nurse Educ*, **8**(3), 33–7.

Weldon, K. (1998) Neurological observations. In: *Neuro-Oncology for Nurses* (ed. D. Guerrero). Whurr, London, pp. 1–28.

Pain management and assessment

Chapter contents

Definition

Pain is not a simple sensation but a complex phenomenon having both a physical and an affective (emotional) component. Because pain is subjective the favoured definition for use in clinical practice, proposed originally by McCaffery (1968), is: 'Pain is whatever the experiencing person says it is, existing whenever the experiencing person says it does'.

Reference material

There are several ways to categorize the types of pain that occur but it is important to recognize that patients may experience both acute and chronic pain. Foley (1998) describes the following types of pain, which are also recognized by McCaffery & Beebe (1989).

Acute pain

The International Association for the Study of Pain (IASP) has defined acute pain as 'pain of recent onset and probable limited duration. It usually has an identifiable temporal and causal relationship to injury or disease' (Ready & Edwards 1992).

Chronic pain

Chronic pain is usually prolonged and defined as pain that exists for more than 3 months (International Association for the Study of Pain 1996). It is often associated with major changes in personality, lifestyle and functional ability (Foley 1998).

In addition, it is essential to mention episodic, incident and breakthrough pains, which are all terms referring to 'a transitory exacerbation of pain experienced by the patient who has relatively stable and adequately controlled baseline pain' (Hanks 1991). The breakthrough pain experienced by the patient is when the regular opioid regimen used for baseline pain fails to provide adequate analgesic cover. During pain assessment it is essential that nurses include exploration of this type of pain.

Assessment of pain

Assessment is a key step in the process of managing pain. The aim of assessment is to identify all the factors – physical and non-physical – that affect the patient's perception of pain. A comprehensive clinical assessment is essential to gain a thorough understanding of the patient's pain and as a means to evaluate the effectiveness of interventions.

Acute pain assessment for surgical patients

For surgical pain to be controlled effectively, pain must be assessed regularly and systematically. The process of pain assessment begins before surgery and continues through to discharge.

Assessment of anxiety, meaning of pain and past pain experience

A number of psychosocial factors influence an individual's pain. Patients may be anxious about the outcome of the surgery or how pain will be controlled, particularly if they have bad memories of previous pain experiences (Audit Commission 1997). Anxiety in turn exacerbates pain by increasing muscle tension. Providing patients with appropriate support and information to address these concerns can reduce both anxiety and postoperative pain (Audit Commission 1997).

Assessment of pre-existing pain

Patients who have been taking regular strong analgesics for a pre-existing chronic pain problem may require higher doses of analgesia to manage an acute pain episode (Macintyre 2001). It is therefore important to take a history of pre-existing pain and analgesic use so that appropriate analgesic measures can be planned in advance of surgery.

Assessment of location and intensity of pain

Location

Many complex surgical procedures involve more than one incision site and the nature and extent of pain at each site may vary. A careful assessment of the location and type of pain is required, because each pain problem may respond to different pain management techniques.

Intensity

As part of the assessment process it is important to assess the intensity of pain. Only then can the effects of any intervention be evaluated and care modified as appropriate. The simplest techniques for pain measurement involve the use of a visual analogue scale, verbal rating scale or numerical rating scale. Using one of these scales, patients are asked to match pain intensity to the scale.

Three principles apply to the use of these scales:

- The patient must be involved in scoring his/her own pain intensity. This is important because professionals frequently underestimate the intensity of a patient's pain (Scott 1994; Field 1996; Drayer *et al.* 1999).
- Pain intensity should be assessed on movement because patients need to be able to move comfortably to prevent immobility and its associated complications, e.g. deep vein thrombosis (Macintyre & Ready 2001).
- It is important to remember that a complete picture of a patient's pain cannot be derived solely from the use of a pain scale (Lawler 1997). Ongoing communication with the patient is required to uncover and manage any psychosocial factors that may be affecting the patient's pain experience.

Chronic pain assessment

The nature of chronic pain means that at times it can be difficult to assess, as patients rarely present with this one symptom. For example, approximately two-thirds of advanced cancer patients will also complain of anorexia, one-half will have a symptomatic dry mouth and constipation, and one-third will suffer nausea, vomiting, insomnia, dyspnoea, cough or oedema (Donnelly & Walsh 1995). It will be clear from these figures that chronic pain assessment cannot be seen in isolation; identification of all related symptoms is of equal importance as they will contribute to a lowered pain threshold (the lowest stimulus intensity at which a person perceives pain) and impaired pain tolerance (the greatest stimulus intensity causing pain that a person is prepared to tolerate) (Grond *et al.* 1996). Seventy-five per cent of cancer patients present with pain, 33% of whom will have pain in three or more sites (Grond *et al.* 1996). Furthermore, chronic cancer pain is often multifocal.

A diagnosis of cancer does not necessarily mean that the malignant process is the cause of the pain. Pain in chronic cancer may be:

- Caused by the cancer itself
- Caused by treatment
- Associated with debilitating disease, such as a pressure ulcer
- Unrelated to either the disease or the treatment, such as headache.

The cause of *each* pain should therefore be identified carefully; many pains unrelated to the cancer will respond to specific treatment. If the pain is due to the cancer,

Table 27.1 Factors affecting pain sensitivity

Sensitivity increased:	Sensitivity lowered:
Discomfort	Relief of symptoms
Insomnia	Sleep
Fatigue	Rest
Anxiety	Sympathy
Fear	Understanding
Anger	Companionship
Sadness	Diversional activity
Depression	Reduction in anxiety
Boredom	Elevation of mood

then it is important to determine the precise mechanism of pain because treatment will vary accordingly.

The perception of painful stimuli will always be modulated by the emotional response to that perception. Changes in mood may alter considerably the experience of pain (McCaffery & Beebe 1989). Gray (2001) noted a link between chronic pain and depression. Social and psychological factors will also affect the severity and perception of pain. Pain assessment needs to acknowledge these facts and particular attention must be paid to factors that will modulate pain sensitivity (Table 27.1).

Assessment tools for acute and chronic pain

Accurate pain assessment is a prerequisite of effective control and is an essential component of nursing care. In the assessment process, the nurse gathers information from the patient that allows an understanding of the patient's experience and its effect on the patient's life. The information obtained guides the nurse in planning and evaluating strategies for care. Pain is rarely static; therefore its assessment is not a one-time process but is ongoing.

Pain assessment is difficult to achieve. For example, the tendency suggested by both research and clinical practice is for the patient not to report any pain or to do so inadequately or inaccurately, minimizing the pain experience (McCaffery & Beebe 1989). Hunt *et al.* (1977) found that nurses tended to overestimate the pain relief obtained from analgesia and underestimate the level of the patient's pain. It has also been suggested that nurses do not possess sufficient knowledge to care for patients in pain (McCaffery & Ferrell 1997; Drayer *et al.* 1999).

Pain charts are useful tools for assisting nurses to assess pain and plan nursing care. They enable pain to be successfully assessed and monitored (Walker 1987; McCaffery & Beebe 1989; Twycross *et al.* 1996) and improve communication between staff and patients (Raiman 1986). Higginson (1998) notes that 'taking assessments directly from the patient is the most valid

way of collecting information on their quality of life'. Encouraging patients to take an active role in their pain assessment by using pain charts helps to increase their confidence and makes them feel part of the pain management process.

Some degree of caution, however, must be exercised with the use of pain charts. The nurse must be careful to select the tool that is most appropriate for a particular type of pain experience. For example, it would not be appropriate to use a pain assessment chart that had been designed for use with patients with chronic pain, to assess postoperative pain. Furthermore, pain charts should not be used totally indiscriminately. Walker *et al.* (1987) found that charts appeared to have little value in cases of unresolved or intractable pain.

The use of pain assessment tools for acute pain has been shown both to increase the effectiveness of nursing interventions and to improve the management of pain (Scott 1994; Harmer & Davies 1998). Several pain assessment tools are available (Kitson 1994). Since many of these focus on assessing the intensity of pain, it is important that nurses do not neglect to combine their use of these tools with an assessment of the patient's psychosocial needs.

The most commonly used pain assessment tools meet the following criteria (Hancock 1996):

- Simplicity – ease of understanding for all the patient groups
- Reliability – reliability of the tool when used in similar patient groups
- Sensitivity – sensitivity of the tool to the patient's pain
- Accuracy – accurate recording of data through patient involvement
- Practicality – a practical tool is more likely to be used by patients and nursing staff.

For practical purposes, a combined pain assessment and observation chart is frequently used in the postoperative period. The Royal Marsden Hospital Postoperative Observation and Pain Assessment Chart is an example of one of these (Fig. 27.1). The patient's assessment of their pain is recorded on the pain scale at the bottom of the chart at the same time that other observations are carried out (usually 2–4 hourly but more frequently if pain is not controlled).

A study was carried out at The Royal Marsden Hospital in order to design a chart for use with patients with chronic cancer pain and to evaluate its effectiveness (Walker *et al.* 1987). The study indicated that the chart was a valuable tool for pain assessment in 98% of cases. The chart has recently been updated following a review by nursing staff at The Royal Marsden Hospital (Fig. 27.2).

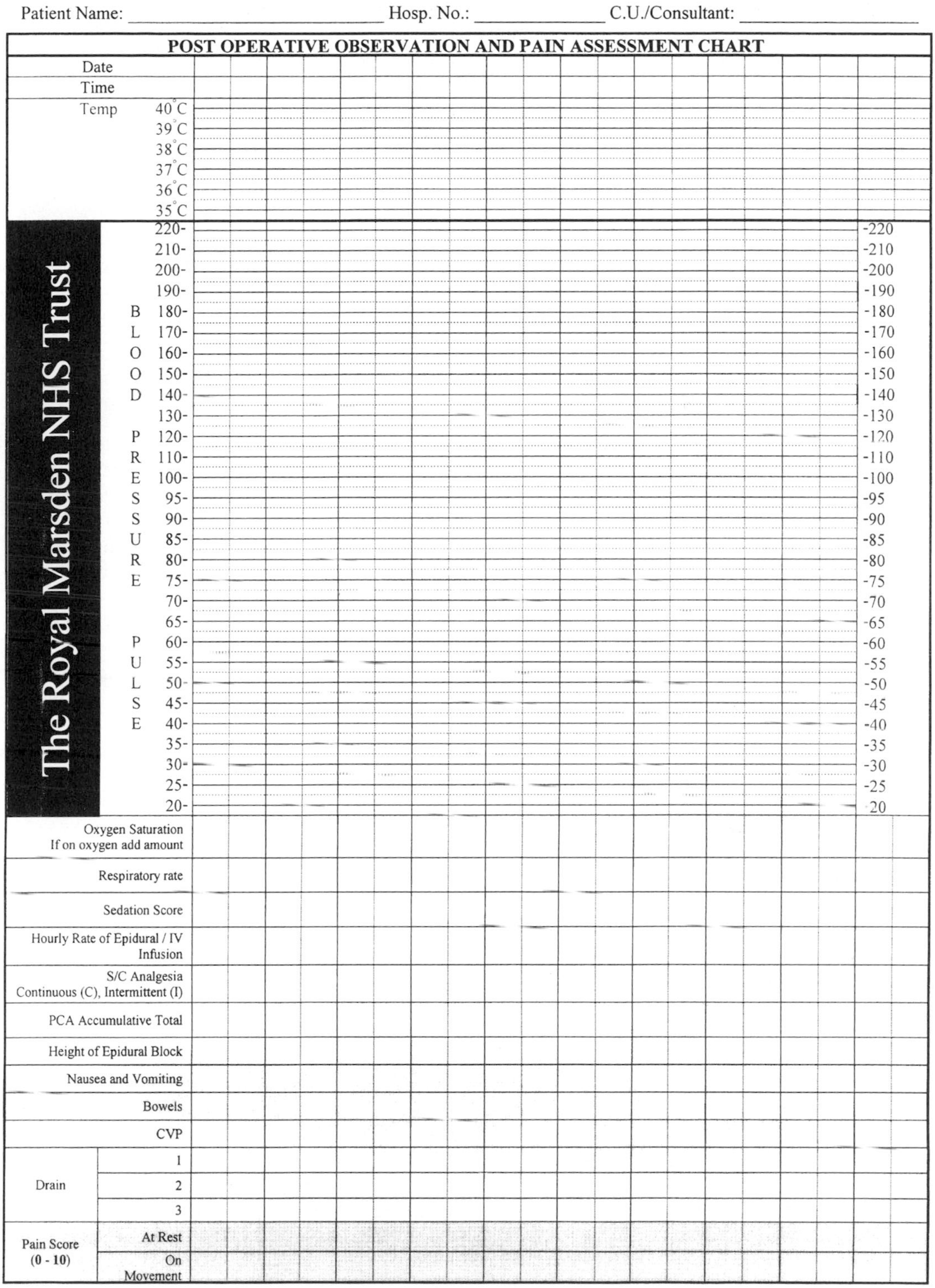

Patient Name: _____ Hosp. No.: _____ C.U./Consultant: _____

POST OPERATIVE OBSERVATION AND PAIN ASSESSMENT CHART																					
Date																					
Time																					
Temp	40°C																				
	39°C																				
	38°C																				
	37°C																				
	36°C																				
	35°C																				

The Royal Marsden NHS Trust

BLOOD PRESSURE / PULSE chart:

220- / -220
210- / -210
200- / -200
190- / -190
B 180- / -180
L 170- / -170
O 160- / -160
O 150- / -150
D 140- / -140
130- / -130
P 120- / -120
R 110- / -110
E 100- / -100
S 95- / -95
S 90- / -90
U 85- / -85
R 80- / -80
E 75- / -75
70- / -70
65- / -65
P 60- / -60
U 55- / -55
L 50- / -50
S 45- / -45
E 40- / -40
35- / -35
30- / -30
25- / -25
20- / -20

Oxygen Saturation If on oxygen add amount																					
Respiratory rate																					
Sedation Score																					
Hourly Rate of Epidural / IV Infusion																					
S/C Analgesia Continuous (C), Intermittent (I)																					
PCA Accumulative Total																					
Height of Epidural Block																					
Nausea and Vomiting																					
Bowels																					
CVP																					
Drain	1																				
	2																				
	3																				
Pain Score (0 - 10)	At Rest																				
	On Movement																				

Figure 27.1 The Royal Marsden Hospital Postoperative Observation and Pain Assessment Chart.

The Royal Marsden NHS Trust
Patient Held Pain Chart

Surname:

Who completed the assessment:
(specify if nurse or family member helped)

First name:

Date of this assessment:

Instructions for use:

1. This chart is for you to complete (you may want your family or a nurse to help you)

2. Work through the questions in section 1 and 2 of the chart. Do ask for help if you are not clear about any of the questions.

3. When you get to section 3 use the instructions at the top of the sheet to help you keep an ongoing record of your pain and the effect of any pain treatments.

Please keep this chart with you because the nurses and doctors who are looking after you will use it to help manage your pain(s)

Section 1: Where is your pain?

Please draw on the body outlines below to show where you feel pain. Label each site A, B, C, etc. or use a different colour

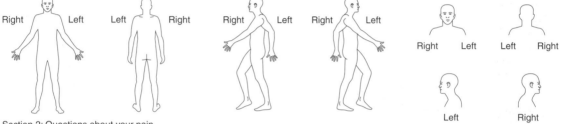

Section 2: Questions about your pain

How would you describe your pain(s) at the site(s) you drew on the body diagram? (e.g. aching, tender, sharp, shooting, burning).

What helps reduce your pain(s) at each site? (e.g. specific drugs, activities or treatments such as massage).

What makes your pain worse at each site? (e.g. specific activity or heat/cold).

How often do you get pain at each site? (e.g. all the time or at different times during the day).

How do you feel when you are in pain and how has it changed your daily activities? (e.g. moving, sleeping).

Section 3: Scoring and recording your pain scores

Pain Scores
0 = No pain
1–4 = Mild pain
5–6 = Moderate pain
7–9 = Severe pain
10 = Worst pain imaginable

Instructions for scoring and recording pain scores

1) In the column marked **Pain scores** use the scoring system shown here to record your pain score(s) at each site (see columns A, B, C, etc.) where you feel pain.
2) Score your pain at regular intervals. Do this before you take your pain treatments (e.g. analgesics/pain medicines, massage) and 30–45 minutes afterwards so that you can see if they have helped.

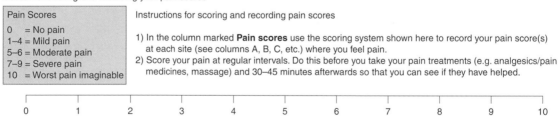

Date	Time	Pain scores Colours or A B C D	Analgesics (pain medicines) Write down any analgesics taken to reduce pain	Other treatments to reduce pain Write down other measures used to reduce pain (e.g. positioning relaxation, massage)	Factors influencing pain Write down any factors influencing pain (e.g. activity, rest) and how they affect the pain	Evaluation and comments Assess or evaluate how well the analgesics or other treatments worked to reduce the pain

Figure 27.2 The Royal Marsden Hospital Chronic Pain Assessment Chart.

The need for effective pain control

There are several reasons why pain needs to be well controlled following surgery, not least that patients have a right to expect good pain control (Audit Commission 1997). Uncontrolled pain can lead to increased anxiety and muscle tension which further exacerbate pain. It can delay the recovery process by hindering mobilization and deep breathing, which increases the risk of a patient developing a deep vein thrombosis, chest infection or pressure ulcer (Macintyre & Ready 2001). With severe pain, activity of the sympathetic nervous system and the neuroendocrine 'stress response' cause platelet activation, changes in regional blood flow and stress on the heart. These can lead to impaired wound healing and myocardial ischaemia (Macintyre & Ready 2001). There is evidence to suggest that in the long term, poorly controlled acute pain may lead to the development of chronic pain. Tasmuth *et al.* (1996) found that patients who went on to develop chronic pain following surgically treated breast cancer remembered having more severe postoperative pain than those women who had no chronic pain.

Management of pain

The control of pain is directed by the 'Analgesic Ladder' which was presented by the World Health Organization in 1996 (Fig. 27.3). The simple principles are such that pharmacological intervention begins on the first step of the ladder and proceeds upwards as and when the pain reaches a higher level and the current analgesia is no longer effective. Analgesia should be administered 'around the clock' (ATC) to enable chronic persistent pain to be controlled. It is important to remember that the patient will experience different types of pain due to different aetiological and physiological changes, manifested through the cancer trajectory (e.g. bone pain,

neuropathic pain). It is important to make an assessment of each pain separately, since the pain may need to be managed in a different manner and one analgesic intervention will rarely be sufficient. Often the best practice is to combine the baseline analgesia with an appropriate adjuvant treatment in order to achieve maximum pain control (Table 27.2).

Oral administration of therapeutic interventions may not always be appropriate. In chronic pain the European Association of Palliative Care (EAPC) recommends that if patients can no longer manage the oral route, the preferred alternative route is subcutaneous, which is simple and less painful than the intramuscular route (Hanks *et al.* 2001).

Accurate ongoing assessment is imperative for efficient and effective pain control.

The management of pain following surgery

Since nurses, surgeons, anaesthetists, pain specialists, pharmacists and physiotherapists are all involved in the management of surgical pain, teamwork is essential. Professionals must reach clear agreement as to their individual roles so that patients receive the best possible

Table 27.2 The use of adjuvant drugs (co-analgesics)

Type	Use	Examples
Non-steroidal anti-inflammatory drugs (NSAID)	Bone pain Muscular pain Inflammation Visceral pain	Diclofenac Naproxen Rofecoxib Celecoxib
Steroids	Pressure Bone pain Inflammation Raised intracranial pressure	Dexamethasone Prednisolone
Tricyclic antidepressants	Neuropathic pain	Amitriptyline
Anticonvulsants		Sodium valproate Carbamazepine Gabapentin
Antibiotics	Infection	Flucloxacillin Trimethoprim
Benzodiazepines	Anxiety	Diazepam
Antispasmodics	Spasms	Baclofen
Bisphosphonates	Bone pain	Sodium clodronate Disodium pamidronate

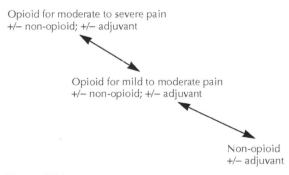

Opioid for moderate to severe pain
+/– non-opioid; +/– adjuvant

Opioid for mild to moderate pain
+/– non-opioid; +/– adjuvant

Non-opioid
+/– adjuvant

Figure 27.3 The Analgesic Ladder. (Modified from World Health Organization 1996.)

care from preadmission through to discharge (Audit Commission 1997).

A wide variety of pharmacological and non-pharmacological techniques are available for the management of surgical pain. The following basic principles apply to their use:

1 Tailor the treatments to:
   (a) Meet individual needs
   (b) Prevent pain, rather than allowing it to become established.
2 Whenever possible, choose the simplest and safest techniques to achieve the desired level of pain relief (McQuay *et al.* 1997).
3 Use the WHO Analgesic Ladder (Fig. 27.3) to select the most appropriate analgesics for mild, moderate and severe acute pain.
4 Choose the most appropriate route for giving analgesia.
5 Combine techniques to provide balanced analgesia and enhance overall pain control (Kehlet 1997).
6 Ensure patients receive regular antiemetics to control postoperative nausea and vomiting. Vomiting increases muscle tension and exacerbates pain.

Acute pain

Pharmacological techniques

Opioid analgesics

Opioids are the first-line treatment for pain that follows major surgery. The key principle for the safe and effective use of opioids is for the dose to be titrated to achieve pain relief while minimizing any unwanted side-effects (McQuay *et al.* 1997; see 'Chronic pain' section for further details on side-effects).

A number of opioids are used for controlling pain following surgery. These include morphine, diamorphine and fentanyl. The most common routes of opioid administration are intravenous, epidural, subcutaneous, intramuscular or oral.

Intravenous analgesia

Continuous intravenous infusions of opioids such as morphine, diamorphine and fentanyl are effective for controlling pain in the immediate postoperative period. Their use is often restricted to critical care units where patients can be closely monitored because of the potential risk of respiratory depression (Macintyre & Ready 2001).

Patient-controlled analgesia (PCA) is an alternative and safer technique for giving intravenous opioids (usually morphine) in the ward environment (Sidebotham *et al.* 1997). With PCA, patients self-administer intermittent

doses of opioids, by using an infusion pump and timing device. When in pain, the patient presses a button connected to the pump and a set dose of opioid is delivered (usually intravenously but it may also be given subcutaneously) to the patient (Macintyre & Ready 2001).

There are a number of advantages of using PCA.

• PCA is more likely to maintain reasonably constant blood concentrations of the opioid within the analgesic corridor. This is the blood level where analgesia is achieved without significant side-effects. The flexibility of PCA helps to overcome the wide interpatient variation in opioid requirements (Macintyre & Ready 2001).
• PCA allows patients to titrate analgesia against daily variations in the pain stimulus (Tye & Gell-Walker 2000). By using a PCA pump, patients can administer analgesia as soon as pain occurs and titrate the dose of analgesia according to increases and decreases in the pain stimulus. This is particularly helpful for controlling more intense pain during movement.
• PCA prevents delays in patients receiving analgesics.

Whilst PCA may be very effective for controlling pain for a number of patients undergoing surgery (Macintyre 2001), it is not suitable for the following groups (Tye & Gell-Walker 2000):

• Patients who are unable to activate the PCA device due to problems with dexterity or visual impairment
• Patients who are unable to understand the concept of PCA, particularly the very young or patients who are confused
• Patients who do not wish to take responsibility for their pain control.

For further details about the use of PCA pumps refer to Ch. 11, Drug administration: delivery (infusion devices).

Epidural analgesia

Low concentrations of local anaesthetics and opioids can be infused directly into the epidural space using a catheter. Giving analgesia epidurally is a particularly valuable technique for the prevention of postoperative pain in patients undergoing major thoracic, abdominal and lower limb surgery. Commonly used opioids for epidural analgesia include fentanyl and diamorphine (Wheatley *et al.* 2001). Further details of this technique are given in Ch. 29, Pain management: epidural analgesia.

Subcutaneous analgesia

Opioids are often given subcutaneously to manage chronic cancer pain. More recently, there has been an increase in the use of subcutaneous opioids for postoperative pain control. Both PCA- and nurse-administered opioid injections of morphine and diamorphine via an indwelling subcutaneous cannula have been used successfully to manage postoperative pain (Vijayan 1997). An advantage of giving analgesia subcutaneously is that it avoids the problems associated with maintaining intravenous access.

Intramuscular analgesia

Until the early 1990s regular 3–4-hourly intramuscular injections of opioids such as pethidine, morphine or preparations containing morphine (Omnopon) were routinely used for the management of postoperative pain. Because alternative techniques such as PCA and epidural analgesia are available, intramuscular analgesia is now used less frequently. Some useful algorithms have been developed to give guidance on titrating intramuscular analgesia (Harmer & Davies 1998; Macintyre & Ready 2001).

Oral analgesia

Oral opioids are used less frequently in the immediate postoperative period because most patients are nil by mouth for a period of time. Often this route is used if patients require strong analgesics following discontinuation of epidural or intravenous analgesia. Morphine is an ideal oral preparation because it is available as a tablet (Sevredol) or an elixir (Oramorph).

Weak opioid and non-opioid analgesics

Paracetamol and paracetamol combinations

The use of non-opioid analgesics such as paracetamol or paracetamol combined with a weak opioid such as codeine is recommended for managing pain following minor surgical procedures or when the pain following major surgery begins to subside (McQuay et al. 1997). Paracetamol can also be given rectally if the oral route is contraindicated.

Paracetamol taken in the correct dose of not more than 4 g per day is relatively free of side-effects. When used in combination with codeine preparations, the most frequent side-effect is constipation.

Tramadol

Another weak opioid, which has been shown to be an effective analgesic for postoperative pain, is tramadol (McQuay & Moore 1998; Reicin et al. 2001). Although tramadol does have some side-effects which include nausea and dizziness, it is free of NSAID side-effects and causes less constipation than codeine preparations and opioids (Bamigbade & Langford 1998).

Non-steroidal anti-inflammatory drugs (NSAIDs)

NSAIDs have been shown to provide better pain relief than paracetamol combinations for acute pain (McQuay et al. 1997). These drugs can be used alone or in combination with both opioid and non-opioid analgesics. Two commonly used NSAIDs are diclofenac, which can be administered either orally or rectally, and ibuprofen, which is available only as an oral preparation. The disadvantage of both of these is that often side-effects such as coagulation problems, renal impairment and gastrointestinal disturbances limit their use. Newer COX 2-specific NSAIDs, such as rofecoxib and celecoxib, have the advantage that they are associated with similar analgesia and anti-inflammatory effects (Reicin et al. 2001) but have no effect on platelets or the gastric mucosa (Rowbotham 2000). As a result coagulation problems and gastrointestinal irritation are likely to be significantly reduced. These drugs will have an important role in the management of both acute and chronic pain in the future.

Nitrous oxide (Entonox)

Inhaled nitrous oxide provides analgesia that is short acting and works quickly. It has a special role in managing pain associated with wound dressings and drain removal (see Ch. 28 on the use of Entonox).

Local anaesthetics

In addition to epidural analgesia, local anaesthetics may be used to block individual or groups of peripheral nerves during surgical procedures and to infiltrate surgical wounds at the end of an operation (Carroll & Bowsher 1993).

Non-pharmacological techniques for acute and chronic pain

Optimal pain control is more likely to be achieved by combining non-pharmacological techniques with pharmacological techniques. Despite the lack of research evidence to support the effectiveness of many non-pharmacological techniques, their benefits to patients and families should not be underestimated.

Psychological interventions

A number of simple psychological interventions can improve a patient's pain control by:

- Reducing anxiety, stress and muscle tension
- Distraction (distraction plays a role in pain management by pushing awareness of pain out of central cognition)
- Increasing control and pain coping mechanisms
- Improving general well-being.

Some simple interventions include the following.

Creating trusting therapeutic relationships

By creating trusting relationships with patients, nurses are instrumental in reducing anxiety and helping patients to cope with pain (Carr & Mann 2000). Nurses can help to create a trusting relationship by:

- Listening to the patient
- Believing the patient's pain experience (Seers 1996)
- Acting as a patient advocate
- Providing patients with appropriate physical and emotional support.

The use of gentle humour
Pasero (1998) suggests that many patients find gentle humour an effective way of coping with pain. Humour may be particularly helpful prior to a painful procedure as it can have a lasting effect. In the clinical setting, humorous tapes, books and videos can be made available for patient use.

Information/education
Patient information/education can make all the difference between effective and ineffective pain relief. Information/ education helps to reduce anxiety (Hayward 1975; Taylor 2001) and enables patients to make informed decisions about their care. Patients should be given specific information about why pain control is important, what to expect in terms of pain relief, how they can participate in their management and what to do if pain is not controlled.

Some caution is required, however, because not all patients respond positively to the same level of information. Patients with high levels of anxiety may find that detailed information can increase their anxiety and influence their pain control. To avoid this patients can be given a choice of whether or not they receive simple or detailed information (Mitchell 1997).

Relaxation
Whilst scientific evidence for the effectiveness of relaxation techniques is limited (Seers & Carroll 1998; Carroll & Seers 1998), a number of studies have shown benefits for patients experiencing pain (Sloman *et al.* 1994; Good *et al.* 1999; Lang *et al.* 2000). Payne (1995) describes several relaxation techniques ranging from simple breathing techniques to progressive muscle relaxation and more complex techniques. One simple relaxation technique script that has been adapted for use at The Royal Marsden Hospital is outlined in Box 27.1. This technique can be taught to patients and used during painful procedures or at times when the patient feels anxious or stressed. Patients should be encouraged to practise the technique to gain mastery.

Music
The use of taped music in the health care setting can also provide relaxation and distraction from pain (Beck 1991; Good 1996; Heiser *et al.* 1997; Good *et al.* 1999).

Box 27.1 Simple relaxation technique script

Please note that breathing during this technique should be normal for the patient in their present condition.

1 Loosen any tight clothing and position yourself comfortably, either lying or sitting. Have your arms and legs uncrossed. Ensure your back and head are well supported.
2 Allow both your hands to rest on your abdomen, one on top of the other. It may be helpful to place a pillow on your lap for your hands to rest on.
3 Gently allow your eyes to close. Breathe normally in and out through your nose if you find this comfortable.
4 As you breathe in, be aware of your abdomen rising gently under your hands (do not force this movement).
5 As you breathe out, be aware of your abdomen relaxing under your hands.
6 Let your shoulders relax and drop down.
7 Let your jaw relax.
8 Now keep your attention softly focused on the rise and fall of your abdomen as this movement follows each breath.
9 Repeat steps 4–8 for between 3 and 5 minutes or longer if appropriate.

During the exercise
As you become aware of any thoughts that arise, let them go and just bring your attention back to the rise and fall of the abdomen. If you are still having difficulty focusing on the technique try saying the following phrases: 'I am relaxed' or 'I feel calm'.

To finish the exercise
Now slowly become aware of your surroundings, stretch out your fingers and toes, gently open your eyes and come back to the room.

Setting up a library of taped music (e.g. easy listening, classical) and having personal stereos available for patient use is a simple way to provide patients with relaxing music.

Art
Art therapies have also been used to assist the patient in moving the focus of attention away from the physical sensation of pain to other aspects of the person (Trauger-Querry & Haghighi 1999). The skills of an art therapist are required to ensure the successful use of this intervention.

Physical interventions

In addition to psychological interventions, a number of physical interventions can be helpful in reducing pain.

Comfort measures
Simple comfort measures such as careful body positioning (for example, supporting a painful arm on a pillow)

and the use of soft and therapeutic mattresses (Ballard 1997) can help to improve patient comfort and pain control.

Exercise

Both passive and active physical exercises may benefit patients by increasing range of motion (Feine & Lund 1997), preventing joint stiffness and muscle wasting which may further compound pain problems. Exercise should always be tailored to the patient's tolerance and stamina. A simple exercise regimen which is practised regularly and supervised by a therapist can help patients feel better and more in control as well as having benefits in terms of pain relief.

Rest

In addition to exercise, teaching patients to rest comfortably in any position when in pain is a meaningful action and the base from which a person can learn to move more easily (O'Connor & Webb 2002). A person with a terminal illness may experience restriction of movement and neuromuscular pain with increased tension. For these patients, learning to rest and letting go of any tension can be helpful. O'Connor & Webb (2002) describe a specific method for resting known as the Feldenkrais method. Using this, a person can be taught how to rest comfortably in any position: this may be lying down, sitting or standing.

Transcutaneous electrical nerve stimulation (TENS)

TENS is thought to work by sending a weak electrical current through the skin to stimulate the sensory nerve endings. Depending on the stimulation parameters used, TENS is thought to modulate pain impulses by closing the gate to pain transmission within the spinal cord by stimulating the release of natural pain-relieving chemicals in the brain and spinal cord (King 1999).

To date there is limited scientific evidence for the effectiveness of TENS. Despite this, many health care professionals use TENS for a variety of chronic pain conditions and support the view that this is a useful form of analgesia (Walsh 1997). In contrast, TENS has not been found to improve the control of acute pain following surgery (McQuay et al. 1997).

Acupuncture

This involves placing fine solid needles into the skin at acupoints or trigger points. Although the exact mechanism of action is unknown, acupuncture is believed to work in part by stimulating release of the body's own natural opioids. Although there is also limited scientific evidence for the pain-relieving effects of acupuncture, largely due to the poorly controlled studies (Ezzo et al. 2000), it is used widely and has an important role in pain management.

Heat therapies

For decades superficial heat therapy has been used to relieve a variety of muscular and joint pains, including arthritis, back pain and period pain. There is much anecdotal and some scientific evidence to support the usefulness of heat as an adjunct to other pain treatments (Akin et al. 2001; Nadler et al. 2002; Welch et al. 2002).

Heat works by:

- Stimulating thermoreceptors in the skin and deeper tissues, thereby reducing the sensitivity to pain by closing the gating system in the spinal cord
- Reducing muscle spasm
- Reducing the viscosity of synovial fluid which alleviates painful stiffness during movement and increases joint range (Carr & Mann 2000).

In the home environment people use a variety of different methods for applying heat therapies, such as warm baths, hot water bottles, wheat-based heat packs and electrical heating pads. In the hospital setting caution is required with this equipment as it does not reach health and safety standards (no even and regular temperature distribution) and there have been incidences of serious burns (Barillo et al. 2000). Carr & Mann (2000) note that heat therapy should not be used immediately following tissue damage as it will increase swelling.

Cold therapies

Cold therapies can also be used to stimulate nerves and modulate pain (Carr & Mann 2000). Cold may be particularly valuable following an acute bruising injury where it can help to reduce inflammation and limit further damage. Cold can be applied in the form of crushed ice or gel-filled cold packs which should be wrapped in a towel to protect the skin from an ice burn.

Chronic pain

Pharmacological techniques

Using the WHO Analgesic Ladder (1996)

The Analgesic Ladder was designed as a framework for the management of chronic pain (Fig. 27.3). There are several drugs available to manage chronic pain and the Analgesic Ladder allows the flexibility to choose from the range according to the patient's requirements and tolerance (Hanks et al. 2001).

Step 1: non-opioid drugs

Examples of non-opioid drugs include paracetamol and aspirin. These drugs are effective in mild to moderate pain, especially musculoskeletal and visceral pain (Twycross & Lack 1990).

Step 2: weak opioids

Examples of weak opioids include co-codamol (codeine 30 and paracetamol 500) and dihydrocodeine (also available in long-acting form). These drugs are used when adequate pain management is not achieved with the use of non-opioids and are usually used in combination formulations. They are equivalent to small doses of strong opioid drugs. It is not recommended to administer another weak opioid from the same group if the drug being used is not controlling the pain. Uncontrolled pain needs to be assessed and managed with the titration of an opioid by moving up the Analgesic Ladder. The exception to this would be if the patient was experiencing intolerable side-effects on the weak opioid and an alternative drug may be beneficial (Hanks 1991).

Tramadol has proved to be useful in the treatment of chronic pain and also has a role in neuropathic pain. It tends to be well tolerated and it is a useful step for those patients who are reluctant to commence morphine (see below), but who have several pain problems. It is available in immediate- and slow-release preparations (Budd 1995; Leppert et al. 2002).

Step 3: strong opioids
Morphine
A large amount of information and research is available concerning morphine and therefore it tends to be the drug of choice within this category (Hanks & Cherny 1998; Hanks et al. 2001). All strong opioids require careful titration from an expert practitioner. It is better to begin with a small dose, usually one that is equivalent to the previous medication, and increase gradually in conjunction with careful assessment of its effectiveness (Hanks et al. 1996, 2001). Titration begins with the immediate-release form which is available in tablet (Sevredol) or elixir (Oramorph) preparations, and once pain control is achieved the patient can be converted to the long-acting sustained release form that acts over a 12- or 24-hour period (MST or MXL respectively).

Breakthrough analgesia is administered using the equivalent 4-hourly dose of the immediate-release form and subsequent adjustments can be made to the long-acting form if the patient is requiring more than three breakthrough doses in a 24-hour period (Hanks et al. 2001).

Patients should be warned of potential side-effects such as constipation, nausea and increased sleepiness, in order to allay any fear. The patient should also be told that nausea and drowsiness are transitionary and normally improve within 48 hours, but that constipation can be an ongoing problem and it is recommended that a laxative should be prescribed at the same time as the opioid is started (Hanks et al. 1996).

Patients often have many concerns about commencing strong drugs such as morphine. Frequent fears centre around addiction and believing that its use signifies the terminal phase of the illness (Twycross 1994; McQuay 1999). Time should be taken to reassure patients and their families and provide verbal and written information.

Many new drugs are now available for use in chronic pain (e.g. oxycodone, hydromorphone) which allow the practitioner to carefully assess the patient on an individual basis and make an informed decision about the most appropriate drug/route to use.

Durogesic (fentanyl)
Fentanyl is a strong opioid, available in a patch, which is recommended in patients who have stable pain requirements. It is reported to have an improved side-effect profile in comparison to morphine (Ahmedzai & Brooks 1997), although some patients experience nausea and mild drowsiness (BMA/Royal Pharmaceutical Society of Great Britain 2002) and occasionally patients may develop a reaction to the adhesive in the patch (Ling 1997). Use of the patch has increased because it allows the patient freedom from taking tablets.

Changing of the patch is recommended every 3 days, and steady plasma levels are reported to be reached after 8–16 hours (Zech et al. 1994), although in some patients it may be necessary to change it more frequently. The patch should be applied to skin that is free from excess hair and any form of irritation and should not be applied to irradiated areas. It is advisable to change the location on the body to avoid an adverse skin reaction. Occasionally difficulties arise relating to the titration of the patch as each patch is equivalent to a range of morphine (see Table 27.3). An immediate-release fentanyl

Table 27.3   Oral morphine conversion to Durogesic (fentanyl patch)

4-hourly oral morphine dose (mg)	Durogesic patch strength (g/hour)	24-hour oral morphine dose (mg)
20	25	135
25–35	50	135–224
40–50	75	225–314
55–65	100	315–404
70–80	125	405–494
85–95	150	495–584
100–110	175	585–674
115–125	200	675–764

lozenge (OTFC) is available for use in breakthrough or incident pain. The advantage is its fast onset via the buccal mucosa (5–15 min) and its short duration (up to 2 hours). It is available in a range of doses (200–1600 μg) but there is no direct relation between the baseline analgesia and the breakthrough dose. Titration can be difficult and lengthy as the recommended starting dose is 200 μg with titration upwards (Portenoy *et al.* 1999).

Fentanyl is also a useful alternative if the patient is experiencing side-effects from diamorphine. Subcutaneous fentanyl is approximately 50–100 times more potent than subcutaneous morphine.

There are potential problems with fentanyl due to dose limitations. The ampoules are available in 50 μg/1 ml. If the dose required is too large a volume to use in the syringe driver, then Alfentanil may be a useful alternative (Dickman *et al.* 2002).

Palladone (hydromorphone)

Palladone (hydromorphone) is mostly used when patients experience unacceptable drowsiness with morphine. It is similar to morphine in its pharmacokinetic profile and it is approximately 5–7.5 times more potent than morphine. It is available in immediate-release and sustained-release preparations and titration occurs in the same manner as morphine (Hays *et al.* 1994).

The side-effects are similar to those of morphine (Ellershaw 1998).

Methadone

Methadone is a drug that has not been used frequently in the management of pain; however, its use is now increasing. The reluctance to use methadone arose from the difficulties experienced in titrating the drug due to its long half-life (15 hours) which caused accumulation to occur, especially in the elderly (Gannon 1997). There are different methods of achieving effective titration (Gannon 1997); for example, one regimen is to calculate one tenth of the total daily dose of morphine (maximum starting dose must not exceed 30 mg). Administer the methadone to the patient on an as-required basis but not within 3 hours of the last fixed dose. The total dose required over a 24-hour period is calculated after 5–6 days, divided and given as a 2 or 3 times daily regimen and this avoids the build-up of methadone within the body (Morley & Makin 1998). Titration is recommended within a hospital setting to ensure accurate administration. This can be difficult for patients because they have to experience pain before they are administered a dose of methadone in the titration period.

Methadone can be a cheap, effective alternative to morphine if titration is supervised by the specialist pain or palliative care team (Gardner-Nix 1996).

Methadone is particularly useful in patients with renal failure. Morphine is excreted via the kidneys and if renal failure occurs this may lead to the patient experiencing severe drowsiness as a result of culmination of morphine metabolites (Gannon 1997).

Oxycodone

Oxycodone is available as an immediate- or sustained-release tablet and titration should occur in the same way as morphine. Oxycodone is a useful opioid for rotation if the patient is experiencing intolerable side-effects from morphine, e.g. excessive drowsiness/nausea (Shah & Hardy 2001).

It has similar properties to morphine, but when adjusted orally it is more potent (1.5–2 times) and it is usually given 6-hourly because of having a plasma half-life of 3.5 hours (Narcessian 1997). It has similar side-effects to morphine, although oxycodone has been found to cause less nausea (Heiskanen *et al.* 1996) and significantly less itchiness (Mucci-LoRusso *et al.* 1998).

Diamorphine

Diamorphine is used parenterally in a syringe driver for the control of moderate to severe pain when patients are unable to take the oral form of morphine. It is calculated by dividing the total daily dose of oral morphine by 3. Breakthrough doses are calculated by dividing the 24-hour dose of diamorphine by 6 and administering on an as-required basis (Twycross 1994).

Alfentanil

Alfentanil is also a useful alternative to diamorphine. The onset of action is rapid owing to a more rapid blood-brain equilibration. It is ten times more potent than diamorphine (i.e. diamorphine 10 mg = alfentanil 1 mg). It is beneficial when high doses are required as it comes in ampoules of 1 mg/2 ml and 5 mg/1 ml and smaller volumes can be used (Hill 1992).

Buprenorphine

Buprenorphine is an alternative strong opioid available in a patch form. The patch has similar advantages to fentanyl but does not contain a reservoir of the drug. Instead it is contained in a matrix form with effective levels of the drug being reached within 24 hours. Titration is recommended with an alternative opioid initially and then transfer to the patch when stable requirements have been reached. The patches are available in three strengths: 35 μg, 52.5 μg and 70 μg.

Conversion is based on the chart supplied by the pharmaceutical company which demonstrates equivalent doses. Buprenorphine is also available as a sublingual tablet which is titrated from 200 μg to 800 μg 6 hourly. Conversion is based on multiplying the total daily dose of buprenorphine by 100 to give the total daily dose of morphine (i.e. 200 μg buprenorphine/8 hourly = 600 μg buprenorphine/24 hours = 60 mg morphine/24 hours) (Budd 2002).

Cannabis

Studies are currently taking place to examine the potential benefits of using cannabis for the management of chronic conditions, e.g. multiple sclerosis and cancer. Good-quality research is sparse (Wall *et al.* 2001) but there are a number of studies that allude to its benefits in managing chronic pain, spasticity and muscle spasms (Martyn 1995; Consroe 1997).

Breakthrough analgesia

'Stat', 'rescue' or 'breakthrough' doses of analgesia are given if the background dose of the drug is not sufficient to adequately control pain levels and an additional dose is required. There should not be a time limit on this type of prescription because it would need to be given when and if the patient demonstrated any signs of discomfort or pain (with the exception of renal failure where dosages would need to be limited).

Breakthrough doses are calculated on a 4-hour equivalence; for example, if a patient was prescribed 60 mg MXL (a long-acting form of morphine given once a day), the equivalent breakthrough dose would be 10 mg of the immediate-release formulation. If several breakthrough doses are required within a 24-hour period, then the background analgesia (long-acting form) would have to be increased (McMillan 2001).

The use of opioids in renal failure

Renal failure can cause significant and dangerous side-effects due to the accumulation of the drug. Basic guidelines for pain management in renal failure include:

- Reduce analgesia dose and/or choose alternative drug
- Avoid sustained-release preparations
- Seek advice from a specialist pain team and/or pharmacist (Farrell & Rich 2000).

Adjuvant drugs (co-analgesics)

Adjuvant drugs are drugs whose primary indication is for conditions other than pain, but which have a role in the management of chronic pain. The action of traditional analgesics has been shown to be enhanced when used in conjunction with adjuvant agents (Bonica 1994). Examples of this category of drugs include NSAIDs, steroids, antibiotics and anticonvulsants (Portenoy 1998).

The World Health Organization Analgesic Ladder recommends the use of these drugs in combination with non-, weak and strong opioids (see Table 27.2).

Cancer treatment interventions

In addition to pharmacological and non-pharmacological strategies, treatment of cancer pain may be managed most effectively with radiotherapy, surgery, chemotherapy, hormonal manipulation and bisphosphonates. Many palliative care units/hospices may not have access to these interventions and, indeed, careful consideration must be given to ensure that the advantages achieved from any proposed treatment are not outweighed by the potential side-effects and consequent poor quality of life. The aim of these treatments would be to reduce the overall size of the tumour(s), and therefore to improve symptom control, and this must be clearly indicated to the patient.

Anaesthetic interventions

Sometimes it is difficult to attain and maintain adequate pain control and it is in situations such as this that anaesthetic interventions may be of benefit.

Effective control can be achieved by epidural and/or local blocks, especially for pelvic pain and postradiation brachial plexopathy. These interventions can be useful, but careful consideration and assessment must be given to the patient's current condition and the prognosis, as many of these treatments can leave the patient severely limited in his or her activities (McQuay 1990; see Ch. 29, Pain management: epidural analgesia).

Conclusion

The management of acute and chronic pain is a constant challenge to the health care professional. Accurate assessment of the type and site of each pain, accompanied by careful monitoring of any intervention, are essential in order to provide care that benefits the patient and does not impinge on his or her quality of life.

Nurses are in an ideal situation to promote a trusting relationship with the patient by encouraging the patient to express any concerns, thus allowing the patient adequate opportunities to work in partnership and be an active participant in his or her pain management programme.

Procedure guidelines: **Patient assessment and preparation before surgery: optimizing pain control**

Procedure

Action	Rationale
1 If patient has had previous surgery, ask for details of: (a) Previous and current pain control methods (pharmacological and non-pharmacological) (b) Effectiveness of these methods (c) Experience of side-effects, such as nausea and vomiting.	To ensure previous experiences are taken into consideration when planning pain control. To allay any fears based on previous experience. To ensure care is planned to minimize side-effects such as nausea and vomiting.
2 Assess patient for pre-existing long-term pain problems. Obtain information on: (a) Pain type, location and intensity (b) Use of analgesics.	To plan in advance of surgery the pain control methods that will be used to manage both the patient's long-term and anticipated postoperative pain.
3 Check patient suitability for various pain control methods, e.g. renal function, clotting abnormalities, dexterity, visual impairment.	To avoid the use of inappropriate pain control methods, e.g. (a) Diclofenac in renal impairment (b) Epidural analgesia with clotting abnormalities (c) PCAs, if lack of dexterity or visual impairment makes the patient incapable of pressing the demand button which is connected to the pump.
4 Liaise with multidisciplinary team and patient to select most appropriate pain control method(s).	To ensure effective collaboration between the patient and team in order to optimize postoperative pain control.
5 Explain and discuss with patient: (a) How pain will be assessed and the use of a pain scale (b) How pain will be controlled (c) Goals for pain control at rest and on movement.	To allay anxiety and promote patient well-being and control. To encourage active involvement in pain control. To give patients a chance to ask questions. To ensure the patient understands the rationale for pain control during deep breathing and movement. This will help prevent postoperative complications, e.g. chest infections.
6 Provide patient with written information about pain control.	To support verbal information.
7 Where appropriate, demonstrate the use of pain control methods before surgery.	To ensure the patient has the skill and knowledge to effectively use the pain control methods chosen, e.g. PCAs.

Procedure guidelines: **Using a chronic pain chart**

Procedure

Action	Rationale
1 Explain the purpose of using the chart to the patient.	To ensure that the patient understands the procedure and gives his/her valid consent and co-operation.
2 Encourage the patient, where appropriate, to identify pain himself/herself.	The body outline (Fig. 27.2) is a vehicle for the patient to describe his/her own pain experience.
3 When it is necessary for the nurse to complete the chart, ensure that the patient's own description of his/her pain is recorded.	To reduce the risk of misinterpretation.
4 (a) Record any factors that influence the intensity of the pain, e.g. activities or interventions that reduce or increase the pain such as distractions or a heat pad.	Ascertaining how and when the patient experiences pain enables the nurse to plan realistic goals. For example, relieving the patient's pain during the night and while he/she is at rest is usually easier to achieve before relief from pain on movement.
(b) Record whether or not the patient is pain free at night, at rest or on movement.	To ascertain an understanding of the experience of pain for the patient.

Procedure guidelines: **Using a chronic pain chart** *(cont'd)*

Action	Rationale
(c) Record frequency of pain, what helps to relieve the pain, what makes the pain worse and how the patient feels when they are in pain.	
5 Index each site (A to D, Fig. 27.2) in whatever way seems most appropriate, e.g. shading or colouring of areas or arrows to indicate shooting pains.	This enables individual pain sites to be located.
6 Give each pain site a numerical value according to the key to pain intensity or the pain scale and note time recorded.	To indicate the intensity of the pain at each site.
7 Record any analgesia given and note route and dose.	To monitor efficacy of prescribed analgesia.
8 Record any significant activities that are likely to influence the patient's pain.	Extra pharmacological or non-pharmacological interventions might be indicated.
Note: fixed times for reviewing the pain have been omitted intentionally to allow for flexibility. It is suggested that, initially, the patient's pain is reviewed by the patient and nurse every 4 hours. When a patient's level of pain has stabilized, recordings may be made less frequently, e.g. 12-hourly or daily. The chart should be discontinued if a patient's pain becomes totally controlled.	

References and further reading

Ahmedzai, F. & Brooks, D. (1997) *Transdermal fentanyl versus oral morphine in cancer pain: preference: efficacy and quality of life.* On behalf of TTS – Fentanyl Comparative Group, Publ. 13, pp. 254–61.

Akin, M., Weingand, K., Hengehold, D., Beth Goodale, M., Hinkle, R. & Smith, R. (2001) Continuous low-level topical heat in the treatment of dysmenorrhea. *Obstet Gynecol*, **97**(3), 343–9.

Audit Commission (1997) *Anaesthesia Under Examination.* Audit Commission, Oxon.

Ballard, K. (1997) Pressure-relief mattresses and patient comfort. *Prof Nurse*, **13**(1), 27–32.

Bamigbade, T. & Langford, R. (1998) Tramadol hydrochloride: an overview of current use. *Hosp Med*, **59**(5), 373–6.

Barillo, D., Centro Coffey, E., Shirani, K. & Goodwin C. (2000) Burns caused by medical therapy. *J Burn Care Rehabil* **21**(3), 269–73.

Beck, S. (1991) The therapeutic use of music for cancer-related pain. *Oncol Nurse Forum*, **18**(8), 1327–37.

BMA/Royal Pharmaceutical Society of Great Britain (2002) *British National Formulary.* Pharmaceutical Press, Oxford.

Bonica, J. (1994) *Effective Pain Management for Cancer Patients.* Simms Medical Systems, Deltec.

Bonica, J., Ventafridda, V. & Twycross, R. (1990) Management of cancer pain. In: *The Management of Pain*, 2nd edn (ed J. Bonica). Lea & Febiger, Philadelphia, pp. 400–460.

Budd, K. (1995) Tramadol – a step towards the ideal analgesia? *Eur J Palliat Care*, **2**(2), 56–60.

Budd, K. (2002) *Evidence-Based Medicine in Practice. Buprenorphine: A Review.* Haywood Medical, London.

Carr, E. (1990) Post-operative pain: patient expectations and experiences. *J Adv Nurs*, **15**(1), 89–100.

Carr, E. & Mann, E. (2000) Managing chronic pain. In: *Pain: Creative Approaches to Effective Management.* Macmillan Press/ Bournemouth University, London, pp. 81–108.

Carroll, D. & Bowsher, D. (1993) *Pain; Management and Nursing Care.* Butterworth-Heinemann, Oxford.

Carroll, D. & Seers, K. (1998) Relaxation for the relief of chronic pain: a systematic review. *J Adv Nurs*, **27**(3), 476–87.

Caunt, H. (1992) Reducing the psychological impact of post-operative pain. *J Nurs*, **1**(1), 13–19.

Coda, B., O'Sullivan, B., Donaldson, G. *et al.* (1997) Comparative efficacy of patient-controlled administration of morphine, hydromorphone, or sufentil for the treatment of oral mucositis following bone marrow transplantation. *Pain*, **72**(3), 333–46.

Consroe, P. (1997) The perceived effects of smoked cannabis on patients with multiple sclerosis. *Eur Neurol*, **38**(1), 44–8.

Dickman, A., Littlewood, C. & Varga, J. (2002) Drug information. In: *The Syringe Driver. Continuous Subcutaneous Infusions in Palliative Care.* Oxford University Press, Oxford, pp. 11–58.

Donnelly, S. & Walsh, D. (1995) The symptoms of advanced cancer. *Semin Oncol*, **22**(2), Suppl 3, 67–72.

Doyle, D., Hanks, G. & MacDonald, N. (eds) (1998) *Oxford Textbook of Palliative Medicine*, 2nd edn. Oxford Medical Publications, Oxford.

Drayer, R.A., Henderson, B.S. & Reidenberg, M. (1999) Barriers to better pain control in hospitalised patients. *J Pain Symptom Control*, **17**(6), 434–40.

Ellershaw, J. (1998) Hydromorphone: a new alternative to morphine. *Prescriber*, **9**(4), 21–7.

Ezzo, J., Berman, B., Hadhazy, V., Jadad, A., Lao, L. & Singh, B. (2000) Is acupuncture effective for the treatment of chronic pain? A systematic review. *Pain*, **86**(3), 217–25.

Farrell, A. & Rich, A. (2000) Analgesic use in patients with renal failure. *Eur J Palliat Care*, **7**(6), 201–5.

Feine, J. & Lund, J. (1997) An assessment of the efficacy of physical therapy and physical modalities for the control of chronic musculoskeletal pain. *Pain*, **71**(1), 5–23.

Field, L. (1996) Are nurses still underestimating patients' pain post-operatively? *Br J Nurs*, **15**(13), 778–84.

Fine, P.G., Marcus, M., De Boer, A.J. & Van der Oord, B. (1991) An open label study of oral transdermal fentanyl citrate (OTFC) for the treatment of breakthrough cancer pain. *Pain*, **45**, 149–53.

Foley, K. (1998) Pain assessment and cancer pain syndromes. In: *Oxford Textbook of Palliative Medicine*, 2nd edn (eds D. Doyle, G. Hanks & N. MacDonald). Oxford Medical Publications, Oxford, pp. 310–31.

Gannon, C. (1997) The use of methadone in the care of the dying. *Eur J Palliat Care*, **4**(5), 152–8.

Gardner-Nix, J. (1996) Oral methadone for managing chronic non malignant pain. *J Pain Symptom Control*, **11**(5), 321–2.

Good, M. (1996) Effects of relaxation and music on postoperative pain: a review. *J Adv Nurs*, **24**, 905–14.

Good, M., Stanton-Hicks, M., Grass, J. *et al.* (1999) Relief of post-operative pain with jaw relaxation, music and their combination. *Pain*, **81**(1–2), 163–72.

Gould, T., Crosby, D., Harmer, M., *et al.* (1992) Policy for controlling pain after surgery: effect of sequential changes in management. *Br Med J*, **305**(6863), 1187–93.

Gray, E. (2001) Linking chronic pain and depression. *Nurs Stand*, **15**(25), 33–6.

Grond, S., Zech, D., Diefenbach, C., Radbruch, I. & Lehmann, K. (1996) Assessment of cancer pain: a prospective evaluation. *Pain*, **64**(1), 107–14.

Hancock, H. (1996) The complexity of pain assessment and management in the first 24 hours after cardiac surgery. *Intens Crit Care Nurs*, **12**(6), 346–53.

Hanks, G. & Cherny, N. (1998) Opioid analgesic therapy. In: *Oxford Textbook of Palliative Medicine*, 2nd edn (eds D. Doyle, G. Hanks & N. MacDonald). Oxford Medical Publications, Oxford, pp. 331–54.

Hanks, G. & Expert Working Group of the European Association for Palliative Care (1996) Morphine in cancer pain: modes of administration. *Br Med J*, **3**(12), 823–6.

Hanks, G.W. (1991) Opioid-responsive and opioid non-responsive pain in cancer. *Br Med Bull*, **47**, 718–31.

Hanks, G.W., De Conno, F., Cherney, N. *et al.* (2001) Morphine and alternative opioids in cancer pain: the EAPC recommendations. *Br J Cancer*, **84**(5), 587–93.

Harmer, M. & Davies, K. (1998) The effect of education, assessment and a standardised prescription on postoperative pain management. *Anaesthesia*, **53**(5), 424–30.

Hays, H. *et al.* (1994) Comparative clinical efficacy and safety of immediate release and controlled release hydromorphone for chronic severe pain. *Cancer*, **74**(6), 1808–16.

Hayward, J. (1975) *Information, A Prescription Against Pain, The Study of Nursing Care*. Research Project, Series 2, (5). RCN, London.

Heiser, R., Chiles, K., Fudge, M. & Gray, S. (1997) The use of music during the immediate postoperative recovery period. *AORN J*, **65**(4), 777–85.

Heiskanen, T., Ruismaki, P. & Kelso, E. (1996) Double blind, randomised repeated dose crossover comparison CR oxycodone and CR morphine tablets in cancer pain; 1 & 2, pharmacodynamic profile. *8th World Congress of Pain*, Vancouver, Abstract 49 & 50.

Higginson, I. (1998) Can professionals improve their assessments? *J Pain Symptom Manage*, **15**(3), 149–50.

Hill, H.F. (1992) Patient controlled analgesic infusions: alfentanil versus morphine. *Pain*, **49**(3), 301–10.

Hunt, J.M. *et al.* (1977) Patients with protracted pain; a survey conducted at the London Hospital. *J Med Ethics*, **3**(2), 61–73.

International Association for the Study of Pain (1996) Classification of chronic pain. *Pain*, Suppl **3**, 51–226.

Kehlet, H. (1997) Multimodal approach to control of postoperative pathophysiology and rehabilitation. *Br J Anaesth*, **78**(5), 606–17.

King, A. (1999) *King's Guide to TENS for Health Professionals*. King's Medical Physio-Med Services, Glossop, Derbyshire.

Kitson, A. (1994) Post-operative pain management: a literature review. *J Clin Nurs*, **3**(1), 7–18.

Lang, E., Bentosch, E., Fick, L. *et al.* (2000) Adjunctive non-pharmacological analgesia for invasive medical procedures: a randomised trial. *Lancet*, **355**(9214), 1486–90.

Lawler, K. (1997) Pain assessment. *Prof Nurs Study*, **13**(1), Suppl, S5–8.

Leppert, W., Luczak, J., Oliver, D. (2002) Tramadol and cancer pain. *Eur J Palliat Care*, **9**(2), 49–51.

Ling, J. (1997) The use of transdermal fentanyl in palliative care. *Int J Palliat Nurs*, **3**(2), 65–8.

Macintyre, P. (2001) Safety and efficacy of patient-controlled analgesia. *Br J Anaesth*, **87**(1), 36–46.

Macintyre, P. & Ready, L. (2001) *Acute Pain Management. A Practical Guide*. W.B. Saunders, London.

Martyn, C. (1995) 'N = 1' cross-over trial using nabilone in a patient with multiple sclerosis. *Lancet*, **345**(8949), 579.

McCaffery, M. (1968) *Nursing Practice Theories Related to Cognition, Bodily Pain, and Man–Environment Interactions*. University of California, Los Angeles.

McCaffery, M. (1990) Nursing approaches to non-pharmacological pain control. *Int J Nurs Stud*, **27**(1), 1–5.

McCaffery, M. & Beebe, A. (1989) *Pain: Clinical Manual for Nursing Practice*. Mosby, St Louis.

McCaffery, M. & Ferrell, B.R. (1997) Nurses' knowledge of pain assessment and management: how much progress have we made? *J Pain Symptom Manage*, **14**(3), 175–88.

McMillan, C. (2001) Breakthrough pain: assessment and management in cancer patients. *Br J Nurs*, **10**(13), 860–6.

McQuay, H. (1990) The logic of alternative routes. *J Pain Symptom Manage*, **5**(2), 75–7.

McQuay, H. (1999) Opioids in pain management. *Lancet*, **353**, 2229–32.

McQuay, H. & Moore, A. (1998) Oral tramadol versus placebo, codeine and combination analgesics. In: *An Evidence Based Resource for Pain*. Oxford University Press, Oxford, pp. 138–46.

McQuay, H., Moore, A. & Justins, D. (1997) Treating acute pain in hospital. *Br Med J*, **314**(7093), 1531–5.

Mitchell, M. (1997) Patients' perceptions of pre-operative preparation for day surgery. *J Adv Nurs*, **26**(2), 356–63.

Morley, J.S. & Makin, M.K. (1998) The use of methadone in cancer pain poorly responsive to other opioids. *Pain Rev*, **5**, 51–8.

Mucci-LoRusso, P., Berman, B., Silberstein, P., Citron, M. & Bressler, L. (1998) Controlled release oxycodone compared with controlled release morphine in the treatment of cancer pain: a randomised, double-blind, parallel group study. *Eur J Pain*, **2**, 239–49.

- Removal of sutures from sensitive areas, e.g. the vulva
- Invasive procedures such as catheterization and sigmoidoscopy
- Removal of radioactive intracavity gynaecological applicators
- Altering the position of a patient who experiences incident pain
- Manual evacuation of the bowel in severe constipation
- Acute trauma, e.g. applying orthopaedic traction following pathological fracture
- Physiotherapy procedures, particularly postoperatively.

Contraindications

Entonox should not be used with any of the following conditions:

- Maxillofacial injuries (BOC 1995), as the patient may not be able to hold the mask tightly to the face or use the mouthpiece adequately. There is a risk of causing further damage to facial wounds and there may also be a significant risk of blood inhalation.
- Head injuries with impairment of consciousness.
- Heavily sedated patients – as they would be unable to breathe in the Entonox on demand and to potentiate sedation further may be hazardous.
- Intoxicated patients – as drowsiness and aspiration would be a hazard in the event of vomiting.
- Pneumothorax, air embolism, bowel obstruction or abdominal distension (BOC 2000). The nitrous oxide constituent of Entonox passes into any air-filled cavity within the body faster than nitrogen passes out. As the gas expands this is likely to result in a build-up of tension, which will increase the patient's symptoms.
- Decompression illness or a recent dive (the 'bends') – as nitrous oxide escapes into the bloodstream and increases the size of the nitrogen bubbles in the tissues.
- Laryngectomy patients – as they will be unable to use the apparatus.
- Temperatures of below $-6°C$ as the gases separate (BOC 1995). If this occurs the cylinders will initially deliver a high concentration of oxygen but will eventually deliver nearly pure nitrous oxide.

Cautions

Prior to Entonox use consideration should be given to the following.

- The high level of oxygen (50%) in Entonox may depress respiration in patients who have chronic obstructive pulmonary disease.

- Entonox should not be used as a replacement for procedures requiring increased levels of medical intervention where intravenous analgesia or general anaesthesia is required.
- As a precaution the British Oxygen Company (BOC 1995) data sheet recommends that patients should avoid driving or operating machinery for 12 hours after Entonox administration.

Reference material

Patient assessment prior to use

The patient's ability to administer Entonox safely and effectively (particularly the very young or old) must be assessed prior to use. Patients should be able to:

- Understand the instructions for Entonox use
- Hold the demand valve to self-administer the gas
- Inhale the gas through the mask or mouthpiece whilst breathing normally (patients who have impaired lung function may not be able to inhale the gas sufficiently to provide adequate analgesia).

Equipment

Cylinders

Two types of Entonox cylinder are available from the BOC: the new light-weight cylinders (available from 2001) and the older cylinders. Both cylinders have blue and white markings on their shoulder.

The new light-weight cylinders have the following advantages:

- They are easier to carry
- They have a live contents gauge
- Changing an empty cylinder is simple because it is not necessary to fit a regulator or use a cylinder key.

Demand apparatus

There are a number of different companies which supply the demand apparatus for self-administered Entonox use (Fig. 28.1a,b).

Use of bacterial filters

Because Entonox equipment is a potential source of cross-infection, bacterial filters should be fitted between the face mask and demand valve (Chilvers & Weisz 2000). Local policies must also be followed for the cleaning/sterilization of equipment between patient use.

Principle of administration

Entonox is designed for self-administration by the patient. This method of administration makes use of a demand unit which safeguards the patient from excess inhalation of Entonox. The demand unit ensures that

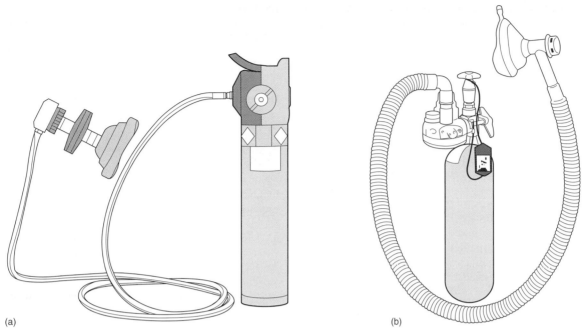

Figure 28.1 (a) Sabre Ease demand apparatus with light-weight cylinder. (b) Ohmeda demand apparatus.

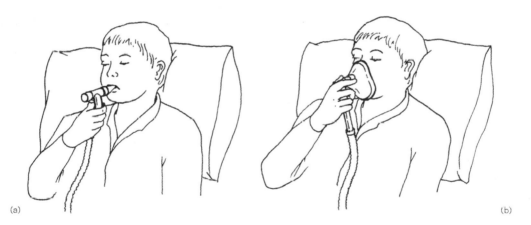

Figure 28.2 A patient administering Entonox (a) through a mouthpiece and (b) through a face mask. (Courtesy of BOC Medical Gases.)

gas can be obtained only by the patient inhaling from the mouthpiece or mask and producing a negative pressure (Fig. 28.2a,b). The gas flow stops when the patient removes the mouthpiece or mask from their face. Therefore, the patient must hold the mask firmly over the face or mouthpiece to the lips to produce an airtight fit and breathe in before the gas will flow. Expired gases escape by the expiratory valve on the handpiece. It is essential to adhere to this method of self-administration as it is then impossible for patients to overdose themselves because if they become drowsy they will relax their grip on the handset and the gas flow will cease when no negative pressure is applied. Since pain is usually relieved with a concentration of 25% nitrous oxide (BOC 1995), continued inhalation does not usually occur. However, should inhalation continue, light anaesthesia supervenes and the mask drops away as the patient relaxes. Entonox may be self-regulated, but additionally may be administered by attendant medical personnel trained in its use, e.g. within obstetric/accident and emergency units, and accident ambulances.

Entonox has an oxygen content two-and-a-half times that of air and is, therefore, a good way of giving extra oxygen as well as providing analgesia.

Duration and frequency of administration

The duration and frequency of Entonox administration should always be tailored to individual patient needs. Because prolonged exposure to Entonox causes inactivation of vitamin B_{12}, impaired folate metabolism and pernicious anaemia (BOC 1995), it is recommended that:

- Entonox is used on a short-term rather than a long-term basis
- Exposure to Entonox should not be for more than 6 hours continuously (BOC 1995)
- If daily use is required for more than 4 days, this should be accompanied by twice-weekly blood tests to check for changes in red and white blood cells (BOC 1995). Consideration should also be given to the administration of B_{12} and folate supplements.

Prescribing of Entonox

In a number of health care settings, nurses, midwives and physiotherapists may be able to administer Entonox without a written prescription from a doctor providing there is a local patient group direction to allow this (see Ch. 9, Drug administration). Where this is the case, Entonox can be used more readily and time is not wasted waiting for a medical prescription.

Staff training

Where Entonox is available for patient use it is important that staff are given appropriate theoretical and practical training (Hollinworth 1995).

Use during pregnancy and lactation

It has been suggested that prolonged exposure to high levels of nitrous oxide may affect a woman's ability to become pregnant (BOC 1995). Mild skeletal teratogenic changes have been observed in pregnant rat embryos when the dam (pregnant mother) has been exposed to high levels of nitrous oxide during the period of organogenesis. However, no increased incidence of foetal malformation has been discovered in eight epidemiological studies and case reports in humans (BOC 1995). No published material shows that nitrous oxide is toxic to the human foetus. Therefore, there is no absolute contraindication to its use in the first 15 weeks of pregnancy.

Complications

Inappropriate inhalation of Entonox will ultimately result in unconsciousness, passing through stages of increasing lightheadedness and intoxication. The treatment is removal to fresh air, mouth-to-mouth resuscitation and, if necessary, the use of an oxygen resuscitator (BOC 1995).

Procedure guidelines: **Entonox administration**

Equipment

1 Entonox cylinder and head.
2 Face mask and/or mouthpiece.

3 Sterile filter.

Procedure

Action	Rationale
1 Explain and discuss the procedure with the patient.	To ensure that the patient understands the procedure and gives his/her valid consent.
2 Turn on the Entonox supply from the cylinder. (If using the older type cylinder the tap should be turned in an anticlockwise direction.)	To ascertain whether there is any Entonox in the cylinder.
3 Examine the gauge to determine how much gas is in the cylinder.	To ensure an adequate supply of gas throughout the procedure.
4 Ensure that the patient is in as comfortable a position as possible.	

*Procedure guidelines: **Entonox administration** (cont'd)*

Action	Rationale
5 Demonstrate how to use the apparatus by holding the mask tightly to your face. Explain to the patient that when the patient breathes in and out regularly and deeply a hissing sound will be heard, indicating that the gas is being inhaled.	To ensure that the patient understands what to do and what to expect before any painful procedure commences.
6 Allow the patient to practise using the apparatus.	To enable the patient to adopt the correct technique and for the nurse to observe the analgesic effect of the gas before the procedure commences.
7 Encourage the patient to breathe gas in and out for at least 2 minutes before commencing any painful procedure.	To allow sufficient time for an adequate circulatory level of nitrous oxide to provide analgesia. (When the patient inhales, gas enters first the lungs then the pulmonary and systemic circulations. It takes 1–2 minutes to build up reasonable concentrations of nitrous oxide in the brain.)
8 During the procedure encourage the patient to breathe in and out regularly and deeply.	To maintain adequate circulatory levels, thus providing adequate analgesia.
9 At the end of the procedure observe the patient until the effects of the gas have worn off.	Some patients may feel a transient drowsiness or giddiness and should be discouraged from getting out of bed until these effects have worn off. It is rare for the patient to experience transient amnesia (BOC 1999).
10 Evaluate the effectiveness of Entonox with the patient throughout, and following procedures, by verbal questioning and encouraging the patient to self-assess the analgesic effect.	To establish whether the Entonox has been a useful analgesic for the procedure. This should then be documented to assist any subsequent procedures, e.g. dressing changes.
11 Turn off the Entonox supply from the cylinder. (If using the older type cylinder the tap should be turned in a clockwise direction. The gauge should read 'Empty' when turned off.)	To avoid potential seepage of gas from the apparatus.
12 Depress the diaphragm under the valve.	To remove residual gas from tubing.
13 Follow local policies/guidelines for the cleaning and sterilization of face mask, expiratory valve and tubing. Filters and mouthpieces should be discarded after use.	To reduce the risk of cross-infection.
14 Record the administration on appropriate documentation.	To promote continuity of care, maintain accurate records and provide a point of reference in the event of any queries.

Problem solving

Problem	Cause	Suggested action
Patient not experiencing adequate analgesic effect.	Entonox cylinder empty. Apparatus not properly connected.	Check before procedure commences.
	Patient not inhaling deeply enough.	Encourage the patient to breathe in until a hissing noise can be heard from the cylinder. Reassess suitability of patient for Entonox use. The patient may not be strong enough to inhale deeply or may have reduced lung capacity.
	Patient inhaling pure oxygen, i.e. cylinder has been stored below −6°C and nitrous oxide has liquified and settled at the bottom of the cylinder. (All cylinders should be stored horizontally at a temperature of 10°C or above for 24 hours before use.)	Initially safe, but later the patient may inhale pure nitrous oxide and be asphyxiated. Discontinue the procedure. Ensure adequate warming of the cylinder and inversion of the cylinder to remix the gases adequately.

Problem solving (cont'd)

Problem	Cause	Suggested action
	Not enough time has been allowed for nitrous oxide to exert its analgesic effect.	Allow at least 2 minutes of Entonox use before commencing the procedure.
Patient experiences generalized muscle rigidity.	Hyperventilation during inhalation.	Discontinue Entonox and allow the patient to recover. Explain the procedure again, stressing deep and regular inspiration. Use a mouthpiece in place of a mask.
Patient unable to tolerate a mask.	Smell of rubber, feeling of claustrophobia.	Use a mouthpiece in place of a mask.
Patient feels nauseated, drowsy or giddy.	Effect of nitrous oxide accumulation.	Discontinue Entonox administration – the effect will then rapidly disappear.
Patient afraid to use Entonox.	Associates gases with previous hospital procedures, e.g. anaesthesia before surgery.	Reassure patient and reiterate instructions for use and short-term effects.

References and further reading

BOC (1995) *BOC Gases Data Sheet: Entonox.* BOC Group, Manchester.

BOC (1999) *Inhalation Pain Control* (video). BOC Gases, Manchester.

BOC (2000) *Entonox: Controlled Pain Relief Reference Guide.* BOC Group, Manchester.

Bruce, E. & Franck, L. (2000) Self-administered nitrous oxide (Entonox) for the management of procedural pain. *Paediatr Nurs*, **12**(7), 15–19.

Chilvers, R. & Weisz, M. (2000) Entonox equipment as a potential source of cross-infection. *Anaesthesia*, **55**(2), 176–9.

Gillman, M. & Lightigfeld, F. (1998) Clinical role and mechanisms of action of analgesic nitrous oxide. *Int J Neurosci*, **93**(1–2), 55–62.

Hollinworth, H. (1995) Nurses' assessment and management of pain at wound dressing changes. *J Wound Care*, **4**(2), 77–83.

Peate, I. & Lancaster, J. (2000) Safe use of medical gases in the clinical setting: practical tips. *Br J Nurs*, **8,9** (4), 231–6.

Pickup, S. & Pagdin J. (2000/2001) Procedural pain: Entonox can help. *Paediatr Nurs*, **12**(10), 33–6.

Street, D. (2000) A practical guide to giving Entonox. *Nurs Times* **96**(34), 47–8.

Pain management: epidural analgesia

Chapter contents

Definition

Epidural analgesia is the administration of analgesics (with or without adjuvants such as corticosteroids and clonidine) into the epidural space. This technique enables analgesics to be injected close to the spinal cord and spinal nerves where they exert a powerful analgesic effect. It is one of the most effective techniques available for the management of acute pain (Macintyre & Ready 2001; Wheatley *et al.* 2001).

Advantages

There are three main advantages in using epidural analgesia.

- It has the potential to provide effective dynamic pain relief for many patients (Wheatley *et al.* 2001).
- Because lower doses of opioids are required to achieve effective analgesia via the epidural route, patients experience a lower incidence of opioid-related side-effects, such as sedation and prolonged ileus.
- There is also evidence that the use of epidural analgesia may reduce the stress response to surgery or trauma, thereby reducing morbidity, recovery time and hospital stay (Kehlet 1997).

Indications

- Provision of analgesia during labour.
- As an alternative to general anaesthesia, e.g. in severe respiratory disease or for patients with malignant hyperthermia.
- Provision of postoperative analgesia. Epidural analgesia has been used since the late 1940s as a method of controlling postoperative pain (Chapman & Day 2001).
- Provision of analgesia for pain resulting from trauma, e.g. fractured ribs, which may result in respiratory impairment due to pain on breathing.

- Management of chronic intractable pain, for example advanced cancer pain where nerves are compressed.
- To relieve muscle spasm and pain resulting from lumbar cord pressure due to disc protrusion or local oedema and inflammation.

Contraindications

These may be absolute or relative.

Absolute

- Patients with coagulation defects, which may result in epidural haematoma formation and spinal cord compression, e.g. iatrogenic (anticoagulated patient) or congenital (haemophiliacs), or thrombocytopenia due to disease or as the result of anticancer treatment (Horlocker & Wedel 1998)
- Local sepsis at the site of proposed epidural injection; the result might be meningitis or epidural abscess formation
- Proven allergy to the intended drug
- Unstable spinal fracture
- Patient refusal to consent to the procedure.

Relative

- Unstable cardiovascular system
- Spinal deformity
- Raised intracranial pressure (a risk of herniation if a dural tap occurs)
- Certain neurological conditions, for example multiple sclerosis, where an epidural may result in an exacerbation of the disease (Hall 2000)
- Unavailability of staff trained in the management of epidural analgesia (Macintyre & Ready 2001). Hall (2000) notes that staff managing patients with epidural analgesia should have undertaken a period of formal training to care for patients safely and competently.

Reference material

Anatomy of the epidural space

The epidural space lies between the spinal dura and ligamentum flavum. The contents of the epidural space include a rich venous plexus, spinal arterioles, lymphatics and extradural fat (Fig. 29.1).

Spinal nerves traverse the epidural space laterally. There are 31 pairs of spinal nerves of varying size. The two main groups of nerve fibres are:

- *Myelinated* – myelin is a thin, fatty sheath which protects and insulates the nerve fibres and prevents impulses from being transmitted to adjacent fibres.

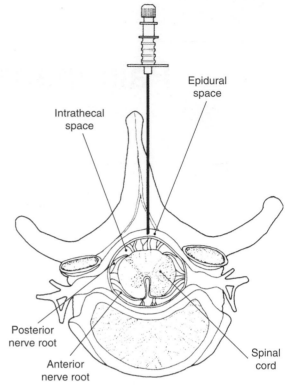

Figure 29.1 Positioning of Tuohy needle. (Courtesy of Crul, B. & Delhaas, E. (1991) Technical complications during long-term subarachnoid or epidural administration of morphine in terminally ill cancer patients. *Regional Anaesthesia*, **16**, 209–13.)

- *Unmyelinated* – delicate fibres, more susceptible to hypoxia and toxins than myelinated fibres.

The spinal nerves are composed of a posterior and anterior root, which join to form a spinal nerve:

- *Posterior root* – transmits ascending sensory impulses from the periphery to the spinal cord.
- *Anterior root* – transmits descending motor impulses from the spinal cord to the periphery by means of its corresponding spinal nerve.

Specific skin surface areas are supplied/innervated by each of the spinal nerves. These skin areas are known as dermatomes (see Fig. 29.2).

Classes of epidural drugs and mechanism of action

Three classes of drugs are commonly used to provide epidural analgesia: opioids, local anaesthetic agents and adjuvant drugs such as corticosteroids and clonidine.

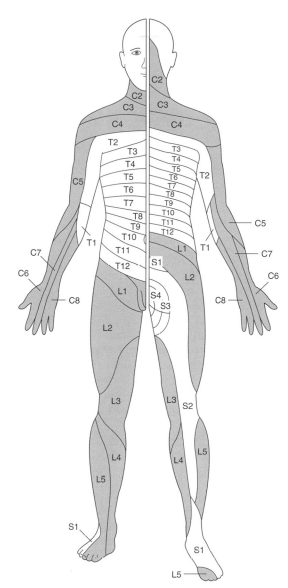

Figure 29.2 Dermatomes. (Redrawn with permission from Walsh, D. (1997) *TENS: Clinical Applications and Related Theory*. Churchill Livingstone, Edinburgh.)

Opioids

Whilst a number of different opioids have been used for epidural analgesia, two of the most commonly used are diamorphine and fentanyl (Cook *et al*. 1997; Romer & Russell 1998; Bannon *et al*. 2001). When either of these opioids is injected into the epidural space, part of the opioid dose:

- Crosses the dura and arachnoid membrane and enters the cerebrospinal fluid (CSF). From the CSF a

proportion of the drug is taken up into the spinal cord and reaches the opioid receptors in the spinal cord. Once bound to the opioid receptors, this results in blocking of pain impulses
- Enters the systemic circulation and contributes to analgesia
- Binds to the epidural fat and does not contribute to analgesia.

Fentanyl differs from diamorphine in that it is more lipid soluble. This means that it passes more easily into the CSF, gaining faster access to the opioid receptors and having a more rapid onset of action. Fentanyl also has a shorter duration of action (1–4 hours) as opposed to diamorphine (6–12 hours) (Macintyre & Ready 2001).

Local anaesthetic drugs

Commonly used local anaesthetic agents include bupivacaine and ropivacaine. When given epidurally, these drugs gain access to the nerve roots and the spinal cord by crossing the dura and subarachnoid membranes (Macintyre & Ready 2001). They inhibit pain transmission by blocking sodium ion channels which are involved in the propagation of electrical impulses along the spinal nerves.

The dose of a local anaesthetic agent will also determine which nerves are blocked. Low concentrations of bupivacaine (e.g. 0.1–0.125%) preferentially block nerve impulses in the smallest diameter nerve fibres, which include the pain and temperature sensory fibres. As the larger diameter motor fibres are less likely to be blocked with concentrations of 0.1–0.125% bupivacaine, leg weakness is avoided and the patient is able to mobilize.

Adjuvant drugs

Corticosteroids

Although not licensed for epidural use, corticosteroid injections are often used to relieve pain caused by inflammatory irritation of nerve roots (Papagelopoulos *et al*. 2001).

Clonidine

Clonidine is a mixed alpha-adrenergic agonist. Although its exact mechanism of action is unknown, clonidine is believed to enhance analgesia provided by epidural opioids and local anaesthetic drugs (Smith & Elliott 2001). Clonidine has a specific role in the management of neuropathic pain in patients with advanced cancer (Mercadante 1999).

Methods of administration

Continuous infusion

Continuous infusions of epidural drugs are the most effective way of providing dynamic pain relief after major surgical procedures (Kehlet & Holte 2001). Continuous

Table 29.1 Optimal catheter location for different surgical sites

Surgical site	Catheter location
Thoracic	T6–T9
Upper abdominal	T7–T10
Lower abdominal	T9–L1
Hip/knee	L1–L4

infusions can be given by either a syringe pump or a designated infusion pump system. The effectiveness of this method of administering drugs is dependent on a number of factors including the combination of drugs used, the position of the epidural catheter and the volume of the local anaesthetic agent infused.

Combination of drugs used
Epidural infusions of local anaesthetic and opioid combinations are commonly used in the UK (Wheatley *et al.* 2001). The rationale behind their combined use is based on the observation that better analgesia is achieved with lower doses of each drug, therefore minimizing drug-related side-effects. Although the solutions used will vary with the clinical situation, common solutions are bupivacaine 0.1–0.125% with 2–4 μg/ml of fentanyl.

Position of epidural catheter
Local anaesthetic drugs block nerve fibres at spinal segments adjacent to their site of administration. To ensure the local anaesthetic agent spreads to the dermatomes or nerves supplying the area of pain (e.g. the surgical site), the tip of the epidural catheter should be placed within the mid-dermatomal distribution of the pain site (see Table 29.1). This achieves optimal analgesia using the least amount of drugs. If the catheter is placed below the dermatomes supplying the pain site then analgesia is likely to be inadequate.

Volume of infusion
As the volume of local anaesthetic agent influences the number of spinal nerves that are blocked, it is important to maintain the hourly infusion rate at a volume which keeps the appropriate nerves blocked.

Bolus injections

Bolus injections of opioids and local anaesthetic agents are used infrequently to manage postoperative pain but are more commonly used for managing labour pain (Grond *et al.* 2000).

Patient-controlled epidural analgesia (PCEA)

The use of PCEA has gained popularity in recent years because it allows patients to control their analgesia. For patients with postoperative or chronic pain, PCEA is used more effectively in combination with a low-dose background infusion (Wheatley *et al.* 2001). This ensures a baseline level of analgesia which can then be supplemented by the patient when required.

Monitoring

When caring for a patient receiving epidural analgesia, it is important to monitor the patient for the following:

- Signs of drug-related side-effects
- Pain intensity
- Signs of complications due to the epidural procedure.

Drug-related side-effects
There are a number of drug-related side-effects associated with epidural opioids and local anaesthetic agents.

Opioids
- *Respiratory depression*: this is due to the action of opioids on the respiratory centre. Respiratory depression may occur at two different time intervals.
  - Early: usually within 2 hours of the opioid injection. This may occur if high blood levels of the opioid follow absorption from the epidural space into the systemic circulation (Macintyre & Ready 2001).
  - Late: this may not be seen for 6–12 hours after an opioid is given. It results from rostral migration of the drug in the CSF to the brainstem and respiratory centre (Macintyre & Ready 2001). This is less likely to occur with lipid-soluble opioids such as fentanyl.
- *Sedation*: although there may be many different causes of sedation, epidural opioids can cause sedation owing to their effect on the central nervous system. Opioid-induced sedation is often an early warning sign of respiratory depression.
- *Nausea and vomiting*: nausea and vomiting is caused by the action of opioids on the vomiting centre in the brainstem and stimulation of the chemoreceptor trigger zone in the fourth ventricle of the brain.
- *Pruritus*: although the exact mechanism is unknown, pruritus is presumed to be centrally mediated and a consequence of activation of opioid receptors in the spinal cord (Sands *et al.* 1998).
- *Urinary retention*: this is due to opioid inhibition of the micturition reflex which is evoked by increases in bladder volume.

Local anaesthetic agents
- *Hypotension*: this can be caused by two mechanisms. Firstly, local anaesthetic agents can spread outside the epidural space, blocking the sympathetic nerves. This results in peripheral vasodilatation and hypotension. It is most likely to occur if a bolus dose of local anaesthetic agent (e.g. 10 ml of 0.25% bupivacaine) is given

to improve pain control (Macintyre & Ready 2001). Secondly, if the local anaesthetic agent spreads above the T4 dermatome (nipple line) the cardio-accelerator nerves may become blocked, leading to bradycardia and hypotension (Macintyre & Ready 2001).

- *Motor blockade*: this will depend on the concentration and total dose of local anaesthetic agent used and the position of the epidural catheter (Hall 2000). Motor blockade occurs when the local anaesthetic agent blocks the larger diameter motor nerves. Leg weakness will occur if the motor nerves supplying legs are blocked.
- *Urinary retention*: as with epidural opioids, blockade of the nerves supplying the bladder sphincter can cause urinary retention.

Routine monitoring of the patient for these side-effects must be carried out to facilitate early management. The patient's blood pressure, respiratory rate and peripheral tissue oxygenation should be monitored continuously initially and then according to local policy and as the patient's condition dictates.

For guidance on managing the side-effects associated with epidural opioids and local anaesthetic agents, see Procedure guidelines.

Pain assessment

Pain should be assessed (at rest and on movement) at the same time that the patient's routine observations are carried out. Simple numerical or verbal rating scales (0–10 where 0 is no pain and 10 is the worst pain imaginable) can be used. It is important to remember that the patient's pain should be controlled to an intensity which allows deep breathing, coughing and mobilization. If pain is not controlled and the infusion has already been titrated according to hospital guidelines, the pain/anaesthetic team should be contacted for advice after checking the following:

- The catheter is still in situ
- There are no leaks within the epidural system
- The height of the epidural block. This will indicate whether the block has fallen below the upper limit of the incision or pain site. To check the height of the block use a small piece of ice or cold solution (ethyl alcohol) – start at the top of the chest above the patient's incision or pain site. Gently dab the ice (or apply the cold solution) down each side of the patient's body (one side and then the other). Use a dermatome map to assess the upper and lower limit where the sensation changes (see Fig. 29.2).

If the height of the block has fallen below the upper limit of the incision or pain site the pain/anaesthetic team may give the patient a bolus dose of local anaesthetic agent to re-establish the block.

Complications of epidural analgesia

As with any invasive technique, epidural analgesia results in potential complications, many of which are rare. They include the following.

Dural puncture

This usually occurs when the dura mater is inadvertently punctured during the placement of the epidural catheter. The incidence of a dural puncture arising during placement of the catheter is approximately 0.32–1.23% (Wheatley *et al.* 2001). The main symptom is a headache, which arises from leakage of cerebrospinal fluid through the dura.

Catheter migration

Catheter migration is extremely rare, occurring in less than 0.2% of patients (Wheatley *et al.* 2001). The catheter may migrate into either a blood vessel or the cerebrospinal fluid. If the catheter migrates into a blood vessel, opioid or local anaesthetic toxicity will occur. Opioid toxicity results in sedation and respiratory depression. Local anaesthetic toxicity results in circumoral tingling, numbness, twitching, convulsions and apnoea. If the catheter migrates into the cerebrospinal fluid the epidural opioids and local anaesthetic agents may reach as high as the cranial subarachnoid space. If this occurs the respiratory muscles are paralysed together with the cranial nerves, resulting in apnoea, profound hypotension and unconsciousness.

Haematoma

An epidural haematoma can arise from trauma to an epidural blood vessel during catheter insertion or removal. Although the incidence of a haematoma occurring is extremely rare, particular care must be taken in patients receiving thromboprophylaxis (see Procedure guidelines for catheter removal). Initial symptoms include back pain and tenderness. As the haematoma expands to compress the nerve roots or the spinal cord, this proceeds to sensory/motor weakness.

Abscess formation

Wheatley *et al.* (2001) note that infection can be introduced into the epidural space from an exogenous source via contaminated equipment or drugs or from an endogenous source, leading to bacteraemia which seeds to the insertion site or catheter tip. Alternatively the catheter can act as a wick through which the infection tracks down from the entry site on the skin to the epidural space. Symptoms include back pain and tenderness accompanied by redness with a purulent discharge from the catheter exit site.

Table 29.2 Epidural analgesia: safety checklist

Checklist	Rationale
Check the prescription and rate of the epidural infusion	To ensure epidural drugs are being administered correctly
Check the epidural infusion/syringe pump extension set is connected to the epidural catheter and not to any other access device	To ensure drugs are administered via the correct route
Check the filter is securely attached to the epidural catheter	To prevent accidental disconnection of the catheter from the filter
Check that the dressing over the epidural catheter exit site is secure	To prevent catheter dislodgement and minimize the risk of contamination of the catheter site

Equipment and prescription safety checks

When a patient is receiving a continuous infusion of epidural analgesia it is advisable to carry out the safety checks given in Table 29.2 at least once per shift.

Epidural analgesia for patients with intractable cancer pain

Epidural analgesia is a well-established technique for managing intractable cancer pain (Mercadante 1999). A number of special considerations apply to the use of epidurals in the chronic pain setting.

Indications

There are three main indications for using epidural analgesia in patients with intractable cancer pain (Mercadante 1999):

* Patients treated with systemic opioids but who suffer from unacceptable side-effects
* Unsuccessful treatment with strong opioids despite escalating doses
* Severe neuropathic pain due to tumour invasion or compression (Smitt *et al.* 1998).

Factors to consider before using epidural analgesia

Prior to using epidural analgesia for intractable cancer pain, the following issues should be addressed with the patient, family and primary health care team.

Patient/family

The concentration of analgesics needed to provide sufficient analgesia for patients with chronic cancer pain is often higher than the concentrations used postoperatively. As a result, drug-related side-effects such as motor weakness and urinary retention can occur. Some patients find these side-effects unacceptable and may prefer to avoid epidural analgesia altogether. A discussion must therefore take place with the patient and family to ensure

that they are aware of these potential side-effects. The patient should also be informed that they will need to spend a period of time in hospital following insertion of the catheter, to allow for dose adjustment and ensure that side-effects are minimized and optimum pain management achieved.

Primary health care team

If it is anticipated that the patient will go home with a continuous epidural infusion, the patient's general practitioner and district nursing team should be consulted at the outset to determine whether they are willing to be involved and/or trained in the management of an epidural.

Arrangements should also be made with the primary health care team for the provision of a suitable epidural pump and the supply of reconstituted syringes/infusion bags.

Drugs and doses

Epidural infusions of local anaesthetic–opioid combinations are frequently used for the management of intractable cancer pain.

Opioids

The most commonly used opioids are morphine and diamorphine. Although there is a lack of consensus over the method of converting from a systemic to an epidural opioid, Mercadante (1999) recommends that if converting from oral morphine, a starting dose of roughly 10% of the oral opioid should be given epidurally and then titrated to effect. For example, if a patient was receiving a total daily dose of 180 mg morphine sulphate orally, this would convert to 18 mg of morphine via the epidural route.

Local anaesthetic drugs

Bupivacaine is the local anaesthetic agent of choice owing to its long duration of action and predominant action on sensory rather than motor fibres (Mercadante 1999). The starting concentration of bupivacaine can range from 0.125% to 0.25% but concentrations of 0.5% may be required to block resistant pain. Concentrations above 0.25% are associated with motor block (weakness) and autonomic block (urinary retention requiring catheterization).

Monitoring

For the first 24 hours after epidural insertion, the patient should be monitored for signs of drug-related side-effects or uncontrolled pain. Intravenous access should be maintained for at least 24 hours so that emergency drugs and fluids can be given if necessary.

After 24 hours, providing the patient's condition is stable, routine monitoring of respiratory rate and cardiac function is not usually required. Ongoing assessment of pain and observation of the catheter exit site (for any signs of infection) should be continued for the duration of epidural analgesia.

Discharge planning

If the patient is to go home with an epidural infusion, discharge planning should begin prior to epidural insertion. Primary care teams, patients and their families will need to be supplied with the appropriate equipment, drugs, catheter filters, information about the infusion pump, how to identify a catheter-related or systemic infection and what to do if pain occurs or complications arise. Contact numbers must be available in case specialist advice is needed.

Minimizing infection

Infection is a complication with long-term epidural analgesia.

Tunnelling the epidural catheter

To minimize the risk of a serious infection (e.g. epidural abscess, meningitis), it is common to tunnel the epidural catheter during insertion. This reduces the speed at which a local infection can spread along the catheter before reaching the epidural space. Once a local infection is suspected at the tunnelled site, treatment with antibiotics should be prompt to prevent a systemic infection.

Epidural filter changes

De Cicco *et al.* (1995) found that the use of bacterial filters during prolonged epidural catheterization maintained an unmodified antimicrobial function for more than 60 days when perfused with reduced volumes of drugs. It is recommended that epidural filters should only be changed every 4–6 weeks unless blocked (De Cicco *et al.* 1995; Mercadente 1999). More frequent filter changes have been associated with an increased risk of microbial colonization as a direct result of the procedure (De Cicco *et al.* 1995).

Procedure guidelines: **Insertion of an epidural catheter**

Note: patients undergoing epidural analgesia should always have a venous access device or an intravenous infusion in situ before the procedure. This is because, although rare, a reaction to the opioid or local anaesthetic solution (e.g. respiratory depression or sympathetic blockade) may require immediate access to the venous system.

Equipment

1 Chlorhexidine in 70% alcohol.
2 Local anaesthetic.
3 Selection of needles and syringes.
4 Sterile dressing pack.
5 Face mask.
6 Tuohy needle or assorted gauge lumbar puncture needles.
7 Epidural catheter.
8 Bacterial filter.
9 Waterproof dressing and plastic adhesive dressing to tape catheter securely.

Procedure

Action	Rationale
1 Explain and discuss the procedure with the patient. If the intention is to provide postoperative analgesia then explanation and consent should have been discussed the day before surgery.	To ensure that the patient understands the procedure and gives his/her valid consent and to ensure patient has time to assess information and ask questions.
2 Assist the patient into the required position: (a) Lying: Patient should be lying comfortably on a firm surface.	To allow identification of the spinal processes and intervertebral discs.

Procedure guidelines: Insertion of an epidural catheter (cont'd)

Action	Rationale
Position pillow under patient's head. On side with knee drawn up to the abdomen and clasped by the hands. Support the patient in this position.	
(b) Sitting: Patient sits on firm surface with arms resting on a table, and with the head resting on the arms.	To ensure maximal widening of the intervertebral spaces which will provide easy access to the epidural space.
3 Support, encourage and observe the patient throughout the procedure.	As the procedure takes place behind the patient, reassurance is very important.
4 Assist the doctor as required. The doctor will proceed as follows:	
(a) Clean the skin with alcohol-based solution (e.g. chlorhexidine in 70% isopropyl alcohol).	To clean skin and minimize risk of contamination.
(b) Identify the area to be punctured and inject the skin and subcutaneous layers with local anaesthetic.	
(c) Introduce Tuohy or spinal needles usually between third and fourth lumbar vertebrae.	
(d) Ensure epidural space has been entered.	To prevent anaesthesia being given directly into spinal cord or intravenously by means of the dural veins.
(e) Inject test dose of drug (may be performed).	To ensure the position of the needle.
(f) Thread epidural catheter through barrel of Tuohy needle.	To facilitate intermittent topping-up of anaesthesia and to allow greater control.
(g) Attach the bacterial filter.	To prevent injection of contaminants into epidural space.
(h) Apply transparent occlusive dressing and tape to the catheter insertion site.	To prevent the catheter being dislodged, to aid visibility and minimize contamination of the site.
(i) Inject solution into epidural space via catheter.	To provide anaesthesia.
5 Position the patient according to the doctor's instructions, tilting if appropriate.	To ensure spread of solution to provide optimum effect.
6 Take vital signs observations: blood pressure and respirations at least every 6 minutes for 30 minutes, and then 15 minutes for next 90 minutes. Take pulse every 15 minutes for 2 hours, or more frequently if the patient's condition dictates.	To monitor for signs of hypotension and respiratory depression.
7 Make the patient comfortable. Usually the patient is nursed flat for the first 3–6 hours, then slowly elevated into a sitting position. Bedclothes should not constrict the feet.	To ensure that any CSF leak is minimized and to prevent the patient developing a headache. To prevent the development of footdrop.
8 Assess pain regularly using a visual analogue scale or pain chart if appropriate. Observe the patient's movements and facial expressions. Discuss insufficient or ineffective analgesia with the anaesthetist.	To ensure optimal pain management and that the patient is involved in his or her pain management.

Problem solving: **Management of side-effects associated with epidural infusions of local anaesthetic agents and opioids**

Problem	Cause	Suggested action
Respiratory depression.	*Increasing age.* Elderly patients are more susceptible to the side-effects of opioids due to age-related alterations in the distribution, metabolism and excretion of drugs.	If respiratory rate falls to 8 breaths a minute or below: Stop the epidural infusion. Summon emergency assistance. Commence oxygen via face mask and encourage the patient to take deep breaths.

Problem solving (cont'd)

Problem	Cause	Suggested action
	Concurrent use of systemic opioids or sedatives. Patients receiving opioids by epidural infusion should not be given opioids by any other route (Macintyre & Ready 2001).	Stay with the patient and monitor respiratory rate and peripheral tissue oxygenation (using a pulse oximeter) continuously. Prepare naloxone 0.4 mg intravenously. If prescribed, give dose according to hospital policy (e.g. 100 μg increments every 3 minutes).
Sedation: *Mild* – patient drowsy but easy to rouse *Severe* – patient difficult to rouse.	See under Respiratory depression, above	If patient has mild sedation, consider reducing the rate of the infusion or the dose of opioid or taking the opioid out of the epidural infusion. If patient is difficult to rouse and opioid toxicity/ overdose is suspected, follow management for respiratory depression.
Hypotension.	Patients with hypovolaemia. Patients with a high thoracic epidural in whom the concentration of local anaesthetic agent and volume of infusion cause blockade of the cardio-accelerator nerves.	If blood pressure falls suddenly: Stop the epidural infusion. Summon emergency assistance. Place the patient flat and elevate legs on 3–4 pillows. Administer oxygen via face mask or nasal cannula. Stay with the patient and monitor blood pressure at 5 minute intervals. Ensure polyfusor of Haemacel or Gelofusine is readily available and use if prescribed by the anaesthetist. Vasoconstrictor agents such as ephedrine or metaraminol may need to be given by the anaesthetic team if hypotension does not respond to a fluid challenge of Haemacel or Gelofusine.
Motor blockade.	More likely to occur when higher concentrations of local anaesthetic agents are given by continuous infusion. If a high concentration of a local anaesthetic agent is administered via a low lumbar epidural catheter then the lumbar motor nerves are likely to be blocked, causing leg weakness.	Do not attempt to mobilize patient if leg weakness is evident. Contact pain or anaesthetic team for advice – reducing the concentration of the local anaesthetic agent or the rate of the epidural infusion may help to resolve this problem.
Nausea and vomiting.	Previous episodes of nausea and vomiting with opioids. Exacerbated by low blood pressure.	Regular administration of antiemetics. Treat other causes, e.g. low blood pressure.
Pruritus (usually more marked over the face, chest and abdomen).	Previous pruritus with opioids.	Administer an antihistamine such as chlorpheniramine (may be contraindicated in patients who are becoming increasingly sedated) or a small dose of naloxone. If pruritus does not resolve consider switching to another opioid or removing the opioid from the epidural infusion.
Urinary retention.	More likely to occur if opioids and local anaesthetic agents are infused in combination.	Catheterize patient.

Problem solving: **Complications of epidural use and management**

Problem	Signs and symptoms	Suggested action
Dural puncture.	Headache.	• Bedrest – headache will be less severe if patient lies flat. Replacement fluids either intravenously or orally to encourage formation of cerebrospinal fluid. Administer analgesics for headache. If headache does not settle, contact the anaesthetic team.
Catheter migration into an epidural blood vessel.	If catheter migrates into a blood vessel signs of opioid or local anaesthetic toxicity can occur: *opioid*: sedation and respiratory depression; *local anaesthetic*: circumoral tingling and numbness, twitching, convulsions and apnoea.	Stop epidural infusion. Contact pain/anaesthetic team or summon emergency assistance. If necessary support ventilation.
Catheter migration across the dura into the CSF.	If catheter migrates into the CSF the analgesic solution may reach as high as the cranial subarachnoid space. If this occurs the respiratory muscles are paralysed together with the cranial nerves, resulting in apnoea, profound hypotension and unconsciousness.	Stop epidural infusion. Summon emergency assistance. Prepare emergency equipment to support respiration and ventilate lungs. Prepare emergency drugs and intravenous fluids and administer as directed. Prepare equipment for intubation.
Epidural haematoma.	Back pain and tenderness and nerve root pain with sensory and motor weakness.	Urgent neurological assessment. CT or MRI scan to accurately diagnose. If a haematoma is diagnosed an urgent decompression laminectomy will be required, otherwise paraplegia may result (Mackenzie *et al*. 1998). * To avoid haematoma on removal of epidural in patients treated with prophylactic anticoagulants see guidelines for timing of removal.
Epidural abscess.	Back pain and tenderness. May have redness and purulent discharge from catheter exit site. May also develop nerve root signs with neuropathic pain and sensory/motor weakness.	If the epidural catheter is still in situ, remove and send tip off for culture and sensitivity. Treat with antibiotics. Carry out CT or MRI scan and refer for urgent neurosurgery to prevent paraplegia (Mackenzie *et al*. 1998).

Procedure guidelines: **Topping up epidural analgesia**

Usually performed by the doctor. Local anaesthetic agents *or* opioids may be given by nursing staff as part of an extended role, according to local policy. This should follow an agreed period of education and supervised practice, which must be documented.

Equipment

1 Antiseptic cleaning agent.
2 Syringes and needles.
3 Drug as prescribed.

4 Water or 0.9% sodium chloride for injection as necessary.
5 Patient's prescription chart.
6 Sterile hub/bung.

Procedure

	Action	Rationale
1	Wash hands with bactericidal soap and water or bactericidal alcohol handrub.	To reduce risk of cross-infection.
2	Check the drug to be administered and diluents, according to policy.	To ensure the correct drug, amount and concentration is administered to the correct patient.

*Procedure guidelines: **Topping up epidural analgesia** (cont'd)*

	Action	Rationale
3	Draw up the drug.	
4	Check patient's nameband against prescription.	To ensure correct patient receives correct drug.
5	Clean the access portal of the bacterial filter.	To prevent the introduction of contaminants and micro-organisms into the epidural space.
6	Inject drug as prescribed.	
7	Make the patient comfortable.	
8	Monitor vital signs, blood pressure and respirations at least every 5 minutes for 30 minutes, then every 15 minutes for 60 minutes. Take pulse if the patient's condition dictates.	To monitor signs of hypotension and respiratory depression.
9	Dispose of the equipment appropriately.	

Procedure guidelines: **Removal of an epidural catheter**

Note: before an epidural catheter is removed it is essential to consider the clotting status of the patient's blood. If the patient is fully anticoagulated a clotting profile must be performed and advice sought from the medical staff as to when the catheter can be removed. If the patient is receiving a prophylactic anticoagulant the following guidelines are recommended (Vandermeulen *et al*. 1994; Horlocker & Wedel 1998).

- Low-dose low molecular weight heparin – if this is given once daily the epidural catheter should be removed at least 12 hours after the last injection or immediately (1–2 hours) prior to the next dose.
- Unfractionated heparin – the epidural catheter should be removed at least 4 hours after the last injection.

Equipment

1 Dressing pack.
2 Skin cleaning agent, e.g. chlorhexidine in 70% alcohol.

3 Occlusive dressing.

Procedure

	Action	Rationale
1	Explain and discuss the procedure with the patient.	To ensure the patient understands the procedure and gives his/her valid consent.
2	Wash hands with bactericidal soap and water or bactericidal alcohol handrub.	To minimize cross-infection.
3	Open dressing pack.	
4	Wash hands and remove tape and dressing from catheter insertion site.	To minimize risk of cross-infection.
5	Gently, in one swift movement, remove the catheter. Check that the catheter is intact by observing marks along the catheter.	To ensure the catheter is removed intact with the minimum of discomfort to the patient.
6	Clean around the catheter exit site using skin cleaning agent.	To minimize contamination of site by micro-organisms.
7	Apply an occlusive dressing and leave in situ for 24 hours. The epidural tip may be sent for culture and sensitivity if infection is suspected, or according to local policy.	To prevent inadvertent access of micro-organisms along the tract.

Procedure guidelines: **Preinsertion management of an epidural for chronic pain**

If the patient is taking a slow-release preparation of morphine, e.g. MST or MXL, they should be converted to immediate-release morphine, either orally, intravenously or as a subcutaneous infusion for 24 hours before the insertion of the catheter. This is in order to minimize the risk of opioid overdose and the risk of respiratory depression. Once it has been decided that the patient is to have an epidural, a decision will need to be made regarding its fixation. As the catheter may need to stay in situ for several weeks/months it will either be tunnelled subcutaneously or anchored in place with medical glue and sutures.

Equipment

1 Chlorhexidine in 70% alcohol.	6 Dressing pack.
2 Syringes and needles.	7 Intravenous administration set.
3 Analgesia as prescribed.	8 Epidural catheter set.
4 0.9% sodium chloride for injection.	9 Suture material.
5 Patient's prescription chart.	10 Transparent dressing.

Procedure

	Action	Rationale
1	Explain and discuss the procedure with the patient and relatives/carers, obtain written consent.	To ensure that the patient understands the procedure and gives his/her valid consent.
2	Check full blood count (FBC) and clotting.	To assess the risk of haemorrhage and/or epidural haematoma.
3	Assess and document patient's current pain: its location, duration, type and intensity of impact.	To obtain baseline information to guide the epidural therapy.
4	Assess and document motor and sensory function.	To obtain baseline information to guide the epidural therapy.
5	Discuss with the patient about the choices they would like to make and their individual goals – expectations of tolerable pain scores and expectations of motor or sensory deficit.	In the chronic pain setting – it may sometimes be necessary to accept reduced independence (motor function) to achieve reasonable pain control.
6	Ensure adequate community support/expertise.	Essential if the patient is to be discharged from hospital.

Procedure guidelines: **Changing the dressing over the epidural exit site**

The dressing over the epidural exit site (e.g. tunnelled exit site) needs to fulfil the following three functions:

1 To help anchor the epidural catheter.
2 To maintain asepsis and minimize the risk of infection.
3 To allow observation of the site without disturbing the dressing.

A transparent occlusive dressing such as Opsite IV 3000 fulfils these functions. Opsite IV 3000 is also moisture responsive and has been found to perform well as an epidural catheter fixation product (Lawler & Anderson 2002). The epidural site should be inspected daily and the dressing changed at least once weekly or more frequently if there is any serous discharge from the site.

Equipment

1 Sterile dressing pack.	3 Occlusive dressing.
2 Skin cleaning agent, e.g. chlorhexidine in 70% alcohol.	

Procedure

	Action	Rationale
1	Explain and discuss the procedure with the patient.	To ensure that the patient understands the procedure and gives his/her valid consent.

*Procedure guidelines: **Changing the dressing over the epidural exit site** (cont'd)*

Action	Rationale
2 Clean trolley (or plastic tray in the community) with chlorhexidine in 70% alcohol with a paper towel.	To provide a clean working surface.
3 Position the patient comfortably on their side or sitting forward so that the site is easily accessible without undue exposure of the patient.	To maintain the patient's dignity and comfort. This is especially important when carers are attending to an area that is not visible to the patient.
4 Prepare trolley or tray with sterile field and cleaning solution.	To minimize risk of infection and ensure equipment available.
5 Remove old dressing and place in disposable bag.	To prevent cross-infection.
6 Wash hands with bactericidal handrub	To minimize the risk of microbial contamination.
7 Observe site for any signs of infection such as redness, swelling or purulent discharge. If any of these are present contact the hospital anaesthetic/pain team for advice.	To ensure careful monitoring of site to minimize the chance of any infection.
8 Clean site with skin cleaning agent.	To minimize the risk of infection.
9 Apply transparent occlusive dressing over the whole area.	To anchor the epidural catheter, minimize the risk of infection and allow observation of the epidural site.
10 Ensure that the patient is comfortable.	
11 Dispose of all material in the clinical waste bag.	To prevent environmental contamination.
12 Wash hands with bactericidal soap and water.	To reduce the risk of cross-infection.

Procedure guidelines: **Postinsertion monitoring of respiratory and cardiac function in chronic pain management**

It should be noted that the monitoring required in this patient group is different to that required in the postoperative setting. In the chronic setting, patients have already been taking opioids and have not received a general anaesthetic and are therefore less likely to suffer respiratory depression or alterations to their blood pressure (De Leon-Casasola *et al.* 1993).

Procedure

Action	Rationale
1 Monitor the patient's respiratory and cardiovascular function whilst in a recovery or high dependency area for 1 hour postinsertion.	To monitor for signs of respiratory depression and hypotension and to allow for immediate intervention where indicated.
2 On return to the ward for a minimum of 4 hours perform hourly assessment of: respiratory rate and SaO_2, blood pressure and pulse.	To monitor for signs of respiratory depression and hypotension and to allow for intervention if indicated.
3 If patient is stable, 4-hourly observations of the above for 24 hours. After 24 hours if patient is stable, monitoring should only be reintroduced if deemed necessary by the multidisciplinary team.	To monitor patient safety whilst minimising invasive procedures in patients with chronic problems.

Pain assessment

Action	Rationale
1 Assess the patient for their comfort/freedom from pain at rest and on movement, utilizing the same tool as used preinsertion.	This allows the practitioner and the patient to make a valid comparison.
2 Pain assessment should be performed by the practitioner and patient/family together.	To gain the patient's trust and to give the patient some control over their quality of life.

Procedure guidelines: **Postinsertion monitoring of respiratory and cardiac function in chronic pain management** *(cont'd)*

	Action	Rationale
3	Pain assessment should be performed initially at least hourly and then a minimum of 4 hourly until the patient and clinician feel that an optimum target has been achieved.	To aid patient comfort and the adjustment of drug dosages.
4	Document pain assessment.	To provide the patient/family with a visual record of achievement and to allow continuity of information for different clinicians.
5	Assess sensory and mobility quality.	Monitor for any loss of sensation, bladder function and motor function.

Procedure guidelines: **Setting up the epidural infusion (utilizing a syringe pump or driver)**

Equipment

1 Chlorhexidine in 70% alcohol.
2 Syringes and needles.
3 Analgesia as prescribed.
4 0.9% sodium chloride for injection.

5 Patient's prescription chart.
6 Dressing pack.
7 Extension set.

Procedure

	Action	Rationale
1	Explain and discuss the procedure with the patient.	To ensure that the patient understands the procedure and gives his/her valid consent.
2	Wash hands with bactericidal soap and water or bactericidal alcohol handrub.	To reduce risk of cross-infection.
3	Check the drugs to be administered and diluents according to policy.	To ensure the correct drugs, amount and concentration are administered to the correct patient.
4	Draw up the drugs and diluent into the syringe, affix drug identification label and attach the extension set.	To ensure safe practice.
5	Draw up 10 ml of 0.9% sodium chloride in a syringe as a flush.	To check patency of the catheter.
6	Clean the access port of the bacterial filter with a swab lightly soaked in chlorhexidine in 70% alcohol. Allow the chlorhexidine solution to air dry.	To minimize the risk of introducing any contaminants and micro-organisms into the epidural space.
7	Inject 0.9% sodium chloride – the catheter has a very narrow gauge so expect some resistance.	To check patency of the catheter before commencing the infusion.
8	Connect the infusion extension set to the filter and commence the infusion.	
9	Commence the infusion at the prescribed rate.	
10	Dispose of used equipment appropriately.	To prevent cross-infection.

Procedure guidelines: **Setting up the epidural infusion (utilizing an ambulatory pump)**

As above except:

Procedure

	Action	Rationale
1	Instil prescribed drugs and diluent into appropriate infusion bag and attach relevant extension set; apply drug information label.	To ensure infusion is ready to connect.

Procedure guidelines: **Setting up an epidural infusion (utilizing an ambulatory pump)** *(cont'd)*

	Action	Rationale
2	Check patency of epidural catheter as above.	
3	Insert the extension set into the pump and prime the extension set following the manufacturer's instructions for use of the pump.	To ensure the set is free from air when the infusion is commenced, thus minimizing the risk of air entering the catheter.
4	Clean the access portal of the bacterial filter with a swab lightly soaked in chlorhexidine in 70% alcohol. Allow the chlorhexidine solution to air dry.	To minimize the risk of introducing any contaminants and micro-organisms into the epidural space via the filter.
5	Attach the extension set to the bacterial filter and start the pump.	To ensure the pump is working and the drugs are being delivered.
6	Place pump and infusion bag into 'carry bag/pouch', ensuring that the tubing is not kinked.	To ensure comfort for the patient and to avoid obstruction to the infusion.

Procedure guidelines: **Discharge planning**

An epidural infusion should not be seen as a barrier to the patient leaving hospital. Patients can be safely managed in the community provided the following areas are addressed.

Procedure

	Action	Rationale
1	Convert patient's infusion to one that requires the minimum of changing, i.e. an infusion bag and ambulatory pump rather than a 20 ml syringe and driver.	This will reduce the workload of the patient/family or district nurse and also minimizes the number of interruptions to the patient circuit, thus minimizing the chance of microbial contamination.
2	Ensure that the patient will not be alone at home.	Epidural catheters can obstruct, become dislodged and the battery can fail on the device – most patients need immediate reassurance and practical help in these situations.
3	Arrange preparation of epidural drug infusion bags, usually in batches to provide enough delivery for one week. This can be arranged at the cancer centre or the referring hospital if they have the appropriate pharmaceutical arrangements.	Pharmacy reconstitution ensures aseptic preparation, thus minimizing the chance of microbial contamination, and reduces the workload and anxiety for family/district nurse. It should also be noted that epidural infusions may contain a combination of drugs and pharmacy reconstitution may help to reduce preparation error.
4	Discuss how the infusion bags will be collected each week; they cannot be posted because they contain drugs that are categorized as controlled drugs.	The method of collection needs to be discussed at an early stage with the family/district nurse to ensure continuity of epidural delivery and avoid any anxiety or delay to discharge.
5	The patient/family should be provided with the following equipment to take home: (a) Spare battery (b) Bottle of bactericidal handrub (c) Bottle of chlorhexidine in 70% alcohol (d) Sterile gauze (e) Syringes and needles (f) Sodium chloride for injection (g) One spare bacterial filter and screw connector (h) One week's supply of reconstituted epidural infusion bags (i) Written advice re contact numbers/troubleshooting and prescription.	To ensure that the first week of therapy continues smoothly. To reduce anxiety and increase patient comfort and trust.
6	Patient/family and district nurse/GP should be taught and trained in the following areas: (a) Setting up the infusion	

Procedure guidelines: **Discharge planning** *(cont'd)*

Action	Rationale
(b) The functions of the ambulatory device, including alarms and visual displays	
(c) Loading the administration set into the pump and priming the set	
(d) Observation of the epidural site for signs and symptoms which would indicate an infection, e.g. redness, tenderness, swelling, leakage or pus	
(e) The prescribed therapy for breakthrough pain	
(f) Troubleshooting (as described below)	
(g) The procedure for obtaining medical/nursing help locally or at the cancer centre 24 hourly and every day of the week	
(h) Dressing of the epidural site.	

Problem solving

The following can be used by nursing staff and then adapted for use by the patient/family.

Problem	Cause	Suggested action
Ambulatory pump auditory alarm.	(a) Battery failure is most likely.	(a) Stop pump, remove old and replace with new battery; ensure battery is fitted up snugly to connections. Turn on pump and ensure light indicator is flashing.
	(b) Catheter occlusion.	(b) Stop pump, draw up 0.9% sodium chloride and flush catheter, if catheter clears reattach pump, press start and ensure light indicator is flashing. If catheter is still obstructed and will not flush, phone cancer centre/GP.
Sudden acute pain.	Catheter obstruction; catheter movement; change in pathology.	Check the catheter for any obvious problems which can be quickly resolved such as catheter disconnection (see 3). If the catheter has blocked or migrated outwards, stop the infusion pump and give the patient a breakthrough dose of analgesia orally or subcutaneously. Inform GP and/or hospital anaesthetic/pain team as soon as possible. If the patient has had an exacerbation of pain due to disease progression, follow advice from hospital team (the infusion rate may require titrating or the concentration of drugs may need to be changed).
Disconnection of epidural catheter from filter.	Patient movement – typically turning in bed at night.	Stop the pump. Wrap the disconnected end of the catheter in a piece of sterile gauze and contact the district nursing/hospital team for advice. Suggested procedure for district nursing/hospital team (see Langevin *et al.* 1996): • Clean approximately 15 cm of the disconnected catheter with chlorhexidine in 70% alcohol. Allow to air dry completely. • Using sterile scissors, cut the cleaned catheter 10 cm away from the contaminated end. • Insert the cleaned end of catheter into a sterile screw connector and catheter filter.

Problem solving (cont'd)

Problem	Cause	Suggested action
		• Change the epidural infusion extension set and recommence infusion.
Redness, swelling or leakage of discoloured fluid from site.	Infection *or* local irritation at site from skin interaction with the plastic catheter.	Contact GP and hospital anaesthetic/pain team. If infection is suspected, the patient should be started on antibiotics to prevent spread of any infection into the epidural space. It may be necessary to remove the catheter if the patient has a temperature, there is pus at the exit site or the patient has back pain.

References and further reading

Audit Commission (1997) *Anaesthesia Under Examination*. Audit Commission, Oxford.

Bannon, L., Alexander-Williams, M. & Lutman, D. (2001) A national survey of epidural practice. *Anaesthesia*, **56**(10), 1021.

Chapman, S. & Day, R. (2001) Spinal anatomy and the use of epidurals. *Prof Nurse*, **16**(6), 1174–7.

Cook, T., Eaton, J. & Goodwin, A. (1997) Epidural analgesia following upper abdominal surgery: United Kingdom practice. *Acta Anaesthesiol Scand*, **41**(1 P +), 18–24.

de Cicco, M., Matovic, M. & Castellani, G. *et al.* (1995) Time-dependent efficacy of bacterial filters and infection risk in long-term epidural catheterisation. *Anesthesiology*, **82**, 765–71.

De Leon-Casasola, O.A., Myers, D.P., Donaparthi, S. *et al.* (1993) A comparison of post-operative epidural analgesia between patients with chronic cancer taking high doses of oral opioids versus opioid-naïve patients. *Anesth Analg*, **76**, 302–7.

Grond, S., Meuser, T., Stute, P. & Gohring, U. (2000) Epidural analgesia for labour pain: a review of availability, current practices and influence on labour. *Int J Acute Pain Manage*, **3**(1), 31–43.

Hall, J. (2000) Epidural analgesia management. *Nurs Times*, **96**(28), 38–9.

Horlocker, T. & Wedel, D. (1998) Spinal and epidural blockade and perioperative low molecular weight heparin: smooth sailing on the Titanic. *Anaesth Analg*, **8**, 1153–6.

Kehlet, H. (1997) Multimodal approach to control postoperative pathophysiology and rehabilitation. *Br J Anaesth*, **78**(5), 606–17.

Kehlet, H. & Holte, K. (2001) Effect of postoperative analgesia on surgical outcome. *Br J Anaesth*, **87**(1), 62–72.

Langevin, P., Gravenstein, N., Langevin, S. & Gulig, P. (1996) Epidural catheter reconnection: safe and unsafe practice. *Anesthesiology*, **85**(4), 883–8.

Lawler, K. & Anderson, T. (2002) Regional trial of five epidural fixation products and a commonly used control. *Pain Network Newsletter*, **Spring**, 6–8.

Macintyre, P. & Ready, L. (2001) Epidural and intrathecal analgesia. In: *Acute Pain Management. A Practical Guide*, 2nd edn. W.B. Saunders, London.

Mackenzie, A.R. *et al.* (1998) Spinal epidural abscess: the importance of early diagnosis and treatment. *J Neurosurg Psychiatry*, **65**(2), 209–12.

Mercadante, S. (1999) Problems of long-term spinal opioid treatment in advanced cancer patients. *Pain*, **79**(1), 1–13.

Papagelopoulos, P., Petrou, H. & Triantafyllidis, P. *et al.* (2001) Treatment of lumbosacral radicular pain with epidural steroid injections. *Orthopedics*, **24**(2), 145–9.

Richardson, J. (2001) Post-operative epidural analgesia: introducing evidence-based guidelines through an education and assessment process. *J Clin Nurs*, **10**(2), 238–45.

Romer, H. & Russell, G. (1998) A survey of the practice of thoracic epidural analgesia in the United Kingdom. *Anaesthesia*, **53**(10), 1016–22.

Sands, R., Yarussi, A. & de Leon-Casasola, D. (1998) Complications and side-effects associated with epidural bupivacaine/morphine analgesia. *Acute Pain*, **1**(2), 43–50.

Smith, H. & Elliott, J. (2001) Alpha$_2$ receptors and agonists in pain management. *Curr Opin Anaesthesiol*, **14**, 513–18.

Smitt, P., Tsafka, A., Teng-van de Zande, F. *et al.* (1998) Outcome and complications of epidural analgesia in patients with chronic cancer pain. *Cancer*, **83**(9), 2015–22.

Vandermeulen, E., Van Aken, H. & Vermylen, J. (1994) Anticoagulants and spinal-epidural anaesthesia. *Anaesth Analg*, **79**(6), 1165–77.

Wheatley, R., Schug, S. & Watson, D. (2001) Safety and efficacy of postoperative epidural analgesia. *Br J Anaesth*, **87**(1), 47–61.

Perioperative care

Chapter contents

Perioperative care refers to the nursing care delivered to a patient before (pre), during (intra) and after (post) surgery.

Preoperative care

Definition

Preoperative care is the preparation and assessment, physical and psychological, of a patient before surgery.

Objectives

Physical

- To minimize postoperative complications, e.g. by teaching the patient deep breathing exercises and their importance to the individual's well-being postoperatively.
- To assess the physical condition of the patient so that potential problems can be anticipated and prevented.
- To ensure that the patient understands the need to be in an optimum physical condition before surgery.

Psychological

- To ensure that the patient understands the nature of the surgery to be undergone.
- To teach the patient what to expect postoperatively, e.g. about any drains, catheters, pumps and monitors that may be necessary afterwards.
- To recognize anxiety and identify and implement useful coping mechanisms.

Reference material

Patient education and postoperative pain

Much research and discussion have been devoted to the subject of postoperative pain and the ways in which preoperative patient education can influence the pain experience. Since pain and anaesthesia are often the patient's greatest fears (Mitchell 2000), it is necessary to address this cause of anxiety in the preoperative period.

Reducing patient anxiety by giving preoperative information has been shown to reduce postoperative pain (Hayward 1975; Beddows 1997). It also results in the patient requiring less analgesia. The reduction of anxiety and promoting postoperative recovery can be achieved in several ways. The fragmentation of nursing care could account for some patient anxiety (Hughes 2002), and preoperative visiting by theatre nurses is being undertaken in many hospitals in order to significantly decrease levels of patient anxiety (Martin 1996). Research has shown that this can assist the patient to manage their anxiety and has the added benefit of improving collaboration between all members of the surgical team, thus ensuring continuity of care for the patient (Martin 1996; Beddows 1997).

Research has shown that preoperative patient education not only meets patients' information needs but also assists patients in reducing their anxiety levels and promotes well-being (Walker 2002). Copp (1988) also found that teaching patients recovery exercises decreased their feelings of helplessness and, therefore, reduced anxiety, and that the use of cognitive coping methods is an effective way of reducing anxiety.

Jackson (1995) suggested that 50% of patients have pain for the 72 hours after surgery. The patient's pain is assessed in recovery where analgesia and antiemetics are administered accordingly. Regular analgesia is prescribed with *pro re nata* (prn; as required) analgesia prescribed for breakthrough. Use of patient-controlled analgesia (PCA) gives the patient a sense of autonomy which may decrease anxiety, and which will in turn influence the patient's pain perception (Field & Adams 2001) (see Ch. 27, Pain assessment and pain management).

Skin preparation

It has long been a tradition that the patient should be shaved preoperatively in the belief that hair removal reduces the incidence of wound infection. Shaving was traditionally done the night before the operation but this method of hair removal can injure the skin and may increase the risk of infection by producing microscopic infected lacerations. Therefore only the area to be incised needs to have hair removed. This should be done with depilatory cream the day before the operation. If this is not possible then shaving should take place in the anaesthetic room immediately preoperatively, using electric clippers (Kjonniksen *et al.* 2002).

Preoperative fasting

Any patient presenting for anaesthesia may have undigested food in the stomach. For elective surgery the patient is usually 'nil by mouth' for long enough to allow the stomach to empty. Research by Chapman (1996) has revealed that patients often did not know why they were fasting, and that they were often deprived of food and drink for longer than the recommended time of 6 hours and maximum time of 12 hours. Patients on an afternoon theatre list were less likely to be starved for as long as those on the morning list, who were frequently starved from midnight.

Stomach emptying on average takes 6 hours for solid food and 2–4 hours for fluids. However, gastric emptying may be delayed by anxiety or the action of some drugs, e.g. opiates (Jester & Williams 1999; O'Callaghan 2002).

Antiembolic stockings

Deep vein thrombosis, if it occurs, is usually diagnosed 3–14 days postoperatively. The incidence is highest in middle-aged and elderly patients, those on prolonged bedrest, and after major surgery of the lower abdomen, pelvis or hip joints. Patients with a history of coronary artery disease are also at risk. Once high-risk patients have been identified, prophylactic treatment can begin.

One such treatment is the use of antiembolic stockings (Jefferey & Nicolaides 1990). There are two lengths of antiembolic stockings: knee high and thigh high. The latter are more difficult to put on and therefore for surgical patients knee high are more suitable (Bryne 2002). Carman & Fernandez (1999) give specific recommendations on a number of issues in venous thromboembolism and one of these is the use of compression stockings. Graduated compression stockings contribute to the prevention of deep vein thrombosis in hospital patients (Campbell 2001). They work by promoting venous flow and reducing stasis (Evans & Read 2001). They increase the velocity of flow not only in the legs but also in the pelvic veins and inferior vena cava (Hayes *et al.* 2002).

During surgery the use of heel supports which reduce the pressure on the calves on the operating table will also encourage venous return. The use of intermittent calf compression air boots which promote venous flow during surgery has also been reported to be effective (Davis & O'Neill 2002). Good pain control will encourage patients to mobilize early and carry out postoperative exercises, which are also important in preventing serious postoperative complications.

Care of the patient with a latex allergy

Natural rubber latex is a durable flexible material composed of natural proteins and added chemicals. In the health care setting natural rubber latex is present in gloves and other medical devices such as catheters and wound drains. Latex allergy results in a reaction to one or more of the components of natural rubber latex.

It is the admitting nurse's responsibility to ensure that the patient assessment includes discussion and documentation of the patient's allergy status and that this information has been communicated to all members of the health care team including theatres, recovery and other areas the patient may attend. The assessment should involve discussion of the following risk factors:

• Is there a history of multiple surgeries beginning at an early age (e.g. spina bifida, urinary malformation)?
• Do you have any food allergies (avocado, chestnut or banana)?

Table 30.1 Symptoms of latex exposure and possible anaphylaxis

The conscious patient	The unconscious patient
Itchy eyes	Facial oedema
Generalized pruritis	Urticaria/rash
Shortness of breath	Skin flushing
Sneezing/wheezing	Bronchospasm
Nausea	Laryngeal oedema
Oedema	Hypotension
Vomiting	Tachycardia
Abdominal cramp	Cardiac arrest
Diarrhoea	
Feeling faint	

• Is there a history of an allergic reaction to latex?
• Have you ever experienced an allergic reaction during an operation?
• Have you ever suffered from itchy skin, skin rash or redness when in contact with rubber products?
• Have you ever suffered skin irritation from an examination by a doctor or dentist wearing rubber gloves?
• Have you ever suffered sneezing, wheezing or chest tightness when exposed to rubber?

Some of the symptoms of exposure to latex are outlined in Table 30.1.

Management of the patient with known latex allergy

Patients identified as having an allergy to natural latex rubber need to be treated in a latex-free environment:

• The patient must be treated in a controlled area with all latex products removed or covered with plastics so that the rubber elements are not exposed.
• All health care staff must be made aware of the adverse reactions that could occur following the patient's exposure to natural rubber latex.
• Where a type I allergy is suspected, suitable clinical management procedures must be ready for use in the event of the patient having a hypersensitivity reaction.
• All health care staff in direct contact with the patient must wear vinyl gloves during procedures and in the vicinity of the patient.

Further guidance may be sought from the Association of periOperative Registered Nurses (AORN) proposed latex guideline at www.aorn.org/proposed/latex.htm (last accessed 5 November 2003).

Procedure guidelines: **Preoperative care**

Equipment

1 Theatre gown.
2 Labelled denture container if necessary.
3 Hypoallergenic tape to cover wedding rings.

4 Any equipment and documents required by law and hospital policy if a premedication has been prescribed.

Procedure

Action	Rationale
1 Ensure the patient is wearing an identification bracelet with the correct information.	To ensure correct identification and prevent possible problems.
2 Assess the preoperative education received by the patient and ensure that it is complete and understood.	To ensure that the patient understands the nature and outcome of the surgery and reduce anxiety and possible postoperative complications.

*Procedure guidelines: **Preoperative care** (cont'd)*

Action	Rationale
3 Record the patient's pulse, blood pressure, respirations, temperature and weight.	To provide data for comparison postoperatively. The weight is recorded so that the anaesthetist can calculate the dose of drugs to be used.
4 Check that the patient has undergone relevant procedures, e.g. X-ray, ECG, blood tests and that these results are included with the patient's notes.	To ensure all relevant information is available to the nurses, anaesthetists and surgeons. Absence of results may delay or cause cancellation of an operation.
5 Instruct the patient on showering or bathing.	To minimize risk of postoperative wound infection.
6 Assist the patient to change into a theatre gown after having a shower.	
7 Long hair should be held back with, for example, a non-metallic tie.	
8 Ensure that patients undergoing major surgery or abdominal/pelvic surgery, the elderly, frail or bedbound patients or those with a previous history of emboli or other high-risk factors have antiembolic stockings applied correctly. The use of intermittent calf compression boots should be considered.	To reduce the risk of postoperative deep vein thrombosis or pulmonary emboli.
9 Complete the preoperative checklist by asking the patient and checking records and notes before giving any premedication.	*Note*: questioning premedicated patients is not a reliable source of checking information as the patient may be drowsy and/or disorientated.
(a) Check when patient last had food or drink and ensure that it was at least 6 h before.	To reduce the risk of regurgitation and inhalation of stomach contents on induction of anaesthetic.
(b) Check whether patient micturated before premedication.	To prevent urinary incontinence and embarrassment. To allow better access to abdominal cavity for abdomen or pelvic surgery if a catheter is not to be used.
(c) Note whether the patient has dental crowns, bridge work or loose teeth.	The anaesthetist needs to be informed to prevent accidental damage. Loose teeth or a dental prosthesis could be inhaled by the patient when an endotracheal tube is inserted.
(d) Ensure prostheses, dentures and contact lenses are removed.	To promote patient safety during surgery, e.g. dentures may obstruct airway, contact lenses can cause corneal abrasions.
(e) Spectacles may be retained until the patient is in the anaesthetic room. Hearing aids may be retained until the patient has been anaesthetized. (These may be left in position if a local anaesthetic is being used.) Any prosthesis should then be labelled clearly and retained in the recovery room.	To allow patient to see and hear, thus reducing anxiety and enabling the patient to understand any procedures carried out.
(f) All jewellery (apart from wedding ring), cosmetics, nail varnish and clothing, other than the theatre gown, are to be removed.	Metal jewellery may be accidentally lost or may be cause of harm to patient, e.g. diathermy burns. Facial cosmetics make the patient's colour difficult to assess. Nail varnish makes the use of the pulse oximeter, used to monitor the patient's pulse and oxygen saturation levels, impossible and masks peripheral cyanosis.
10 Valuables should be placed in the hospital's custody and recorded according to the hospital policy.	To prevent loss of valuables.
11 Check the consent form is correctly completed, signed and dated.	To comply with legal requirements and hospital policy.
12 Check the operation site is marked correctly.	To ensure the patient undergoes the correct surgery for which he/she has consented.

*Procedure guidelines: **Preoperative care** (cont'd)*

Action	Rationale
13 Check that the patient has undergone preanaesthetic assessment by the anaesthetist.	To ensure that the patient can be given the most suitable anaesthetic.
14 Give the premedication, if prescribed, in accordance with the anaesthetist's instructions and conforming to legal requirements and hospital policy.	Different drugs may be prescribed to complement the anaesthetic to be given, e.g. temazepam to reduce patient anxiety by inducing sleep and relaxation.
15 Advise the patient to remain in bed once the premedication has been given and to use the nurse call system if assistance is needed.	To reduce the risk of accidental patient injury as the premedication may make the patient drowsy and disorientated.
16 Ensure the patient is supported fully on the canvas, especially the head, when transferred from the ward bed to the trolley.	To reduce the risk of injury to the neck, etc., during transfer from the ward to the operating theatre.
17 Ensure that all relevant information, e.g. X-rays, notes, blood results, accompany the patient to the operating theatre.	To prevent delays which can increase the patient's anxiety, and to ensure that the anaesthetist and surgeon have all the information they require for the safe treatment of the patient.
18 The patient should be accompanied to the theatre by a ward nurse who remains until the patient is anaesthetized.	To reduce the patient's anxiety.
19 The ward nurse should give a full handover to the anaesthetic nurse or operating department assistant on arrival of the patient at the anaesthetic room.	To ensure the patient has the correct operation. To ensure continuity of care by exchanging all relevant information.

Intraoperative care

Definition

Intraoperative care is the physical and psychological care given to the patient in the anaesthetic room and theatre until transferral to the recovery room.

Objectives

- To ensure that the patient understands what is happening at all times in order to minimize anxiety.
- To ensure that the patient has the surgery for which the consent form was signed.
- To ensure patient safety at all times and minimize postoperative complications by:
  - (a) Giving the required care for the unconscious patient.
  - (b) Ensuring no injury is sustained from hazards associated with the use of swabs, needles, instruments, diathermy and power tools.
  - (c) Minimizing postoperative problems associated with patient positioning, such as nerve or tissue damage.
  - (d) Maintaining asepsis during surgical procedures to reduce the risk of postoperative wound infection in accordance with hospital policies on infection control.

Reference material

Diathermy

Diathermy is used routinely during many operations to control haemorrhage by cauterizing blood vessels or cutting or fulgerizing body tissues. Diathermy is potentially hazardous to the patient if used incorrectly. It is important that all theatre nurses know how to test and use all diathermy equipment in their department to prevent patient injury (Aigner *et al.* 1997; Wicker 2000; Molyneux 2001).

The main risk when using diathermy is of thermoelectrical burns. The most common cause is incorrect application of the patient plate or a break in the connecting lead (Aigner *et al.* 1997). If this occurs when using an isolated diathermy machine then the current output will stop. However, if a grounded diathermy machine is used then the electrical current will find an alternative route back to the diathermy machine (Wainwright 1988). If the patient is in contact with any metal, e.g. on the operating table (Wicker 1997) then loss of plate contact using a grounded unit could result in a serious burn.

Other causes of burns include skin preparation solutions or other liquids pooling around the plate site (Fong *et al.* 2000). With alcohol-based skin preparations especially, the skin should be allowed to dry before diathermy is used, as the alcohol can ignite (Fong *et al.*

2000). If the patient's position is changed during the operation the patient plate should be rechecked to ensure that it is still in contact and that the connecting clamp or lead is not causing pressure in the new position.

Use of diathermy and the plate position should be noted on the nursing care plan, and the patient's skin condition should be checked postoperatively.

Patient positioning

The position of the patient on the operating table must be such as to facilitate access to the operation site(s) by the surgeon, taking into account the patient's airway, monitoring equipment or intravenous choices. It should not compromise the patient's circulation, respiratory system or nerves. The patient's positioning will be dependent upon the type of surgery performed and accessibility for the anaesthetist. However, the safety of the patient in relation to their position remains the responsibility of the whole theatre team (AORN 2001). Preoperative assessment will identify patients with particular needs which may be influenced by factors such as weight, nutritional state, age, skin condition and pre-existing disease. All these factors may indicate the need for extra precautions during positioning. Consideration by and the co-operation of all theatre personnel can help prevent many of the preoperative complications related to intraoperative positioning (McEwen 1996; AORN 2001).

All equipment that may be needed to support the patient during surgery, e.g. the table, arm supports, lithotomy poles and securing straps, should be checked to ensure that they are in working order, clean and free from sharp edges. Metal parts that may come into contact with the patient should be covered as there is an increased risk of burns if diathermy is used (Aigner et al. 1997). Padding should be placed at the patient's elbows and heels, and pillows positioned between the legs if the patient is lying in a lateral position. Special consideration should also be given to vulnerable points or areas such as heels, elbows, ears, the head, back and sacrum.

When a patient is transferred between the trolley or bed and operating table, adequate personnel should be present to ensure patient and staff safety (AORN 2001). It is recommended that an approved rolling or sliding device is used to transfer patients from trolley to operating table, in compliance with legislation on manual handling. Safe manual handling and the safety of the patient depend on the participation of the correct number of staff in the specified handling manoeuvre.

All movements of the limbs of the unconscious patient should take into account the anatomy and natural planes of movement of that limb to avoid stretching and pressure on the related nerve planes (AORN 2001). Hyperabduction of the arm when placed on a board, for example, could stretch the brachial plexus, causing some postoperative loss of sensation and reduced movement of the forearm, wrist and fingers. The ulnar and radial nerves may be affected by direct pressure as a result of insufficient padding on arm supports or lack of care when inserting poles into the canvas and hitting the elbows.

Pre-existing conditions such as backache or sciatica can be exacerbated, particularly if the patient is in the lithotomy position as the sciatic nerve can be compressed against the poles (AORN 2001). Most postoperative palsies are due to improper positioning of the patient on the operating table (Ulrich et al. 1997).

Control of infection and asepsis in operating theatres

The term asepsis means the absence of any infectious agents. The aseptic technique is the foundation on which contemporary surgery is built (Gruendemann & Meeker 1983). The aim of operating theatres is to provide an area free from infectious agents. Large quantities of bacteria are present in the nose, mouth, on the skin, hair and on the attire of personnel; therefore people entering the operating theatres wear clean scrub suits and lint-free surgical hats to eliminate the possibility of these bacteria, hair or dandruff being shed (Tammelin et al. 2000). Sterile gowns and gloves are worn to prevent cross-infection. Well-fitting shoes with impervious soles should be worn and regularly cleaned to remove splashes of blood and body fluids (Woodhead et al. 2002). Face masks are worn to prevent droplets falling from the mouth into the operating field. The extent to which face masks are capable of preventing droplet spread is disputed (Lipp & Edwards 2002). It is, however, accepted that masks offer protection to the wearer from blood splashes and for safety reasons should be worn by the scrub team.

Presurgical hand washing is essential to the maintenance of asepsis in the operating theatre. New research has recommended a 1-minute hand wash with a non-antiseptic soap followed by hand rubbing with liquid aqueous alcoholic solution, prior to each surgeon's first procedure of the day. Before any other procedure the process should be repeated. This has been shown to be as effective as traditional hand scrubbing with antiseptic soap in preventing surgical site infections (Parienti et al. 2002). However, the traditional 3-minute first scrub of the day is recommended for all intermediate, major and complex cases. The closed method of donning sterile surgical gloves is preferred.

Surgical gloves have a dual role, acting as a barrier for personal protection from patients' blood and other exudate and preventing the bacterial transfer from the surgeon's hand to the operating site. It has been suggested that double gloving significantly reduces the number of perforations to the innermost glove in low-risk surgical patients, thus reducing infection rates during surgical procedures (Tanner & Parkinson 2002).

Universal precautions should be taken in theatres to minimize the risk of infection from blood and body fluids. These include the wearing of gloves, masks, barrier gowns and aprons. Protective eyewear or face shields should be worn during procedures likely to cause splashes or droplets of blood or generate bone chips (Tokars *et al.* 1995). Instruments must be handled carefully, and needle holders and forceps used to manipulate sutures to minimize the risk of needlestick or sharps injury.

Laparoscopic surgery

Laparoscopy has evolved from a diagnostic modality into a widespread surgical technique. Advantages for the patient include: a shorter stay in hospital, reduced postoperative pain and a shorter recovery period. However, this technique is not without its complications (O'Malley & Cunningham 2001). Laparoscopic surgery is now common in operating departments, and it is important that potential complications are identified and steps taken to minimize risk to the patient, both during surgery and in the recovery period. Patients should be prepared psychologically and physically for an open procedure, which may be undertaken under certain circumstances.

Instruments and supplies for an open procedure must be readily available in the operating theatre.

Laparoscopy involves insufflation of the abdomen with carbon dioxide (CO_2). Prolonged insufflation can cause hypothermia since although the gas temperature in the hose equals room temperature, the temperature in the abdomen can decrease to 27.7°C due to high gas flow and the large amounts of gas used (Jacobs *et al.* 2000). Sharma *et al.* (1997) refer to the increased risk of hypercarbia and surgical emphysema during insufflation with CO_2. Careful monitoring and recording of the patient's vital signs, including oxygen saturation and expiratory gas levels, are therefore essential during laparoscopy.

Haemorrhage can occur during the procedure and may be difficult to detect because surgeons have a limited view of the area being operated upon. Electrosurgical injuries to organs may occur as a result of capacitive coupling (Wu *et al.* 2000) (capacitive coupling is the transfer of electrical currents from the active electrode through coupling of stray currents into other conductive surgical equipment). Theatre staff must be aware of potential complications and ensure that equipment is used safely and according to the manufacturer's instructions.

The equipment used for laparoscopic surgery is very specialized and can be daunting for theatre staff. The Association of periOperative Registered Nurses (AORN 2000) recommends that all equipment is regularly and competently maintained and a maintenance record kept in a log. Policies and procedures should be developed for the checking procedure, and all staff thoroughly instructed in the operation of laparoscopic equipment.

Procedure guidelines: **Intraoperative care**

Procedure

Action	Rationale
1 Greet the patient by name. Confirm with the ward nurse that it is the correct patient for the scheduled operation.	To make the patient feel welcome. To ensure that the patient is safeguarded against problems related to misidentity.
2 Identify the patient by checking the name bracelet and number against the patient's notes and the operating list.	Questioning the premedicated patient can be unreliable (AORN 2001).
3 Examine the preoperative checklist.	To ensure that all of the listed measures have been completed and that any additional information has been recorded.
4 Check that the blood results, X-rays, etc., are present in the patient's notes.	To ensure that all of the required results are available for the medical team's use.
5 Maintain a calm, quiet environment and explain all the procedures to the patient.	To reduce anxiety and enhance the smooth induction of anaesthesia.
6 When the patient is anaesthetized ensure that the eyes are closed and hypoallergenic tape is applied.	To prevent corneal damage due to drying or accidental abrasion.

*Procedure guidelines: **Intraoperative care** (cont'd)*

Action	Rationale
7 Ensure that there are adequate staff to transfer the patient to the operating table. Ensure the brakes on the trolley and operating table have been applied. Ensure the patient's head and limbs are supported when transferring to the operating table.	To ensure that the patient receives no injury during the transfer.
8 Check with anaesthetist before moving patient.	To ensure that the airway is protected.
9 Ensure all limbs are supported and secure on the table. Ensure adequate padding and cushioning of bony prominences. The patient's position will be dictated by the nature of the surgery but must take into account the requirements of the anaesthetist and the physical, psychological and social needs of the patient.	If the patient is unconscious and unable to maintain a safe environment, support is necessary to prevent injury. The patient is especially at risk from damage due to pressure and stretching, so measures to maintain the skin's integrity are vital. Nerve damage due to compression or stretching must be prevented.
10 Ensure the patient is covered by the gown or blanket. These items should only be removed immediately before surgery.	To maintain the patient's dignity. To help prevent a reduction in body temperature or accidental hypothermia.
11 Use a warm air mattress on the operating table. Ensure all fluids used are warmed if possible.	To help maintain the patient's body temperature and prevent postoperative complications due to hypothermia.
12 Ensure all the equipment to be used is checked and in working order before the operating list commences, including suction, the anaesthetic machine, medical gases, monitoring equipment, diathermy and operating table.	To prevent accidental injury due to faulty equipment and to ensure all equipment necessary to the patient's treatment is present.
13 Ensure diathermy patient plate is attached securely in accordance with the manufacturer's instructions and hospital policy.	To ensure that no injury is sustained from the use of diathermy during surgery.
14 Follow hospital policy for the checking of swabs, needles and instruments.	To ensure that swabs, needles and instruments are accounted for at the end of the operation.
15 Follow hospital policy for the disposal of sharps and clinical waste.	To reduce the risk of injury to the patient and staff.
16 Ensure the surgeon is informed that the number of swabs, needles and instruments is correct.	It is the responsibility of the nurse and surgeon to check that nothing is accidentally left inside the patient on completion of surgery.
17 The scrub nurse accompanies the patient with the anaesthetist to the recovery area. A handover is given that includes:	To ensure continuity of care of the patient.
(a) What procedure was performed	To ensure that the recovery nurse has all the information required to assess the patient's recovery needs.
(b) The presence, position and nature of any drains, infusions or intravenous or arterial devices	
(c) Information including allergies or pre-existing medical conditions, such as diabetes mellitus	To assist the recovery nurse in the assessment of postoperative problems with which the patient may present.
(d) The patient's cardiovascular state and pattern of anaesthesia used	
(e) Specific instructions from the anaesthetist for postoperative care	
(f) Information about any anxieties of the patient expressed before surgery such as a fear of not waking after anaesthesia or fear about coping with pain	To ensure appropriate action can be taken as the patient regains consciousness and to enable an assessment of the efficacy of nursing interventions used.
(g) All information is to be recorded on the theatre nursing care plan.	To provide a written record of nursing intervention for use by recovery staff and ward nursing staff.

Postanaesthetic recovery

Definition

Postanaesthetic recovery involves the short-term critical care required by patients during their immediate post-operative period until they are stable, conscious and orientated.

Indication

All patients undergoing surgery and anaesthesia.

Reference material

The postanaesthetic recovery room is an area within the operating department specifically designed, equipped and staffed for the support, monitoring and assessment of patients through the reversing stages of anaesthesia.

The recovery period is potentially hazardous. Therefore, when the patient arrives in the postanaesthetic recovery room, individual nursing care is required until patients are able to maintain their own airway (AAGBI 2002). While the majority of patients can be expected to achieve uneventful recovery, 24% of all patients have complications (Hines *et al.* 1992). Although nausea and vomiting are high on the list of complications (Jolley 2001), the most notable are respiratory and circulatory complications. Obstruction of the upper airway is the most common respiratory complication in the immediate postoperative period. Close observation and appropriate action can prevent the sequence of respiratory obstruction resulting in hypoxia leading to cardiac arrest (Peskett 1999).

Guedel's classification of general anaesthesia

Guedel first published his systemization of the signs of inhalation anaesthesia, based on the description of patients under open-drop ether anaesthesia in 1920. Current practice does not depend on the use of a single agent administered in this way and the effects of opiates and muscle relaxants will affect the signs of the stages of anaesthesia as formulated in his classification. However, the system can still be used as a framework within which to assess the progress of postanaesthetic recovery as long as other factors influencing the return of consciousness are taken into consideration (Table 30.2). With modern anaesthetic agents particulary propofol (Diprivan), rapid and symptom-free recovery from anaesthesia is seen and the frequency of nausea and vomiting, headaches and confusion/restlessness has been shown to be reduced (Sneyd *et al.* 1998). This type of anaesthetic is commonly used in day surgery.

Assessment for discharge

The length of any patient's stay in the recovery room is dependent on the patient's condition and the rate at which that patient returns to a physical, mental and emotional state where he or she can be left unattended between routine observations.

Minimum criteria for discharge are:

- The patient is conscious and orientated and all protective reflexes have returned to normal.
- Respiratory function is adequate and good oxygenation is being maintained.
- Pulse and blood pressure are within normal preoperative limits on consecutive observation.
- There is no persistent or excessive bleeding from wound or drainage sites.
- Patients with urinary catheters have passed adequate amounts of urine (more than 0.5 ml/kg/hour) (Eltringham *et al.* 1989).
- Satisfactory analgesia and antiemetics have been provided for the patient, as prescribed by the anaesthetist.
- Body temperature is at least 36°C (Kean 2000).

Table 30.2   Guedel's classification of general anaesthesia (Guedel 1937; Lunn 1982)

Stage I	Analgesia or the stage of disorientation from induction of anaesthesia to loss of consciousness
Stage II	Excitement: reflexes remain and coughing, vomiting and struggling may occur; respiration can be irregular with breath-holding
Stage III	Surgical anaesthesia, divided into four planes:
	Plane I – eyelid reflex lost, swallowing reflex disappears, marked eyeball movement but loss of conjunctival reflex
	Plane II – eyeball movement ceases, laryngeal reflex lost although inflammation of the upper respiratory tract increases reflex irritability, corneal reflex disappears, secretion of tears increases, respiration automatic and regular, movement and deep breathing as a response to skin stimulation disappears
	Plane III – diaphragmatic respiration, progressive intercostal paralysis, pupils dilated and light reflex abolished. The laryngeal reflex lost in plane II can still be initiated by stimuli arising in the anus or cervix
	Plane IV – complete intercostal paralysis to diaphragmatic paralysis
Stage IV	Medullary paralysis with respiratory arrest and vasomotor collapse as a result of anaesthetic overdose

Wherever possible, a prior knowledge of patients gained from preoperative contact is of great value in assessing their return to a normal state. It also has the advantage of helping their orientation to time and place, as familiarity generates a degree of security and confidence.

Local and regional anaesthesia

Patients having surgical procedures performed under local or spinal anaesthesia, whether intra- or extra- (epi) dural, will require a period of postoperative observation, although the priorities of their care will be geared towards different considerations, such as hypotension, headaches and dizziness (AAGBI 2002).

Layout of equipment

While a greater part of the nursing procedures carried out in the recovery room will of necessity be of a routine and repetitive nature, the reason for their performance is for the detection of potential as well as actual complications and the initiation of appropriate interventions. The need for speed, efficiency and economy of movement is essential when time becomes a critical factor in the ultimate safety of the patient. Thus, the basic equipment for monitoring airway maintenance and assisted ventilation must be available at the patient's head in each recovery bay. Equipment must be arranged for ease of

access and always be clean and in full working order. Further support equipment should be available centrally, whenever possible being stored on trolleys for ease of transportation (AAGBI 2002).

Summary

Postanaesthetic care can best be described and understood as a series of many nursing procedures performed in sequence and simultaneously on patients who are in an artificially induced and traumatized condition. These patients will display varying degrees of responsiveness and physical and emotional states. It is important to establish a rapport with each individual to prevent the feeling of 'conveyor-belt processing' and gain the patient's confidence and co-operation. It is also necessary to understand that when emerging from the final stage of anaesthesia, some patients can behave in an emotional and disinhibited fashion, at variance with their normal behaviour (Eckenhoff *et al.* 1961). These displays are always transient and fortunately patients seldom have any recollection of them. Most patients will have an uneventful recovery following surgery. However, recovery can be adversely affected by the extent and length of both surgery and anaesthesia; in some situations the recovery period can only be deemed uneventful with the benefit of hindsight. Physical and psychological recovery can be unpredictable at times.

Procedure guidelines: **Postanaesthetic recovery**

Equipment

1 Theatre trolley bed, which must incorporate the following features:
   (a) Oxygen supply.
   (b) Trendelenburg tilt mechanism.
   (c) Adjustable cot sides.
   (d) Adjustable back rest.
   (e) Brakes.
   (f) Radio translucency.
2 Basic equipment required for each patient:
   (a) Oxygen supply, preferably wall-mounted with tubing, face masks (with both fixed and variable settings), a T-piece system and full range of oropharyngeal and nasopharyngeal airways.
   (b) Suction – regulatable with tubing, and a range of nozzles and catheters.
   Note: spare oxygen cylinders with flowmeters and an electrically powered portable suction machine should always be available in case of pipeline failure.
   (c) Sphygmomanometer and stethoscope. Automatic blood pressure recorders are a valuable means of saving time and of minimizing disturbance to patients, especially those in pain or disorientated, and leaving the nurse's hands free to attend to other needs. However, such equipment can be non-functioning in certain cases, e.g. shivering or profoundly bradycardic patients, and is subject to electrical and mechanical failure.
   (d) Pulse oximeter, whenever possible.
   (e) Miscellaneous items: receivers, tissues, disposable gloves, sharps container and waste receptacle.

*Procedure guidelines: **Postanaesthetic recovery** (cont'd)*

3 Essential equipment centrally available for respiratory and cardiovascular support:
  (a) Self-inflating resuscitator bag, e.g. Ambu bag and/or Mapleson C circuit with face mask.
  (b) Full intubation equipment: laryngoscopes with spare bulbs and batteries, range of endotracheal tubes, bougies and Magill's forceps, syringe and catheter mount.
  (c) Anaesthetic machine and ventilator.
  (d) Wright respirometer.
  (e) Cricothyroid puncture set.
  (f) Range of tracheotomy tubes and tracheal dilator.
  (g) Intravenous infusion sets and cannulae, range of intravenous fluids.
  (h) Central venous cannulae and manometer.
  (i) Emergency drug box – contents in accordance with current hospital policy.
  (j) Defibrillator.
4 Standard equipment for routine nursing procedures.

Procedure

The following recommended actions are not necessarily listed in order of priority. Many will be carried out simultaneously and much will depend on the patient's condition, surgery and level of consciousness. All actions must be accompanied by commentary and explanation regardless of the apparent responsiveness, as the sense of hearing returns before the patient's ability to respond (Levinson 1965).

Action	Rationale
1 Assess the patency of the airway by feeling for movement of expired air.	To determine the presence of any respiratory depression or neuromuscular blockade. Observe chest and abdominal movement, respiratory rate, depth and pattern (Drummond 1991).
(a) Listen for inspiration and expiration. Apply suction if indicated. Observe any use of accessory muscles of respiration and check for tracheal tug.	To ensure absence of material in the airway, i.e. blood, mucus, vomitus. To ascertain absence of laryngeal spasm.
(b) If indicated, support the chin with the neck extended.	In the unconscious patient the tongue is liable to fall back and obstruct the airway, and protective reflexes are absent.
(c) Apply a face mask and administer oxygen at the rate prescribed by the anaesthetist. If an endotracheal tube or laryngeal mask is in position, check whether the cuff or mask is inflated and administer oxygen by means of a T-piece system.	To maintain adequate oxygenation. Oxygen should be administered to all patients in the recovery room (Nimmo *et al.* 1994).
(d) Observe skin colour and temperature. Check the colour of lips and conjunctiva, then peripheral colour and perfusion.	Central cyanosis indicates impaired gaseous exchange between the alveoli and pulmonary capillaries. Peripheral cyanosis indicates low cardiac output (Nimmo *et al.* 1994).
2 Feel the pulse. The patient's position will probably mean that the head, carotid, facial or temporal arteries will offer the easiest access. Note the rate, rhythm and volume, and record.	To assess cardiovascular function and establish a postoperative baseline for future observations.
3 Obtain full information about anaesthetic technique, potential problems and the patient's general medical condition.	To plan subsequent treatment.
4 Obtain full information about the surgical procedure and any drains, packs, blood loss and specific postoperative instructions.	To ensure intervention is based on informed observation.
Note: the information gained from points 3 and 4 will be recorded on the anaesthetic chart and the nursing care document, but an initial verbal handover will ensure that there is no delay in providing care that may be needed before all relevant information can be gathered from documentation.	
5 Take and record blood pressure on reception and at a minimum of 5-minute intervals. Record the pulse and respiratory rate at the same interval unless patient's condition dictates otherwise.	To enable any fluctuations or gross abnormalities in observations to be established quickly. Accurate records are of medicolegal importance in the event of an inquiry.

*Procedure guidelines: **Postanaesthetic recovery** (cont'd)*

Action	Rationale
6 Hypothermia. Check the temperature of the patient, especially those who are at high risk of hypothermia, e.g. the elderly, children, those who have undergone long surgery or where large amounts of blood or fluid replacement therapy have been used. Check patients who are shivering, restless, confused or with respiratory depression (hypothermia interferes with the effective reversal of muscle relaxants: Bowers Feldman 1988). Use 'space' (reflective) blankets and extra blankets to warm the patient.	More than 90% of patients undergoing surgery experience some degree of postoperative hypothermia (Fallacaro *et al.* 1986; White *et al.* 1987). The symptoms of hypothermia can mimic those of other postoperative complications, which may result in inappropriate treatment. Some of the symptoms such as shivering put an increased demand on cardiopulmonary systems as oxygen consumption is increased (Bowers Feldman 1988). Other complications such as arrhythmias or myocardial infarct can result (Bales 1988), and the longer the duration of the postoperative hypothermia, the greater the patient mortality (Crayne *et al.* 1988).
7 Check wound site(s) and observe dressings and any drains. Note and record drainage.	To be aware of any changes or bleeding and take appropriate action, e.g. inform the surgeon.
8 Ensure any intravenous infusions are running at the prescribed rate. Check the prescription chart for any medications prescribed for administration during the immediate postoperative period.	To ensure correct treatment is given.
9 Remain with the patient at all times. Assess level of consciousness during reversing stages of anaesthesia, observing for returning reflexes, i.e. swallowing, tear secretion and eyelash and lid reflexes and response to stimuli – both physical (*not* painful) and verbal (do not shout).	To ascertain progress towards normal function.
10 Orientate the patient to time and place as frequently as is necessary.	To alleviate anxiety, provide reassurance, and gain the patient's confidence and co-operation. Premedication and anaesthesia can induce a degree of amnesia and disorientation.
11 Suction of the upper airway is indicated if gurgling sounds are present on respiration and if blood secretions or vomitus are evident or suspected, and the patient is unable to swallow or cough either at all or adequately. Suction must be applied with care to avoid damage to mucosal surfaces and further irritation or initiation of a gag reflex or laryngeal spasm.	Foreign matter can obstruct the airway or cause laryngeal spasm in light planes of anaesthesia. It can also be inhaled when protective laryngeal reflexes are absent. Vagal stimulation can induce bradycardia in susceptible patients (Atkinson *et al.* 1982, p. 819).
12 Endotracheal suction is performed following the same procedure as that for suction of tracheostomy tubes. (For further information see the procedure on tracheostomy, Ch. 41, Tracheostomy care.)	To maintain the patency of the tube and remove secretions.
13 Give mouth care. (For further information, see Procedure guidelines, Ch. 32, Personal hygiene: mouth care.)	Preoperative fasting, drying gases and manipulation of lips, etc., leave mucosa vulnerable, sore and foul tasting.
14 After regional and/or spinal anaesthesia, assess the return of sensation and mobility of limbs. Check that the limbs are anatomically aligned.	To prevent inadvertent injury following sensory loss.

Problem solving

Note: no observation of cardiovascular function is informative when taken in isolation. Full assessment must be made of respiratory function in conjunction with observations of pulse, blood pressure, emotional state and significant medical history.

Problem	Cause	Suggested action
Airway obstruction.	Tongue occluding the airway.	Support chin forward from the angle of the jaw. If necessary insert a Guedel airway. Use a nasopharyngeal airway if the teeth are clenched or crowned.

Problem solving (cont'd)

Problem	Cause	Suggested action
	Foreign material, blood, secretions, vomitus.	Apply suction. Always check for the presence of throat pack.
	Laryngeal spasm.	Increase the rate of oxygen. Assist ventilation with an Ambu bag and face mask. If there is no improvement, inform anaesthetist and have intubation equipment ready. Offer the patient reassurance.
Hypoventilation.	Respiratory depression from opiates, inhalations, agents, barbiturates.	Inform the anaesthetist and have available naloxone (opiate antagonist) and doxapram (respiratory stimulant). *Note*: if naloxone is given it can reverse the analgesic effects of opiates and has a duration of action of only 20–30 minutes. The patient must be observed for signs of returning hyperventilation (Nimmo *et al.* 1994).
	Decreased respiratory drive from a low partial pressure of carbon dioxide ($PaCO_2$), loss of hypoxic drive in patients with chronic pulmonary disease.	With chronic pulmonary disease, give oxygen using, e.g. a Venturi mask with graded low concentrations (Atkinson *et al.* 1982).
	Neuromuscular blockade from continued action of non-depolarizing muscle relaxants, potentiation of relaxants caused by electrolyte imbalance, impaired excretion with renal or liver disease.	Inform the anaesthetist, have available neostigmine and glycopyrolate, or atropine potassium chloride and 10% calcium chloride. Often the degree of blockade is mild and will wear off in minutes without treatment, but it is extremely frightening and patients will need continuous reassurance that their condition is not unnoticed and is resolving and that they will not be left alone.
Hypotension.	Hypovolaemia.	Take central venous pressure (CVP) readings if catheter is in place. Give oxygen. Lower the head of the trolley unless contraindicated, e.g. hiatus hernia, gross obesity. Check the record of anaesthetic agents used which might cause hypotension, e.g. enflurane, halothane, beta-blockers, nitroprusside, opiates, droperidol, sympathetic blockade following spinal anaesthesia. Check the peripheral perfusion. If the CVP is low, increase intravenous infusion unless contraindicated, e.g. congestive cardiac failure. Check drains and dressings for visible bleeding and haematoma. Inform the anaesthetist or surgeon.
Hypertension.	Pain, carbon dioxide retention.	Treat pain with prescribed analgesia. Pain from certain operation sites can also be alleviated by changing the patient's position.
	Distended bladder.	Offer a bedpan or urinal.
	Some anaesthetic drugs.	Check the prescription chart for those patients on regular antihypertensive therapy. If the situation is not resolved inform the anaesthetist.
Bradycardia.	Very fit patient, opiates, reversal agents, beta-blockers, pain, vagal stimulation, hypoxaemia from respiratory depression.	Check the prescription chart and anaesthetic sheet. Connect the patient to the ECG monitor to exclude heart block. Inform the anaesthetist.

Problem solving (cont'd)

Problem	Cause	Suggested action
Tachycardia.	Pain, hypovolaemia, some anaesthetic drugs, septicaemia, fear, fluid overload.	Provide analgesia. Check the anaesthetic chart. Connect the patient to the ECG monitor to exclude ventricular tachycardia.
Pain.	Surgical trauma, worsened by fear, anxiety and restlessness.	Provide prescribed analgesia and assess its efficacy. Reassure and orientate the patients, who can be unaware that surgery has been performed, in which case their pain is more frightening. Try positional changes where feasible, e.g. experience has shown that after breast surgery some relief can be obtained from raising the back support by 20–40°; patients with abdominal or gynaecological surgery can be more comfortable lying on their side; elevate limbs to reduce swelling where appropriate. Unless significant relief is obtained, inform the anaesthetist.
Nausea and vomiting.	Opiates, hypotension, abdominal surgery, pain; some patients are prone to vomiting.	Offer antiemetics if the patient is conscious. Encourage slow, regular breathing. If the patient is unconscious, turn onto the side, tip the head down and suck out pharynx, give oxygen. *Note*: have wire-cutters available if the jaws are wired.
Hypothermia.	Depression of the heat-regulating centre, vasodilatation, following abdominal surgery, large infusions of blood and fluids.	Use extra blankets or a 'space blanket'. Monitor the patient's temperature.
Shivering.	Some inhalational anaesthetics, especially halothane, hypothermia.	Give oxygen, reassure the patient and take patient's temperature.
Hyperthermia.	Infection, blood transfusion reaction.	Give oxygen, use a fan or tepid sponging if this is warranted.
	Malignant hyperpyrexia.	Medical assessment of antibiotic therapy. Malignant hyperpyrexia is a medical emergency and a malignant hyperpyrexia pack with the necessary drugs should be readily available.
Oliguria.	Mechanical obstruction of catheter, e.g. clots, kinking.	Check the patency of the catheter.
	Inadequate renal perfusion, e.g. hypotension, systolic pressures under 60 mmHg, hypovolaemia, dehydration.	Take blood pressure and CVP if available. Increase intravenous fluids. Inform the anaesthetist.
	Renal damage, e.g. from blood transfusion, infection, drugs, surgical damage to the ureters.	Refer to the anaesthetist or surgeon.

Procedure guidelines: **Postoperative recovery**

Procedure

After discharge from the recovery room to the ward, the nursing care given during the postoperative period is directed towards the prevention of those potential complications resulting from surgery and anaesthesia which might be anticipated to develop over a longer period of time.

Consideration of the psychological and emotional aspects of recovery will of necessity be altered by the changed state of consciousness, awareness and knowledge of patients and their differing responses to surgery, diagnosis and treatment.

Potential respiratory complications

Action	Rationale

1 Observe respirations, noting rate and depth and any presence of dyspnoea or orthopnoea.
  (a) Observe chest movement for equal, bilateral expansion.
  (b) Observe colour and perfusion.
  (c) Position the patient to facilitate optimum lung expansion and reinforce preoperative teaching of deep breathing exercises and coughing.
	Respiratory function postoperatively can be influenced by a number of factors: increased bronchial secretions from inhalation anaesthesia; decreased respiratory effort from opiate medication; pain or anticipation of pain from surgical wounds; surgical trauma to the phrenic nerve; pneumothorax as a result of surgical or anaesthetic procedures. All factors limiting the adequate expansion of the lung and the ejection of bronchial secretions will encourage the development of atelectasis and consolidation of the affected lung tissue.

2 Change position of patients on bedrest every 2–3 hours.	To prevent and monitor formation of pressure sores and tissue viability.
3 Provide adequate prescribed analgesia.	Patients in pain are more likely to be disorientated and show signs of high blood pressure and tachycardia (Nimmo *et al.* 1994).
4 Record temperature and pulse. If sputum produced, observe nature and quantity for culture.	If infection follows there may be a rise in temperature, pulse and respiratory rate.

Potential circulatory problems
Deep venous thrombosis and pulmonary embolus

Action	Rationale
1 Encourage early mobilization where patient's condition allows. For patients on bedrest, encourage deep breathing and exercises of the leg – flexion/extension and rotation of the ankles.	Patients are at increased risk of developing deep venous thrombosis as a result of muscular inactivity, postoperative respiratory and circulatory depression, abdominal and pelvic surgery, prolonged pressure on calves from lithotomy poles, etc., increased production of thromboplastin as a result of surgical trauma, pre-existing coronary artery disease.
2 Where worn, ensure that antiembolic stockings are of the correct size and fit smoothly.	Incorrect sizing causes swelling and bruising to ankles and can constrict blood supply.
3 Advise against crossing of legs or ankles.	To prevent constriction of blood supply and swelling.
4 Record temperature.	
5 Report any complaints of calf or thigh pain to medical staff.	To monitor for signs of deep vein thrombosis.
6 Observe for any dyspnoea, chest pain or signs of shock.	To monitor for signs of pulmonary embolism.

Haemorrhage

Action	Rationale
1 Observe dressings, drains and wound sites, and quantity and nature of drainage. Observe pulse, blood pressure, respirations and colour.	Early haemorrhage may occur as the patient's blood pressure rises. Record postoperatively re-establishing blood flow or blood as a result of the slipping of a ligature or the dislodging of a clot.
2 Observe wound for redness, tenderness and increased temperature.	Secondary haemorrhage may occur after a period of days as a result of infection and sloughing.

Potential fluid and electrolyte imbalance and malnutrition

Action	Rationale
1 Maintain accurate records of intravenous infusions, oral fluids, wound and stoma drainage, nasogastric drainage, vomitus, urine and urological irrigation.	Preoperative fasting and dehydration, increased secretion of antidiuretic hormone, blood loss and paralytic ileus all contribute to potential fluid and electrolyte imbalance. Vomiting and stasis of intestinal fluid may lead to potassium depletion.
2 Observe nature and quantity of all drainage, aspirate, faeces, etc.	To monitor and replace fluid loss.

Procedure guidelines: Postoperative recovery (cont'd)

Action	Rationale
3 Give prescribed antiemetics if nausea or vomiting occur.	
4 Observe state of mouth for coating, furring and dryness.	To maintain oral hygiene and to assess for thrush and hydration.
5 Encourage oral fluids as soon as the patient is able to take them unless the nature of the surgery contraindicates this.	To encourage hydration, and promote diuresis and digestion.
6 Encourage early resumption of diet.	Return to an adequate nutritional state is necessary for wound healing (see Ch. 47, Wound Management); it is particularly important that diabetic patients should return to their pre-operative insulin/diet regime to avoid increased risk of metabolic disturbance.

Potential problem of pain

Action	Rationale
1 Observe the patient, noting physiological signs indicative of pain, e.g. sweating, tachycardia, hypotension, pallor or flushed appearance.	These are the first indications of pain related to intraoperative trauma and postoperative complications.
2 Note restlessness, immobility and facial expressions.	Continuous severe pain can cause restlessness, anxiety, insomnia and anorexia, and may thus interfere with recovery by impeding deep breathing, mobilization and nutrition.
3 Listen to the patient and ascertain the location and nature of the pain. If necessary, use a pain scale chart (see Ch. 27, Pain management and assessment).	Communication skills are necessary for the effective assessment and alleviation of pain as there may be multiple contributory factors, both physical and emotional in origin.
4 Administer prescribed analgesia and observe effect.	To relieve and control pain and if necessary to review pain relief available.
5 Try changing position of patient. Give attention, information and reassurance; assist with relaxation exercises.	To promote comfort and reduce anxiety due to pain.

References and further reading

Aigner, N., Fialko, C., Fritz, A., Winks, O. & Zoch, G. (1997) Complications in the use of diathermy. *Burns*, **23**, 256–64.

AORN (2000) Recommended practices for safety through identification of potential hazards in the perioperative environment. *AORN*, **72**(4), 690–8.

AORN (2001) Recommended practices for positioning the patient in the perioperative practice setting. *AORN*, **73**(1), 231–8.

Association of Anaesthetists of Great Britain and Ireland (AAGBI) (2002) *Immediate Postanaesthetic Recovery*. Association of Anaesthetists of Great Britain and Ireland, London.

Atkinson, R.S. *et al.* (1982) *A Synopsis of Anaesthesia*, 9th edn. John Wright, Bristol.

Bales, R. (1988) Hypothermia, a postoperative problem that's easy to miss. *Reg Nurse*, **51**(4), 42–3.

Beddows, J. (1997) Alleviating pre-operative anxiety in patients: a study. *Nurs Stand*, **11**(37), 35–8.

Bowers Feldman, M.E. (1988) Inadvertent hypothermia, a threat to homeostasis in the postanaesthetic patient. *J Postanaesth Nurs*, **3**(2), 82–7.

Bryne, B. (2002) Deep vein thrombosis prophylaxis: the effectiveness and implications of using below knee or thigh length graduated compression stockings. *J Vasc Nurs*, **20**(2), 53–9.

Campbell, S. (2001) Review: graduated compression stockings prevent deep venous thrombosis in patients who are in hospital. *Evidence-Based Nurs*, **4**(1), 20.

Carman, T.L. & Fernandez, B.B. (1999) Issues and controversies in venous thromboembolism. *Cleve Clin J Med*, **66**(2), 113–23.

CEPOD (2002) *Report of the National Confidential Inquiry into Perioperative Deaths*. CEPOD, London.

Chapman, A. (1996) Current theory and practice: a study of pre-operative fasting. *Nurs Stand*, **10**(18), 33–6.

Copp, G. (1988) Intra-operative information and pre-operative visiting. *Surg Nurse*, **1**(2), 27–8.

Crayne, H.E. *et al.* (1988) Thermoresuscitation for postoperative hypothermia using reflective blankets. *AORN J*, **47**(1), 222–3, 226–7.

Davis, P. & O'Neill, C. (2002) The potential benefits of intermittent pneumatic compression in the prevention of deep venous thrombosis. *J Orthopaed Nurs*, **6**(2), 95–100.

Drummond, G.B. (1991) Keep a clear airway. *Br J Anaesth*, **66**, 153–66.

Eckenhoff, J.E., Kneale, D.H. & Dripps, R.D. (1961) The incidence and aetiology of postanaesthetic excitement. *Anaesthesiology*, **22**, 667.

Eltringham, R. *et al.* (1989) *Post-Anaesthetic Recovery: A Practical Approach*, 2nd edn. Springer, Berlin.

Evans, D. & Read, K. (2001) Graduated compression stockings for the prevention of post-operative venous thromboembolism. *Best Practice*, **5**(2), 1–6.

Fallacaro, M. *et al.* (1986) Inadvertent hypothermia – etiology, effects and preparation. *AORN J*, **44**(1), 54–61.

Field, L. & Adams, N. (2001) Pain management 2: the use of psychological approaches to pain. *Br J Nurs*, **10**(15), 971–4.

Fong, E.P., Tan, W.T. & Chye, L.T. (2000) Diathermy and alcohol skin preparations – a potential disastrous mix. *Burns*, **26**(7), 673–5.

Gruendemann, B. & Meeker, H.M. (1983) *Alexander's Care of the Patient in Surgery*, 7th edn. Mosby, St Louis.

Guedel, A.E. (1937) *Inhalation Anaesthesia: A Fundamental Guide*. Macmillan, New York.

Hayes, C.A., Lehman, J.M. & Castonguay, P. (2002) Graduated compression stocking: updating practice, improving compliance. *Med Surg Nurs*, **11**(4), 163–6, 167.

Hayward, J. (1975) *Information: A Prescription Against Pain*. Royal College of Nursing (Research Series), London.

Hines, R., Beresh, P.G., Watrous, G. *et al.* (1992) Complications occurring in the postanaesthesia care unit: a survey. *Anaesth Analg*, **74**, 503.

Hughes, S. (2002) The effects of giving patients pre-operative information. *Nurs Stand*, **16**(28), 33–7.

Jackson, J. (1995) Acute pain: its physiology and the pharmacology of analgesia. *Nurs Times*, **91**(16), 27–8.

Jacobs, V.R., Morrison, J.E., Mundhenke, C., Golombeck, K. & Jonat, W. (2000) Intraoperative evaluation of laparoscopic insufflation technique for quality control in the OR. *J Soc Laparoendoscopic Surg*, **4**(3), 189–95.

Jefferey, P.C. & Nicolaides, A.N. (1990) Graduated compression stocking in the prevention of post-operative deep vein thrombosis. *Br J Surg*, **77**(4), 380–3.

Jester, R. & Williams, S. (1999) Pre-operative fasting: putting research into practice. *Nurs Stand*, **13**(39), 33–5.

Jolley, S. (2001) Managing post-operative nausea and vomiting. *Nurs Stand*, **15**(40), 47–52.

Kean, M. (2000) Adult/elderly care nursing. A patient temperature audit within a theatre recovery unit. *Br J Nurs*, **9**(3), 150–6.

Kjonniksen, I., Andersen, B.M., Sondenaa, V.G. & Segadal, L. (2002) Preoperative hair removal – a systematic literature review. *AORN*, **75**(5), 928–34, 936, 938.

Lipp, A. & Edwards, P. (2002) Disposable surgical face masks for preventing surgical wound infection in clean surgery. *Cochrane Library*, 2002 (1).

Lunn, J.N. (1982) *Lecture Notes on Anaesthetics*, 2nd edn. Blackwell Scientific Publications, Oxford.

Martin, D. (1996) Pre-operative visits to reduce patient anxiety: a study. *Nurs Stand*, **10**(23), 33–8.

McEwen, D.R. (1996) Intra-operative positioning of surgical patients. *AORN*, **63**(6), 1059–63, 1066–79; quiz 1080–6.

Mitchell, M. (2000) Nursing interventions for pre-operative anxiety. *Nurs Stand*, **14**(37), 40–3.

Molyneux, C. (2001) Open forum. Electrosurgery policy… 'Electrosurgery in perioperative practice'. *Br J Periop Nurs*, **11**(10), 424.

Nimmo, W.S. *et al.* (eds) (1994) *Anaesthesia*, 2nd edn. Blackwell Science, Oxford.

O'Callaghan, N. (2002) Pre-operative fasting. *Nurs Stand*, **16**(36), 33–7.

O'Malley, C. & Cunningham, A.J. (2001) Physiologic changes during laparoscopy. *Anesthesiol Clin North Am*, **19**(1), 1–19.

Parienti, J.J., Thibon, P. & Heller, R. *et al.* (2002) Hand-rubbing with an aqueous alcoholic solution vs. traditional surgical hand-scrubbing and 30-day surgical site infection rates: a randomised equivalence study. *JAMA*, **288**(6), 722–7.

Peskett, M.J. (1999) Clinical indicators and other complications in the recovery room or post anaesthetic care unit. *Anaesthesia*, **54**(12), 1143–9.

Rothrock, J.C. (2002) *Alexander's Care of the Patient in Surgery*, 12th edn. Mosby, London.

Sharma, K.C., Kabinoff, G., Ducheine, Y., Tierney, J. & Brandstetter, R.D. (1997) Laparoscopic surgery and its potential for medical complications. *Heart Lung: J Acute Crit Care*, **26**(1), 52–67.

Sneyd, J.R., Carr, A., Byrom, W.D. & Bilski, A.J. (1998) A meta-analysis of nausea and vomiting following maintenance of anaesthesia with propofol or inhalational agents. *Eur J Anaesthesiol*, **15**(4), 433–45.

Tammelin, A., Domicel, P. & Hambraeus, A. (2000) Dispersal of methicillin-resistant *Staphylococcus epidermidis* by staff in an operating suite for thoracic and cardiovascular surgery: relation to skin carriage and clothing. *Hosp Infect*, **44**(2), 119–26.

Tanner, J. & Parkinson, H. (2002) Double gloving to reduce surgical cross-infection. *Cochrane Library*, **1**(3).

Tokars, J.I., Culver, D.H. & Mendelson, M.H. *et al.* (1995) Skin and mucous membrane contacts with blood during surgical procedures: risk and prevention. *Epidemiology*, **16**(12), 703–11.

Ulrich, W. *et al.* (1997) Damage due to patient positioning in anaesthesia and surgical medicine. *Anaesthesiol Intens Med Notfallmed Schmerzther*, **32**(1), 4.

Wainwright, D. (1988) Diathermy – how safe is it? *Natl Assoc Theatre Nurses News*, **25**(1), 7–8.

Walker, J.A. (2002) Emotional and psychological preoperative preparation in adults. *Br J Nurs*, **11**(8), 567–75.

White, H.E. *et al.* (1987) Body temperature in elderly surgical patients. *Res Nurs Health*, **10**(5), 317–21.

Wicker, C.P. (1997) Electrosurgery. In: *Principles of Safe Practice in the Operating Theatre*. National Association of Theatre Nurses, Harrogate.

Wicker, P. (2000) Back to basics. Electrosurgery in perioperative practice. *Br J Periop Nurs*, **10**(4), 221–6.

Woodhead, K., Taylor, E. & Bannister, G. (2002) Behaviours and rituals in the operating theatre: a report from the Hospital Infection Society Working Party on Infection Control in Operating Theatres. *Hosp Infect*, **51**(4), 241–55.

Wu, M.P., Ou, C.S., Chen, S.L., Yen, E.Y. & Rowbotham, R. (2000) Complications and recommended practices for electrosurgery in laparoscopy. *Am J Surg*, **179**(1), 67–73.

31

Personal hygiene: eye care

Chapter contents

Definition

Eye care is the practice of assessing, cleaning or irrigating the eye and/or the instillation of prescribed ocular preparations.

Indications

Eye care may be necessary under the following circumstances:

- To relieve pain and discomfort
- To prevent or treat infection
- To prevent further injury to the eye
- To detect disease at an early stage
- To detect drug-induced toxicity at an early stage
- To prevent damage to the cornea in sedated or unconscious patients
- To maintain contact lenses and care for false eye prostheses (Cloutier 1992; Ashurst 1997; Cunningham & Gould 1998).

Reference material

If able, and after appropriate instruction, patients should be encouraged to carry out many of the procedures involved in eye care themselves. However, in the case of postoperative, very ill or unconscious patients, it is often the nurse who is responsible for eye care. A poor eye care technique may lead to the transmission of infection from one eye to the other or the development of irreversible damage to the eye (Ashurst 1997; Cunningham & Gould 1998). In some cases this can lead to loss of sight.

Anatomy and physiology

The eye consists of three main areas: the orbit, the globe (eyeball) and the extrinsic structures. The orbit, or socket, is formed by seven bones of the skull and is lined with fat; it supports and protects the globe and its accessory structures and provides attachments for the ocular muscles. The globe itself can be divided into three layers (Fig. 31.1):

- The outer layer or fibrous tunic, composed of the cornea and sclera
- The middle layer or vascular tunic, composed of the choroid, ciliary body and iris
- The inner layer or nervous tunic, composed of the retina.

The function of the outer layer is protective and gives shape to the eyeball. The middle layer contains the globe's vascular supply and is darkly pigmented. The inner layer contains the light-sensitive cells know as the rods and cones and is also the site of the macula lutea (yellow spot) and central fovea (area of highest visual acuity). Extrinsic structures of the eye include the eyelids, eyelashes, eyebrows and lacrimal (tear) apparatus. These structures protect the globe from external injury (SoftKey Multimedia 1995). The blood vessels inside the eye may be readily viewed with an ophthalmoscope and examined for changes due to systemic diseases, such as diabetes or hypertension, or local disease processes, such as senile macular degeneration (Tortora & Grabowski 2002).

The optic nerve which deals with vision (cranial nerve II) exits the eye to the side of the macula lutea at an area called the optic disc or blind spot. The optic nerve passes from the orbit, through the optic foramen and into the brain. The two separate optic nerves meet at the optic chiasma and in this area some optic nerve fibres cross over to the opposite side of the brain. The nerves then continue along the optic tracts and terminate in the thalamus. From there projections extend to the visual areas in the occipital lobe of the cerebral cortex (Tortora & Grabowski 2002) (Fig. 31.2). An additional blind spot, or scotoma, may be indicative of a brain tumour. For example, in pituitary gland tumours it is common to develop bilateral defects in the field of vision due to invasion of the optic chiasm (Wickham & Rohan 1997).

The inside of the globe is divided into two chambers by the lens: the anterior cavity, anterior to the lens, and the vitreous chamber, posterior to the lens. The anterior cavity is divided into the anterior chamber and the posterior chamber by the iris. It contains a clear, watery fluid called the aqueous humour. The vitreous chamber is filled with a jelly-like substance called the vitreous body or vitreous humour. Together these two fluid-filled cavities help maintain the shape of the eyeball and the intraocular pressure (Marieb 2001; Tortora & Grabowski 2002) (see Fig. 31.5).

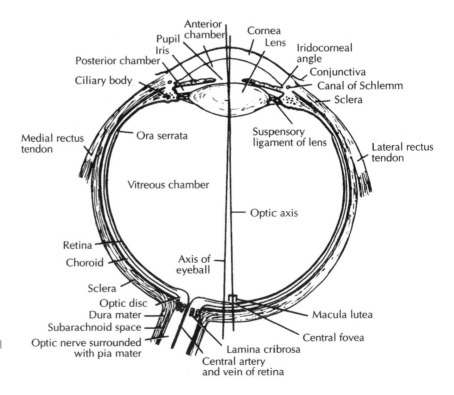

Figure 31.1 Horizontal section through eyeball at level of optic nerve. Optic axis and axis of eyeball are included.

The aqueous humour is continuously secreted by the choroid plexus of the ciliary process (a part of the ciliary body) located behind the iris. This fluid then permeates the posterior chamber, passing between the lens and the iris, and flows through the pupil into the anterior chamber. From the anterior chamber the aqueous humour drains into the scleral venous sinus (canal of Schlemm) (see Fig. 31.7) and is absorbed back into the blood stream. The aqueous humour is the principal source of nutrients and waste removal for the lens and cornea, as these structures have no direct blood supply. If the outflow of aqueous humour is blocked, excessive intraocular pressure may develop, leading to the disease process known as glaucoma. This excess pressure can cause degeneration of the retina and blindness. The vitreous humour, unlike the aqueous humour, is produced during foetal development and is never replaced (Marieb 2001; Tortora & Grabowski 2002).

Tears are produced in the lacrimal glands located at the upper, outer edge of the eye (see Fig. 31.6). They are excreted onto the upper surface of the globe and washed over the globe by the action of blinking. The function of tears is to clean, moisten and lubricate the globe and eyelids. Tears also provide antisepsis as they contain an enzyme called lysozome that is able to rupture the cell membranes of some bacteria leading to their lysis and death (Tortora & Grabowski 2002).

The tears collect in the nasal canthus (inner, medial aspect of the eye) where they drain into the upper and lower lacrimal puncti. The puncti are small openings leading to the lacrimal canaliculi (or canals), these in turn drain into the lacrimal sac. From here the tears pass into the nasolacrimal duct and empty into the nasal cavity (Soft Key Multimedia 1995; Marieb 2001; Tortora & Grabowski 2002).

General principles of eye care

Aseptic technique is necessary only in certain circumstances, for example, when the eye is damaged or following ophthalmic surgery.

Position of patient

The patient should be sitting or lying with his or her head tilted backwards and chin pointing upwards. This allows for easy access to the eyes and is usually a good position for patient comfort and compliance.

Position of light source

A good light source is necessary prior to commencing eye care procedures to enable careful assessment of the eyes and to avoid damage to their delicate structures. The light source should be positioned above and behind the nurse. It should never be allowed to shine directly into the patient's eyes, as this will be extremely uncomfortable for the patient.

Instillation of drops

Most types of drops are instilled into the upper rim of the inferior fornix (i.e. just inside the lower eyelid) (see Fig. 31.3), as the conjunctiva in this area is less sensitive than that overlying the cornea. Also, the drops will run into the pocket of the inferior fornix preventing immediate loss of

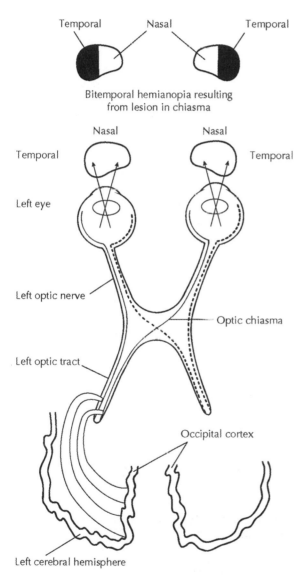

Figure 31.2 Visual pathways and visual fields.

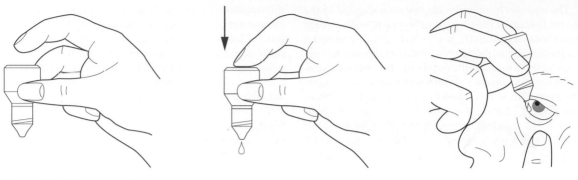

Figure 31.3 How to instil eye drops.

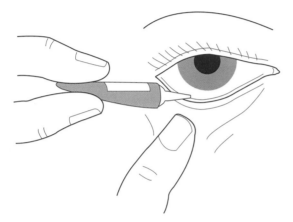

Figure 31.4 How to instil eye ointment.

the drops into the nasolacrimal drainage system. Exceptions to this installation technique are as follows:

- *Drugs used to lubricate the cornea*: oil-based drops produce less corneal reaction than aqueous ones as they do not feel as cold to the cornea when administered. They may therefore be instilled directly into the inferior fornix.
- *Anaesthetic drops*: the first drop should be instilled into the inferior fornix for absorption and then directly onto the cornea one drop at a time until the patient is no longer able to feel the drops.
- *Drops used to treat the nasal passages*: these should be instilled at the nasal canthus end of the eye.

The number of drops instilled depends on the type of solution used and its purpose. Usually, one drop only is ordered and will be sufficient if it is instilled in the correct manner. The exceptions to the 'one-drop' rule are:

- *Oil-based solutions*: these are used for lubricating the eyeball. Usually one drop is instilled and repeated as required.

- *Anaesthetic drops*: it is usual to instil two or three drops at a time. This is repeated until the drop cannot be felt on the eye.

The dropper should be held as close to the eye as possible without touching either the lids or the cornea. This will avoid corneal damage and reduce the risk of cross-infection. If the drop falls from too great a height it is difficult to control and will also be uncomfortable for the patient. The eye should be closed for as long as possible after application, preferably for 1–2 minutes.

A variety of droppers and bottles are available for the instillation of eye preparations. These include pipettes, bottles incorporating pipettes, plastic bottles with a dropper attachment and single dose packs. Pipettes are easy to use but need to be dried and sterilized between doses. Plastic bottles can be squeezed and so avoid the need for a pipette and they are also cheaper than glass bottles with a dropper. Each patient should have their own, individual eye drop container and single dose containers should be used for all patients in eye clinics or in accident and emergency departments (British National Formulary 2002).

Instillation of ointments

Ointments are also applied to the upper rim of the inferior fornix using a similar technique to eye drops (see Fig. 31.4). A 2 cm line of ointment should be applied from the nasal canthus outwards. Similarly to the instillation of eye drops, the nozzle should be held approximately 2.5 cm above the eye to avoid contact with the cornea and eyelids.

Contact lenses and eye preparations

Contact lenses may affect the distribution and absorption of eye preparations. Some drugs and preservatives in eye preparations may accumulate in soft hydrogel lenses and induce a toxic reaction. For these reasons

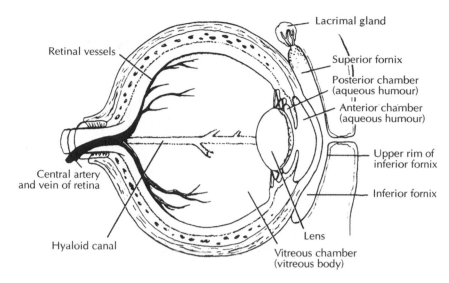

Figure 31.5 Anterior cavity in front of lens is incompletely divided into anterior chamber (anterior to iris) and posterior chamber (behind iris), which are continuous through pupil. Aqueous humour, which fills the cavity, is formed by ciliary processes and reabsorbed into venous blood by the canal of Schlemm.

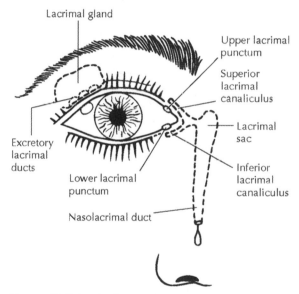

Figure 31.6 Lacrimal apparatus.

contact lenses should be removed prior to instillation of eye drops or ointments and not worn for the period of treatment (British National Formulary 2002). Eye drops can be instilled over rigid contact lenses (BNF 2002).

Care of contact lenses

Contact lenses are thin, curved discs made of hard or soft plastic or a combination of both. Hard contact lenses are made of a rigid plastic that does not absorb water or saline solutions and can be worn for a maximum of 12–14 hours continuously. Soft contact lenses are more pliable and can be worn for up to 30 days and cleaned once weekly. Gas-permeable lenses are a combination of both and permit oxygen to reach the cornea, providing greater comfort, and can be left in for several days.

Most people look after their own contact lenses. Cleaning depends on the type of lenses used – manufacturers provide specific instructions for the care of their products. They should be stored in a container with slots for R and L eye, so they can be worn in the correct eye. Seriously ill patients should have their lenses removed and stored correctly until they can reinsert their own lenses. Contact lenses are stored in a sterile solution, usually sodium chloride, when they are not in the eye. This helps to lubricate the lens and enable the lens to glide over the cornea, reducing the risk of injury (Kozier *et al.* 1998).

Eye irrigation

The most common use of eye irrigation is for the removal of caustic substances from the eye, e.g. domestic cleaning agents or medications, particularly cytotoxic material. This should be done as soon as possible to minimize damage. The procedure is also used as a preoperative preparation or to remove infected material. The fluids most commonly used are sterile 0.9% sodium chloride, 'for irrigation', or sterile water, 'for irrigation'. In an emergency tap water may be used (McConnell 1991). The volume used will vary depending on the degree of contamination; copious amounts are needed for corrosive chemicals and smaller volumes for removal of eye secretions.

Care of the insensitive eye

If the eye-blink reflex is absent the eye's surface will dry out, causing irreversible corneal damage. The cornea may become ulcerated or infected, leading to scarring and possibly loss of vision. This is a particular problem in the sedated, ventilated or unconscious patient. When the patient has lost this protective reflex, the nurse must institute measures to maintain eye moisture and corneal integrity. The surface of the eye and surrounding structures should be keep clean and moist by gentle cleaning with sterile 0.9% sodium chloride and, when necessary, the instillation of lubricating preparations. If there is no eye-blink reflex the eyelids should be kept closed by the use of hypoallergenic tape or by the application of hydrogel sheet preparations, e.g. Geliperm. If the eyes become infected the relevant medication should be prescribed and administered (Ashurst 1997).

With each of these measures care must be taken not to spread infection between the eyes. Any alteration to the appearance of the eye must be reported to the doctor.

Artificial eyes

These are made of glass or plastic; some are permanently implanted. Most people who have artificial eyes care for themselves. If the patient is unconscious it is not necessary to remove them regularly for cleaning.

Eye medications

Drugs may be given either systemically or topically to exert an effect on the eye. However, if given systemically the prescribing doctor needs to take account of the physiological barrier and the blood–aqueous barrier which exists within the eye and which is selective in allowing drugs to pass into the intraocular fluids. Permeability of this barrier may be altered in inflammatory conditions and following paracentesis (removal of excess fluid with a needle or cannula).

Medications applied locally meet some resistance at the barrier presented by the lacrimal system (tear film barrier). A further barrier is that of the cornea which is selectively permeable and only allows the passage of water and not drugs. However, the corneal resistance may alter if there is damage to the corneal epithelium. Many drugs will produce a similar effect on both the healthy and diseased eye. Drugs for use in the eye are usually classified according to their action.

Mydriatics and cycloplegics

These drugs cause pupil dilation and produce their effects by paralysing the ciliary muscle, stimulating the dilator muscle of the pupil or by a combination of both

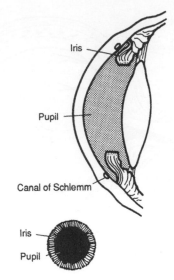

Figure 31.7 Effect of mydriatics.

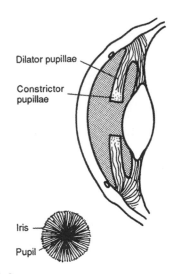

Figure 31.8 Effect of miotics.

(Fig. 31.7). They are used mainly for diagnostic purposes and most have an anticholinergic action. The most commonly used preparations are cyclopentolate hydrochloride, tropicamide and atropine (BNF 2002).

Miotics

These drugs produce their effects by contracting the ciliary muscle and constricting the pupil (Fig. 31.8). Miotics help in the drainage of aqueous humour and are used primarily in the treatment of glaucoma. Examples are pilocarpine and carbachol (BNF 2002).

Local anaesthetics

These render the eye and the inner surfaces of the lids insensitive. They are used before minor surgery, removal of foreign bodies and tonometry (measurement of intraocular pressure). The most widely used eye anaesthetics are oxybuprocaine and amethocaine. Cocaine is no longer used as an eye anaesthetic due to corneal toxicity and the possibility of patients developing an idiosyncrasy to it and suddenly collapsing (BNF 2002).

Anti-inflammatories

Anti-inflammatory drugs include steroids, antihistamines, lodoxamide and sodium cromoglycate. The most commonly used steroid preparations are dexamethasone, prednisolone and betamethasone (British National Formulary 2002).

Corticosteroid eye drops should be used with caution as they can cause a gradual rise in intraocular pressure in a small percentage of people (especially if they have a history of glaucoma).

Antibacterials/antivirals/antifungals

Antibacterials and antivirals can be used for the active treatment of infections or as prophylactic treatment for eye surgery, after removal of a foreign body or following an eye injury. Antibiotic preparations in common use are chloramphenicol, neomycin and framycetin. Aciclovir is the only antiviral available as an eye preparation (BNF 2002). Antifungal preparations are not available so the patient has to be referred to a specialist centre.

Artificial tears

Artificial tears are used when there is a deficiency in natural tear production. This can be due to a disease process, postradiotherapy treatment, as a side-effect of certain drugs and when the eye-blink reflex is absent. These artificial lubricants commonly contain hypromellose or hydroxyethylcellulose (BNF 2002). Additionally, pilocarpine can be given orally. The severity of the problem and the patient's choice will determine the treatment.

Toxic effects of common systemic drugs on the eye

As the eye may be the first place to show signs of systemic disease, so some systemic drugs may show their toxic effects in the eye. These effects range from pruritis, irritation, redness, epiphora (excess tear production with overflow), photophobia and blepharoconjunctivitis (inflammation of the eyelids and conjunctiva), to disturbance of vision (Cloutier 1992). Particular effects of specific drugs are listed below.

- *Methotrexate and related antimetabolites*: these drugs can affect the meibomian glands (specialized sebaceous glands in the eyelids), causing blepharoconjunctivitis. They may also induce photophobia, epiphora, periorbital oedema and conjunctival hyperaemia.
- *5-Fluorouracil (5-FU)*: 5-FU can cause canalicular fibrosis and oculomotor disturbances (probably secondary to a local neurotoxicity affecting the brainstem).
- *Antihistamines*: these drugs decrease tear production and may lead to 'dry eye', especially in patients with Sjögren's syndrome (a wasting disease of the salivary glands), ocular pemphigus (rare, autoimmune disease of the skin), those who wear contact lenses and in the elderly.
- *Tamoxifen*: this drug can cause subepithelial whirl-like deposits in the cornea, and retinal lesions.
- *Indomethacin*: this can cause corneal deposits and retinal pigmentary toxicity.
- *Oral contraceptives*: these can stimulate corneal steeping and intolerance to contact lenses.
- *Atropine, scopolamine and belladonna-like substances*: such drugs cause mydriasis (widening of the pupil) and cycloplegia (paralysis of the ciliary muscle that moves the iris) (Martin 1996).
- *Corticosteroids*: prolonged use of corticosteroids produces posterior subcapsular cataracts.
- *Chloramphenicol*: chloramphenicol treatment can lead to optic neuritis.
- *Ethambutol*: this drug can cause damage to the optic nerve.
- *Rifampicin*: stains soft contact lenses.
- *Digoxin*: in overdose results in blurred vision and yellow/green vision.
- *Oxygen*: in neonates, high concentrations for a long period can cause retrolental fibroplasia (abnormal proliferation of fibrous tissue behind the lens causing blindness) (Martin 1996).

Tumours of the eye

There are a number of tumours associated with the eye and they may involve the orbit, globe or extrinsic structures. To appreciate the spread of disease and clinical features associated with eye tumours, it is important to be aware of the relationship between the eye and other local structures. The anterior cranial fossa lies superiorly, the nasal cavity and ethmoid labyrinth medially, the maxillary antrum inferiorly and the infratemporal and middle cranial fossa laterally to the eye (Tortora & Grabowski 2002).

Tumours of the orbit

While orbital tumours are rare, primary and metastatic lesions do occur. However, metastases are more likely to arise in the globe than in the orbit. The most common primary tumours of the orbit are rhabdomyosarcoma in children and lymphoma in adults. Occurring less often are meningiomas, soft tissue sarcomas and nerve sheath tumours (including optic nerve gliomas) (Henderson 1980; Char 1993; Souhami & Tobias 1998). Development of metastases in the orbit is indicative of a primary tumour elsewhere in the body. Metastases may vary from a rapidly developing mass, often invading local soft tissues and bone, to slow scarring of the soft tissues of the eye. The primary tumours most likely to develop orbital metastases arise in the thyroid, bronchus, breast, prostate, kidney and skin (Tijl *et al.* 1992; Souhami & Tobias 1998).

Signs and symptoms

Most orbital tumours push the eye away from its normal visual axis in a sagittal or vertical plane. In almost all cases the direction of displacement is opposite to the growing tumour (Moeloek 1993). Lack of room for growth due to the rigid bony cavity causes the eye to protrude (proptosis), often to a large degree. The average volume of the orbital cavity is 24 ml and an increase in volume of only 4 ml will produce 6 mm of proptosis. Therefore proptosis, with signs of diplopia (double vision), is the main clinical feature of orbital tumours and this can be a very disfiguring and distressing symptom for the patient (Tijl *et al.* 1992; Char 1993; Moeloek 1993; Souhami & Tobias 1998). It should be noted that bilateral proptosis is most commonly related to hyperthyroidism (Leitman 1988).

If the tumour involves the muscles of the eye it may cause ophthalmoplegia (paralysis of the eye muscles); this may also occur if cranial nerve III is involved. Chemosis (swelling of the conjunctiva) may occur and, in conjunction with an infection, may be misdiagnosed as cellulitis. In addition, panophthalmitis (inflammation of the interior of the eye) can develop and may lead to perforation of the globe and unilateral blindness. This is common with advanced tumours (Souhami & Tobias 1998).

Visual changes can occur with tumours that involve the optic nerve or its sheath, or that press against its surface externally. Diplopia, excess tear production, a visible mass, ptosis (drooping of the upper eyelid), epiphora and pain are other clinical features of orbital tumours (Tijl *et al.* 1992; Char 1993; Moeloek 1993; Souhami & Tobias 1998).

Tumours of the globe

Retinoblastoma (malignant tumour of the retina) and malignant melanoma are the most common tumours occurring in the globe. Melanoma occurs most often in adults and retinoblastoma is generally a disease of childhood, with most cases presenting before the age of 5. Forty percent of retinoblastomas are hereditary and 60% are spontaneous (non-hereditary). Retinoblastoma has a good prognosis, with a 5-year survival rate of over 90% (Goddard *et al.* 1999). The most common site for melanoma of the globe is in the vascular tunic (choroid, ciliary body and iris). There are about six cases per million a year and the majority (85%) occur in the choroid. Because this layer of the eye is very vascular, metastases are common and suggest a poor prognosis. Melanomas of the iris and ciliary body are usually diagnosed earlier as they are more visible, whereas choroidal tumours may remain undiagnosed for some time unless they cause a disturbance in the visual field, for example if they are in the macula lutea or cause retinal detachment. As the choroid is a common site of secondary deposits from cutaneous melanoma, the possibility of the tumour being metastatic and not a primary must be ruled out (Souhami & Tobias 1998; National Cancer Institute 1999a,b).

Melanoma and squamous cell carcinoma (SCC) are occasionally found in the conjuctiva. Conjunctival melanoma has a good overall prognosis with about 75% of patients surviving for over 5 years; however for patients presenting with large lesions the risk of disseminated disease is high. A precancerous lesion known as ocular melanosis can occur in the conjunctiva and this must be differentiated from a true melanoma. These lesions should be managed by careful observation, as a malignant change can develop but may take many years to do so. The early diagnosis of conjunctival SCC is important and with the correct treatment there is generally a good prognosis (Souhami & Tobias 1998).

Tumours of the extrinsic structures

Basal cell carcinoma (BCC) and SCC are fairly common tumours of the eyelid, particularly in the elderly. The lower eyelid and inner canthus are the areas most commonly affected (Finger 2000; Lindgren *et al.* 1998; Souhami & Tobias 1998). BCC grows slowly and rarely metastasizes; however, it can spread by direct growth into adjacent structures such as the orbit and, ultimately, even the brain. SCC has a similar epidemiology to BCC but it grows more rapidly and may metastasize to regional lymph nodes, particularly in the neck. Metastatic SCC carries a poor prognosis (National Cancer Institute 1999d).

Investigations

Comprehensive clinical examination by a specialist consultant is imperative. Additional investigations include:

- Histology
- Computed tomography (CT)

- Magnetic resonance imaging (MRI)
- Orbital venography
- Carotid angiography
- Ultrasound.

The last three techniques have become less popular with the advent of CT and MRI (Lund 1987). Histological confirmation of the tumour type should be performed if possible, by either biopsy or cytology. Care needs to be taken during these procedures as tumour spillage, haemorrhage and blindness are potential risks with either method of sampling. If the tumour is encapsulated it is suggested that it be excised in entirety (Souhami & Tobias 1998).

Treatment

The treatment of any eye malignancy is always based on the principle of curing the disease and preserving sight. In the instance of large or invasive tumours this is not always possible so the aim then is to maintain a suitable cosmetic appearance. Clinicians should be reminded that any decision on preservation of the orbital contents must be based on a clear and unemotional decision that will not compromise the overall prognosis (Lund 1987). It should also be remembered that the patient must make the final decision on treatment. In order to make this decision the patient must be fully informed and aware of all treatment or non-treatment options available to them, and the likely outcome of each option.

Rhabdomyosarcomas are usually treated with radiotherapy and adjuvant chemotherapy with good results (National Cancer Institute 1999c). The standard treatment for orbital lymphoma is radiotherapy alone (Souhami & Tobias 1998). Orbital metastases are treated according to the type of primary tumour. With metastatic breast cancer, radiotherapy is given in the first instance with chemotherapy and hormonal therapy also used if proven effective. Prostate cancer is generally radiosensitive, therefore radiotherapy is used to treat orbital deposits. Radiotherapy is again used for thyroid secondaries and may be an external beam or in the form of radioactive iodine (Tijl *et al.* 1992). These are usually palliative measures and are only appropriate if the patient is well enough to tolerate them. They can help to preserve vision, reduce pain and, consequently, improve quality of life.

Treatment of retinoblastoma will depend on the size of the tumour. Small tumours may be controlled with ablative therapies (cryotherapy or photocoagulation, for example), brachytherapy ('short distance' therapy, see Ch. 34, Radioactive source therapy: sealed sources) or external beam radiotherapy. If the tumour is large, radiotherapy is often combined with adjuvant

chemotherapy, giving a 5-year survival rate of about 75%. When the tumour is very extensive and/or the eye is beyond the point of useful recovery then enucleation (removal of the globe) is considered the treatment of choice (Souhami & Tobias 1998; National Cancer Institute 1999b). If there is local spread of the tumour then adjuvant chemotherapy is indicated (Goddard *et al.* 1999). The management of ocular melanoma has recently changed from the use of extensive surgery, usually enucleation, to a more conservative approach of close observation and intervention only if symptoms develop. This approach is commonly taken in elderly patients. When treatment is needed, the choice again depends on the size of the tumour. The approach is the same as for retinoblastoma, with surgical excision, ablative therapies and local irradiation being the mainstays of treatment for small tumours. For larger tumours enucleation is usual, possibly in conjunction with preoperative external beam radiotherapy (Souhami & Tobias 1998; National Cancer Institute 1999a).

The most common treatments for SCC and BCC of the external eye are surgery or ablative therapies and radiotherapy, either alone or in combination. Early diagnosis of conjunctival melanoma and SCC is essential as small lesions may be effectively treated by radiotherapy, conserving the eye and preserving vision. Surgical excision followed by brachytherapy is also a common treatment for these lesions (Souhami & Tobias 1998; National Cancer Institute 1999d).

Any tumour of the eye may necessitate enucleation if it is very large or has local extension, if the optic nerve is involved or retinal detachment has occurred. It may also be necessary for the control of pain or if secondary glaucoma has developed. However, minimally invasive tumours of the orbit that do not involve the ocular muscles may be resected without enucleation and any defect to the periosteum reconstructed using the temporalis facia. This procedure is usually followed by postoperative radiotherapy (Goldberg & Cantore 1997).

Summary

Like most disfigurements of the head and neck, orbital tumours are also difficult to camouflage. Commonly patients will wear tinted glasses, or wear an eye pad/protector so that it looks more like protection from an eye injury rather than camouflage of a tumour. Eye patches are occasionally worn, but most patients feel that this is indicative of eye loss.

Patients with orbital disease need skilled emotional support. This is particularly true if the disease is inoperable and/or end stage. The tumour may be exophytic, proptosed or causing splaying of the nasal and ethmoid bones. Such disfiguring complications may lead to social isolation, avoidance and despair. These patients not only live with disfigurement and dysfunction, but also the threat to their survival from the disease process. It is suggested that eye tumours, for example childhood retinoblastoma (National Cancer Institute 1999b) and choroidal melanoma (Foss *et al.* 1999), be treated at specialist centres for the optimal prognostic outcome. Nursing and medical staff in these centres are more likely to have the experience and knowledge required in dealing with these relatively rare and demanding disease processes and their consequences. In addition, they may be more aware of community support networks and can ensure that, when necessary, patients are referred to an appropriate specialist prosthetic department.

Primarily, the nurse will be involved in helping the patient cope with the diagnosis and treatment of their disease, care of the eye (or cavity if enucleation has been performed) and any prostheses the patient has had fitted. Reintegration into the community and workplace must be followed up closely through outpatient clinics or via telephone contact to help reduce any feelings of isolation and abandonment once discharged from hospital. Further nursing interventions include observation and early detection of any eye irregularities and clinical management of symptoms. This will involve assessment and management of pain (see Ch. 27, Pain assessment and pain management), maintaining the eye in a clean and comfortable state and administering eye preparations as prescribed. The eye may need to be covered for protection, patient comfort or as a means of camouflage.

Procedure guidelines: **Eye swabbing**

Equipment

1   Sterile dressing pack.

2   Sterile 0.9% sodium chloride for irrigation or sterile water for irrigation.

Procedure

Action	Rationale
1 Explain and discuss the procedure with the patient.	To ensure that the patient understands the procedure and gives his/her valid consent.
2 Assist the patient into the correct position: (a) Head well supported and tilted back. (b) Preferably the patient should be in bed or lying on a couch.	The patient needs to be discouraged from flinching or making unexpected movements and so should be in the most comfortable position possible at the start of the procedure.
3 Ensure an adequate light source, taking care not to dazzle the patient.	To enable maximum observation of the eyes without causing the patient harm or discomfort.
4 Wash hands thoroughly using bactericidal soap and water or bactericidal alcohol handrub, then dry hands.	To reduce the risk of cross-infection.
5 Always treat the uninfected or uninflamed eye first.	To reduce the risk of cross-infection.
6 Always bathe lids with the eyes closed first.	To reduce the risk of damaging the cornea.
7 Using a slightly moistened low-linting swab, ask the patient to look up and gently swab the lower lid from the nasal corner outwards. Use an aseptic technique for the damaged or postoperative eye.	If the swab is too wet the solution will run down the patient's cheek. This increases the risk of cross-infection and causes the patient discomfort. Swabbing from the nasal corner outwards avoids the risk of swabbing discharge into the lacrimal punctum, or even across the bridge of the nose into the other eye. Aseptic technique reduces the risk of cross-infection.
8 Ensure that the edge of the swab is not above the lid margin.	To avoid touching the sensitive cornea.
9 Using a new swab each time, repeat the procedure until all the discharge has been removed.	To reduce risk of cross-infection.

*Procedure guidelines: **Eye swabbing** (cont'd)*

Action	Rationale
10 Gently swab the upper lid by slightly everting the lid margin and asking the patient to look down. Swab from the nasal corner outwards and use a new swab each time until all discharge has been removed.	To effectively remove any foreign material from the eye. To reduce the risk of cross-infection.
11 Once both eyelids have been cleaned and dried, make the patient comfortable.	
12 Remove and dispose of equipment.	
13 Wash hands.	To reduce the risk of cross-infection.
14 Record the procedure in the appropriate documents.	To monitor trends and fluctuations.

Note: for information about obtaining an eye swab for pathological investigations, see the appropriate section in Ch. 39, Specimen collection.

Procedure guidelines: **Eye swabbing for comatose patients**

Equipment

1 Sterile dressing pack.
2 Sterile low-linting gauze.
3 Sterile 0.9% sodium chloride or sterile water for irrigation.

Procedure

Action	Rationale
1 Explain the procedure to the patient.	Hearing is often still present in unconscious patients so it is good practice to explain the procedure.
2 Wash hands thoroughly using bacterial soap and water or bactericidal alcohol handrub, then dry hands.	To reduce the risk of cross-infection.
3 Always treat the uninfected or uninflamed eye first.	To reduce the risk of cross-infection.
4 Always bathe lids with the eyes closed first.	To reduce the risk of damaging the cornea.
5 Use a new piece of gauze for each wipe.	To prevent spreading infection from one eye to the other.
6 Ensure that the edge of the swab is not above the lid margin.	To avoid touching the sensitive cornea.
7 Swab inner to outer canthus.	To prevent debris being washed into the nasolacrimal duct.
8 Instil ophthalmic ointment as prescribed, into lower lids.	To keep eyes moist.
9 Close eyes and apply mineral oil to lids.	To protect and lubricate skin.
10 If corneal reflexes are absent, apply soaked saline pads and affix with hypoallergenic tape.	To protect and prevent dryness.
11 Remove and dispose of equipment.	
12 Wash hands.	To reduce the risk of cross-infection.
13 Record the procedure in the appropriate documents.	To monitor trends and fluctuation.

Procedure guidelines: **Care of artificial eyes**

Equipment

1 Sterile dressing pack.
2 Sterile 0.9% sodium chloride for irrigation.

3 Low-linting gauze.

Procedure

Removal of artificial eye

Action	Rationale
1 Explain and discuss the procedure with the patient.	To ensure that the patient understands the procedure and gives his/her consent.
2 Wash hands thoroughly using bactericidal soap and water or bactericidal alcohol handrub.	To reduce the risk of cross-infection.
3 Wearing gloves and with the dominant hand, gently pull the eyelid downwards and exert slight pressure below the eyelid to overcome the suction, enabling the prosthesis to be removed.	
4 Clean the eye socket with sterile 0.9% sodium chloride and low-linting gauze.	
5 Clean the eye with sterile 0.9% sodium chloride.	

Insertion of artificial eye

Action	Rationale
1 Explain and discuss the procedure with the patient.	To ensure that the patient understands the procedure and gives his/her consent.
2 Wash hands thoroughly using bactericidal soap and water or bactericidal alcohol handrub.	To reduce the risk of cross-infection.
3 Wearing gloves and with the dominant hand, gently lift up the upper eyelid and pull down the lower eyelid. With the other hand, hold the prosthesis between the thumb and index finger and gently insert it.	

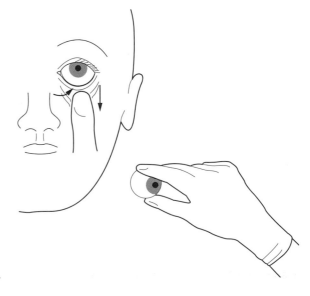

Figure 31.9 Removing an artificial eye.

Procedure guidelines: **Care of contact lenses**

Procedure

Removal of hard contact lenses

Action	Rationale
1 Explain and discuss the procedure with the patient.	To ensure that the patient understands the procedure and gives his/her consent.
2 Wash hands thoroughly using bactericidal soap.	To reduce the risk of cross-infection.
3 Wearing gloves, separate the eyelids using the thumb of each hand. Keeping the eyelid stationary, lift the bottom edge of the lens and remove.	
4 Store lenses in the appropriate solution as recommended by the manufacturers and ensure lenses are placed in the correct left and right storage pots.	To prevent deterioration and contamination.
5 Refer to manufacturer's instructions for further storage information, particularly if patient will not be using the lenses for a lengthy period of time.	To prevent deterioration and growth of organisms.

Removal of soft contact lenses

Action	Rationale
1 Explain and discuss the procedure with the patient.	To ensure that the patient understands the procedure and gives his/her consent.
2 Wash hands thoroughly using bactericidal soap.	To reduce the risk of cross-infection.
3 Wearing gloves, gently pinch the lens between the thumb and index finger.	To encourage the lens to fold together, allowing air to enter underneath the lens for easy removal.
4 Store lenses in the appropriate solution as recommended by the manufacturers and ensure lenses are placed in the correct left and right storage pots.	To prevent deterioration and contamination.
5 Refer to manufacturer's instructions for further storage information, particularly if patient will not be using the lenses for a lengthy period of time.	To prevent deterioration and growth of organisms.

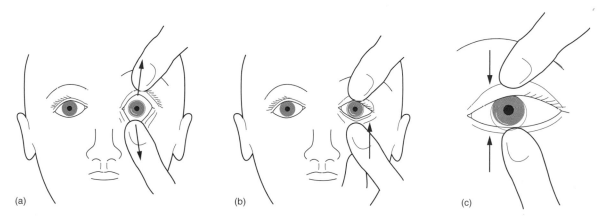

(a)   (b)   (c)

Figure 31.10 Removing hard contact lenses.

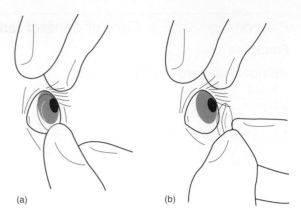

Figure 31.11 (a) Moving a soft lens down the interior part of the sclera. (b) Removing a soft lens by pinching it between the pads of the thumb and index finger.

(a)   (b)

Procedure guidelines: **Instillation of eye drops**

Equipment

1 Sterile dressing pack.
2 Sterile 0.9% sodium chloride for irrigation or sterile water for irrigation.

3 Appropriate eye drops. (Any preparation must be checked against the doctor's prescription.)
4 Low-linting swab.

Procedure

Action	Rationale
1 Explain and discuss the procedure with the patient.	To ensure that the patient understands the procedure and gives his/her valid consent.
2 If there is any discharge, proceed as for eye swabbing.	To remove any infected material and thus ensure adequate absorption of the drops.
3 Consult the patient's prescription sheet, and ascertain the following: (a) Drug (b) Dose (c) Date and time of administration (d) Route and method of administration, including which eye the drops are prescribed for (e) Expiry date on bottle (f) Validity of prescription (g) Signature of doctor.	To ensure that the patient is given the correct drug in the prescribed dose in the correct eye, and that the drug has not expired.
4 Assist the patient into the correct position, i.e. head well supported and tilted back.	To ensure that drops are instilled into the pocket of the inferior fornix and to avoid excess solution running down the patient's cheek.
5 Wash hands thoroughly using bactericidal soap and water or bactericidal alcohol handrub, and dry them.	Asepsis is essential when the patient has a damaged eye or has just had an operation on the eye. Infection can lead to loss of an eye.
6 Place a wet low-linting swab on the lower lid against the lid margin and gently pull down to evert the lower eyelid.	To absorb any excess solution which may be irritating to the surrounding skin and open the inferior fornix.
7 Ask the patient to look up immediately before instilling the drop.	This opens the eye and allows the drop to be instilled into the upper rim of the inferior fornix. If drop instilled too soon, the patient may blink as the drop is instilled.

*Procedure guidelines: **Instillation of eye drops** (cont'd)*

Action	Rationale
8 Ask the patient to close the eye. Keep the wet low-linting swab on the lower lid.	To ensure absorption of the fluid and to avoid excess running down the cheek.
9 Make the patient comfortable.	
10 Remove and dispose of equipment.	
11 Wash hands with bactericidal soap and water.	To reduce the risk of cross-infection.
12 Complete the patient's recording chart and other hospital and/or legally required documents.	To maintain accurate records. To provide a point of reference in the event of any queries. To prevent any duplication of treatment.

Procedure guidelines: **Instillation of eye ointment**

Equipment

1 Sterile dressing pack.
2 Sterile 0.9% sodium chloride for irrigation or sterile water for irrigation.

3 Appropriate eye ointment. (Any preparation must be checked against the doctor's prescription.)
4 Low-linting swab.

Procedure

Action	Rationale
1 Explain and discuss the procedure with the patient.	To ensure that the patient understands the procedure and gives his/her valid consent.
2 If there is any discharge, and to remove any previous application of ointment, proceed as for eye swabbing.	To remove any infected material and previous ointment to allow for absorption of ointment.
3 Consult the patient's prescription sheet, and ascertain the following: (a) Drug (b) Dose (c) Date and time of administration (d) Route and method of administration, including which eye the ointment is prescribed for (e) Expiry date on bottle (f) Validity of prescription (g) Signature of doctor.	To ensure that the patient is given the correct drug in the prescribed dose in the correct eye, and that the drug has not expired.
4 Wash hands thoroughly using bactericidal soap and water or bactericidal alcohol handrub.	To reduce the risk of cross-infection.
5 Place a wet low-linting swab on the lower lid against the lid margin.	To absorb excess ointment which may be irritating to the surrounding skin.
6 Slightly evert the lower lid by pulling on the low-linting swab. Ask the patient to look up immediately before applying the ointment.	To allow the application to be made inside the lower lid into the lower fornix.
7 Apply the ointment by gently squeezing the tube and, with the nozzle 2.5 cm above the eye, drawing a line along the inner edge of the lower lid from the nasal corner outwards.	To reduce the risk of cross-infection, contamination of the tube and trauma to the eye.
8 Ask the patient to close the eye and remove excess ointment with a new wet low-linting swab.	To avoid excess ointment irritating the surrounding skin.
9 Warn the patient that, when the eye is opened, vision will be a little blurred for a few minutes.	To prepare patient and to avoid anxiety.
10 Make the patient comfortable.	

Procedure guidelines: **Instillation of eye ointment** *(cont'd)*

Action	Rationale
11 Remove and dispose of equipment.	
12 Wash hands with bactericidal soap and water.	To reduce the risk of cross-infection.
13 Complete the patient's recording chart and other hospital and/or legally required documents.	To maintain accurate records. To provide a point of reference in the event of any queries. To prevent any duplication of treatment.

Procedure guidelines: **Eye irrigation**

Equipment

1 Sterile dressing pack.
2 Sterile 0.9% sodium chloride for irrigation or sterile water for irrigation (in an emergency tap water may be used).
3 Receiver.
4 Towel.
5 Plastic cape.
6 Irrigating flask.
7 Warm water in a bowl to heat irrigating fluid to tepid temperature.
8 Anaesthetic drops.

Procedure

Action	Rationale
1 Explain and discuss the procedure with the patient.	To ensure that the patient understands the procedure and gives his/her valid consent.
2 Instil anaesthetic drops if required (proceed as for instillation of eye drops).	To avoid any discomfort.
3 Prepare the irrigation fluid to the appropriate temperature.	Tepid fluid will be more comfortable for the patient. The solution should be poured across the inner aspect of the nurse's wrist to test the temperature.
4 Assist the patient into the appropriate position: (a) Head comfortably supported with chin almost horizontal (b) Head inclined to the side of the eye to be treated.	To avoid the solution running either over the nose into the other eye or out of the affected eye and down the side of the cheek.
5 Wash hands using bactericidal soap and water or bactericidal alcohol handrub, and dry.	To reduce risk of cross-infection.
6 If there is any discharge proceed as for eye swabbing.	To prevent washing the discharge down the lacrimal duct or across the cheek.
7 Ask the patient to hold the receiver against the cheek below the eye being irrigated.	To collect irrigation fluid as it runs away from the eye.
8 Position the towel and plastic cape.	To protect the patient's clothing.
9 Hold the patient's eyelids apart, using your first and second fingers, against the orbital ridge.	The patient will be unable to hold the eye open once irrigation commences.
10 Do not press on the eyeball.	To avoid causing the patient discomfort or pain.
11 Warn the patient that the flow of solution is going to start and pour a little onto the cheek first.	To allow time for adjustment to feeling of water flow.
12 Direct the flow of the fluid from the nasal corner outwards.	To wash away from the lacrimal punctum and prevent contaminating other eye.
13 Ask the patient to look up, down and to either side while irrigating.	To ensure that the whole area is washed.
14 Evert lids while irrigating.	To ensure complete removal of any foreign body.
15 Keep the flow of irrigation fluid constant.	To ensure swift removal of any foreign body.
16 When the eye has been thoroughly irrigated, ask the patient to close the eyes and use a new swab to dry the lids.	For patient comfort.

*Procedure guidelines: **Eye irrigation** (cont'd)*

Action	Rationale
17 Take the receiver from the patient and dry the cheek.	To prevent spillage of receiver contents and promote patient comfort.
18 Make the patient comfortable.	
19 Remove and dispose of equipment.	
20 Wash hands with bactericidal soap and water.	To reduce the risk of cross-infection.
21 Complete the patient's recording chart and other hospital and/or legally required documents.	To maintain accurate records. To provide a point of reference in the event of any queries. To prevent any duplication of treatment.

References and further reading

Ashurst, S. (1997) Nursing care of the mechanically ventilated patient in ITU: 1. *Br J Nurs*, **6**(8), 447–54.

BMA (2002) *British National Formulary* (BNF) No. 44. British Medical Association, London.

Char, D.H. (1993) Management of orbital tumours. *Mayo Clin Pract*, **68**, 1081–96.

Cloutier, A.O. (1992) Ocular side-effects of chemotherapy: nursing management. *Oncol Nurs Forum*, **8**(19), 1251–9.

Cunningham, C. & Gould, D. (1998) Eyecare for the sedated patient undergoing mechanical ventilation: the use of evidence-based care. *Int J Nurs Stud*, **35**, 32–40.

Finger, P.T. (2000) Tumour location affects the incidence of cataract and retinopathy after ophthalmic plaque radiation therapy. *Br J Ophthalmol*, **84**(9), 1068–70.

Foss, A.J.E., Cree, I.A., Dolin, P.J. *et al.* (1999) Modelling uveal melanoma. *Br J Ophthalmol*, **83**, 588–94.

Goddard, A.G., Kingston, J.E. & Hungerford, J.L. (1999) Delay in diagnosis of retinoblastoma: risk factors and treatment outcome. *Br J Ophthalmol*, **83**(12), 1320–3.

Goldberg, S.H. & Cantore, W.A. (1997) Tumours of the orbit. *Curr Opin Ophthalmol*, **815**, 51–6.

Henderson, J.W. (1980) Metastatic carcinoma. In: *Orbital Tumours*, 2nd edn (ed. J.W. Henderson). Decker, New York, pp. 451–71.

Kozier, B., Wilkinson, J.M., Erb, G. & Blais, K. (1998) Assisting with hygiene. In: *Fundamentals of Nursing: Concepts, Process, Practice*. Longman, California, pp. 729–84.

Leitman, M.W. (1988) *Manual for Eye Examination and Diagnosis*, 3rd edn. Medical Economics Body, New Jersey.

Lindgren, G., Diffey, B.L. & Larko, O. (1998) Basal cell carcinoma of the eyelids and solar ultraviolet radiation exposure. *Br J Ophthalmol*, **82**(12), 1412–5.

Lund, V.J. (1987) The orbit. In: *Otolaryngology*, 5th edn (ed. A.G. Kerr). Butterworth, London.

Marieb, E.N. (2001) *Human Anatomy and Physiology*, 5th edn. Benjamin Cummings, San Francisco.

Martin, E.A. (1996) *Concise Colour Medical Dictionary*. Oxford University Press, Oxford.

McConnell, E.A. (1991) How to irrigate the eye. *Nursing*, **91**, March, 28.

Moeloek, N.F. (1993) Updates in orbital tumours. *Eye Sci*, **9**(1), 40–4.

National Cancer Institute (1999a) Intraocular melanoma. http://cancernet.nci.nih.gov/clinpdq/soa/intraocular_melanoma physician.html

National Cancer Institute (1999b) Retinoblastoma. http://cancernet.nci.nih.gov/clinpdq/soa/retinoblastoma physician.html

National Cancer Institute (1999c) Childhood rhabdomyosarcoma. http://cancernet.nci.nih.gov/clinpdq/soa/childhood_rhabdomyosarcoma_physician.html

National Cancer Institute (1999d) Skin cancer. http://cancernet.nci.nih.gov/clinpdq/soa/skin_cancer_physician.html

SoftKey Multimedia (1995) *BodyWorks 5.0 for Windows* CD-ROM. SoftKey International, Cambridge, Massachusetts.

Souhami, R. & Tobias, J. (1998) *Cancer and its Management*. Blackwell Science, Oxford.

Tijl, J. *et al.* (1992) Metastatic tumours to the orbit – management and prognosis. *Graefe's Arch Clin Exp Ophthalmol (Amsterdam)*, **230**, 527–30.

Tortora, G. & Grabowski, S. (2002) *Principles of Anatomy and Physiology*, 9th edn. John Wiley, New York.

Wickham, R. & Rohan, K. (1997) Endocrine malignancies. In: *Cancer Nursing: Principles and Practice*, 4th edn (eds S.L. Groenwald, M. Hansen Frogge, M. Goodman, *et al.*). Jones and Bartlett, Sudbury, Massachusetts, pp. 1055–81.

Personal hygiene: mouth care

Chapter contents

Definition

Mouth care (oral hygiene) is defined as the scientific care of the teeth and mouth (Thomas 1997). The aims of oral care are to:

- Keep the mucosa clean, soft, moist and intact and to prevent infection
- Keep the lips clean, soft, moist and intact
- Remove food debris as well as dental plaque without damaging the gingiva
- Alleviate pain and discomfort and enhance oral intake
- Prevent halitosis and freshen the mouth (Daeffler 1980).

Reference material

Anatomy and physiology

The mouth is the oval cavity at the anterior end of the digestive tract (Mosby 1997). It consists of the mouth cavity (cavum oris proprium) and the vestibule (vestibulum oris), which is bounded by the lips and cheeks, and the gums and teeth. The oral cavity is lined with moist stratified epithelium consisting of 15–20 layers of cells (Porter 1994). It is an area of rapid replication designed to meet the constant demands of activities such as chewing and talking (Porter 1994). The tongue forms the greater part of the floor of the oral cavity.

The mouth has three main functions: (1) ingestion of food and water; (2) communication; and (3) breathing (with the nasal cavity) (Lippold & Winton 1972).

The mouth is lubricated by secretions from the salivary glands: parotid, submandibular and sublingual. Approximately 1.5 litres of saliva are produced each day (Torrance 1990). The functions of saliva are both protective and digestive in nature.

Predisposing factors to poor oral health are:

- Inability to take adequate fluids leading to dehydration and dryness of mucosa
- Poor nutritional status leading to poor cellular repair and vitamin deficiencies
- Insufficient saliva production leading to infection and dryness of the mucosa
- Major intervention altering oral status – surgery, radiotherapy or chemotherapy causing structural changes
- Lack of knowledge or motivation towards maintaining oral hygiene (Trenter & Creason 1986).

Oral complications

Oral complications manifest as pain, ulcers, infection, bone and dentition changes, bleeding and functional disorders affecting verbal and non-verbal communication, chewing and swallowing, taste and respiration (Porter 1994). Stomatitis (inflammation of the oral cavity) results from damage to the mucous membrane (Holmes 1990). It may be induced by trauma, infection or by factors that decrease the proliferation rate of the cells (e.g. chemotherapy and radiotherapy). Xerostomia is an alteration in the production of saliva. Salivary function can be reduced or even destroyed by radiation (Beck 1996; Porter 2000) as the salivary glands are highly sensitive to radiation (Carl 1983). Radiotherapy may also cause damage to the bone and dentition. Long-term damage may result in severe osteoradionecrosis (Yusef & Bakri 1993).

The oral cavity harbours many varieties of bacteria which do not normally pose any problems (Clarke 1993). However, immunosuppression and systemic treatments such as cytotoxic therapy and antifungal therapy may increase the pathogenicity of these organisms leading to local infection. Common organisms include *Pseudomonas*, *Klebsiella*, *Escherichia coli* and *Candida* species (Porter 1994). Local infection may lead to systemic or secondary infection such as septicaemia or pneumonia.

Mouth care

Mouth care involves oral assessment, appropriate frequency of care and the use of oral care tools and agents.

Oral assessment

Oral assessment is required in planning effective care (Eilers *et al.* 1988). Thorough assessment of the oral cavity is required to: (1) provide baseline data; (2) monitor response to therapy; and (3) identify new problems as they arise (Holmes & Mountain 1993).

A number of oral assessment tools have been developed. Holmes & Mountain (1993) evaluated three

oral assessment guides for reliability, validity and clinical usefulness. In their conclusion they showed a preference for that developed by Eilers *et al.* (1988), but stressed that further work is required to develop a tool that is entirely satisfactory for use in clinical practice and future research.

Andersson *et al.* (1999) tested Eiler's oral assessment guide with minor amendments for patients undergoing high-dose chemotherapy treatment. The guide was found to be a reliable and clinically useful tool for assessing the oral cavity status and determining changes. The authors suggest that once the changes have been identified, other methods may be required in order to make a complete diagnosis.

Frequency of care

Ginsberg (1961) concluded that the incidence of oral complications was reduced by the frequency of care rather than the agents employed. However, since then there has been little research to indicate the most effective frequency. Studies have reported various suggested time intervals including 2 hourly, 4 hourly and after meals (Ginsberg 1961; Howarth 1977; Beck 1979; Dudjak 1987).

Following a review of the work performed by Howarth (1977), Dudjak (1987) and Beck (1979), Krishnasamy (1995) recommends the following:

- 4-hourly care will reduce the potential for infection from micro-organisms.
- 2-hourly care will reduce mouth care problems and ensure patient comfort.
- 1-hourly care is recommended for patients requiring oxygen therapy, those who are mouth breathing, who have an infected mouth or are unconscious.

There is clearly a need for further research.

Oral care tools

A number of different oral care tools have been reported in the literature including toothbrush, foamstick, dental floss and gauze. The most appropriate tool should be determined by its efficacy together with its potential to damage the gingiva. The use of the toothbrush is well supported by the literature (Clay 2000; Xavier 2000). The foamstick, however, can cause less trauma, particularly when oral care includes free flaps and skin grafts (Hahn & Jones 2000) or oral bleeding occurs as a result of thrombocytopenia (Walton *et al.* 2002). Unquestionably, the toothbrush is the most effective at removing debris from the teeth and gums, including plaque (Pearson 1996; Xavier 2000; Pearson & Hutton 2002). Borowski *et al.* (1994) showed that intensive oral hygiene such as dental treatment, gingival and tooth brushing, during aplasia, does not increase the percentage of documented septicaemia. It has been found that this is superior to limited oral care, which excluded gingival and tooth brushing during periods of aplasia. Care must be taken to ensure that the toothbrush is kept free from infection as toothbrushes have been shown to harbour organisms such as group A beta-haemolytic streptococci, staphylococci, *Candida* and *Pseudomonas*. These have been found to contribute to persistent oropharyngeal infections (Taji & Rogers 1998; Brook & Gober 1998).

Oral care agents

The choice of an oral care agent is dependent on the aim of care. The agent may be used to remove debris and plaque, prevent superimposed infection, alleviate pain, stop bleeding, provide lubrication or to treat specific problems (Porter 1994). A wide variety of agents are available and should be determined by the individual needs of the patient together with a detailed nursing assessment. The agents described below comprise those included in *The Royal Marsden Hospital Trust Prescribing Guidelines for Mouth Care* (2002).

Chlorhexidine gluconate

Chlorhexidine is a compound with broad-spectrum antimicrobial activity that results in binding to and sustained release from mucosal surfaces (Ferretti *et al.* 1987). It has been shown to protect the patient from infection and to aid resolution of existing infections (Ferretti *et al.* 1987) and causes a reduction in soft tissue disease and oral microbial burden. It is effective against both anaerobes and aerobes as well as *Candida* (Mandel 1988; Walker 1988) and its efficacy is dose related (Addy & Moran 1991). Efficacy has been shown in doses of 0.01–0.2%. However, Foote *et al.* (1994) identified that patients receiving chlorhexidine mouthwash while undergoing radiation therapy showed a trend to develop more mucositis than those receiving a placebo mouthwash, leading to the hypothesis that chlorhexidine may be detrimental in this clinical setting.

In a study of 222 outpatients, Dodd *et al.* (1996) found that chlorhexidine as a mouthwash was no more effective than water in preventing chemotherapy-induced mucositis. Ferretti *et al.* (1990) found that prophylactic chlorhexidine mouthwashes reduce microbial flora in patients undergoing intensive chemotherapy and radiotherapy, but only reduce oral mucositis in those undergoing intensive chemotherapy. However, more research needs to be done within this area.

Fluconazole

Fluconazole is an orally absorbed antifungal azole which is soluble in water. It has been demonstrated to be effective in the treatment of candidosis of the oropharynx, oesophagus, urinary tract and a variety of deep tissue sites (Brammer 1990).

Sucralfate

Barker *et al.* (1991) showed that consistent daily oral hygiene and use of a mouth-coating agent such as sucralfate in patients receiving radiotherapy results in less pain and may reduce weight loss and interruption of radiation therapy because of severe mucositis. Reduction in pain and increase in oral intake have also been shown in patients with chemotherapy-induced ulcerating or erythematous mucositis taking oral sucralfate (Adams *et al.* 1986).

Chiara *et al.* (2001) performed a pilot study to assess the efficacy of sucralfate gel for the treatment of chemotherapy-induced mucositis and found that the gel did not demonstrate any significant advantage over the placebo used. Further research is therefore needed.

Nystatin

Nystatin is the best known and most commonly used antifungal agent (Campbell 1995). It is an antifungal antibiotic that is used as an oral suspension (Campbell 1995). Barkvoll *et al.* (1989) showed in their *in vitro* study that combinations of nystatin and chlorhexidine gluconate were not effective against *Candida albicans* and recommended that the most efficient treatment plan must be restricted to the use of one of these drugs alone. *The Royal Marsden Hospital Trust Prescribing Guidelines for Mouth Care* (2002) suggested that it is logical to leave a time interval of 15–30 minutes between administration of each agent.

Fluoride

Fluoride helps to prevent and arrest tooth decay, especially radiation caries, demineralization and decalcification. Following its use no food or fluids should be taken for at least 30 minutes in order for it to work (Myers & Mitchell 1988).

Artificial saliva

Saliva substitutes duplicate the properties of normal saliva (Kusler & Rambur 1992). They buffer the acidity of the mouth and lubricate the mucous membranes (Heals 1993).

Maintaining good oral hygiene

- Clean teeth with toothpaste and toothbrush after meals.
- Use chlorhexidine gluconate 0.2% 5 ml, four times a day diluted in 100 ml of water, which should be retained in the mouth for at least 1 minute before discarding.

Problems

Oral candidiasis

Prophylaxis

Nystatin mouthwash 1 ml used four times a day. This should be rinsed around the mouth and retained for at least 1 minute before swallowing. Dentures must be removed prior to rinsing. One millimetre of nystatin oral suspension should be added to the water to soak acrylic dentures (Lloyd, cited in Walton *et al.* 2002). A time interval of 15–30 minutes should be allowed between administration of chlorhexidine and nystatin to ensure efficacy.

Treatment

Surgical patients
    First-line: Nystatin 5 ml four times a day
    Second-line: Fluconazole 50 mg tablet or sugar-free suspension, daily for 7 days
Radiotherapy/chemotherapy patients
    First-line: Fluconazole 50 mg orally, daily for 7 days. Use 100 mg IV daily if patients cannot tolerate oral therapy
    Second-line: Fluconazole 200–400 mg IV, daily until able to tolerate oral therapy.

Painful mouth

First-line

Aspirin mouthwash four times a day (1–2 × 300 mg soluble tablets) used as mouthwash for oral cavity or a gargle for the oropharynx, mixed with lemon or raspberry mucilage to aid adherence of aspirin to the mucosa when treating the hypopharynx. Paracetamol is an alternative if aspirin is contraindicated (e.g. in clotting disorders).

Second-line

Lignocaine 2% gel applied four times a day for pain relief of mucositis or ulceration. For extensive mucositis use lignocaine spray; this can, however, cause a secondary numbing effect on the throat, producing an aspiration pneumonitis if patients are not informed of the delay required before recommencing diet and fluids (Toth & Frame 1983). Sucralfate suspension 5 ml, four times a day rinsed around the mouth and swallowed. Owing to its coating action, sucralfate must be used last in the oral care medication sequence otherwise it will block the effect of any topical agent (Toth *et al.* 1996). The sucralfate coating may mask mucosal infections (e.g. candidiasis) so there should be close monitoring for signs and symptoms of an infection during its use (Toth *et al.* 1996).

Third-line

Low-dose opiates by oral, subcutaneous or intravenous route.

Reduced salivary flow

Sodium fluoride (e.g. Fluorigard) mouthwash used after breakfast and subsequent cleaning of teeth and use of chlorhexidine mouthwash. No other mouthwash should be used for at least 1 hour after use as its action may be affected. Fluoride gel (e.g. Gel-Kam) should be brushed on the teeth last thing at night.

Treatment of dry mouth

Artificial saliva (e.g. Saliva Orthana), two or three sprays up to four times daily or as often as necessary.

Advances in mouth care

The last few years have seen advances in the management of oral complications. Much of the research has arisen from the dental literature and may need to be researched in the cancer arena.

Local delivery of antimicrobials

Periodontitis is a bacterial infection which often appears in local areas within the oral cavity. Local antimicrobial delivery systems such as tetracycline fibre, doxycycline polymer, chlorhexidine chip, minocycline ointment and metronidazole gel are now available and aim to deliver high concentrations of antimicrobials directly to the site of the infection (Killoy 1998). These systems are currently used predominantly in the treatment of chronic inflammatory periodontal diseases.

Autologous saliva

Sreebny *et al.* (1995) investigated the use of autologous saliva in patients undergoing radiation for head and neck cancer. Their study showed them that it was feasible to collect saliva from patients prior to receiving radiation, sterilize it and ensure that it retained its protective properties. Saliva could then be stored in a saliva bank for use in post-radiation xerostomia.

Growth factors

Studies have been carried out to determine the efficacy of colony stimulating factors such as granulocyte colony-stimulating factor (G-CSF) and granulocyte-macrophage colony-stimulating factor (GM-CSF) on the incidence of oral mucositis. Nicolatou *et al.* (1998) showed that the local administration of GM-CSF significantly reduced and almost healed radiation-induced mucositis in 14 out of 17 patients during radiotherapy. This supports the findings of Kannan *et al.* (1997) who also suggest that further study in randomized double-blind trials is warranted. Rovirosa *et al.* (1998) also showed that GM-CSF was effective in the control of pain, oral intake and weight loss. It has been shown that by giving transforming growth factor (TGF)-beta 3, a potent negative regulator of epithelial and haemopoietic stem cell growth, it is possible to temporarily arrest oral mucosal basal cell proliferation and provide a safe and effective intervention for patients who undergo aggressive regimens of cancer therapy (Spijkervet & Sonis 1998).

Mascarin *et al.* (1999) investigated the effect of subcutaneous G-CSF on 26 patients with head and neck cancer undergoing hyperfractionated radiotherapy. Whilst G-CSF reduced the number of treatment breaks associated with radiotherapy, it did not appear overall to improve mucositis. Similarly, Makkonen *et al.* (2000) compared subcutaneous GM-CSF and sucralfate mouthwashes to sucralfate mouthwashes for 40 head and neck cancer patients undergoing radiotherapy. There was no evidence to suggest that subcutaneous GM-CSF reduces the severity of radiation-induced mucositis. Sprinzl *et al.* (2001) compared a once-daily GM-CSF mouthwash with a conventional mouthwash for 35 patients with head and neck cancer for radiochemotherapy-induced oral mucositis. The topical use of GM-CSF as a mouthwash had no clinical benefit over the conventional mouthwash. Clearly further research is still required.

Chlorhexidine chewing gum

Smith *et al.* (1996) showed that the use of a chlorhexidine chewing gum was as effective to oral hygiene and gingival health as a 0.2% chlorhexidine mouthwash. Teeth staining, a common side-effect of chlorhexidine mouthwash, was less with the gum than with the mouthwash, although this was not statistically significant.

Pilocarpine

This has been shown to improve saliva production and relieve symptoms of xerostomia after radiation of head and neck cancer. As a cholinergic drug the minor side-effects associated with its use were limited to sweating (Johnson *et al.* 1993).

Cryotherapy

Dose (1992) found that using ice chips within the oral cavity decreased the incidence of 5-fluorouracil (5-FU) induced stomatitis. 5-FU has a relatively short half-life so by reducing the blood supply to the oral mucosa by application of cold before, during and after systemic bolus administration of the drug, the amount of 5-FU taken up by the cells can be reduced, thereby reducing cellular damage.

Mahood *et al.* (1991) found that when patients received cryotherapy (ice chips) at the time of chemotherapy administration, mucositis toxicity scores were decreased. Dalberg & Sorensen (1996) summarize their literature review by suggesting that cryotherapy does reduce the frequency and grade of stomatitis during chemotherapy but the optimal use as a supportive measure is not yet identified – further evaluations are required.

Tumours of the oral cavity

Clinical presentation

Tumours of the oral cavity include a spectrum of benign, premalignant and malignant lesions which usually present as exophytic swellings, mucosal thickenings or painful ulcerative tumours. Benign tumours such as fibromas, granulomas and adenomas of the tongue and buccal mucosa are slow growing, rarely ulcerate except if they are situated on the lateral border of the tongue when they may be traumatized by the teeth, and are easily excised. Premalignant lesions include leukoplakia, erythroplakia and chronic hyperplastic candidiasis, but there are other oral conditions such as lichen planus and submucous fibrosis which may be associated with a higher incidence of oral cancer.

Malignant tumours of the mouth are most commonly squamous cell carcinomas arising from the mucosal surface. The most frequent sites are the lateral border of the tongue and the anterior floor of the mouth which, because of their position, often present early. More posterior lesions on the tongue and tonsil produce rather vague symptoms of throat discomfort and may not be diagnosed until they are more advanced, although earlier detection may be predicted by astute investigation of a suspicious lump in the upper neck which is a common presentation of a metastatic cervical lymph node from this site.

The most common aetiological factor in squamous carcinoma of the oral cavity is tobacco which may be taken in several different forms, often associated with excessive alcohol intake. In Western countries where cigarette smoking is the most frequent causative factor, cancers of the upper aerodigestive tract account for about 10% of all cancers, but in the Asian subcontinent where chewing of tobacco and betel nut is common, the incidence is in the region of 40%. Alcohol is a synergistic factor which increases the mucosal absorption of carcinogens which are more soluble in alcohol than in normal aqueous mucus or saliva.

Management

The only curative treatments for squamous carcinoma of the oral cavity are surgery and radiotherapy. These modalities may be combined with postoperative radiotherapy in more advanced tumours depending on the histology and its potential for invasion and spread to the neck. Alternatively brachytherapy with iridium wire implants may be used for early lesions confined to the tongue, although this technique is not recommended for lesions that encroach near the alveolus because of the risk of radionecrosis.

Surgery

Early tumours of the tongue and oral cavity may cause only minimal ulceration or discomfort to the patient, but as they become more advanced they will cause major symptoms due to fungation, trismus, bleeding, foul odour due to secondary infection, loss of eating ability and cosmetic deformity. Temporary limited control of these symptoms may be achieved by basic oral hygiene with the use of oral douches and systemic metronidazole, which is an excellent deodorizer for these tumours. The use of tranexamic acid often minimizes the risk of bleeding in haemorrhagic tumours (Sindet-Pedersen & Steubjerg 1986; Waly 1995).

Surgical resection of the tumour, however, provides the most reliable way of removal of the disease, together with any local lymph node metastases. This may be achieved in the small tumour with laser excision and primary closure or leaving the wound open to allow secondary healing. Regular douching of the open wound will help to prevent secondary infection. Alternatively, reconstruction of the remaining tongue with a free radial forearm flap can be achieved with good success and functional rehabilitation.

Malignant tumours of the upper jaw may require partial or total maxillectomy and this operation results in a defect in the palate and maxilla which usually is filled with a complex upper denture prosthesis. This needs to be taken out daily for regular douching and cleaning of the cavity to prevent secondary infection.

Radiotherapy

Treatment with radiotherapy involves implantation of the tumour with iridium afterloading wires and/or external beam irradiation. Local mucositis and ulceration of the mucosa and skin occur frequently towards the end of treatment and are managed by local mouthcare treatment to keep the mouth clean and comfortable. Radionecrosis of the mandible may occur after irradiation which results in exposure of an area of bone in the floor of mouth. This must be kept clean with regular douching, preferably with a pulsating 'water-pick'. Often this will eventually heal after sequestration of the devascularized piece of bone.

Chemotherapy

Chemotherapy is not a curative treatment for squamous carcinoma of the oral cavity and pharynx. However, it may be used as adjuvant therapy to help eliminate microscopic disease or as neo-adjuvant treatment prior to radiotherapy or surgery (Jones & Gore 1995). More commonly chemotherapy is used in palliative treatment of recurrent inoperable disease or metastases. This often successfully palliates disease-related symptoms and affords the patient some quality of life.

Summary

It is essential that consideration is given to those patients at risk of potential isolation, social ostracism and prejudice if lesions are visible and if halitosis is evident. Good oral hygiene will help to minimize complications related to infection, foul odour, bleeding and pain. This in turn will facilitate patient comfort especially where oral prostheses are worn. A comfortable mouth will not only assist with appetite and food intake but also help the patient feel more sociable and confident. Sexual relationships can also be disrupted in this group of patients as the mouth plays an important role in oral stimulation and sexual expression. To achieve optimum oral status for each individual patient, it is vital that the nurse uses all resources available and involves members of the multidisciplinary team (clinical nurse specialist, dentist, dental hygienist, maxillofacial prosthodontist, pharmacist, pain control team, speech and language therapist, and dietitian). Any oral regimen must be evaluated frequently for efficacy and the patients should know how to access members of the team for advice and support, especially on discharge, for continuity of care given.

Procedure guidelines: **Mouth care**

Equipment

1 Clean tray.
2 Plastic cups.
3 Mouthwash or clean solutions.
4 Appropriate equipment for cleaning.
5 Clean receiver or bowl.
6 Paper tissues.
7 Wooden spatula.
8 Small-headed, soft toothbrush.
9 Toothpaste.
10 Disposable gloves.
11 Denture pot.
12 Small torch.

Items 1–11 may be left in the patient's locker when appropriate, and should be cleaned, renewed or replenished daily.

Procedure

Action	Rationale
1 Explain and discuss the procedure with the patient.	To ensure that the patient understands the procedure and gives his/her valid consent.
2 Wash hands with bactericidal soap and water/ bactericidal alcohol handrub and dry with paper towel. Put on disposable gloves.	To reduce the risk of cross-infection.

*Procedure guidelines: **Mouth care** (cont'd)*

Action	Rationale
3 Prepare solutions required.	Solutions must always be prepared immediately before use to maximize their efficacy and minimize the risk of microbial contamination.
4 If the patient cannot remove their own dentures, using a tissue or piece of gauze, grasp the upper plate at the front teeth with the thumb and second finger and move the denture up and down slightly (Kozier *et al.* 1998). Lower the upper plate, remove and place in denture pot.	Removal of dentures is necessary for cleaning of underlying tissues. A tissue or topical swab provides a firmer grip of the dentures and prevents contact with the patient's saliva. The slight movement breaks the suction that secures the plate.
5 Lift the lower plate, turning it so that one side is lower than the other, remove and place in denture pot (Kozier *et al.* 1998).	Lifting the lower plate at an angle helps removal of the denture without stretching the lips.
6 Remove a partial denture by exerting equal pressure on the border of each side of the denture (Kozier *et al.* 1998).	Holding the clasps could result in damage or breakage.
7 Inspect the patient's mouth with the aid of a torch and spatula.	The mouth is examined for changes in condition with respect to moisture, cleanliness, infected or bleeding areas, ulcers, etc.
8 Using a soft, small toothbrush and toothpaste (or foamstick if the gingiva is damaged) brush the patient's natural teeth, gums and tongue.	To remove adherent materials from the teeth, tongue and gum surfaces. Brushing stimulates gingival tissues to maintain tone and prevent circulatory stasis.
9 Hold the brush against the teeth with the bristles at a 45° angle. The tips of the outer bristles should rest against and penetrate under the gingival sulcus. Then move the bristles back and forth using a vibrating motion, from the sulcus to the crowns of the teeth (Kozier *et al.* 1998). Repeat until all teeth surfaces have been cleaned. Clean the biting surfaces by moving the toothbrush back and forth over them in short strokes.	Brushing loosens and removes debris trapped on and between the teeth and gums. This reduces the growth medium for pathogenic organisms and minimizes the risk of plaque formation and dental caries. Foamsticks are ineffective for this.
10 Give a beaker of water or mouthwash to the patient. Encourage patient to rinse the mouth vigorously then void contents into a receiver. Paper tissues should be to hand. If the patient is immunosuppressed do not allow to rinse directly into a sink.	Rinsing removes loosened debris and toothpaste and makes the mouth taste fresher. The glycerine content of toothpaste will have a drying effect if left in the mouth. Reservoirs of stagnant water may harbour *Pseudomonas* bacteria.
11 If the patient is unable to rinse and void, use a rinsed toothbrush to clean the teeth and moistened foamsticks to wipe the gums and oral mucosa. Foamsticks should be used with a rotating action so that most of the surface is utilized.	To remove debris as effectively as possible.
12 Apply artificial saliva to the tongue if appropriate and/or suitable lubricant to dry lips.	To increase the patient's feeling of comfort and well-being and prevent further tissue damage.
13 Clean the patient's dentures on all surfaces with a denture brush or toothbrush. Hold dentures over a sink of water in case they are dropped (Clay 2000; Curzio & McCowan 2000). Check the dentures for cracks, sharp edges and missing teeth (Curzio & McCowan 2000). Rinse them well and return them to the patient.	Cleaning dentures removes accumulated food debris which could be broken down by salivary enzymes to products which irritate and cause inflammation of the adjacent mucosal tissue. Some commercial denture cleaners may have an abrasive effect on the denture surface. This then attracts plaque and encourages bacterial growth.
14 Dentures should be removed at night and placed in a suitable cleaning solution (Sweeney *et al.* 1995; Clay 2000).	

*Procedure guidelines: **Mouth care** (cont'd)*

Action	Rationale
15 Dentures should be soaked in diluted antifungal for 4–6 hours daily if oral *Candida* species are present.	Soaking in diluted antifungal reduces the risk of reinfecting the mouth with infected dentures.
16 Floss teeth (unless contraindicated, e.g. clotting abnormality) once in 24 hours using lightly waxed floss (Clay 2000). To floss the upper teeth, use your thumb and index finger to stretch the floss and wrap one end of floss around the third finger of each hand. Move the floss up and down between the teeth from the tops of the crowns to the gum and along the gum lines wherever possible. To floss the lower teeth, use the index fingers to stretch the floss.	Flossing helps to remove debris between teeth.
17 Discard remaining mouthwash solutions.	To prevent the risk of contamination.
18 Clean and thoroughly dry the toothbrush.	
19 Wash hands with soap and water or alcohol handrub and dry with paper towel.	To reduce the risk of cross-infection.

Problem solving

Problem	Cause	Suggested action
Dry mouth.	Inadequate hydration.	Monitor fluid balance and increase fluid intake where necessary.
	Impaired production of saliva, e.g. as a consequence of radiotherapy or chemotherapy.	Apply artificial saliva to the oral cavity as required. Give the patient ice cubes to suck.
	Presence of specific stressors, e.g. mouth breathing, oxygen therapy, no oral intake, intermittent oral suction.	Inspect the mouth frequently, e.g. half-hourly. Swab mucosa with water.
Dry lips.	As above.	Smear a thin layer of appropriate lubricant.
Thick mucus.	Postoperative closure of a tracheostomy. Radiotherapy. Poor swallowing mechanism.	Use sodium bicarbonate solution in the mouth care procedure. Rinse the mouth afterwards with water or 0.9% sodium chloride.
Patient unable to tolerate toothbrush.	Pain, e.g. postoperatively; stomatitis.	Use foamsticks to clean the patient's gums and mucosa. 0.9% sodium chloride is advisable as a cleaning agent. For severe pain use an anaesthetic mouth spray or mouthwash before giving mouth care.
Toothbrush inappropriate or ineffective.	Infected stomatitis. Accumulation of dried mucus, new lesions, blood or debris.	As above and take a swab of any infected areas for culture before giving mouth care.

References and further reading

Adams, S.C. *et al.* (1986) Evaluation of sucralfate as a compound oral suspension for the treatment of mucositis. *Proc Annu Meeting Am Soc Clin Oncol*, **5**, 257.

Addy, M. & Moran, J. (1991) The effect of some chlorhexidine containing mouth rinses on salivary bacterial counts. *J Clin Periodontol*, **18**, 90–93.

Andersson, P., Persson, L., Hallberg, I.R. & Renvert, S. (1999) Testing an oral assessment guide during chemotherapy treatment in a Swedish care setting: a pilot study. *J Clin Nurs*, **8**, 150–8.

Barker, G. *et al.* (1991) The effects of sucralfate suspension and diphenhydramine syrup plus kaolin-pectin on radiotherapy-induced mucositis. *Oral Surg Oral Med Oral Pathol*, **71**(3), 288–93.

Barkvoll, P. *et al.* (1989) Effect of nystatin and chlorhexidine digluconate on *Candida albicans*. *Oral Surg Oral Med Oral Pathol*, **67**, 279–81.

Beck, S. (1979) Impact of a systemic oral protocol on stomatitis after chemotherapy. *Cancer Nurs*, **2**(5), 185–99.

Beck, S.L. (1996) Mucositis. In: *Cancer Symptom Management*, (eds S. Groenwald, M. Hansen-Frogge & C. Henke-Yarbro). Jones & Bartlett, Massachusetts.

Borowski, B., Benhamou, E., Pico, J.L. *et al.* (1994) Prevention of oral mucositis in patients treated with high dose chemotherapy and bone marrow transplantation: a randomised controlled trial comparing two protocols of dental care. *Eur J Cancer Oral Oncol*, **30B**(2), 93–7.

Brammer, K.W. (1990) Management of fungal infection in neutropenic patients. *Haematol Blood Transf*, **33**, 546–50.

Brook, I. & Gober, A.E. (1998) Persistence of group A beta-hemolytic streptococci in toothbrushes and removable orthodontic appliances following treatment of pharyngotonsillitis. *Arch Otolaryngol Head Neck Surg*, **124**(9), 993–5.

Campbell, S. (1995) Treating oral candidiasis. *Nurse Prescriber*, June, 12–13.

Carl, W. (1983) Oral complications in cancer patients. *Am Fam Physician*, **27**, 161–70.

Chiara, S., Nobile, M.T., Vincenti, M. *et al.* (2001) Sucralfate in the treatment of chemotherapy-induced stomatitis: a double-blind, placebo-controlled pilot study. *Anticancer Res*, **21**, 3707–10.

Clarke, G. (1993) Mouth care in the hospitalized patient. *Br J Nurs*, **2**(4), 221–7.

Clay, M. (2000) Oral health in older people. *Nurs Older People*, **12**(7), 21–5.

Curzio J. & McCowan, M. (2000) Getting research into practice: developing oral hygiene standards. *Br J Nurs*, **9**(7), 434–8.

Daeffler, R. (1980) Oral hygiene measures for patients with cancer. II. *Cancer Nurs*, December, 427–31.

Dalberg, J. & Sorensen, J.B. (1996) Cryotherapy (oral cooling) as prevention of chemotherapy-induced stomatitis. A literature review. *J Cancer Care*, **5**, 131–4.

Dodd, M.J., Larson, P.L., Dibble, S.L. *et al.* (1996) Randomized clinical trial of chlorhexidine versus placebo for prevention of oral mucositis in patients receiving chemotherapy. *Oncol Nurs Forum*, **23**(6), 921–7.

Dose, A.M. (1992) *Cryotherapy for prevention of 5 fluorouracil induced mucositis. Cancer nursing, changing frontiers*. Proc 7th Int Conf Cancer Nursing, August.

Dudjak, L. (1987) Mouth care for mucositis due to radiation therapy. *Cancer Nurs*, **10**, 131–40.

Eilers, J. *et al.* (1988) Development, testing and application of the oral assessment guide. *Oncol Nurs Forum*, **15**(3), 325–30.

Ferretti, G. *et al.* (1987) Chlorhexidine for prophylaxis against oral infections and associated complications in patients receiving bone marrow transplants. *J Am Dent Assoc*, **114**(4), 461–7.

Ferretti, G.A., Raybould, T.P., Brown, A.T. *et al.* (1990) Chlorhexidine prophylaxis for chemotherapy- and radiotherapy-induced stomatitis: a randomised double-blind trial. *Oral Surg Oral Med Oral Pathol*, **69**(3), 331–7.

Foote, R.L., Loprinzi, C.L., Frank, A.R. *et al.* (1994) Randomized trial of a chlorhexidine mouthwash for alleviation of radiation-induced mucositis. *J Clin Oncol*, **12**(12), 2630–3.

Ginsberg, M. (1961) A study of oral hygiene nursing care. *Am J Nurs*, **61**, 67–9.

Hahn, M.J. & Jones, A. (2000) Mouth care. In: *Head and Neck Nursing*. Churchill Livingstone, London, pp. 35–57.

Heals, D. (1993) A key to wellbeing: oral hygiene in patients with advanced cancer. *Prof Nurse*, March, 391–8.

Holmes, S. (1990) *Cancer Chemotherapy. Lisa Sainsbury Foundation*. Austen Cornish, London, pp. 180–1.

Holmes, S. & Mountain, E. (1993) Assessment of oral status: evaluation of three oral assessment guides. *J Clin Nurs*, **2**, 35–40.

Howarth, H. (1977) Mouth care procedures for the very ill. *Nurs Times*, **73**, 354–5.

Johnson, J.T., Feretti, G.A., Nethery, W.J. *et al.* (1993) Oral pilocarpine for post irradiation xerostomia in patients with head and neck cancer. *N Engl J Med*, **329**(6), 390–5.

Jones, A.L. & Gore, M.E. (1995) Medical treatment of malignant tumours of the mouth, jaw and salivary glands. In: *Malignant Tumours of the Mouth, Jaws and Salivary Glands*, 2nd edn (eds J.D. Langdon & J.M. Henk). Edward Arnold, London, pp. 123–35.

Kannan, V., Bapsy, P.P., Anantha, N. *et al.* (1997) Efficacy and safety of granulocyte macrophage-colony stimulating factor (GM-CSF) on the frequency and severity of radiation mucositis in patients with head and neck carcinoma. *Int J Radiat Oncol Biol Phys*, **37**(5), 1005–10.

Killoy, W.J. (1998) Chemical treatment of periodontitis: local delivery of antimicrobials. *Int Dent J*, **3** Suppl, 305–15.

Kozier, B., Erb, G., Blais, K. & Wilkinson, J.M. (1998) Assisting with hygiene. In: *Fundamentals of Nursing: Concepts, Process & Practice*. Longman, California, pp. 729–84.

Krishnasamy, M. (1995) Oral problems in advanced cancer. *Eur J Cancer Care*, **4**, pp. 173–7.

Kusler, D.L. & Rambur, B.A. (1992) Treatment for radiation-induced xerostomia: an innovative remedy. *Cancer Nurs*, **15**(3), 191–5.

Lippold, A.J.C. & Winton, F.R. (1972) *Hearing and Speech Human Physiology*. Churchill Livingstone, Edinburgh, pp. 443–64.

Mahood, D.J., Dose, A.M., Loprinzi, C.L. *et al.* (1991) Inhibition of fluorouracil-induced stomatitis by oral cryotherapy. *J Clin Oncol*, **9**(3), 449–52.

Makkonen, T.A., Minn, H., Jekunen, A., Vilja, P., Tuominen, J. & Joensuu, H. (2000) Granulocyte macrophage-colony stimulating factor (GM-CSF) and sucralfate in prevention of radiation-induced mucositis: a prospective randomised study. *Int J Radiat Oncol Biol Phys*, **46**(3), 525–34.

Mandel, I. (1988) Chemotherapeutic agents for controlling plaque and gingivitis. *J Clin Periodontol*, **15**, 488–98.

Mascarin, M., Franchin, G., Minatel, E. *et al.* (1999) The effect of granulocyte colony-stimulating factor on oral mucositis in head and neck cancer patients treated with hyperfractionated radiotherapy. *Oral Oncol*, **35**, 203–8.

Miller, M. & Kearney, N. (2001) Oral care for patients with cancer: a review of the literature. *Cancer Nurs*, **24**(4), 241–54.

Mosby (1997) *Mosby's Medical, Nursing and Allied Health Dictionary*, 5th edn. Mosby, London.

Myers, R.E. & Mitchell, L.D. (1988) Fluoride for the head and neck radiation patient. *Military Med*, **153**(8), 411.

Nicolatou, O. *et al.* (1998) A pilot study of the effect of granulocyte-macrophage colony-stimulating factor on oral mucositis in head and neck cancer patients during X-radiation therapy. *Int J Radiat Oncol Biol Phys*, **42**(3), 551–6.

Pearson, L.S. (1996) A comparison of the ability of foam swabs and toothbrushes to remove dental plaque: implications for nursing practice. *J Adv Nurs*, **23**(1), 62–9.

Pearson, L.S. & Hutton, J.L. (2002) A controlled trial to compare the ability of foam swabs and toothbrushes to remove dental plaque. *J Adv Nurs*, **39**(5), 480–9.

Porter, H.J. (1994) Mouth care in cancer. *Nurs Times*, **90**(14), 27–9.

Porter, H. (2000) Oral care. In: *Nursing in Haematological Oncology* (ed. M. Grundy). Harcourt, London.

Rovirosa, A., Ferre, J. & Biete, A. (1998) Granulocyte macrophage-colony stimulating factor mouthwashes heal oral ulcers during head and neck radiotherapy. *Int J Radiat Oncol Biol Phys*, **41**(4), 747–54.

Royal Marsden Hospital (2002) *The Royal Marsden Hospital Prescribing Guidelines for Mouth Care*. Drugs and Therapeutic Advisory Committee, September. The Royal Marsden Hospital, London.

Sindet-Pedersen, S. & Steubjerg, S. (1986) Effect of local antifibrinolytic treatment with tranexamic acid in hemophiliacs undergoing oral surgery. *J Oral Maxillofac Surg*, **44**(9), 903–9.

Smith, A.J., Moran, J., Dangler, L.V. *et al.* (1996) The efficacy of an anti-gingivitis chewing gum. *J Clin Periodontol*, **23**(1), 19–23.

Spijkervet, F.K. & Sonis, S.T. (1998) New frontiers in the management of chemotherapy-induced mucositis. *Curr Opin Oncol*, **10**(Suppl 1), S23–7.

Sprinzl, G.M., Galvan, O., de Vries, A. *et al.* (2001) Local application of granulocyte-macrophage colony stimulating factor (GM-CSF) for the treatment or oral mucositis. *Eur J Cancer*, **37**, 2003–9.

Sreebny, L.M., Zhu, W.X. & Meek, A.G. (1995) The preparation of an autologous saliva for use with patients undergoing therapeutic radiation for head and neck cancer. *J Oral Maxillofac Surg*, **53**(2), 131–9.

Sweeney, M.P., Shaw, A., Yip, B. & Bagg, J. (1995) Oral health in elderly patients. *Br J Nurs*, **4**(20), 1204–8.

Taji, S.S. & Rogers, A.H. (1998) ADRF Trebitsch Scholarship. The microbial contamination of toothbrushes. A pilot study. *Aust Dent J*, **43**(2), 128–30.

Thomas, C.L. (1997) *Taber's Cyclopedic Medical Dictionary*, 18th edn. F.A. Davis, Philadelphia.

Torrance, C. (1990) Oral hygiene. *Surg Nurse*, **15**, 16–20.

Toth, B.B. & Frame, R.T. (1983) Dental oncology. *Curr Probl Cancer*, **10**, 7–35.

Toth, B.B., Chambers, M.S. & Fleming, T.C. (1996) Prevention and management of oral complications associated with cancer therapies: radiotherapy/chemotherapy. *Texas Dent J*, **June**, 23–9.

Trenter, P. & Creason, N.S. (1986) Nurse administered oral hygiene: is there a scientific basis? *J Adv Nurse*, 11, 323–31.

Walker, C. (1988) Microbial effects of mouth rinses containing antimicrobials. *J Clin Periodontol*, **15**, 499–505.

Walton, J.C., Miller, J. & Tordecilla, L. (2002) Elder oral assessment and care. *ORL Head Neck Nurs*, **20**(2), 12–19.

Waly, N.G. (1995) Local antifibrinolytic treatment with tranexamic acid in hemophiliac children undergoing dental extractions. *Egypt Dent J*, **41**(1), 961–8.

Xavier, G. (2000) The importance of mouth care in prevention. *Nurs Stand*, **14**(18), 47–51.

Yusef, Z.W. & Bakri, M.M. (1993) Severe progressive periodontal destruction due to radiation tissue injury. *J Periodontol*, **64**(12), 1253–8.

Personal hygiene: skin care

Chapter contents

Definition

Personal hygiene is the physical act of cleaning the body to ensure that the skin, hair and nails are maintained in an optimum condition (DoH 2001). The prevention of infection is also pertinent and will be referred to within the text (see Ch. 5, Barrier nursing).

Reference material

'Cleanliness is not a luxury in a highly developed country, it is ... a basic human right' (Young 1991). When an individual becomes ill, he or she may depend on others to perform this elementary intervention. If this occurs, it is important that the nurse is able to appropriately observe and assess the patient.

Hygiene is a personal entity and everyone will have their own individual requirements and standards of cleanliness. In this way, 'nurses must take care not to impose their own norms on patients and clients and should respect their autonomy in decisions concerning care' (Spiller 1992). When assessing personal considerations, the patient's religious and cultural beliefs should be taken into account. Personal hygiene is individual to that person and is also based on family influences, peer groups, economic and social factors. Various examples of this will be given throughout the text.

In Western culture, privacy is of the utmost importance and considered to be a basic human right. In some cultures, modesty is crucial, e.g. for Muslims, and can cause problems in the hospital setting (Neuberger 1987). Patients will feel a great deal of embarrassment having to depend on another person to help/assist them with this extremely private act and consideration should be given to their personal needs (Wagnild & Manning 1985; Spiller 1992). It is therefore surprising to find that such little reference is made to these elements in the literature. The nurse's role is 'the maintenance of an acceptable level of cleanliness' (Young 1991) which promotes 'comfort, safety and well-being' for the patient. Frequently, the time taken to attend to personal hygiene will provide ample opportunity for communication. Wilson (1986) states:

> '… a bedbath facilitates listening and enables the nurse to pick up cues to a patient's anxieties and fears. It provides the time and opportunity for the nurse to offer support and encouragement when difficult situations have to be confronted, solutions sought and decisions made.'

This also focuses on the nurse's ability to 'be with the patient' as well as 'doing things for the patient' (Campbell 1984) and is part of the essence of nursing care (Kitson 1999). This derives from theorists such as Henderson (1966) and Nightingale (1969) focusing on the aspect of patient-centred care or holistic care. This is essential when thinking of the personal hygiene of patients as it is about the uniqueness of patients, their needs and how they wish to be treated.

It is during the delivery of personal hygiene that the nurse is able to demonstrate a wide range of skills such as communication, observation and caring for the patient. This can be the most significant social interaction of the day for the patient, as the nurse develops a deeper understanding of the patient's personality and needs, providing a personal bond between the nurse and patient (Hector & Touhy 1997).

Health care assistants with a recognised qualification such as a National Vocational Qualification (NVQ) can complement the role of the qualified nurse in the implementation of planned care.

Nursing models, which provide a conceptual framework for practice, all make some reference to meeting the patient's hygiene needs. Roper *et al.* (1981) adapted Henderson's original concept of nursing (Henderson 1966) to develop a model reflecting the activities of daily living.

Another example was given by Orem (1980) who focused on the ability of the patient to self-care and refers to the universal self-care requisites of the 'condition of the skin, nails and hair' and the 'usual patterns of hygiene'. The assessment process will show if there is a 'deficit' and then an appropriate nursing intervention can result.

The assessment should allow the nurse to carry out the appropriate intervention(s) and evaluate the effectiveness of care given.

Clinical benchmarking is a valid framework by which nurses can establish and share best practice throughout the work environment. Three *Essence of Care* benchmarks – hygiene, self-care and privacy and dignity – are important to consider when reviewing patient hygiene.

- All patients are assessed to identify the advice and/or assistance required in maintaining and promoting their individual personal hygiene.
- Planned care is negotiated with patients and/or their carers and is based on assessment of their individual needs.
- Patients have access to an environment that is safe and acceptable to the individual.
- Patients are expected to supply their own toiletries but single-use toiletries are provided until they can supply their own.
- Patients have access to the level of assistance that they require to meet their individual personal hygiene (DoH 2001).

Areas of care

Skin care

Maintaining the skin's integrity is essential to the prevention of infection and the promotion of health. The skin has several functions:

- Maintenance of temperature
- Protection
- Excretion
- Sensation.

It is made up of three layers: the epidermis, dermis and the deep subcutaneous layer.

The *epidermis* is the outer coating of the skin and contains no blood vessels or nerve endings. The cells on the surface are continually being rubbed off and replaced by new cells which have arisen from deeper layers. The epidermis has hairs, sweat glands and the ducts of sebaceous glands passing through it.

The *dermis* is the thicker layer which contains blood vessels, nerve fibres, sweat and sebaceous glands and lymph vessels. It is made up of white fibrous tissue and yellow elastic fibres which give the skin its toughness and elasticity.

The *subcutaneous layer* contains the deep fat cells (areolar and adipose tissue) and provides the heat regulation factor for the body. It is also the support structure for the outer layers of the skin (Ross & Wilson 1998).

The skin will go through many changes in the course of development, e.g. temperature, texture, elasticity, and has a great ability to adapt to changes in the environment and stimuli. Its integrity, continuity and cleanliness are essential to maintain its physiological functions.

In elderly people the skin structure becomes thinner and the growth of epidermal and dermal cells slows down. This results in the skin becoming drier and increasingly brittle, thus leading to an increased risk of tissue breakdown (see Ch. 47, Wound management). The skin will also become more permeable to infection (Armstrong-Esther 1981), so extra care and vigilance should be taken when washing and drying elderly patients.

An initial assessment using observational skills is essential to ascertain the skin's general condition. Several factors may influence the appearance of the tissue:

- Hydration state – dehydration will cause loss of elasticity and drying of the skin. Oedema will cause stretching and thinning of the skin.
- The individual's age, health and mobility status (Gooch 1989), e.g. presence of pressure ulcers (see Ch. 47, Wound management).
- Treatment therapies, e.g. radiotherapy (skin may become moist and cracked), chemotherapy (some cytotoxic agents such as methotrexate can cause erythematous rashes), and continuous infusions of 5-fluorouracil (5-FU) can cause a condition called palmar–plantar erythrodysesthesia syndrome which presents with cracking and epidermal sloughing of the palms and soles (Lokich & Moore 1984). A low platelet count can lead to an increased risk of bruising and a decrease in the white blood cells can influence the rate of healing. Steroids may cause the skin to become papery and fragile. (See Ch. 34, Radioactive source therapy: sealed sources, and Ch. 47, Wound management.)
- Any concurrent skin conditions, e.g. eczema, psoriasis.

Frailty and the presence of pressure ulcers, redness, abrasions, cuts, papery skin and open wounds should prompt the nurse to take extra care in the bathing procedure. Involving patients in their care plans ensures that correct and/or preferred lotions are used. For example, some people prefer not to apply soap to the facial area and others will need to use a particular soap which does not contain perfumes. Persistent use of some soaps can alter the pH of the skin, leading to drying and cracking (Gooch 1989). In addition, patients may like to use moisturizers and this should be respected and applied accordingly. Care should be taken with skin folds and crevices, paying particular attention to thorough drying of the areas and observing for any breaks in the skin.

Frequently, patients may have intravenous devices and wound drains inserted as part of their therapy and these should be handled with caution to prevent the hazards of introducing infection or of 'pulling' the tubes.

Patients who require assistance may be able to have a bath or shower depending on their level of dependence. Alternatively, assistance with care may occur by the bedside or in bed as 'bed bathing'. When practising bed bathing the nurse informs the patient of his/her plan of care, seeking consent from the patient or patient's family/carer, especially if hoists, slides or transfers sheets are to be used. The nurse must also respect cultural and religious factors, privacy and dignity at all times, e.g. some people prefer to sit under running water as opposed to sitting in a bath (Sampson 1982).

Perineal/perianal care

When the nurse is performing care for the perineal/perianal area, the patient may experience emotions such as embarrassment or humiliation. Care should be taken to maintain privacy at all times, especially with regard to cultural beliefs.

It is important to be meticulous with this area, especially for those people who may be prone to infection (see Ch. 16, Elimination: urinary catheterization).

Problems arising from treatment therapy, for example radiotherapy, fistulae, diarrhoea, constipation and urinary tract infections, require additional vigilance with cleanliness and patients should be encouraged at every opportunity to perform this themselves (see Ch. 34, Radioactive source therapy: sealed sources; Haisfield Wolfe 1998).

Ideally, perineal hygiene should be attended to after the general bath or, at the very least, the water and wipes should be changed and clean once utilized (Gooch 1989; Gould 1994) due to the large colonies of bacteria that tend to live in or around this area (Gould 1994). It is generally acknowledged that soap and lotions administered improperly to the perineum/perianal area can cause irritation and infection (Heidrick *et al.* 1984; Ravnskov 1984; Charmorro 1990). Many nurses will use soap or a similar chemical derivative in order to promote and ensure thorough cleaning, but frequently lack of knowledge can lead to further problems and discomfort for the patients (Lindell & Olsson 1989). It is suggested that warm water alone be used to avoid irritating the mucous membranes which become sensitive during the ageing process.

Hair care

The way a person feels is often related to their appearance. Hair care can be complex – consideration should be given to the patient's personal preferences.

Washing of the hair can be difficult if a patient is bedbound, but there are several ways to manage this. To wash a patient's hair, move the patient to the top of the bed and hang their head over the end. (For an illustration of this procedure see Baker *et al.* 1999.) The patient's condition must be assessed before performing this task; for example, it would not be appropriate for patients with head and neck or spinal injuries. Shampooing frequency depends on the patient's well-being and his/her hair condition. Referral to a hairdresser may also be appropriate.

Grooming the hair provides an ideal opportunity to observe for dandruff, psoriasis, flaky skin and head lice. Head lice are extremely infectious so it is imperative to treat the hair with a medicated shampoo from the pharmacy as soon as possible. Hospital policy/protocol should be followed regarding the disposal of infected linen. Towel drying of hair should occur. Hairdryers can be used with the consent of the patient. Hairdryers should be checked for safety by the hospital electrician.

A patient's cultural and religious beliefs should always be taken into consideration when attending to hair. Some religions do not allow hair washing or brushing, while others may require the hair to be covered by a turban. Similarly, in some countries facial hair is significant and should never be removed without the patient's/relatives' consent. Always establish any preferences before beginning care.

In the oncology setting chemotherapy is an established treatment and some cytotoxic drugs can cause alopecia (loss of hair). The patient's physical, psychological and social needs are affected by the loss of hair. Special care and skilled advice are required regarding the adjustment to hair loss. Referral to the hospital surgical appliance officer is appropriate to discuss the choice and fitting of a wig. A shampoo with a neutral pH is recommended for patients who are at risk of alopecia. Prevention of alopecia is discussed further in Ch. 38, Scalp cooling.

Care of the beard and moustache is also important. Excess food can often become lodged here so regular grooming is essential for hygiene and comfort purposes. Beard trimmers can be used as appropriate.

Care of the nails and feet

The feet and nails require special care in order to avoid pain and infection occurring. Nails should be trimmed correctly. Specialist advice from a chiropodist can be useful. Chronic diseases such as diabetes and the long-term use of steroids can result in problems such as pressure ulcers, breakdown of the skin integrity and delays in the healing process. Special attention should be paid to cleaning the feet and in between the toes to avoid any fungal infection. Powders and creams are available that help with the treatment of infections and odour management.

Care of the ears and nose

Lack of attention to cleaning the ears and nose can lead to impairment of the senses. Usually these small organs require minimal care, but observation for a buildup of wax in the ears and deposits in the nose is essential to maintain patency.

Special care should be taken to avoid damage to the aural cavity or ear drum. Clean area with cotton wool or gauze and warm water. Towel dry.

Patients undergoing enteral feeding and oxygen therapy should have regular nasal care to avoid excessive drying and excoriating of the delicate air passages. Gentle cleaning of the nasal mucosa with wool/gauze and water is recommended and application of a thin coating of a water-based lubricant to prevent discomfort can be beneficial. Patients who have had piercing of the ears or nose will require cleaning of the holes to avoid the risk of infection. Gently cleaning around the piercing area. Cotton wool/gauze and warm water should be used. Towel dry area. Observe for inflammation or oozing. If this occurs, inform the patient and doctor. Remove device on consent of the patient if inflammation or oozing occurs.

Eye care

Specific aspects of eye care, e.g. irrigation, are referred to in Ch. 31, Personal hygiene: eye care.

In general, the eye structure and delicate surface are protected by the tears that maintain the eye's moistness, but in a patient who is unconscious, drying of the eye may occur (Ross & Wilson 1998). Gentle cleaning with low-linting gauze and 0.9% sodium chloride will be sufficient to prevent infection and will keep the eyes moist. The eye is an important organ of communication and consideration should always be given to a patient's sight aids, e.g. glasses, contact lenses. Assistance may be required to help clean these aids and advice regarding the most appropriate method should be sought, preferably from the patient.

Some patients may have an artificial eye and care should be taken to ensure this remains clean. Advice regarding the ideal method of removal and insertion should be sought.

Mouth care

Mouth care, e.g. cleaning and infection control, is referred to in Ch. 32, Personal hygiene: mouth care.

Summary

Personal hygiene of patients is an integral part of the role of the nurse, creating a bond with the patient. In doing this, the nurse is able to spend time with his/her patient listening to issues, concerns or fears the patient may have regarding admission, treatment, discharge planning or prognosis. This may decrease patient barriers, building a therapeutic relationship.

The patient is an individual who will depend on others to assist them in times of ill health; however, considerable thought should be given to individual preferences.

Comfort, cleanliness, availability of washing facilities, privacy and assistance from nurses were expressed as being important in providing hygiene care by patients in a recent ward audit (unpublished) at The Royal Marsden Hospital.

The world of nursing, though, is ever changing, and there is a risk that activities such as attending to the personal hygiene of patients may become devalued or just another routine. Personal hygiene is considered part of the essence of care which nurses should never treat as ritualistic.

It is clearly evident from the lack of research that more work is required in this area to improve and raise standards of patient care.

Procedure guidelines: **Bed bathing a patient**

Procedure

Prior to each part of the procedure, explain and obtain agreement from the patient. The procedure can allow time and opportunity for communication between the nurse and the patient. Planned care is negotiated with the patient and is based on assessment of their individual needs. Planned care should be documented and changed according to the patient's/carer's needs on a daily basis. Before commencing this procedure, read the patient's care plan, manual handling documentation and risk assessment to gain knowledge of safe practice.

Action	Rationale
1 Assess patient's needs, addressing religious and cultural beliefs.	To plan care.
2 Plan care with the patient and family/friend if desired. Note personal preferences, including hair-washing requirements.	To encourage participation and independence. To ensure patient comfort during procedure.
3 Offer patient urinal, bedpan or commode.	To reduce any disruption to procedure and prevent any discomfort.
4 Collect all equipment by bedside: • Clean bed linen. • Bath towels. • Laundry skip, applying local guidelines for soiled and/or infected linen. • Flannels, preferably disposable. • Toiletries, as preferred by patient. • Clean clothes as desired. • Wash bowl and warm water; ensure bowl is cleaned with hot soapy water before use.	To minimize time away from patient during procedure. Disposable flannels are preferable as this reduces the risk of infection. To meet patient preference during procedure.
5 Ensure area around bed is private and draught free.	To maintain safe environment and promote privacy and dignity.
6 Wash hands; use disposable gloves and aprons according to local guidelines.	To minimize risk of cross-infection.
7 Assist patient with removal of clothing, cover patient with bath towel or fleece and fold back bedclothes.	To maintain privacy and dignity and body temperature.
8 Ask patient whether they use soap on the face, wash, rinse and dry face, neck and ears.	To promote cleanliness and independence.
9 Wash, rinse and dry top half of body, starting with the side furthest away from you. Care needs to be taken not to wet drains/dressings and IV devices. Apply toiletries as required.	To promote patient well-being and cleanliness and reduce the risk of cross-infection.
10 Change the water, put on your disposable gloves. Inform the patient that you are going to wash around	To reduce risk of infection and to maintain a safe environment.

*Procedure guidelines: **Bed bathing a patient** (cont'd)*

Action	Rationale
the genitalia, gain verbal consent from the patient or ask the patient if they wish to wash this area themselves. Using a separate flannel or wipe, wash around the area, then dry the area. Remove gloves, dispose as per hospital policy. If there is an indwelling catheter, put on your gloves and wash the tubing away from the genitalia area, dry tubing and remove gloves as per hospital policy. (Patients may prefer to do this themselves.) When washing this area, remember female patients wash from the front to back. Male patients should draw back the foreskin if uncircumcised when washing the penis.	
11 Assist male patients with facial shaving as desired.	To promote positive body image.
12 Change water and gloves, ensuring patient has nurse call bell within reach.	To maintain cleanliness, preserving dignity and privacy.
13 Wash, rinse and dry legs, starting with the side furthest away from you. Assess the need for possible chiropody referral. Wash back, then using disposable flannel wash sacral area, observing pressure areas. Cover areas that are not being washed.	To prevent and treat pressure ulcers, ensuring appropriate referrals are made.
14 Replace clothes and change bottom sheet whilst patient is being turned, if they are to remain in bed. Ensure a minimum of two nurses are present during procedure.	To reduce unnecessary activity for patient and nurse. To maintain safety of patient and safe manual handling, following risk assessment.
15 Provide appropriate equipment and assist patient, if required, to brush teeth and/or rinse mouth.	To maintain good oral hygiene.
16 Dry and comb patient's hair as desired.	To enhance patient comfort. To promote positive body image.
17 Remake top bedclothes.	
18 Help patient to sit or lie in desired position.	To enhance patient comfort and reduce risk of pressure ulcers.
19 Remove equipment from bedside; replace patient's possessions in their appropriate place. Place locker, bedside table and call bell within reach.	To maintain a safe environment and promote patient independence.
20 Remove apron and gloves and dispose of them according to local rules.	To prevent cross-infection.
21 Wash hands.	
22 Document any changes in planned care.	To provide recorded documentation of care and aid in communication to the multiprofessional team.

References and further reading

Armstrong-Esther, C.A. (1981) Skin introduction. *Nursing*, Series 1, 1115.

Baker, F., Smith, I. & Stead, I. (1999) Practical procedures for nurses: no. 22.1. *Nurs Times Suppl*, **95**(5), 3–9.

Campbell, A. (1984) Nursing, nurturing and sexism. In: *Moderated Love: A Theology of Professional Care*. SPCK, London.

Charmorro, T. (1990) Cancer of the vulva and vagina. *Semin Oncol Nurs*, **6**(3), 198–205.

DoH (2001) *Essence of Care*. Stationery Office, London.

Gooch, J. (1989) Skin hygiene. *Prof Nurse*, October, 13–17.

Gould, D. (1994) Helping the patient with personal hygiene. *Nurs Stand*, **8**(34), 30–32.

Haisfield Wolfe, M.E. (1998) Providing effective perineal–rectal skin care to patients with cancer. *Oncol Nurs Forum*, **25**(3), 472.

Hector, L.M. & Touhy, T.A. (1997) The history of the bath: from art to task? Reflections for the future. *J Gerontol Nurs*, **23**(5), 7–15.

Heidrick, F.E., Beurg, A.O. & Bergman, J. (1984) Clothing factors and vaginitis. *J Family Pract*, **19**(4), 491–4.

Henderson, V. (1966) *The Nature of Nursing*. Collier Macmillan, London.

Kitson, A. (1999) The essence of nursing. *Nurs Stand*, **13**(23), 42–6.

Lindell, M. & Olsson, H. (1989) Lack of care givers' knowledge causes unnecessary suffering in elderly patients. *J Adv Nurs*, **14**, 976–9.

Lokich, J.J. & Moore, C. (1984) Chemotherapy associated palmar plantar erythrodysesthesia syndrome. *Ann Intern Med*, **101**, 798–800.

Neuberger, J. (1987) *Caring for Dying People of Different Faiths*, 2nd edn. Mosby, London, p. 26.

Nightingale, F. (1969) *Notes on Nursing*. Dover Publications, New York.

Orem, D. (1980) *Nursing – Concepts of Practice*, 2nd edn. McGraw Hill, New York.

Ravnskov, U. (1984) Soap is the major cause of dysuria. *Lancet*, **5**, 1027.

Roper, N. *et al.* (1981) *Learning to Use the Process of Nursing*. Churchill Livingstone, Edinburgh.

Ross, J. & Wilson, K. (1998) *Foundations of Anatomy and Physiology*. Churchill Livingstone, Edinburgh.

Sampson, C. (1982) *The Neglected Ethic; Religious and Cultural Factors in the Care of Patients*. McGraw-Hill, London, p. 36.

Spiller, J. (1992) For whose sake – patient or nurse? *Prof Nurse*, April, 431–4.

Wagnild, G. & Manning, R.W. (1985) Convey respect during bathing procedures. *J Gerontol Nurse*, **11**(12), 6.

Wilson, M. (1986) Personal cleanliness. *Nursing*, **3**(2), 80–2.

Young, L. (1991) The clean fight. *Nurs Stand*, **5**(35), 54–5.

34

Radioactive source therapy: sealed sources

Chapter contents

Sealed radioactive source therapy

Definition

Sealed radioactive sources are usually powders or solids enclosed in a casing which is inserted into the patient. Generally, there is little risk of spreading radioactive contamination from these sources, unless the casing is cracked during sterilization. Radioactive iridium-198 is a solid metal which may be made into alloy wires and used for direct insertion into tissues or cavities. Although not sealed in a metal casing, the methods applied to the use of sealed sources are also applied to this substance. The principles of radiation protection – distance, time and shielding, which minimize personal exposure to radiation – must be applied when working with sealed sources to ensure that all unnecessary exposure is avoided (Morris 2001).

Indications

Permanent or temporary insertions of small, sealed sources are used to deliver very high doses of radiation into tumours or tumour-bearing tissue while giving rapidly diminishing doses to adjacent structures. This will limit the damage caused to normal tissue (Harrison 1997). A specific dose of radiation will be received by the cancer. This is delivered continuously over a period of minutes, hours or days.

Reference material

Measures of radiation

Ionizing radiation is the term used to describe energetic particles (e.g. alpha, beta) or electromagnetic waves with a wavelength of no more than 100 nanometres because they are capable of producing ions by ejecting electrons from their atoms (DoH 2000).

Radiation kills by causing ionization within living cells. The activity of radioisotopes was at one time measured in millicuries (mc), but the standard unit is now the becquerel (Bq). A becquerel is the Système International (SI) unit of activity and is 1 disintegration per second.

$$k \text{ (kilo)} = 1 \times 10^3$$
$$M \text{ (mega)} = 1 \times 10^6, \text{ e.g. megabecquerel (MBq)}$$
$$G \text{ (giga)} = 1 \times 10^9$$

The half-life of a radioactive substance is the time taken for it to decay to half its original number of radioactive atoms. The sensitive target appears to be deoxyribonucleic acid (DNA) in the nucleus of the cell. The ionizing radiation thus passes through the cells and tissues, and the dose of radiation received is measured in terms of energy absorbed. The unit of absorbed dose is the gray:

$$100 \text{ centigray (cGy)} = 1 \text{ gray (Gy)}$$

For the purposes of radiation protection of staff and patients, the dose to the whole body must be known. Whereas the absorbed dose is measured in gray, the dose to the whole body is measured in sieverts. For instance, for staff over 18 who are not pregnant, wearing a monitoring badge to monitor exposure to radiation, the annual dose limit is 20 millisieverts, but doses allowed to staff should be kept below 6 millisieverts where practicable (DoH 1999).

Ionizing radiation regulations

The use of ionizing radiation is governed by strict regulations. The Ionising Radiations Regulations 1999 place duties on employers and employees to ensure the safe use of ionizing radiations in the workplace (DoH 1999). The Ionising Radiation (Medical Exposure) Regulations 2000 lay down basic measures for the health protection of individuals undergoing medical exposures. These regulations require medical exposures to ionizing radiations to be justified and authorized and the doses received by the individuals must be kept as low as reasonably practicable (ALARP) and within recommended limits (DoH 2000). The Medicines (Administration of Radioactive Substances) Regulations 1978 impose duties on those responsible for administering radioactive substances. A patient may receive a radioactive substance provided the patient's medical consultant has obtained a certificate from the Department of Health to enable them to administer that substance (DoH 1978).

To help ensure compliance with the regulations the following must be in place.

- The area in which work with ionizing radiation is undertaken must be designated as a controlled area if special procedures are required to restrict significant exposures (i.e. 6 mSv per year) or to reduce the probability and magnitude of radiation accidents occurring. The area may otherwise need to be designated as a supervised area if a person may be exposed to more than 1 mSv per year.
- Local rules must be written for each controlled or supervised area.
- Staff monitoring must be performed in controlled areas.
- A Radiation Protection Adviser must be appointed to provide advice on all aspects of radiation protection.
- Radiation Protection Supervisors must be appointed for all controlled areas to ensure that the local rules for their area are being followed.
- Protocols and procedures must be written for all medical exposures to ionizing radiation.
- Practitioners (persons who justify and authorize the medical exposure) and operators (persons who undertake any practical aspect of the medical exposure) must be appointed and they must comply with the written protocols and procedures.
- Referrers (persons who refer patients for examination or treatment) must be identified.
- Staff training must be provided. This must include adequate theoretical knowledge and practical experience to ensure both their own and the patients' safety.
- Patients must be given adequate information so that they may give informed consent for therapy exposures to ionizing radiation.
- Patients must receive adequate instructions to ensure they fully understand the restrictions associated with their treatment.
- Visitors must receive adequate information to ensure they understand the restrictions and the risks associated with their potential exposure to ionizing radiation from the radioactive substances administered to patients.
- A quality assurance programme must be established to ensure that the policies, procedures and protocols are being performed satisfactorily and comply with agreed standards.
- A quality control clinical audit must be undertaken to ensure the quality assurance programme is followed.

Patient assessment

All patients who have been referred for treatment with radioactive sources must be assessed by the interdisciplinary staff associated with their treatment to ensure the treatment being planned will be successful (see 'Preparation of the patient' below). This assessment should establish that the patient can understand and is able to follow the restrictions imposed by the treatment.

Difficulties understanding the spoken word, being deaf or hard of hearing, being partial or totally sightless, having problems feeding or walking, being incontinent or being in need or in receipt of psychological or psychiatric support, will all require extra time being spent with the patient. Patients with these difficulties will need to be assessed to ensure they are suitable for sealed radioactive source therapy, as it is essential that the radiation restrictions necessary for these treatments will not cause the patients any physical or psychological problems (Montgomery *et al.* 1997). The assessment would normally be initially undertaken in the outpatient department and then on admission to the ward. If potential problems are indicated during the assessment, the doctor responsible for the patient should be informed and the nursing and physics staff involved with the treatment should be asked for help and advice.

Use of contamination monitor

Waste and equipment must be monitored before being removed from controlled areas where patients have received or are receiving therapy using interstitial or intracavitary sealed sources. This monitoring will establish that sources, which might have been dislodged from the patient, are not present amongst the items being removed. Before using a contamination monitor it is important to check that the monitor batteries are fully charged. The background reading on the monitor must then be noted before undertaking the monitoring. The background must be reasonably low (normally less than 10 counts per second), otherwise it will be difficult to detect small levels of radioactivity present on the item being monitored. If the background reading immediately outside the treatment room is found to be high it will be necessary to monitor the items further away where the background is lower. Items should be monitored by passing the monitor's probe over each item, while watching for fluctuations in the count rate. If an item is found to be contaminated (indicated by a sustained increase in count rate), it should either be returned to a safe location in the treatment room or set aside in a designated area while help is sought from the patient's doctor and from the physics department.

Incident procedure

If an accident or incident has occurred or if one is suspected, the immediate priority is to ensure the safety of patients, staff and visitors and take whatever action is practicable to prevent further damage or injury (see Procedure guidelines: Care of patients with insertions of sealed radioactive sources). As soon as immediate care has been provided, all accidents, untoward incidents and near misses, irrespective of severity, must be reported on an incident report form. Proactive and reactive risk management processes are important. These processes should identify areas of potentially higher risk or allow lessons to be learnt from past incidents and accidents. This will allow the implementation of appropriate action plans to reduce the probability and/or severity of an incident occurring or recurring.

Radioactive isotopes used as sealed sources

Most radioactive isotopes used as sealed sources for brachytherapy emit both beta (β) and gamma (γ) radiation. Brachytherapy is where there is a very short distance between the radiation source and the tumour. It is either intracavitary, where radioisotope sources are placed in pre-existing body cavities, such as the uterine cavity or vagina, or interstitial, where radioisotope sources are inserted directly into the tissues in tubes or needles (Blake *et al.* 1998).

The radiation useful in treating malignant disease includes X-rays, produced artificially by electron bombardment of a metal target, and gamma rays, a natural emission in the nuclear decay of radioisotopes. They are sometimes referred to as 'photon' radiation. Beta particles are also capable of ionization; these are distinguishable from electromagnetic radiation by their characteristic of carrying a negative electrical charge. Beta particles result when a neutron within the nucleus disintegrates to form a proton and an electron. The electron is ejected from the nucleus, producing beta radiation (IPEM/RCN 2002).

Caesium-137

Caesium-137 is a radioisotope that can be used in the form of interstitial implants or in intracavitary applicators. It has a half-life of 30 years and has largely replaced radium as a source of brachytherapy.

Oral implants

Caesium-137 can be used in a needle-like implant that is inserted directly into the tissue surrounding the tumour. This is a fairly common treatment for early lesions of the cheek, lip and anterior two-thirds of the tongue. If bone involvement is suspected, e.g. in the mandible, alternative external treatment will be given.

The sources (Fig. 34.1) are inserted in theatre under a general anaesthetic. They are inserted individually in a predetermined pattern so that the implant covers the whole growth, with a safety margin of at least 1 cm. Each needle is positioned by pushers so that its eye, through which silk is threaded, is just visible beneath the mucosal surface. Each silk is then stitched to the tongue with a single suture. When all the needles have

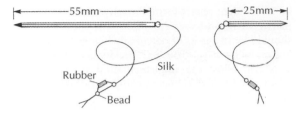

Figure 34.1 Caesium-137 needles.

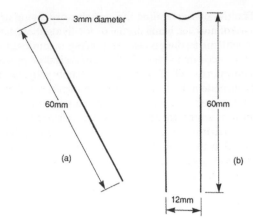

Figure 34.2 Iridium-192 pins. (a) Iridium single pin. (b) Iridium hair pin.

been inserted, the silks are counted and gathered together. They are threaded through a piece of rubber to prevent friction and trauma to the mouth. The silks are strapped to the cheek to prevent any needle being swallowed should it work loose. Small beads are attached to the ends of the threads to facilitate counting the needles. X-rays are always taken to check the positions of the needles and to enable estimation of the dose distribution.

Gynaecological applicators

Caesium-137 can be used in applicators. The most common malignancies treated by the use of radioactive applicators are tumours of the female genital tract. Intracavitary applicators are used which deliver a high dose to the region of the cervix, the paracervical tissue, the upper part of the vagina and the uterine body.

Iridium-192

Iridium-192 is a radioisotope which can be used in the form of pins or wires in interstitial therapy (Krull *et al.* 1999). Its half-life is 74.2 days. Iridium-192 is used because of the low energy of its gamma emission compared to caesium, which simplifies radiation protection, and because in the form of a platinum–iridium alloy it can be drawn into thin flexible wires. The wires consist of an active platinum–iridium alloy core encased in a sheath of platinum 10 μm thick, which screens out the beta radiation from the iridium-192.

Iridium-192 can now be made with a very high specific activity, that is, in a very radioactive form. High activity sources of iridium are used in high dose-rate remote afterloading systems, which reduce the amount of radiation to which clinical oncologists and other staff are exposed.

Iridium-192 implants are used under the following circumstances:

- As a treatment for small primary lesions, for example, tongue or breast lesions.
- As a 'boost' dose after external radiotherapy for larger primary tumours or where nodes are also involved.
- To treat recurrence (Shasha *et al.* 1998; Smith *et al.* 2000).

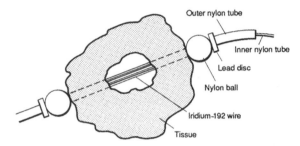

Figure 34.3 Iridium-192 wire in polythene cannula. Typical assembly in tissue.

Iridium-192 hair pin and single pin types of implants are usually used intraorally (Fig. 34.2). They are slotted into tissue using steel guides to obtain accurate alignment. Radiological examination is used to check the position of the guides before the iridium is inserted. The pins are held in place by sutures.

The staff of the physics department are normally responsible for calculating how long a radioactive implant is to stay in place. This is usually about 6 days, depending on the size of the tumour. Removal is carried out in theatre by the clinical oncologist.

Iridium-192 wires are usually used for head and neck, breast or lesions of vulva or perineum (Fig. 34.3). Polythene or metal cannulae are inserted under a general anaesthetic. In the case of breast lesions, both ends of each tube protrude through the skin. Correct alignment is established often with the aid of a Perspex template which fits over the breast and holds the metal cannulae in the correct alignment. In the case of vulval or perineal insertions, only one end of the tube protrudes. For these, alignment of the sources may be achieved by using a Perspex template and vaginal obturator.

The iridium wire source is afterloaded, usually on the ward, and the wires are held in the cannulae with crimped lead washers (see Fig. 34.3). The tiny size of the high activity iridium-198 source in high dose rate machines may allow some interstitial brachytherapy to be given as a few treatments of several minutes each, in contrast to the single treatment of many hours' duration which is necessary with low-activity iridium wire (Hath 1993).

The clinical oncologist is responsible for calculating how long a radioactive implant should stay in place. This is usually for 3–6 days, depending on the size of the tumour. Removal of the implant is usually carried out on the ward.

Interstitial perineal template

Iridium-192 interstitial brachytherapy can be used to treat locally advanced or recurrent tumours (Nag *et al.* 1997; Gupta *et al.* 1999).

Interstitial brachytherapy is a suitable alternative to standard intracavitary brachytherapy where the patient is considered unsuitable because the dose distribution may be suboptimal (Nag *et al.* 1998). Side-effects expected are similar to those from afterloading techniques and are considered to be dose related (Charra *et al.* 1998; Gupta *et al.* 1999). Late side-effects such as fistulae and bowel complications requiring surgery have been documented in some patients.

In a study to evaluate the long-term efficacy and safety of transperineal interstitial implant for advanced pelvic malignancy (Hughes-Davies *et al.* 1995), it was found that this treatment offered a modest chance of cure for women with advanced pelvic malignancy. However, it causes significant late morbidity, with major bowel complications found in 17% of patients without locally recurrent disease.

The device itself consists of two acrylic cylinders and an acrylic template with an array of holes that serve as guides for trocars and a cover plate (Fig. 34.4). The cylinders are usually placed in the vagina but can also be used in the rectum for rectal tumours. They are then fastened to the template, so that a fixed geometric relationship among the tumour volume and normal structures, i.e. bladder and rectum, is produced. This ensures that the source placement is preserved throughout the course of the implantation (Martinez *et al.* 1985). The iridium wire is then manually afterloaded and held in place with a crimped washer to prevent movement of the source during treatment (see Fig. 34.3).

Nursing care is similar to the care that patients receive for intracavitary brachytherapy (see Guidelines).

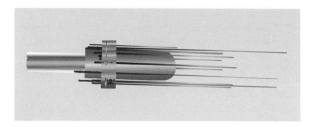

Figure 34.4 Interstitial perineal template device.

Iodine-125

Seeds of iodine-125 have replaced those of gold-198 which was used for many years after the withdrawl of radon seeds on the grounds of safety. The half-life of iodine-125 is 60 days. Some therapists believe that there is a radiobiological advantage to this long half-life in treating slowly growing tumours such as carcinoma of the prostate (Blank *et al.* 2000).

Seeds are inserted into the tissue that is to be irradiated under ultrasound or image intensifier control. The patient requires a general anaesthetic for the insertion.

Because the energy of the gamma-ray emission from iodine-125 is very low compared with that from gold-198, large numbers of seeds are required, which means that more precautions must be taken in order to achieve a regular geometrical arrangement to ensure satisfactory distribution of the dose.

Application of sources

Small sealed sources inserted into the body may take the form of:

- *Intracavitary applicators*, i.e. sources that are placed in natural cavities and usually held in place by packing.
- *Interstitial implants*, i.e. sources that are inserted directly into the tumour-bearing tissue.

(*Note*: sources held in plastic surface applicators or moulds are applied directly to superficial cancers.)

Intracavitary applicators and interstitial implants can be used in three forms:

- The source is preloaded in the applicator before it is placed in the patient for a fixed length of time, e.g. caesium-137 needles and iridium-192 hair pins.
- Permanent insertion in the case of iodine-125 seeds, which, once inserted, would be difficult to remove.
- Afterloading systems – where the applicator is placed in position and the radioactive source is inserted when the position of the applicator and the condition of the patient are satisfactory. Insertion of the sealed source can be undertaken manually in the case of

iridium-192 wires or by remote control as in the case of the low dose rate Selectron machine and the high dose rate microSelectron machine.

Afterloading techniques have the advantage of allowing the source carrier to be accurately positioned (Teruya *et al.* 2002), and for the sources to be withdrawn to a radiation-proof safe during patient care, sparing staff from radiation exposure.

The proportions of radioisotope (initially radium and latterly caesium) within the intrauterine tube and the vaginal ovoids were calculated to give a constant dose rate to a geometrical point A when using different lengths of intrauterine tube and different sizes of vaginal ovoids. This constancy of dose rate when using applicators of different sizes is an important aspect of the Manchester system.

Active sources

The radioisotope initially used for intracavitary brachytherapy was radium. Radium has been replaced by caesium, but the hazards of handling active sources have largely led to the development of afterloading techniques minimizing source handling and staff exposure.

Afterloading brachytherapy

The basis of afterloading brachytherapy is that applicators are placed within the cervix and vaginal fornices, and that the radioisotope is only introduced into these when the applicators are correctly positioned, check radiographs have been taken and the patient is comfortable and in a protected environment. The sources may then be inserted either manually or by remote control. Manual methods are common and have the advantage of being cheap, but do not entirely protect staff as the sources have to be inserted by staff and cannot be removed for short periods while a patient's needs are attended to. Remote systems have the advantage of complete protection of staff, but have the disadvantage of high cost and the need for interlocking mechanisms. These ensure that the correct source has been inserted into the correct applicator for the programmed length of time.

Remote afterloading systems allow the dose rate of brachytherapy to be increased. Classically, the dose rate with the Manchester system was approximately 50 cGy/hour to point A. With modern engineering methods, caesium pellets can be produced which will allow a dose rate of between 150 and 200 cGy/hour to point A. Many systems now use sources that allow a higher than standard dose rate to be delivered. This has the advantage of reducing treatment time (Kuipers *et al.* 2001).

If the concept of increasing dose rate is taken further, high dose rate brachytherapy, delivering doses at rates in excess of 1 Gy/minute to point A, offers the possibility of very short treatment times. This allows complete geometrical stability of the applicator during the treatment and makes a higher patient throughput possible. However, there is considerably less time for repair of radiation damage to normal tissues in a high dose rate treatment and, therefore, such treatments have to be fractionated over several days, in contrast to the continuous treatment given by a low dose rate brachytherapy implant. High-dose brachytherapy produces survival rates comparable to low-dose brachytherapy (Lorvidhaya *et al.* 2000), although complications can occur (Wang *et al.* 1997).

Intracavitary applicators

Intracavitary applicators are inserted under a general anaesthetic, and the position of the applicator is checked by X-ray before the patient returns to the ward. A urinary catheter is also inserted in theatre to reduce the risk of the sources becoming dislodged by the patient when micturating.

Several different types of applicator are available and choice is usually determined by the site of the tumour, the anatomy of the patient and the preference of the treatment centre. The most commonly used types of applicator are described below (also see Fig. 34.5).

Manchester applicator

Manchester applicators in their original form were live sources enclosed in intrauterine tubes of varying lengths and vaginal applicators (ovoids) of varying sizes. The applicators were inserted under general anaesthetic and held in place by a gauze pack. More recently, the applicators have been modified for either manual or remote afterloading at either low or high dose rate, but the principle of the three applicator system remains. Removal of the applicators or, if still used, the live sources is carried out on the ward and may require administration of Entonox as analgesia.

Stockholm applicator

This is used for carcinoma of the body of the uterus or cervix. Usually a uterine tube and two vaginal packets are inserted. Occasionally, if the vaginal vault is small, one packet is omitted or replaced by a vaginal tube. The radioactive material is held in place with a proflavine-soaked gauze pack. It is usually left in place for 22 hours. Tubes and packets have strings attached for removal and colour-coded beads indicate which should be removed first (Wang & Lo 1970).

Modified Stockholm applicator

This is used for carcinoma of the body of the uterus and cervix. It consists of a uterine tube and a square box which connect together by a point and a hole. The vagina is

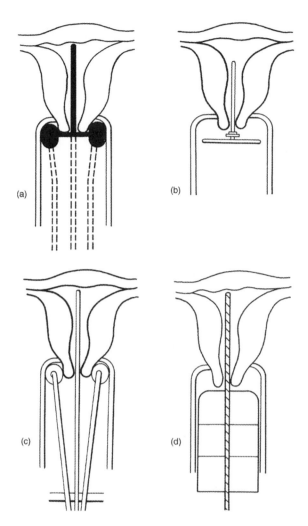

Figure 34.5 Gynaecological caesium applicators. Arrangement of brachytherapy sources in the uterus and vagina for treatment of cervical carcinoma. Sources may be active or, more usually these days, afterloaded into applicators along catheters protruding from the vagina. (a) Manchester applicator. (b) Modified Stockholm applicator. (c) Fletcher applicator. (d) Dobbie applicator.

then packed with gauze saturated with proflavine. They are usually left in place for 20 hours. The box should be removed first.

Fletcher applicator
This is used for carcinoma of the corpus or cervix, but the patient needs to have a fairly capacious vaginal vault. Hollow applicators, a uterine tube and two vaginal ovoids are inserted in theatre and loaded with the radioactive sources later, on the ward, by the radiotherapist. The apparatus is held in place with a proflavine

pack. Long ends project through the vulva so that after-loading can be carried out. These insertions are usually left in place for 60–72 hours. No strings are needed as the apparatus itself projects from the vulva.

Dobbie applicator
This is used to irradiate the whole vagina. A Perspex cylindrical applicator, with radioactive sources in the centre, is inserted into the vagina and sutured in place to the vulva. It may be used with low or high dose rate sources. Strings are attached to the applicator for removal.

Manual afterloading systems
Manual afterloading systems are largely being replaced by remote systems, but they are still used in a few centres and are widely used in developing countries.

The plastic applicator tubes follow the pattern of the Manchester system with an intrauterine tube and two vaginal ovoids. The plastic tubes are designed to be disposed of after a single use. Insertion of the tubes takes place under general anaesthetic, after which confirmatory X-rays are taken with dummy sources in place. As with the classical Manchester system there are varying lengths of intrauterine tube and sizes of ovoids.

If the X-rays are satisfactory and the dosimetry has been calculated, the radioactive caesium sources are introduced on their carrying rods using long-handled forceps. Once in place a silver metal cap is screwed over the end of the plastic tube to hold the sources securely.

Manual afterloading does not permit, for reasons of staff safety, the use of high activity sources and treatment may last many hours or even several days. When treatment is complete the caps are removed from the tubes and the sources are withdrawn and placed immediately in a lead storage vessel. The plastic applicator tubes are then removed.

It is particularly important to observe for displacement or extrusion of the applicator tubes over the long treatment times. It is customary to mark the thigh level with the end of the applicator tubes and to compare this alignment at regular intervals as the treatment progresses. In addition, the silver metal caps should be monitored regularly for any loosening or displacement.

Remote afterloading

Definition

Remote-controlled afterloading machines transfer active sources from a radiation-proof safe to the patient only when it is safe to do so.

Indications

Remote-controlled afterloading machines are gradually replacing conventional intracavitary caesium applicators as well as other manual and mechanical afterloading techniques.

The low dose rate Selectron is used predominantly for the treatment of gynaecological cancers. While the high dose rate microSelectron is also regularly used in the treatment of gynaecological cancers, in some cases it may also be useful in the treatment of bronchial or oesophageal or other intraluminal carcinomas (Sannazzari *et al.* 1998).

Reference material

The low dose rate (LDR) Selectron

The Selectron unit comprises a lead-shielded safe containing caesium-137 sources in the form of small spherical pellets, a microprocessor, keyboard, display unit and printer (Fig. 34.6). Leading from the Selectron unit are either three or six flexible plastic transfer tubes corresponding to numbered treatment channels. Each tube ends in a fragile plastic catheter which is inserted into the appropriately numbered applicator and secured by a coupling device. The unit has a supply of compressed air and it is air pressure that the system uses to transfer the sources from the safe within the unit to the applicators along the connecting tubes. Operation of the unit is initiated from a remote-control unit situated outside the protected treatment area. Together, these components form the basis of the remote-controlled afterloading system (Blake *et al.* 1998).

The Selectron provides an accurate and safe method of radiotherapy treatment for cancers of the cervix, uterus and upper part of the vagina.

The advantages of the Selectron system are threefold:

- Remote afterloading eliminates contact with radioactive material and protects personnel.
- It allows highly accurate dosimetry.
- The activity of the caesium-137 sources is such (up to 1.5 GBq) that treatment times for patients are considerably shorter than with conventional techniques.

Patients have hollow, lightweight stainless steel applicators positioned in the operating theatre under a general anaesthetic. These are usually modified Manchester or Fletcher type applicators consisting of a uterine tube and two vaginal ovoids held in place with a proflavine-soaked vaginal packing. However, several other applicators are available. Accurate positioning of the applicators is confirmed by taking X-rays with

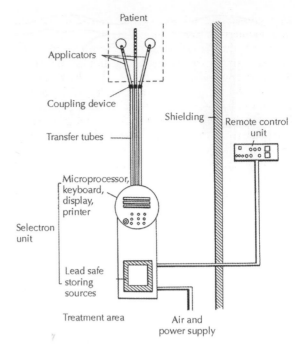

Figure 34.6 Selectron unit.

dummy sources in situ and the optimum source configuration is selected, taking account of individual anatomical variations.

The Selectron is programmed by the physicist. For each treatment channel being used, active source pellets are interspersed with inactive stainless steel spacer pellets to achieve the desired dose distribution. The treatment time required to reach the prescribed dose is also entered. With a six-channel Selectron unit it is possible to treat two patients with three applicators each simultaneously. The radiotherapist is responsible for connecting the transfer tubes to the applicators. The transfer tubes are led over a bed bracket which supports the weight of the tubes and prevents traction being applied to the applicators in the patient. If the wrong catheter is connected to the applicator, the system will fail to operate.

Operating the Selectron

Treatment is commenced by activation of the remote control unit when all staff have left the treatment area. While treatment is in progress it can be interrupted and restarted from the remote control unit by pressing the stop and start buttons. The display panel indicates which channels are being used for treatment and which are unused with red and green lights respectively. The time of the longest treatment is displayed in decimal hours and a telephone intercom system, for example, allows for communication with the patient without the need to interrupt treatment.

Interrupting the treatment by pressing the green stop button results in the sources being withdrawn into the Selectron unit and stops the timer. This allows nursing staff to enter the treatment area in safety and give routine or specific care to the patient. Pressing the red start button transfers the sources back into the applicators and restarts the timer. The red lights demonstrate that the channels are operating again satisfactorily.

The system has built-in safety features. In the event of a failure in the system, treatment stops automatically. An audible and visual alarm at the remote control unit alerts staff to a problem and indicates whether this is a fault related to the air or power supply, the pellets or the timer. There is an optional nurse station display unit with a similar alarm indicator which also emits an audible signal when treatment has been interrupted. This helps to prevent treatment being inadvertently left interrupted for long periods.

A record of any break in treatment is shown on the print-out from the unit itself, together with any programming or system fault. These appear as an error code and can be identified by reference to the Selectron user's manual.

At the end of the treatment time, all sources will be withdrawn automatically from the applicators back into the Selectron unit. When two patients are being treated simultaneously termination of the treatment of one patient may be some time before that of the other. This means the timer will register the longer treatment time, but the indicator lights for the channels used for the first patient will have changed from red to green.

Additional safety features include a door switch facility to retract sources immediately if the door to the treatment area is opened when treatment is in progress, and/or Geiger dose meters visible when entering the treatment area and approaching the patient, which indicate when there are radioactive sources either in the patient or in the connecting tubes.

The high dose rate (HDR) microSelectron

The operating principles of the HDR microSelectron are similar to those of the low dose rate Selectron. Low dose rate Selectron applicators are afterloaded with active sources interspersed with inactive spacers to produce the correct isodose pattern. HDR microSelectron machines, on the other hand, achieve the desired isodose pattern with a single iridium-192 source which moves within the applicators and stops at preset positions for predetermined dwell times.

The HDR microSelectron delivers radiation at approximately 100 times the rate of the LDR Selectron and treatment times are therefore much shorter. It has the added advantage of applicators with a smaller diameter which can be put in place under local anaesthetic in the outpatients' department and is a suitable alternative for patients who may not be able to tolerate the demands of LDR (Stitt 1999).

Once in position, HDR microSelectron intracavitary applicators are fixed to the treatment couch by means of an adjustable clamp (Jones *et al.* 1999). Movement of the applicators is therefore minimal and dosimetry calculations accurately represent actual treatment (Jones *et al.* 1999). In addition, more constant and reproducible geometry of source positioning is possible (Jones *et al.* 1999).

Treatment protocols generally consist of two treatments but can involve as many as five. Following explanation and support for the patient, the procedure is carried out under local anaesthetic (Stitt 1999). For the first treatment a urinary catheter is passed and the balloon inflated with dilute contrast medium. Check radiographs are taken once the applicator tubes are in place to collect information which is fed into the Selectron planning computer and used to calculate the treatment time.

The HDR microSelectron follows the same principles for programming and treatment as the LDR Selectron. When treatment is complete the applicators and catheter are removed and the patient is free to go home. A case report found that patients undergoing treatment with HDR microSelectron for gynaecological cancer found the experience acceptable (Tan *et al.* 1996).

Adequate preparation of the patient is essential. Montgomery *et al.* (1997) suggest that time spent preparing the patient increases tolerance of the implant procedure, and that badly prepared patients may be more anxious and less able to follow instructions. An assessment of patients' physical and emotional needs must be made prior to each treatment to identify whether any aspect of the treatment is problematic.

The advantages of the HDR microSelectron are four-fold:

- The shorter treatment time reduces variations in the patient's position and allows more accurate dosimetry (Jones *et al.* 1999).
- Treatment lasts only minutes, minimizing the need for immobilization and reducing discomfort and the risk of complications associated with bed-rest.
- Treatment can be offered on an outpatient basis with a consequent reduction in cost (Pinilla 1998).
- As an alternative to LDR, which may be more suitable for some patients.

Complications of intracavitary radiotherapy for gynaecological cancers

Radiation-induced early complications of intracavitary treatment are generally mild. They include, during treatment, pain and nausea (Rollison & Strang 1995) and following treatment, radiation-induced fatigue, diarrhoea, urinary frequency, dysuria, vaginal discharge and perineal irritation (Christman et al. 2001). Severe reactions are rare, but may include severe or prolonged proctitis in patients with pre-existing bowel disease, and urgency and freqency of micturition, nocturia and dysuria. Late complications may include bowel and bladder strictures, ulceration and, occasionally, fistula formation. One study found that 38% of patients developed rectal and 11% bladder complications following HDR microSelectron therapy (Wang et al. 1997).

Preparation of patient

Information about radiation therapy should be given to patients and carers when therapy is first discussed to allay fears and misconceptions about radiotherapy. Verbal information should be reinforced with written material to prepare the patient, reduce anxiety and promote coping. A contact name and telephone number are useful for patients who wish to obtain further information at a later date.

Information for gynaecological patients receiving radiotherapy can be divided into three categories: disease and treatment, short- and long-term side-effects and sexuality.

All patients should have a thorough nursing assessment undertaken to assess their suitability for the treatment, both in the outpatients department and on admission to the ward. This will ensure that they are able to comply with the demands of the treatment. Any doubt due to the patient's physical or psychological problems and concerns can then be discussed with the patient and their medical team. This will allow for action to be taken, either to improve the patient's general condition so they are suitable for treatment or to postpone or cancel the radioactive sealed source therapy in favour of a more suitable treatment option (Velji & Fitch 2001).

LDR often follows 5 weeks of external beam radiotherapy of the pelvis (Petereit et al. 1998). This may mean that patients are already experiencing a number of symptoms at the time of the planned sealed source therapy. These may include radiation-induced enteritis, nausea, fatigue and skin reactions. Management of these symptoms may be required before LDR can be considered.

Prior to the procedure, it should be explained to patients that they will require an indwelling catheter and will be connected to the Selectron unit with flexible plastic tubes. Patients should be prepared for the noises made by the Selectron system, especially when sources are being transferred in and out of the applicators. Some patients may find the prospect of treatment alarming (Gosselin & Waring 2001) and may prefer to receive regular sedation for the duration of treatment. Patients' movements will need to be restricted during their treatment and they will be required to lie flat to maintain the pelvis in roughly the same position. This is to ensure that there is no significant movement of the applicators. The patient may be allowed to have a maximum of two pillows to support their head if this improves their comfort during treatment. Where practicable, the patient should be closely monitored during treatment. This can be achieved by the use of CCTV, telephone or intercom access for the patient and nurse, and a nurse call system, all of which provides further reassurance for patients.

Vaginal care following intracavitary treatment

Because the vaginal canal is included in the radiation field, vaginal stenosis, fibrosis, loss of elasticity and lubrication, and a decrease in sensation may develop after treatment if prophylactic measures are not taken (Muscari Lin et al. 1999).

To help prevent changes due to radiation, women who are sexually active should continue to have regular intercourse after any discomfort caused by an acute radiation reaction has resolved. Alternatively, a dilator can be used to keep the vagina open and stretched. Water-soluble lubricants may alleviate the dry mucosa, and hormone therapy, if appropriate, may be given orally or vaginally to increase natural lubrication (Blake et al. 1998).

Women can consider using a dilator once treatment has been completed for 2–6 weeks. Initially, the dilator should be inserted into the vagina daily for 5–10 minutes (removing and reinserting three or four times). A water-soluble lubricant should be used to ensure ease of insertion (Robinson et al. 1999). Following advice from a doctor or nurse specialist, frequency of dilatation can be reduced to between three times and once per week. However, dilatation should continue for life if the patient wishes to maintain vaginal patency (Fraunholz et al. 1998). Dilatation should maintain vaginal patency and allow follow-up vaginal examination and smears to be performed without undue discomfort. It should also help comfortable resumption of intercourse.

Some clinical oncologists additionally recommend douching during radiotherapy and following brachytherapy, continuing for up to 8 weeks, to avoid infections and the formation of adhesions. Douching can be seen as controversial due to a theoretical risk of causing tumour cells to be transported and lodged further away from the site of the original tumour. The decision to use douching should therefore be made in discussion with the patient, her consultant and clinical nurse specialist. Douching should not be carried out, however, if there is a risk of haemorrhage from a persistent tumour (Blake et al. 1998).

Patients are encouraged to douche once a day using a disposable douche and tap water. Douching should continue until symptoms have resolved and advice has been given by a doctor or nurse specialist.

Follow-up care

Remote-controlled afterloading brachytherapy is a safe and effective treatment for cervical cancer, and has the added advantage of eliminating radiation exposure to staff, visitors and other patients (Rogers et al. 1999). However, side-effects can occur (Lorvidhaya et al. 2000), including complications to the bladder (Katz et al. 2001), rectum (Uno et al. 1998; Davis et al. 2000) and vagina (Bergmark et al. 1999) and signs and symptoms associated with menopause in premenopausal women (Muscari Lin et al. 1999). A 20-year evaluation of the long-term survival and safety of interstitial and intracavitary brachytherapy in the treatment of carcinoma of the cervix found a reasonable chance of cure with acceptable morbidity (Syed et al. 2002).

In a study by Cull et al. (1993), women with cervical cancer reported the concerns they had, including the fear of recurrent disease. These women felt that they required more information about cancer, its treatment and how they could help themselves to cope with their illness. The authors suggest that the emotional status of women with cervical cancer could be improved by giving more attention to their psychological concerns. This is supported by a study to evaluate patient disclosure of psychosocial problems, where a 51% disclosure rate was found. These authors suggest that disclosure can be increased by adding one or two questions about mood

and interpersonal problems into more general conversation (Robinson & Roter 1999), and emphasize the need for nurses to assess their patients carefully.

Teruya et al. (2002) found that all patients included in a retrospective review of HDR microSelectron therapy had vaginal mucosal changes, but had no complaints regarding sexual functioning. Cancer treatment can cause persistent changes to the vagina which results in considerable distress by compromising sexual activity (Bergmark et al. 1999); patients need to be reassured that many women regain their capacity for sexual activity and enjoyment. Sexual counselling may improve outcome. Counselling should focus on self-esteem, body image and sexuality (Farrell 2002). Although vaginal dilatation is widely recommended to maintain vaginal health and good sexual functioning, it appears that compliance is poor. However, this can be improved when the patient is given assistance in overcoming her fears and taught how to use the dilator (Robinson et al. 1999).

Male partners of women with cancer reported difficulty in knowing how to behave and how to communicate with their partners (Lalos et al. 1995). Almost all male partners were given the news of the diagnosis exclusively by their ill partner, which provoked feelings of anger and bitterness (Lalos 1997). Coping improved if the men were integrated in the patient's care from the time the diagnosis of cancer was made (Lalos et al. 1995).

Discharge of the patient

Patients are usually discharged on the day of completion of brachytherapy. They must void urine normally following removal of the urinary catheter. Patients are sometimes unsteady on their feet after prolonged bed rest and may require assistance. They should be informed that normal bowel actions may not return for a day or so; advice on managing diarrhoea or constipation should be given. Light spotting or discharge from the vagina is normal. If patients experience pain or any more marked bleeding, hospital staff should be contacted immediately. Symptoms of urinary tract infection such as dysuria and/or elevated temperature should also be reported.

Procedure guidelines: **Care of patients with insertions of sealed radioactive sources**

Action	Rationale
1 Before treatment begins, ensure the room is set up appropriately. This includes placing a lead pot and	To reduce unnecessary time spent in the room once patient returns from theatre.

Procedure guidelines: **Care of patients with insertions of sealed radioactive sources** *(cont'd)*

Action	Rationale
long-handled forceps in the room to hold any dislodged sources.	
2 Switch on controlled arca radiation warning light outside the room and check it is working correctly.	To warn staff, visitors and other patients of the radiation risk and to ensure only trained personnel enter the room.
3 Place radiation warning notice outside patient's room.	To ensure only authorized personnel enter the room.
4 Place lead shields in position at the door. All staff entering the room should work behind the lead shield when in close contact with the patient.	To reduce radiation exposure of staff in close contact with the patient.
5 When transferring patients from theatre to ward, the nurse and porter should remain at the head and foot of the bed and at least 120 cm from the centre of the bed in the event of any delay in the transfer. If the source is intraoral, the nurse should stand at the foot of the bed.	To minimize the risk of exposure to radiation.
6 A yellow radiation hazard board should accompany the patient back from theatre. This must remain at the bottom of the bed or outside the cubicle until the source is removed.	To alert everybody that the patient has a radioactive source.
7 Nursing staff must calculate the time allowed with the patient in any 24-hour period. This time should be written on the yellow warning notice on the bed or cubicle door.	To minimize exposure to radiation.
8 A contamination monitor should be available on the ward.	To monitor radioactivity if a dislodged source is suspected, e.g. in the bed linen.
9 Whilst one nurse should be responsible for planning the nursing care of the patient, the time spent with the patient should be shared between all suitably trained nurses and all time spent in performing nursing procedures must be kept to a minimum. Only those staff whose presence is necessary should spend time with the patient.	To minimize the risk of overexposure to radiation.
10 Every nurse must wear a radiation badge above the level of the lead shield.	To record the extent of exposure to radiation.
11 All bed linen and waste materials removed from the patient area should be monitored before being removed from the ward.	To prevent loss of an accidentally dislodged source.
12 If a source becomes dislodged, use the long-handled forceps to put the source into a lead pot. Care should be taken not to damage the source. It must never be handled directly with the fingers.	To minimize the dose of radiation received.
13 Visitors must seek permission each time they wish to enter the room. Visitors must remain at least 120 cm away from the patient. Visitors must always sit behind one of the bed shields. The visit should not last longer than the time shown on the warning notice. No children or pregnant women are allowed to visit.	To minimize the risk of overexposure to radiation.
14 When the patient needs to visit another department, for example to X-ray, the following must be ensured:	In order that medical care can continue to be provided while the patient is receiving radioactive sealed source therapy.
(a) That the receiving department is aware of the hazard of exposure to radioactivity.	To allow the appointment to be made when the department is quiet, thus ensuring waiting time is kept to a minimum and to minimize exposure to others.

*Procedure guidelines: **Care of patients with insertions of sealed radioactive sources** (cont'd)*

Action	Rationale
(b) One porter and a nurse should accompany the patient in a wheelchair; two porters and a nurse should accompany the patient on a trolley. In the event of any delays, the nurse and porters should remain at the head and foot of the bed and at least 120 cm from the centre of the bed; if the source is intraoral, the nurse should stand at the foot of the bed.	To minimize the risk of exposure of staff to radiation.
(c) A radiation warning hazard sign should accompany the patient.	To warn all staff that the patient has a radioactive source in situ.
(d) Unless the patient is likely to be in the department for a long time the nurse and porter should stay with the patient.	To ensure time distance, shielding and segregation restrictions are maintained.
(e) If the source becomes dislodged during transfer, the porter must ring the switchboard who will send out an emergency call to the physics department. The nurse must ensure the area around the patient is kept clear of other patients, staff and visitors.	To minimize the risk of exposure to radiation.
A member of staff from the ward should take a lead pot, forceps and a monitor to the nurse who will place the source in the lead pot and monitor the area to ensure it is free of radioactivity.	To contain the radioactive source and minimize risk of exposure.
(f) The Radiation Protection Adviser and supervisor should be informed of incident.	To evaluate the incident, and to prevent it recurring.
15 *In the event of a cardiac arrest*, an Ambu bag or similar device must be used, and the physics department must be informed immediately.	To minimize exposure.
16 *In the event of a fire*, the fire policy must be followed. Following evacuation, the appropriate distance between the radioactive patient and other staff should be maintained; help should be sought from the physics department.	To minimize exposure.
17 *In the event of a patient's death* Remove sources:	Remove radioactivity to allow last offices to be undertaken as normal.
(a) The radiation sources should be removed by the radiotherapist. Inform the physics department.	
Non-removable sources:	
(a) When a source cannot be removed, e.g. iodine-125 seeds, inform the physics department immediately.	In order for the physics department staff to begin making the necessary arrangements for removal of the body to the mortuary. Arrangements would include: segregated refrigerator, warning notices and use of body bag to contain seeds if they became dislodged.
(b) The body should be placed in a body bag.	
(c) Transfer of the body should be arranged by the physics department.	The physics staff will supervise the transfer of the body.
18 *In the event of bleeding*, in order to stem bleeding in the vicinity of the implant, apply pressure using at least four thick dressing pads. The padding should only be compressed for 15 minutes by any single person.	To minimize exposure.
19 In the event of a confused or agitated patient, premature removal of sources may be required.	To prevent overexposure to radiation of the nurses attending the patient, as well as to prevent the patient removing or dislodging sources.

Procedure guidelines: **Care of patients with insertions of sealed radioactive sources** *(cont'd)*

Action	Rationale
20 Only staff who have received training and have been authorized may enter a controlled area. A list of suitably trained staff should be kept by the domestic and catering managers and by the ward's local Radiation Protection Supervisor. A domestic or catering supervisor should undertake tasks if the ward-based employee is not trained.	To keep all radiation exposure as low as can be reasonably achievable.
Domestic and catering staff should not remove items such as cleaning equipment and crockery until it has been monitored by a nurse and deemed safe.	To prevent sources being removed from the room before it is safe to do so.

Procedure guidelines: **Care of patients with intraoral sources**

Preparation of patient

Dental assessment of the patient is usually carried out before oral brachytherapy so that caries, mouth infections and dental extractions may be dealt with in case of the oral blood supply being impaired by the treatment. The patient is usually admitted 24 hours before the implant, during which time the nature of the procedure and the implications of having a radioactive source should be explained to the patient. The patient will be nursed in a single controlled room away from other patients to reduce the amount of radiation exposure to other people. Only staff and visitors authorized to enter the controlled area should go into the room. Written arrangements for entering the room should be contained within the local rules and should be displayed at the door of the room.

Action	Rationale
1 Encourage frequent mouth care. The patient should void the solution into a bowl and not into a handbasin.	To reduce the risk of infection. To prevent the loss of a dislodged source.
2 Provide a soft, puréed or liquid diet.	To reduce the risk of the patient biting into the source or tongue. Eating is often difficult when implants are present.
3 Avoid spicy and/or hot foods. Discourage the patient from smoking and/or drinking alcohol.	To prevent exacerbation of local reaction or soreness.
4 Encourage ingestion of carbonated drinks.	To alleviate dryness.
5 Provide crushed ice for the patient to suck and/or soluble aspirin as a mouthwash.	To minimize oral pain and discomfort.
6 Give steroids as prescribed.	To prevent and/or minimize swelling.
7 Provide writing equipment for the patient.	To reduce the need for oral communication. This is liable to increase soreness and alter the distribution of the sources.
8 Provide paper tissues and a bowl for saliva.	The patient may have difficulty in swallowing due to soreness and oedema.
9 The sources should be checked at regular intervals, e.g. at the beginning of a span of duty.	To make sure that the sources have not become dislodged.
10 The patient should be confined to the room and only leave when necessary, e.g. to visit the X-ray department.	To minimize the risk of radiation exposure to other people on the ward.

Discharge of the patient

The patient is usually discharged the day after the removal of the implant. The patient should be warned about the painful local reaction that may be experienced due to rapid cell breakdown induced by the radiation. In order to minimize the risk of infection or soreness, the patient should be taught how to care for the treated area, e.g. oral toilet 4-hourly when awake and after meals.

Procedure guidelines: **Care of patients with manually and afterloaded iridium and caesium gynaecological sources**

Preparation of patient

The patient is usually admitted 12–48 hours before the procedure so that any preanaesthetic investigations may be performed. Full bowel prep with a low-residue diet will reduce the chance of the patient having a bowel action while the sources are in place, which could dislodge the sources. Some patients, however, have diarrhoea on admission due to previous radiotherapy and will need regular medication, such as codeine phosphate, both before and during the application of the sources. A full explanation should be given to the patient along with information about the implications of having a radioactive source inside her and informed consent obtained. The patient should be bathed before any premedication is administered.

Action	Rationale
1 The patient must remain in bed in a recumbent or semi-recumbent position while the applicators or implants are in place.	To prevent the applicators becoming dislodged or changing their position in relation to the internal organs.
2 Log rolling from side to side is permitted and should be encouraged if the patient is at risk of developing a pressure sore.	To promote comfort and to relieve prolonged pressure on any one area.
3 On return from theatre, the following should be checked:	
(a) The sanitary towel	To secure the position of the sanitary towel.
(b) Disposable pants in position	To ensure that urine is draining freely.
(c) Urinary catheter in correct position and draining satisfactorily.	
4 Observe for any blood or other discharge from the vagina.	To monitor haemorrhage, shock and other postoperative complications.
Ensure routine postoperative observations are performed until patient is stable. Continue to monitor temperature and pulse throughout treatment, at least 2 hourly.	
5 Administer prescribed analgesics, antiemetics and antidiarrhoeal agents.	For the patient's comfort.
6 Encourage fluid intake as soon as the patient is allowed to drink.	
(a) Encourage a fluid intake of 50–100% a day over and above the patient's normal intake.	To ensure adequate hydration. To reduce the risk of urinary tract infection.
(b) A low-residue diet may be taken. Liaise with dietitian regarding suitable supplements.	To prevent the stimulation of a bowel action.

Procedure guidelines: **Removal of gynaecological caesium and iridium wires**

The removal of applicators is usually performed by suitably qualified and competent nursing staff or a clinical oncologist.

Equipment

1 Sterile gynaecological pack containing large receiver, green towel, paper towel, long dissecting forceps, sanitary towel, cotton wool balls.
2 Equipment for the administration of Entonox.
3 Solutions of choice for swabbing, e.g. 0.9% sodium chloride.
4 Gloves.
5 Sterile scissors or stitch cutter.
6 Contamination monitor.
7 Lead pot.
8 Alcoholic handrub.

*Procedure guidelines: **Removal of gynaecological caesium and iridium wires** (cont'd)*

Procedure

Action	Rationale
1 Explain and discuss the procedure with the patient.	To ensure that the patient understands the procedure and gives her valid consent.
2 Check the date and time for removal on the form that was received from the physics department when sources were inserted.	The accurate timing of the removal is essential for the administration of the correct therapeutic dose of radiation.
3 Check that any pre-removal drugs (e.g. sedatives, analgesics) have been administered.	
4 Check, with another nurse, the exact time of removal and the number of applicators.	To reduce the risk of error.
5 Ensure that:	
(a) The lead shield is suitably positioned beside the patient.	To shield the nurse from exposure to radiation.
(b) The lead pot is also suitably positioned with the lid removed.	So that sources can be placed in the pot immediately after removal.
6 Begin the administration of Entonox at least 2 minutes before commencing the procedure.	To allow time for the effects of the gas to be felt. (For further information on Entonox administration, see Ch. 28.)
7 Prepare a trolley, clean hands, put on gloves and open the pack before going to the bedside.	Although this is a clinically clean, not an aseptic procedure, hands should still be cleaned before every patient contact. To reduce the time spent in close proximity to the source, all preparation of equipment should be undertaken away from the patient.
8 Working from behind the lead shield, assist the patient into the dorsal position with knees apart. Remove the sanitary towel.	To obtain access to the sources.
9 Remove any sutures, if present. Remove the vaginal packing.	
10 Remove the caesium sources in reverse order of insertion. Contact the clinical oncologist immediately if difficulty is encountered in removing a source.	To prevent damage to the vagina.
Place the removed sources in a lead pot immediately and cover with the lid.	To contain radioactivity.
11 Remove the lead pot to a designated area, e.g. an isotope sluice or safe. Ensure that the lid of the pot or the sluice door is locked.	To remove the radioactive source from the ward area. To prevent unauthorized access to the source.
12 Monitor the patient's level of radioactivity.	To ensure that no sources remain inside the patient.
13 Remove gloves, clean hands then put on clean pair of gloves.	To reduce the risk of contamination from gloves that may have become contaminated whilst handling the lead pot.
14 Remove the urinary catheter.	The urinary catheter is no longer required.
15 Swab the vulva and perineal area with a solution such as 0.9% sodium chloride. Ensure that the patient has a clean sanitary towel in position and is made comfortable.	To promote patient hygiene and comfort.
16 Monitor the bed linen, paper bags, vaginal packing and other waste material. (Two nurses should monitor the patient independently.)	To ensure that no source has been lost or remains inside the patient.
17 The patient should remain in bed until the physics department staff or other suitably trained staff member are satisfied that all sources are accounted for.	To ensure that all sources have been accounted for before the patient moves around.
18 Remove the radiation warning notice.	

Problem solving

Problem	Cause	Suggested action
Patient has a bowel action.		Inform the radiotherapist.
Patient removes source herself.	Confusion, e.g. postanaesthetic.	Using long-handled forceps place the source in the lead container or safe. Inform the radiotherapist and the physics department.
Pyrexia.	Pelvic cellulitis or abscess. Reaction to the proflavine pack. Urinary infection. Physiological reaction to the breakdown of the tumour. Chest infection. Peritonitis due to perforation of the uterus.	If the patient's temperature remains over 37.5°C for two consecutive readings, inform the radiotherapist. The source may have to be removed if the pyrexia persists.

Procedure guidelines: **Care of patients undergoing Selectron treatment**

Action	Rationale
1 Ensure written consent has been obtained.	To ensure patient fully understands and agrees to the treatment planned.
2 Ensure thorough nursing assessment of patient has been undertaken by nursing staff.	To ensure patient is suitable and will comply with treatment restrictions.
3 Ensure full preoperative medical assessment has been undertaken, for example baseline blood tests, ECG and X-ray.	To ensure patient is fit for treatment.
4 Administer antidiarrhoeal drugs the night before treatment. Patient to be monitored and if necessary treatment provided for radiation-induced enteritis.	To prevent bowel action dislodging applicators during treatment.
5 Nurse the patient on a pressure-relieving mattress or with a foam wedge under her buttocks or a pillow under knees to alter position.	To promote comfort and to relieve backache since rolling is not permitted.
6 Ensure the plastic transfer tubes are supported securely in the bed bracket, leaving slight slack.	To enable the patient to change position slightly without putting traction on the applicators.
7 Limit the frequency and duration of interruption to treatment. Visitors are discouraged unless the patient is markedly distressed.	To prevent unnecessary prolongation of treatment time.
8 Check patient's physical and psychological condition at least 2 hourly.	To monitor for haemorrhage, shock or other postoperative complications.
(a) Temperature, pulse and vaginal loss.	
(b) Contents of catheter drainage bag.	To ensure urine is draining freely.
(c) Assist patient to adjust her position.	To promote comfort and relieve prolonged pressure on any one area.
9 Check position of applicators. Marking the position of the applicators on the patient's legs can assist the checking of their position.	To ensure no movement of the applicators has occurred.
10 Administer prescribed analgesics, antiemetics, antidiarrhoeal and sedative agents as appropriate and evaluate effect.	To promote the patient's comfort and well-being.
11 Encourage fluid intake as soon as the patient is able to drink.	To ensure adequate hydration and reduce the risk of urinary tract infection.
12 If the patient wishes to eat, a light, low-residue diet may be taken. Ideally food should be chosen which is easy to eat lying down.	To prevent stimulation of a bowel action.

Procedure guidelines: **Removal of Selectron applicators**

If two patients are being treated simultaneously, removal of the applicators may be delayed until both patients have finished treatment, depending on the individual treatment times. Monitor remaining treatment time of the second patient, to ensure that the applicators of both patients can be removed at the first possible opportunity.

Equipment

As for removal of other gynaecological applicators, see Procedure guidelines: Removal of gynaecological caesium and iridium wires, p. 601 (items 1–7) plus:
  8 Rubber caps for the applicators.

Procedure

Action	Rationale
1 Check treatment has been terminated by: (a) Ensuring the appropriate channel lights are green (b) Ensuring the time display on the Selectron unit reads zero for the appropriate channels (c) Ensuring the print-out indicates treatment has stopped for those channels.	The applicators should be removed only on completion of treatment.
2 Check that the closed-circuit television camera is not focused on the patient.	To ensure privacy.
3 Explain and discuss the procedure with the patient.	To ensure that the patient understands the procedure and gives her valid consent.
4 Ensure any pre-removal drugs have been administered.	To allow analgesic or sedative to be effective.
5 Assist the patient into a comfortable position with her knees apart.	To allow access to the applicators.
6 Uncouple the plastic transfer tubes by rotating the black coupling anticlockwise in the direction of the arrow and very carefully store the tubes on the plastic supporting mantle attached to the Selectron unit.	To prevent the plastic catheter becoming damaged or kinked.
7 Place rubber caps on the ends of the applicators.	To ensure no fluid or debris is allowed to enter the applicator tubes.
8 Commence administration of Entonox (see Ch. 28) at least 2 minutes before removal of the applicators.	To allow the effect of the gas to be felt.
9 Prepare the equipment and put on gloves.	The procedure is clinically clean and not aseptic.
10 Remove the vulval dressing pads, any sutures and vaginal packing.	These must be removed before the applicators can be eased out.
11 Dismantle the applicators by loosening the screws holding them together.	To promote ease of removal.
Remove the uterine tube first, ensuring it is taken out complete with its small white flange, followed by the ovoids.	To prevent the flange being left in the patient's vagina.
12 Remove the catheter, swab the vulval area and ensure the patient has a clean sanitary pad and a fresh sheet.	To promote cleanliness and patient comfort.
13 The patient can then be assisted into a comfortable position and is permitted up to have a bath.	The patient is reassured that the procedure has been completed, that she is no longer radioactive and can resume normal activities.
Applicators are retained carefully for cleaning in accordance with local policies.	

Problem solving

See also 'Problem solving' for conventional gynaecological sources, p. 603.

Problem	Cause	Suggested action
Patient removes the applicators herself.	Confusion, e.g. postanaesthetic.	Check room for any sources that may have escaped, using contamination monitor. Sources that have escaped should be placed in lead pots using long-handled forceps. Remove applicators completely if partially removed.
Applicator is partially dislodged.	Patient may have moved too much or too vigorously.	Interrupt treatment. Inform physicist and radiotherapist. The applicator may have to be removed as above.
Alarm sounding at nurse station.	Treatment has been interrupted and inadvertently left off.	Check patient is unattended and recommence treatment.
Sources are not transferred to the applicators.	Incorrect coupling or loose connection.	Check print-out to identify which channel is at fault. Tighten appropriate coupling device.
Alarm activated at remote control unit.	Failure in the system.	Check the error code on the print-out with the Selectron user's manual. Rectify as indicated in the manual or seek technical assistance from the physics department.
Pellets stuck in the applicator or transfer tubing.	A damaged or kinked catheter.	A risk assessment to be completed regarding the likelihood of this occurrence (see example risk assessment).

Procedure guidelines: **Care of patients with radioactive seeds (e.g. iodine-125)**

Preparation of the patient

The patient is usually admitted at least 1 day before treatment: patients should be nursed ideally in a single room but, more importantly, in a bed away from the main thoroughfare.

Seeds are implanted permanently into the tissue and therefore the patient must agree to stay in hospital until the physics staff state that the radioactivity is at a legally permissible level for discharge.

Breast and lymph node implantation

	Action	Rationale
1	Leave the dressing securely in position unless special instructions are given by the radiotherapist.	Sources may become detached, dressings will prevent them from becoming lost.
2	If dressing becomes dislodged, leave it at the bedside, preferably in a lead pot, and inform the physics staff.	If sources have became detached and are in the dressings physics staff will take the necessary action.
3	If there is any possibility that the sources have become detached, inform physics department staff immediately and do not remove anything from the room.	It is important that the source is not lost as this could result in contamination of the environment. The patient's total dose will be altered and the medical staff will need to be informed.

Lung implantation

	Action	Rationale
1	Check all sputum and drainage from the chest with the contamination monitor. If no radioactivity is found the sputum and drainage may be disposed of in the usual way unless special instructions are given by the physics department or radiotherapy staff.	To check for radioactivity in case any sources are coughed up or expelled in the drainage.

Procedure guidelines: Care of patients with radioactive seeds (e.g. iodine-125) (cont'd)

Action	Rationale
2 If radioactivity is detected, inform physics department staff immediately. Save the sputum or drainage for them to deal with.	To prevent contamination of the hospital environment.

Bladder and prostate implantation

Action	Rationale
1 Check all urine with the contamination monitor. If no radioactivity is found the urine may be disposed of in the usual way.	To check for radioactivity in case any sources are expelled in the urine.
2 If radioactivity is detected, inform physics staff immediately and save urine for them to deal with.	To prevent contamination of the hospital environment.
3 Leave suspect urine in a safe place at the bedside, e.g. under the bed.	To prevent accidental disposal.

Procedure guidelines: **Care of patients with breast sources**

Preparation of patient

The patient will usually be admitted for local excision of the breast tumour and an axillary clearance. Drains are inserted and these are usually removed before the iridium wire sources are loaded 24–48 hours after surgery. When the sources are loaded, the patient should be nursed in a single room.

Action	Rationale
1 Leave any dressing undisturbed for the duration of treatment.	To minimize the time spent in proximity to the patient.
2 Confine the patient to the room.	To minimize the risk of radiation to other people on the ward.
3 Administer prescribed analgesia as required throughout the treatment period and before removal.	For the patient's comfort.

Discharge of the patient

The patient should normally be discharged the day after the removal of the implant. The patient should be warned about the painful local reaction which she may experience due to the rapid cell breakdown induced by the radiation. In order to minimize the risk of infection or soreness, the patient should be taught how to care for the treated area.

Procedure guidelines: **Interstitial perineal template (Hammersmith hedgehog)**

Care of patient with interstitial perineal template with insertion of radioactive sources (iridium-192). Please also refer to care of patients with insertions of sealed radioactive sources.

Action	Rationale
1 Perform full preoperative nursing assessment (see Ch 1, Context of care, and Ch 30, Preoperative care).	To ensure patient is suitable for anaesthetic/spinal anaesthetic and suitable for treatment.
2 Assess for previous medical problems: (a) Deep vein thrombosis/pulmonary embolism (b) Psychological problems (c) Fear of isolation (d) Pressure sores (e) Back problems (f) Any physical condition which may prevent patient from lying flat, e.g. chronic obstructive pulmonary disease, respiratory/cardiac problems.	To ensure patient can comply with approx. 5–7 days of complete bedrest in semi-recumbent position. See Fig. 34.7.

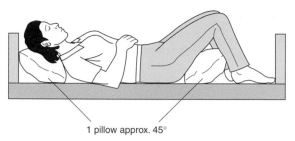

1 pillow approx. 45°

One pillow under head and a second
under knees. Knees to be slightly apart

Figure 34.7 Semi-recumbent position to be adopted
during interstitial perineal template therapy.

*Procedure guidelines: **Interstitial perineal template (Hammersmith hedgehog)** (cont'd)*

Action	Rationale
3 Ensure informed consent has been obtained. Check patient's understanding of planned treatment.	To ensure that the patient understands the radiation protection restrictions associated with this treatment and the nature and outcome of surgery, to reduce anxiety and postoperative complications.
4 Offer further explanation, verbal and written information.	Important that patient fully understands the planned treatment to ensure compliance with treatment.
5 Bowel preparation	
(a) Ensure preoperative bowel preparation is carried out. *Note*: Consultant preference will dictate what bowel preparation is used. Generally this is either:	Treatment time is 5–7 days. Bowel action may dislodge applicator. Patient comfort is improved if bowel evacuation complete preoperatively.
• Bowel prep, e.g. Citramag given to ensure thorough bowel evacuation. Patient starts clear fluids while on bowel prep or	
• A low-residue diet is commenced 2 days before treatment and phosphate enema is given the night before and on morning of surgery.	Low-residue/light diet to prevent bowel stimulation, to prevent bloating and discomfort from constipation.
(b) For duration of treatment, patient to receive codeine phosphate regularly to induce constipation. During treatment, patients to take a low-residue or light diet.	To reduce the likelihood of a bowel action which could cause the applicators to be moved.
(c) Encourage good fluid intake, IV fluids if necessary.	To ensure adequate hydration.
(d) Doctors and physics department to be contacted if patient has bowel action.	To assess whether applicators have been dislodged.
6 Observations	
(a) Observations to be performed 2–4 hourly as patient's condition dictates during treatment.	To observe for bleeding/hemorrhage/ infection/reaction to treatment.
(b) Observe wires to check number and position.	To observe for accidental movement of wires, to prevent inappropriate treatment to surrounding tissues.
(c) Ensure legs parted slightly using pillows to position.	Facilitates observation.
(d) Monitor skin integrity around iridium wires.	Radiation skin reaction can occur and medical/nursing intervention may be required to relieve symptoms and promote comfort.
(e) Monitor vaginal bleeding, changing pads as necessary.	Bleeding may occur which may require medical/nursing intervention to stop the bleeding.
(f) Monitor pain and if necessary, provide prescribed analgesia and assess efficacy.	To minimize pain.
(g) Monitor for nausea and vomiting and if necessary, provide prescribed antiemetics and assess efficacy.	To promote patient comfort.

*Procedure guidelines: **Interstitial perineal template (Hammersmith hedgehog)** (cont'd)*

Action	Rationale
(h) Monitor for deep vein thrombosis. Ensure TED stockings are correctly fitted unless otherwise indicated. Deep vein thrombosis prophylaxis may be prescribed (e.g. Fragmin). Encourage gentle leg exercises, but avoid excessive movement.	To prevent deep vein thrombosis.
(i) Monitor pressure areas.	To prevent development of pressure sores.
(j) Patients can be log rolled onto side to allow assessment of pressure areas and hygiene needs and to relieve pressure areas.	To promote patient comfort.
7 Ensure access to radio, telephone, TV with remote control, books, etc.	To help patient deal with isolation by maintaining contact with outside world; prevent boredom.
8 Following removal of interstitial perineal template:	
(a) Encourage vulval douching/vaginal douching after removal of template. Use hairdryer to dry area.	To facilitate good hygiene and comfort and to prevent infection. Hairdryer helps limit friction which can cause more discomfort.
(b) Catheter to be removed after treatment.	
(c) Ensure normal urination recommences.	To ensure that retention of urine has not occurred following removal of catheter.
9 Encourage vaginal dilating 4–6 weeks post procedure (length depending on postoperative recovery) to be reassessed in the outpatient department.	To prevent vaginal stenosis, so facilitating patient comfort for future pelvic examinations and sexual intercourse.

Useful websites

www.doh.gov.uk/irmir.htm
www.legislation.hmso.gov.uk/si/si1999/19993232.htm
legislation.h,so.gov.uk/si/si2000/20001059.htm
Training available on the web:
www.iaea.or.at/ns/rasanet/training/index.htm

References and further reading

Bergmark, K. *et al.* (1999) Vaginal changes and sexuality in women with a history of cervical cancer. *N Engl J Med*, **340**(18), 1383–9.

Blake, P.R. *et al.* (1998) *Gynaecological Oncology*. Oxford University Press, Oxford.

Blank, L.E., Gonzalez, D., De Reijke, T.M. *et al.* (2000) Brachytherapy with transperineal [125]iodine seeds for localized prostate cancer. *Radiother Oncol*, **57**(3), 307–13.

Charra, C., Roy, P., Coquard, R., Romestaing, P., Ardiet, J.M. & Gerard, J.P. (1998) Outcome of treatment of upper third vaginal recurrences of cervical and endometrial carcinomas with interstitial brachytherapy. *Int J Radiat Oncol Biol Phys*, **40**(2), 421–6.

Christman, N.J., Oakley, M.G. & Cronin, S.N. (2001) Developing and using preparatory information for women undergoing radiation therapy for cervical or uterine cancer. *Oncol Nurs Forum*, **28**(1), 93–8.

Cull, A. *et al.* (1993) Early stage cervical cancer: psychosocial and sexual outcomes of treatment. *Br J Cancer*, **68**(6), 1216–20.

Davis, C.S., Zinkard, J.E. & Fitch, M.I. (2000) Cancer treatment induced menopause: meaning for breast and gynaecological cancer survivors. *Can Oncol Nurs*, **10**(1), 14–21.

DoH (1978) *The Medicine (Administration of Radioactive Substances) Regulations*. HMSO, London.

DoH (1999) *The Ionising Regulations No. 3232*. Stationery Office, London.

DoH (2000) *The Ionising Radiation (Medical Exposure) Regulations No. 1059*. Stationery Office, London.

Farrell, E. (2002) Premature menopause. 'I feel like an alien'. *Aust Fam Physician*, **31**(5), 419–21.

Fraunholz, I.B., Schopohl, B. & Bottcher, H.D. (1998) Management of radiation injuries of vulva and vagina. *Strahlenther Onkol*, **174**(3), 90–2.

Gosselin, T.K. & Waring, J.S. (2001) Nursing management of patients receiving brachytherapy for gynaecologic malignancies. *Clin J Oncol Nurs*, **5**(2), 59–63.

Gupta, A.K., Vicini, F.A., Frazier, A.J. *et al.* (1999) Iridium-192 transperineal intersitial brachytherapy for locally advanced or recurrent gynaecological malignancies. *Radiat Oncol Biol Phys*, **43**(5), 1055–60.

Harrison, L.B. (1997) Application of brachytherapy in head and neck cancer. *Semin Surg Oncol*, **13**(3), 177–84.

Hath, R. (1993) New direction in radionuclide sources for brachytherapy. *Semin Radiat Oncol*, **3**(4), 278–89.

Hughes-Davies, L., Silver, B. & Kapp, D.S. (1995) Parametral interstitial brachytherapy for advanced or recurrent pelvic malignancy: the Harvard/Standard experience. *Gyneocol Oncol*, **58**(1), 24–7.

IPEM/RCN (Institute of Physics and Engineering in Medicine/ Royal College of Nursing) (2002) Radiation. In: *Ionising Radiation Safety: A Handbook for Nurses*. York Publishing, York, pp. 1–7.

Jones, B., Pryce, P.L., Blake, P.R. & Dale, R.G. (1999) High dose brachytherapy practice for the treatment of gynaecological cancers in the UK. *Br J Radiol*, **72**(856), 371–7.

Katz, A., Njuguna, E., Rakowsky, E. *et al.* (2001) Early development of vaginal shortening during radiation therapy for endometrial or cervical cancer. *Int J Gynecol Cancer*, **11**(3), 234–5.

Krull, A., Friedrich, R.E., Schwarz, R. *et al.* (1999) Interstitial high dose rate brachytherapy in locally progressive or recurrent head and neck cancer. *Anticancer Res*, **19**(4A), 2695–7.

Kuipers, T., Hoekstra, C.J., Van't Riet, A. *et al.* (2001) HDR brachytherapy applied to cervical carcinoma with moderate lateral expansion: modified principles of treatment. *Radiother Oncol*, **58**(1), 25–30.

Lalos, A. (1997) The impact of diagnosis on cervical and endometrial cancer patients and their spouses. *Eur J Gynaecol Oncol*, **18**(6), 513–19.

Lalos, A. *et al.* (1995) Experience of the male partner in cervical and endometrial cancer – a prospective interview study. *J Psychosom Obstet Gynaecol*, **16**(3), 153–65.

Lorvidhaya, V., Tonusin, A., Changwiwit, W. *et al.* (2000) High-dose-rate afterloading brachytherapy in carcinoma of the cervix: an experience of 1992 patients. *Int J Radiat Oncol Biol Phys*, **46**(5), 1185–91.

Martinez, A., Edmundson, G.K., Cox, R.S., Gunderson, L.L. & Howes, A.E. (1985) Combination of external beam irradiation and multiple-site perineal applicator (MUPIT) for treatment of locally advanced or recurrent prostatic, anorectal and gynecologic malignancies. *Int J Radiat Oncol Biol Phys*, **11**(2), 391–8.

Montgomery, C., Lydon, A. & Lloyd, K. (1997) Psychological distress among cancer patients and informed consent. *J Psychosom Res*, **46**(3), 241–5.

Morris, S. (2001) Radiation protection. Brachytherapy equipment. In: *Radiotherapy Physics and Equipment*. Churchill Livingstone, Edinburgh.

Muscari Lin, E., Aikin, J.L. & Good, B.C. (1999) Premature menopause after cancer treatment. *Cancer Pract*, **7**(3), 114–21.

Nag, S., Martinez-Monge, R., Capeland, L.J., Vacarello, L. & Lewandowski, G.S. (1997) Perineal template interstitial brachytherapy salvage for recurrent endometrial adenocarcinoma metastatic to the vagina. *Gynecol Oncol*, **66**(1), 16–19.

Nag, S., Martinez-Monge, R., Selman, A.E. & Copeland, L.J. (1998) Interstitial brachytherapy in the management of primary carcinoma of the cervix and vagina. *Gynecol Oncol*, **70**(1), 27–32.

Petereit, D.G., Sarkaria, J.N. & Chappell, R.J. (1998) Perioperative morbidity and mortality of high dose rate gynecologic brachytherapy. *Int J Radiat Oncol Biol Phys*, **42**(5), 1025–31.

Pinilla, J. (1998) Cost minimization analysis of high-dose-rate low-dose-rate brachytherapy in endometrial cancer. Gynecology Tumor Group. *Int J Radiat Oncol Biol Phys*, **42**(1), 87–90.

Robinson, J.W. & Roter, D.L. (1999) Psychosocial problem disclosure by primary care patients. *Soc Sci Med*, **48**(10), 1353–62.

Robinson, J.W., Faris, P.D. & Scott, C.B. (1999) Psychoeducational groups increase vaginal dilation for younger women and reduce fears for women of all ages with gynecological carcinoma treated with radiotherapy. *Int J Radiat Oncol Biol Phys*, **44**(3), 497–506.

Rogers, C.L., Freel, J.H. & Speiser, B.L. (1999) Pulsed low rate brachytherapy for uterine cervix carcinoma. *Int J Radiat Oncol Biol Phys*, **43**(1), 95–100.

Rollison, B. & Strang, P. (1995) Pain, nausea and anxiety during intra-uterine brachytherapy of cervical carcinomas. *Support Care Cancer*, **3**(3), 205–7.

Sannazzari, G.L., Ruo Redda, M.G., Rampino, M. & Verna, R. (1998) Brachytherapy and local control. *Rays*, **23**(3), 427–38.

Shasha, D., Harrison, L.B. & Chiu-Tsao, S.T. (1998) The role of brachytherapy in head and neck cancer. *Semin Radiat Oncol*, **8**(4), 270–81.

Smith, R.V., Krevitt, L., Yi, S.M. & Beitler, J.J. (2000) Early wound complications in advanced head and neck cancer treated with surgery and Ir-192 brachytherapy. *Laryngoscope*, **110**(1), 8–12.

Stitt, J.A. (1999) High dose rate brachytherapy in the treatment of cervical carcinoma. *Hematol Oncol Clin North Am*, **13**(3), 585–93.

Syed, A.M., Puthawala, A.A., Abdelaziz, N.N. *et al.* (2002) Long term results of low-dose-rate interstitial–intracavitary brachytherapy in treatment of carcinoma of the cervix. *Int J Radiat Oncol Biol Phys*, **54**(1), 67–78.

Tan, L.T., Jones, B., Freestone, G. & Dale, R.G. (1996) Case report: low-dose-rate and high-dose-rate intracavitary brachytherapy in a patient with carcinoma of the cervix. *Br J Radiol*, **69**(817), 84–6.

Teruya, Y., Sakumoto, K., Moromizato, H. *et al.* (2002) High-dose intracavitary brachytherapy for carcinoma in situ of the vagina occurring after hysterectomy: a rational prescription of radiation dose. *Am J Obstet Gynecol*, **187**(2), 360–4.

Uno, T. *et al.* (1998) High dose rate brachytherapy for carcinoma of the cervix: risk factors for late rectal complications. *Int J Radiat Oncol Biol Phys*, **40**(3), 615–21.

Velji, K. & Fitch, M. (2001) The experience of women receiving brachytherapy for gynecologic cancer. *Oncol Nurse Forum*, **28**(4), 743–51.

Wang, C.C. & Lo, H.H. (1970) A modified Stockholm radium applicator for the treatment of carcinoma of the uterine cervix. *Radiology* **96**(3), 631–4.

Wang, C.J., Leung, S.W., Chen, H.C. *et al.* (1997) High-dose-rate brachytherapy (HDR-IC) in treatment of cervical carcinoma: 5-year results and implication of increased low-grade rectal complications on initiation of an HDR-IC fractionation scheme. *Int J Radiat Oncol Biol Phys*, **38**(2), 391–8.

35

Radioactive source therapy and diagnostic procedures: unsealed sources

Chapter contents

Definition

Unsealed radioactive sources are radionuclides supplied in liquid or colloidal form, systemically administered orally or by injection. They are used in the diagnosis and treatment of disease (IPEM/RCN 2002).

Definition of terms

1 *Radiopharmaceutical*: this is a specially formulated sterile compound consisting of two main components: the pharmaceutical, which primarily determines the distribution profile of the compound around the body's organs, and a radionuclide, which enables the distribution of the radiopharmaceutical to be determined (Walker & Jarritt 1998).

2 *Radionuclide*: a nuclide of an element which possesses an unstable configuration of protons and neutrons within the nucleus, and which achieves stability by undergoing a radioactive decay process (Walker & Jarritt 1998).

3 *Imaging*: images that show the distribution of radiopharmaceutical within the patient and are obtained using a gamma camera.

4 *Scanning*: the measurement of the distribution of radioactivity over an area of the body by counting the rate at which the radiation is received (count rate) by a detector moved over the body surface (Walker & Jarritt 1998).

5 *Radiation protection adviser*: this is an individual who meets the HSE's criteria for competence (Ionising Radiations Regulations 1999 (IRR99) (regulation 2)). A radiation employer must appoint a radiation protection adviser in writing to advise him on the observance of the IRR99 (regulations 13(1), (2)) (DoH 1999).

6 *Radiation protection supervisor*: this is a person appointed for the purpose of securing compliance with the IRR99 in respect of work carried out in any area subject to local rules (IRR99 regulation 17(4)).

7 *Controlled area*: this is any area where the effective dose to a person working in the area is likely to exceed 6 millisieverts (mSv) per year or an equivalent dose greater than three-tenths of any relevant dose limit (IRR99 regulation 16(1)). Entrance to controlled areas is restricted to classified workers and those entering under written arrangements (IRR99 regulation 18(2)).

8 *Supervised area*: this is any area not designated as a controlled area where any person is likely to receive an effective dose greater than 1 mSv per year or an equivalent dose greater than one-tenth of any relevant dose limit (IRR99 regulation 16(3)).

9 *Local rules*: these are documents that identify the key working instructions intended to restrict any exposure in controlled or supervised areas (IRR99 regulation 17(1), Approved Code of Practice (section 272)).

10 *Written arrangements*: these detail the conditions for access into controlled areas for non-classified employees to ensure adequate restriction of their exposure to ionizing radiation (IRR99 regulation 18(3), Guidance (section 314)).

11 *Classified persons*: these are employees who are likely to receive an effective dose in excess of 6 mSv per year or an equivalent dose which exceeds three-tenths of any relevant dose limit (IRR99 regulation 20).

12 The Ionising Radiation (Medical Exposure) Regulations *(IRMER) practitioner*: this is a registered medical practitioner, dental practitioner or other health professional who is entitled in accordance with the employer's procedures to take responsibility for an individual medical exposure (IRMER regulation 2) (DoH 2000).

13 *IRMER operator*: this is any person who is entitled, in accordance with the employer's procedure, to carry out practical aspects of medical exposures (IRMER regulations 2, 3).

14 *IRMER referrer*: this is a registered medical practitioner, dental practitioner or other health professional who is entitled in accordance with the employer's procedures to refer individuals for medical exposure to a practitioner (IRMER regulation 2).

15 *Radiation employer*: this is an employer who carries out work with ionizing radiation or who intends to carry out such work (IRR regulation 2).

Reference material

Unsealed sources are used to concentrate a radioisotope in a particular part of the body. Unsealed sources carry an additional risk of environmental contamination and therefore protective measures are required to prevent contamination of staff, visitors, other patients and the environment (Wootton 1993). For example, unsealed sources may concentrate in body fluids, which will then contain radioactivity, and when eliminated reduce the amount of radioactivity in the patient (Martin & Harbinson 1997), but increase the risk of contamination to staff and the environment.

Radionuclides used for diagnosis of disease in the nuclear medicine department and four unsealed sources will be discussed here.

Radionuclides used in the nuclear medicine department

Unsealed radionuclides are used in nuclear medicine for the diagnosis and treatment of disease, using both imaging and non-imaging investigations. The important properties that make them useful for diagnostic purposes include:

• The physical half-life
• Decay characteristics
• Ease of incorporation into radiopharmaceuticals
• Availability of radionuclide.

A desirable radionuclide should have a half-life just long enough to allow for the preparation, administration and concentration in the region of interest, but short enough for radiation to effectively disappear after the test (Walker & Jarritt 1998). Imaging studies commonly performed in a nuclear medicine department include:

• Assessment of structures and/or function of organs
• Sites of infection
• Presence of tumours.

Common non-imaging studies include investigations into red cell mass and plasma volume, gastrointestinal tract and renal function.

Radiopharmaceuticals are legally categorized as prescription only medicines (POMs), and, in addition to the standard legislation surrounding the administration of such drugs, are subject to regulations related to their radioactive content. In the UK, a statutory committee called the Administration of Radioactive Substances Advisory Committee (ARSAC) has been established to give ionizing radiation advice to health ministers and to manage the certification process for administration of radiopharmaceuticals. This committee issues certificates which authorize individuals to administer radiopharmaceuticals to patients. It also lists the maximum permissible doses of radioactivity that may be administered to adult patients, and appropriately reduced adult doses for children, according to a child's body weight or body surface area.

A radionuclide investigation involves administration of the appropriate radiopharmaceutical, and dynamic imaging or waiting a predetermined time to allow the dose to be taken up in the organ to be investigated. The patient is then positioned and is required to keep still during the scan, because movement causes artefacts which reduce diagnostic accuracy. The scan may last 15–60 minutes (Perkins 1995). Most procedures require little physical patient preparation (Table 35.1).

Five unsealed sources will be discussed:

- Rhenium-186 hydroxyethylidene diphosphonate (Re186 HEDP), used in the treatment of bone metastases
- Iodine-131 (I-131), used in the treatment of thyroid disorders
- Meta-iodobenzylguanidine (mIBG), used in the treatment and diagnosis of neuroblastoma and other neuroectodermal tumours
- Monoclonal antibodies labelled with iodine-131, used in the treatment of recurrent cystic glioblastoma
- Sentinal node biopsy using technetium-99m colloid.

Rhenium-186 hydroxyethylidene diphosphonate (Re186 HEDP)

Definition

Rhenium-186 forms a stable diphosphonate chelate with hydroxyethylidene diphosphonate (HEDP) forming rhenium-186 hydroxyethylidene diphosphonate (Re186 HEDP). The linking of the radionuclide rhenium-186 to a suitable chemical compound produces a radiopharmaceutical which is localized in metastatic foci in bone (O'Sullivan *et al.* 2002). Rhenium-186 HEDP is a beta-gamma-emitting radionuclide with a maximum beta energy of 1.07 MeV (megaelectron volts), and has a gamma ray emission of 137 keV (Maxon *et al.* 1992).

The beta particles travel only short distances and, therefore, their energy deposition is localized in metastatic foci in bone, delivering a therapeutic radiation dose directly to the metastases while delivering a much lower dose to normal bone marrow. Because Re186 HEDP also emits gamma rays, which can be located by diagnostic imaging techniques, it is possible to verify its location in areas of metastatic disease, and to measure the dose of radiation delivered to the tumour and bone marrow (McEwan 1998).

Use

Bone metastases are a common presentation of prostate, breast, lung and renal cancers, leading to various complications including pain, fractures and hypercalcaemia as well as reduced performance and quality of life

(Serafini 2001), and are a significant cause of morbidity (McEwan 1997). Eighty per cent of those patients with prostate cancer who develop clinical metastases will have bone metastases (Scher 2002), in spite of conventional therapy (Di Lorenzo *et al.* 2003). Pain control is important; one study using Re186 HEDP to treat patients with bone metastases found a 67.5% improvement in pain (Kucuk *et al.* 2000).

It is estimated that the leading site of new cancers is the prostate. It is also the second leading cause of cancer death by gender in the USA (Jemal *et al.* 2002). Man's cumulative lifetime risk of developing prostate cancer is approximately 6.25% and the cumulative risk of death from prostate cancer is 2% (Rietbergen *et al.* 1999). Studies using Re186 HEDP as targeted radiotherapy have shown that it can significantly reduce pain, improve quality of life, reduce management costs and may slow the progression of painful metastatic lesions (McEwan 2000).

Re186 HEDP has advantages over conventional external beam radiotherapy because it is tumour specific with relative sparing of surrounding healthy tissue (O'Sullivan *et al.* 2002). While thrombocytopenia is a dose-limiting but short-lasting (O'Sullivan *et al.* 2002) toxicity, leucopenia is less severe (de Klerk *et al.* 1994), although in a study by Holle (1997) an 87% response rate was achieved with no myelosuppressive effects. It is also possible to adjust the dosage to each patient to avoid unacceptable toxicity (de Klerk *et al.* 1996) or to use autologous peripheral blood stem cell rescue (O'Sullivan *et al.* 2002). A mild transient increase in pain may occur within a few days of administering Re186 HEDP (Serafini 2001).

Re186 HEDP is administered by intravenous injection by an IRMER operator. Because Re186 HEDP is excreted in the urine, urinary catheterization is carried out prior to treatment to ensure that the bladder remains empty and the radiation dose to the bladder is minimized. Therefore caution must be exercised when emptying the catheter bag (see 'Preparation of therapy room', below). Because the half-life of Re186 HEDP is only 90 hours patients only need to be segregated for a few days after it has been administered. In one study all patients were discharged within 4 days (O'Sullivan *et al.* 2002).

The Re186 HEDP treatment programme for carcinoma of prostate involves the following.

Preparation of patient prior to admission

- Complete assessment as an outpatient.
- At least 3 weeks before treatment: G-CSF growth factor (10 µg/kg) given over 4 days as an outpatient.
- At least 2 weeks before treatment: harvest of stem cells.

Admission and inpatient stay

- Admitted for up to 4 days into a controlled area.
- Re186 HEDP given intravenously on admission.
- Analgesics administered for initial increase in bone pain.

Following discharge of patient

- Fourteen days post treatment: stem cells reinfused as a day patient.
- Analgesics administered as required for the expected initial increase in bone pain.

Table 35.1 Radionuclide investigations

Investigation/target organ	Radiopharmaceutical	Procedures and clinical interventions
Imaging studies		
Bone scan		
Used to assess bone function in which malignancy, fractures and diseases such as osteomalacia and Paget's disease can be diagnosed (Murray 1998)	Technetium (^{99m}Tc) phosphate and phosphonate compounds, including methylene diphosphonate (MDP) and hydroxymethylene diphosphonate (HDP)	Patient to drink 5–6 cups of fluid and to empty bladder regularly while waiting for scan. This is to enhance soft tissue clearance and minimize absorbed radiation dose to the bladder
Renogram (dynamic renal study)		
Used to assess renal function by monitoring clearance of radiopharmaceutical via kidneys (Testa & Prescott 1996)	^{99m}Tc MAG$_3$ Benzoylmercaptoacetyltriglycine ^{99m}Tc DTPA Diethylenetriamine pentaacetic acid	Patients to drink approximately 600 ml of fluid and to empty bladder prior to scan, which takes approximately 1 hour. Intravenous diuretic is to be administered to patient during the scan to diagnose obstructive uropathy (Russell 1998)
Static renal study		
Used to assess size, shape and position and function of kidneys (Testa & Prescott 1996). Used to diagnose renal scarring in children (Oei 1998)	^{99m}Tc DMSA Dimercaptosuccinic acid	No preparation
Perfusion lung scan		
Used to assess blood supply to alveolar tree. Provides complementary information to a ventilation lung scan. Used to diagnose pulmonary embolism (Palla *et al.* 1995)	^{99m}Tc MAA Macroaggregated albumin	Radiopharmaceutical is administered as a slow bolus intravenous injection. Patient to lie supine and breathe deeply while injection is being given. This is to enhance even distribution of MAA through lung capillary bed. If patient is pregnant, administered activity needs to be reduced
Ventilation lung scan		
Provides complementary information to a perfusion lung scan in diagnosis of pulmonary embolism. Used to assess patency of airways	^{99m}Tc Technegas, ^{99m}Tc aerosol, ^{81m}Kr gas, ^{133}Xe gas (Owunwanne *et al.* 1995)	A chest X ray performed within the preceding 24 hour is required prior to scan, to assist with interpretation of lung scan. Patient breathes the radiopharmaceutical through a special mouthpiece while scan is being performed
Cardiac studies – perfusion imaging		
Used to assess areas of viable perfused myocardium. This is a two-part test with myocardial perfusion monitored under stress and subsequently at rest (Pennell 1998). Stress may be exercise or pharmocologically induced (Nowotnik 1995). Often performed on patients with suspected coronary artery disease, recent myocardial infarction or those who have undergone coronary artery bypass surgery	^{99m}Tc MIBI, ^{99m}Tc tetrafosmin, ^{201}Tl thallous chloride	Patient needs to be closely monitored during postexercise period because there is the potential risk of triggering a myocardial infarction after stress. This test is usually performed within a cardiology unit with appropriately trained personnel and equipment. Patient is usually kept in the department until he/she has been assessed by a clinician

(continued)

Table 35.1 Radionuclide investigations (*continued*)

Investigation/target organ	Radiopharmaceutical	Procedures and clinical interventions
Cardiac – left ventricular ejection fraction (LVEF)/multiple gated acquisition scan (MUGA) Used to evaluate cardiac function in patients prior to and during courses of chemotherapy containing cardiotoxic agents (Owunwanne *et al.* 1995)	^{99m}Tc labelled red blood cells	Current weight of patient is required for calculation of dose of a red bood cell labelling agent, which ensures red blood cells are labelled with required radioactivity (Rigo & Braot 1998). This volume calculated is then administered intravenously 20–30 minutes prior to scan. Patient lies supine for 30–40 minutes
Thyroid scan May be used to confirm presence of one or more nodules within the thyroid, or to identify functional characteristics of nodule(s) (Clark 1998)	^{99m}Tc pertechnetate, ^{123}I/^{124}I/^{131}I sodium iodide	Patient to avoid foods containing iodine (including seasalt, seafood, cod liver oil, mineral tablets and kelp) for 3 days prior to test. These foods decrease uptake of radiopharmaceutical within thyroid bed. Patient to discontinue thyroid medication for between 3 days and 3 weeks prior to test, depending on specific instructions given by clinician
Parathyroid scan Used to diagnose parathyroid adenomas in patients with primary hyperparathyroidism (O'Doherty & Coakley 1998a)	^{99m}Tc pertechnetate, ^{201}Tl thallous chloride	This is a two-part test, comprising a thyroid scan which is completed prior to the parathyroid scan. Patient should follow instructions for thyroid test
Tumour imaging Used to differentiate between metabolically active tumours and space-occupying lesions, or for the diagnosis of unknown primary tumours	^{18}F FDG 2-Fluorodeoxyglucose	Patient to fast for up to 6 hours prior to injection, with only water to be taken. Patients may experience a metallic taste in the mouth immediately after administration. Waiting interval between injection and scan is 30 minutes, scan being performed with a positron emission tomography (PET) camera
Used to diagnose infection and diagnose and stage cancers such as lung, Hodgkin's disease and lymphomas (Van der Wall & McLaughlin 1998)	^{67}Ga gallium citrate	Due to excretion of gallium citrate via the GI tract, patients should be given laxatives or encouraged to increase fibre and fluid intake to avoid constipation. There are specific radiation protection precautions to be adhered to
Used to diagnose and assess patients with neuroectodermal tumours including phaeochromocytomas, neuroblastomas, carcinoid, medullary thyroid cancers and paragangliomas (Hoefnagel & Lewington 1998)	^{123}I mIBG meta-iodobenzylguanidine	Patient must take Lugol's iodine or potassium iodide for 2 days prior to and for 3 days after day of administration. mIBG may cause hypertension and is administered slowly over a 10-minute period. On occasions, patients may experience some discomfort at the injection site. This may be relieved by applying heat to the area of discomfort and reducing rate of infusion. For paediatric patients, it is preferable to administer mIBG via a central venous catheter. Some drugs that act on the adrenergic system may interfere with uptake of mIBG

(*continued*)

Table 35.1 Radionuclide investigations (*continued*)

Investigation/target organ	Radiopharmaceutical	Procedures and clinical interventions
Often used in conjunction with mIBG scans to assist with localization of the primary tumour and sites of metastatic spread in the aforementioned diseases (Bomanji *et al.* 1995)	^{111}In Octreotide DTPA-D-Phe-1-Octreotide	Patients with insulinoma should have their blood sugar levels monitored pre- and post-injection. An intravenous solution containing glucose should be available in case of hypoglycaemia. Patients should be encouraged to increase fluid and fibre intake to avoid constipation
Sites of infection To identify areas of lymphocyte localization in patients with either acute or chronic inflammatory infections	Labelled white blood cells	50 ml of blood is taken from patient using a 19 G needle. Labelled blood is reinjected after approximately 2 hours, following which patient is scanned later the same day and/or the following day
Gastrointestinal tract To determine cause of gastrointestinal bleeding, including Meckel's diverticulum (Maurer 1998a)	^{99m}Tc pertechnetate	Patients (usually children) need to fast for 4–6 hours before scan; adults to fast from midnight
Non-imaging studies *Kidney function* Measurement of glomerular filtration rate (GFR) provides an assessment of renal function. Often used in renal transplant patients, in compromised renal function due to long-term use of certain drugs (e.g. cyclosporin) or in patients with systemic lupus erythematosus (Valdes Olmos 1998). Oncology patients often have renal function assessed prior to chemotherapy, particularly if regimen includes platinum-based cytotoxic agents	^{51}Cr EDTA Ethylenediaminetetra-acetic acid	Renal clearance of administered radiopharmaceutical is assessed from residual radioactivity in blood samples taken from patient at either 3 hours, or at 2, 3 and 4 hours postinjection. Patient's height and weight are required to enable GFR to be calculated accurately. It is important that no hydration or blood products are commenced during the test as this may alter results of test
Red cell mass/plasma volume Often used to diagnose polycythaemia vera in patients with cardiovascular disease (Rigo & Braot 1998)	^{125}I human serum albumin, ^{51}Cr or ^{99m}Tc labelled red blood cells	10 ml of blood is taken from patient using a 19 G needle. Labelled blood is reinjected after approximately 1.5 hours, following which patient's blood is taken at 10-minute intervals for 40 minutes. Patient's height and weight are recorded

Iodine-131

Definition

Radioactive iodine-131 is a beta-gamma emitter with a half-life of 8 days, and is used mainly in the form of iodide solution. The beta radiation gives a high, local dose in iodine concentrating tissue. The gamma component is useful for external measurement and scanning (Pointon 1991).

Use

Approximately 900 new cases and 250 deaths are recorded in England and Wales every year due to thyroid cancer, making it the commonest malignant endocrine tumour. However, this only represents about 1% of all malignancies (BTA/RCP 2002). Four variables result in a poor prognostic impact on thyroid cancer. These are extremes of age, male gender, poorly differentiated histological feature of the tumour and tumour stage. The choice of treatment also influences prognosis (Mazzaferri & Jhiang 1994). The use of total thyroidectomy and iodine-131 ablation for the treatment of thyroid cancers has improved outcomes (Kendall-Taylor 2002).

Thyroid tissue selectively concentrates iodide, which enables iodine-131 to be used in the diagnosis and treatment of thyroid disorders. These patients usually have a good prognosis (Harmer 1996):

- Thyrotoxicosis. Usually treatments of between 75 and 400 megabecquerels (MBq) activity of iodine-131 can be given, often on an outpatient basis.
- Well-differentiated thyroid cancers (papillary and follicular) and metastases that function similarly to the thyroid tissue. Treatment is usually on an inpatient basis because of the higher activities involved.

Iodine-131 is normally administered as a capsule taken orally by the patient, followed by a hot drink. It can also be administered in liquid form either intravenously or orally.

Treatment programme for carcinoma of the thyroid

Surgical removal of the thyroid

Normal thyroid tissue concentrates iodine more efficiently than malignant tissue, and some malignant tissues concentrate iodine-131 only after removal of normal tissue. It is recommended, therefore, that a surgical near-total thyroidectomy is performed before administration of iodine-131 (Beasley *et al.* 2002).

Iodine-131 treatment

This is one of the most specific therapies available that has few adverse effects (O'Doherty & Coakley 1998b). Following thyroidectomy an ablation dose of, typically, 3 GBq of iodine-131 is administered to ablate the remnants of thyroid tissue. Further treatments of 5.5 GBq may be necessary to destroy deposits in local lymph nodes and distant metastases. Following treatment, patients will be followed up as outpatients (Pacini *et al.* 2002).

Preparation of patient before admission

- *Twenty-one days before admission*: patients taking tetraiodothyronine (T_4) (thyroxine) must stop taking this medication.
- *Ten days before admission*: patients taking triiodothyronine (T_3) must stop taking this medication.
- *Three days before admission*: occasionally, to enhance the uptake of iodine-131, three daily injections of thyroid-stimulating hormone are administered.

Principles of protection policies

Iodine-131 is excreted rapidly in patients who have had a thyroidectomy via all body fluids, especially the urine. In those patients who have not undergone thyroidectomy, excretion is rapid initially, slowing as the iodine-131 is bound by the thyroid tissue. Consequently, great care must be taken with all body fluids, especially during the first few days.

Meta-iodobenzylguanidine (mIBG)

Definition

mIBG is a synthetic physiological guanethidine analogue which is structurally similar to both the neurotransmitter hormone nonadrenaline (norepinephrine) and the ganglionic blocking drug guanethidine. mIBG will localize in a wide variety of neuroendocrine tumours including neuroblastomas and phaeochromocytomas yet in relatively few normal cells (Lashford *et al.* 1991).

mIBG can be linked to iodine-131 and iodine-123 (a radionuclide) to produce the radiopharmaceutical I-131 mIBG or I-123 mIBG. A radiopharmaceutical is a radionuclide linked to a suitable chemical compound whose biochemical properties allow the radionuclide to be localized in the desired tissue (Shapiro *et al.* 1999).

Use

Neuroblastoma is the most common extracranial solid tumour of childhood and accounts for 8–10% of all childhood cancers. However, treatment success rates remain poor (Okuyama *et al.* 2002).

I-131 mIBG can be used as a safe, effective, non-invasive method of localizing both primary and metastatic neuroendocrine tumours (Okuyama *et al.* 2002). Therapeutic doses of I-131 mIBG can be given to patients in whom standard surgical and chemotherapeutic treatments have failed to control primary tumours, or can be used as an adjuvant to these treatments to prevent recurrence of the tumour (Fielding *et al.* 1991). In the treatment of neuroblastoma, response rates of 75% can be initially achieved using induction chemotherapy and stem cell rescue, although only 25% of patients will survive long term (Meller 1997). I-131 mIBG has been found to be equally effective but with considerably less toxicity (Hoefnagel *et al.* 1995).

Prior to therapy patients undergo scanning investigations using a tracer dose of I-123 or I-131 mIBG which allows calculation of the treatment dose. Therapeutic doses of I-131 mIBG are custom-synthesized for each patient and kept chilled or frozen from the time of synthesis until the dose is administered to reduce the risk of autoradiolysis. The solution is thawed and infused intravenously over 30–60 minutes using a shielded delivery system. During infusion pulse and blood pressure are monitored (Barry *et al.* 1990).

Side-effects include anorexia and mild nausea and vomiting, which can be controlled with antiemetics and an adequate intake of fluids. Little specific organ toxicity other than myelosuppression has been seen (Matthay *et al.* 2001).

Preparation of patient

To prevent the uptake of any free iodine-131, the uptake of radioactive iodine by the thyroid gland is blocked by giving patients excess oral iodine continually from 3 days before until 3 weeks after administration of mIBG for therapy doses, while for diagnostic investigations Lugol's iodine is taken over 5 days, commencing 2 days before the injection of I-123 mIBG.

As mIBG stimulates noradrenaline, drugs that act as antagonists (e.g. phenothiazines) are contraindicated during treatment (Shulkin & Shapiro 1990).

Monoclonal antibodies labelled with iodine-131 for recurrent cystic glioblastoma

Definition

Monoclonal antibodies specific to glioma antigens can be radiolabelled with iodine-131 and administered as therapy for patients with cystic gliomas (Bigner *et al.* 1995). The tumour is targeted by the monoclonal antibodies which deliver the radiation dose to the tumour. Because the antibodies are specific to glioma tissue, the exposure of normal tissues is limited (Bigner *et al.* 1995).

An antibody is a protein which is produced as a result of the introduction of an antigen. It has the ability to combine with the antigen that stimulated its production. Monoclonal antibodies are identical copies of a single antibody (Stites & Terr 1991). It is possible to produce monoclonal antibodies that are specific to tumour cells, which can be labelled with a radioisotope. When administered to the patient, the labelled monoclonal antibody seeks, attaches itself to, and then as the radioisotope decays, emitting radiation, it destroys malignant cells which carry the appropriate specific antigen (Bigner *et al.* 1995).

Use

High-grade malignant gliomas are at present not curable with conventional treatment (surgery, radiotherapy and chemotherapy) (Hammoud *et al.* 1996). Small studies of monoclonal antibodies labelled with iodine-131 administered intrathecally have shown that some patients have a significant and lasting therapeutic response without significant immediate or lasting toxicity (Moseley *et al.* 1990).

The procedure consists of surgically inserting a catheter into the tumour, and then administering a diagnostic dose of monoclonal antibody labelled with iodine-124. Following positron emission tomography (PET), a technique for imaging the distribution of radiolabelled pharmaceuticals (Horwich 1995), it is possible to calculate the therapeutic dose of antibody labelled with iodine-131. The therapeutic dose is administered slowly into the catheter by the patient's physician.

Following administration, it is important to carry out careful neurological observations to identify complications related to placement of the catheter, allergic reactions to the monoclonal antibody labelled with iodine-131 or possible toxicities associated with instillation of intracystic therapies.

The principles of radiation protection must be followed. Education and support for patients and carers are particularly important because of the poor survival rate of patients with gliomas (Cokgor *et al.* 2000).

Radioactive sentinel node biopsy using technetium-99m colloid

Sentinel node biopsy involves the use of technetium-99m colloid, a radiopharmaceutical, which is injected prior to the patient going to theatre. This nuclear medicine procedure assists the surgeon by identifying the nodes, thereby making removal of axillary sentinel lymph nodes easier and more accurate.

Sentinel lymph nodes receive drainage from the breasts (Kamm 1999). By undertaking biopsies of these nodes, the surgeon can predict the cancer status of all nodes in the axillary region. This procedure allows for accurate diagnosis of the patient cancer status, as well as avoiding unnecessary axillary dissection (Kellar 2001), as axillary dissection can cause serious complications such as lymphoedema, scarring, numbness, pain and psychological distress (Zack 2001). Accurate diagnosis prevents understaging and inadequate treatment (Spillane & Sacks 2000).

During the procedure all staff must wear their film badges and those handling the specimen must wear finger dosimeters. The theatre door should be labelled with a warning controlled area sign and disposable drapes and gowns should be used. The specimen should be placed in a screwtop container, which is labelled with the radioactive symbol and the details recorded in the log book. The specimen is then stored for 48 hours, after which time it is sent to histopathology in the normal way. The radioactive label is removed in histology after one week when the specimen is then considered nonradioactive.

On completion of the procedure, the used drapes, gown and gloves should be placed in a clinical waste bag and the environment and waste monitored to ensure no contamination is present. Any contaminated items should be marked radioactive and stored in a secure store, usually for one week, until sufficient radioactive decay has occurred. Only then should the warning symbols be removed and the waste disposed of in the normal way.

On returning to the ward, the patient is cared for as described later.

Principles of radiation protection

Radiation protection is based on three principles.

- *Justification:* no practice should be adopted unless its introduction produces a net benefit.
- *Optimization:* all exposure shall be As Low As Reasonably Practicable (ALARP).
- *Limitation:* the dose equivalent to staff and menbers of the public shall not exceed the dose limits.

The Ionising Radiation Regulations 1999, which came into force in 2000, set down requirements for the use of ionizing radiation and are enforced by the Health and Safety Executive (HSE).

The regulations require that radiation safety standards be maintained. Requirements for procedures involving unsealed sources include:

- Those administering radioactive material must hold an approved Administration of Radioactive Substances Advisory Committee (ARSAC) certificate.
- Administration of therapeutic and diagnostic radioactive substances can only be carried out in centres with appropriate facilities (Cormack *et al.* 1998).
- Risk assessments must be carried out prior to work with ionizing radiation.
- All controlled areas will have warning notices to restrict entry.
- All controlled and supervised areas have local rules, summarizing the arrangements for controlling work with ionizing radiation. The Radiation Protection Supervisor ensures the local rules are followed.
- Visitors are restricted. Doses received by relatives/friends of patients undergoing treatment or examination with ionizing radiation are restricted to the doses allowed to members of the public unless they are classified as comforters and carers when different rules and restrictions apply.
- Exposure is controlled by the use of time, distance and shielding.
- Personal protective clothing including gloves, aprons and overshoes used to limit the risk of contamination.
- Procedures are in place for reporting incidents (RIDDOR 1995).
- Adequate training is provided and only trained staff are allowed to work unsupervised.
- No pregnant or breastfeeding staff to enter the controlled area.
- Quality assurance initiatives have to be undertaken; these include clinical audit of procedures and standards.

Controlled area

The entrance to the controlled area must be marked with a warning sign. Information is displayed to indicate the following:

- The radioactive material and activity administered.
- Essential nursing procedures should only be carried out and unnecessary time must not be spent in close proximity to the patient while the sign is displayed.

Appropriate barriers, i.e. lead shields, should be placed at the entrance to:

- Prevent inadvertent entry by unauthorized personnel
- Reduce radiation exposure to visitors and staff.

Patients treated with unsealed radioactive sources should be confined to their rooms, except for special medical or nursing procedures, when they must be accompanied by suitably trained staff.

Therapeutic unsealed sources generate a significant amount of liquid radioactive waste. This can be from the patient's shower and toilet. However, the amount of radioactive waste that enters the sewage system is governed by local regulations. Multiple holding tank systems can be employed where waste can be held to allow decay to occur before being released into the main waste drainage system (Leung & Nikolic 1998).

Film badges

Film badges should be worn at all times when on duty. A digital dosimeter should be used when ongoing immediate dose records are required.

Contamination control

With unsealed sources, it is important to guard against contamination of both personnel and the hospital environment by the correct use of protective gloves, gowns and overshoes. The patient's body fluids are highly radioactive, especially in the days immediately after iodine-131 has been administered. Any action that is likely to cause contamination of personnel, for example the application of cosmetics, eating, drinking or smoking when the health care worker's hands are contaminated with radioactivity, is prohibited.

In the event of any incident involving radioactive material, the physics department must be advised immediately, even if the incident occurs outside normal working hours.

Preparation of therapy room

Equipment

Equipment should be kept to a minimum. It must be checked to ensure that it is in working order, as maintenance staff will only be allowed into the room in exceptional circumstances.

Bed linen and disposable items (gloves, aprons, overshoes, cutlery and crockery) should be kept in a utility room or anteroom along with the patient's treatment chart and a radiation monitor.

Personal items

Nurses should be sensitive to the psychological implications for patients of being labelled 'radioactive' and confined in isolation. Although patients may want to bring some personal belongings with them, they should be advised to keep these to a minimum, as items may become contaminated and need to be stored until radioactivity has decayed.

Protective floor covering

Plastic-backed absorbent paper, kept in place by adhesive tape, is used to retain accidental urine spills or splashes on the floor immediately surrounding the toilet. Each patient is assessed to decide whether further floor covering is necessary, e.g. catheterized patients will require floor covering below the catheter bag.

Cleaning the treatment room

During occupancy of the treatment room by the patient, cleaning of the room is kept to a minimum and should be supervised by the physics staff. After the patient is discharged, monitoring and any necessary decontamination of the room will be arranged by the physics department, which will inform the relevant personnel when this has been completed. Only then may the room be entered and thoroughly cleaned.

Preparation of patient

Consent

Careful preparation of the patient before the administration of unsealed source therapy is essential. Fully prepared, knowledgeable patients and visitors are the key to radiation safety and contamination control (Stajduhar *et al.* 2000; Thompson 2001). Incidents and accidents are less likely to occur if the patient fully understands the reasons for the restrictions being undertaken.

Patients are required to sign a consent form agreeing to treatment, following a full explanation from the treating clinician. This is to comply with medical, ethical and legal requirements and local hospital policy. Consent is usually obtained in the outpatient clinic before ordering the radioactive material.

On admission

Before the administration of unsealed sources, any symptoms of diarrhoea or constipation must be remedied. Diarrhoea could result in contamination of the treatment area. Constipation not only inhibits the elimination of radioactivity but also could obscure radiological investigations, e.g. scanning.

Patients and relatives should be educated about the principles of radiation protection and the procedures with which the patient has to comply while in isolation. Psychosocial and physical needs must be addressed which require a collaborative approach between patients and nurses (Stajduhar *et al.* 2000). It is important to identify potential anxieties before administration while the nurse is able to reassure the patient and is unconstrained by time limits.

The patient must also agree to stay in hospital until the physics department advises that the level of radioactivity permits discharge.

Discharge of patient

A patient should not be discharged from hospital until the activity retained has fallen below recommended levels. This level will depend on several factors, including:

- Mode of transport on leaving hospital
- Journey time involved
- Personal circumstances, e.g. young children or pregnant women at home.

Patients will be assessed individually for radiation clearance by the physics department before discharge. The treating physician will then be advised of the results of the assessment. Advice will be given to patients on issues such as return to work and visits to public places. Patients who are discharged will be given appropriate information in the form of an instruction card carrying details of precautions to be taken. This card must be signed by the treating clinician or the physics department staff.

It must be emphasized that this card must be carried and the instructions followed until the latest date shown so that, for instance, staff would be alerted should the patient be readmitted to hospital. Additional verbal instructions may be necessary.

Regulations

Ionising Radiation Regulations (1999). Stationery Office, London.

Web resources

Regulations and guidance available on the web:
www.legislation.hmso.gov.uk/si/si1999/19993232.htm
The Ionising Radiation Regulations 1999 (SI 1999 No. 3232).
www.legislation.hmso.gov.uk/si/si2000/20001059.htm
The Ionising Radiation (Medical Exposure) Regulations 2000 (SI 2000 No. 1059).

Procedure guidelines: **Care of the patient before administration of iodine-131**

	Action	Rationale
1	Explain and discuss the procedure with the patient.	To ensure that the patient understands the procedure and gives his/her valid consent.
2	The patient is to be fasted for 2 hours before and after administration of an iodine-131 dose. Offer a light diet for the remainder of the day.	To reduce the risk of nausea and/or vomiting.
3	Administer a prophylactic antiemetic 30 minutes before scheduled administration of the dose.	To prevent nausea and vomiting.
4	Check that the preparation of the room and the patient is complete. Ensure that any surplus items have been removed.	To prevent contamination of extraneous equipment.
5	Remove jewellery except wedding rings.	Jewellery may become contaminated.

Procedure guidelines: **Care of the patient receiving iodine-131 thyroid treatment**

	Action	Rationale
1	Explain and discuss the procedure with the patient.	To ensure that the patient understands the procedure and gives his/her valid consent.
2	Assist the patient to remove dentures/bridges, if dose is administered in liquid form.	To prevent radioactive material being trapped behind dental plates.
3	The patient swallows the capsule or drinks the iodine-131 through a straw, physically directed by an authorized physicist in the presence of the clinician directing treatment.	Drinking through a straw reduces the amount of radioactive material left around the mouth. To meet current regulations.
4	Offer the patient a drink of water to rinse out the mouth. (This must be swallowed.) Assist the patient to replace dentures.	To remove any iodine-131 from inside the mouth.
5	Physics staff place the radiation warning sign at the entrance to the therapy room.	To identify the room as a controlled area.

Procedure guidelines: **Care of the patient receiving iodine-131 mIBG treatment**

	Action	Rationale
1	Explain and discuss the procedure with patient and/or parents if the patient is a child.	To ensure that the patient and/or parents understands the procedure and gives his/her consent.
2	Apply a vital signs monitor with a variable time setting mode to the patient that will be visible to staff from outside the room.	Following the administration of mIBG, a transient rise in blood pressure and pulse may occur.

*Procedure guidelines: **Care of the patient receiving iodine-131 mIBG treatment** (cont'd)*

	Action	Rationale
3	Check that the patient has been cannulated or, for children, a central venous device is in place, and commence prescribed intravenous fluids 4 hours before iodine-131 mIBG administration.	To ensure safe administration of mIBG and adequate hydration.
4	The clinician will set up iodine-131 mIBG infusion and give it over 30–60 minutes.	To minimize transient rise in blood pressure and pulse.
5	Monitor blood pressure and pulse at least: (a) Every 5 minutes during infusion (b) Every 10 minutes for the first 45 minutes postinfusion (c) Hourly for 4 hours (d) Four-hourly; or more frequently if required. (e) Monitor whole body retention measurements as directed by physics.	To detect and monitor any change.
6	Continue intravenous hydration for 24 hours post-infusion and simultaneously encourage oral fluids.	To increase the urinary output and elimination of radioactivity from the bladder.

Procedure guidelines: **Care of the patient after administration of unsealed source therapy**

Entering the room

	Action	Rationale
1	Collect digital dosimeter, record reading before entering and on leaving room.	Digital dosimeter provides ongoing and immediate indication of the amount of exposure received.
2	Put on disposable gloves.	To prevent contamination of the hands.
3	Put on disposable overshoes.	To prevent spread of contamination outside the treatment area.
4	Put on a suitable protective gown: (a) Long-sleeve cotton gown, e.g. for lifting patient	To protect against low levels of contamination, e.g. from the patient's skin.
	(b) Disposable plastic apron, e.g. for dealing with vomit or incontinence.	To protect against high levels of contamination.
5	Plan work before entering the controlled area and then work quickly and efficiently, keeping within the time allowance stated.	To minimize radiation exposure, as consistent with good nursing care.
6	Only use disposable crockery and cutlery to present meals to patients. Remove all fruit stones and fish and meat bones from diet.	China crockery and cutlery may become contaminated. Uneaten food and disposable cutlery and crockery are disposed of in a macerator. Fruit stones and bones will block the macerator.

Maintaining patient comfort and hygiene

	Action	Rationale
1	Encourage the patient to shower frequently, at least once a day.	To reduce any radioactive perspiration on the skin.
2	Encourage the patient to wash the hands thoroughly after each possible contact with bodily fluids, e.g. cleaning teeth, going to the toilet.	To remove radioactivity from the hands.
3	The patient should regularly remove any dentures and clean under running water.	To remove radioactive saliva from around dentures.

Procedure guidelines: **Care of the patient after administration of unsealed source therapy** *(cont'd)*

Action	Rationale
4 The patient should regularly remove any contact lenses and rinse in their usual cleaning fluid.	To remove any radioactive tears from lenses.
5 Encourage a good fluid intake of between 2 and 3 litres per day.	To increase the urinary output and elimination of radioactivity from the bladder.
6 Ensure that the patient has own personal toilet facilities and flushes the toilet twice after use.	To reduce contamination of others and of the environment. Urine of patients treated with iodine-131 is initially highly radioactive.
7 Bedbound patients should be catheterized before the dose is given. Empty the catheter bag every 4–6 hours, or more frequently if necessary.	Catheterization reduces the nursing time spent with the patient and the likelihood of contamination. Frequent emptying of the bag reduces the radiation level in the room.
8 If the patient requires a bedpan or urinal, this item must be kept solely for this patient's use. The bedpan or urinal must be handled carefully and the contents disposed of in the patient's toilet, which is flushed twice. The bedpan or urinal may be washed in the bedpan washer. It should be sealed in a plastic bag for the journey to and from the sluice.	To reduce contamination of the environment and of other patients and staff.
9 If leakage occurs from injection sites, wound sites, etc., the nurse should contact the medical staff and the physics department immediately. Any contact with the dressing should be done with long-handled forceps.	It must be remembered that all body fluids are potentially radioactive.
10 Gloves and a protective gown must be worn whenever handling soiled bed linen.	To prevent contamination.
11 All used linen must be deposited in a special bag provided for this purpose.	Used linen must be monitored for contamination before going to the laundry.
12 Collection of laboratory specimens should, if possible, be deferred. If collections are unavoidable, a radiation warning sticker must be attached to the specimen and request card and the specimen delivered to the laboratory following consultations with the physics department.	To reduce the risk of contamination of the laboratory and its staff.

Visitors

Action	Rationale
1 Visiting time is limited as advised by the physicist during the first day following administration of an unsealed source.	The patient is highly radioactive during this period.
2 On subsequent days, visiting is unlimited, providing visitors remain outside the room behind the lead screen, the exception being parents of young children who will need to be authorized by the physics department.	To minimize the exposure of visitors to radiation.
3 Physical contact with the patient or bed linen is not allowed as protective clothing is not available to visitors.	To prevent contamination of visitors.
4 Children under 16 years of age and pregnant women will be discouraged from visiting.	Radiation exposure of children and the unborn must be kept as low as practicable.

On leaving the room

Action	Rationale
1 Remove overshoes, taking care not to touch the shoes worn underneath.	These are removed first while gloves are still being worn to prevent the spread of contamination to hands or the floor outside the room.

*Procedure guidelines: **Care of the patient after administration of unsealed source therapy** (cont'd)*

Action	Rationale
2 Remove the plastic apron, by holding the front of apron and breaking the neck and waist ties.	
3 Remove gloves by peeling them off the hands, taking care not to touch the outside surfaces with bare hands, and discard them in the clinical waste bag provided.	To prevent transfer of contamination from the gloves' outer surfaces to the hands.
4 Wash hands thoroughly using soap and water.	To remove any contamination.
5 Use the radiation monitor each time when leaving the room and monitor for contamination of the hands, feet and clothing. If contamination has occurred, inform the physics department immediately and follow the decontamination procedure.	To ensure that the nurse is not contaminated.
6 The physics department will advise if further whole body monitoring is required.	To check for internal or external contamination.

Procedure guidelines: **Care of the patient receiving unsealed sources for diagnostic investigations**

Action	Rationale
1 Explain and discuss the procedure with the patient, and, if relevant, with the relative accompanying the patient.	To ensure the patient is physically and psychologically prepared for the procedure and understands the procedure and gives his/her informed consent.
2 Preparation of patients (special considerations):	
(a) Provide effective pain control for those patients with pain.	Patients should be pain free so that immobility during scan time can be maintained.
(b) Pregnant women will generally not be scanned. When essential tests must be undertaken, the patient must sign a consent form and receive a reduced dose of radionuclide.	To avoid unnecessary irradiation to the abdominal/pelvic region which will include the embryo or foetus.
(c) The person accompanying the patient should not be pregnant, or bring young children or babies with them.	To avoid unnecessary exposure in the time period immediately after the radionuclide administration.
(d) In women of reproductive age, the possibility of pregnancy must be excluded and the patient asked if her menstrual period is late. Patients receiving I-131 or other radioactive agent with a long half-life should not become pregnant for a minimum of 3 months (Sharp *et al.* 1998).	To avoid unnecessary irradiation to the abdomen of a women who may be pregnant.
(e) With breastfeeding mothers, seek advice from the radiation protection adviser.	Radioactivity can be excreted in breast milk. Therefore breastfeeding may need to be suspended and the mother encouraged to avoid unnecessary cuddling of the child during this time.
(f) If the patient is incontinent, incontinence pads should be worn and universal precautions are to be adopted.	To limit the spread of contamination. Disposable gloves and apron should be worn and handwashing performed following patient contact, as these will prevent contamination of staff in close contact with the patient.
(g) Empty urine bags regularly.	To remove the radioactivity from the patient area.
(h) Debilitated patients may require prolonged close contact. Nursing staff should share the care of these patients, by regular rotation of staff.	To keep doses to staff as low as possible, by avoiding prolonged exposure to any one member of staff.
3 Administering radionuclides:	
(a) Follow guidelines for drug administration in Ch. 9.	To comply with national and professional guidelines for the administration of drugs.

Procedure guidelines: **Care of the patient receiving unsealed sources for diagnostic investigations** (cont'd)

Action	Rationale
(b) Follow for guidelines aseptic technique in Ch. 4.	To reduce the risk of contamination.
(c) Follow radiation protection precautions, which include:	To reduce the possible contamination of self and the environment.
• Wear thermoluminescent (TLD) finger-dose meter and film badge.	To measure radiation doses received by member of staff.
• Wear disposable gloves and plastic apron, which are discarded after use.	To reduce the risk of contamination.
• Draw up the dose behind a lead shield, and place the syringe in a lead syringe shield.	To reduce exposure to radiation.
• Dispose of all used syringes and needles in a designated radioactive sharps disposal bin which is stored within a lead shield.	To contain radioactivity and allow safe disposal.
• Wash hands at end of procedure.	To remove any possible radioactive contamination.
• Place yellow identity bracelet on the wrists of all inpatients, complete information card with the details of when precautions can be discontinued. Give the completed information card to the patient or the nurse accompanying the patient.	The yellow wrist band will provide visual warning to inform all health care workers of the patient's recent diagnostic investigation. The information card will inform ward staff of restrictions related to managing a patient, as well as when measures that have to be adopted in the event of the patient vomiting or being incontinent can be discontinued. The card also states where to obtain help and advice related to the patient's diagnostic investigation.
• Monitor hands at end of procedure and before leaving the room.	To check for possible radioactive contamination.
• Monitor the room for radioactive contamination at the end of each day or if contamination may have occurred.	To establish whether contamination has occurred.
4 Avoid urine, faecal and blood sample collection for laboratories other than nuclear medicine, for 24 hours. If collection is unavoidable, a radiation warning sticker must be attached to the specimen and request card, and the specimen taken to the laboratory under the supervision of the physics departmental staff (see Ch. 39, Specimen collection).	To prevent contamination of the laboratory and its staff, as specimens taken within 24 hours of some scans may contain radioactivity.
5 Avoid bone marrow and stem cell harvests for 24 hours. Seek advice from the physics department.	Cells may contain radioactivity.
6 Seek advice from physics staff if the patient is to undergo a procedure in the operating theatre within 24 hours of a scan.	To prevent theatre equipment from becoming contaminated with radioactivity.
7 Place soiled bed linen used within the first 24 hours of certain scans, e.g. bone scan, within a purple plastic bag and inform the physics departmental staff.	To prevent contamination of the environment.

Procedure guidelines: **Emergency procedures**

In an emergency, the safety and medical care of the patient must take precedence over any potential radiation hazards to staff. Written radiation safety instructions must be available in all radiation areas where an emergency may arise. These instructions must contain a detailed description of how to manage a patient in the event of a medical emergency and the action required in other emergency situations, such as fire. The course of action in an emergency procedure depends on local circumstances and the nature of the emergency.

An incident occurring within the first 24 hours of iodine-131 being administered is obviously a greater hazard than a similar incident on the day of discharge. Movement of the patient to other wards or areas, e.g. X-ray or CCU, must only be undertaken following the physics department's advice.

Procedure guidelines: Emergency procedures (cont'd)

Major spillage of radioactive body fluids, i.e. incontinence and/or vomiting

	Action	Rationale
1	Inform the physics department immediately.	So that the physics department can advise on radiation protection as soon as possible.
2	If physics department staff are not immediately available, use a radiation monitor to assess the extent of the spillage.	To define extent of contamination and determine what further measures need to be taken.
3	Put some absorbent material on top of all the radioactive wet area.	To absorb contamination.
4	Any waste that cannot be flushed down the toilet or macerated must be placed in a purple polythene bag and the physics staff informed.	To prevent contamination of the environment.
5	Follow the advice of the physics department staff in clearing the spillage.	To prevent spread of contamination.

Contamination of bare hands

	Action	Rationale
1	Wash hands in warm soapy water, paying special attention to the areas around the fingernails, between the fingers and on the outer edges of the hands. Continue washing until contamination is below the permissible limits indicated by local monitoring protocols.	To remove radioactive material from any areas where it might be trapped.
2	If the skin is broken in a contamination accident, wash thoroughly under running water, opening the edges of the cut. This should be continued until physics department staff can demonstrate that no residual radioactivity remains in the wound.	To stimulate bleeding and permit thorough flushing of the cut.

Death

	Action	Rationale
1	Inform the physics department immediately.	So that the physics department staff can begin making the necessary arrangements for removal of the body to the mortuary.
2	Two nurses wearing gloves, plastic aprons, gowns and overshoes should perform last offices. All orifices must be packed carefully. Any vomit, blood, faeces or urine must be cleaned from the body.	To avoid contamination with body fluids. Minimal handling of the body reduces the risk of contamination.
3	The body should be totally enclosed in a plastic body bag.	To avoid contamination of the porters and the mortuary staff.
4	Transfer of the body should be arranged with the physics department.	The physics department will supervise the transfer of the body.

Cardiac arrest

	Action	Rationale
1	The switchboard must be told to inform the physics department as soon as possible after alerting the emergency resuscitation team.	So that the physics department can advise on radiation protection as soon as possible.
2	Do not use mouth-to-mouth resuscitation. All areas must be supplied with an Ambu bag for this purpose.	Mouth-to-mouth contact could result in contamination of the resuscitator.
3	Overshoes, gloves and gowns must be put on as soon as it is practically possible.	To minimize personal contamination.

Procedure guidelines: **Emergency procedures** *(cont'd)*

Action	Rationale
4 All emergency equipment must be monitored and decontaminated as necessary before being returned to general use.	To prevent contaminated equipment leaving the controlled area.

Fire

1 Every effort should be made to contact the physics department without compromising the patient's safety.	To help in the evacuation of the patients treated with iodine-131.
2 Following evacuation, patients treated with iodine-131 should be kept at a distance from other patients and staff.	To minimize exposure of others to radiation.

References and further reading

Barry, L. *et al.* (1990) Radioiodinated metaiodobenzylguanidine (MIBG) in the management of neuroblastomas. In: *Neuroblastoma Tumor Biology and Therapy* (ed. C. Pochedly). CRC Press, Boston.

Beasley, N.J., Lee, J., Eski, S. *et al.* (2002) Impact of nodal metastases on prognosis in patients with well-differentiated thyroid cancer. *Arch Otolaryngol Head Neck Surg*, **128**(7), 825–8.

Bigner, D.D., Brown, M.T., Coleman, R.E. *et al.* (1995) Phase 1 studies of treatment of malignant gliomas and neoplastic meningitis with 131-I radiolabelled monoclonal antibodies anti-tenascin 81C6 and anti-chondroitin proteoglycan sulfate Mel-14F[ab'] 2 – a preliminary report. *J Neuro-Oncol*, **24**(1), 109–22.

Bomanji, J.B., Britton, K.E. & Clarke, S.E.M. (1995) *Oncology, Clinicians' Guide in Nuclear Medicine* (ed. P.J. Ell). British Nuclear Medicine Society, London.

BTA/RCP (British Thyroid Association/Royal College of Physicians) (2002) *Guidelines for the Management of Thyroid Cancer in Adults*. Royal College of Physicians, London.

Clark, S.E.M. (1998) Radioiodine therapy of the thyroid. In: *Nuclear Medicine in Clinical Diagnosis and Treatment*, 2nd edn (eds I.P.C. Murray & P.J. Ell). Churchill Livingstone, Edinburgh.

Cokgor, I., Akabani, G., Kuan, C.T. *et al.* (2000) Phase 1 trial results of iodine-131 labelled antitenascin monoclonal antibody 81c6 treatment of patients with newly diagnosed malignant gliomas. *J Clin Oncol*, **18**(22), 3862–72.

Cormack, J., Towson, J.E.C. & Flower, M.A. (1998) Radiation protection and dosimetry in clinical practice. In: *Nuclear Medicine in Clinical Diagnosis and Treatment*, 2nd edn (eds I.P.C. Murray & P.J. Ell). Churchill Livingstone, Edinburgh.

De Klerk, J.M. *et al.* (1994) Evaluation of thrombocytopenia in patients treated with rhenium-186-HEDP: guidelines for individual dosage recommendations. *J Nucl Med*, **35**(9), 1423–8.

De Klerk, J.M. *et al.* (1996) Bone marrow absorbed dose of rhenium-186 HEDP and the relationship with decreased platelet counts. *J Nucl Med*, **37**(1), 38–41.

Di Lorenzo, G., Autorino, R., Ciardiella, F. *et al.* (2003) External beam radiotherapy in bone metastatic prostate cancer: impact on patient's pain relief and quality of life. *Oncol Rep*, **10**(2), 399–404.

DoH (1999) *The Ionising Regulations No. 3232*. Stationery Office, London.

DoH (2000) *The Ionising Radiation (Medical Exposure) Regulations No. 1059*. Stationery Office, London.

Fielding, S.L. *et al.* (1991) Dosimetry of 131-I mIBG for treatment of resistant neuroblastoma: results of a UK study. *Eur J Nucl Med*, **18**, 308–16.

Hammoud, M.A., Sawaya, R., Shi, W. *et al.* (1996) Prognostic significance of preoperative MRI scans in glioblastoma multiforme. *J Neuro Oncol*, **27**(1), 65–73.

Harmer, C.L. (1996) Radiotherapy in the management of thyroid cancer. *Ann Acad Med Singapore*, **25**(3), 413–19.

Hoefnagel, C.A. & Lewington, V.J. (1998) mIBG therapy. In: *Nuclear Medicine in Clinical Diagnosis and Treatment*, 2nd edn (eds I.P.C. Murray & P.J. Ell). Churchill Livingstone, Edinburgh.

Hoefnagel, C.A., De Kraker, J., Valdes Olmos, R.A. & Voute, P.A. (1995) 131-I mIBG as a first line treatment in advanced neuroblastoma. *J Nucl Med*, **39**(4), Suppl 1, 61–4.

Horwich, A. (ed.) (1995) *Oncology: A Multidisciplinary Textbook*. Chapman & Hall Medical, London.

IPEM/RCN (Institute of Physics and Engineering in Medicine/Royal College of Nursing) (2002) Procedures involving radiation. In: *Ionising Radiation Safety. A Handbook for Nurses*. York Publishing, York, pp. 17–32.

Jemal, A., Thomas, A., Murray, T. & Thun, M. (2002) Cancer statistics 2002. *CA Cancer J Clin*, **52**(1), 23–47.

Kamm, B.L. (1999) Current techniques in sentinel node mapping. *Radiol Technol*, **70**(4), 323–33.

Kellar, S.J. (2001) Sentinel lymph node biopsy for breast cancer. *AORN*, **74**(2), 197–201.

Kendall-Taylor, P. (2002) Managing differentiated thyroid cancer. *Br Med J*, **324**(7344), 988–9.

Kucuk, N.O., Ibis, E., Aras, G. *et al.* (2000) Palliative analgesic effects of Re-186 HEDP in various cancer patients with bone metastases. *Ann Nucl Med*, **14**(4), 239–45.

Lashford, L.S., Hancock, J.P. & Kemshead, J.T. (1991) Metaiodobenzylguanidine (Mibg) update and storage in the human neuroblastoma cell line SK-N-BE(2C). *Int J Cancer*, **47**(1), 105–9.

Leung, P.M. & Nikolic, M. (1998) Disposal of therapeutic 131-I waste using a multiple holding tank system. *Health Phys*, **75**(3), 315–21.

Martin, A. & Harbinson, S. (1997) *An Introduction to Radiation Protection*. Chapman & Hall Medical, London.

Matthay, K., Panina, C., Huberty, J. *et al.* (2001) Correlation of tumor and whole body dosimetry with tumor response and toxicity in refractory neuroblastoma treated with (131)I-mIBG. *J Nucl Med*, **42**(11), 1713–21.

Maurer, A.H. (1998) Gastrointestinal bleeding. In: *Nuclear Medicine in Clinical Diagnosis and Treatment*, 2nd edn (eds I.P.C. Murray & P.J. Ell). Churchill Livingstone, Edinburgh.

Maxon, H.R. *et al.* (1992) Rhenium-186 hydroxyethylidene diphosphonate for the treatment of painful osseous metastases. *Semin Nucl Med*, **22**(1), 33–40.

Mazzaferri, E.L. & Jhiang, S.M. (1994) Long term impact of initial surgical and medical therapy on papillary and follicular thyroid cancer. *Am J Med*, **97**(5), 418–28.

McEwan, A.J. (1997) Unsealed source therapy of painful bone metastases: an update. *Semin Nucl Med*, **27**(2), 165–82.

McEwan, A.J. (1998) Palliation of bone pain. In: *Nuclear Medicine in Clinical Diagnosis and Treatment*, 2nd edn (eds I.P.C. Murray & P.J. Ell). Churchill Livingstone, Edinburgh.

McEwan, A.J. (2000) Use of radionuclides for the palliation of bone metastases. *Semin Radiat Oncol*, **10**(2), 103–14.

Meller, S. (1997) Targeted radiotherapy for neuroblastoma. *Arch Dis Child*, **77**(5), 389–91.

Mosely, R.P., Davies, A.G., Richardson, R.B. *et al.* (1990) Intrathecal administration of 131-I radiolabelled monoclonal antibody as a treatment for neoplastic meningitis. *Br J Cancer*, **62**(4), 637–42.

Murray, I.P.C. (1998) Bone scintigraphy: the procedure and interpretation. In: *Nuclear Medicine in Clinical Diagnosis and Treatment*, 2nd edn (eds I.P.C. Murray & P.J. Ell). Churchill Livingstone, Edinburgh.

Nowotnik, D.P. (1995) *Textbook of Radiopharmacy*, 2nd edn (ed. C.B. Sampson). Gordon and Breach, Switzerland, pp. 40–1.

O'Doherty, M.J. & Coakley, T.J. (1998a) Parathyroid imaging. In: *Nuclear Medicine in Clinical Diagnosis and Treatment*, 2nd edn (eds I.P.C. Murray & P.J. Ell). Churchill Livingstone, Edinburgh.

O'Doherty, M.J. & Coakley, A.J. (1998b) Drug therapy alternatives in the treatment of thyroid cancer. *Drugs*, **55**(6), 801–812.

Oei, H.Y. (1998) Dynamic and static renal imaging. In: *Nuclear Medicine in Clinical Diagnosis and Treatment*, 2nd edn (eds I.P.C. Murray & P.J. Ell). Churchill Livingstone, Edinburgh.

Okuyama, C., Ushijima, Y., Kubota, T. *et al.* (2002) Utility of follow up studies using meta-[123-I]iodobenzylguanidine scintigraphy for detecting recurrent neuroblastoma. *Nucl Med Commun*, **23**(7), 663–72.

O'Sullivan, J.M., McCready, V.R., Flux, G. *et al.* (2002). High activity Rhenium-HEDP with autologous peripheral blood stem rescue: a phase I study in progressive hormone refractory prostate cancer metastatic to bone. *Br J Cancer*, **86**(11), 1715–20.

Owunwanne, A., Patel M. & Sadek, S. (1995) *The Handbook of Radiopharmaceuticals*. Chapman & Hall Medical, London, pp. 73–6.

Pacini, F., Capezzone, M., Elisei, R. *et al.* (2002) Diagnostic 131-iodine whole body scan may be avoided in thyroid cancer patients who have undetectable stimulated serum Tg levels after initial treatment. *J Clin Endocrinol Metabol*, **87**(4), 1499–501.

Palla, A., Tumeh, S.S. & Giuntini, C. (1995) Perfusion lung imaging. In: *Principles and Practice of Nuclear Medicine* (eds P.J. Early & D.B. Sodee). Mosby, St Louis.

Pennell, D.J. (1998) Cardiac stress. In: *Nuclear Medicine in Clinical Diagnosis and Treatment*, 2nd edn (eds I.P.C. Murray & P.J. Ell). Churchill Livingstone, Edinburgh.

Perkins, A.C. (1995) *Nuclear Medicine Science and Safety*. John Libby, London.

Pointon, R.C.S. (1991) *The Radiotherapy of Malignant Disease*. Springer, London.

RIDDOR (1995) *The Reporting of Injuries, Diseases and Dangerous Occurrences Regulations*. HMSO, London.

Rietbergen, J.B., Hoedemaeker, R.F., Kruger, A.E. *et al.* (1999) The changing pattern of prostate cancer at the time of diagnosis. Characteristics of screen detected prostate cancer in a population based screening study. *J Urol*, **161**(4), 1192–8.

Rigo, P. & Braot, S.H. (1998) Radiopharmaceuticals for the study of the heart. In: *Nuclear Medicine in Clinical Diagnosis and Treatment*, 2nd edn (eds I.P.C. Murray & P.J. Ell). Churchill Livingstone, Edinburgh.

Russell, C. (1998) Measurement and interpretation of renal transit times. In: *Nuclear Medicine in Clinical Diagnosis and Treatment*, 2nd edn (eds I.P.C. Murray & P.J. Ell). Churchill Livingstone, Edinburgh.

Scher, H.I. (2002) Prostate carcinoma. *Cancer*, **97**(S3), 758–71.

Serafini, A.N. (2001) Therapy of metastatic bone pain. *J Nucl Med*, **42**(6), 895–906.

Shapiro, B., Fig. L., Gross, B. *et al.* (1999) Neuroendocrine tumours. In: *Nuclear Oncology* (eds B. Shapiro, L. Fig & B. Gross). Springer, Berlin.

Sharp, C., Shrimpton, J.A. & Bury, R.F. (1998) *Diagnostic Medical Exposures: Advice on Exposure to Ionising Radiation During Pregnancy*. National Radiological Protection Board, Didcot.

Shulkin, B.L. & Shapiro, B. (1990) Radioiodinated MIBG in the management of neuroblastoma. In: *Neuroblastoma Tumor Biology and Therapy* (ed. C. Pochedly). CRC Press, Boston.

Smart, R.C. (1998) Intestines evaluation of absorption. In: *Nuclear Medicine in Clinical Diagnosis and Treatment*, 2nd edn (eds I.P.C. Murray & P.J. Ell). Churchill Livingstone, Edinburgh.

Spillane, A.J. & Sacks, N.P. (2000) Role of axillary surgery in early breast cancer: review of the current evidence. *Aust NZ J Surg*, **70**(7), 515–24.

Stajduhar, K.I., Neithercut, J., Chu, E. *et al.* (2000) Thyroid cancer: patients' experience of receiving iodine-131 therapy. *Oncol Nurs Forum*, **27**(8), 1213–18.

Stites, D.P. & Terr, A.I. (1991) *The Basis of Human Immunology*. Prentice-Hall International, London.

Testa, H.J. & Prescott, M.C. (1996) *Nephrourology, Clinician's Guide in Nuclear Medicine* (ed. P.J. Ell). British Nuclear Medicine Society, London.

Thompson, M.A. (2001) Radiation safety precautions in the management of the hospitalized 131-I therapy patient. *Nucl Med Technol*, **29**(2), 61–6.

Valdes Olmos, R.A. (1998) Functional analysis of cancer therapy effects in other organs. In: *Nuclear Medicine in Clinical Diagnosis and Treatment*, 2nd edn (eds I.P.C. Murray & P.J. Ell). Churchill Livingstone, Edinburgh.

Van der Wall, H. & McLaughlin, A.F. (1998) Gallium scintigraphy in tumor diagnosis and management. In: *Nuclear Medicine in Clinical Diagnosis and Treatment*, 2nd edn (eds I.P.C. Murray & P.J. Ell). Churchill Livingstone, Edinburgh.

Walker, B. & Jarritt, P. (1998) Basic physics of nuclear medicine. In: *Nuclear Medicine in Clinical Diagnosis and Treatment*, 2nd edn (eds I.P.C. Murray & P.J. Ell). Churchill Livingstone, Edinburgh.

Wootton, R. (1993) *Radiation Protection of Patients*. Cambridge University Press, Cambridge.

Zack, E. (2001) Sentinel lymph node biopsy in breast cancer: scientific rational and patient care. *Oncol Nurs Forum*, **28**(6), 997–1005.

36

Renal replacement therapy: peritoneal dialysis and continuous venovenous haemodiafiltration

Chapter contents

Definition

Renal replacement therapies such as peritoneal dialysis, haemodialysis and continuous filtration methods are interventions used when patients have inadequate renal function and can no longer filter the blood and excrete waste products. This malfunction may be temporary, as in acute renal failure, or permanent when patients are in end-stage renal failure (ESRF).

Reference material

In health the kidneys are the main excretory organ of the body. Every day they filter approximately 200 litres of fluid from the blood. This fluid contains toxins, metabolic waste and excess ions and leaves the body as urine. As the kidneys excrete this fluid they are maintaining the volume and electrolyte balance of the blood by balancing water and salts, and the pH of the blood by balancing acids and bases (Marieb 2001).

When renal replacement therapy is required the kidneys are temporarily replaced by using an alternative membrane or filter. In peritoneal dialysis (PD) the membrane used is the peritoneum itself; in all other forms of renal replacement therapy an artificial membrane or filter is used. Therefore renal replacement therapies may be instituted when the patient is in ESRF, the main causes of which are diabetes, uncontrolled hypertension, glomerulonephritis, polycystic kidney disease and trauma (Marieb 2001). For ESRF the therapies of choice will be transplant, where possible, haemodialysis or PD.

In the setting of a critical illness acute renal failure can be caused by a number of insults to the body, including sepsis, nephrotoxic drugs or other compounds, severe burns, hypovolaemic shock, tumour lysis syndrome and multiorgan failure (Block & Manning 2002). When the patient is critically ill and in acute renal failure haemodynamic instability is common and life threatening so the treatment of choice in this setting is continuous venovenous haemodiafiltration (CVVHDF) (Toft *et al.* 1999).

Types of renal replacement therapy

There are three main types of therapy available:

- Haemodialysis
- Peritoneal dialysis
- Continuous filtration and diafiltration methods.

The choice of therapy will depend first on whether the patient's kidneys are likely to recover and second on their current condition. If the patient is in ESRF then the optimum therapy is a renal transplant; however, the need for organs constantly outpaces the supply and many patients require haemodialysis while they are awaiting a transplant (Briggs *et al.* 1997). Haemodialysis is usually performed 2–3 times a week either in a regional renal centre or in the patient's home. The patient is connected up to a renal dialysis machine via an arteriovenous shunt which is formed usually between the artery and vein at their wrist (Marieb 2001). For these patients each day's treatment takes about 4–8 hours and patients have to adhere to a special diet and a restricted fluid intake (Oreopoulos 1998).

Many patients elect to utilize PD as opposed to haemodialysis in the chronic setting as when it is working effectively, it has less impact on their quality of life than haemodialysis. As PD and the slow continuous filtration methods of renal replacement therapy are used outside specialist centres, they will be described in greater detail.

Peritoneal dialysis (PD)

Indications

Patients and their clinicians may select PD for the following reasons:

- Widespread availability
- Technical simplicity
- The greater stability of biochemical parameters
- The use of continuous ambulatory peritoneal dialysis (CAPD) devices means that the patient can remain ambulant, at home and achieve greater independence (Oreopoulos 1998)
- Because the patient can use PD every day or every night, they have greater freedom with diet and fluid intake and often feel better (CANUSA 1996)
- Low maintenance costs mean this is an affordable treatment in most health care settings (CANUSA 1996).

However comparison studies on survival, morbidity, hospitalization and quality of life between patients receiving haemodialysis and CAPD have not been able to demonstrate significant differences. Local circumstances and the patient's individual clinical needs should therefore be addressed in deciding which therapy to choose (Selgas *et al.* 2001).

Reference material

In 1926 Rosenak, basing his work on that of Ganter, saw the possibility of using the peritoneum of humans as a dialysing membrane (Blumenkrantz & Roberts 1979). Gunther is described as the first to introduce 2 litres of fluid into the peritoneal cavity of a patient with acute renal failure (Oreopoulos 1998). The use of PD steadily increased and in 1959 came the introduction of commercial dialysis solutions and tubing. The 1960s saw advances made in the catheters designed by Tenckhoff, thus ensuring the long-term access needs of patients on PD. The technique of CAPD is attributed to Popovich *et al.* (1978). In the middle to late 1980s the Italian group described the use of the Y set for PD, a technique that, whilst modified, is still widely used today (Buoncristiani 1989). In the 1990s the first papers were published highlighting that malnutrition is a significant problem for over 40% of patients on CAPD (Jones 1994; CANUSA 1996).

In the late 1980s the technique of haemodialysis had been introduced and towards the late 1990s the first papers comparing outcomes from the two techniques were published (Bloembergen *et al.* 1995; Fenton *et al.* 1997; Selgas *et al.* 2001). Finally between 1997 and 2000 the first standardized guidelines for the treatment of PD were developed. These clinical practice guidelines bring together the work of many expert groups under the auspices of the National Kidney Foundation of the United States and cover areas such as haemodialysis, PD, vascular access, anaemia and nutrition (KDOQI 2000).

Anatomy and physiology

The peritoneum in the abdominopelvic cavity is the most extensive of the body's serous membranes. In adults it has a surface area of approximately $2.2\,\text{m}^2$. The peritoneum consists of two layers:

- The visceral peritoneum that covers the surface of most of the digestive organs
- The parietal peritoneum that lines the body wall.

Although the peritoneum has these two layers they are continuous with each other and surround the peritoneal cavity. The peritoneal cavity is a narrow potential

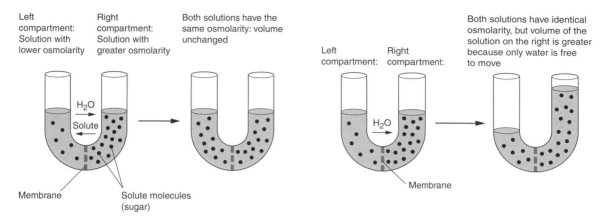

Figure 36.1 Influence of membrane permeability on diffusion and osmosis. (a) Membrane permeable to both solute molecules and water. (b) Membrane impermeable to solute molecules, permeable to water. (Redrawn from Marieb 2001, with permission.)

space containing fluid secreted by the serous membranes. This serous fluid is used to lubricate the mobile digestive organs, allowing them to glide easily across one another and along the body wall as they perform their digestive functions. The visceral peritoneum is formed of areolar connective tissue covered with mesothelium, which is a single layer of squamous epithelial cells (Marieb 2001).

The process of osmosis and diffusion and solution concentrations

Osmosis is the process by which a solvent such as water diffuses through a selectively permeable membrane. Osmosis will occur whenever the water concentration is different on either side of the membrane. When the concentration on either side of the membrane is equal, osmosis will cease.

Diffusion refers to the tendency of molecules or solutes to scatter evenly throughout their environment. All molecules possess kinetic energy and are in constant motion. Molecules generally move away from areas where they are in higher concentrations to areas where their concentration is lower. Therefore molecules diffuse along their concentration gradient.

Finally filtration is the process by which water and solutes are forced through a membrane by fluid or hydrostatic pressure (Marieb 2001) (see Fig. 36.1).

All types of renal replacement therapy rely on osmosis, diffusion and to some degree filtration.

The osmotic pressure of dextrose is utilized in PD to remove water and solutes from the patient. The composition of most commercially available peritoneal dialysis solutions falls into one of the following three groups.

1 The solution's electrolyte content approximates to normal extracellular fluid, i.e. its potassium concentration is 4 mmol/l and its glucose concentration is 1.3–1.5%.
2 As solution 1, but contains no potassium.
3 Hypertonic solution with a glucose concentration of 6.3% and the same potassium concentration as solution 1.

The ideal PD solution is one that does not affect the structure and function of the peritoneum. Research into new solutions has focused on two areas: an improved more biocompatible osmotic agent, and a better pH and buffer (Mahon 2002). A new two-chamber solution bag has recently been developed with the top chamber containing a solution of dextrose, calcium chloride and magnesium chloride. The bottom chamber contains a solution of sodium bicarbonate, sodium lactate and sodium chloride. When the seal between the two chambers is broken the contents are mixed together and can be infused into the patient. Decisions concerning which solutions to use will depend on the clinical needs of the patient and whether they are sensitive to lactate buffered solutions (Carrasco et al. 2001; Mahon 2002).

Dialysis cycle

Normally, a cycle consists of three steps (Fig. 36.2).

Step 1 (inflow)

The dialysis solution at body temperature is infused into the peritoneal cavity to initiate the dialysis. The fluid infuses by gravity and its rate can be controlled by raising or lowering the container in relation to the patient's abdomen or by releasing or compressing the occluding clamp on the tubing.

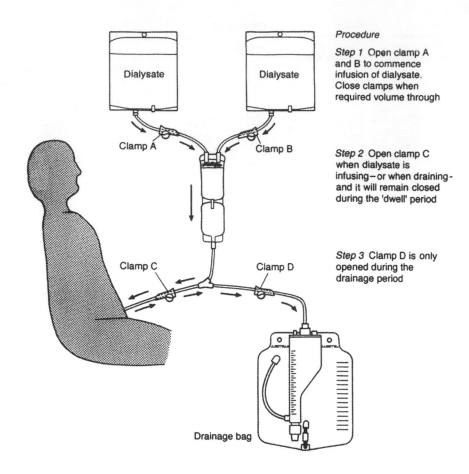

Dialysate

Dialysate

Clamp A

Clamp B

Clamp C

Clamp D

Drainage bag

Procedure

Step 1 Open clamp A and B to commence infusion of dialysate. Close clamps when required volume through

Step 2 Open clamp C when dialysate is infusing – or when draining – and it will remain closed during the 'dwell' period

Step 3 Clamp D is only opened during the drainage period

Figure 36.2 Using the Y-type administration set for peritoneal dialysis.

Step 2 (dwell time)

The dwell time is the time that the fluid remains in the peritoneal cavity to allow for equilibration. Different dwell times may be established to remove substances of differing molecular weights. The dwell time is relevant to the molecular weight of the solute and how much needs to be removed.

Step 3 (drainage)

The drainage stage is that of emptying the equilibrated solution from the peritoneal cavity to complete dialysis or to prepare for the infusion of fresh solution. Drainage is also dependent on gravity.

Technique

In PD the patient's own peritoneum is used as the dialysing membrane. A cuffed long-dwelling dialysis catheter is introduced into the lower abdomen through the rectus muscle and is secured with three purse-string sutures (Stegmayr 2002). A Y set is then connected to the dialysis catheter and iso-osmotic fluid is introduced

into the peritoneal cavity. The fluid is left to equilibrate for 15–60 minutes in acute therapy and several hours in chronic treatments; this is known as the 'dwell time'. The fluid is then allowed to drain out through the same dialysis catheter and the procedure is repeated. The cycles are repeated until the patient's blood biochemistry has returned to agreed parameters. For PD to achieve maximum efficacy, fresh solutions must be instilled at equilibration to prevent reabsorption of water and uraemic toxins (Marieb 2001).

Continuous renal replacement therapy (CRRT)

Reference material

The use of CRRT has increased markedly since the late 1980s with advances in technology that have ensured safe user-friendly devices. In many critical care units CRRT can now be provided by critical care or appropriately trained nurses. The main advantage of CRRT for the

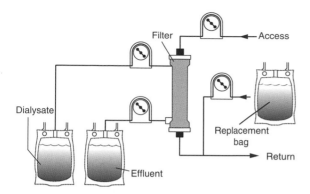

Figure 36.3 Continuous haemodiafiltration provides solute and fluid removal by diffusion and convection. The integral blood pump means that high-volume ultrafiltration is achieved. Diafiltration is achieved by infusing dialysate countercurrent to blood.

acutely ill patient is its ability to provide excellent clearance of solutes and water whilst avoiding the haemodynamic instability that can result from haemodialysis, although more research is needed in this area (Kellum *et al.* 2002). CRRT can also be instituted in a patient who has a lowered mean arterial pressure, a condition which is common in critical care. Finally with the newer CRRT devices, critical care nurses can safely institute and monitor therapy.

Continuous arteriovenous haemofiltration (CAVH) and continuous venovenous haemodiafiltration (CVVHDF) are used more than the filtration methods, with CVVHDF being the most common as it has the advantage that only one vessel needs to be cannulated. As CVVHDF is the therapy with the widest application to a variety of clinical situations, it is examined in greater detail here.

CVVHDF

CVVHDF combines convection and diffusion. The convection of ultrafiltration utilizes a large hydrostatic pressure gradient which means that 1–2 litres of fluid an hour can be removed from the patient via the filter. Removal of the solutes (i.e. urea, creatinine and potassium) is achieved by blood flow through the filter, while

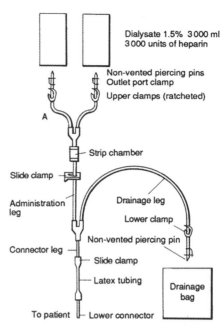

Figure 36.4 Peritoneal dialysis system set-up. (Courtesy of Abbott Renal Care.)

dialysate is administered in a countercurrent flow (Murray & Hall 2000) (Fig. 36.3).

Manufacturers of CRRT devices supply biocompatible filters with different clearance specificities. Generally the filters clear molecules with small and medium size molecular weights but there are high-flux filters being tested which may be useful in the treatment of severe sepsis (Cole *et al.* 2001).

Because the patient's blood flows through an extracorporeal circuit and over a filter, there is a danger of blood clotting in the circuit. Unless the patient is auto-anticoagulated, an anticoagulant should be administered continuously.

Note: because the filters used in CVVHDF filter out some drugs it is essential to calculate concomitant drug therapy utilizing the literature available (Tsubo *et al.* 2001). Some drugs are effectively cleared by the filter while others are only partially cleared (Pittrow & Penk 1998; Bunn & Ashley 1999).

Procedure guidelines: **Peritoneal dialysis (see Fig. 36.4)**

Equipment

1 Dialysis Y-type administration set and drainage bag.
2 Sterile paracentesis abdominus set containing forceps, scalpel, topical swabs, towels, suturing equipment.

3 Sterile gown, gloves.
4 Peritoneal catheter stylet or trocar and drainage bag.
5 Local anaesthetic (1–2% lidocaine).

Procedure guidelines: Peritoneal dialysis (cont'd)

6 Syringe, needle.
7 Chlorhexidine in 70% alcohol.

8 Supplementary drugs as prescribed.
9 Peritoneal dialysis fluid, as prescribed, warmed to 36°C.

Procedure

Action	Rationale
1 Explain and discuss the procedure with the patient. An acutely ill patient may be confused and restless, but every effort should be made to ensure the patient is informed.	To ensure that the patient understands the procedure and gives his/her valid consent. Some hospitals require a patient to sign a consent form before the procedure can be carried out.
2 Ask the patient to micturate and defecate before the procedure begins.	To avoid perforation of the bladder and/or rectum when the trocar is introduced into the peritoneum.
3 Record the patient's vital signs before the procedure begins.	To assess physical/psychological state and to monitor changes.
4 Weigh the patient before the procedure begins and then daily.	To assess hydration and to monitor any fluid losses.
5 Assist the patient to lie in the semi-recumbent position.	To ensure that the patient is in the safest position for the insertion of the trocar.
6 Continue to observe and reassure the patient throughout the procedure.	To assess and monitor any physical/psychological changes.
7 Assist the doctor as required.	To facilitate a smooth and effective procedure for the patient.

Insertion of catheter

Action	Rationale
1 Using aseptic technique, the abdomen is prepared and local anaesthetic injected subcutaneously.	To reduce the risk of contamination and infection. To minimize the pain of the incision.
2 A small incision is made in the abdominal wall 3–5 cm below the umbilicus. The trocar is inserted through the incision. The patient is asked to raise their head from the pillow after the trocar is introduced.	This tightens the abdominal muscles and permits easier penetration of the trocar without danger of injury to the internal organs.
3 When the peritoneum is punctured, the trocar is directed to the left side of the pelvis. The stylet is removed and the catheter is inserted through the trocar and gently manoeuvred into position.	To prevent the omentum from adhering to the catheter or occluding its opening.
4 Once the trocar is removed, the skin may be sutured and a sterile dressing placed around the catheter.	To prevent the loss of the catheter in the abdomen. To prevent leakage of peritoneal fluid onto the surrounding skin.
5 The tubing is flushed with the dialysis fluid.	To prevent air from entering the peritoneal cavity.

Preparation of dialysis fluid

Action	Rationale
1 Wash hands with bactericidal soap and water or bactericidal alcohol handrub. Proceed using aseptic technique.	To reduce risk of infection.
2 The dialysis fluid should have been warmed to body temperature (36°C).	For the patient's comfort. To prevent abdominal pain. Heating causes dilatation of the peritoneal vessels and increases clearance of urea. Cold fluid would decrease rate of removal of large molecular solutes and can cause abdominal cramp pain.
3 Add any drugs, e.g. heparin, to the dialysis fluid if prescribed.	Heparin prevents fibrin clots from occluding the catheter.
4 Attach the dialysis fluid to the administration set via Luer–Lok connections.	
5 Attach the administration set to the catheter connection.	

*Procedure guidelines: **Peritoneal dialysis** (cont'd)*

Action	Rationale
6 Allow the dialysis fluid to flow freely into the peritoneal cavity. (This normally takes from 5 to 10 minutes.)	To ascertain whether the catheter is in the required position. The flow should be steady and brisk. If not, the tip of the catheter may be buried in the omentum or it may have been occluded by a blood clot.
7 Allow fluid to remain in the peritoneal cavity for the prescribed time. Prepare the next exchange while the first container of fluid is in the peritoneal cavity.	The fluid must remain in the peritoneal cavity for the prescribed dwell time so that potassium, urea and other waste products may be removed. The solution is most effective over the first 5–10 minutes when the concentration gradient is at its greatest (De Fijter *et al.* 1994).
8 Unclamp the peritoneal drainage tube. Drainage time will vary with each patient but, on average, should be completed in 10 minutes.	To rid the body of the required products. The abdomen is drained by a siphon effect through the closed system. Drainage is normally straw-coloured.
9 Clamp off the drainage tube when outflow ceases and begin infusing the next exchange, again using aseptic technique.	To enable the next cycle to begin. To reduce the risk of local and/or systemic infection.
10 Record the following: (a) Time of commencement and completion of each exchange and the start and finish of the drainage stage (b) Amount of fluid infused and recovered (c) Fluid balance after each complete exchange (d) Any medication added to the dialysis fluid.	To detect and monitor trends and fluctuations and to identify any outflow obstruction.
11 Take and record the vital signs: (a) Blood pressure and pulse every 15 minutes during the first exchange and hourly thereafter, depending on the patient's condition. (b) Temperature every 4 hours, or more frequently if condition demands.	Hypotension may be indicative of excessive fluid loss due to the glucose concentration of the dialysis fluid. Changes in pulse may indicate impending shock or overhydration. To monitor for any signs of infection. Infection is more likely to become evident after dialysis has been discontinued.
12 Record fluid balance accurately.	To prevent complications such as circulatory overload and hypertension that may occur if most of the fluid is not recovered during the drainage stage. The fluid balance should be about even or show slight fluid loss, unless the reason for treatment was to remove excess fluid.
13 Dialysis is usually continued until blood chemistry levels are satisfactory.	The duration of dialysis is related to the severity of the condition and the size and weight of the patient. The usual time is about 12–36 hours, giving between 24 and 28 exchanges.
14 Ensure that the patient is comfortable during dialysis by attending to pressure area care and altering the patient's position as required. Assist the patient to sit in a chair for short periods as their condition allows.	The period of dialysis is lengthy and often exhausts the patient.
15 Send a daily specimen of peritoneal fluid for microscopy and culture.	To monitor for any infections.

Problem solving

Problem	Cause	Suggested action
Peritonitis, indicated by fever, persistent abdominal pain and cramping, abdominal fullness, abdominal rigidity, slow dialysis	Poor aseptic technique during catheter insertion or dialysis, or poor nutritional/ immune state.	If peritonitis is suspected, notify the doctor immediately. Send a peritoneal fluid sample to the laboratory for fluid analysis, culture and sensitivity testing,

Problem solving (cont'd)

Problem	Cause	Suggested action
drainage, cloudy and offensive-smelling drainage, swelling and tenderness around the catheter and increased white blood cell count.		Gram staining and cell count. Antibiotics may be prescribed by the doctor either locally or systemically in severe cases. Monitor vital signs; careful pain control is required.
Infection at the site of entry, indicated by redness, swelling, rigidity, tenderness and purulent drainage around the catheter.	Poor aseptic technique during catheter insertion or dialysis, or incomplete healing around the site of entry.	Notify a doctor. Obtain a specimen of the drainage fluid and send it to the laboratory. Antibiotics and pain control may be prescribed as above. Monitor vital signs.
Subcutaneous tunnel infection with cuffed catheter indicated by redness, rigidity and tenderness over subcutaneous tunnel.	Poor aseptic technique during catheter insertion or dialysis, or incomplete healing in subcutaneous tunnel.	Notify a doctor. Antibiotics may be prescribed as above. Monitor vital signs.
Perforation of the bladder or the bowel, indicated by signs and symptoms of peritonitis, bright yellow dialysis fluid drainage (if bladder is perforated) or faeces in drainage (if bowel is perforated).	Catheter inserted when the patient had a full bladder or bowel.	If perforation is suspected, stop dialysis and notify a doctor immediately. Monitor vital signs. Only minimal oral fluids should be given in case surgery is required.
Bleeding through the catheter.	Minor trauma to the abdomen or minor trauma to the subcutaneous tunnel (with a cuffed catheter) or perforation of a major abdominal blood vessel during surgery.	Bleeding usually stops spontaneously. If it does not, notify the doctor, who may order blood transfusions. One-litre hourly dialysis exchanges may be ordered until the drainage fluid is clear.
Dialysis fluid leaking around the catheter.	Excessive instillation of dialysis fluid. Incomplete healing around the cuff of the catheter. Catheter obstruction. Catheter dislodged or positioned improperly.	Instil less dialysis fluid at exchanges. Drain the patient's abdomen completely during outflow. Use small volumes of dialysis fluid in exchanges through a new catheter. Irrigate the catheter with sterile 0.9% sodium chloride solution. Inform a doctor, who will replace the catheter or revise its position surgically.
Kinking of the cuffed catheter.	Subcutaneous tunnel too short or scarring in the subcutaneous tunnel.	Inform a doctor, who will remove the catheter and implant a new one.
Lower back pain.	Pressure and weight of dialysis fluid in the abdomen (particularly so in CAPD patients).	Doctor may order analgesics. Exercises to strengthen the patient's muscles and improve posture may also be ordered.
Abdominal or rectal pain (with possible referred pain in shoulder).	Improperly positioned catheter tip causing irritation.	Catheter position to be revised surgically.
	Dialysis fluid accumulating under the diaphragm.	Drain the abdomen completely during outflow.
	Dialysis fluid not at 36°C. With 2 litres of 6.36% solution, severe shoulder pain can occur.	Ensure that the fluid is infused at the correct temperature. If hypertonic dialysis fluid is used, only one container should be used per cycle.
	If air enters the peritoneal cavity, pain may occur.	Maintain a closed system.
Paralytic ileus indicated by sharp pain in abdomen, constipation, abdominal distension, nausea and vomiting, and diarrhoea.	Catheter manipulated excessively during insertion.	Notify the doctor immediately as signs and symptoms may indicate peritonitis. Administer fluids and electrolytes as prescribed. If general condition allows,

Problem solving (cont'd)

Problem	Cause	Suggested action
		encourage patient to walk, unless advised otherwise by the doctor. Prepare the patient for surgery, as advised by the doctor. The condition may disappear spontaneously after 12 hours.
Cramping.	Dialysis fluid warmer or cooler than 36°C.	Adjust the temperature of the dialysis fluid to 36°C before infusion.
	Too rapid infusion or drainage.	Decrease the infusion or drainage rate to a speed the patient can tolerate.
	Pressure from excess dialysis fluid in the abdomen.	Infuse less dialysis fluid at exchanges to a total volume that the patient can tolerate.
	Chemical irritation.	Use a dialysis fluid with a dextrose concentration lower than 7%.
	Air in the abdomen.	Clamp off the dialysis tubing before the dialysis fluid empties completely into the abdomen.
Excessive fluid loss.	Use of dialysis fluid with too great a dextrose concentration for the patient or inadequate sodium intake or inadequate fluid intake.	Monitor the patient's weight and blood pressure. Ensure that the patient is receiving dialysis fluid with the correct dextrose concentration. The doctor may prescribe a reduced dextrose concentration.
Fluid overload.	Use of dialysis fluid with an osmotic pressure that is too low for the patient or excessive sodium intake or excessive fluid intake.	Monitor the patient's weight and blood pressure. The doctor will order a reduced fluid and sodium intake. The doctor may also order increased use of dialysis fluid with a 4.25% dextrose concentration.
Metabolic disturbance usually affects plasma levels of glucose, potassium or sodium.	Continued use of inappropriate dialysate fluid.	Monitor relevant plasma levels pre- and postdialysis. If patient has pre-existing diabetes mellitus or insulin deficiency, insulin dosage should be titrated carefully.
Respiratory difficulties.	Pressure from the fluid in the peritoneal cavity and upward displacement of the diaphragm or 'splinting' of the diaphragm resulting in shallow breathing.	Elevate the head of the bed. Encourage breathing exercises and coughing. Involve the physiotherapist to establish respiratory care.

Procedure guidelines: **Preparation of equipment for CVVHDF utilizing a CVVHDF device**

Note: when using the CVVHDF method of filtration, the venous access is obtained by the insertion of a double- or triple-lumen catheter. This will be inserted into a central vein, usually the internal jugular, subclavian or femoral vein. The catheter will then be flushed with a heparinized solution and capped off ready to commence CVVHDF.

Equipment

1 Volumetric infusion pump × 1.
2 CVVHDF machine.
3 Set of dialysate tubing and filter.
4 10 ml Luer–Lok syringe × 2.

5 Plastic clamps × 3.
6 Gloves.
7 Chlorhexidine 0.5% in 70% alcohol.
8 Low-linting gauze swabs.

*Procedure guidelines: **Preparation of equipment for CVVHDF utilizing a CVVHDF device** (cont'd)*

Procedure

Action	Rationale
1 Discuss patient's condition with the multidisciplinary team and establish treatment plan.	To ensure all medical and nursing teams are aware of patient's biochemistry and haematological profiles and the plan for treatment.
2 Collect all equipment together as above.	To ensure that all the equipment is available before commencing the procedure.
3 Instill 5000 units heparin (or as per manufacturer's instructions) into 1 litre of 0.9% sodium chloride.	To anticoagulate the tubing and the filter to provide prophylaxis against clotting in the extracorporeal circuit.
4 Load the CVVHDF device following the automated instructions on the electronic screen of the device.	To form the CVVHDF circuit.
5 When the circuit has been primed, ensure that the patient is ready for connection to the CVVHDF device.	The first 15–30 minutes can cause a period of cardiovascular instability and it is therefore important to ensure that the patient is comfortable (i.e. does not want to use the commode) and ready to commence therapy.

Procedure guidelines: **Commencement of CVVHDF**

Procedure

Action	Rationale
1 Explain and discuss the procedure with the patient and his/her family.	To ensure that the patient understands the procedure and gives his/her valid consent.
2 Ensure that all information concerning the patient's blood biochemistry, full blood count and clotting profile is available.	To have a baseline from which to work and to monitor any change in the patient.
3 Ensure that the patient's mean arterial pressure is above 60 mmHg or that physician's guidelines have been agreed.	During the first 2 hours of CVVHDF there is usually a large fluid drainage, which can result in a sudden drop in blood pressure.
4 Ensure that baseline recordings of weight, temperature, heart rate, blood pressure, respiratory rate, tissue oxygen saturation (SaO$_2$) and central venous pressure (CVP) have been recorded.	To have a baseline from which to work and to monitor any change in the patient.
5 Ensure that the patient is attached to a haemodynamic monitor.	CVVHDF can cause cardiac instability, although this is rare (Toft *et al.* 2000).
6 Ensure that a treatment programme has been agreed with the multidisciplinary team and review regularly.	To ensure that the plan for cycling and the total fluid removal has been discussed and that it is altered according to patient status.
7 Prepare the appropriate fluid replacement.	There is a rapid fluid loss with CVVHDF and patients often require replacement of this loss.
8 Prepare a sterile field and apply gloves.	To reduce the risk of infection and provide universal protection for the nurse.
9 While keeping the patient's catheter clamped, remove the injection caps from both lumens and clean the lumens with chlorhexidine in 70% alcohol.	To prevent haemorrhage and to reduce the risk of infection
10 Flush each lumen with heparinized saline.	To ensure that the patient's catheter is patent.
11 Apply plastic clamps to the patient ends of the red and blue tubing and separate from each other. Clean the ends of the tubing with chlorhexidine in 70% alcohol.	To prevent air entering the tubing and to reduce the risk of infection.
12 Connect red tubing to the red lumen and blue tubing to the blue lumen of the catheter.	To complete patient circuit.

Procedure guidelines: **Commencement of CVVHDF** *(cont'd)*

Action	Rationale
13 Undo catheter clamps and plastic clamp on tubing.	To ensure free flow.
14 Ensure that there are no clamps left closed and that all connections are secure.	To ensure that there is no obstruction to flow and no risk of fluid leakage.
15 Turn on machine and start blood pump at 75–100 ml/hour.	To commence CVVHDF at a gentle speed.
16 Observe the patient and monitor the dialysis circuit carefully.	To ensure that any alteration in patient condition is noted immediately.
17 If everything is stable, increase speed to appropriate level, probably between 100 and 150 ml/hour.	To ensure good filtration.
18 Commence dialysate fluid infusion at appropriate rate, usually between 1 and 2 litres/hour.	To provide the counter-current and achieve movement of solutes.
19 Continue monitoring patient with continuous ECG, heart rate, rhythm, BP, CVP, SaO_2 and respiratory rate hourly or more frequently if required.	To ensure any change in patient condition is noted immediately and dealt with as appropriate.
20 Maintain accurate fluid balancing.	To ensure patient is protected from large positive or negative fluid shifts.
21 Send regular blood samples for biochemical analysis.	To adjust dialysate fluid and electrolyte replacement therapy as appropriate.
22 Send regular blood samples for clotting profile.	To provide appropriate anticoagulant therapy.
23 Ensure patient tubing and circuit are easily visible and free from obstruction.	To protect patient from sudden disconnection or obstruction to tubing.
24 Review patient's condition regularly with multidisciplinary team.	To ensure optimum patient monitoring and evaluation of care to enable appropriate treatment.
25 Ensure optimum recording in documentation of venous pressure, pump speeds and drainage.	To ensure information exchange between members of the nursing team.

References and further reading

Block, C.A. & Manning, H.L. (2002) Prevention of acute renal failure in the critically ill. *Am J Respir Crit Care Med*, **165**(3), 320–4.

Bloembergen, W.E., Port, F.K., Mauger, E.A. & Wolfe, R.A. (1995) A comparison of mortality between patients treated with hemodialysis and peritoneal dialysis. *J Am Soc Nephrol*, **6**(2), 177–83.

Blumenkrantz, M.J. & Roberts, M. (1979) Progress in peritoneal dialysis: an historical prospective. *Contrib Nephrol*, **17**, 101–10.

Briggs, J.D., Crombie, A., Fabre, J., Major, E., Thorogood, J. & Veitch, P.S. (1997) Organ donation in the UK: a survey by a British Transplantation Society working party. *Nephrol Dialysis Transplant*, **12**(11), 2251–7.

Bunn, R. & Ashley, C. (1999) *The Renal Drug Handbook*. Radcliffe Medical Press, Oxford.

Buoncristiani, U. (1989) The Y set with disinfectant is here to stay. *Peritoneal Dialysis Int*, **9**(3), 149–50.

CANUSA (Canada–USA Peritoneal Dialysis Study Group) (1996) Adequacy of dialysis and nutrition in continuous peritoneal dialysis: association with clinical outcomes. *J Am Soc Nephrol*, **7**(2), 198–207.

Carrasco, A.M., Rubio, M.A.B., Tomero, J.A.S. *et al.* (2001) Acidosis correction with a new 25 mmol/l bicarbonate/15 mmol/l lactate peritoneal dialysis solution. *Peritoneal Dialysis Int*, **21**, 546–53.

Chitalia, V.C., Almeida, A.F., Rai, H. *et al.* (2002) Is peritoneal dialysis adequate for hypercatabolic acute renal failure in developing countries? *Kidney Int*, **61**(2), 747–57.

Cole, L., Bellomo, R., Journois, D., Davenport, P., Baldwin, I. & Tipping, P. (2001) High volume haemofiltration in human septic shock. *Intensive Care Med*, **27**, 978–86.

de Fijter, C.W., Oe, L.P., Nauta, J.J. *et al.* (1994) Morbidity associated with continuous cyclic compared with continuous ambulatory peritoneal dialysis. *Ann Intern Med*, **120**(4), 264–71.

Fenton, S.S., Schaubel, D.E., Desmeules, M. *et al.* (1997) Hemodialysis versus peritoneal dialysis: a comparison of adjusted mortality rates. *Am J Kidney Dis*, **30**(3), 334–42.

Ford-Martin, P.A. (1999) Dialysis, kidney. In: *Gale Encyclopedia of Med*. Gale Research, Michigan.

Hyman, A. & Mendelssohn D.C. (2002) Current Canadian approaches to dialysis for acute renal failure in the ICU. *Am J Nephrol*, **22**(1), 29–34.

Jones, M.R. (1994) Etiology of severe malnutrition: results of an international cross-sectional study in continuous ambulatory peritoneal dialysis patients. *Am J Kidney Dis*, **23**(3), 412–20.

KDOQI (Kidney Disease Outcomes Quality Initiative) (2000) The National Kidney Foundation – DOQI – Clinical Practice Guidelines. www.kidney.org

Kellum, J.A., Angus, D.C., Johnson, J.P. *et al.* (2002) Continuous versus intermittent renal replacement therapy: meta-analysis. *Intens Care Med*, **28**(1), 29–37.

Mahon, A. (2002) Advances in bicarbonate peritoneal dialysis solutions. www.nephronline.org/management/advances. Accessed 08/05/2002.

Marieb, E.N. (2001) The urinary system. In: *Human Anatomy and Physiology*, 5th edn. Benjamin Cummings, New York, pp. 1004–39.

Murray, P. & Hall, J. (2000) Renal replacement therapy for acute renal failure. *Am J Respir Crit Care Med*, **162**, 777–81.

Oreopoulos, D.G. (1998) Shaping the future of peritoneal dialysis. Satellite Symposium, 18th International CAPD Meeting, Nashville, Tennessee, USA, pp. 1–10.

Pittrow, L. & Penk, A. (1998) Pharmacokinetics and dosage of fluconazole in continuous haemofiltration and haemodialysis. *Mycoses*, **41**, Suppl 2, 86–8.

Popovich, R.P., Moncrief, J.W., Nolph, K.D., Ghods, A.J., Twardowski, Z.J. & Pyle, W.K. (1978) Continuous ambulatory peritoneal dialysis. *Ann Intern Med*, **88**(4), 449–56.

Schaubel, D.E., Blake, P.G. & Fenton, S.S. (2001) Trends in CAPD technique failure: Canada, 1981–1997. *Peritoneal Dialysis Int*, **21**(4), 365–71.

Selgas, R., Cirugeda, A., Fernandez-Perpen, A. *et al.* (2001) Comparisons of hemodialysis and CAPD in patients over 65 years of age: a meta-analysis. *Int Urol Nephrol*, **33**(2), 259–64.

Stegmayr, B. (2002) Various clinical approaches to minimise complications in peritoneal dialysis. *Int J Artif Organs*, **25**(5), 365–72.

Toft, P., Felding, M. & Tonnesen, E.K. (2000) Continuous veno-venous hemodiafiltration in critically ill patients with acute renal failure. *Ugeskr Laeger*, **162**(20), 2868–71.

Toft, P., Kehler, D., Brandslund, I. & Tonnsen, E. (1999) The immunological effects of continuous veno-venous haemodiafiltration in critically ill patients. *Critical Care*, **3**, 159–65.

Tsubo, T., Sakai, I., Okawa, H., Ishihara, H. & Matsuki, A. (2001) Ketamine and midazolam kinetics during continuous hemodiafiltration in patients with multiple organ dysfunction syndrome. *Intensive Care Med*, **27**(6), 1087–90.

Respiratory therapy

Chapter contents

Definition

The principle of respiratory therapy is the administration of oxygen by an appropriate delivery system – nasal cannulae, mask, non-invasive or invasive ventilation – in order to correct impaired oxygenation.

Indications

- Respiratory failure, of which there are two types:
  - *Type 1*, referred to as hypoxaemic respiratory failure (failure to oxygenate the tissues). The PaO_2 is $<8\,kPa$ (60 mmHg) while the carbon dioxide (PCO_2) is normal or low. Common causes include infective conditions, pneumonia, pulmonary oedema and adult respiratory distress syndrome.
  - *Type 2*, referred to as hypercapnic (raised carbon dioxide) or respiratory pump failure. Alveolar ventilation is insufficient to excrete carbon dioxide accompanied by hypoxaemia (deficiency of oxygen in the arterial blood). The PCO_2 is $>6\,kPa$ (45 mmHg). Common causes include COPD, chest wall deformities, respiratory muscle weakness (Guillain–Barré syndrome), drug overdose and chest injury.
- Acute myocardial infarction
- Cardiac failure
- Shock–haemorrhagic, bacteraemic and cardiogenic
- Conditions in which there is a reduced ability to transport oxygen, e.g. anaemia
- During anaesthesia
- Postoperatively
- Sleep apnoea.

Reference material

Physiology (see also Ch. 25, Observations)

The respiratory system consists of a gas exchange system (the lungs) and a ventilatory pump (respiratory muscles and thorax). The major function of the respiratory system is the adequate delivery of oxygen to and elimination of carbon dioxide from the cells via the blood. Failure to carry out this function results in respiratory failure. Oxygen must be continuously available to all cells of the body. Oxygen enters the body by the lungs, is transferred by the blood to the tissues and then to the cells where it is consumed by the mitochondria to provide energy for metabolism (energy is in the form of adenosine triphosphate (ATP); this is required for various chemical and mechanical processes in the body).

Under normal conditions energy is provided by oxygen – aerobically. If oxygen is unavailable anaerobic respiration (without oxygen) will take place. This is an inefficient way for metabolism to occur, with the formation of lactic acid. Accumulation of lactic acid can result in a metabolic acidosis, which can lead to cell death.

If a defect occurs physiologically or mechanically at any point in the oxygen delivery pathway, normal oxygenation can be reduced or impaired, causing tissue damage or cell death (West 1995; Oh 1997; Kumar & Clarke 1998; Pierson 2000; Hess 2000; Berne & Levy 1998; Marieb 2001; Tortora & Grabowski 2000; Guyton 2000).

There are three separate components to oxygenation: oxygen uptake, oxygen transportation and oxygen utilization. *Oxygen uptake* is the process of extracting oxygen from the environment. *Oxygen transportation* is the mechanism by which the uptake of oxygen results in delivery of oxygen to the cells. *Oxygen utilization* is the metabolic need for molecular oxygen by the cells of the body.

In order for oxygenation to take place there needs to be an adequate cardiac output.

Oxygen uptake

The atmosphere is composed of several gases:

- Oxygen 21%
- Carbon dioxide 0.03%
- Nitrogen 79%
- Rare gases 0.003%.

Inspired air at sea level has a total atmospheric pressure of 760 mmHg. Each gas exerts its own pressure (partial pressure):

- Oxygen $0.21 \times 760 = 159$ mmHg (21 kPa)
- Carbon dioxide $0.03 \times 760 = 22.8$ mmHg (3.0 kPa)
- Nitrogen $0.79 \times 760 = 600$ mmHg (80 kPa).

As inspired air enters the respiratory tract it encounters water vapour present in the upper airways which warms and humidifies it. Water vapour exerts its own partial pressure of 47 mmHg. The partial pressure of the water vapour must be subtracted from the total atmospheric

Table 37.1 Oxygen cascade. Pressure gradients for oxygen transfer from inspired gas to tissue cells

	mmHg	kPa
Inspired air	150	20
Alveolar	103	13.7
Arterial	100	13.3
Capillary	51	6.8
Tissue	20	2.7
Mitochondrial	1–20	0.13–1.3

pressure to give a corrected atmospheric pressure and partial pressure of each gas:

- Corrected total atmospheric $760 - 47 = 713$ mmHg
- Oxygen $0.21 \times 713 = 150$ mmHg (20 kPa)
- Carbon dioxide $0.03 \times 713 = 21$ mmHg (2.8 kPa).

As oxygen continues to pass down the respiratory tract to the alveolus it encounters carbon dioxide leaving the respiratory tract which also exerts a partial pressure, equal to 40 mmHg. This in turn must be subtracted to determine the correct values. Oxygen has a corrected value of $150 - 40 = 110$ to 100 mmHg (14.6 to 13.3 kPa).

Movement of gases is by diffusion. Diffusion is the movement of gas molecules from an area of relatively high partial pressure to one of lower partial pressure.

Diffusion of oxygen takes place from the alveolus into the pulmonary capillaries and movement of carbon dioxide from the capillary into the alveolus. From the alveolus the oxygen diffuses from the capillaries into the tissues and mitochondria of the cells (Fig. 37.1).

The alveolar oxygen partial pressure is higher than the arterial oxygen partial pressure in order to push the oxygen through the alveolar membrane into the interstitial spaces and from there into the pulmonary capillaries. Oxygen continues to diffuse from the capillaries into the tissues then to the mitochondria of the cells for metabolism (Carpenter 1991; Oh 1997; Pierce 1995; Esmond 2000; Berne & Levy 1998; Marieb 2001; Tortora & Grabowski 2000; Guyton 2000).

Oxygen transportation

Oxygen is carried in the blood in two ways:

- *Dissolved in the plasma (serum)*: only 2–3% is carried in this way as oxygen is not very soluble (Aherns & Tucker 1999; Marieb 2001). This is measured as the PaO_2. There is 0.003 ml of blood for each 1 mmHg partial pressure oxygen. At 100 mmHg partial pressure, only 0.3 ml of oxygen would be carried per 100 ml of plasma.

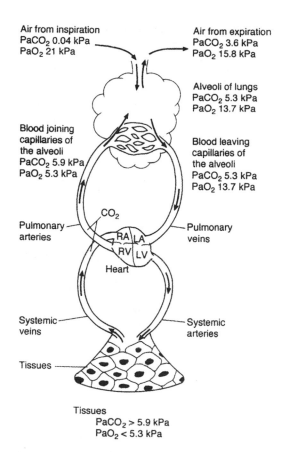

Air from inspiration
PaCO$_2$ 0.04 kPa
PaO$_2$ 21 kPa

Air from expiration
PaCO$_2$ 3.6 kPa
PaO$_2$ 15.8 kPa

Alveoli of lungs
PaCO$_2$ 5.3 kPa
PaO$_2$ 13.7 kPa

Blood joining
capillaries of
the alveoli
PaCO$_2$ 5.9 kPa
PaO$_2$ 5.3 kPa

Blood leaving
capillaries of
the alveoli
PaCO$_2$ 5.3 kPa
PaO$_2$ 13.7 kPa

CO$_2$

Pulmonary
arteries

Pulmonary
veins

RA LA
RV LV
Heart

Systemic
veins

Systemic
arteries

Tissues

Tissues
PaCO$_2$ > 5.9 kPa
PaO$_2$ < 5.3 kPa

Figure 37.1 Gas movement in the body is facilitated by partial pressure differences. Top of figure illustrates pressure gradients that facilitate oxygen and carbon dioxide exchange in the lungs. Bottom of figure shows pressure gradients that facilitate gas movements from systemic capillaries to tissues.

- *Bound to haemoglobin in the red blood cells*: 95–98% of oxygen is carried in this way and is measured as the percentage of oxygen saturated (SaO$_2$). Each gram of haemoglobin can carry 1.34 ml of oxygen per 100 ml blood.

Haemoglobin is composed of haem (iron) and globulin (protein). Each haemoglobin molecule has four binding sites each able to carry one molecule of oxygen. A haemoglobin molecule is said to be fully saturated with oxygen when all four haem sites are attached to oxygen. When fewer than four are attached the haemoglobin is said to be partially saturated. Oxygen saturation gives the percentage of the sites which are loaded.

The bond between haemoglobin and oxygen is affected by various physiological factors that shift the oxygen dissociation curve to the right or left (see Fig. 37.2).

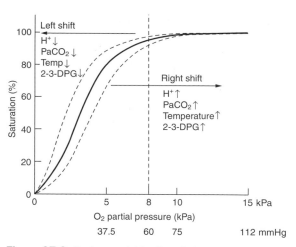

Figure 37.2 Oxyhaemoglobin dissociation curve. With a PaO$_2$ of 8 kPa and more, saturations will remain high (flat portion of curve). NB The middle dark line is the normal position of the curve.

Oxyhaemoglobin curve shift to the right

When a shift occurs to the right there is reduced binding of oxygen to haemoglobin and oxygen is given up more easily to the tissues. The saturation will be lower.

Factors that cause the curve to shift to the right are:

- Increase in body temperature
- Increase in hydrogen ion content (acidaemia) known as the Bohr effect
- Increase in carbon dioxide
- Increase in 2-3-DPG (2-3-DPG is an enzyme found in the red blood cells that affects haemoglobin and oxygen binding).

Oxyhaemoglobin curve shift to the left

When a shift occurs to the left there is an increase in the binding of oxygen to the haemoglobin, oxygen is given less easily to the tissues and cellular hypoxia can occur.

Factors that cause the curve to shift to the left are:

- Decrease in body temperature
- Decrease in hydrogen ion content (alkalaemia)
- Decrease in carbon dioxide
- Decrease in 2-3-DPG.

Oxygen utilization

The relationship between the PaO$_2$ and the SaO$_2$ is represented as the oxygen dissociation curve. Oxygen uptake in the lungs is shown by the upper flat part of the curve. When the PaO$_2$ is between 8.0 and 13.3 kPa (60–100 mmHg) the haemoglobin is 90% or more saturated with oxygen. At this point of the curve, large changes in the PaO$_2$ lead to small changes in the SaO$_2$

of haemoglobin, because the haemoglobin is almost completely saturated. Release of oxygen to the tissues is shown by the lower part of the curve. There is easy removal of oxygen from the haemoglobin for use by the cells. It is at this part of the curve that small changes in the PaO_2 cause major changes in the SaO_2. This is important clinically.

A patient's oxygen level must be kept at 8 kPa (60 mmHg). Below this level desaturation can occur at a rapid rate, resulting in tissue hypoxia and cell death.

Oxygen consumption

At rest the normal oxygen consumption is approximately 200–250 ml/minute. As the available oxygen per minute in a normal man is about 700 ml, this means there is an oxygen reserve of 450–500 ml/minute. Factors that increase the above consumption of oxygen include fever, sepsis, shivering, restlessness and increased metabolism (Oh 1997). It is difficult to say at which absolute level oxygen therapy is necessary as each situation should be judged by the requirements for oxygen and the availability of oxygen. Therefore, all of the above information needs to be taken into account together with the measurement of the arterial blood gases.

Generally, additional oxygen will be required when the PaO_2 has fallen to 8 kPa (60 mmHg) or less (Oh 1997). Oxygen saturation level in the tissues can be measured using a pulse oximeter, which works by emitting narrow shafts of red and infrared light through the tissue of a finger, toe or earlobe. Different amounts of light rays are absorbed by the arterial blood depending on its saturation with oxygen. The final oxygen saturation (SaO_2) is then calculated by computer (Ehrhardt & Graham 1990).

Hazards of respiratory therapy

Carbon dioxide narcosis

Carbon dioxide is the chemical that most directly influences respiration by its direct effect on the efficiency of alveolar ventilation. The normal partial pressure of carbon dioxide in the blood is 4.0–6.0 kPa (30–45 mmHg). When this level rises, the pH of the cerebrospinal fluid drops which in turn causes excitation of the central chemoreceptors, and hyperventilation occurs (Marieb 2001).

In people who always retain carbon dioxide, and are therefore usually hypercapnic because of chronic pulmonary disease such as chronic bronchitis, the chemoreceptors are no longer sensitive to a raised level of carbon dioxide. In these cases the falling PaO_2 becomes the principal respiratory stimulus (the hypoxic drive) (Marieb 2001). Therefore, if a high level of supplementary oxygen was delivered to such patients, severe respiratory depression would ensue and ultimately unconsciousness and death.

Oxygen toxicity

Pulmonary toxicity following prolonged higher percentages of oxygen therapy is recognized clinically, but there is still much to be learnt about the condition. The degree of injury is related to the length of time of exposure and percentage of oxygen to which the individual is exposed. The pattern is one of decreasing lung compliance as a result of a sequence of events, tracheal bronchial inflammation, haemorrhagic interstitial and intra-alveolar oedema, leading ultimately to fibrosis (Pierce 1995; Oh 1997; Pierson 2000).

Where possible, long periods (i.e. 24 hours or more) of oxygen therapy above 50% should be avoided.

Retrolental fibroplasia

Retrolental fibroplasia is a disease affecting premature babies that weigh under 1200 g (about 28 weeks' gestation) if they are exposed to high concentrations of oxygen within the first 3–4 weeks of life. It appears that the oxygen stimulates immature blood vessels in the eye to vasoconstrict and obliterate, which results in neovascularization, accompanied by haemorrhage, fibrosis and then retinal detachment and blindness (Pierce 1995; Oh 1997).

General considerations

- Oxygen is an odourless, tasteless, colourless, transparent gas that is slightly heavier than air.
- Oxygen supports combustion; therefore there is always a danger of fire when oxygen is being used. The following safety measures should be remembered:
  (a) Oil or grease around oxygen connections should be avoided.
  (b) Alcohol, ether and other inflammatory liquids should be used with caution in the vicinity of oxygen.
  (c) No electrical device must be used in or near an oxygen tent.
  (d) Oxygen cylinders should be kept secure in an upright position and away from heat.
  (e) There must be no smoking in the vicinity of oxygen.
  (f) A fire extinguisher should be readily available.
  (g) Care should be taken with high concentrations of oxygen when using the defibrillator.

Equipment necessary to administer respiratory therapy

Any oxygen delivery system will include these basic components:

- Oxygen supply, from either a piped supply or a portable cylinder. All medical gas cylinders have to conform to a

standardized colour coding: oxygen cylinders are black with a white shoulder and are labelled 'Oxygen' or 'O$_2$'.
- A reduction gauge – to reduce the pressure to that of atmospheric pressure.
- Flowmeter – a device that controls the flow of oxygen in litres per minute.
- Tubing – disposable tubing of varying diameter and length.
- Mechanism for delivery – a mask or nasal cannulae.
- Humidifier – to warm and moisten the oxygen before administration.
- Water trap if humidifier in use.

Oxygen delivery systems

Simple semi-rigid plastic masks (Fig. 37.3)

Simple semi-rigid plastic masks are low-flow masks which entrain the air from the atmosphere and therefore are able to deliver a variable oxygen percentage (anything from 21 to 60%) (see Table 37.2). Large discrepancies between the delivered fractional inspired oxygen (FiO$_2$) and the actual amount received by the patient will occur, dependent on the patient's rate and depth of breathing.

Nasal cannulae catheter (Fig. 37.4)

Nasal cannulae consist of two prongs that are inserted inside the anterior nares and supported on a light frame. Advantages to the patient are that they have access to their face and are able to eat, drink and communicate. Nasal cannulae catheters provide an alternative to a mask, but again there are great discrepancies between the delivered FiO$_2$ and the actual oxygen percentage received by the patient. When used at low flow rates, for example 2 litres/minute, they are well tolerated and afford the patient more freedom than a mask. At high flow rates, above 8 litres/minute, they may cause discomfort and dryness of the nasal mucosa leading to crusting of secretions and epistaxis (Pierce 1995). Nasal cannulae cannot be attached satisfactorily to an external humidification device (see Table 37.3).

Partial rebreathing masks

These are similar to the simple semi-rigid plastic masks with the addition of a reservoir bag. The reservoir bag allows the oxygen delivered to increase beyond 60%. During inspiration the patient draws air and oxygen from the mask, bag and through the holes in the side of the mask. When the patient expires the initial one third of the expired gases will flow back into the reservoir bag. The expired gas is rich in oxygen and contains very little carbon dioxide. The patient is able to breathe the previously expired gas along with the oxygen from the source.

Note: if the oxygen flow is too low the carbon dioxide can accumulate in the reservoir bag and fail to meet the

Table 37.2 Approximate oxygen concentration related to flow rates of semi-rigid masks

Oxygen flow rate (l/min)	% Oxygen delivered
2	24
4	35
6	50
8	55
10	60
12	65
15	70

Table 37.3 Oxygen flow rates for nasal cannulae

Oxygen flow rate (l/min)	% Oxygen delivered
1	24
2	28
3	32
4	36
5	40
6	44

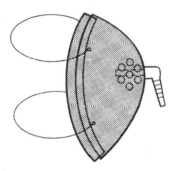

Figure 37.3 Semi-rigid plastic mask.

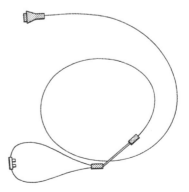

Figure 37.4 Nasal cannula.

patient's requirement, resulting in an increase in carbon dioxide (Pierce 1995).

Non-rebreathing mask

Oxygen delivery of greater than 80% can be achieved. The semi-rigid mask has the addition of a reservoir bag with a one-way valve between the reservoir bag and mask, preventing accumulation of expired gases in the reservoir bag and retention of carbon dioxide (Pierce 1995).

Fixed performance masks or high-flow masks (Venturi-type masks) (Fig. 37.5)

With fixed performance masks it is possible to achieve an unvarying mixture of gases and a known concentration of oxygen using the high air flow oxygen enrichment principle. These masks derive their name from the Venturi barrel in which a relatively low flow rate of oxygen is forced through a narrow jet. There are side holes in the barrel and this jet causes the air to be drawn in at a high rate. As the mixture of gas created is at a flow rate above that of inspiration, the mixture will be constant (Foss 1990). There are many Venturi-type masks available, but the larger-capacity masks are the most accurate and therefore the safest when a known concentration of oxygen is required or when efficient elimination of carbon dioxide is essential, for example, to provide respiratory therapy for the patient with chronic respiratory disease (Fell & Boehm 1998).

Table 37.4 Fixed performance mask oxygen flow rates

Oxygen flow rate (l/min)	% Oxygen delivered
2	24
6	31
8	35
10	40
15	60

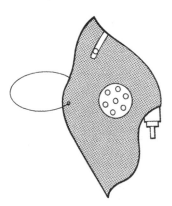

Figure 37.5 High-flow mask.

Tracheostomy mask

Tracheostomy masks perform in a similar way to the simple semi-rigid plastic face mask, outlined above. The mask is placed over the tracheostomy tube or stoma (see also Ch. 41, Tracheostomy care).

T-piece circuit

The T-piece circuit is a simple, large-bore, non-rebreathing circuit which is attached directly to an endo-tracheal or tracheostomy tube. Humidified oxygen is delivered through one part of the T, and expired gases leave through the other part. This device may be used as part of the weaning process when a patient has been ventilated previously by a mechanical ventilator (Oh 1997).

Domiciliary oxygen and portable oxygen

Some patients are so disabled by chronic respiratory disease that they require continual supplementary oxygen at home. Low-flow oxygen given over a period of time improves the prognosis of some patients (Benditt 2000).

Long-term oxygen may be prescribed for treatment of chronic obstructive pulmonary disease (COPD), cystic fibrosis, interstitial lung disease, neuromuscular and skeletal disorders, pulmonary hypertension and palliation in lung cancer. Long-term oxygen may be provided in the form of cylinders. The problem with this supply is that the cylinders need changing frequently. Oxygen condensers (concentrators) are far more economical than cylinders. A condenser consists of a compressor powered by electricity. The condenser works by drawing in room air that is passed through a bacterial filter and a sieve bed. The sieve bed contains zeolite which has an affinity with nitrogen and when under pressure works by removing nitrogen and other gases, concentrating oxygen and delivering it through a meter at the front of the compressor.

The oxygen can be delivered to the patient by nasal cannulae or mask (Esmond 2000).

Liquid oxygen

The use of liquid oxygen in a portable cylinder has been developed for portable oxygen delivery. The patient is provided with a large tank in their own home from which smaller cylinders can be filled.

Paediatric circuits

A child's compliance with oxygen masks or cannulae may be limited, requiring other devices to be used. Some examples of these are:

* *Headbox or hood.* Oxygen can be delivered to infants and small children using a headbox or hood. The clear plastic box is fitted carefully over the child's head, encasing the head and neck. It is essential to monitor

the oxygen concentration near the face to enable an accurate assessment of FiO_2 (Oh 1997).

- *Oxygen tent/cot.* An oxygen tent can be used to supply oxygen therapy to larger children. The child is placed in a clear plastic tent which fits over the bed. The humidified oxygen supply is then directed into the tent. The advantages with the oxygen tent are that the child has freedom from any device over the face, and high degrees of humidity can be reached which may be especially useful in obstructive conditions, e.g. croup (Allan 1988). The main disadvantages are the difficulty in maintaining a constant oxygen concentration (Oh 1997) and decreased access to the child for the family and carers.

Continuous positive airway pressure (CPAP)

Definition

CPAP therapy is the maintenance of a positive airway pressure greater than ambient pressure throughout inspiration and expiration. It can be delivered through a face mask, nasal mask or mouthpiece, or through an endotracheal or tracheostomy tube (Oh 1997).

Indications

- In acute respiratory failure in a spontaneously breathing patient who is able to maintain his or her own airway
- As a method of weaning a patient from mechanical ventilation
- After major surgery as a means of improving gaseous exchange
- As a supportive measure in patients where intubation and mechanical ventilation are not considered appropriate (Greenbaum *et al.* 1976)
- Acute hypoxia with a normal $PaCO_2$
- Acute respiratory distress syndrome (ARDS)
- Postoperatively (following major abdominal or thoracic surgery) prophylactically to prevent atelectasis
- Pulmonary oedema
- In patients with sleep apnoea
- In neonates with respiratory distress syndrome/hyaline membrane disease.

Reference material

Use of the CPAP circuit dates back at least to 1912, when Bunnell used a primitive circuit during thoracic surgery. The first recorded use in intensive care was by Poulton

and Oxon in 1936. In the 1940s increased interest in CPAP was prompted by research into respiratory support in high altitude flying. Further developments occurred in the 1950s and 1960s, and in 1976 Greenbaum *et al.* reported the use of CPAP with a face mask in ARDS. In 1972 Williamson & Modell successfully used CPAP for selected spontaneously breathing patients with acute respiratory failure.

The aim of CPAP therapy is to improve gas exchange (oxygen and carbon dioxide) within the lungs and improve the work of breathing. CPAP is able to do this by:

- Increasing the functional residual capacity (FRC), which is the amount of gas left in the lungs at the end of normal expiration which is available for pulmonary gas exchange. In acute lung injury where gaseous exchange is severely inhibited CPAP increases the FRC by improving ventilation in poorly or non-ventilated alveoli (Miller & Semple 1991).
- Improving the ventilation/perfusion ratio. Decreased intrapulmonary shunting with hypoxia could cause ventilation to the lungs to be reduced or blood flow to them impaired. Intrapulmonary shunting can then occur with underventilation of the lungs. CPAP helps to decrease the intrapulmonary shunting by improving the ventilation to perfusion mismatch (Lenique *et al.* 1997).
- Improved lung compliance (elasticity) of the lungs. In respiratory failure the lungs become much stiffer and less compliant and breathing can become more difficult. Reduction in lung volume below a certain level results in airway collapse and underventilation. The pressure required to overcome this can be achieved by CPAP.
- Increasing lung volume (alveolar volume) for gaseous exchange to take place. The factors above enable the work of breathing to be reduced plus a decrease in the percentage of oxygen that might be required.

Disadvantages of CPAP therapy

- With any circuit that includes the use of positive end expiratory pressure (PEEP) there is the possibility of reduction in cardiac output; however, spontaneous ventilation decreases both the incidence and severity of this complication (Oh 1997).
- There is a danger of vomiting and aspiration of gastric contents due to gastric insufflation, although this is minimized when used in awake patients, or by the insertion of an oro/nasogastric tube (Schumaker *et al.* 1996).
- Damage to skin integrity due to pressure from the tightly fitting face mask; the sites particularly vulnerable are the bridge of the nose and over the ears.

Non-invasive ventilation

Non-invasive ventilation refers to mechanical ventilatory support applied without an artificial airway (endotracheal tube or tracheostomy). It can be delivered to the patient via a nasal or face mask. The patient must be conscious and co-operative for this type of ventilation to be effective. It is particularly useful in patients with chronic respiratory disease:

- In restrictive pulmonary disease, e.g. muscular dystrophy
- In progressive neuromuscular disease, e.g. motor neurone disease
- In obstructive pulmonary disease, e.g. COPD, bronchiectasis, cystic fibrosis
- In nocturnal hypoventilation
- In patients with acute exacerbation of chronic respiratory disease
- In patients where endotracheal intubation and ventilation may not be considered appropriate or where difficulties may be anticipated in weaning a patient from a ventilator.

Non-invasive ventilators generally fall into two categories:

- Pressure preset machines
- Volume preset machines (Esmond 2000).

Mechanical ventilation

A mechanical ventilator is a device used to replace or assist breathing in order for satisfactory gas exchange to take place. The decision to ventilate a patient will be made after careful clinical examination including assessment of respiratory mechanics, oxygenation and ventilation.

Ventilators are able to control tidal volume, respiratory rate, time of inspiration against time of expiration, inspired flow rate and inspired oxygen concentration (West 1995; Pierce 1995; Hinds 1997; Oh 1997).

Ventilators are divided into two main categories: negative pressure ventilators and positive pressure ventilators.

Negative pressure ventilators

These devices are now rarely used. They mimic normal breathing (negative pressure) and are known as iron lungs. The patient is enclosed in an airtight tank and a negative pressure is created by a separate pump which causes the alveolar pressure to fall within the lungs so a pressure gradient results, with air flowing into the lungs along the pressure gradient in order for ventilation to take place. An adaptation from the tank ventilator is the cuirass shell, which surrounds the thorax and abdomen, which works on the same principle. The rare use of these devices would be in patients with chronic respiratory

failure (neuromuscular disease, skeletal deformity or sleep-related respiratory problems).

Positive pressure ventilators

These devices provide a satisfactory gas exchange when inflating the lungs with a positive pressure via an endotracheal tube or tracheostomy.

Positive pressure ventilators have four main functions to perform during each respiratory cycle:

- Inflate the lungs
- Cycle from inspiration to expiration
- Allow expiration to take place
- Cycle from expiration to inspiration.

They have a driving mechanism and can cycle from one phase of the respiratory cycle to another by a preset pressure, preset time or preset volume.

Varying modes of ventilation can be used:

- IMV (intermittent mandatory ventilation)
- Pressure support
- Pressure control
- SIMV (simulated intermittent mandatory ventilation)
- CPAP (continuous positive airway pressure).

Hyperbaric respiratory therapy

Hyperbaric respiratory therapy is used mainly in the treatment of carbon monoxide poisoning, burns, gas gangrene, skin lesions, soft tissue injury, decompression sickness (the bends) and in multiple sclerosis. The therapy is designed to give 100% oxygen at a range of pressures greater than atmospheric pressure. Oxygen is dissolved in the plasma, increasing the oxygen tension in the tissues (Oh 1997).

Humidification

Humidity is the amount of water vapour present in a gas. The terms used to define humidity are absolute humidity, maximum capacity and relative humidity. Absolute humidity is the mass of water vapour that a given volume of gas can carry at a set temperature. When a gas is at its maximum capacity it is said to be fully saturated. Relative humidity is the ratio of the absolute humidity to the maximum capacity.

The warmer the gas, the more vapour it can hold but if the temperature of the gas falls, water held as vapour will condense out of the gas into the surrounding atmosphere.

In normal health the nasal passages and upper airways are able to warm, moisten and filter the inspired gases very effectively. The process of humidification is necessary to compensate for the normal loss of water from the respiratory tract which, under resting conditions, is about 250 ml per day. This can increase in patients who are unwell.

Normal room air has an approximate temperature of 22°C with a relative humidity of 50% and a water content of 10 mg H_2O. For effective gas exchange to occur in the lungs, the air would need to be at a temperature of 37°C with 100% humidity and a water content of 44 mg H_2O per litre by the time it reaches the bifurcation in the trachea, which is referred to as the isothermic point.

When the temperature falls below 37°C and humidity falls below 100% several changes take place in the airways. The respiratory tract is lined with ciliated epithelial cells that secrete mucus. Each cell has about 200 hair-like structures known as cilia, whose role is to remove unwanted mucus and secretions. With a drop in temperature and humidity, the mucus that collects in the airways thickens and movement of the cilia is reduced. If there is no improvement the mucus will become thicker and immobile; the cilia will also lose their mobility so clearance of all secretions will stop and infection can set in.

If there is a continuing lack of humidity further damage occurs. The cilia can break off, causing damage to the mucosal lining of the respiratory tract. The isothermic point of saturation moves from the bifurcation of the trachea to a lower point in the lungs, resulting in further damage which can lead to collapse of the alveoli, decrease in lung function and hypoxaemia (Carroll 1997; Fell & Boehm 1998; Ward & Park 2000).

Inhalation of oxygen used during respiratory therapy, which is a dry gas, can cause evaporation of water from the respiratory tract and lead to the consequences above if humidification is not provided.

In patients who are intubated or have a tracheostomy the natural pathway of humidification is bypassed.

Methods of humidification

Many devices can be used to supply humidification; the best of these will fulfil the following requirements:

- The inspired gas must be delivered to the trachea at a room temperature of 32–36°C with 100% humidity and should have a water content of 33–43 g/m³ (Oh 1997).
- The set temperature should remain constant; humidification and temperature should not be affected by large ranges of flow.
- The device should have a safety and alarm system to guard against overheating, overhydration and electric shocks.
- It is important that the appliance should not increase resistance or affect the compliance of respiration.

Table 37.5 A comparison of devices for humidification

Device	Advantages	Disadvantages
HME	Simple Cheap Short term	Inadequate humidity Risk of airway obstruction Can become waterlogged Infection risk
Cold water humidifier	Simple Cheap	Inadequate humidity Infection risk
Hot water humidifier	Delivers maximal humidification	Infection risk Overhumidification Risk of aspiration water/drowning Excessive condensation in circuit Overheating causing damage to trachea Resistance in circuit Restriction of gas flow

- It is essential that whichever device is selected, wide-bore tubing (elephant tubing) is used to allow efficient formation of water vapour.

Devices for humidification

- *Heat and moisture exchanger (HME)*. In this situation an HME performs the function of the nose and pharynx in conditioning the inspired air. It retains heat and moisture in the expired air and returns them to the patient in the next inspired breath. Many HMEs contain a bacterial filter.

  The HME consists of spun, pleated, highly thermal conductive material. It can be used in a self-ventilating patient with a tracheostomy who is being weaned from oxygen (Fig. 37.6a). It is also known as an artificial or 'Swedish' nose. It can also be used in ventilated patients, inserted between the patient's airway and the ventilator circuit (Fig. 37.6b).
- *Cold water bubble humidifier*. This device delivers partially humidified oxygen that is about 50% relative humidity. Gas is either forced across or bubbled through water at room temperature (Fig. 37.6c). Its use is not advised as it is so inefficient (Oh 1997).
- *Water bath humidifiers*. With these devices, inspired gas is forced over or through a heated reservoir of water (Fig. 37.6d). To achieve an adequate humidity for the patient, the water bath must reach a set temperature. The gas will then cool as it moves down the breathing circuit to the patient, and a relative humidity of 100% will be reached. Hot water bath humidifiers are therefore very efficient and useful in the care of the immobile patient, particularly to humidify when the

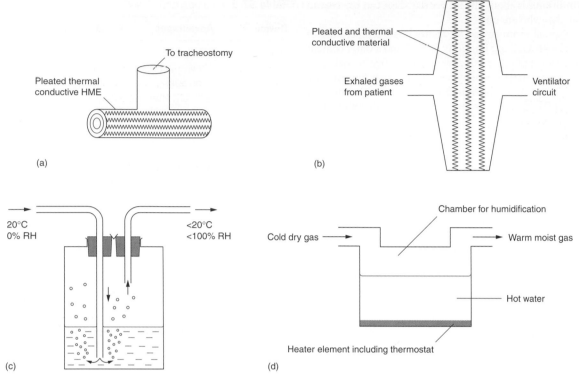

Figure 37.6 (a) Heat and moisture exchanger. (b) Cross-section of an HME used with a ventilator circuit. (c) Cold water bubble humidifier. (d) Hot water bath humidifier.

patient is receiving mechanical ventilatory support. However, they have four main disadvantages:

(a) Danger of overheating and causing damage to the trachea
(b) Their efficiency can alter with changes in gas flow rate, surface area and the water temperature
(c) Condensation and collection of water in the oxygen delivery tubes
(d) The possibility of microcontamination of stagnant water (Tinker & Zapol 1992).

• *Aerosol generators.* These devices are not governed by temperature, but provide microdroplets of water suspended in the gas (Oh 1997). The gas provided through aerosol devices can be very highly saturated with water. There are three main types of aerosol humidifier:

(a) Gas-drive nebulizer
(b) Mechanical (spinning disc) nebulizer
(c) Ultrasonic nebulizer.

These devices are useful for the spontaneously breathing patient with chronic chest disease.

Procedure guidelines: **Pre-continuous positive airway pressure (CPAP)**

Procedure

Action	Rationale
1 Explain the principle of CPAP to the patient and where possible show the patient the CPAP system.	To minimize anxiety and aid in patient compliance.
2 Observe and record the following:	
(a) Patient's respiratory function and his or her ability to maintain own airway	To obtain a baseline of respiratory function.
(b) Colour, skin, etc.	To observe for any change in respiratory function.

Procedure guidelines: Pre-continuous positive airway pressure (CPAP) (cont'd)

Action	Rationale
(c) Respiratory rate (d) Oxygen saturation.	
3 Check if arterial catheter is in situ.	In order to take a sample for gas analysis.
4 Observe and record the patient's cardiovascular function, including: (a) Heart rate (b) Blood pressure (c) Central venous pressure (if patient has a central line).	To obtain a baseline in order to assess any change in conditions (see Ch. 25, Observations).
5 Accurate assessment of fluid balance including: • Input • Output • Overall fluid balance • Daily weight if appropriate (patient sufficiently mobile).	To obtain a baseline of fluid balance. To enable assessment of dehydration or fluid overload.
6 Assess patient's conscious level.	To obtain a baseline and to be able to assess for change in condition (see Ch. 26, Observations: neurological).
7 Assess patient's level of anxiety and compliance with treatment (the patient's ability to cope with the treatment).	To enable an assessment to be made and, where necessary, a referral to medical staff.

Procedure guidelines: **Setting up continuous positive airway pressure (CPAP)**

Equipment

1 Oxygen supply.
2 Compressed air supply.
3 Flow generator.
4 Oxycheck.
5 Prepared CPAP circuit.
6 Y-connector.
7 T-piece.

8 Humidifier.
9 Temperature probe.
10 Water trap.
11 CPAP mask/nasal mask.
12 Headstrap.
13 PEEP valves (2.5/5.0/7.5/10.0 cm).

Procedure

Action	Rationale
1 Set up CPAP circuit.	
2 Ensure patient is in a comfortable position, sitting up in bed, well supported by a pillow.	To promote comfort and aid lung expansion and breathing.
3 Ensure patient is comfortable in surrounding environment.	To promote comfort and aid in compliance with using CPAP.
4 Explain to patient how the mask is to be applied. Apply mask gently, applying pressure as the patient adapts to the tight-fitting mask. Hold mask until patient is comfortable and settled.	To relieve anxiety and to reassure patient. To aid patient's compliance with CPAP.
5 Once the patient is settled with mask, apply the headstrap. Ensure mask and headstrap are comfortable for the patient; alter position as required.	To retain mask in place and aid patient comfort.
6 Ensure a good seal and that no leaks are present.	To ensure a tight seal in order that the system functions optimally.
7 Apply protective field dressing around vulnerable pressure points: nose, ear, back of head and neck.	To alleviate pressure and prevent tissue breakdown.
8 Give further explanation to family/next of kin of how CPAP works and the importance of their presence and participation in communication.	To relieve anxiety and support and reassure family and patient.

Problem guidelines: **Pre-continuous positive airway pressure (CPAP)** *(cont'd)*

Action	Rationale
9 Reassure the patient constantly.	
10 Discuss with doctor use of medication that might aid the patient in compliance with CPAP therapy.	To relieve patient anxiety and promote co-operation.

Procedure guidelines: **Humidification**

Various humidifiers exist. Select the system most appropriate for the patient.

Procedure

Action	Rationale
1 Discuss with the team the choice of system to be used.	The most appropriate device is selected to meet the patient's needs.
2 Explain to patient the reason for use of the humidifier and how it works.	So patient understands what is happening and thus to help the patient tolerate the humidification.
3 Prepare the device to be used. (a) Some circuits are ready prepared with humidifier. (b) Prepare humidifier and circuit. Humidifier/wide-bore oxygen tubing: ensure minimal length of tubing, water trap and mask.	
4 Once circuit is set up, run system to check it is functioning correctly and the circuit is intact.	To ensure that oxygen is being delivered through the circuit as set. To ensure the system is humidifying the oxygen and that no leaks exist.
5 If hot water system is in use check it is running within recommended temperature range.	To ensure no damage to the patient's lungs if temperature above range.
6 Ensure water is present in water source of system; do not allow to run dry.	Aid adequate delivery of humidity to the patient. Prevent damage to the humidifier.
7 Ensure circuit tubing is positioned below patient.	To ensure collection of humidity in the circuit is able to drain into the water trap or circuit rather than into the patient.
8 Ensure the patient finds the humidification comfortable.	
9 Continually check running of system.	To ensure the system is functioning adequately and delivering humidity.
10 Ensure the patient is well informed and continuously reassured. The patient may find the system noisy and may be distressed by excessive moisture in the circuit.	
11 Change the humidification and circuit on a weekly basis.	

Problem solving: **Oxygen therapy by nasal cannulae or oxygen mask**

Problem	Cause	Suggested action
Maintenance of airway.	Position of patient. Airway secretions.	Position patient properly. Encourage patient to cough and expectorate if able or remove secretions by suction if patient unable to do so.
Maintenance of adequate oxygenation.	Inadequate oxygen delivery, patient's condition deteriorating. More breathless. Oxygen saturation decreased. Deteriorating blood gases.	Assess level of oxygen support required in liaison with doctor. Increase oxygen delivery.
Dry mouth.	Oxygen therapy drying mouth.	Add humidification to the circuit (see Procedure guidelines: Humidification). Give regular mouth care.

Problem solving: Oxygen therapy by nasal cannulae or oxygen mask (cont'd)

Problem.	Cause	Suggested action
Nasal cannulae or mask discomfort.	Position or use of cannulae and oxygen mask.	Ensure correct placement.
Development of pressure points on nose/ears.	Incorrect placement of cannulae support or mask headstrap.	Change position of cannulae or mask. Apply padding around headstrap or to bridge of nose to relieve pressure.
Intolerance of oxygen therapy.	Fear and anxiety. Confusion. Hypoxia.	Assess patient for change. Ensure continual reassurance given to patient. Ensure patient remains orientated to the environment and oxygen device. If intolerant of mask, nasal cannulae may be tolerated. If hypoxic, oxygen may need to be increased.
Communication.	Mask makes communication difficult; patient may not hear carer and nurse may not hear patient.	Assist patient to move around bed area if not able to go far. Mobilize patient with portable oxygen cylinder if appropriate.
Inability to maintain personal hygiene.	Immobility. On bedrest. Mask restricting independence.	Provide reassurance for patient to remain independent where able. Allow them to carry out their own hygiene if able or to help patient with hygiene if not.
Maintenance of safety.	Detachment of oxygen from flow meter. Kinked or looped oxygen tubing. Mask removed by patient.	Ensure oxygen attached to flow meter. Check patient regularly. Ensure no kinks or loops arise. Ensure patient is attached to oxygen.
Documentation.	Rapidly changing situation.	Ensure all changes to oxygen therapy or patient are documented in nursing care plan.

Problem solving: **CPAP**

Problem	Cause	Suggested action
Maintenance of airway.	Deteriorating respiratory function. Physical tiring.	Continuously monitor respiratory function: skin colour; breathing pattern; respiratory rate; oxygen saturation; blood gases if arterial catheter in situ. Report changes to medical or anaesthetic staff.
Cardiovascular instability.	Hypotension. Arrhythmias. Decreasing central venous pressure. Decreasing cardiac output due to CPAP.	Continuously monitor cardiovascular function: heart rate; blood pressure. Continuously monitor central venous pressure. Report changes to medical staff.
Dehydration	Decreased oral intake. Decreased circulating volume. Nausea and vomiting.	Maintain an accurate fluid balance chart measuring input and output of both oral and intravenous fluids and urinary output. Take into account fluid loss from vomit/ diarrhoea or wound drainage. Check overall balance on an hourly basis. Report to medical staff who may order intravenous fluid therapy. Prescribe antiemetic.
Fluid overload: May present with pulmonary oedema. Retention of urine.	Sepsis. Cardiac failure.	Observe and assess patient. Maintain accurate fluid balance chart. Report to medical staff, who may order a diuretic. Undertake further assessment of fluid balance. Catheterize patient if unable to pass urine. Carry out accurate assessment of output.

*Problem solving: **CPAP** (cont'd)*

Problem	Cause	Suggested action
Inadequate dietary intake.	Gastric distension due to CPAP. Loss of appetite. Difficulty in eating; distress caused by respiratory status and CPAP. Nausea and vomiting	Encourage diet and oral supplementary fluids. If unable to take orally, refer to dietitian and doctor; an alternative method of feeding may be considered, e.g. nasogastric feeding and intravenous feeding (TPN). Administer antiemetic. Encourage and reassure patient.
Aspiration, if unable to maintain own airway.	Inability to maintain own airway. Continuous pressure from CPAP system. Insufflation of air.	Observe and assess patient closely. After discussion with medical staff the following actions should be considered: insert nasogastric tube; use clear CPAP mask.
Gastric distension and discomfort may cause nausea and vomiting.	Continuous pressure from CPAP system. Insufflation of air.	Encourage patient to belch to relieve air if it aids comfort. Insert nasogastric tube.
Dry mouth.	CPAP system utilizes a very high oxygen flow which has a drying effect.	Carry out regular mouth care (see Ch. 32, Personal hygiene: mouth care). Give patient regular sips of water, ice to suck or drinks as patient is able to take. Humidify, as in CPAP circuit.
Eyes: Dry Sore	Mask – air leak. High flow oxygen.	Ensure mask is well sealed with no leaks. Apply pressure-relieving padding around mask. Apply regular eye care (see Ch. 31, Personal hygiene: eye care).
Conjunctival oedema.	Facial pressure from mask – causing oedema.	Adjust mask to facial contour. Alter and position mask as comfortable. Loosen mask every couple of hours to relieve pressure. Position padding around the headstrap to relieve pressure.
Tissue integrity problems with sacrum, elbows, heels.	Continued bedrest. Difficulty in moving. Fear of moving.	Change patient's position in bed regularly. Nurse patient on alternate sides. Patient may sit out of bed if able. Consider alternative pressure-relieving mattress if patient immobile or has high Waterlow score (see Ch. 47, Wound management).
Mask incorrectly sealed.		Alter mask position to correct and ensure comfort. Ensure mask is correct size. Alter position to ensure correct seal.
Anxiety.	Tight-fitting mask. Feeling of claustrophobia and isolation. Fear of dying.	Reassure patient. Inform patient that nurse is present at all times and able to see patient. Inform patient of any changes taking place. Communicate with the patient's family, keep them informed and involve them in care and communication with patient. Inform doctor of patient's anxiety level. Administer anxiolytic agent if required.
Maintenance of safety of patient and environment.		Ensure nurse present with patient at all times.
Communication.		Observe patient and CPAP system closely to ensure equipment is working adequately and there is no failure of the system.

Problem solving: **CPAP** *(cont'd)*

Problem	Cause	Suggested action
Inability to communicate effectively.		Reassure patient and ensure he or she is comfortable.
Mask restriction.		Encourage patient to communicate and explain how he or she can use letterboard to do so.
Feeling of isolation.		Reassure patient.

References and further reading

Aherns, T. & Tucker, K. (1999) Pulse oximetry. *Crit Care Clin North Am,* **11**(1), 87–97.

Allan, D. (1988) Making sense of oxygen delivery. *Nurs Times,* **83**(18), 40–2.

Allison, R.C. (1991) Initial treatment of pulmonary oedema: a physiological approach. *Am J Med Sci,* **302**(6), 385–91.

Ball, C. (1999) Optimising oxygen delivery: haemodynamic workshop, part 1. *Intensive Crit Care Nurs,* **15**, 371–3.

Ball, C. (2000a) Optimising oxygen delivery: haemodynamic workshop, part 2. *Intensive Crit Care Nurs,* **16**, 33–44.

Ball, C. (2000b) Optimising oxygen delivery: haemodynamic workshop, part 3. *Intensive Crit Care Nurs,* **16**, 84–7.

Beaumont, M., Le Jeune, D., Mariotte, H. & Lotaso, F. (1997) Effects of chest wall counter pressure on lung mechanics under high level CPAP in humans. *J Physiol,* **83**(2), 591–8.

Benditt, J.W. (2000) Adverse effects of low flow oxygen therapy. *Respir Care* **45**(1), 54–80.

Berne, R.M. & Levy, M.N. (1998) *Physiology,* 4th edn. Mosby, St Louis.

Byron Brow, C.W. & Dracup, K. (2000) Too much of a good thing. *Am J Crit Care,* **9**(5), 300–2.

Carroll, P. (1997) Pulse oximetry at your fingertips. *RN,* May, 31–5.

Carpenter, D. (1991) Oxygen transport in the blood. *Crit Care Nurse,* **11**(9), 20–31.

Carroll, P. (1997) When you want humidity. *RN,* May 31–5.

Cooper, N. (2002) Oxygen therapy: myths and misconceptions. *Care Crit Ill,* **18**(3), 74–7.

Coull, A. (1992) Making sense of pulse oximetry. *Nurs Times,* **88**(32), 42–3.

Dunn, L. & Chrisholm, H. (1998) Oxygen therapy. *Nurs Stand,* **13**(7), 57–64.

Ehrhardt, B.S. & Graham, M. (1990) Making sense of oxygen delivery. *Nursing* (US), March, 50–4.

Esmond, G. (2000) *Respiratory Nursing.* Baillière Tindall, London.

Fell, H. & Boehm, M. (1998) Easing the discomfort of oxygen therapy. *Nurs Times,* **94**(38), 56–8.

Foss, M.A. (1990) Oxygen therapy. *Prof Nurse,* January, 180–90.

Goldhill, D. (2001) Postoperative oxygen. *Care Crit Ill,* **17**(5), 154–5.

Greeg, R.W. *et al.* (1990) Continuous positive airway pressure by face mask in *Pneumocystis carinii* pneumonia. *Crit Care Med,* **18**(1), 21–4.

Greenbaum, D.M., Synder, J.V., Grenvik, A.K.E. & Safar, P. (1976) Continuous positive airways pressure without tracheal intubation in spontaneously breathing patients. *Chest,* **69**, 615–20.

Guyton, A. (2000) *A Textbook of Medical Physiology,* 10th edn. W.B. Saunders, Philadelphia.

Hess, D. (2000) Detection and monitoring of hypoxaemia and oxygen therapy. *Respir Care,* **45**(1), 65–80.

Hinds, C.J. (1997) *Intensive Care. A Concise Textbook,* 2nd edn. Baillière Tindall, London.

Keen, A. (2000) Continuous positive airway pressure in the intensive care unit: uses and implications for nursing management. *Nurs Crit Care,* **5**(3), 137–41.

Keilty, S.E. & Bott, J. (1992) Continuously positive airway pressure. *Physiotherapy,* **78**(2), 90–2.

Kumar, P. & Clark, C. (1998) *Clinical Medicine,* 4th edn. W.B. Saunders, London.

Lenique, F., Habis, M., Lofasof, F. *et al.* (1997) Ventilatory and haemodynamic effects of continuous positive airway pressure in heart failure. *Am J Respir Crit Care Med,* **155**, 500–5.

Marieb, E.N. (2001) *Human Anatomy and Physiology,* 5th edn. Benjamin Cummings, New York.

Miller, R. & Semple, S. (1991) Continous positive airway pressure ventilation for respiratory failure associated with *Pneumocystis carinii* pneumonia. *Respir Med,* **85**, 133–8.

Oh, T.E. (1997) *Intensive Care Manual.* Butterworths, Sydney.

Petty, T.L. (2000) Historical highlights of long-term oxygen therapy. *Respir Care,* **45**(1), 29–38.

Pierce, L.N.B. (1995) *Guide to Mechanical Ventilation and Intensive Respiratory Care.* W.B. Saunders, London.

Pierson, D.J. (2000) Pathophysiology and clinical effects of chronic hypoxia. *Respir Care,* **45**(1), 39–51.

Place, B. (1998) Pulse oximetry in adults. *Nurs Times,* **94**(50), 48–9.

Romand, J.A. & Donald, E. (1995) Physiological effects of continuous positive airway pressure ventilation in the critically ill. *Care Crit Ill,* **11**(6), 239–42.

Schumaker, W.C., Ayres, S.M., Grevik, A. & Holbrook, P.R. (1996) *Textbook of Critical Care.* W.B. Saunders, Philadelphia, pp. 628–952.

Tinker, J. & Zapol, W. (1992) *Care of the Critically Ill Patient.* Springer, New York.

Tortora, G.J. & Grabowski, S.R. (2000) *Principles of Anatomy and Physiology,* 9th edn. John Wiley, New York.

Ward, B. & Park, G.R. (2000) Humidification of inspired gases in the critically ill. *Clin Intensive Care,* **11**(4), 169–76.

West, J.B. (1995) *Pulmonary Pathophysiology: The Essentials.* Williams & Wilkins, Baltimore.

Williamson, D.C. & Modell, J.H. (1972) Intermittent continuous airways pressure by mask – its use in the treatment of atelectasis. *Arch Surg,* **177**, 970–2.

Scalp cooling

Chapter contents

Definition

Scalp cooling is a method of preventing chemotherapy-induced alopecia. It acts by reducing the temperature of the scalp, causing the blood vessels supplying the hair follicles to constrict; this decreases the amount of drug that can pass to the hair follicles, thus reducing the cellular uptake of the drug and the degree of hair loss.

Indications

The effectiveness of scalp cooling has been demonstrated satisfactorily with doxorubicin, epirubicin, docetaxel and paclitaxel (Dean *et al.* 1979; Robinson 1987; Lemanager *et al.* 1995; Katsimbri 2000). Patients receiving other cytotoxic drugs which may cause alopecia, such as vindesine and vincristine, have undergone the procedure, although there are insufficient data to evaluate its effectiveness with these drugs. However, scalp cooling requires the consultant's permission as the procedure may protect micrometastases in the scalp from chemotherapy, especially where there is the possibility of circulating cancer cells, e.g. in cases of leukaemia and lymphoma (Witman *et al.* 1981). In spite of this, scalp cooling has been used successfully in patients with relapsed lymphoma (Purohit *et al.* 1992). Dean *et al.* (1983), drawing on evidence from 7800 women with breast cancer, found that only two experienced recurrence of disease on the scalp, suggesting that the risk of scalp metastases was minimal. They concluded that scalp cooling should not be contraindicated and could be used routinely with a wide variety of solid tumours. Nevertheless, patients with advanced metastatic disease have been found to develop scalp metastases during scalp cooling and Middleton *et al.* (1985) argued strongly against the use of scalp cooling in this group. Other studies have found no scalp metastases at follow-up (Ron *et al.* 1997). The potential risk of scalp metastases, albeit remote, should be addressed and demands discussion by health care professionals and patients (Peck 2000; Batchelor 2001).

The issues relating to scalp metastases are controversial. This dilemma, along with the media coverage regarding preventive measures for chemotherapy-induced alopecia (Carr 1998; Kendell 2001), have led some practitioners to question whether scalp cooling should be offered. Patients have highlighted how they feel about hair loss (Carr 1998) and also the need to provide more comfortable and effective scalp cooling in all cancer units and centres (Wilson 1994). In addition, an extensive review of the literature concluded that scalp cooling was effective and should be offered to all patients for whom it was appropriate (Crowe *et al.* 1998; Batchelor 2001). This was supported by the views of many nurses who felt that the use of scalp cooling with chemotherapy protocols which are associated with hair loss can effectively prevent alopecia and result in improved quality of life for patients (Lemanager *et al.* 1998). Patients also feel it is worthwhile regardless of how successful it is (Dougherty 2002).

Reference material

Alopecia is a common consequence of many chemotherapeutic regimens and is one of the most devastating effects of cancer chemotherapy (Pickard-Holley 1995; Williams *et al.* 1999). It has been identified as such a devastating prospect that some patients may refuse to accept treatment (Williams *et al.* 1999). Hair loss can also result in changes to the patient's body image (Freedman 1994) which may not be improved by the regrowth of hair (Munstedt *et al.* 1997).

Prevention of chemotherapy-induced alopecia

Several techniques have been tested to prevent chemotherapy-induced hair loss, the first being scalp tourniquets. These were used to minimize the contact the drug had with the hair follicles by occluding, using pressure, the superficial blood vessels supplying the scalp (Maxwell 1980). However, while some investigators found scalp tourniquets effective, others reported this method to be time-consuming, uncomfortable or ineffective (Parker 1987). Research findings indicate that scalp hypothermia may be simpler, less traumatic and more effective as a means of preventing alopecia when compared with the scalp tourniquet (David & Speechley 1987). Scalp cooling has an advantage over the scalp tourniquet in that it inhibits the cellular uptake of a drug that is temperature dependent (Dean *et al.* 1979).

More recently, biological methods of preventing hair loss have focused on promoting hair growth or protecting the hair follicles (Batchelor 2001). For example:

- Minoxidil 2% topical solution applied twice a day (Shapiro & Price 1998)

- Topical topitriol (Hidalgo *et al.* 1999)
- Application of a steroid 5-alpha reductase inhibitor (Uno & Kurata 1993)
- Immunosuppressive immunophilin ligands such as cyclosporin (Maurer *et al.* 1997), immunomodulators, AS101 (Sredni *et al.* 1996), CDK2 inhibitors (Davis *et al.* 2001) and P53 (a mediator of cellular response which is essential for chemotherapy-induced hair loss) (Vladimir *et al.* 2000).

The scientific rationale for scalp cooling

The rationale is based on characteristics of hair growth, the effect of cytotoxic drugs on hair follicles, physiological changes in scalp circulation and pharmacokinetics (Keller & Blausey 1988). Ninety per cent of all scalp hair is in an active phase of growth. The growth phase is characterized by significant mitotic activity, thus rendering the hair bulb especially sensitive to chemotherapeutic agents (Parker 1987). Scalp hypothermia produces changes in the scalp circulation by causing vasoconstriction of superficial vessels. Decreased blood flow to the scalp reduces the amount of the drug reaching the hair follicles and thus minimizes damage to the scalp hair (Kennedy *et al.* 1983; Parker 1987). Its success is also related to the metabolic effects of cooling, i.e. slowing the metabolic rate (Bulow *et al.* 1985), and it also appears that the degree of hair loss is temperature dependent. In order to prevent alopecia the temperature of the scalp must be reduced to at least 24°C but preferably 22°C (Gregory *et al.* 1982). Caps have to be kept in a freezer in order to reach temperatures of −18 to −20°C (Anderson *et al.* 1981; Kennedy *et al.* 1983; Giacone *et al.* 1988). Then when the cap is placed on the head the scalp temperature will drop from 37°C to 23–24°C within the first 15 minutes (Guy *et al.* 1982; Tollenaar *et al.* 1994). This is why a preinjection scalp cooling time of 20–30 minutes is said to be required (Anderson *et al.* 1981; Kennedy *et al.* 1983; Satterwhite & Zimm 1984; Middleton *et al.* 1985; Robinson 1987; Giacone *et al.* 1988).

Scalp cooling has been used in an attempt to reduce hair loss with palliative whole-brain radiotherapy. However, a pilot study (Shah *et al.* 2000) found that all patients still lost their hair and there was evidence that the cold cap application increased the dose of radiotherapy to the scalp.

Types of drugs

Doxorubin is commonly used in cancer chemotherapy and has a uniquely short half-life of approximately 30 minutes (compared to other drugs, such as cyclophosphamide which has a plasma half-life of over

6 hours) (Priestman 1989). This factor makes prophylactic scalp cooling feasible because it need only be utilized during peak plasma levels (Cline 1984). This is particularly important since doxorubicin results in a consistently high incidence of alopecia (80–90% of all patients), often leading to total hair loss (Dean *et al.* 1983). The involvement of doxorubicin, whether used alone or in combination, is a feature of most of the reported scalp cooling studies. In some studies, there was less success in maintaining hair with increasing doses of doxorubicin and/or liver metastases (Dean *et al.* 1983; David & Speechley 1987), but this may be resolved by extending the time the cap remains in place following chemotherapy administration.

Scalp cooling has also been used during the administration of epirubicin, as a single agent, with good results (Robinson 1987), although doses may influence outcomes (Adams *et al.* 1992). Subsequent studies have investigated combination regimens containing epirubicin and other drugs such as cyclophosphamide and 5-fluorouracil, with results of mild to moderate hair loss. However, when intravenous cyclophosphamide is added to any single agent anthracycline, the success rate is reduced from 80% of patients keeping most of their hair to about 50–60% of patients (Middleton *et al.* 1985; David & Speechley 1987). Some authors have therefore concluded that when combinations of cyclophosphamide and anthracyclines are given, scalp cooling had no place at all (Tollenaar *et al.* 1994). The group of drugs known as the taxanes also have the unfortunate side-effect of total alopecia; however, evidence has been produced to show that using scalp cooling in patients receiving docetaxel and paclitaxel can prevent complete hair loss (Lemanager *et al.* 1995, 1997; Katsimbri 2000; MacDuff *et al.* 2003).

Techniques

Homemade caps

Most of the studies that used an ice cap method of scalp cooling used a 'homemade' or commercial cap (Anderson *et al.* 1981; Dean *et al.* 1983; David & Speechley 1987; Lemanager *et al.* 1997).

Initially scalp cooling was achieved using crushed ice in plastic bags (Dean *et al.* 1979). A study of the efficacy of using a moulded prefrozen ice cap handmade from cryogel bags was conducted at The Royal Marsden Hospital (Anderson *et al.* 1981). David & Speechley (1987) confirmed that severe alopecia was consistently prevented in patients on doxorubicin alone (70%), with encouraging results for patients on other combinations of cytotoxic drugs.

Cryogel caps

The first commercial cap (Kold Kap) was successful in reducing hair loss, particularly with higher doses of doxorubicin (Dean *et al.* 1983). A three-layer cap (inner cotton, middle cryogel, outer lamb's wool) was also reported to prevent total hair loss (Howard & Stenner 1983). However, Wheelock *et al.* (1984) found that most patients suffered from severe hair loss even with the use of the Kold Kap. The most recent work has involved the use of cryogel caps such as the Chemocap and Penguin caps, which have been used for patients receiving single agents and combinations of anthracyclines (Peck 2000; Katsimbri 2000; Christodoulou *et al.* 2002) as well as in the use of docetaxel (Lemanager *et al.* 1995, 1997).

A large (170 patients) randomized study comparing Chemocap with the gelpack method found no statistical difference in efficacy between the two caps but Chemocap was shown to be more comfortable and offered a better fit, as well as being easier to use (Dougherty 2002).

Scalp cooling machines

Attempts have been made to produce an alternative type of cap that would improve effectiveness of scalp cooling, in particular to achieve a temperature that ensures a sufficiently low and constant reduction in scalp temperature that would endure during the entire procedure. Two types of scalp cooling machine have been designed: (1) refrigerated cooling systems where liquid coolant is pumped via a cap and maintains a more reliable temperature. Guy *et al.* (1982) reported encouraging results when the thermocirculator was first introduced, although Tollenaar *et al.* (1994) found that when used with patients receiving fluorouracil, epirubicin and cyclophosphamide (FEC), there was still a 50% chance of total alopecia occurring. The other scalp cooling machines appear to provide a more comfortable and effective system, e.g. Paxman and digitized systems (Ridderheim *et al.* 2003). (2) The use of refrigerated air passed over the patient's scalp via a hair-drying helmet was reported to be beneficial in over 50% of patients, with most experiencing no hair loss or slight hair loss and six requiring a wig (Symonds & McCormick 1986). However, other authors found that the system was only successful at lower doses of epirubicin (Adams *et al.* 1992).

There have also been good results using an electrically cooled cap in patients receiving CMF (cyclophosphamide, methotrexate and fluorouracil) chemotherapy (Ron *et al.* 1997).

Despite the large number of studies on scalp cooling they are difficult to compare with one another, owing to the multiple variables – different types of scalp cooling caps, varying methods of applying the caps, different chemotherapy regimens, tools for assessment of hair loss and who performs the assessment. Also sample numbers are often small and few studies are randomized or have a control group.

Factors which influence success

The success of all these methods in preventing hair loss varies and the amount of hair loss experienced by the patient is dependent on a number of factors:

- Involvement of the liver with metastatic disease leads to elevated plasma levels of doxorubicin for a longer period. Extension of the cooling period does not seem to improve the results (Satterwhite & Zimm 1984).
- Inadequate cooling because of exceptionally thick hair may lead to partial loss. It has been demonstrated that maximum cooling occurs 20 minutes after the cap has been placed in position. The weight of the cap (as well as the temperature) may be a factor, as this ensures that the contact is maintained over the complete scalp (Hunt et al. 1982). Success does not appear to be dose dependent, as was first thought (David & Speechley 1987; Dougherty 2002).
- It seems likely that when anthracyclines are used in combination with other drugs that cause alopecia (e.g. etoposide and cyclophosphamide) the success rate is not as high as with anthracyclines alone (Middleton et al. 1985).

Patient selection

All patients with solid tumours receiving doxorubicin, epirubicin or docetaxel as a single agent or in combination should be offered scalp cooling. However, scalp cooling should not be offered to:

- Patients with haematological disease unless the consultant feels it is appropriate to offer scalp cooling on the basis of quality of life
- Patients receiving drugs that cause hair loss, e.g. vincristine, where there is no research or evidence of the effectiveness of scalp cooling
- Patients who have already received a first course of chemotherapy which may induce hair loss but who were not offered or declined scalp cooling.

Patients must consent when they have been fully informed about the nature and length of the procedure, the chances of success and, where appropriate, the risk of scalp metastases (Peck 2000). Scalp cooling can be a long and uncomfortable procedure and should not be offered unless it is beneficial or the patient insists on undergoing the procedure even after a full explanation regarding the lack of any benefit. Patients must also be informed that they may discontinue the procedure at any time if they find it too physically or psychologically traumatic (Tierney 1987) or if they fail to retain hair.

Research shows that scalp cooling can be very distressing (Tierney et al. 1989) although patients still find it a worthwhile procedure to undergo regardless of whether or not it is successful and would have it again if necessary (Dougherty 1996, 2002). It has also been shown that the severity and distress associated with hair loss may be less for those who use scalp cooling (Protiere et al. 2002). Patients have reported adverse effects during and following treatment such as headaches, claustrophobia and ice phobias (Tierney et al. 1989; Dougherty 2002). Nurses need to understand the meaning that hair loss has for the patient. Alopecia can cause depression, loss of self-confidence and humiliation – it is a very visible sign of cancer.

Patients who have relapsed and are undergoing further chemotherapy which causes alopecia may find the loss of hair a second time to be more devastating (Gallagher 1996). It is important therefore to ensure that if a patient fails to retain hair or decides not to undergo scalp cooling, adequate time is spent helping the patient to adapt to the hair loss physically, psychologically and socially. It is recommended that nursing interventions be directed towards helping the patient and family to adapt to alopecia by using patient education, available resources and supportive listening (Pickard-Holley 1995). This can be partly achieved by ensuring that the patient sees the surgical appliance officer as soon as possible, in order to obtain a wig that can be matched to the patient's desired hair style and colour. Advice can be given on hair care and various ideas of hats, turbans and scarves, and reinforced with a hair care information booklet (Pickard-Holley 1995; Batchelor 2001).

Procedure guidelines: **Scalp cooling**

Equipment

1 A scalp cooling cap, e.g. Chemocap.
2 Overcap.
3 Skin protection, e.g. gauze, cotton wool pads.

4 Comfortable chair (recliner) or bed.
5 Extra pillows and blankets as required.

*Procedure guidelines: **Scalp cooling** (cont'd)*

Procedure

Action	Rationale
1 Before beginning, it is important to explain and discuss the procedure fully with the patient. Explain that the coldest and most uncomfortable time is the first 15 minutes after the cap has been applied. The patient should understand that the scalp cooling can be discontinued at any time and that it will not jeopardize the chemotherapy.	To ensure that the patient understands the procedure and what the success rate is likely to be depending on the type of chemotherapy regimen he/she is receiving. Patients who have undergone scalp cooling highlighted this as important knowledge to share when first undergoing scalp cooling (Dougherty 2002). To ensure that the patient gives his/her valid consent and knows that if the scalp cooling does not work, he/she can obtain a wig.
2 Check the cap has been in the freezer for a minimum of 12 hours (temperature −25 to −32°C).	To ensure the cap is cold enough to be effective.
3 Place the cap on the patient's head, making sure it fits closely and covers the whole hairline.	To ensure cooling over the head, including all the hair roots.
4 Apply the overcap to the patient's head.	To ensure even and close contact of the cap to the scalp.
5 Place protection in any areas where the cap touches the skin.	To prevent cold injury and improve the patient's comfort.
6 Place a pillow behind the patient's head if required.	To provide support for the patient's head and neck and to reduce the effect of the heaviness of the cap (approximately 2–3 kg).
7 Offer the patient the use of a blanket.	To provide the patient with some protection against the feeling of cold.
8 Leave the patient for at least 15 minutes before injection of the drug.	To obtain initial cooling of the scalp.
9 Administer the drug by intravenous injection as per prescription.	To administer treatment as appropriate.
10 The cap must be changed after 30 minutes regardless of the stage of administration.	To maintain adequate cooling.
11 If a drug takes longer than 30 minutes to administer the cap will need to be changed after 1 hour and then every hour thereafter depending on the type of drug.	To maintain adequate cooling.
12 On completion of the drug (i.e. the one likely to cause alopecia, e.g. doxorubicin), leave the patient for a further 45 minutes.	To maintain cooling until the plasma levels of drug have fallen (Hunt *et al.* 1982).
13 When sufficient time has elapsed, remove the cap.	To prevent damage to the scalp and hair.
14 Encourage the patient to rest, if desired.	To prevent faintness due to the cap being lifted off.
15 Wash the cap, dry and store on cardboard insert.	To minimize cross-infection and to maintain shape.
16 Ensure the patient is given the booklet 'Hair care and hair loss' (Patient information series).	To reinforce verbal information given during procedure.

Problem solving

Problem	Cause	Suggested action
Inadequate cooling.	Poorly fitting cap. Cap not sufficiently cooled.	Follow the procedure carefully. Ensure the cap size is correct and that the hair roots are covered. Ensure the cap is changed at correct times. Check the cap has been cooled to the correct temperature.
Excess cooling.	Thin hair.	Use plenty of gauze between the cap and scalp. If it is still painful then discontinue the procedure.

Problem solving (cont'd)

Problem	Cause	Suggested action
Complaints of headache.	Weight and coldness of cap.	Provide physical support to the neck and shoulders and blankets as required.
Distressed patient.	Claustrophobia.	Support and reassure the patient. If necessary, remove the cap.
	Ice phobia.	Be aware of this possible problem; encourage the patient to discuss feelings.
Hair loss.	Scalp cooling was not successful.	Offer the patient the opportunity to discontinue the scalp cooling. Make arrangements for the patient to see the appliance officer and obtain a wig. Discuss care of hair and scalp and give patient information booklet.

References and further reading

Adams, L. *et al.* (1992) The prevention of hair loss from chemotherapy by the use of cold air scalp cooling. *Eur J Cancer Care*, **15**, 16–18.

Anderson, J. *et al.* (1981) Prevention of doxorubicin-induced alopecia by scalp cooling in patients with advanced breast cancer. *Br Med J*, **282**, 423–4.

Batchelor, D. (2001) Hair and cancer chemotherapy. *Eur J Cancer Care*, **10**, 147–63.

Bulow, J. *et al.* (1985) Frontal subcutaneous blood flow and epi- and subcutaneous temperatures during scalp cooling in normal man. *Scand J Clin Lab Invest*, **45**, 505–8.

Burdine, S.A. (2001) *Who Needs Hair – The Flipside of Chemotherapy*. Saba Books, Florida.

Carr, K. (1998) How I survived the fall out. *You Magazine, Mail on Sunday*, 10 May, 61–7.

Christodoulou, C. *et al.* (2002) Effectiveness of the MSC cold cap system in the prevention of chemotherapy induced alopecia. *Oncology*, **62**(2), 97–102.

Cline, B.W. (1984) Prevention of chemotherapy-induced alopecia; a review of the literature. *Cancer Nurs*, June, 221–8.

Crowe, M., Kendrick, M. & Woods, S. (1998) *Is scalp cooling a procedure that should be offered to patients receiving alopecia induced chemotherapy for solid tumours?* Proceedings of 10th International Conference on Cancer Nursing, Jerusalem, Abstract, p. 64.

David, J.A. & Speechley, V. (1987) Scalp cooling to prevent alopecia. *Nurs Times*, **83**(32), 36–7.

Davis, S.T. *et al.* (2001) Prevention of chemotherapy induced alopecia in rats by CDC inhibitors. *Science*, **5**(291), 25–6.

Dean, J.C. *et al.* (1979) Prevention of doxorubicin-induced hair loss with scalp hypothermia. *N Engl J Med*, **301**, 1427–9.

Dean, J.C. *et al.* (1983) Scalp hypothermia: a comparison of ice packs and the Kold Kap in the prevention of doxorubicin-induced alopecia. *J Clin Oncol*, **1**(1), 33–7.

Dougherty, L. (1996) Scalp cooling to prevent hair loss in chemotherapy. *Prof Nurse*, **11**(8), 1–3.

Dougherty, L. (2002) A study to compare two methods of scalp cooling to prevent chemotherapy induced alopecia. Paper given at 12th ISCCN Conference, Wembley, August.

Freedman, T.G. (1994) Social and cultural dimensions of hair loss in women treated with breast cancer. *Cancer Nurs*, **174**, 334.

Gallagher, J. (1996) *Women's experiences of hair loss associated with chemotherapy – longitudinal perspective*. Proceedings of 9th International Conference on Cancer Nursing, Brighton, Abstract, p. 52.

Gallagher, J. (1997) Chemotherapy induced hair loss – impact on a woman's quality of life. *Qual Life*, **5**(4), 75–8.

Giacone, G. *et al.* (1988) Scalp hypothermia in the prevention of doxorubicin induced hair loss. *Cancer Nurs*, **11**(3), 170–3.

Gregory, R.P. *et al.* (1982) Prevention of doxorubicin induced alopecia by scalp hypothermia: relation to degree of cooling. *Br Med J*, **284**, 1674.

Guy, R. *et al.* (1982) Scalp cooling by thermocirculator. *Lancet*, 24 April, 937–8.

Hidalgo, G.M. *et al.* (1999) A phase I trial of topical topitriol. *Anticancer Drugs*, **10**(4), 393–5.

Howard, N. & Stenner, R.W. (1983) Technical notes – an improved 'ice cap' to prevent alopecia caused by adriamycin (doxorubicin). *Br J Radiol*, **56**, 963–4.

Hunt, J. *et al.* (1982) Scalp hypothermia to prevent adriamycin-induced hair loss. *Cancer Nurs*, **5**(1), 25–31.

Katsimbri, P. (2000) Prevention of chemotherapy induced alopecia using an effective scalp cooling system. *Eur J Cancer Care*, **36**, 766–71.

Keller, J.F. & Blausey, L.A. (1988) Nursing issues and management in chemotherapy-induced alopecia. *Oncol Nurs Forum*, **15**(5), 603–7.

Kendell, P. (2001) Magic gel that helps cancer patients hold onto their hair. *Daily Mail*, 6 January.

Kennedy, M. *et al.* (1983) The effects of using Chemocap on occurrence of chemotherapy induced alopecia. *Oncol Nurs Forum*, **10**(1), 19–24.

Lemanager, M. *et al.* (1995) Docetaxel induced alopecia can be prevented. *Lancet*, **346**, 371–2.

Lemanager, M. *et al.* (1997) Effectiveness of cold cap in the prevention of docetaxel induced alopecia. *Eur J Cancer*, **33**(2), 297–300.

Lemanager, M. *et al.* (1998) Alopecia induced by chemotherapy – a controllable side effect. *Oncol Nurs Today*, **3**(2), 18–20.

MacDuff, C., MacKenzie, T., Hutcheon, A. *et al.* (2003) The effectiveness of scalp cooling in preventing alopecia for patients receiving epirubicin and docetaxel. *Eur J Cancer Care*, **12**, 154–61.

Maurer, M. *et al.* (1997) Hair growth modulation by topical immunophilin ligands. *Am J Pathol*, **150**(4), 1433–41.

Maxwell, M.B. (1980) Scalp tourniquets for chemotherapy-induced alopecia. *Am J Nurs*, **5**, 900–2.

Middleton, J. *et al.* (1985) Failure of scalp hypothermia to prevent hair loss when cyclophosphamide is added to doxorubicin and vincristine. *Cancer Treat Rep*, **69**(4), 373–5.

Molassiotis, A. (2003) A multicentre study to determine the efficacy and patient acceptability of the Paxman scalp cooler to prevent hair loss in patients receiving chemotherapy. *Eur J Oncol Nurs*, in press.

Munstedt, K. *et al.* (1997) Changes in self concept and body image during alopecia induced cancer chemotherapy. *Support Care Cancer*, **5**, 139–43.

Parker, R. (1987) The effectiveness of scalp hypothermia in preventing cyclophosphamide induced alopecia. *Oncol Nurs Forum*, **14**(6), 49–53.

Peck, H.J. (2000) Evaluating the efficacy of scalp cooling using Penguin cold caps. *Eur J Cancer Care*, **4**(4), 246–8.

Pickard-Holley, S. (1995) The symptom experience of alopecia. *Semin Oncol Nurs*, **11**(4), 235–8.

Priestman, T.J. (1989) *Cancer Chemotherapy: An Introduction*, 3rd edn. Springer, Berlin.

Protiere, C., Evans, K., Camerlo, J. *et al.* (2002) Efficacy and tolerance of a scalp cooling system for prevention of hair loss and the experience of breast cancer patients treated by adjuvant chemotherapy. *Support Care Cancer*, **10**, 529–37.

Purohit, O.P. *et al.* (1992) A six week chemotherapy regimen for relapsed lymphoma efficacy results and the influence of scalp cooling. *Ann Oncol*, **3**(Suppl 5), 126.

Ridderheim, M., Bjurburg, M. & Gustavsson, A. (2003) Scalp hypothermia to prevent chemotherapy-induced alopecia is effective and safe: a pilot study of a new digitized scalp-cooling system used in 74 patients. *Support Care Cancer*, **11**, 371–7.

Robinson, M.H. (1987) Effectiveness of scalp cooling in reducing alopecia caused by epirubicin treatment of advanced breast cancer. *Cancer Treat Rep*, **71**, 913–14.

Ron, I.G. *et al.* (1997) Scalp cooling in the prevention of alopecia in patients receiving depilating chemotherapy. *Support Care Cancer*, **5**, 136–8.

Satterwhite, B. & Zimm, S. (1984) The use of scalp hypothermia in the prevention of doxorubicin-induced hair loss. *Cancer*, **54**, 34–7.

Shah, N. *et al.* (2000) A pilot study to assess the feasibility of prior scalp cooling of palliative whole brain radiotherapy. *Br J Radiol*, **73**, 514–16.

Shapiro, J. & Price, V.H. (1998) Hair regrowth: therapeutic agents. *Dermatol Clin*, **16**(2), 341–56.

Sredni, B. *et al.* (1996) The protective role of the immunomodulator AS101 against chemotherapy induced alopecia: studies on humans and animals. *Cancer Res*, **65**, 97–103.

Symonds, R.P. & McCormick, C.V. (1986) Adriamycin alopecia prevented by cold air scalp cooling. *Am J Clin Oncol*, **9**(5), 454–7.

Tierney, A.J. (1987) Preventing chemotherapy-induced alopecia in cancer patients: is scalp cooling worthwhile? *J Adv Nurs*, **12**, 303–10.

Tierney, A.J. *et al.* (1989) *A Study to Inform Nursing Support of Patients Coping with Chemotherapy for Breast Cancer*. Report prepared for the Scottish Home and Health Department.

Tollenaar, R.A.E.M. *et al.* (1994) Scalp cooling has no place in the prevention of alopecia in adjuvant chemotherapy in breast cancer. *Eur J Cancer*, **30A**(10), 1448–53.

Uno, H. & Kurata, S. (1993) Chemical agents and peptide affect hair growth. *J Invest Dermatol*, **101**(1), 143–8S.

Vladimir, A.B. *et al.* (2000) P53 is essential for chemotherapy induced hair loss. *Cancer Res*, **60**, 5002–6.

Wheelock, J.B. *et al.* (1984) Ineffectiveness of scalp hypothermia in the prevention of alopecia in patients treated with doxorubicin and cisplatin combinations. *Cancer Treat Rep*, **68**, 1387–8.

Williams, J. *et al.* (1999) A narrative study of chemotherapy induced alopecia. *Oncol Nurs Forum*, **26**(9), 1463–8.

Wilson, C. (1994) The ice cap that could help save your hair. *Daily Mail*, 20 September, 36–7.

Witman, G. *et al.* (1981) Misuse of scalp hypothermia. *Cancer Treat Rep*, **65**(5–6), 507–8.

39

Specimen collection for microbiological analysis

Chapter contents

Definition

Specimen collection is the collection of a required amount of tissue or fluid for laboratory examination, to allow for the isolation and identification of micro-organisms that cause disease, and to determine their antimicrobial sensitivity to guide the doctor with the selection of appropriate antimicrobial therapy (Mims *et al.* 1998).

Indications

Specimen collection is required when microbiological, biochemical or other laboratory investigations are indicated. Nursing staff should be able to identify the need for microbiological investigations and, if appropriate, initiate the taking of specimens (Papasian & Kragel 1997). Specimen collection is often a first crucial step in investigations that define the nature of the disease and determine diagnosis and the mode of treatment.

The clinical microbiology laboratory plays a fundamental role in the diagnosis of infection. Its importance increases in immunosuppressed patients because the usual signs and symptoms may be absent (Shelton 1999) and because infection is the cause of significant morbidity and mortality (Sandin & Rinaldi 1996).

Reference material

General principles

Successful laboratory diagnosis depends on the collection of specimens at the appropriate time, using the correct technique and equipment and transporting them to the designated laboratory safely without delay. For this to be achieved, good liaison is essential between medical, nursing, portering and laboratory staff.

The first step in the accurate diagnosis of infectious disease is to obtain adequate specimens for microbiological examination. Therefore the sample must be

(Shanson 1999). There are three main laboratory techniques available for the diagnosis of viral infections (Baker *et al.* 1998):

- Direct microscopy
- Culture (isolation of growth in living cell systems)
- Serology.

For culture specimens the use of viral transport media and speed of delivery to the laboratory are important as viruses do not survive well outside the body. With good liaison, the nursing personnel should obtain the specimen when the laboratory staff have the transport ready to take it to the virus laboratories. If delays occur, the specimen should be refrigerated at a temperature of 4°C, but never frozen in normal refrigerator freezers, where the temperature is around −20°C, as viruses may die rapidly at this temperature (Shanson 1999).

The time at which specimens are collected for viral investigations is important. Many viral illnesses have a prodromal phase during which the multiplication and shedding of the virus are at a peak and the patient is most infectious (Mims *et al.* 1998). Immunocompromised patients are particularly susceptible to viral respiratory tract infections. When an upper respiratory specimen is collected it is important to ensure the recovery of respiratory epithelial cells from the lining of the upper part of the nasal passage. To obtain an adequate number of cells nasopharyngeal swabs, aspirates and washes need to be undertaken correctly (Storch 2000). To aid the retrieval of cells from higher up the nasal passage, equipment such as a filling tube (Kwill®), a wide-bore bladder syringe or a cut-down suction catheter to instil the 0.9% sodium chloride can be used.

Serological

Serological testing for the presence of antigens and antibodies is used when it is not possible to isolate the organism from the patient's tissue easily. By demonstrating serum antibodies to suspected organisms it is inferred that the patient is, or has been, infected with the organism. A single test is inadequate as if the titres (the concentration of the substance being measured) are raised it is impossible to determine whether this is due to past or present infection. Two tests need to be carried out, both of which involve the collection of 10 ml of blood once at the beginning of the illness and again 10–14 days later. If a rising titre level is demonstrated it suggests the patient's infection is current (Mims *et al.* 1998).

Mycosis

Although many pathogenic fungi will grow on ordinary bacteriological culture media, they grow better and with less risk of bacterial overgrowth on special mycological media. The presence of fungi in clinical specimens is difficult to interpret, as *Candida albicans*, for example, is commonly present in the upper respiratory, alimentary and female genital tract and on the skin of healthy people (Baker *et al.* 1998).

Mycobacteriological

For further information, please refer to the procedure on tuberculosis (see Ch. 5, Barrier nursing).

Protozoa

Most protozoa do not cause disease, but those that do, e.g. malaria, make a formidable contribution to human illness (Armitage & King 2000). Laboratory investigations depend on direct microscopy which necessitates specimens being delivered to the laboratory as quickly as possible, while the protozoa are mobile and therefore visible.

Blood

Blood specimens are obtained for several reasons:

- To indicate relatively common disorders
- To make a diagnosis
- To follow the course of a disease
- To regulate therapy and drug dosage (Weinstein 2000).

Wherever possible, blood should be obtained peripherally (see Ch. 45, Venepuncture). Blood samples can be obtained from central venous access devices (CVAD); however, the device must then be flushed directly after obtaining the blood sample to avoid an occlusion (Gabriel 1999) (see Ch. 44, Vascular access devices).

Blood cultures

Bacteraemia and fungaemia are frequent complications in immunocompromised and critically ill patients. Ideally, the causative agent should be readily identified to facilitate timely treatment to promote the patient's recovery (Henker 2000). Accurate and speedy microbiological detection of infection using blood cultures is of paramount importance to determine the cause and guide the treatment (see Ch. 5, Barrier nursing). Success in gaining information from blood cultures relies on the accurate timing of the specimen and obtaining the correct volume of blood. Most bacteraemias are intermittent, so blood cultures should be taken when the signs of infection are present (Gill *et al.* 2000). These may include fever, chills, rigors, changes in mental status and lethargy (Shelton 1999).

Blood for culture should be sampled before administration or modification of antibiotic therapy, as antibiotics may delay or prevent bacterial growth, causing false negative results (Engervall & Bjorkholm 1996; Higgins 2000).

Failure to use aseptic technique when obtaining blood cultures can result in diagnosis of a pseudobacteraemia, due to contamination of the culture by bacteria originating outside the patient's bloodstream. This could result in inappropriate antibiotic therapy being administered and a significant waste of health care resources (Jumaa & Chattopadhyay 1994).

The needle used to obtain blood for culture investigation should be changed prior to the inoculation of the blood into the blood culture bottle. This is because studies have indicated an increase in contamination rates when the needle is not changed (Spitalnic et al. 1995).

CVAD-related infection and its associated morbidity and mortality are often underestimated in clinical practice (Elliott 1993). A fever of unknown origin does not always indicate that a CVAD should be immediately removed (Goodwin & Carlson 1993). When it is suspected that the CVAD is the source of infection, a blood culture sample must be obtained from both the device and a peripheral vein (Gabriel 1999). If there are signs of infection, e.g. redness and/or discharge around the site of insertion, a swab should also be taken for microbiological culture. This will then confirm or eliminate the CVAD as the cause of infection.

Some catheters facilitate microbial adherence, which will increase in proportion to the time the catheter is in situ (Henderson 2000). However, Wormser et al. (1990) suggest that if an aseptic technique is used to obtain blood from a catheter that has been in place for a relatively short time then reliable results can still be achieved.

Quantitative analysis of drugs in blood

Therapeutic drug monitoring by blood analysis is important to determine the correct optimal dosage, while avoiding dangerous side-effects. For most drugs used in clinical practice this type of monitoring is unnecessary. However, there are a limited number of drugs that must be frequently monitored in clinical practice. These include: lithium, digoxin, theophylline, phenytoin and a number of antibiotics, for example the aminoglycoside antibiotics and vancomycin (Higgins 2000).

The aminoglycoside antibiotics and vancomycin possess a narrow therapeutic range, so if the serum levels are too low the efficacy of the drug is decreased (Tam et al. 1999). However, these antibiotics are potentially nephrotoxic and ototoxic and therefore all patients receiving these drugs should have serum sent regularly for antimicrobial assay (Downie et al. 2000). The primary purpose is to avoid toxic accumulation, but it is also important to obtain good therapeutic levels, particularly

in patients with a Gram-negative sepsis (Shirrel et al. 1999).

Analysis involves laboratory testing of blood serum. Although this knowledge can be gained from random sampling, most benefit will be obtained by the correct timing of sample collection. This will provide a direct relationship to drug administration, and therefore give the correct interpretation of the serum concentration results.

Ideally, a trough sample just before the next scheduled dose, plus a peak level at a set time following the administration of the drug, will provide the most useful information (Mims et al. 1998). Abnormally elevated drug levels may be obtained if the blood samples are taken from a CVAD through which the drug has been administered. This is more likely if the catheter has not been flushed correctly following administration of the drug (Johnston & Messina 1991) or the first 10 ml of blood has not been discarded. Occasionally the CVAD may have to be used, for example, for paediatric patients or when only poor or limited venous access is available. If a multilumen CVAD is in place, a different lumen from the one used to administer the drug must be used to obtain the blood specimen. If scrupulous attention to policy is adhered to, blood levels obtained from CVAD can compare favourably with specimens taken from peripheral veins (Shulman et al. 1998).

If blood samples have to be taken from a CVAD because peripheral vein access is not available, this information must be written onto the microbiology request card (Shulman et al. 1998).

A 6-year audit of gentamicin drug monitoring to establish optimal regimens found that in those patients who achieved therapeutic drug levels, the average duration of antibiotic therapy was statistically shorter than in those patients who failed to achieve therapeutic peak concentrations. During this audit, 7% of patients' blood levels was found to be in the toxic range. This audit indicated that drug monitoring leads to improved drug administration (Ismail et al. 1997) by preventing toxicity and improving outcome.

In the procedure guidelines below two examples of drug analysis have been discussed; the laboratory will supply specific times for blood sampling for other drugs.

For further information on the collection of blood see the procedure for venepuncture (Ch. 44).

Urine

Urine is normally sterile, while the distal urethra of both men and women is normally colonized with a large number of bacteria (Gill et al. 2000) and even a carefully taken urine specimen may contain a few bacteria. As urine is such a good culture medium, any bacteria present at the time of collection will continue to multiply in the specimen container, resulting in a falsely raised bacteriuria (Higgins 1995, 2000), which will then result in misleading information (Gill *et al.* 2000).

It was thought that cleaning of the area around the urinary meatus prior to the collection of a midstream specimen of urine would reduce genital secretion contamination by removing loose epithelial cells and adherent bacteria. However, studies have suggested that such cleaning makes no difference to contamination rates (Holliday *et al.* 1991), although perineal and penile cleaning may be of benefit to those patients whose personal hygiene is poor. Patients should, however, be encouraged to wash their hands prior to collecting a 'clean catch' midstream urine specimen (Higgins 2000). Female patients should be instructed to part the labia while passing urine to avoid contamination (Graham & Galloway 2001).

The principle for obtaining midstream collection of urine is that any bacteria present in the urethra are washed away in the first portion of urine voided (Higgins 2000).

Procedure guidelines: **Specimen collection**

Procedure

Action	Rationale
1 Explain and discuss the procedure with the patient and ensure privacy while the procedure is being carried out.	To ensure that the patient understands the procedure and gives his/her valid consent.
2 Wash hands using bactericidal soap and water or bactericidal alcoholic handrub before and after obtaining specimen.	Hand washing greatly reduces the risk of infection transfer.
3 On completion of procedure, place specimens and swabs in the appropriate, correctly labelled containers.	To ensure that only organisms for investigation are preserved.
4 Dispatch specimens promptly to the laboratory with the completed request form.	To ensure the best possible conditions for any laboratory examinations.

Eye swab

Action	Rationale
1 Using either a plastic loop or a cotton wool-covered wooden stick, hold the swab parallel to the cornea and gently rub the conjunctiva in the lower eyelid.	To ensure that a swab of the correct site is taken. To avoid contamination by touching the eyelid.
2 If possible, smear the conjunctival swab on an agar plate at the bedside.	Eye swabs are often unsatisfactory because of the action of tears, which contain the enzyme lysozyme which acts as an antiseptic. Conjunctival scrapings are preferable. This procedure is usually performed by medical staff.

Nose swab

Action	Rationale
1 Moisten the swab beforehand with sterile water.	To prevent discomfort to the patient. The healthy nose is virtually dry and a dry swab may cause discomfort.
2 Move the swab from the anterior nares and direct it upwards into the tip of the nose (Fig. 39.1).	To swab the correct site and to obtain the required sample.
3 Gently rotate the swab.	

Perinasal swab (for whooping cough)

Action	Rationale
1 Using a special soft-wire mounted swab, pass it along the floor of the nasal cavity to the posterior wall of the nasopharynx (Fig. 39.1).	To minimize trauma to nasal tissue. To obtain a swab from the correct site.
2 Rotate the swab gently.	

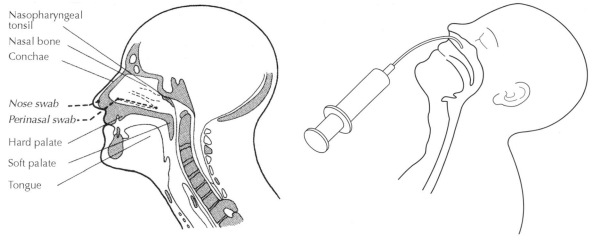

Figure 39.1 Area to be swabbed when sampling the nose.

Figure 39.2 Nasopharyngeal specimen collection. Nasal wash: syringe method.

Procedure guidelines: Specimen collection (cont'd)

Nasopharyngeal specimen collection: Nasal wash: syringe method (Fig. 39.2)

Equipment

1 5 ml 0.9% sodium chloride.
2 5 ml syringe or wide-bore bladder syringe.
3 Filling tube (or cut-off tip from a suction catheter if using 5 ml syringe).
4 Viral transport medium (VTM) (if required by laboratory).
5 Specimen container.

Procedure

Action	Rationale
1 Fill a syringe with 0.9% sodium chloride and attach a filing tube to the syringe tip.	To facilitate instillation of 0.9% sodium chloride high into the patient's nostril.
2 (a) Ask the patient to tilt their head slightly back whilst sitting upright.	To promote the flow of 0.9% sodium chloride into the nostril.
(b) Quickly instil 0.9% sodium chloride into one nostril.	To facilitate maximum recovery of epithelial cells.
3 (a) Aspirate the recoverable nasal specimen.	Recovery must occur immediately as the instilled saline will rapidly drain.
(b) Alternatively, where appropriate, patients may tilt head forward and gently push the fluid out of the nostril into the specimen container.	To allow specimen to drain into suitable sterile container. Patient may feel more comfortable.
4 If aspirated: inject aspirated specimen from syringe into suitable dry, sterile container or one containing viral transport medium, according to virology laboratory requirements.	To ensure a good-quality specimen is transported safely to the laboratory.
5 Repeat procedure on other nostril.	To promote optimal combined specimen.

Nasopharyngeal specimen collection: Vacuum-assisted nasal aspirate method (Fig. 39.3)

Equipment

1 Suction pump.
2 Sterile suction catheter.
3 Mucus trap (i.e. Lukens tube).
4 Viral transport medium (VTM) (if required by laboratory).

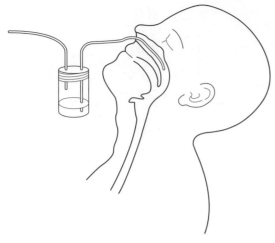

Figure 39.3 Nasopharyngeal specimen collection.
Vacuum-assisted nasal aspirate method.

Table 39.1 Catheter sizes and suction pressures

Patient age	Catheter size (French)	Suction pressure (mmHg)
Premature infant	6	80–100
Infant	8	80–100
Toddler/preschooler	10	100–120
School age	12	100–120
Adolescent/adult	14	120–150

Procedure guidelines: **Specimen collection** *(cont'd)*

Procedure

Action	Rationale
1 Attach mucus trap to suction pump and appropriate sized catheter (Table 39.1), leaving wrapper on suction catheter.	To ensure catheter stays clean while getting equipment ready.
2 Turn on suction and adjust to suggested pressure (Table 39.1).	To ensure suction machine is working correctly and pressure is set at the appropriate level.
3 Without applying suction, insert catheter into the nose, directed posteriorly and towards the opening of the external ear. *Note:* depth of insertion necessary to reach posterior pharynx is equivalent to distance between anterior naris and external opening of ear.	To prevent damaging the nasopharynx. To minimize patient discomfort.
4 Apply suction. Using a rotating movement, slowly withdraw catheter. *Note:* catheter should remain in nasopharynx no longer than 10 seconds.	To prevent damaging nasopharynx.
5 Hold trap upright to prevent secretions from going into pump.	To prevent loss of specimen.
6 Rinse catheter (if necessary) with approximately 20 ml viral transport medium.	To ensure maximum recovery of epithelial cells.
7 Disconnect suction; connect tubing to arm of mucus trap to seal.	To prevent contamination and/or loss of specimen.

Sputum

Action	Rationale
1 Use a specimen container that is free from organisms of respiratory origin. This need not, therefore, be a sterile container.	Sputum is never free from organisms since material originating in the bronchi and alveoli has to pass through the pharynx and mouth, areas that have a normal commensal population of bacteria.

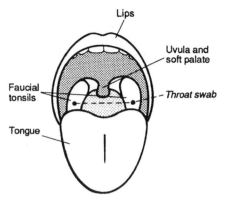

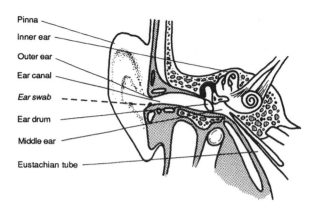

Figure 39.4 Area to be swabbed when sampling the throat.

Figure 39.5 Area to be swabbed when sampling the outer ear.

*Procedure guidelines: **Specimen collection** (cont'd)*

Action	Rationale
2 Care should be taken to ensure that the material sent for investigations is sputum, not saliva.	To obtain the required sample.
3 Encourage patients who have difficulty producing sputum to cough deeply first thing in the morning. Alternatively, a physiotherapist should be called to assist.	To facilitate expectoration.
4 Send any sputum specimen to the laboratory immediately.	The bacterial population alters rapidly and rapid dispatch should ensure accurate results.

Throat swab

Action	Rationale
1 Ask the patient to sit in such a position that he/she is facing a strong light source. Depress the patient's tongue with a spatula.	To ensure maximum visibility of the area to be swabbed. The procedure is one that is likely to cause the patient to gag and the tongue will move to the roof of the mouth, contaminating the specimen.
2 Quickly, but gently, rub the swab over the prescribed area, usually the tonsillar fossa or any area with a lesion or visible exudate (Fig. 39.4).	To obtain the required sample.
3 Avoid touching any other area of the mouth or tongue with the swab.	To prevent contamination by other organisms.

Ear swab

Action	Rationale
1 No antibiotics or other chemotherapeutic agents should have been used in the aural region 3 hours before taking the swab.	To prevent collection of traces of such therapeutic agents.
2 Place the swab into the outer ear as shown in Fig. 39.5. Rotate the swab gently.	To avoid trauma to the ear. To collect any secretions.

Wound swab

Action	Rationale
1 Take any swabs required before cleaning procedure begins.	To collect the maximum number of micro-organisms and to prevent collection of any therapeutic agents that may be employed in the dressing procedure.

Procedure guidelines: Specimen collection (cont'd)

Action	Rationale
2 Rotate the swab gently.	To collect samples. It is preferable to send samples of purulent discharge instead of swabs.

Note: the use of disposable gloves is recommended in the following procedures in order to prevent cross-infection.

Vaginal swab

Action	Rationale
1 Introduce a speculum into the vagina to separate the vaginal walls. Take the swab as high as possible in the vaginal vault.	To ensure maximum visibility of the area to be swabbed. To ensure that the swab is taken from the best site. If infection by *Trichomonas* species is suspected, a charcoal-impregnated swab is recommended as this organism survives longer in this medium.

Penile swab

Action	Rationale
1 Retract prepuce.	To obtain maximum visibility of area to be swabbed.
2 Rotate swab gently in the urethral meatus.	To collect any secretions.

Rectal swab

Action	Rationale
1 Pass the swab, with care, through the anus into the rectum.	To avoid trauma. To ensure that a rectal and not an anal sample is obtained.
2 Rotate gently.	To avoid trauma.
3 In patients suspected of suffering from threadworms, take the swab from the perianal region.	Threadworms lay their ova on the perianal skin.

Faeces

Action	Rationale
1 Ask the patient to defecate into a clinically clean bedpan.	To avoid unnecessary contamination from other organisms.
2 Scoop enough material to fill a third of the specimen container using a spatula or a spoon, often incorporated in the specimen container.	To obtain a usable amount of specimen. To prevent contamination.
3 Examine the specimen for such features as colour, consistency and odour, and record your observations.	To monitor any fluctuations and trends.
4 Segments of tapeworm are seen easily in faeces and any such segments should be sent to the laboratory for identification.	Unless the head is dislodged, the tapeworm will continue to grow. Laboratory confirmation of the presence of the head is essential.
5 Patients suspected of suffering from amoebic dysentery should have any stool specimens dispatched to the laboratory immediately.	The parasite causing amoebic dysentery exists in a free-living non-motile cyst. Both are characteristic in their fresh state but are difficult to identify when dead.

Urine

Action	Rationale
1 Specimens of urine should be collected as soon as possible after the patient wakens in the morning and at the same time each morning if more than one specimen is required.	The bladder will be full as urine has accumulated overnight. If specimens are taken at other times, the urine may be diluted. All specimens will be comparable if taken at the same time each morning.
2 Dispatch all specimens to the laboratory as soon after collection as possible.	Urine specimens should be examined within 2 hours of collection or 24 hours if kept refrigerated at a temperature of 4°C. At room temperature overgrowth will occur and lead to misinterpretation.

*Procedure guidelines: **Specimen collection** (cont'd)*

Midstream specimen of urine: male

Action	Rationale
1 Retract the prepuce and clean the skin surrounding the urethral meatus with soap and water, 0.9% sodium chloride solution or a solution that does not contain a disinfectant.	To prevent other organisms contaminating the specimen. Disinfectants may irritate or be painful to the urethral mucous membrane.
2 Ask the patient to direct the first and last part of his stream into a urinal or toilet but to collect the middle part of his stream into a sterile container.	To avoid contamination of the specimen with organisms normally present on the skin.

Midstream specimen of urine: female

Action	Rationale
1 If necessary, clean the urethral meatus with soap and water, 0.9% sodium chloride solution or a solution that does not contain a disinfectant.	To prevent other organisms contaminating the specimen. Disinfectants may irritate or be painful to the urethral mucous membrane.
2 (a) Use a separate cotton-wool swab for each swab. (b) Swab from the front to the back.	To prevent cross-infection. To prevent perianal contamination.
3 Ask the patient to micturate into a bedpan or toilet. Encourage patient to spread labia with one hand while micturating.	To avoid contamination of the specimen with organisms normally present on the skin.
4 Place sterile receiver or a wide-mouthed container under the stream of urine and remove before micturation finishes.	To prevent contamination of specimen.
5 Transfer the specimen into a sterile container.	

Specimen of urine from an ileal conduit

For further information see the relevant section in the procedure on stoma care (Ch. 15).

Catheter specimen of urine

For further information see the relevant section in the procedure on urinary catheterization (Ch. 16).

24-hour urine collection

Action	Rationale
1 Request the patient to void the bladder at the time appointed to begin this procedure. Discard this specimen.	To ensure the urine collected is that produced in the 24 hours stated.
2 All urine passed in the next 24 hours is collected In a large specimen bottle. The final specimen is collected at exactly the same time the bladder was voided 24 hours earlier.	Body chemistry alters constantly. A 24-hour collection will accommodate all the variables within a representative period.
3 Care must be taken to ensure the patient understands the procedure in order to eliminate the risk of an incomplete collection.	A 24-hour collection will not be obtained if one sample is lost, and the results will be invalid.

Semen

Action	Rationale
1 Sexual intercourse should not have taken place for 3–4 days before the specimen is collected.	To ensure the sperm count will be at maximum levels. It takes between 3 and 4 days for the sperm count to return to normal after ejaculation.
2 A fresh masturbated specimen must be collected in a sterile container and delivered to the laboratory within 2 hours of the collection of the specimen.	Sperm will die if there is a delay in testing. Specimens must not be collected in a condom as sperm die when in contact with materials such as rubber.

Procedure guidelines: Specimen collection (cont'd)

Cervical scrape

Action	Rationale
1 The ideal time for smear testing is mid-cycle.	To allow for accuracy of results as the cervix is usually free of contamination from menstrual flow at this time.
2 The menses should be avoided.	This is less uncomfortable for the patient.
3 The smear must be taken before a vaginal examination is carried out.	To ensure that normal tissue samples are obtained.
4 Label the ground glass end of the slide with the patient's name.	To ensure patient identification.
5 Expose the cervix by using a dry speculum or one moistened with warm tap water.	To ensure maximum visibility. Greasy lubricants inhibit specimen collection.
6 Using the bilobed end of the cervical spatula, scrape firmly but gently around the squamocolumnar junction of the cervix. If the os is splayed open or scarred, a wider sweep with the broad end of the spatula may be necessary.	To obtain a usable amount of specimen.
7 Smear both sides of the spatula evenly on the slide with one stroke from each side of the spatula.	To ensure complete specimens.
8 Fix immediately.	To preserve the specimen and ensure accurate results.
9 Allow the fixing agents to dry.	Dry specimens are less likely to be damaged.
10 Place the slides in a transport container.	To safeguard delicate glass slides.
11 Small endocervical lesions, which could be missed by the use of a spatula, may be sampled using an endocervical plastic brush (Singer *et al.* 1994).	This brush with its narrow tip can be inserted into the cervical canal, improving the quality of smear taken from the endocervix (Barton & Jenkins 1989).
12 Identify the lesion and insert and gently rotate the brush in the cervical canal.	To obtain a usable amount of specimen.
13 Withdraw the brush and gently smear the brush evenly on the slide (treat slide as above; see 8, 9 and 10).	To ensure a complete specimen.
14 Send, with a completed cervical cytology request form, to the appropriate laboratory.	

Procedure guidelines: **Analysis of drug levels in blood**

Procedure

Action	Rationale
1 Following venepuncture guidelines (see Ch. 45), withdraw 10 ml of blood and place in appropriate blood specimen container.	To ensure blood is obtained correctly and safely.
2 Clearly label blood specimen container 'pre-drug administration blood'.	To ensure that there is no confusion between the pre-drug and post-drug serum level specimens.
3 Administer intravenous antibiotic as patient's prescription states (following procedure for administration of drugs; see Ch. 9) via patient's established vascular access device.	To continue with patient's prescribed drug regimen.
4 One hour after administration of drug withdraw 10 ml of blood to obtain specimen for clotted sample to provide peak-level serum following venepuncture guidelines (Ch. 45). Clearly label blood specimen container 'post-drug administration blood'.	Time gap allows for even distribution of the drug through the blood and for peak blood levels to be achieved.

*Procedure guidelines: **Analysis of drug levels in blood** (cont'd)*

Action	Rationale
5 Rarely but occasionally when only poor and limited venous access is available, the blood specimens may have to be obtained from the patient's existing device.	The possibility of these specimens being contaminated with residue drug is high.
The device must be flushed thoroughly before taking the blood sample (see Ch. 44, Vascular access devices).	Contamination can be reduced by thorough flushing of the device.
The blood specimen container and request form must be labelled to indicate this deviation from the usual procedure.	The clinician interpreting the result will then be aware of the method of obtaining the blood specimen.

References and further reading

Armitage, K.B. & King, C.H. (2000) Malaria. In: *Principles and Practice of Infectious Diseases* (eds G. Mandell, J. Bennett & R. Dolin). Churchill Livingstone, Philadelphia.

Baker, F.J., Silverton, R.E. & Pallister, C.J. (1998) Microbiology. In: *Introduction to Medical Laboratory Technology*. Butterworth Heinemann, Oxford, pp. 251–325.

Barton, S. & Jenkins, D. (1989) An exploration for the problems of the false negative cervical smear. *Br J Obstet Gynaecol*, **96**, 492–9.

Bille, J. (2000) Microbiologic diagnostic procedures. In: *Management of Infection in Immunocompromised Patients* (eds M. Glauser & P. Pizzo). W.B. Saunders, London.

Downie, G., Mackenzie, J. & Williams, A. (2000) Drug treatment of infections. In: *Pharmacology and Drug Management for Nurses*. Churchill Livingstone, Edinburgh, pp. 189–206.

Elliott, T.S.J. (1993) Line-associated bacteraemias. *Commun Dis Rep*, **3**(7), R91–6.

Ellorhorst-Ryan, J.M. (2000) Infection. In: *Cancer Nursing: Principles and Practice* (eds S. Groenwald, M. Frogge, M. Goodman & C. Yarbro). Jones and Bartlett, Boston.

Engervall, P. & Bjorkholm, M. (1996) Infections in neutropenic patients II: management. *Med Oncol*, **13**(1), 63–9.

Finegold, S.M. (2000) Anaerobic bacteria: general concepts. In: *Principles and Practice of Infectious Diseases* (eds G. Mandell, J. Bennett & R. Dolin). Churchill Livingstone, Philadelphia.

Gabriel, J. (1999) Long-term central venous access. In: *Intravenous Therapy in Nursing Practice* (eds L. Dougherty & J. Lamb). Churchill Livingstone, Edinburgh.

Gilchrist, B. (2000) Taking a wound swab. *Nurs Times*, **96**(4), 2.

Gill, D. (1999) Stool specimen part 1. *Nurs Times*, **95**(25), 1–2.

Gill, D. (1999) Stool specimen part 2. *Nurs Times*, **95**(26), 1–2.

Gill, V.J., Fedorko, D.P. & Witebsky, F.G. (2000) The clinician and the microbiology laboratory. In: *Principles and Practice of Infectious Diseases* (eds G. Mandell, J. Bennett & R. Dolin). Churchill Livingstone, Philadelphia.

Gold, H.S. & Eisenstein, B.I. (2000) Introduction to bacterial diseases. In: *Principles and Practice of Infectious Diseases* (eds G. Mandell, J. Bennett & R. Dolin). Churchill Livingstone, Philadelphia.

Goodwin, M. & Carlson, I. (1993) The peripherally inserted catheter: a retrospective look at 3 years of insertions. *J Intravenous Nurs*, **12**(2), 92–103.

Graham, J.C. & Galloway, A. (2001) The laboratory diagnosis of urinary tract infections. *J Clin Pathol*, **54**, 911–19.

Health Services Advisory Committee (1991) *Safety in Health Services Laboratories: The Labelling, Transport and Reception of Specimens*. Stationery Office, London.

Health Services Advisory Committee (1998) *Safe Working and Prevention of Infection in Clinical Laboratories*. Stationery Office, London.

Henderson, D.K. (2000) Bacteraemia due to percutaneous intravenous devices. In: *Principles and Practice of Infectious Diseases* (eds G. Mandell, J. Bennett & R. Dolin). Churchill Livingstone, Philadelphia.

Henker, R. (2000) Infection control. Use of blood cultures in critically ill patients. *Crit Care Nurs*, **20**(1), 45–9.

Higgins, C. (1995) Microbiological examination of urine in urinary tract infection. *Nurs Times*, **91**(11), 33–5.

Higgins, C. (2000) Microbiology testing. In: *Understanding Laboratory Investigations*. Blackwell Science, Oxford, pp. 295–325.

Holliday, G., Strike, P.N. & Masterton, R.G. (1991) Perineal cleansing and mid stream urine specimen in ambulatory women. *J Hosp Infect*, **18**(1), 71–5.

Hopkins, S.J. (1999) Antibiotics and other anti-infective chemotherapeutic agents. In: *Drugs and Pharmacology for Nurses*. Churchill Livingstone, Edinburgh.

Ismail, R. *et al.* (1997) Therapeutic drug monitoring of gentamicin: a 6-year follow-up audit. *J Clin Pharm Ther*, **22**(1), 21–5.

Johnston, J.B. & Messina, M. (1991) Erroneous laboratory values obtained from central catheters. *J Intraven Nurs*, **14**(1), 13–15.

Jumaa, P.A. & Chattopadhyay, B. (1994) Pseudobacteraemia. *J Hosp Infect*, **27**(3), 167–77.

Kiehn, T.E., Ellner, P.D. & Budzko, D. (1989) Role of the microbiological laboratory in care of the immunosuppressed patient. *Rev Infect Dis*, **11**(Suppl 7), S1706–10.

Macleod, J.A. (1992) Collecting specimens for the laboratory tests. *Nurs Stand*, **6**(20), 36–7.

Magadia, R.R. & Weinstein, M.P. (2001) Laboratory diagnosis of bacteremia and fungemia. *Infect Dis Clin North Am*, **15**(4), 1009–24.

Mead, M. (1999) High vaginal swab. *Practice Nurse*, **17**(9), 642.

Mims, C.A. *et al.* (1993) *Medical Microbiology*. C.V. Mosby, St Louis.

Mims, C.A. *et al.* (1998) General principles and specimen quality. In: *Medical Microbiology*. Mosby, St Louis, pp. 157–62.

O'Grady, N.P. *et al.* (1998) Practice guidelines for evaluating new fever in critically ill adult patients. *Clin Infect Dis*, **26**(5), 1042–59.

Papasian, C.J. & Kragel, P.J. (1997) The microbiology laboratory's role in life-threatening infections. *Crit Care Nurse*, **20**(3), 44–59.

Parini, S. (2000) How to collect specimens. *Nursing*, **30**(5), 66–7.

Reeves, D.S. (1980) Therapeutic drug monitoring of aminoglycoside antibiotics. *Infection*, **8**(Suppl 3), S313–20.

Sandin, R.L. & Rinaldi, M. (1996) Special consideration for the clinical microbiology laboratory in the diagnosis of infections in the cancer patient. *Infect Dis Clin North Am*, **10**(2), 413–30.

Shanson, D.C. (1999) Use of the microbiology laboratory – general principles. In: *Microbiology in Clinical Practice*. Butterworth Heinemann, Oxford, pp. 24–36.

Shelton, B.K. (1999) Sepsis. *Semin Oncol Nurs*, **15**(3), 209–21.

Shirrel, D.J., Gibbar-Clements, T., Dooley, R. & Free, C. (1999) Understanding therapeutic drug monitoring. *Am J Nurs*, **99**(1), 42–4.

Shulman, R.J. *et al.* (1998) Central venous catheter versus peripheral veins for sampling blood levels of commonly used drugs. *J Parenteral Enteral Nutr*, **22**(4), 234–7.

Singer, A. *et al.* (1994) *Lower Genital Tract Pre-cancer*. Blackwell Science, Oxford.

Spitalnic, S.J., Woolard, R.H. & Mermel, LA. (1995) The significance of changing needles when inoculating blood cultures: a meta-analysis. *Clin Infect Dis*, **21**(5), 1103–6.

Storch, G.A. (2000) Specimen collection and transport. In: *Diagnostic Virology*. Churchill Livingstone, New York, pp. 295–325.

Tam, V.H., Moore, G.E., Triller, D.M. & Briceland, L.L. (1999) Vancomycin peak serum concentration monitoring. *J Intravenous Nurs*, **22**(6), 336–42.

Thomson, R.B. (2002) Use of microbiology laboratory tests in the diagnosis of infectious diseases. In: *Expert Guide to Infectious Diseases* (ed. J. Tan). American College of Physicians, Philadelphia.

Thys, J.P., Jacobs, F. & Bye, B. (1994) Microbiological specimen collection in the emergency room. *Eur J Emerg Med*, **1**(1), 47–53.

Weinstein, S.M. (2000) Laboratory tests. In: *Plumer's Principles and Practice of Intravenous Therapy*. J.B. Lippincott, Philadelphia, p. 69.

Wilson, J. (2001) Understanding the microbiology laboratory. In: *Infection Control in Clinical Practice*. Baillière Tindall, Edinburgh, pp. 17–28.

Wilson, M.L. (1996) General principles of specimen collection. *Clin Infect Dis*, **22**(5), 766–77.

Wormser, G.P. *et al.* (1990) Sensitivity and specificity of blood cultures obtained through intravenous catheters. *Crit Care Nurs*, **18**(2), 152–6.

40

Spinal cord compression management

Chapter contents

Definition

Spinal cord compression is the compression of the spinal cord and nerve roots.

Reference material

Spinal cord compression (SCC) can be caused by disease processes as well as extradural or intradural tumours. The resulting signs and symptoms depend on the spinal tracts involved. When the nerve roots are affected, the clinical manifestation can be motor, sensory or a combination of both. Symptoms that relate to compression of the spinal cord itself are termed 'myelopathy', whilst those that relate to compression of the nerve root(s) are known as 'radiculopathy'.

Spinal cord compression, whatever its aetiology, is always a neurological and/or oncological emergency. Prompt action is therefore required in both the diagnosis and its management so as to prevent further neurological deterioration, which can make the difference between the patient being paralysed or functionally independent. As such, the maintenance of neurological function is paramount in order to ensure an improvement in the patient's quality of life. The management goal is therefore to relieve pain, preserve or restore neurological function and allow for early mobilization.

Patients at risk of SCC should be made aware of the danger signs that may require immediate action. Therefore professionals have a responsibility to ensure their own awareness of SCC and take prompt and appropriate action as require (British Association of Surgical Oncology 1999).

In the context of cancer therapy and rehabilitation, the management of SCC differs from that of the young individual whose spinal cord has been damaged as a result of trauma and although many problems will be similar for both groups of patients, this chapter will deal mainly with the former.

Incidence and aetiology

The spine is the most common site for bone metastases. It is estimated that 3–5% of patients with cancer and 10–15% of patients with spinal metastases may develop compression during the course of their illness (Hillier & Wee 1997), while approximately 5% of patients with systemic cancer will have SCC on autopsy (Posner 1995). Primary tumours of the spinal cord are relatively uncommon, while secondary involvement of the central nervous system is more common (Sharpe 1998). In the adult population, approximately 50% of all metastases in the spine causing epidural SCC arise from breast, lung or prostate carcinoma. In children, the primary pathology is usually Ewing's sarcoma, neuroblastoma, osteogenic sarcoma or rhabdomyosarcoma (Britton & Ng 1998).

In SCC there is oedema and decreased blood supply to the spinal cord and mechanical damage to the neural tissue, which can lead to a hemiparesis or hemiplegia (Dyck 1991).

Classification

Causes of spinal cord compression include the following.

- Acute or chronic infection – this can be intradural or extradural.
- Degenerative processes, such as prolapsed vertebral disc, spondylosis.
- Haematoma – traumatic, spontaneous or related to congenital abnormality, e.g. arteriovenous malformation. These can be extra/intradural or intramedullary.
- Cystic lesion, e.g. syringomyelia, generally intramedullary but may also occur intra/extradurally.
- Trauma, e.g. fractures of the spine which may compress or actually sever the cord.
- Tumours (see below).

Tumours of the spine are classified according to their relationship to the dura and the spinal cord itself (Addison & Shah 1998):

- Extradural lesions, that is, lesions of the osseous spine, epidural space and paraspinal soft tissues; these tumours compress the dural and spinal cord.
- Intradural extramedullary lesions, which are inside the dura but outside the spinal cord.
- Intramedullary lesions, which are within the spinal cord (Britton & Ng 1998).

The majority of extradural tumours are metastatic in nature. Intradural extramedullary tumours are evenly divided between the primary and metastatic tumours, while intradural intramedullary tumours are most often primary gliomas.

The speed of onset of SCC can vary considerably, depending on the cause. For example, with trauma this can occur immediately whilst with tumours, the signs and symptoms may be evident several weeks before cord compression actually occurs (Held & Peahota 1993).

Clinical presentation

Clinical presentation of SCC correlates with the spinal tracts involved and includes the following.

- *Pain*. This is usually the earliest presenting symptom. The onset of pain is usually mild and becomes more severe with time. However, the absence of pain does not mean an absence of SCC (Posner 1995).
- *Motor deficits*, that is, weakness of the extremities. Motor deficits may progress to ataxia, loss of co-ordination and paralysis. The specific neurological findings depend on the level of the cord lesion (Keller & Benton 2001).
- *Sensory loss*. This may include decreased sensation to pain and temperature, pins-and-needles and numbness of the toes and fingers. These symptoms can ascend to the level of SCC (Held & Peahota 1993). It is worth noting that sensory complaints without pain are rare with SCC (Posner 1995).
- *Autonomic nervous system problems*. These include the symptoms of constipation and urinary retention. Often, constipation is aggravated in those patients receiving opiates.

Early diagnosis is essential in order to ensure prompt treatment. The success of treatment is dependent on the patient's general condition and mobility. Studies indicate that patients who are not mobile at presentation do not generally regain the ability to walk (Held & Peahota 1993; Ingham *et al.* 1993).

Investigations

Investigations for SCC can include plain X-rays (cervical, lumbar and thoracic), bone scans, computed tomography (CT) and magnetic resonance imaging (MRI). Such investigations are often dependent on what imaging techniques are available. However, if available, MRI is the investigation of choice (Britton & Ng 1998). This is because MRI is more sensitive in detecting small CNS metastases that can be missed with other imaging methods. Autopsy studies suggest that about 25% of spinal lesions are not identifiable by plain X-rays (Posner 1995).

At present, one of the disadvantages of MRI is slower image acquisition; it can take up to four times as long to image a patient with suspected SCC compared with CT scans. The MRI scanner is a more enclosed space than the CT scanner. This, coupled with the time taken for the scan, needs to be considered for those patients with pain. Appropriate analgesia should therefore be provided.

It is important that there is a clear established route of rapid diagnosis and management for the optimum treatment of SCC. This should include appropriate radiological imaging as well as appropriate referral to a neurosurgical and/or oncological centre. To facilitate expert medical/clinical or surgical oncology assessment, there may be a need for the transfer of images (e.g. scans) to a regional cancer centre (British Association of Surgical Oncology 1999).

Treatment

Treatment should be commenced as soon as possible once a diagnosis has been established to maximize recovery chances and minimize functional deficits (Janjan 1996). Treatment can be a combination of steroids, surgery, radiotherapy and/or chemotherapy. For those patients presenting with pain, proper analgesia coupled with steroids should also be considered as an integral part of treatment. If motor function has already been lost, despite treatment, it is unlikely to be regained. However, early treatment may help to restore bladder and/or bowel control.

Steroids

Steroids are used primarily for the control and reduction of brain and spinal cord oedema (Posner 1995; Keller & Benton 2001). Steroids have both glucocorticoid (anti-inflammatory) and mineralocorticoid (water and mineral) effects. Glucocorticoid side-effects include diabetes, osteoporosis, Cushing's syndrome and neuropsychiatric effects, to name a few. Mineralocorticoid side-effects include hypertension, sodium and water retention and potassium loss (BNF 2002). Steroid side-effects are numerous and mostly unpleasant, many of which can take weeks to months to subside after completion of therapy (Evans & Guerrero 1998).

Surgery

Surgery, in the form of laminectomy to decompress the spinal cord or vertebral body resection to allow for removal of the tumour, can be considered. The surgical approach for spinal tumours depends on whether the tumour is extradural, intradural or intramedullary (Addison & Shah 1998). Where bone has been eroded or removed, extensive surgical instrumentation devices may be required to maintain the stability of the spine and to allow early mobilization.

Other factors that need to be taken into account are the patient's age, his or her performance status, as well as any other pre-existing medical condition. In the context of malignant disease, radiation and steroids are often preferred treatments over surgery because of the added risk of surgery in patients with advanced metastatic cancer (Peterson 1993). However, with the increasing skill of interventional radiologists and pathologists, diagnoses are increasingly being made by needle aspirates (Keller & Benton 2001), thus avoiding surgery.

Radiotherapy

Radiotherapy alone is used for patients with radiosensitive cancer, lesions below the conus medullaris, slow onset of compression, medical contraindications to surgery or surgically unapproachable tumours (Keller & Benton 2001). Radiotherapy should be commenced immediately once SCC has been diagnosed to prevent further neurological deterioration. Those patients who have had surgery will also require radiotherapy. However, patients with complete paralysis rarely respond to radiotherapy (Hillier & Wee 1997).

Chemotherapy

For patients with SCC from chemoresponsive tumours, such as small cell lung cancer and lymphomas, treatment with the cytotoxic drug appropriate for the tumour may be considered (Guerrero 1998).

Rehabilitation

Rehabilitation must commence on diagnosis and must encompass the skills of various professionals. No one professional intervention would be wholly effective in isolation (Robinson 1998). An effective team does not just provide a better programme for the patient's rehabilitation needs but also very importantly allows for colleague support and advice from other team members when dealing with complex cases (Robinson 1998).

In the context of SCC due to metastatic cancer, the rehabilitation team should take a palliative care approach as this group of patients generally have a poor prognosis. The emphasis should therefore be on the improvement of quality of life, not just for the patient but also for those managing his or her care. Home adaptation, appropriate lifting, special mattresses and wheelchairs may be indicated and therefore the involvement of the primary health care, palliative care teams and social services should be sought at an early stage of care. Their psychosocial and sexual needs also need to be addressed and both the patient and family provided with appropriate counselling if and when required. Families should be encouraged to participate in care, where appropriate or acceptable to the patient, whether the patient is in hospital or at home, and techniques such as the management of indwelling catheters, bowel care and appropriate

scheduling of medication should be taught. Such measures are important in order to encourage independence and avoid the development of future crisis. This should also ensure that families feel that they have been consulted and involved in care throughout the illness experience. Such involvement may help family members when coping with future bereavement.

Procedure guidelines: **Care of patients with spinal cord compression**

Initial care

Action	Rationale
1 Explain and discuss the proposed procedure(s) with the patient.	To ensure the patient understands the procedure and gives his/her consent.
2 Ensure adequate psychological and physical preparation for tests and procedures by giving accurate explanations and instructions.	To ensure that patient is informed of any procedures and possible action plans. To decrease pain which may be associated with anxiety.
3 Reinforce that the aim of any intervention is to relieve pain and to restore function if possible (Wilkowski 1986; Hillier & Wee 1997).	To provide hope (that is realistic).
4 Assist with and explain details of ongoing investigations, e.g. X-rays, bone scan, CT and/or MRI scan.	To ensure that the patient understands and is aware of each stage of the procedure as it occurs and to decrease anxiety.

Moving and handling

Action	Rationale
1 Ensure that assessment for manual handling is carried out (see Ch. 23).	To maintain staff and patient safety. To avoid any unnecessary risk to the patient of further complications resulting from injury.
2 Always, until otherwise determined by the medical team, treat the patient as if they have an unstable spine. Maintain patient on bedrest, maintain neutral spinal alignment. When patient needs to be moved use sufficient staff to perform 'log roll' technique to avoid any twisting to the spine (Dyck 1991). If a hard collar is indicated this should be fitted by an appropriately trained professional.	To stabilize any vertebral instability and prevent further damage to the vertebrae and spinal cord. The fragile status of the affected vertebra(e) may result in a crush fracture to the body of the vertebrae and/or spinal cord compression.
3 A comprehensive assessment of the patient's condition and ability to mobilize should be conducted by the multiprofessional team including the physiotherapist, medical team, nurse and, importantly, the patient. All these individuals should be involved in decisions and discussions regarding moving and handling.	Individual risk assessment and agreeing safest practice require a multiprofessional perspective which should additionally cover patient transfers, positioning and mobilization. This approach may assist the patient with pain control and comfort.
4 If patient has impaired mobility then antiembolic stockings should be applied. Low molecular weight heparin may be used depending on physician preference and whether surgery is a treatment option.	To reduce complications of immobility such as risk of deep vein thrombosis.
5 The appropriateness of using a low air loss mattress should be considered on an individual basis in line with Waterlow or other assessment score balanced with the risk of further cord damage (Hatcliffe & Dawe 1996) (see Ch. 43).	To reduce risk of pressure sore formation as patients with sensory deficits may not detect pain or pressure associated with formation of pressure ulcers. There is no research evidence to indicate whether a firm or pressure-relieving device is more appropriate for the care of patients with

*Procedure guidelines: **Care of patients with spinal cord compression** (cont'd)*

Action	Rationale
	spinal cord compression, but mattresses are best avoided in patients with unstable spines, as further damage could occur. Neutral alignment and appropriate methods of repositioning should always be utilized to prevent secondary damage.

Assessment

Action	Rationale
1 Monitor and document respiratory function and vital signs for complications such as respiratory failure, spinal shock (see Ch. 25, Observations, and Ch. 37, Respiratory therapy). Refer abnormal findings to medical team and other relevant professionals, e.g. physiotherapists.*	To provide information with regard to the patient's condition and to ensure treatment and care are planned and implemented. Spinal shock requires immediate review by the medical team. These complications are more commonly associated with spinal injury patients, but may also exist in spinal cord compression patients. * Assisted coughing by appropriately trained professionals may be required to prevent chest infection.
2 (a) Assess, monitor and document the patient's neurological function such as limb strength, sensation, bladder and bowel function.	To establish baseline of deficit and to detect deterioration at the earliest opportunity. Initial sensory loss may be subtle before progressing to numbness and immobility.
(b) Early urinary catheterization is often indicated after a documented assessment of related sensation and function, e.g. urgency, frequency, retention with or without pain (see Ch. 16).	Early autonomic dysfunction results in constipation and urinary retention. More advanced dysfunction results in bladder and bowel incontinence and carries poor prognosis for return to normal function (Held & Peahota 1993).
3 If urinary catheterization is appropriate, conduct procedure using aseptic technique; provide and teach regular catheter care (see Ch. 16).	To allow voiding of urine. To reduce risk of infection.
4 Monitor blood chemistry and patient for signs of hypercalcaemia, such as confusion, drowsiness and lethargy. If Ca^{2+} is elevated then intravenous hydration and medication to lower the serum calcium may be indicated. Monitor and care for vascular devices (see Ch. 44).	To correct fluid and electrolyte imbalance. Elevated calcium levels may be associated with bone metastasis causing the spinal cord compression. To promote patient's safety and comfort.
5 Assess patient's pain (see Ch. 27). This should include factors such as duration, location, type, intensity and quality of pain.	To assist in identifying possible level of spinal cord involvement and to assist in the appropriate prescribing of analgesia and interventions designed to minimize pain. Information concerning pain will provide an indication of underlying pathology. For example, local pain occurs over the area of the tumour and may be constant. Radicular pain (pain caused by nerve root compression) may travel down the extremity associated with the area of compression and may be worsened by sneezing, coughing or straining. Thoracic pain is often described as a tight band around the chest or upper abdomen. Medullary pain is referred pain, which is often described as 'burning' or 'shooting' in nature and may be poorly localized.
Document on pain assessment chart.	To provide for continuity of care, accurate documentation and for future review. To ensure pain assessment and analgesic requirements are reviewed on a regular basis, as patient's needs may alter as treatment and rehabilitation progress. To allow for comparative reassessment and evaluation of interventions.
If required, administer analgesia as prescribed, noting effects and any side-effects; report to medical team as necessary. Consider use of non-pharmacological	Adequate pain control is essential for comfortable mobilization. Relaxed muscles will facilitate better movement. Narcotics are not always sufficient to control

Procedure guidelines: **Care of patients with spinal cord compression** *(cont'd)*

Action	Rationale
interventions such as relaxation, therapeutic massage and adjusting patient's position.	nerve root pain and additional medications prescribed by experts in pain control, such as anticonvulsants, steroids and tricyclic antidepressants, may help to ease pain (Hillier & Wee 1997). The role of complementary therapies has yet to be explored fully, but they may prove useful in reducing pain in particular patients.
6 Assess patient's and relatives' understanding of any information given to them. Facilitate family discussion on treatment options with other members of the medical/surgical teams.	For some patients and their families, spinal cord compression may be a first diagnosis of cancer, for others it may signify the progression of their disease. It is essential for the team to be honest but tactful, for example when asked about the return of motor function.
7 Consider referral to another health care professional to increase support available to patient and their family, e.g. clinical nurse specialist/nurse consultant, counsellor or spiritual leader (hospital chaplain).	To provide a patient-centred, holistic approach to care.

Treatment(s)

Action	Rationale
1 *Neurosurgery*. If the patient undergoes neurosurgery, provide appropriate pre- and postoperative care (e.g. breathing exercises, pain management, log-rolling, recording of vital signs and neurological function, bowel and bladder care) (see Ch. 30, Perioperative care).	Surgery in the form of a decompression laminectomy and debulking of tumour, with or without the stabilization of metal rods or bone graft, may be a treatment option (Dyck 1991; Hickey 1997) and is influenced by: (a) The site of the tumour (b) The degree of spinal instability (c) The likely prognosis (d) The extent of spinal disease. Many postoperative measures concerning monitoring of spinal cord compression remain the same as during presurgery. This can be the case for days or weeks postsurgery.
2 *Radiotherapy*. If the patient requires radiotherapy:	Radiotherapy alone is effective in over 85% of cases of spinal cord compression and is used in combination with steroids (see steroid section below).
(a) Prepare patient to receive radiotherapy by providing written and verbal information and education (RMH Radiotherapy booklet, Patient Information Series).	Radiotherapy may also be used in combination with surgery, depending on location and extent of neurological compromise (Janjan 1996). Radiotherapy may be commenced as an emergency treatment to preserve as much neurological function as possible (Kirkbridge 1995).
(b) Prepare patient for daily treatments.	Radiotherapy is generally administered to a total dose of 20 Gy in 5 fractions (usually fractions are daily). Higher total doses of radiotherapy can only be tolerated by the spinal cord when small fractions of radiation are separated by 24 hours (Kirkbridge 1995).
(c) Monitor and manage side-effects (administering treatment, such as drugs as prescribed) depending on area affected as follows: • Skin – erythema over treated area (see Ch. 47, Wound management). • Oesophagitis – administer analgesia and antacids as prescribed/required: provide a soft diet. • Nausea and vomiting – administer antiemetics as prescribed/required (Twycross & Lack 1998).	Radiation field usually extends to vertebral bodies above and below the spinal cord compression. A number of symptoms may occur as a result of using radiotherapy and as a particular consequence of the area irradiated, that is the cervical/thoracic/lumbar area of the spine. Nausea, vomiting, diarrhoea and dysuria occur as the result of irradiation to the thoracic/lumbar spine (Kirkbridge 1995).

*Procedure guidelines: **Care of patients with spinal cord compression** (cont'd)*

Action	Rationale
• Diarrhoea – provide a low-fibre diet; administer as prescribed antidiarrhoeal agents, e.g. Imodium (see Ch. 13, Elimination: bowel care). • Dysuria – exclude urinary tract infection by culturing MSU and increase fluid intake. • Fatigue – provide and encourage rest periods.	The development of fatigue may be related to radiobiological action, with metabolites from cell destruction and normal tissue damage accumulating to give rise to fatigue (Faithfull 1998).
3 *Chemotherapy.* If the patient requires chemotherapy, where appropriate, assist the patient's understanding with information regarding the rationale for chemotherapy and possible side-effects (see Ch. 10, Drug administration: cytotoxic drugs).	Chemotherapy may be administered if extradural spinal cord compression is present, e.g. lymphoma, myeloma, teratoma, but also in cases where SCC is the first presentation of cancer (Held & Peahota 1993). Each case is assessed individually for appropriateness of treatment. Side-effects will impact on the rehabilitation process, due to fatigue, bone marrow depression, skin fragility, constipation, altered appetite.

Rehabilitation care

Action	Rationale
1 Begin rehabilitation as soon as possible, taking into consideration any limitations associated with the stability of the spine and pain present.	If the spine is not stable and medical stabilization procedures are inappropriate the patient may need to have completed radiotherapy (to reduce tumour mass and improve pain) before mobilization; close liaison with the medical, physiotherapy and occupational therapy team is necessary to plan appropriate mobilization.
2 Refer the patient to the appropriate multiprofessional team member. This should include: **(a)** Physiotherapist **(b)** Occupational therapist **(c)** Social worker **(d)** Community liaison nurse specialist **(e)** Dietitian **(f)** Specialist palliative care physicians and nurses.	Nurses play a key role in facilitating effective teamwork. The successful delivery of rehabilitation demands excellent internal organization and multidisciplinary approaches (Carson *et al.* 1997).
Ensure that regular multidisciplinary team meetings are held to assess the patient's progress.	To ensure a continuous and consistent approach to individual patient care.
3 Ensure that goals set are short term and attainable so as to achieve the best possible quality of life.	To fully involve patient in the proposed care plan and to ensure that progress is within patient's limitations. If spinal cord compression is the result of metastatic disease, then rehabilitation would take a functional approach, as the patient may survive for months depending on the primary cancer type and histology, etc. However, the patient's psychological status must always be taken into account and referral for counselling instigated if and when appropriate. Goals are based on a patient's entire situation and lifestyle (Hunter 1998).
A rehabilitation programme with regular assessment and intervention should be initiated.	To restore confidence and self-esteem, to give structure to the patient's day and to increase understanding of realistic aims of rehabilitation.
Goals need to be flexible.	The degree of patient functioning cannot always be anticipated (Cooper 1997).
4 Assess and monitor patient's and family's psychological status and adaptation to diagnosis and implications on lifestyle. Encourage patient to express feelings. Do not give false reassurance but communicate empathy for	Rehabilitation starts with helping the patient to confront the existence of a disability and may continue as the grief process proceeds. Feelings of helplessness, hopelessness and depression are common. Bedbound patients become

*Procedure guidelines: **Care of patients with spinal cord compression** (cont'd)*

Action	Rationale
patient's feelings. Promote the use of a variety of coping techniques. Cultivate a positive and realistic outlook on life (Davidhizar 1997).	withdrawn and lose motivation (Hillier & Wee 1997). The degree of the patient's motivation will influence the rehabilitation process (Davidhizar 1997). The skill in managing this condition is to provide care without sacrificing patient autonomy and control.
5 Maximize potential for mobilization by the following.	
(a) Work as an integral part of the rehabilitation team to ensure that rehabilitation is continuous.	To maintain and increase patient's independence in activities requiring motor performance. To help patient to adjust and adapt to altered mobility. To facilitate participation in social and occupational activities.
(b) Assist the patient to perform an active or passive range of movement exercises, based on physiotherapy assessment, patient's assistance and instructions.	Active and passive range of movement exercises help to prevent complications associated with decreased movement and will also increase muscle strength. However, joint damage, due to decreased or absent sensation, is possible with these exercises.
(c) Reinforce transfer techniques proposed and formulated by the physiotherapist and occupational therapist.	To ensure safety of patient and nursing team and to ensure consistency of approach across the multidisciplinary team.
(d) A home assessment may be needed to ensure that correct equipment is fitted appropriately (Borgman-Gainer 1996).	For safety and independence (Hillier & Wee 1977).
6 Monitor pressure areas continuously; it may be necessary to provide a therapeutic mattress and cushions as well as appropriate manual handling equipment.	It is essential to be aware that this group of patients differ from spinal injury patients, due to immunosuppressive treatments and overall physical condition. The predisposition to shearing forces and pressure sores may be greater (Cooper 1997).
7 Assess and promote optimal urinary elimination handling equipment.	To establish degree of bladder function and to retrain bladder function. The degree of bladder dysfunction depends on the degree of damage to the sensory and motor tracts of the spinal cord, which send messages between the bladder and the supraspinal centre. The presence of spinal shock, autonomic neurogenic bladder, sensory paralytic bladder and motor paralytic bladder influences management techniques.
Insert indwelling catheter or teach intermittent catheterization to the patient or relative/carer if appropriate.	Catheterization may be necessary to assist with elimination for those patients who experience a loss of bladder motor function (Pires 1996). Long-term catheterization may be an option and will require significant patient/family teaching (see Ch. 16, Elimination: urinary catheterization).
If the patient is incontinent, treat sensitively and promote hygiene and skin integrity.	The patient may be very embarrassed and upset by this condition. To minimize the risk of any associated complications.
8 Promote and encourage optimal bowel care (see Ch. 13, Eliminaton: bowel care).	Bowel activity is influenced by decreased mobility, spinal innervation, narcotics and other analgesics as well as anorexia (Gender 1996). If patient is incontinent, promote dignity and physical hygiene.
9 Acknowledge and assess effects of diagnosis and disability on sexual function. Facilitate discussion with patient and partner, if appropriate.	Sexuality is often overlooked by professional carers who are focusing on the more obvious physical effects of spinal cord compression, rather than the psychological issues (Hillier & Wee 1997).
10 Begin discharge planning as soon as level of functioning is ascertained. Work closely with the rehabilitation team and the patient and family in conjunction with GPs and community teams, hospitals, hospices, voluntary services and charitable organizations (see Ch. 8, Discharge planning).	To offer realistic care packages to enable the patient to return home quickly where appropriate. The co-ordination required to discharge and support these patients at home is complex and challenging (Hillier & Wee 1997).

Problem solving

Problem	Cause	Preventive action	Suggested action
Altered respiratory status.	Diaphragmatic paralysis can be associated with cervical and/or thoracic spine involvement (NB: breathing pattern may be altered due to pain).	Monitor respiratory rate and pattern when recording vital signs on admission. Assess patient and establish baseline measurement for comparison with future measurements. Encourage patient to report any altered sensation or difficulty with breathing in order to note and report any changes immediately.	Respiratory function monitoring should be recorded and documented as often as clinical assessment demands. Ensure patient is given the opportunity to make an informed decision about their future management should respiratory failure result, e.g. appropriateness of ventilation in critical care against the prognosis of their disease process. If the patient is for full resuscitation, early communication with critical care and anaesthetic staff is essential, as this event necessitates urgent transfer for assisted ventilation. However, if the emphasis of treatment is palliative, mechanical ventilation may not be deemed appropriate by the patient and/or the multidisciplinary team. Always provide the patient and family with information and support.
Neurogenic or 'spinal' shock, characterized by hypotension and bradycardia (NB: spinal shock is rare in patients with SCC and more common in patients with spinal injury associated with cord transection).	Spinal shock is caused by a disruption of sympathetic outflow and manifests as low vascular resistance with increased intravascular capacity. The patient is functionally hypovolaemic even if no blood has been lost (Barker 1995).	Care with manual handling to prevent further injury to spine as outlined previously.	Assess vital signs and ensure medical team are contacted urgently. Carry out intravenous fluid resuscitation to correct any hypovolaemia (NB: fluid overload may precipitate pulmonary oedema, particularly as fluid volume has not been lost). Central venous access for drug administration and fluid monitoring is indicated. Inotropes such as ephedrine or adrenaline may be necessary. Bladder catheterization to assess fluid volume status (Barker 1995). The patient should be cared for in a high dependency or critical care unit.
'Autonomic dysreflexia' is a medical emergency and is indicated by an acute rise in blood pressure (systolic pressure can exceed 200), bradycardia, severe headache and visual blurring, flushing above injury level and pallor below. Seizures are also possible.	Complication associated with compression of spinal cord at T6–8 or higher, caused by an imbalance between sympathetic and parasympathetic response and usually triggered by an internal stimulus, such as a distended bladder or bowel and/or pressure sores.	If left untreated, condition may be lethal due to cerebral haemorrhage and thus the first line of treatment is prevention or removal of the stimulus (i.e. drainage of distended bladder, prevention of pressure sore, prevention of constipation, etc.). The medical team should be informed immediately.	Ensure a vasodilator is used, e.g. glyceryl trinitrate or captropril oral medication. The patient should be reassured and kept as calm as possible. NB: if blocked urinary catheter is suspected change indwelling catheter immediately. Do not attempt a bladder lavage as fluid may be retained. Refer to local spinal injury unit for advice.

Problem solving (cont'd)

Problem	Cause	Preventive action	Suggested action
Low blood pressure.	Dehydration associated with nausea and vomiting (possibly associated with hypercalcaemia).	Maintain appropriate fluid intake. Administer prescribed antiemetics as and when required.	Monitor blood chemistry profile. Alert medical team to changes in patient's condition.
Raised blood pressure.	Pain and anxiety.	Provide interventions to avoid or minimize pain.	Evaluate patient's pain management. Refer patient for psychological support if appropriate.
Urgency to eliminate urine.	Presence of indwelling catheter and/or urinary infection.	Maintain catheter care. Avoid blocked catheter. Maintain fluid chart.	Consider the removal of indwelling catheter if appropriate. Assess the degree and type of sensation present, e.g. distension. Establish a timed voiding schedule and teach behavioural techniques such as pelvic floor exercises and relaxation exercises.
Constipation in complete spinal cord injuries.	Absent anal sphincter reflex.	Daily per rectum check to monitor return of reflex (usually about 48 hours after SCC). If stool present then gentle digital manual evacuation should be undertaken.	On return of reflex alternate-day microenema or bisocodyl suppositories with gentle digital manual evacuation.
In complete lesions below T12, reflex bowel emptying will not be possible.	Interruption of sacral reflex arc.	Patient will require daily gentle manual evacuation.	Seek advice from local specialist spinal centre on regimen and fibre/'laxative' options.
In lesions above T12, reflex bowel emptying may be possible.	Sacral reflex arc spared.	Regular timed routine involving alternate-day regimen of microenema or glycerin/bisocodyl suppositories and possibly manual evacuation.	As above.
Nurse may be anxious about performing manual evacuation.	Unfamiliar technique.	Ensure training for nurses is available in this essential technique and explain consequence for patient if constipation is not managed appropriately. Liaise with medical staff.	Consult any local policy/procedure manual. Seek advice from local spinal centre or continence expert and refer to RCN (2000) *Digital Rectal Examination*.

References and further reading

Addison, C. & Shah, S. (1998) Neurosurgery. In: *Neuro-Oncology for Nurses* (ed. D. Guerrero). Whurr, London, pp. 124–50.

Barker, S.J. (1995) Anaesthesia in the high-risk patient. In: *Textbook of Critical Care*, 3rd edn (eds W.C. Shoemaker, M.A. Ayres, A. Grenvik & P.R. Holbrook). W.B. Saunders, Philadelphia.

BNF (British National Formulary) (2002) British Medical Association and Royal Pharmaceutical Society of Great Britain, London.

Borgman-Gainer, M.F. (1996) Independent function: movement and mobility. In: *Rehabilitation Nursing: Process and Application*, 2nd edn (ed. S. Hoeman). Mosby, New Jersey, pp. 225–69.

Brada, M., Collins, V.P., Dorwand, N.L. & Thomas, D.G.T. (2001) Tumours of the brain and spinal cord in adults. In: *The Oxford Textbook of Oncology*, 2nd edn (eds R. Souhami, I. Tannock, P. Hohenberger & C. Horiojt). Oxford University Press, London.

British Association of Surgical Oncology (1999) The management of metastatic bone disease in the United Kingdom. The Breast Speciality Group of the BASO. *Eur J Surg Oncol*, **25**(1), 3–23.

Britton, J. & Ng, V. (1998) Clinical neuro-imaging. In: *Neuro-Oncology for Nurses* (ed. D. Guerrero). Whurr, London, pp. 81–123.

Carson, M., Williams, T., Everett, A. & Barker, S. (1997) The nurse's role in the multidisciplinary team. *Eur J Palliat Care*, **4**(3), 96–8.

Cooper, J. (1997) Occupational therapy in specific symptom control and dysfunction. In: *Occupational Therapy in Oncology and Palliative Care* (ed. J. Cooper). Whurr, London, pp. 59–87.

Davidhizar, R. (1997) Disability does not have to be the grief that never ends: helping patients adjust. *Rehabil Nurs*, **22**(1), 32–5.

Dyck, S. (1991) Surgical instrumentation as a palliative treatment for spinal cord compression. *Oncol Nurs Forum*, **18**(3), 515–21.

Evans, C. & Guerrero, D. (1998) Medication used in the symptom management of CNS tumours. In: *Neuro-Oncology for Nurses* (ed. D. Guerrero). Whurr, London, pp. 201–20.

Faithfull, S. (1998) Fatigue in patients receiving radiotherapy. *Prof Nurse*, **13**(7), 459–61.

Gender, A.R. (1996) Bowel regulation and elimination. In: *Rehabilitation Nursing: Process and Application*, 2nd edn (ed. S. Hoeman). Mosby, New Jersey, pp. 452–75.

Guerrero, D. (1998) Radiotherapy. In: *Neuro-Oncology for Nurses* (ed. D. Guerrero). Whurr, London, pp. 151–78.

Harrison, P. (2000) *Managing Spinal Injury: Critical Care*. Spinal Injuries Association, London.

Harrison, P. (2000) *The First 48 Hours. The Initial Management of People with Actual or Suspected Spinal Cord Injury from Scene of Accident to Accident and Emergency Department*. Spinal Injuries Association, London.

Hatcliffe, S. & Dawe, R. (1996) Monitoring pressure sores in a palliative care setting. *Int J Palliat Nurs*, **2**(4), 182–6.

Held, J.L. & Peahota, A. (1993) Nursing care of the patient with spinal cord compression. *Oncol Nurs Forum*, **20**(10), 1507–16.

Hickey, J.V. (1997) Vertebral and spinal cord trauma. In: *The Clinical Practice of Neurological and Neurosurgical Nursing*, 4th edn. Lippincott, London.

Hillier, R. & Wee, B. (1997) Palliative management of spinal cord compression. *Eur J Palliat Care*, **4**(6), 189–92.

Hunter, M. (1998) Rehabilitation in cancer care: a patient-focused approach. *Eur J Palliat Care*, **7**(7), 85–7.

Ingham, J., Beveridge, A. & Cooney, N.J. (1993) The management of spinal cord compression in patients with advanced malignancy. *J Pain Symptom Manage*, **8**(1), 1–7.

Janjan, N.A. (1996) Radiotherapeutic management of spinal metastases. *J Pain Symptom Manage*, **11**(1), 47–56.

Keller, J.W. & Benton, J.B. (2001) Oncologic emergencies. In: *Clinical Oncology: A Multidisciplinary Approach for Physicians and Students* (ed. P. Rubin). W.B. Saunders, London.

Kirkbridge, P. (1995) The role of radiation therapy in palliative care. *J Palliat Care*, **11**(1), 19–26.

Lindsay, K.W. & Bone, I. (1997) *Neurology and Neurosurgery Illustrated*. Churchill Livingstone, Edinburgh.

Peterson, R. (1993) A nursing intervention for early detection of spinal cord compressions in patients with cancer. *Cancer Nurs*, **16**(2), 113–16.

Pires, M. (1996) Bladder Elimination and Continence. In: *Rehabilitation Nursing: Process and Application*, 2nd edn (ed. S. Hoeman). Mosby, New Jersey, pp. 417–45.

Posner, J. (1995) *Neurologic Complications of Cancer*. F.A. Davis, Philadelphia.

RCN (2000) *Digital Rectal Examination*. RCN, London.

Robinson, S. (1998) Multidisciplinary teamwork. In: *Neuro-Oncology for Nurses* (ed. D. Guerrero). Whurr, London, pp. 221–52.

Sharpe, G. (1998) Pathological and clinical aspects of CNS tumours. In: *Neuro-Oncology for Nurses* (ed. D. Guerrero). Whurr, London, pp. 66–80.

Twycross, R. & Lack, I. (1998) Nausea and vomiting in advanced cancer. *Eur J Palliat Care*, **5**(2), 39–45.

Wilkowski, J. (1986) Spinal cord compression; an oncologic emergency. *J Emerg Nurs*, **12**(1), 9–12.

41

Tracheostomy care and laryngectomy voice rehabilitation

Tracheostomy care

A tracheostomy is an artificial airway that bypasses the body's natural protective mechanism of the upper airway. Airway management is a key component of caring for a patient with an artificial airway. It is therefore paramount that nurses are aware of the principles and procedures specific to tracheostomy management.

The care of patients with a tracheostomy varies from one hospital to another. The changing of a tracheostomy tube will usually be undertaken by a doctor or a trained nurse who has been instructed in this procedure.

Definition

A tracheostomy is the creation of an opening into the trachea through the neck. A tube is then inserted to help facilitate breathing and the removal of secretions (O'Toole 1992).

A tracheostomy tube is curved to accommodate the anatomy of the trachea. Tracheostomy tubes are available in different designs. Some have both an outer and an inner cannula. The outer cannula maintains the patency of the airway while the inner cannula, which fits snugly inside the outer cannula, can be removed for cleaning without disturbing the stoma site.

Tubes are now manufactured from plastic and some have an inflatable cuff that holds the tube in place. This prevents the flow of air around the outside of the cannula, allowing for more effective ventilation, and prevents the aspiration of liquids into the trachea (O'Toole 1992).

Indications

Tracheostomy may be carried out:

- To provide and maintain an airway for respiratory support
- To enable the aspiration of tracheobronchial secretions

- To bypass any upper respiratory tract obstruction
- To aid in weaning patients from ventilatory support.

Reference material

Types of tracheostomy

Temporary

A temporary tracheostomy (Fig. 41.1b) is performed for patients as an elective procedure, e.g. at the time of major surgery such as a partial glossectomy.

Permanent

A permanent tracheostomy is the creation of a tracheostomy following a total laryngectomy (Fig. 41.1c). The top three tracheal cartilages are brought to the surface of the skin and sutured to the neck wall to form a stoma. The 'end' tracheostomy is permanent and the rigidity of the tracheal cartilage keeps the stoma open. The patient will breathe through this stoma for the remainder of his/her life. As a result, there is no connection between the nasal passages and the trachea.

Emergency

A tracheostomy may be performed as an emergency procedure when a patient has an obstructed airway. Among the more common conditions causing obstruction are trauma to the airway or neck, poisoning, infections or neoplasms.

Percutaneous

This technique enables the pretracheal tissues to be incised under local anaesthesia. A sheath is inserted into the trachea between the cricoid and the first tracheal ring or between the first and second rings. The trachea is dilated with forceps or a conical dilator, which is then slipped over a guidewire, ready for a tracheostomy tube to be inserted. One advantage of this method is that it can be performed within a critical care unit rather than a theatre (Scanlan *et al.* 1999; Sykes & Young 1999).

Surgical

This procedure is often performed under a general anaesthetic, although it can be carried out using local anaesthetic. An incision is made in the neck over the second or third tracheal ring. The thyroid isthmus is divided (to reduce the risk of bleeding) and the tracheostomy tube is inserted. As little cartilage as possible should be removed, in order to promote better closure after extubation (Scanlan *et al.* 1999; Sykes & Young 1999).

Mini-tracheostomy

Unlike the previous two techniques, which enable oxygen therapy and mechanical ventilation to be given, this method is used only when frequent tracheal suctioning is required. The mini-tracheostomy tube has a small internal diameter, often only 4 mm. This tube is inserted under local anaesthetic, either via a surgical incision or with the use of a guidewire (Sykes & Young 1999).

Types of tracheostomy tube

Experience has shown that the choice of tracheostomy tube depends on the type of operation performed. The patient's ability to tolerate the tube depends on various external factors. A selection of tubes is listed below.

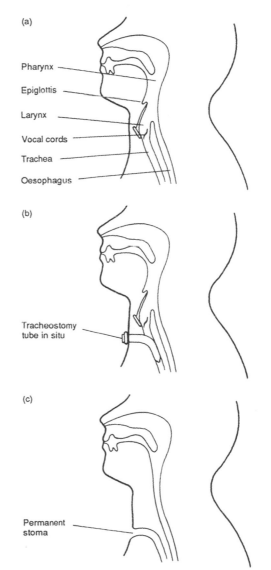

Figure 41.1 (a) Anatomy of the head and neck. (b) Temporary tracheostomy. (c) Permanent tracheostomy (total laryngectomy).

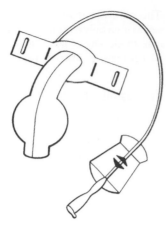

Figure 41.2 Portex cuffed tube.

Portex cuffed tracheostomy tube

This is a disposable plastic tracheostomy tube with an introducer and inflatable cuff to give an airtight seal (Fig. 41.2). It is available with or without an inner tube. The cuff prevents blood from reaching the lungs and the seal facilitates ventilation at the time of surgery.

It is an anaesthetic tube which is usually in situ for 24–48 hours. Depending on the patient's condition and the operation performed, the Portex tube will be removed and the stoma left exposed, e.g. total laryngectomy, or a more suitable sturdier tube will be inserted, such as a Shiley tracheostomy tube.

Shiley plain tracheostomy tube (Fig. 41.3a)

This is a plastic tube with an introducer and two inner tubes. One inner tube has an extension at its upper aspect. This facilitates connection to other equipment, e.g. speaking valves.

This tube is usually used for the following reasons:

- To keep the tracheostomy tract patent if the patient is going to have further surgery
- In place of a metal tracheostomy tube if the patient is going to have radiotherapy to the neck area when a metal tube would cause tissue reaction (Holmes 1996)
- For a laryngectomy patient who has a benign or malignant stenosis of the trachea and requires a longer tube than the regular length laryngectomy tube to keep the stenosis patent.

Shiley cuffed tracheostomy tube (Fig. 41.3b)

This is a plastic tube with an introducer and one inner tube. The inner tube has an extension at its upper aspect to facilitate connection to other equipment. The outer tube has an inflatable cuff to give an airtight seal. The cuff prevents secretions from reaching the lungs. The seal facilitates ventilation.

This is often used for the immediate postoperative phase, i.e. 24–72 hours. The use of tracheostomy tubes with smaller cuff volumes has enabled the intracuff pressure to be used as a measure when applied to the tracheal mucosa (Sykes & Young 1999). For those patients who require a cuffed tracheostomy tube for lengthy periods, a cuff manometer should be used to check cuff pressure. In order to prevent tracheal injury or aspiration, cuff pressures should be maintained between 18 and 20 mmHg (Crimlisk *et al.* 1996).

Shiley fenestrated tube (Fig. 41.3c)

This is a plastic tube with an introducer and two inner tubes. One inner tube has an extension at its upper end to facilitate connection to other apparatus. The other inner tube has a fenestration in the middle which, when inserted, lines up with the fenestration in the outer tube. This is to encourage the passage of air and secretions into the oral and nasal passages. It is useful when attempting to encourage a return to normal function following long-term use of a temporary tracheostomy.

The fenestrations enable this type of tube to be most suitable for the weaning method. A cap is inserted onto the tube, occluding the artificial airway. This enables the patient to become used to breathing via the oral and nasal passages again. The cap can be left in situ for certain periods of time until the patient can tolerate the tube occluded for a full uninterrupted 24 hours. Only then can removal of the entire tube, known as decannulation, be considered (Bull 1996).

Shiley cuffed fenestrated tube (Fig. 41.3d)

This is a plastic tube with an introducer and two inner tubes. One inner tube has an extension at its upper aspect to facilitate connection to other apparatus, while the other has a fenestration midway down the tube. This tube can also be occluded with a cap, to assess the patient's oral and nasal airway, first ensuring that the cuff has been completely deflated and that the fenestrated inner tube is in situ. The outer tube has a fenestration in the middle of the cannula, again to encourage a return to normal function. The outer tube also has an inflatable cuff to give an airtight seal. The cuff prevents secretions from reaching the lungs. This tube is useful for patients with swallowing problems but who are starting to return to normal function.

Jackson's silver tracheostomy tube

This is a silver tube with an introducer and inner tube (Fig. 41.4a). The inner tube is locked in position by a small catch on the outer tube and may be removed and cleaned as necessary without disturbing the outer tube.

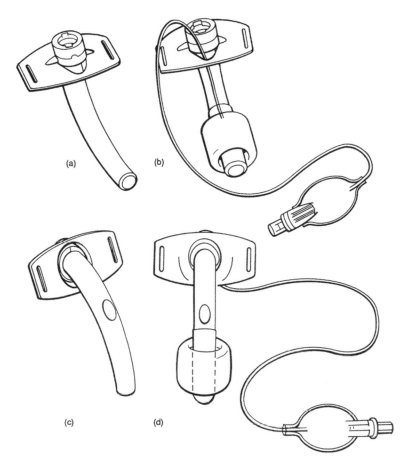

Figure 41.3 Shiley's tracheostomy tubes. (a) Shiley plain tube. (b) Shiley cuffed tube. (c) Shiley plain fenestrated tube. (d) Shiley cuffed fenestrated tube.

Negus's silver tracheostomy tube

This is a silver tracheostomy tube with an introducer and a choice of inner tubes, with and without speaking valves (Fig. 41.4b). The outer tube does not have a safety

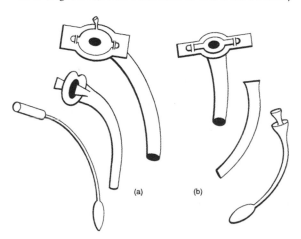

Figure 41.4 (a) Jackson's silver tube. (b) Negus's silver tube.

catch, consequently the inner tube may be coughed out inadvertently.

Kapitex Bivona Hyperflex tube

This is a silicone, wire-reinforced cuffed tracheostomy tube (Fig. 41.5). It has an adjustable flange and is a longer length tube, thereby accommodating unusual airway anatomy. The cuff is totally flat when deflated, which makes the insertion and removal less traumatic. An introducer is provided to aid insertion. It is essential that tracheostomy care is maintained scrupulously in order to prevent obstruction as no inner tube is provided with this product.

Speaking valve

This is a plastic device with a two-way valve which fits onto the extended aspects of the Shiley inner tube (Fig. 41.6a). When breathing, the valve stays open but when the patient attempts to speak the valve closes, thus redirecting air up through the normal air passages and allowing the production of voice.

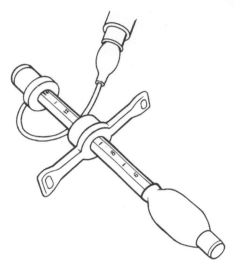

Figure 41.5 Kapitex Bivona Hyperflex cuffed tracheostomy tube.

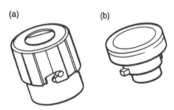

Figure 41.6 (a) Rusch speaking valve. (b) Decannulation plug.

Kapitex Tracoetwist fenestrated tube

This is a plastic tube with an introducer and two inner tubes (Fig. 41.7). One of these inner tubes has an extension at its upper end to facilitate connection to other apparatus. The other inner tube has a fenestration midway down the tube. The outer tube also has a fenestration consisting of a series of small holes. This helps to reduce the risk of granulation tissue growing through the fenestration and enables suction catheters to slide down the tube more easily when performing suction. The neck plate or flange moves in a vertical and horizontal direction enabling the plate to move as the patient moves. An inner tube with integrated speaking valve can be ordered separately.

A variety of other tubes are available in this series, including both cuffed and plain tracheostomy tubes.

Decannulation plug

This is a small plastic plug which fits into the outer fenestrated tube (Fig. 41.6b). It is used to encourage patients to breathe via the oral and nasal air passages before removal of the tracheostomy tube. Alternatively,

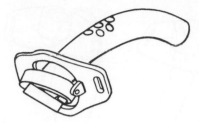

Figure 41.7 Kapitex Tracoetwist fenestrated tube.

a small plastic plug (Kapitex) or a blind hub (Shiley) can be fitted into or over the inner fenestrated tube. This is particularly useful for patients who are still producing tenacious secretions as the plug or hub can be removed to enable the inner tube to be cleaned.

Colledge silver laryngectomy tube

This is a silver laryngectomy tube with an introducer (Fig. 41.8a). It is often used to dilate a laryngectomy stoma which has stenosed. These tubes can be cleaned, autoclaved and reused.

Shiley laryngectomy tube

This is a plastic tube with an introducer and inner tube (Fig. 41.8b). It is shorter in length than a tracheostomy tube, thereby conforming to the slightly shorter trachea in the patient who has undergone a total laryngectomy. The inner tube may be removed and cleaned frequently without disturbing the outer tube. It is sometimes worn postoperatively while the stoma is healing to help facilitate a good shaped stoma.

Shaw's silver laryngectomy tube

This is a silver laryngectomy tube with an introducer and an inner tube beyond both lower and upper aspects of the outer tube (Fig. 41.8c). Thus pressure dressings may be secured without occluding the stoma. The silver catch on the outer tube keeps the inner tube in position.

Stoma button

This is a soft Silastic 'button' (Fig. 41.8d). It may be used in place of a laryngectomy tube. It is very light and comfortable to wear and can be used in conjunction with a Blom–Singer speaking valve. In order to facilitate the use of the Blom–Singer speaking valve a diamond-shape is cut out of the Silastic.

Laryngectomy tube

This is a slightly opaque Silastic tube which is longer in length in comparison to the stoma button. These tubes are 36 and 55 mm in length and are available in a variety of different sizes (Fig. 41.8e). This tube is most suitable for patients who experience a degree of stenosis further

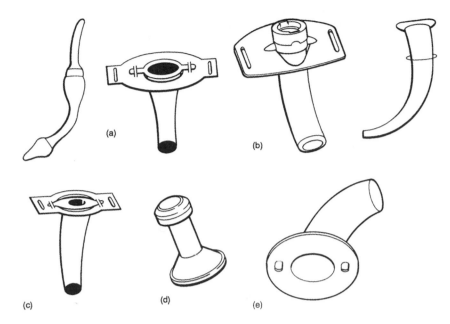

Figure 41.8 Tubes for permanent tracheostomies.
(a) Colledge silver tube.
(b) Shiley laryngectomy tube.
(c) Shaw's laryngectomy tube.
(d) Stoma button.
(e) Laryngectomy tube.

down the trachea (see 'Stoma buttons and vents' later in this chapter for further information).

Heat and moisture exchange (HME) filters

Following laryngectomy, patients lose normal nasal airway functions. The air they breathe is no longer warmed, humidified and filtered by the nasal passages as they now breathe directly in and out of the tracheostome. The result of this is an increase in secretions which have to be coughed up out of the trachea. The amount of secretions produced will vary from patient to patient but is greater in the immediate and early postoperative period and gradually improves over the ensuing months. Patients find that any sharp change in temperature stimulates excessive mucus production (Mathieson 2001).

Prior to the development of HME filters, patients coped with this by spraying the tracheostomal area with water, using a Roger's spray or equivalent and wearing either a small foam pad, a 'bib' or specially designed cravat or scarf over the stoma. However, over the past few years there have been a number of developments in the availability of HME filters for laryngectomy patients (Young *et al.* 2002). HME filters are available on prescription and while there are a number of different designs, as with the voice prostheses, the basic principle remains the same and selection criteria depend upon individual need and preference.

HME filters consist of a self-adhesive baseplate which is placed around the stoma and a specially treated foam filter which is clipped into the centre. This enables the patient to breathe more easily while the air is warmed, humidified and filtered by the foam. For a minority of patients who cannot tolerate the baseplate on the skin or maintain a good seal, the filter section can also be clipped into a flexible silastic laryngectomy tube, vent or stoma button.

It is the role of the clinical nurse specialist and/or speech and language therapist to assess and fit the HME filter in the initial stages of care.

General care of tracheostomy patients

- When caring for a tracheostomy patient the following should always be at the bedside or accessible if the patient is self-caring or ambulant:
  (a) Humidified oxygen with tracheostomy mask
  (b) Suction machine with a selection of suction catheters
  (c) Sterile water or a covered bowl of sodium bicarbonate (1 teaspoon to 500 ml of sterile water) can be used to help clear suction tubing of secretions after suctioning has been performed (Serra 2000)
  (d) Clean disposable gloves (Hooper 1996) and individually packaged, sterile, disposable gloves (Ward *et al.* 1997)
  (e) Disposable plastic apron and eye protection (Ward *et al.* 1997)
  (f) Two cuffed tracheostomy tubes, one the same size as the patient is wearing, the other a size smaller, in the event of an emergency tracheostomy tube change

(g) One 10 ml syringe to inflate cuff on tracheostomy tube

(h) Tracheal dilators, in the event of tracheostomy tube falling out or being removed and inability to insert another tube. Tracheal dilators can be used to keep stomal opening patent until medical assistance arrives.

- Tracheostomy tube changes are mostly dependent on the type of secretions the patient has, for example, a patient with copious, tenacious secretions will need a daily tube change, sometimes twice a day, as this will be the only way of ensuring that the stoma and tube are free from any accumulation of secretions. If the patient has minimal secretions then the necessity to change the tube decreases until some patients need to have their tube changed only weekly.

Sometimes if the patient has a wound area up to the stoma edge, the tracheostomy tube has to be removed to gain access for cleaning the wound and observing its general status.

The tracheostomy dressing can be renewed without removing the tube which should be done twice a day or more frequently if necessary (Serra 2000). Changing the dressing will help prevent secretions around the outside of the stoma from becoming dry and possibly blocking the tube. Furthermore, this will minimize the risk of skin excoriation and wound breakdown (Minsley & Wrenn 1996).

Tracheostomy suctioning

Tracheostomy suctioning is performed to maintain a clear airway and optimize respiratory functions, for example alveolar ventilation and gas exchange. Suctioning via a tracheostomy is performed when patients are unable to clear their own secretions. Some patients, however, may be able to clear their secretions into the tracheostomy tube by means of expectorating, thus reducing the need for suctioning.

Indications for suctioning

The use of routine suctioning should be avoided and an assessment of the patient's chest condition should be carried out instead. Inspection, auscultation, percussion and palpation will help to determine the following:

- Patient's ability to clear his or her own secretions
- Location of any secretions
- Whether these secretions could be reached by the catheter
- How detrimental these secretions might be for the patient (Pryor & Prasad 2001; Hough 2001).

Despite the benefits of suctioning, this action can also be hazardous for the patient.

- *Hypoxia*: the act of suctioning reduces vital lung volume from the lungs and upper airways. Each suctioning procedure should last no more than a breath cycle, about 10–15 seconds. Any longer than this may cause hypoxia. Ventilator disconnection or the removal of the oxygen supply will also add to the risk of hypoxia prior to suctioning. Within a critical care setting this risk can be avoided by hyperoxygenating the lungs with 100% oxygen, either manually or via a ventilator (Glass & Grap 1995; Hough 2001).
- *Mucosal trauma*: an incorrect choice of catheter, poor technique and the use of an excessively high suction pressure may all lead to mucosal trauma. The recommended suction pressure is 60–150 mmHg or 8–20 kPa (Pryor & Prasad 2001).
- *Cardiac arrhythmias*: arrhythmias may be brought about by the onset of hypoxaemia or a vasovagal reflex instigated by tracheal stimulation by the catheter (MacIntyre & Branson 2001).
- *Raised intracranial pressure*: this may occur if the suction catheter causes excessive tracheal stimulation and result in coughing and an increase in the patient's intrathoracic pressure, both of which compromise cerebral venous drainage (Pryor & Prasad 2001).
- *Infection risk*: both care giver and patient are at risk of infection when suctioning is performed. Research has shown that bacteria can be introduced during tracheostomy suctioning if a contaminated suction catheter is used (Brown 1982; Gibson 1983). Griggs (1998) highlights that using sterile catheters, combined with a non-touch suction technique and sterile gloves, should minimize the risk of infection. However, the question of whether to use boxed non-sterile gloves for suctioning has not been resolved. Rossoff *et al.* (1993) point out that boxed gloves are often contaminated before they are used, while other studies show a general consensus that boxed non-sterile gloves are no more likely to introduce infection than sterile ones (Griggs 1998; MacIntyre & Branson 2001).

The DoH (2001) suggest that a risk assessment of suctioning should be carried out so that the related risks to patients and health care practitioners can be assessed, thus establishing whether sterile or non-sterile gloves are required. If contact with a sterile piece of equipment during an aseptic technique is likely to occur, then the risk assessment would conclude that sterile gloves are required.

A number of standard principles have been highlighted by the DoH (2001):

- Gloves should be worn as single-use items, conform to Conformité Européene (CE) standards and be of an acceptable quality.

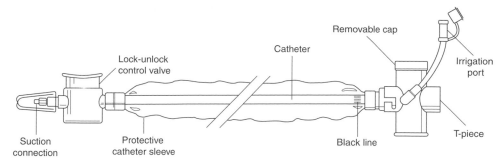

Figure 41.9 Components of a closed-circuit catheter. The control valve locks the vacuum on or off. The catheter is protected inside an airtight sleeve. A T-piece connects the device to the tracheal tube. The irrigation port allows saline instillation for irrigating the patient's airway or for cleaning the catheter (Hough 2001).

- Powdered and polythene gloves should not be used in health care activities.
- Alternatives to natural rubber latex gloves must be available for use by practitioners and patients with latex sensitivity.

Suction catheters

Suction catheters are now made from polyvinyl chloride and do not require any lubrication. Multihole catheters are often preferred over single-hole catheters as these dissipate the focus of suction pressure, making it less likely for the mucosa to be sucked into the catheter. Furthermore, multihole catheters produce a cushion of air at the tip, thus preventing the catheter coming into contact with the tracheal mucosa (Griggs 1998). Choosing the correct suction catheter size depends on the size of the tracheostomy tube. As a guide, the diameter of the suction catheter should be half of the tracheostomy tube size (Griggs 1998; Hough 2001).

Within a critical care setting, a closed-circuit suction system is an alternative method to the open suction system for patients being mechanically ventilated. This closed system has the catheter sealed in a protective plastic sleeve, which is connected permanently into a standard ventilator circuit thus preventing the catheter becoming contaminated (Fig. 41.9). This also reduces the number of times the patient is disconnected from the ventilator, avoiding further hypoxia and cross-infection. Other patient groups who may benefit from its use include those who are immunosuppressed, actively infectious patients or those who require high levels of positive end-expiratory pressure (PEEP).

Resuscitation

In the event of a patient with a tracheostomy needing resuscitation, the nurse should ensure that the tracheostomy is clear then connect an artificial ventilation device (for example, an Ambu-bag with a connector or catheter mount attached) to the tracheostomy tube in order to perform manual ventilation. She should ensure that the cuff of the tracheostomy tube is inflated to prevent air leakage, thus ensuring adequate oxygenation and ventilation.

Laryngectomy voice rehabilitation

Definition

A voice prosthesis is a one-way silicone valve that slots into a surgically created fistula reconnecting the trachea to the pharynx following surgical removal of the larynx. The valve, once fitted, allows air to be directed from the lungs and trachea into the pharynx when the patient wishes to speak. This airflow causes the pharyngeal muscles to vibrate, producing the sound or voice for speech. Since the valve is one-way it also prevents food and drink passing from the pharynx into the trachea and down the airway. A valve which begins to leak food and/or drink may be defective, worn-out or ill-fitting.

The fistula for the voice valve may be created at the time of the total laryngectomy operation. Hence the terms primary surgical voice restoration (at the time of laryngectomy) and secondary surgical voice restoration (i.e. procedure carried out later) are used.

Reference material

Voice prostheses for patients undergoing laryngectomy have been available in Britain since the early 1980s (Blom & Singer 1980). There are a number of different types of prosthesis on the market, including Blom–Singer, Bivona, Provox and Gröningen. All work according to

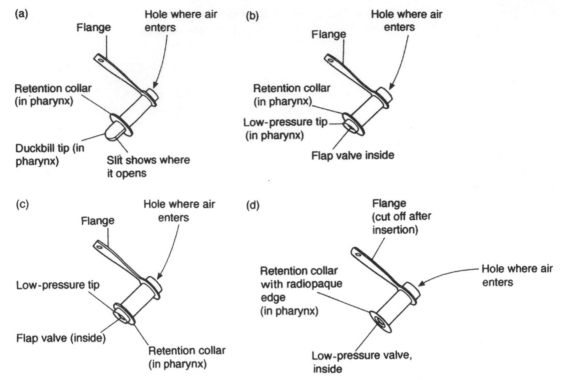

Figure 41.10 Laryngectomy voice rehabilitation. (a) Duckbill valve. (b) Low-pressure valve, 16 Fr gauge. (c) Low-pressure valve, 20 Fr gauge. (d) Indwelling valve, 20 Fr gauge.

the same principle. The Blom–Singer prosthesis, developed in the USA by Eric Blom, a speech pathologist, and Mark Singer, an otolaryngologist, will be described in detail here.

Types of valve (Fig. 41.10)

Although there are many different makes of voice valve, most have a diameter of either 16 or 20 Fr. All makes of valve are available in a series of different lengths (1.4–3.6 cm) to fit the depth of the tracheopharyngeal wall, which varies from patient to patient. Initially, the patient should be measured and fitted with a prosthesis by an experienced and specialized practitioner who will select the most suitable type of valve, taking into account the patient's fitness and individual needs.

Duckbill valve/Blom–Singer type voice prosthesis

This prosthesis is named after its design: the valved end of the prosthesis opens like a duck's bill to allow air to pass into the pharynx. Talking with the prosthesis requires a little more effort than talking prior to laryngectomy. The device has a rounded end, making it easy to insert, and is less susceptible to infection by *Candida albicans* than the low-pressure model. The duckbill valve requires

more effort to use than the low-pressure type as it creates greater resistance to the airflow.

Low-pressure valve/Blom–Singer type voice prosthesis

The Blom–Singer low-pressure device has a flatter posterior aspect than the duckbill with a small hinged flap acting as the one-way valve. It can sometimes be more difficult to insert, though recent gel cap insertion techniques help to minimize problems. Its design makes it more susceptible to infection with *C. albicans*. Talking with the prosthesis requires approximately the same amount of effort as talking prior to laryngectomy.

Low-pressure valve/Blom–Singer type voice prosthesis (20 Fr gauge)

This is a special wide-diameter prosthesis recommended for patients with specialized needs. The decision to fit this lies with the specialist ENT doctor and/or specialist speech and language therapist.

Indwelling valve/Blom–Singer type voice prosthesis (20 Fr gauge)

The main advantage of this valve is that it can last for about 6 months, providing the patient uses prophylactic antifungal treatment to counteract fungal infection of the valve. It has to be inserted and removed by a specialist speech and language therapist, ENT doctor experienced in fitting and managing voice prostheses or a nurse trained in the procedure.

Economy duckbill valve/Bivona type voice prosthesis (economy)

This is another duckbill valve, similar to the Blom–Singer device. It is made of flesh-tone silicone and is available in a full range of sizes, including the extra long 4 cm size.

Bivona type voice prosthesis (ultra-low resistance)

The Bivona ultra-low voice prosthesis functions with little resistance like the Blom–Singer type, low-pressure model. The valved part of the prosthesis is a small, blue, hinged flap within the main body of the device. The posterior aspect is hooded to divert food and drink away. This device is susceptible to infection by *C. albicans*.

Provox type indwelling voice prosthesis

This device is more difficult to insert as it has to be passed through the mouth and pharynx. This can be done under local anaesthetic, although for some patients a general anaesthetic is preferable. Once inserted it remains in place for an average of 4–6 months. This device is susceptible to infection by *C. albicans*. The Provox 2 voice prosthesis has more recently become available and can be inserted and removed via the tracheostoma. It has a wider diameter than the Blom–Singer type prosthesis.

Gröningen type voice prosthesis

In most cases this prosthesis is inserted under general anaesthetic. It is currently used at only one centre in the UK. Once inserted it remains in place for approximately 6 months. This device is susceptible to infection by *C. albicans*.

Stoma buttons and vents

To prevent stenosis of the stoma created for the voice prosthesis, patients may need to wear a stoma button, especially in the first few weeks after surgery. Although the stoma would not close completely, it may become so narrow that breathing is restricted and care of the voice prosthesis difficult.

Stoma buttons, made of soft Silastic, are available in a range of diameters: 10, 12 and 14 mm. For patients with voice prostheses, 12 or 14 mm is most suitable, so that the stoma is wide enough for the patient to clean the prosthesis. If a voice prosthesis is used with a stoma button, a hole is cut in the button to allow air to pass through the valve during speech. An experienced, specialized practitioner is required to adapt the button in this way. (For further information see 'Stoma button', above.)

Bivona type vent and Forth Medical type laryngectomy tube for use with a voice prosthesis

These devices are made of a softer plastic than the traditional Shiley type laryngectomy tube, making them more comfortable and more appropriate for long-term use (beyond the postoperative period and on a continuing basis providing they are kept clean). Some patients find the stoma consistent enough in diameter to dispense completely with a vent or button some 6 months to 1 year after the laryngectomy. Other patients need to continue wearing either a vent or a button all the time. They are available in a range of three diameters, and two different lengths: 36 or 55 mm. If a voice prosthesis is used at the same time as either of these two devices, an aperture is made in the upper side to allow air to pass through the valve. The Forth tube is made with an indentation to mark the site of the aperture.

Indications for replacing a voice prosthesis

- *Voice prosthesis showing signs of wear and tear.* In most cases, experience indicates that a voice prosthesis will last for 6–8 weeks. After that time patients may find it harder to use it to make voice, when previously they had no difficulty. This deterioration is gradual.
- *Voice prosthesis is leaking.* Valves are made of silicone and are therefore susceptible to fungal infection by *C. albicans*. Micro-organisms burrow into the silicone and interfere with the functioning of the posterior (internal) end of the prosthesis. The effect of this is to cause saliva and drinks to leak in small drops through it, causing the patient to cough. Leakage such as this is a very common problem and can shorten the life of the prosthesis considerably.
- *Drink and/or food are leaking around the valve.* This problem is less common. It indicates that the diameter of the fistula has become greater than the diameter of the valve, probably as a result of infection. A specialist speech and language therapist or a nurse or doctor with the ENT training required to fit and manage voice prostheses should be contacted for advice.
- *Patient cannot make any sound with the voice prosthesis.* It is possible that patients may suddenly find that they can no longer make any sound with the prosthesis, or sound may be intermittent. The prosthesis must be removed and inspected, and almost certainly needs to be changed. A specialist speech and language therapist, or a nurse or doctor with the ENT training required to fit and manage voice prostheses should be contacted for advice.

Indications for replacing a 'lost' or dislodged voice prosthesis

The voice prosthesis is held in position by a silicone retention collar which is an integral part of the whole device. It is therefore possible for it to become accidentally dislodged. Patients are told that this might happen, and shown how to insert a Jacques 14 Fr red rubber catheter or a white Silastic 14 Fr Foley catheter through the

fistula to keep it open. If patients are able to perform this procedure when a voice prosthesis is accidentally dislodged, the fistula remains open and a new prosthesis is inserted after removal of the catheter. If the voice prosthesis is ejected and the patient is unable to insert a catheter satisfactorily a speech and language therapist or doctor with experience in fitting and managing voice prostheses should be contacted for advice.

Procedure guidelines: **Changing a tracheostomy dressing**

Equipment

1 Sterile dressing pack.
2 Tracheostomy dressing or a keyhole dressing.
3 Cleaning solution, such as 0.9% sodium chloride.

4 Tracheostomy tape.
5 Bactericidal alcohol handrub.

Procedure

Action	Rationale
1 Explain and discuss the procedure with the patient.	To ensure that the patient understands the procedure and gives his/her valid consent.
2 Screen the bed or cubicle.	To ensure the patient's privacy.
3 Wash hands using bactericidal soap and water or bactericidal alcohol handrub, and prepare the dressing tray or trolley.	To minimize the risk of infection.
4 Perform the procedure using aseptic technique.	To minimize the risk of infection.
5 Remove the soiled dressing from around the tube, clean around the stoma with 0.9% sodium chloride using low-linting gauze.	To reduce the risk of fragments entering the altered airway and to remove secretions and any crusts.
6 Replace with a tracheostomy dressing or a comfortable keyhole dressing.	To ensure the patient's comfort. To avoid pressure from the tube.
7 Renew tracheostomy tapes, checking that one finger can be placed between the tapes and neck.	To secure the tube. To ensure that the tapes are not too tight or too loose, thus decreasing the chance of necrosis caused by excessive pressure from the tapes.

Procedure guidelines: **Suctioning a patient with a tracheostomy**

Equipment

1 Suction machine (wall source or portable).
2 Aero-flow sterile suction catheters (assorted sizes; see action 5).
3 A selection of gloves (sterile or non-sterile clean boxed gloves).
4 Jug of sodium bicarbonate solution (1 teaspoon in 500 ml sterile water). The receptacle must be sterile

initially and changed every 24 hours (Ward *et al*. 1997) to prevent the growth of bacteria.
5 Disposable plastic apron.
6 Eye protection, e.g. goggles.
7 Bactericidal alcohol handrub.

Procedure

Action	Rationale
1 Nurses and patients should use a 0.9% sterile sodium chloride nebulizer 2 hourly or more frequently as prescribed, if secretions are tenacious.	Suctioning may not be as effective if the secretions become too tenacious or dry. A 0.9% sterile sodium chloride nebulizer will assist in loosening dry and thick secretions (Hough 2001).

Procedure guidelines: **Suctioning a patient with a tracheostomy** *(cont'd)*

Action	Rationale
2 Suctioning should be taught if the patient is able to perform his/her own suction. Otherwise inform the patient what is to be done.	To obtain the patient's co-operation and to help him or her relax. The procedure is unpleasant and can be frightening for the patient. Reassurance is vital. Self-control of the patient's suction is preferable if the patient is able to manage it.
3 Wash hands with bactericidal soap and water or bactericidal alcohol handrub, and put on a disposable plastic apron, and eye protection.	To minimize the risk of cross-infection. Some patients may accidently cough directly ahead at the nurse; standing to one side with tissues at the patient's tracheostomy minimizes this risk.
4 Check that the suction machine is set to the appropriate level.	Recommended suction pressure is 60–150 mmHg or 8–20 kPa for adults (Pryor & Prasad 2001). Sputum which is more tenacious requires more powerful suction, the maximum level being 200 mmHg. If pressures up to and above 200 mmHg are used, then vacuum-interrupted suctioning techniques are recommended to prevent pressure buildup should the catheter become occluded (Young 1984). The use of excessive high pressure may result in mucosal trauma of the main bronchi.
5 Select the correct size catheter. As a guide, the diameter of the suction catheter should be half the tracheostomy tube size (Griggs 1998; Hough 2001).	The size of suction catheter is dependent on tenacity and volume of secretions, that is, the thicker the secretions and the larger the volume, the greater the bore of the tube (Hough 2001). This ensures that hypoxia does not occur while suctioning.
6 Open the end of the suction catheter pack and use the pack to attach the catheter to the suction tubing. Keep the rest of the catheter in the sterile packet.	To reduce the risk of transferring infection from hands to the catheter and to keep the catheter as clean as possible.
7 For new surgically formed tracheostomy and laryngectomy stomas, use an individually packaged, sterile, disposable glove on the hand manipulating the catheter (Ward *et al.* 1997). (A clean disposable glove can be used on the other hand.) Clean, disposable gloves can be used for subsequent admissions or for established stomas.	Gloves minimize the risk of infection transfer to the catheter or from the sputum to the nurse's hands.
8 Withdraw the catheter from the sleeve and introduce the catheter to about one third of its length and apply suction by placing the thumb over the suction port control.	Gentleness is essential; damage to the tracheal mucosa can lead to trauma and respiratory infection. The catheter should go no further than the carina to prevent trauma.
9 Withdraw the catheter gently with a rotating motion. Do not suction the patient for more than one breath cycle, 10–15 seconds (MacIntyre & Branson 2001).	To remove secretions from around the mucous membranes. Prolonged suctioning may result in acute hypoxia, cardiac arrhythmias, mucosal trauma, infection and the patient experiencing a feeling of choking.
10 Wrap catheter around gloved hand, then pull back glove over soiled catheter, thus containing catheter in glove, then discard.	Catheters are used only once to reduce the risk of introducing infection.
11 Rinse the suction tubing by dipping its end into the jug of sterile water or sodium bicarbonate solution and applying suction until the solution has rinsed the tubing through.	To loosen secretions that have adhered to the inside of the tube.
12 If the patient requires further suction, repeat the above actions using new gloves and a new catheter.	
13 Repeat the suction until the airway is clear.	

Humidification

Definition

Humidification can be defined as increasing water content, the moisture or dampness in the atmosphere or a gas (Hough 2001; Pryor & Prasad 2001). In health, inspired air is filtered, warmed and moistened by the ciliated lining, and mucus is produced in the upper respiratory pathways. Because the upper respiratory pathways are bypassed in patients with a tracheostomy, they need artificial humidification to ensure that these pathways remain moist (Pryor & Prasad 2001).

Procedure guidelines: **Humidification**

Procedure

Action	Rationale
1 Fill a suitable nebulizer with sterile water and attach it to the oxygen or air supply, then set the gas rate for the liquid to form into humidification droplets. Continuous hot water humidification is needed for the first 48 hours of a newly formed tracheostomy (Hough 2001).	Constant humidification is required while the new stoma adapts to the outside environment (especially for laryngectomy patients). Humidification also prevents the formation of crusts which are liable to obstruct the airway. The use of sterile water reduces the risk of infection (Hough 2001). Any liquid remaining after 24 hours should be replaced.
2 For patients in cubicles, a room humidifier may be placed at the bedside.	

Subsequent care

Action	Rationale
1 Give humidified oxygen as required. Usually, patients need about 10–15 min of humidification every 4 hours. This may be adapted according to the patient's needs, e.g. throughout the night, according to time.	Patients begin to adapt to breathing through their tracheostomy after the first 24–48 hours. Some humidification is required according to individual needs and to prevent crust formation in the airway.
2 If the patient does not require oxygen, blow humidifiers may be used.	These provide humidified air without the need for an oxygen supply.
3 Provide laryngeal stoma protectors, Laryngofoam, Buchanan bib, Romet and heat and moisture exchangers.	To protect and humidify the airway.

Procedure guidelines: **Changing a tracheostomy tube**

With a newly formed tracheostomy, tube changing should be avoided where possible for the first 2 or 3 days to enable the tract to become well established (Bull 1996).

Equipment

1 Sterile dressing pack.
2 Tracheostomy dressing or a keyhole dressing.
3 Tracheostomy tape.
4 Cleaning solution, such as 0.9% sodium chloride.
5 Barrier cream.
6 Lubricating jelly.
7 Disposable plastic apron.
8 Bactericidal alcohol handrub.
9 Eye protection.

Procedure

Action	Rationale
1 Explain and discuss the procedure with the patient.	To ensure that the patient understands the procedure and gives his/her valid consent.

Procedure guidelines: Changing a tracheostomy tube (cont'd)

Action	Rationale
2 Wash hands using bactericidal soap and water or bactericidal alcohol handrub, and prepare a dressing trolley.	To minimize the risk of contamination.
3 Screen the patient's bed.	To ensure the patient's privacy.
4 Perform the procedure using clean technique.	To minimize the risk of contamination.
5 Assist the patient to sit in an upright position, supported by pillows with the neck extended.	To ensure the patient's comfort and to maintain a patent airway. If the neck is not extended, skin folds may occlude the tracheostomy when the tube is removed.
6 Remove the dressing pack from its outer wrappings and open the tracheostomy dressing.	Technique should be clean to reduce the risk of cross-infection.
7 Put on a disposable plastic apron.	
8 Clean hands with bactericidal alcohol handrub.	
9 Put on clean disposable plastic gloves.	To prevent infection.
10 Prepare the tracheostomy tube as outlined in steps 11–14.	So that the tube is ready for immediate insertion when required.
11 Thread on piece of tape through the slits in the flanges so that the tape passes behind the flange next to the stoma.	The tape is kept behind the flange to prevent it occluding the passage of air into the tracheostomy tube.
Alternatively, secure tracheostomy ties to both flanges.	These are made of Velcro and are more comfortable to wear and easy to adjust.
12 Put the tracheostomy dressing around the tube.	To prevent abrasion of the patient's skin by the tube.
13 Lubricate the tube sparingly with a lubricating jelly.	To facilitate insertion.
14 Remove the soiled tube from the patient's neck while asking the patient to breathe out.	Conscious expiration relaxes the patient and reduces the risk of coughing. Coughing can result in unwanted closure of the tracheostomy.
15 Clean around the stoma with 0.9% sodium chloride and dry gently. Apply barrier cream with topical swabs. (An aqueous cream may be used if the patient is having the site irradiated.)	To remove superficial organisms and crusts. Skin around the stoma is at risk of breakdown due to the constant presence of moisture in this area (Serra 2000). Meticulous skin care is therefore essential in order to prevent infection.
16 Insert a clean tube with introducer in place, using an 'up and over' action.	Introduction of the tube is less traumatic if directed along the contour of the trachea.
17 Remove the introducer immediately.	The patient cannot breathe while the introducer is in place.
18 Place the inner tube in position.	The inner tube can be changed as necessary when the outer tube is in position, thus minimizing the risk of trauma to trachea and stoma. The quantity of secretions present will determine the frequency with which the inner tube is changed.
19 Tie the tape securely at the side of the neck.	To secure the tube. Place the tie in an accessible place, at the same time ensuring that it will not cause discomfort to the patient.
20 Remove gloves and ask the patient to breathe out onto the palm of your hand.	Flow of air will be felt if the tube is in the correct position.
21 Ensure that the patient is comfortable.	
22 Clear away the trolley and equipment.	
23 Clean the soiled tube under running water, in line with the manufacturer's recommendations. If the tube is very soiled then use sodium bicarbonate to remove debris. The tube must be rinsed thoroughly and stored dry at the patient's bedside.	To remove debris that may occlude the tube and/or become a source of infection.

Note: plastic tubes should not be soaked in solutions as there is a danger that the material may absorb the solution which could then cause irritation of the trachea.

Problem solving

Problem	Cause	Suggested action
Profuse tracheal secretions.	Local reaction to tracheostomy tube.	Suction frequently, e.g. every 1–2 hours.
Lumen of tracheostomy tube occluded.	Tenacious mucus in tube.	Use 0.9% sodium chloride nebulizers, heat and moisture exchangers and suction. Change the inner tube regularly, e.g. 1–3-hourly.
	Dried blood and mucus in the tube, especially in the postoperative period.	Provide humidified air. (For further information, see 'Procedure guidelines: Humidification', above.)
Tracheostomy tube dislodged accidentally.	Tapes not secured adequately.	Put in spare tube. This should be clean and ready at the bedside. *Note*: tracheal dilators must be kept at the bedside of patients with tracheostomies.
Unable to insert clean tracheostomy tube.	Unpredicted shape or angle of stoma.	Remain calm since an outward appearance of distress may cause the patient to panic and lose confidence. Lubricate the tube well and attempt to reinsert at various angles. If unsuccessful, attempt to insert a smaller-size tracheostomy tube. If this is impossible, keep the tracheostomy tract open using tracheal dilators and inform the doctor.
	Tracheal stenosis due to patient coughing, patient being very anxious or because the tube has been left out too long.	Insert a smaller-size tracheostomy tube. If insertion still proves difficult, do not leave the patient but ask for a tube to be brought to the bed. Keep the tracheostomy patent with tracheal dilators if stenosis is pronounced until the tube is reinserted.
Tracheal bleeding following or during change of the tube.	Trauma due to suction or to the tube being changed. Presence of tumour. Granulation tissue forming in fenestration of tube.	Change the tube as planned if bleeding is minimal. For profuse bleeding, insert a cuffed tube and inflate. Inform the doctor. Perform tracheal suction to remove the blood from the trachea.
Infected sputum.	Nature of surgery and condition of patient often predispose to infection.	Encourage the patient to cough up secretions and/or suction regularly. Change the tube and clean the stoma area frequently, e.g. 4-hourly. Protect permanent stomas with a bib or gauze. Following result of sputum specimen, commence appropriate antibiotics as needed.

Procedure guidelines: **Changing a Blom–Singer type non-indwelling voice prosthesis**

Nurses must wear gloves and eye protection (to prevent phlegm/blood entering the eyes) when carrying out this procedure. The area must be well lit to illuminate the stoma.

Equipment

1 Clinically clean tray or receiver.
2 Correct replacement voice prosthesis and introducer.
3 Red rubber Foley catheter (16 Fr gauge).
4 White plastic stent or dilator with correct diameter.

5 Lubricant jelly, e.g. KY jelly or similar.
6 Tissues.
7 Blenderm transparent hypoallergenic tape or Micropore tape.

Procedure

Action	Rationale
1 Explain and discuss the procedure with the patient.	To ensure that the patient understands the procedure and gives his/her valid consent.
2 Settle the patient in a chair and arrange lighting to illuminate stoma.	To ensure the patient is comfortable and well supported.
3 Place a little lubricating jelly on the tip of the red rubber catheter and/or stent, and on the voice valve and introducer.	To ease insertion.
4 Ask the patient to keep his/her lips apart as the old valve is removed; hold flange where it joins the body of the valve.	To minimize amount of saliva entering fistula and reduce the risk of coughing.
5 Swiftly insert red rubber catheter (or dilator) 20 cm into the fistula.	To keep fistula open. To ascertain the shape and direction of the fistula.
6 Place valve on introducer, securing with flange.	To prevent valve dislodging from introducer during insertion.
7 Remove catheter or stent and replace with valve. A slight click will be felt as the retention collar on the valve passes into the pharynx.	To insert valve.
8 Check valve is correctly inserted by pulling it gently: it will move slightly, then resist.	To ensure valve is correctly positioned.
9 Place 5 cm length of Blenderm tape over flange to secure it to the patient's neck.	To keep flange neatly out of way.

References and further reading

Blom, E.D. & Singer, M. (1980) An endoscopic technique for the restoration of voice after laryngectomy. *Ann Otol Rhinol Laryngol*, **89**(6), 529–33.

Brown, I. (1982) Trach care? Take care – infection on the prowl. *Nursing*, **6**, 70–1.

Bull, P.D. (ed.) (1996) *Lecture Notes on Diseases of the Ear, Nose and Throat*, 8th edn. Blackwell Science, Oxford, pp. 172–80.

Crimlisk, J.T., Horn, M.H., Wilson, D.J. & Marino, B. (1996) Artificial airways: a survey of cuff management practices. *Heart Lung J Acute Crit Care*, **25**(3), 225–35.

Day, T., Wainwright, S.P. & Wilson-Barnett, J. (2001) An evaluation of a teaching intervention to improve the practice of endotracheal suctioning in intensive care units. *J Clin Nurs*, **10**(5), 682–96.

DoH (2001) Standard principles for preventing hospital-acquired infections. *J Hosp Infect*, **47**(Suppl), S21–37.

Fiorentini, A. (1992) Potential hazards of tracheostomy suctioning. *Intensive Crit Care Nurs*, **8**(4), 217–26.

Gibson, I.M. (1983) Tracheostomy management. *Nursing*, **2**(18), 538.

Glass, C. & Grap, M. (1995) Ten tips for safe suctioning. *Am J Nurs*, **5**(5), 51–3.

Griggs, A. (1998) Tracheostomy: suctioning and humidification. *Nurs Stand*, **13**(2), 49–56.

Holmes, S. (1996) *Radiotherapy. Radiation Induced Side Effects*. Austin Cornish, London, pp. 67–78.

Hooper, M. (1996) Nursing care of the patient with a tracheostomy. *Nurs Stand*, **10**(34), 40–3.

Hough, A. (2001) *Physiotherapy in Respiratory Care. An Evidence-Based Approach to Respiratory and Cardiac Management*, 3rd edn. Nelson Thornes, Cheltenham.

MacIntyre, N.R. & Branson, R.D. (2001) *Mechanical Ventilation*. W.B. Saunders, Philadelphia.

Mathieson, L. (2001) Physiological effects of laryngectomy. In: *The Voice and Its Disorders*. Whurr, London, pp. 597–600.

Minsley, M.A.H. & Wrenn, S. (1996) Long-term care of the tracheostomy patient from an outpatient nursing perspective. *ORL Head Neck Nurs*, **14**(4), 18–22.

O'Toole, M. (ed.) (1992) *Miller-Kean Encyclopedia and Dictionary of Medical, Nursing and Allied Health*, 5th edn. W.B. Saunders, Philadelphia.

Pryor, J.A. & Prasad, S.A. (2001) *Physiotherapy for Respiratory and Cardiac Problems: Adult and Paediatric*, 3rd edn. Churchill Livingstone, Edinburgh.

Rossoff, L.J., Lam, S., Hilton, E., Borenstein, M. & Isenberg, H.D. (1993) Is the use of boxed gloves in an intensive care unit safe? *Am J Med*, **94**(6), 602–7.

Scanlan, C.L., Wilkins, R.L. & Stoller, J.K. (1999) *Fundamentals of Respiratory Care*, 7th edn. Mosby, St Louis.

Serra, A. (2000) Tracheostomy care. *Nurs Stand*, **14**(42), 45–55.

Sykes, K. & Young, J.D. (1999) *Respiratory Support in Intensive Care*. BMJ Books, London.

Ward, V., Wilson, J., Taylor, L., Cookson, B. & Glynn, A. (1997) Supplement to *Hospital-Acquired Infection: Surveillance, Policies and Practice. Preventing Hospital-Acquired Infection. Clinical Guidelines*. Public Health Laboratory Service, London.

Wood, C. (1998) Can nurses safely assess the need for endotracheal suction in short term ventilated patients, instead of using routine techniques? *Intensive Crit Care Nurs*, **14**(4), 170–8.

Wood, C. (1998) Endotracheal suctioning: a literature review. *Intensive Crit Care Nurs*, **14**(3), 124–36.

Young, C. (1984) Recommended guidelines for suction. *Physiotherapy*, **70**(3), 106–8.

Young, P. *et al.* (2002) Breathing easy after laryngectomy. *Bull R Coll Speech Lang Ther*, September, 602.

42

Transfusion of blood, blood products and blood substitutes

Chapter contents

Definition

A transfusion consists of the administration of whole blood or any of its components to correct or treat a clinical abnormality.

Reference material

Blood donation and testing

Safety of both the donor and the potential recipient is an important criterion in the selection of blood donors. As well as microbiological testing of the donated blood, reliance is placed on the donor to answer questions on his or her general health, medical history and any drugs taken (Dacie & Lewis 1994). Prevention of transmission of infection is determined by donor selection criteria and laboratory testing. In the UK, all blood donations are tested for infections, which could be passed on to the recipient. Bacterial, parasitic and viral infections can be transmitted by blood components. Recently there have been concerns about the possibility of transmitting variant Creutzfelt-Jakcob disease (vCJD) during transfusion of plasma products. However, there is no evidence that the disease is transmitted by transfusion because currently there is no screening test capable of detecting vCJD (Mollison *et al.* 1997).

Following donation, blood products have varying shelf lives. Red blood cell products have a shelf life of 35 days if kept at 4°C (McClelland 2001), whereas platelets can only be stored for up to 96 hours at room temperature after donation and concentration (McClelland 2001).

Cross matching: ABO and Rh

Landsteiner in 1901 discovered that human blood groups (the ABO system) existed and this marked the beginning of safe blood transfusion (Porter 1999). There are four main blood groups: A, B, AB and O. These are based on antigens on the red cells and antibodies in the serum.

There is racial variation in the frequency of these within a population (Porter 1999). Apart from the ABO system, most of the other red cell antigens are detected by antibodies stimulated by transfusion or pregnancy (Porter 1999). The introduction of cells carrying A or B antigens results in immediate intravascular lysis in anyone with IgM antibodies to these antigens (Mollison *et al.* 1997).

In 1940 the rhesus system was discovered. This is the second most important system in transfusion therapy (Mollison *et al.* 1997) and is also an antigen found on the red cell. Transfusion of positive cells will result in immunization and the appearance of anti-D antibodies (Hoffbrand *et al.* 2001).

Full laboratory compatibility testing for cross matching of red blood cell transfusion can usually be done within 1 hour (Hoffbrand & Pettit 1994; Table 42.1).

Blood groups in haemopoietic stem cell transplantation

The human leucocyte antigen (HLA) is used to determine compatibility for organ transplantation including bone marrow and peripheral blood stem cells. Unfortunately, because ABO blood groups and HLA tissue types are determined genetically, it is not uncommon to find a well-matched HLA donor who is ABO incompatible with the recipient. Major transfusion reactions can be avoided by red cell and/or plasma depletion of the donor cells in the laboratory before reinfusion (Mollison *et al.* 1997). Very occasionally, if the recipient has a very high titre of anti-A or anti-B lytic antibody and the donor marrow or peripheral blood stem cells are blood group A, B or AB, then plasmapheresis of the recipient is performed to lower the titre of this antibody to safe limits. This is necessary because it is not possible to remove all the red cells from the donor product and those remaining may cause a major transfusion reaction in this situation (Mollison *et al.* 1997).

Indications

The range of products currently available, those most widely used, indications for use and recommendations for administration are listed in Table 42.1.

It may be unnecessary to correct a cytopenia or clotting deficiency to normal levels. Instead, physiological levels should be restored (Kickler & Ness 1993). A rise of approximately 10 g/l of haemoglobin may be expected from each transfused unit of red blood cells (Davies & Brozovic 1990).

Delivery of blood and blood products

The transfusion of stored blood exposes the patient to the possible infusion of particulate matter, such as clumps of white blood cells, fibrin, disintegrating platelets and small clots (Porter 1999). After transfusion this may result in clinical problems including non-haemolytic febrile reactions and respiratory impairment caused by pulmonary microemboli. These problems are more commonly associated with large transfusions of 6 units and above.

The variable size (between 10 and 200 μm) and number of microaggregates are dependent on two main factors:

- The storage time: in general the older the blood the more microaggregates it contains.
- The anticoagulant used to prevent the blood clotting.

Inline blood filters

Filters are used to remove microaggregates and leucocytes present in the blood to be transfused.

Microaggregate filters

Microaggregate or microparticle filters are used mainly to filter out red cell debris, platelets, white blood cells and fibrin strands that have clumped together. The filter compartment of commonly used blood administration sets will only remove particles of 170–200 μm and above.

Leucocyte depletion filters

Sensitization from white cells or HLA antigens present in transfusion products is a major problem for recipients, as they can cause minor or major adverse reactions. Specific filters are designated for the transfusion of red cells, platelets or fresh frozen plasma (FFP). Leucodepletion of all blood products at source is now standard practice in the UK (Williamson *et al.* 1999). Bedside filters have been withdrawn from the clinical area. There is no additional benefit of bedside filtration of leucocyte-depleted blood components as it will have the detrimental effect of reducing the volume of blood component transfused (McClelland 2001). Leucocyte depletion techniques aim to prevent or delay the onset of non-haemolytic febrile transfusion reactions.

Blood warming devices

The warming of blood and blood products is not recommended as it is of limited benefit and potentially dangerous. Use of blood warmers is only indicated when:

- Massive, rapid transfusion could result in cooling of cardiac tissue, causing dysfunction. In an adult if the rate of transfusion is greater than 50 ml/kg per hour, or in children if the rate is greater than 15 ml/kg per hour, blood warming devices should be used (McClelland 2001).
- Frozen plasma or other components are prescribed and must be thawed before administration.

Table 42.1 Blood and blood products used for transfusion

Type	Description	Indications	Cross-matching	Shelf life	Average infusion time	Technique	Special considerations
Whole blood	Complete unadulterated blood, approx. 510 ml including anticoagulant	To restore blood volume lost due to massive, acute haemorrhage whatever the cause	Must be compatible with recipient ABO and Rh type	35 days at 2–6°C (dependent on coagulant)	2–4 hours/unit	Give via a blood administration set	If loss and replacement exceed twice the blood volume, abnormalities of haemostasis may occur
Plasma reduced blood (packed red blood cells)*	Whole blood minus approx. 200 ml plasma, and anticoagulant; haematocrit 60–65%	To correct red blood cell deficiency and improve oxygen carrying capacity of the blood	ABO and Rh	21 days at 2–6°C	2–4 hours/unit	As above	–
Red cells in optimal additive solutions	Red cells minus all plasma: 100 ml fluid used as replacement to give optimal red cell preservation; haematocrit 60–65%	As above	ABO and Rh	53 days at 2–6°C	1–2 hours/unit	As above	An example of a replacement solution is 0.9% sodium chloride/adenine/glucose/mannitol
Concentrated red cells*	Plasma removed to produce a haematocrit of 70% plus	To correct anaemias when expansion of blood volume will not be tolerated	ABO and Rh	21 days at 2–6°C	1–2 hours/unit	As above	Availability varies, usually only used in infants (McClelland 2001)
Washed red blood cells*	Red cells centrifuged free of plasma and resuspended in 0.9% sodium chloride	To increase red cell mass and prevent tissue antigen formation in: 1 Immunosuppressed patients 2 Patients with previous transfusion reactions	ABO and Rh	Use within 12 hours or preferably, immediately	1–2 hours/unit	As above	–
Frozen red blood cells	1 Cells from normal healthy donor with very rare blood group	To treat transplant patients or patients with atypical antibodies which react with almost the entire population	ABO and Rh	Stored frozen cells: 3 years. Use within 12 hours of thawing	2–3 hours/unit	As above	Available from a few centres. Freezing process and recovery are time consuming and expensive

(continued)

Table 42.1 Blood and blood products used for transfusion (*continued*)

Type	Description	Indications	Cross-matching	Shelf life	Average infusion time	Technique	Special considerations
	2 Patient's own cells taken in anticipation of later illness (autologous blood transfusion)	To increase safety of transfusion therapy					
Leucocyte-poor blood	Red cells from which accompanying leucocytes have been removed	To prevent further reactions in patients who have had febrile attacks when receiving whole or plasma reduced blood	ABO and Rh	2–6°C. Time stated on pack. Usually within 12 hours of preparation, preferably immediately	2–3 hours/unit	As above	Frozen red cells may be used as an alternative
White blood cells (leucocyte concentrate)†	Mainly granulocytes obtained by leucophoresis or by 'creaming off' the buffy layers from packs of fresh blood	To treat patients with life-threatening granulocytopenia, e.g. due to chemotherapy	ABO and HLA (human leucocyte group A antigen)	24 hours after collection. Stored at 5°C	60–90 minutes/unit	Administer via a blood administration set. Usually 1 unit only	White blood cell infusion induces fever, may cause hypotension, rigors and confusion. Treat symptoms and reassure patient. Preparation may be irradiated to prevent initiation of graft-versus-host (GVH) disease in bone marrow transplant patients. *Do not give* to patients receiving amphotericin B. Indications for granulocyte transfusions should be when possible benefits are thought to outweigh considerable hazards of the treatment option (Brozović *et al.* 1998)
Platelets*	Platelet sediment from platelet-rich plasma, resuspended in 40–60 ml plasma	To treat thrombocytopenia due to 1 Decreased production 2 Increased destruction 3 Functionally abnormal platelets	ABO and rhesus compatibility preferred	Up to 5 days after collection at 22°C, with continuous gentle agitation; best within 6 hours	20–30 minutes/unit	Administration using a platelet administration set. Use a new set for each transfusion. Do not use micro-aggregate filters	General guide to use: 1 Count less than 10×10^9/litre 2 Count $10–20 \times 10^9$/litre with haemorrhage and/or persistent pyrexia 3 Count $20–50 \times 10^9$/litre or on chemotherapy may need platelets

Product	Description	Indications	Compatibility	Storage	Rate	Administration	Notes
		4 Dilutional problems following massive transfusions 5 DIC (critically ill patients receiving supportive therapies such as ventilation/ haemofiltration)					
Plasma: fresh or fresh frozen (FFP)	Citrated plasma separated from whole blood. All coagulation factors preserved for several months	To treat a clotting factor deficiency, when specific concentrates are unavailable or precise deficiency is unknown, e.g. DIC	ABO compatibility; Rh preferred	Fresh: within 4 hours after collection. FFP: 1 year at 30°C Use immediately after thawing (McClelland 2001)	15–45 minutes/ unit (approx. 200 ml)	Administer rapidly via a blood administration set	FFP should be considered if patient has received more than 6 units of blood to prevent dilutional hypocoagulability
Albumin 4.5% (plasma protein fraction)	Solution of selected proteins from pooled plasma in a buffered, stabilized 0.9% sodium chloride diluent. Usually 400-ml bottle	To treat hypovolaemic shock or hypoproteinaemia due to burns, trauma, surgery or infection. Note: current medical opinion is altering regarding the use of plasma rich products and potential relationship and risks with vCJD and other infective agents	Unnecessary	5 years at 2°C, 3 years at 25°C; do not expose to light	30–60 minutes/unit	Administer via a standard solution administration set	Heated at 60°C for 10 hours to inactivate hepatitis virus. The solution should be crystal clear with no deposits
Salt-poor human albumin 20%	Heat-treated, aqueous, chemically processed fraction of pooled plasma	To treat hypovolaemic shock or hypoproteinaemia due to burns, trauma, surgery or infection. To maintain appropriate electrolyte balance. Note: current medical opinion is altering regarding the use of plasma rich products and potential	Unnecessary	5 years at 2°C, 3 years at 25°C; store in the dark	30–60 minutes/unit	Administer via a blood administration set undiluted or diluted with 0.9% sodium chloride or 5% glucose solution. Slower administration is advised if a cardiac disorder is present to avoid gross fluid shift	Heated at 60°C for 10 hours to inactivate hepatitis virus. The solution should be crystal clear with no deposits

(continued)

Table 42.1 Blood and blood products used for transfusion (*continued*)

Type	Description	Indications	Cross-matching	Shelf life	Average infusion time	Technique	Special considerations
		relationship and risks with vCJD and other infective agents					
Factor VIII (cryoprecipitates, dried anti-haemophilic globulin concentrates)	Cold-insoluble portion of plasma recovered from FFP – amount of factor VIII varies. Potency in freeze-dried concentrates can be assayed more reliably	To control bleeding disorders due to lack of factor VIII or fibrinogen, e.g. haemophilia, von Willebrand's disease	ABO compatibility between donor plasma and recipient's red blood cells	Cryoprecipitates at −30°C for 1 year. Use immediately after thawing. Freeze-dried concentrates at +4°C. Reconstitute at room temperature and use immediately	15–30 minutes via infusion, 10–15 minutes via intravenous push	Administer rapidly via syringe or blood administration set.	Heat treated at 80°C for 72 hours to eliminate risk of hepatitis or HIV contamination, as multiple donors and imported for preparation; limited availability
Dried factor IX concentrate	Preparation contains factor IX, prothrombin and factor X. Some may contain factor VII	To correct bleeding disorders due to lack of these factors, e.g. Christmas disease	Unnecessary	Refer to specific expiry dates	15–30 minutes	Administer via a blood administration set. Dose varies	As above. Limited availability

*Most commonly used blood products.
†See Leucocyte depletion.
DIC: Disseminated intravascular coagulation.

- Transfusion is required by patients with cold agglutination disease.
- Exchange transfusion is indicated in the newborn (Weinstein 2000).
- Transfusion of cryopreserved stem cells (blood or marrow).

Both water baths and dry heat blood warmers are available. However, whichever device is chosen the temperature should be maintained below 38°C. Warming in excess of this can cause haemolysis of red cells and can denature proteins while increasing risks of bacterial infection (see manufacturer's guidelines).

Blood products must NOT be warmed by improvization such as putting the pack into hot water, in a microwave or on a radiator, as uncontrolled heating can damage the contents of the pack (McClelland 2001). Whenever there is water, there is a risk of bacterial contamination of blood products, particularly with *Pseudomonas*. For the patient this could result in a fatal systemic infection. Therefore certain safety measures must be adhered to:

- Water baths must be drained after each use and must be stored dry and empty.
- The blood warmer should be drained after each use and must be stored dry and empty.
- When needed they should be refilled with sterile water.
- A protective sterile over-bag to thaw blood and blood products reduces the entry of contaminants through microscopic punctures or breaks in the seal.
- The blood product should be used immediately after it has been thawed.

All devices should be serviced at per hospital health and safety policies, Medicines and Health Care Products Regulatory Agency (MHRA) and manufacturers' guidelines.

Transfusion reactions

Knowledge in the field of immunohaematology continues to grow with improvements in collection and storage methods, which aim to increase the safety of transfusion therapy. Yet risks still exist with the infusion of any blood product; therefore the importance of complying with National Transfusion Policies is critical for the safe administration of all blood products (Cook 1997a,b). Transfusion reactions are either immunological or non-immunological and can be either immediate or delayed.

- *Immunological*: this is the body's response to foreign proteins, or an antigen/antibody reaction from red blood cells, platelets or plasma proteins.

- *Non-immunological*: these are reactions caused by external factors where an antigen/antibody reaction is not present.

Immediate reactions

These reactions can happen in minutes or hours after transfusion therapy.

Acute haemolytic reactions

These are directly related to incompatibilities in the ABO blood group system. Antigen/antibody reactions occur when the recipient's antibodies react with donor erythrocytes. This reaction causes a cascade of events within the recipient. The complement system is activated, causing intravascular haemolysis and the kinin system produces bradykinin, which increases capillary permeability, dilates arterioles and subsequently causes a drop in systemic blood pressure. The coagulation system is also activated and stimulates the intrinsic clotting cascade, causing small clots and triggering disseminated intravascular coagulation (DIC). DIC can lead to formation of thrombi within the microvasculature and can be fatal (Hillyer 2001).

Signs and symptoms
Chills, facial flushing, pain/oozing at cannula site, burning along the vein, chest pain, lumbar or flank pain, or shock (Hillyer 2001). Patients often express a feeling of doom, which may be associated with cytokine activity. Haemolytic shock can occur after only a few millilitres of blood has been infused.

Action
Stop infusion immediately, maintain patency of venous access device and contact medical personnel immediately. Check patient identity against donor unit. Treatment is often vigorous to reverse hypotension, and aid adequate renal perfusion and renal flow to reduce potential damage to renal tubules, and appropriate therapy for DIC reactions (Provan *et al.* 1998). Heparin therapy is controversial in the event of DIC, because of the underlying causative factors and existing bleeding problems. It is important to remember that most acute haemolytic reactions are preventable, as they are usually caused by clerical error or checking errors at the bedside (McClelland 2001).

Anaphylactic reactions

These are rare and usually occur after only a few millilitres of blood or plasma has been infused.

Signs and symptoms
Bronchial spasm, respiratory distress, abdominal cramps, shock and potential loss of consciousness.

Action
Stop infusion and begin immediate resuscitation of the patient (Shamash 2002).

Acute respiratory distress syndrome (ARDS)
Where recipients receive large amounts of red blood cells, the microaggregate debris, which forms during storage, can lead to pulmonary insufficiency, and this in turn can be fatal (Porter 1999).

Air embolism
Air embolism remains a risk with any intravenous therapy (Shamash 2002).

Circulatory overload
Circulatory overload can occur when blood or any of its components are infused rapidly or administered to a patient with an increased plasma volume, causing hypervolaemia. Patients at risk are those with renal or cardiac deficiencies, the young and elderly (Weinstein 2000).

Signs and symptoms
An alteration in vital signs, dyspnoea, constriction of the chest, coughing and a change in pallor (Hoffbrand *et al.* 2001).

Action
Stop infusion immediately and contact medical colleagues. This complication is preventable by ensuring accurate monitoring during infusion of blood or any of its components, especially in at-risk recipient groups, such as the critically ill, neonates and young children (McClelland 2001).

Febrile non-haemolytic reactions
These reactions are due to the recipient's antileucocyte antibody response to the transfusion of cellular components such as donor leucocytes. Specific patient groups are at risk of greater sensitization to leucocytes, for example, critically ill patients, those receiving anticancer therapies or patients requiring multiple transfusion therapy (Williamson *et al.* 1999).

Signs and symptoms
Facial flushing, palpitations, chest tightness, and increase in body temperature with associated chills and/or rigors, and a rapid pulse.

Action
Administer antipyretic agents such as paracetamol (Contreras & Mollison 1998). Notify medical colleagues and document reaction.

Hypothermia
Infusing large quantities of cold blood rapidly can cause hypothermia. Patients likely to suffer from this reaction are those who have suffered massive blood loss due to trauma, haemorrhage, clotting disorders or thrombocytopenia (Porter 1999).

Signs and symptoms
Alteration in vital signs, changes in pallor and observed chills.

Action
Use a blood warmer.

Sepsis
This is caused when bacteria enter the blood or blood product that is to be infused. Bacteria can enter at any point from the time of collection, during storage through to administration to the patient. Organisms implicated in transfusion-related sepsis include Gram-negative *Pseudomonas, Yersinia* and *Flavobacterium* (Provan *et al.* 1998).

Signs and symptoms
Fever, hypotension, tachycardia and septic shock.

Action
Notify medical colleagues immediately, correct hypotension, take blood cultures and commence intravenous antibiotics.

Transfusion-related acute lung injury (TRALI)
This is caused by antileucocyte antibodies reacting against donor leucocytes. This reaction can result in 'leucoagglutination'. Leucoagglutinins can in turn become trapped in the pulmonary microvasculature, causing severe respiratory distress without evidence of circulatory overload or cardiac failure (Contreras & Mollison 1998).

Signs and symptoms
Respiratory distress, chills and fever, cyanosis and hypotension.

Action
Discontinue transfusion and notify medical colleagues immediately; begin respiratory supportive treatment.

Urticaria
This is an uncommon reaction caused by the recipient reacting to protein in donor plasma (Davies & Williamson 1998).

Signs and symptoms
Localised erythema, hives and itching.

Action
Stop infusion and administer prescribed antihistamine therapy. The infusion can then be recommenced. However, if symptoms continue with either a body rash and/or fever, the infusion should be discontinued.

Delayed effects

Some of these reactions can occur days, months or even years after a transfusion.

Citrate toxicity

This is a problem associated with the infusion of large quantities of whole blood and/or FFP. Citrate binds with the calcium in the blood to interrupt the clotting cascade and this may lead to hypocalcaemia (Porter 1999).

Signs and symptoms
Tingling in extremities, muscle cramps, hypotension, possible convulsions and cardiac arrest.

Action
Slowing the infusion rate may relieve symptoms. Calcium therapy may be required. Check for abnormal blood chemistry and administer calcium chloride or calcium gluconate solutions as prescribed. Monitor the recipient closely for any alteration in vital signs.

Delayed haemolytic reactions

These reactions are caused when immune antibodies react to a foreign antigen. Reactions are classified as primary or secondary. A *primary* reaction is often mild, occurring days or weeks after initial transfusion, and may be indicated by no clinical alteration in haemoglobin following transfusion therapy (Cook 1997a). *Secondary* reactions occur with re-exposure to the same antigen, and on rare occasions may be associated with ABO incompatibilities (Cook 1997a).

Signs and symptoms
Fever, mild jaundice and unexplained decrease in haemoglobin value (McClelland 2001).

Action
Antiglobulin testing.

Hyperkalaemia

Hyperkalaemia is a rare complication associated with trauma and the subsequent infusion of large quantities of blood. Potassium is known to leak out of red cells during storage, thereby increasing circulatory levels in recipients receiving blood products (Cook 1997b). The process is exacerbated if products are kept too long at room temperature or gamma irradiated (Davies & Williamson 1998). From starting the infusion to completion, the infusion should take a maximum of 4 hours (McClelland 2001).

Signs and symptoms
Irritability, anxiety, abdominal cramps, diarrhoea and weakness in the extremities (Cook 1997b).

Action
Notify medical colleagues and administer corrective drugs as prescribed.

Iron overload

A unit of blood contains 250 mg iron, which the body is unable to excrete, and as a result patients receiving large volumes of blood are at risk of iron overload (Davies & Williamson 1998).

Signs and symptoms
Poor growth, pigment changes, hepatic cirrhosis, hypoparathyroidism, diabetes, arrhythmia, cardiac failure and death.

Action
Administer desferrioxamine, which induces iron excretion (BMA & RPS, 2003).

Transfusion-associated graft-versus-host disease (TAGVHD)

Although this is a rare complication, it presents serious complications for recipients, and is often fatal. It is usually caused by the infusion of immunocompetent T lymphocytes in blood and blood products to severely immunocompromised recipients. The donor T lymphocytes engraft and multiply, react against the foreign tissue of the host/recipient and cause TAGVHD (Davies & Williamson 1998).

It is not commonly associated with FFP or cryoprecipitate. Onset can be from 4 to 30 days after transfusion.

Signs and symptoms
High fever followed by nausea and vomiting, generalized erythroderma, and profuse diarrhoea. Morbidity and mortality is 75–90% of affected patients, with infection and bone marrow suppression the main causes of death (McClelland 2001).

Preventive measures
Irradiation (25 gray) of blood and blood products, to inactivate T lymphocytes (McClelland 2001). This is especially important in the following recipients:

- Foetuses receiving intrauterine transfusions
- Patients undergoing or who have undergone blood or bone marrow progenitor cell transplantation
- Immunocompromised recipients.

Infectious complications of blood, blood products and blood substitutes

Bacterial infections

Contamination of blood, blood products and blood substitutes can occur during donation, collection, processing, storage and administration. Despite strict guidelines and procedures, the risk of contamination remains. Most common contaminating organisms are skin contaminants such as staphylococci, diphtheroids and micrococci, which enter the blood at the time of venesection (Barbara & Contreras 1998; Provan *et al.* 1998).

Signs and symptoms
Signs and symptoms are usually quick to develop and include chills and rigors, fever, nausea, vomiting, pain and hypotension, and can be fatal (Shamash 2002).

Note: bacterial contamination can present an identical clinical picture to acute haemolytic transfusion reactions.

Action
Stop the transfusion, treat symptoms, take blood cultures and administer prescribed antibiotics.

Viral infections

Viruses transmissible via blood transfusions can be either plasma borne or cell associated (Barbara & Contreras 1998; Williamson *et al.* 1998). Plasma-borne viruses include hepatitis B, hepatitis C, hepatitis A (rarely), serum parvovirus B19, and human immunodeficiency viruses (HIV-1 and HIV-2). Cell-associated viruses include cytomegalovirus (CMV), Epstein–Barr virus, human T-cell leukaemia/lymphoma viruses (HTLV-1/HTLV-2) and HIV-1/HIV-2.

Human T-leukaemia/lymphoma virus type 1 (HTLV-1)
HTLV-1 is an oncogenic retrovirus, associated with the white cells that cause adult T-cell leukaemia, and is connected with several neuromuscular wasting syndromes. The enzyme-linked immunosorbent assay (ELISA) has been recommended because of concerns relating to the transmission of the virus via blood transfusion, and the associated long incubation period of adult T-cell leukaemia. In the UK there is mandatory testing for HTLV (*Guidelines for the Blood Transfusion Service in the UK*; Joint Executive Committee 2001).

Cytomegalovirus (CMV)
CMV is classified as part of the herpes family and hence has the ability to establish latent infection with reactivation during periods of immunosuppression (Barnes 1992; Barbara & Contreras 1998). Approximately 50% of the population in the UK has antibodies to CMV. Therefore it is recognized that the virus may be transmitted by transfusion, although it poses little threat to immunologically intact recipients. However, CMV infection in vulnerable patient groups can cause significant morbidity and mortality, e.g. CMV pneumonitis carries an 85% mortality rate in blood and bone marrow transplant recipients (Mollison *et al.* 1997). Screening of donors and the use of CMV-seronegative or leucocyte-depleted blood and blood products are seen as essential for neonates and immunocompromised recipients who have tested negative to CMV (Prentice *et al.* 1998).

Hepatitis B (HBV)
Screening for hepatitis B surface antigen in donor blood (HBsAg) is mandatory as approximately 1 in 23 000 donations in the UK is detected as having HBsAg (Hewitt & Wagstaff 1998).

Hepatitis C (HCV)
Screening for hepatitis C using the ELISA is mandatory in the UK. Hepatitis C is transmitted primarily via contact with blood or blood products (Friedman 2001).

Human immunodeficiency virus (HIV-1 and HIV-2)
HIV is a retrovirus that infects and kills helper T cells also known as CD4-positive lymphocytes. Transmission of the virus can be via most blood products including red cells, platelets, fresh frozen plasma, and factor VIII and IX concentrates. These viruses are not known to be transmitted in albumin, immunoglobulins or antithrombin III products (Barbara & Contreras 1998). The retrovirus invades cells and slowly destroys the immune system, rendering the individual susceptible to opportunistic infections. Since 1983, when it was recognized that the virus could be transmitted via transfusion, actions were developed to safeguard blood supplies from transmitting the virus that caused AIDS. These include careful screening of donors and testing of donated blood.

Other infective agents

Parasites
Plasmodium falciparum is the most dangerous of the human malarial parasites (Barbara & Contreras 1998). Prevention is by questioning of donors about foreign travel, especially those who have visited areas in which the disease is endemic (Porter 1999).

Prion diseases
Known as transmissible spongiform encephalopathies (TSEs), these are a rare group of conditions which cause progressive neurodegeneration in humans and some animal species. Prion diseases are believed to be caused by the presence of an abnormal form of a cellular protein (Aguzzi & Collinge 1997; Barbara & Contreras 1998; Vamvakas 1999). These abnormal proteins have an altered cellular shape, and become infectious and multiply by converting normal cellular protein to the irregular form. This irregular form is resistant to digestion and breakdown and, once accumulation occurs, can result in the formation of plaque in brain tissue. Transmission is thought to be by direct contact with infected brain or lymphoreticular tissue (Aguzzi & Collinge 1997; Barbara & Contreras 1998; Vamvakas 1999).

1 Prion diseases in animal species:
   (a) Scrapie, a disease of sheep
   (b) Bovine spongiform encephalopathy (BSE)
   (c) Feline spongiform encephalopathy (FSE)
   (d) Chronic wasting disease of deer, mule and elk
2 Prion diseases in humans:
   (a) Sporadic – classic Creutzfeldt–Jakob disease (CJD)
   (b) Inherited – CJD, Gerstmann–Sträussler– Scheinker disease, fatal familial insomnia (FFI)
   (c) Acquired – kuru, variant (vCJD).

There is evidence to suggest that in TSEs, of which vCJD is one, leucocytes, particularly lymphocytes, are the key cells in the transportation of the putative infectious agent to the brain (Aguzzi & Collinge 1997; Bradley 1999). Leucodepletion of all blood and blood components is viewed as a sensible yet precautionary action to reduce any risk of blood-borne infection. All products in the UK are now leucodepleted at source. Currently, all plasma products are brought in from the USA, except FFP and cryoprecipitate which are leucodepleted at source in the UK.

Modified techniques in blood transfusion therapy

Conservation of blood and blood products is now an important issue in medical practice, as awareness increases of the associated risks involved with allogeneic blood transfusions (Chernow et al. 1996; Nelson 1998).

Autologous transfusions

Autologous transfusion is the collection, filtration and reinfusion of one's own blood, making the donor and recipient the same person. It is intended to avoid transmission of infection from the current method of allogeneic red blood cell transfusions (Brown 1998; Gillian & Thomas 1998; van Duijn et al. 1998; Nelson 1998). There are four methods of collecting:

- A pre-deposits programme, which collects blood prior to an operation (Provan et al. 1998)
- Haemodilution, where blood is collected and stored until the end of a surgical procedure, then reinfused into the patient
- Intraoperative salvage, which involves collecting blood from an operation site, washing and anticoagulating the blood, then returning it to the patient during or at the end of the surgical procedure. This method is commonly used in cardiovascular, hepatic, neurological, orthopaedic and thoracic surgery, including transplants (Provan et al. 1998; Weinstein 2000). Postoperative complications can occur from infusion of shed blood; therefore strict medical indications for reinfusion are necessary (Dinse & Deusch 1996; Oeltjen & Santrach 1997; Provan et al. 1998; Porter 1999)
- Postoperative salvage, whereby shed blood is collected from patients following cardiac, orthopaedic, plastic surgery or trauma, making this a safe, simple and cost-effective technique (Porter 1999).

Programmes such as these have been developed to conserve blood and prevent such reactions as iso-immunization and the transmission of infective agents. Administration procedures and monitoring of recipients remain the same as with allogeneic transfusions (Lee & Napier 1990; Dinse & Deusch 1996; Oeltjen & Santrach 1997; Gillian & Thomas 1998; Provan et al. 1998; Porter 1999; Weinstein 2000).

Irradiation of blood and blood products

Irradiation of blood and blood products is used to prevent the transfusion of cells/viruses capable of replication. In immunocompromised recipients, especially transplant patients, lymphocytes may proliferate and have the potential to cause graft-versus-host disease or rejection of transplanted organs. Irradiated products may also be used routinely in patients who are undergoing bone marrow suppressive or ablative therapies (McClelland 2001).

Infusion of cryopreserved bone marrow and peripheral blood stem cells

Stem cells from either the bone marrow or peripheral blood are cryopreserved between collection (harvesting) and reinfusion. Stem cells can be either an autologous or an allogeneic transfusion. Thawing of the cells is carried out using a large-volume water bath. Care should be taken as heating may cause cellular damage, and there is an increased risk of bacterial contamination. Aseptic techniques should be adopted during administration to reduce any possibility of contamination in a recipient group that is already immunocompromised (McClelland 2001).

Red cell substitutes

Minimizing the use of allogeneic blood would both benefit recipients and aid transfusion services where demand often outweighs supplies (Garwood & Knowles 1998). Currently, clinical trials are in progress using haemoglobin and perfluorochemical-based materials. However, their circulatory survival times are short and therefore they remain a poor substitute for the treatment of chronic anaemia. It is anticipated that red blood cell substitutes for use in transfusion medicine and other related biomedicine will emerge once they are immunologically inert, isotonic and safe (Lowe 1998; Urbaniak & Robinson 1998; Porter 1999).

Problem solving

Nurses involved in the transfusion of blood and/or blood products need to develop knowledge and skills to ensure safe administration and effective nursing care of those receiving transfusion therapy. The transfusion of any blood product carries with it the potential of reaction and risk (Cook 1997a; Porter 1999).

Safety checks prior to commencing any blood therapy

In 1996, the Serious Hazards of Transfusion (SHOT) initiative was launched to monitor the incidence of non-infectious hazards of transfusion occurring in UK hospitals (Higgins 2000). SHOT has revealed that every year 100–150 patients receive the wrong blood because of human error at some stage of the transfusion process, including:

1 Withdrawal of the wrong blood unit from the refrigerator (Higgins 2000)
2 Wrong labelling of patient samples for pretransfusion testing

3 Errors in the laboratory
4 Failure of some aspect of the bedside checking process, such as failure to properly identify patient.

1 Check that the product has been stored correctly as per national transfusion guidelines (McClelland 2001).
2 Check patient's name, date of birth, hospital reference number, expiry of product, irradiation and CMV status (specific to immunocompromised recipient groups) with cross-match form and the prescription chart.
3 Check patient consent or, in the case of patients less than 16 years, parental consent. Potential risks should be highlighted to the patient that disease transmission cannot be ruled out despite transfusion policies and practices.

4 Ensure product is administered via the correct administration set (see Table 42.1).
5 Record baseline observations prior to administration. Check pulse and temperature 15 minutes after starting each unit of blood, observe the patient throughout the transfusion, and repeat blood pressure, pulse and temperature on completion of transfusion (McClelland 2001).
6 Blood transfusions should be completed within 4 hours. Administration sets should be changed after every second unit of blood.

Problem	Cause	Prevention	Action
Infusion slows or stops.	Venous spasm due to cold infusion.		Apply warm compress to dilate the vein and increase the blood flow.
	Occlusion.	Ensure flow is maintained.	Flush gently with 0.9% sodium chloride and resume infusion. Consider resiting.
Elevated temperature after the commencement of a unit of blood, with temperature falling if the blood is slowed.	Pyrogenic reaction.	Observation of the patient's temperature, pulse and blood pressure during the transfusion dependent on patient's condition and especially at the start of each unit. If patient has had multiple transfusions or experienced this type of reaction previously, ensure that 'cover' of hydrocortisone and chlorpheniramine is prescribed and administered before commencement of therapy.	Slow blood transfusion rate. Inform medical staff.
A high temperature associated with fever and rigor during a transfusion.	White cell antibody reaction.	Observation as above.	Stop transfusion. Maintain patency of device by flushing with 0.9% sodium chloride. Inform medical staff.
Slightly elevated temperature with associated rash, may be severe with oedema round the eyes and	Allergic reaction to protein in the plasma.	Observation as above. Ensure patient is aware of symptoms to report, e.g. appearance of a rash or breathlessness. Close	If mild, slow the rate of transfusion. Inform medical staff. If severe, stop transfusion. Change administration set and commence infusion of 0.9% sodium chloride to keep vein open, or

Problem solving (cont'd)

Problem	Cause	Prevention	Action
larynx and shortness of breath.		observation of patient for swollen eyes and signs of breathlessness.	flush device and discontinue any infusion. Lie patient flat, treat as for shock. Inform medical staff.
Patient complains of feeling hot, with chest and abdominal pain. Fall in blood pressure; patient's temperature subnormal at first and later rising to a pyrexia.	Infection introduced either from bacteria in the blood or during insertion of vascular access device or administration set change.	Adhere to strict aseptic technique when handling the blood bags and intravenous device. Use blood within 30 minutes of removal from refrigerator. Regular observations, as above.	Stop transfusion. Change administration set and commence infusion of 0.9% sodium chloride slowly to keep vein open. Inform medical staff and institute prescribed treatment, e.g. steroids, antibiotics.
		Adhere to recommended delivery time for each unit of blood; discard if hanging more than 4 hours (McClelland 2001).	Return remaining blood for examination by the bacteriology department.
Patient complaining of feeling a hot flush along the vein, facial flushing and lumbar pain. The patient may become shocked with a fall in the blood pressure and the urine output may fall.	Blood not cross-matched. Urgent cross-match completed and blood not fully compatible.	Ensure blood cross-matching forms are completed correctly. If taking blood sample, check carefully that the name, date of birth and number on the form match the patient. Ensure that a unit is checked against the cross-match form for blood group, patient's name, patient's number, ward, Rh factor, unit number of blood, when blood taken, and expiry date. Begin transfusion slowly and observe the patient carefully at the start of each unit.	Stop transfusion. Change administration set and commence infusion of 0.9% sodium chloride to keep vein open. Lay patient flat and treat as for shock. Inform medical staff.

References and further reading

Aguzzi, A. & Collinge, J. (1997) Post exposure prophylaxis after accidental prion inoculation. *Lancet*, **350**, 1519.

Barbara, J.A.J. & Contreras, M. (1998) Infectious complications of blood transfusion: bacteria and parasites. In: *ABC of Transfusion*, 3rd edn (ed. M. Contreras). British Medical Journal Publishing, London.

Barnes, R. (1992) Infections following bone marrow transplantation. In: *Bone Marrow Transplantation in Practice* (eds J. Treleavan & J. Barrett). Churchill Livingstone, Edinburgh, pp. 281–8.

Bradley, R. (1999) BSE transmission studies with particular reference to blood. *Dev Biol Standard*, **99**, 35–40.

BMA & RPS (2003) *British National Formulary*. British Medical Association and The Royal Pharmaceutical Society of Great Britain, London.

Brown, P. (1998) Transmission of spongiform encephalopathy through biological products. *Dev Biol Standard*, **93**, 73–8.

Chernow, B., Jackson, E., Miller, J.A. & Wiese, J. (1996) Blood conservation in acute care and critical care. *Am Assoc Crit Care Nurses*, **7**(2), 191–7.

Contreras, M. & Mollison, P.L. (1998) Immunological complications of transfusion. In: *ABC of Transfusion*, 3rd edn (ed. M. Contreras). British Medical Journal Publishing, London.

Cook, L.S. (1997a) Blood transfusion reactions involving an immune response. *J Intraven Nurs*, **20**(1), 5–14.

Cook, L.S. (1997b) Non-immune transfusion reactions: when type and crossmatch aren't enough. *J Intraven Nurs*, **20**(1), 15–22.

Dacie, J.V. & Lewis, S.M. (1994) Red cell-group antigens and antibodies. In: *Practical Haematology*. Churchill Livingstone, Edinburgh, p. 445.

Davies, S. & Brozovic, M. (1990) Transfusion of red cells. In: *ABC of Transfusions* (ed. M. Contreras). British Medical Journal Publications, London, pp. 9–24.

Davies, S.C. & Williamson, L.M. (1998) Transfusion of red cells. In: *ABC of Transfusion*, 3rd edn (ed. M. Contreras). British Medical Journal Publishing, London.

Dinse, H. & Deusch, H. (1996) Sepsis following autologous blood transfusion. *Anaesthetist*, **45**(5), 460–3.

Friedman, D. (2001) Hepatitis. In: *Handbook of Transfusion Medicine*. Academic Press, New York, p. 275.

Garwood, P.A. & Knowles, S.E. (1998) Supply and demand of blood and blood components. In: *ABC of Transfusion*, 3rd edn (ed. M. Contreras). British Medical Journal Publishing Group, London.

Gillian, J. & Thomas, D.W. (1998) Autologous transfusion. In: *ABC of Transfusion*, 3rd edn (ed. M. Contreras). British Medical Journal Publishing, London.

Hewitt, P.E. & Wagstaff, W. (1998) The blood donor and tests on donor blood. In: *ABC of Transfusion*, 3rd edn (ed. M. Contreras). British Medical Journal Publishing, London.

Higgins, C. (2000) The risks associated with blood and blood product transfusion. *Br J Nurs*, **9**(22), 2281–9.

Hillyer, D. (2001) Granulocytes. In: *Handbook of Transfusion Medicine*. Academic Press, New York, p. 63.

Hoffbrand, A.V. & Pettit, J.E. (1994) *Essential Haematology*, 3rd edn. Blackwell Science, Oxford.

Hoffbrand, A.V., Pettit, J.E. & Moss, P.A.H. (2001) *Essential Haematology*. Blackwell Science, Oxford.

Joint Executive Committee, National Blood Service (2001) *Guidelines for the Blood Transfusion Services in the United Kingdom*, 5th edn. Stationery Office, London.

Kickler, T.S. & Ness, P.M. (1993) Blood component therapy. In: *Hematological and Oncological Emergencies* (ed. W.R. Bell). Churchill Livingstone, Edinburgh, pp. 125–40.

Lee, D. & Napier, J.A.F. (1990) Autologous transfusion. In: *ABC of Transfusions* (ed. M. Contreras). British Medical Journal Publications, London, pp. 18–21.

Lowe, K.C. (1998) Red cell substitutes. In: *ABC of Transfusion*, 3rd edn (ed. M. Contreras). British Medical Journal Publishing, London.

McClelland, B.D.L. (2001) *Handbook of Transfusion Medicine*. Stationery Office, London.

Mollison, P.L., Engelfriet, C.P. & Contreras, M. (1997) *Blood Transfusion in Clinical Medicine*. Blackwell Science, London.

Nelson, C.L. (1998) Use of allogeneic transfusions (editorial). *Clin Orthopaed*, December (357), 2–3.

Oeltjen, A.M. & Santrach, P.J. (1997) Autologous transfusion techniques. *J Intraven Nurs*, **20**(6), 305–10.

Porter, H. (1999) Blood transfusion therapy. In: *Intravenous Therapy in Nursing Practice* (eds L. Dougherty & J. Lamb). Churchill Livingstone, Edinburgh.

Prentice, G., Grundy, J.E. & Kho, P. (1998) Cytomegalovirus. In: *The Clinical Practice of Stem Cell Transplantation* (eds J. Barrett & J. Treleaven). Isis Medical Media, Oxford.

Provan, D., Chisholm, M., Duncombe, A., Singer, C. & Smith, A. (1998) *Oxford Handbook of Clinical Haematology*. Oxford University Press, Oxford.

Shamash, J. (2002) Blood counts. *Nurs Times*, **98**(45), 23–6.

Urbaniak, S.J. & Robinson, E.A. (1998) Therapeutic apheresis. In: *ABC of Transfusion*, 3rd edn (ed. M. Contreras). British Medical Journal Publishing Group, London.

Vamvakas, E.C. (1999) Risk of transmission of Creutzfeldt–Jakob disease by transfusion of blood, plasma, and plasma derivatives. *J Clin Apheresis*, **14**(3), 135–43.

van Duijn, C.M., Delasnerie-Laupretre, N., Masullo, C. *et al.* (1998) Case–control study of the risk factors of Creutzfeldt–Jakob disease in Europe during 1993–95. EU Collaborative Study Group of Creutzfeldt–Jakob disease. *Lancet*, **351**(9109), 1081–5.

Weinstein, S. (2000) *Plumer's Principles and Practices of Intravenous Therapy*, 7th edn. Lippincott, Philadelphia.

Williamson, L.M., Lowe, S., Love, E. *et al.* (1998) *Serious Hazards of Transfusion (SHOT). Summary of Annual Report* 1996–97. SHOT Office, Manchester.

The unconscious patient

Chapter contents

Definition

Consciousness is a state of awareness of self, environment and one's response to that environment. To be fully conscious means that the individual appropriately responds to the external stimuli. An altered level of consciousness represents a decrease in this full state of awareness and response to environmental stimuli (Boss 1998).

Unconsciousness is a physiological state in which the patient is unresponsive to sensory stimuli and lacks awareness of self and the environment (Hickey 2003a). There are many central nervous system conditions that can result in the patient being in an unconscious state. The depth and duration of unconsciousness span a broad spectrum of presentations from fainting, with a momentary loss of consciousness, to prolonged coma lasting several weeks, months or even years.

Unconscious patients can experience a myriad of altered consciousness experiences that can be grouped into five categories: unconsciousness, inner consciousness, perceived unconsciousness, distorted unconsciousness and paranoid experiences (Lawrence 1995).

If the patient is unconscious and in the terminal phase of the illness, then the focus will be on the general care of any person who is dying. Care of the dying encompasses more than pain and symptom management. One of the keys to success will be an attitude of partnership between the caring team, the patient and the family (Twycross 1997).

The nurse often cares for those who are unconscious for prolonged periods of time. In addition to managing the primary neurological problem, the nurse must also incorporate a rehabilitation framework to maintain intact function, prevent complications and disabilities, and restore lost function to the maximum that is possible. Total care of the patient involves communicating with families and friends on a regular basis to ensure they are supported and are able to participate in patient care if they wish to, and if this is appropriate.

Reference material

Certain neurological problems exist or have the potential to develop when the brain is affected by a pathological condition, irrespective of the cause of that condition. These common problems include development of a coma state, increased intracranial pressure, seizure and headache (Boss 1998). Being aware of what the unconscious patient may be experiencing will add to the ongoing holistic approach to the needs of the patient physically, psychologically and spiritually.

Assessment of level of consciousness

There are many methods of assessing and recording a patient's level of consciousness. The Glasgow Coma Scale (GCS) is a validated tool for the assessment of unconscious patients (Jennett & Teasdale 1974) and the most common internationally used assessment scale (Hickey 2003a). However, studies suggest that examination techniques and correct evaluation of patient responses for the GCS should be taught in detail to ensure accuracy of rating by nurses (Juarez & Lyons 1995; Heron *et al.* 2001). In a retrospective analysis, Price *et al.* (2000) found that it might not be appropriate to use the GCS as a neurological assessment tool in ventilated and sedated patients (see Ch. 26, Observations: neurological).

Ethical considerations

There are many ethical considerations when nursing the unconscious patient, e.g. consent, organ donation, advance directives and termination of life support. It is not within the scope of this manual to discuss these in detail. However, consenting adults who lack capacity, e.g. unconscious patients, can be given treatment under the doctrine of necessity under common law (Leung 2002).

Advance directives enable people to document their wishes regarding treatment in the event of their being unable to make decisions about their medical and nursing care. Nevertheless, in practice these may be difficult to interpret and of little value in the acute setting (Travis *et al.* 2001; Leung 2002).

Physiological changes in the unconscious patient

The physiological changes that occur in unconscious patients will depend on length of immobility, cause of unconsciousness, outcome and quality of care. It is not only being unconscious that will have a deleterious effect on the body but also drugs, e.g. some muscle relaxants such as those used in intensive care, can contribute to muscle weakness, raised intraocular and intracranial pressure, electrolyte imbalances and airway tone (Booij 1996). Unconsciousness can lead to changes and problems for the patient, which have implications for nursing interventions. The discussion below is not exhaustive but offers an insight into the effects of unconsciousness on the main systems of the body.

Immobility

The human body is designed for physical activity and movement. Therefore any lack of exercise, regardless of reason, can result in multisystem deconditioning and anatomical and physiological changes. Involvement of a physiotherapist for passive exercises early in the period of unconsciousness may help in the prevention of further complications.

- *Decreased muscle strength*: the degree of loss varies with the particular muscle groups and the degree of immobility. The antigravitational muscles of the legs lose strength twice as quickly as the arm muscles and recovery takes longer.
- *Muscle atrophy*: this alludes to loss of muscle mass. When the muscle is relaxed, it atrophies about twice as rapidly as in a stretched position. As increased muscle tone prevents complete atrophy, patients with upper motor neurone disease lose less muscle mass than those with lower motor neurone disease (Hickey 2003b).

Gastrointestinal function

Gastric complications can develop in the unconscious patient for a variety of reasons. Gastric ulcers, bleeding, constipation and faecal impaction can be identified as causing symptomatic problems in the unconscious patient. Nutrition is commonly provided by enteral tube feeding (see Ch. 24, Nutritional support) which does not generally stimulate peristalsis. Loose stool can be a result of poorly tolerated enteral feeding or antibiotics. In contrast to this, some pharmacological interventions can lead to constipation, It is imperative that a diagnosis is made to differentiate between true diarrhoea and faecal impaction as they can occasionally be misinterpreted as being one and the same thing (see Ch. 13, Elimination: bowel care).

Genitourinary function

An unconscious state can induce urinary incontinence or retention of urine. The unconscious patient is at risk of two problems: urinary tract infections and kidney or bladder stones. On admission an unconscious patient will usually have an indwelling catheter (see Ch. 16, Elimination: urinary catherization). This is necessary for accurate fluid monitoring and to prevent skin breakdown.

Respiratory function

Owing to the positioning of the unconscious patient, the abdominal muscles predominate in maintaining breathing. All lung volumes decrease except for tidal volume, which can cause partial or complete collapse of lung units, leading to atelectasis, as well as poorly ventilated and overperfused areas which can lead to hypoxia. In addition, atelectasis and hypostatic pneumonia can occur as a result of accumulation of mucous secretions (Hickey 2003b).

In unconscious patients monitoring of rate, rhythm and pattern of breathing is important, particularly in patients with neurological problems as this can indicate level of brain dysfunction (Boss 1998).

Cardiovascular function

Immobility can cause changes in cardiovascular function, for example increased cardiac workload, decreased cardiac output and decreased blood pressure. In addition, the positioning of the unconscious patient causes central fluid shift, from the legs to the thorax and head, so the head of the unconscious patient with raised intracranial pressure may need to be elevated to 30° (Hickey 2003b).

The risk of deep vein thrombosis and pulmonary embolism is increased in the unconscious patient. This is due to several factors: blood pooling in the legs, hypercoagulability and prolonged pressure from immobility in bed (Hickey 2003b).

Impaired tissue integrity

Skin

Direct pressure to the skin and friction during movement of patients are two of the most common causes of injury to the skin that can result in pressure ulcers. Correct moving and handling of the patient will minimize the risk of pressure ulcer formation (see Ch. 23, Moving and handling). Other contributing factors include incontinence, profuse perspiration, poor nutrition and obesity (Hickey 2003b). Use of special beds may be required depending on individual assessment. Skin integrity should be assessed using the Waterlow Scale (see Ch. 47, Wound management).

Eyes

The blink reflex is absent in the unconscious patient and tear production may be reduced (Carpenito 2002). Assessment of the eyes for signs of oedema, irritation, corneal drying or abrasions is essential. Application of an eye patch may protect the eye from injury (Hickey 2003b) (see Ch. 31, Personal hygiene: eye care).

Mouth

The lips, oral mucosa and tongue must be assessed for signs of dryness, irritation and infection (see Ch. 32, Personal hygiene: mouth care).

Self-care

The unconscious patient will require nursing care for all self-care needs. The nurse's role is to ensure that the patient is clean and comfortable.

Fluid/electrolyte imbalance

Serum electrolytes will require regular monitoring in the acute period of unconsciousness. Monitoring of fluid balance is important and correct fluid balance will assist in the prevention of deep vein thrombosis, pulmonary embolism, pressure ulcers and constipation.

Procedure guidelines: **Care of the unconscious patient**

Equipment

1 Airway of correct size.
2 Suction.
3 Oxygen mask.
4 Intravenous infusion equipment.
5 Personal hygiene equipment (measures for eye, oral and catheter care).
6 Cotsides (to be assessed on an individual basis, according to hospital policy).
7 Observation charts (neurological, fluid balance).
8 Feeding equipment.
9 Pen torch.

Procedure

Action	Rationale
1 Introduce yourself. Call the patient by their preferred name, as discussed with family/carer. Explain each procedure before starting.	Hearing often remains intact and recognition of a familiar word may assist in orientation of the unconscious patient.

Procedure guidelines: **Care of the unconscious patient** *(cont'd)*

Action	Rationale
2 Orientate the patient to day, date, time and place.	To promote orientation.
3 Remove all dental prostheses and note caps and crowns. Insert airway as appropriate. Monitor rate, rhythm and pattern of breathing.	To obtain and maintain clear airway. To assess condition of oral cavity. To assess breathing pattern and note changes.
4 Monitor vital signs. Monitor electrolytes and full blood count as appropriate. Administer intravenous fluids as prescribed. Monitor fluid balance.	To note changes in condition and act according to changes. To monitor changes in electrolytes and act accordingly. To maintain fluid balance.
5 Position in lateral or semi-prone position (unless intubated).	To prevent occlusion of airway by tongue falling back against pharyngeal wall.
(a) Head – ensure neutral position, supported by pillow, towel roll or soft collar.	Prevents hyperflexion, airway obstruction and impeding venous drainage from the brain.
(b) Elevate the head of the bed by 10–30°.	Facilitates drainage of secretions from the mouth. To encourage drainage of respiratory secretions and prevent pooling in throat.
(c) Trunk – ensure spine alignment, using pillows as support.	To promote comfort and maintain proper alignment of the body.
(d) Upper limb – bring the uppermost arm forward in front of the patient. Bend the elbow slightly, but keep the wrist extended, and support the arm on a pillow. Bring the lower arm alongside the face with the palm facing upwards.	
(e) Lower limbs – flex the uppermost leg and bring it forward. Support on pillows. Keep the lower leg extended straight and in line with the spine. Make sure the uppermost leg does not rest on the lower leg.	To prevent internal rotation of the hip. To avoid pressure ulcers on bony prominences.
(f) Consult with physiotherapist/anaesthetist about positioning/exercises to enhance pulmonary function.	To optimize respiratory function and prevent atelectasis and hypostatic pneumonia.
(g) Consult with physiotherapist regarding passive exercises for limbs. Monitor colour, temperature and pulses of limbs.	To prevent deep vein thrombosis formation and to recognize early signs of limb deformity.
(h) Apply antiembolic stockings as appropriate.	To prevent deep vein thrombosis formation.
6 Perform neurological assessment as frequently as patient condition dictates using GCS or appropriate tool (see Ch. 26, Observations: neurological).	To note changes in patient's condition and respond appropriately.
7 Assess skin integrity using Waterlow Scale or appropriate tool. Change position every 2 hours or sooner if condition indicates (see Ch. 23, Moving and handling and 47, Wound management).	To prevent and monitor for signs of pressure ulcers.
8 Carry out oral care as frequently as patient's condition indicates (see Ch. 32, Personal hygiene: mouth care).	To maintain a clean and healthy mouth and to promote comfort.
9 Carry out eye care as frequently as patient's condition indicates. Place eye patch if appropriate (see Ch. 31, Personal hygiene: eye care).	To prevent corneal scratches, dryness or ulceration, which can lead to blindness.
10 Assess bowel pattern as per hospital policy (colour, frequency, consistency and size).	To prevent diarrhoea, constipation, abdominal discomfort and bloating and to promote comfort.
11 Catheterize as per hospital policy (see Ch. 16, Elimination: urinary catherization).	To promote comfort and prevent stasis of urine, infection and renal calculi.
12 Position changes as indicated by condition of patient and type of pressure-relieving mattress available. Passive exercises as discussed with physiotherapist.	To prevent complications associated with bedrest, e.g. pressure sores, DVT. To prevent muscle wasting and contractures.

Conclusion

For the nurse, caring for the unconscious patient is a major challenge. The preservation of life and avoidance of further disabilities are priorities of care, but the psychological effects on the patient's family and carers also require sensitivity and open communication. Patients' psychological needs should be addressed and Leigh (2001) suggests that these can be met through communication about their environment and through touch. There is evidence that unconscious patients are aware of what is happening to them and can hear conversations during care episodes (Lawrence 1995; Jacobson 2000). It is important that nurses caring for unconscious patients are aware of this and communicate with the patient in a caring and sensitive manner.

References and further reading

Booij, L. (1996) Muscle relaxants and concurrent diseases. In: *Neuromuscular Transmission* (eds L. Booij, R. Jones, A. Aitkenhead & P. Foex). BMJ Books, London.

Boss, B.J. (1998) Nursing management of adults with common neurologic problems. In: *Adult Health Nursing* (eds B. Gauntlett & J. Myers). Mosby, St Louis.

Carpenito, L.J. (2002) *Nursing Diagnosis: Application to Clinical Practice*, 9th edn. Lippincott, Philadelphia.

Heron, R., Davie, A., Gilles, R. & Courtney, M. (2001) Interrater reliability of the Glasgow Coma Scale scoring among nurses in sub-specialities of critical care. *Aust J Crit Care*, **14**(3), 100–5.

Hickey, J.V. (2003a) Neurological assessment. In: *The Clinical Practice of Neurological and Neurosurgical Nursing*, 5th edn. Lippincott, Williams and Wilkins, Philadelphia, pp. 159–84.

Hickey, J.V. (2003b) Management of the unconscious neurological patient. In: *The Clinical Practice of Neurological and Neurosurgical Nursing*, 5th edn. Lippincott, Williams and Wilkins, Philadelphia, pp. 345–57.

Jacobson, A.F. (2000) Caring for unconscious patients. *Am J Nurs*, **100**(1), 69.

Jennett, B. & Teasdale, G. (1974) Assessment of coma and impaired consciousness. A practical scale. *Lancet*, **ii**, 81–3.

Juarez, V.J. & Lyons, M. (1995) Interrater reliability of the Glasgow Coma Scale. *J Neurosci Nurs*, **27**(5), 283–6.

Lawrence, M. (1995) The unconscious experience. *Am J Crit Care*, **4**(3), 227–32.

Leigh, K. (2001) Communicating with unconscious patients. *Nurs Times*, **97**(48), 35–6.

Leung, W.C. (2002) Consent to treatment in the A&E department. *Accident Emerg Nurs*, **10**, 17–25.

Price, T., Miller, L. & Descissa, M. (2000) The Glasgow Coma Scale in intensive care: a study. *Crit Care Nurs*, **5**(4), 170–3.

Travis, S., Mason, J., Mallett, J. & Laverty, D. (2001) Guidelines in respect of advance directives. *Int J Palliat Nurs*, **7**(10), 493–500.

Twycross, R. (1997) General principles. In: *Symptom Management in Advanced Cancer*. Radcliffe Medical Press, Oxford, pp. 1–11.

Vascular access devices: insertion and management

Chapter contents

Definition

A vascular access device (VAD) is a device that is inserted into either a vein or an artery, via the peripheral or central vessels, to provide for either diagnostic (blood sampling, central venous pressure (CVP) reading) or therapeutic (administration of medications, fluids and/or blood products) purposes. There is now a comprehensive range of VADs available which allow for patients' device, therapy and quality of life needs. Table 44.1 summarizes descriptions of the main types of VADs.

Reference material

Principles of care

Regardless of the type of VAD used, the principles of care for the device remain the same:

- To prevent infection
- To maintain a 'closed' intravenous system with few connections to reduce risk of contamination
- To maintain a patent device
- To prevent damage to the device and associated intravenous equipment.

Each of these principles will be discussed generally and then in more detail under each type of access device.

Prevention of infection

Aseptic technique and compliance with recommendations for equipment and dressing changes are essential if microbial contamination is to be prevented (Wilson 2001; Rickard 2001; Mermel *et al.* 2001; DoH 2001; Jackson 2001; Parker 2002; RCN 2003) (see Ch. 4, Aseptic technique). Whenever the insertion site is exposed or the intravenous system is broken, aseptic technique should be practised. Where blood or body fluids may be present, gloves should be worn to comply with safe practice (Rowley 2001).

Table 44.1 Vascular access devices

Type of device	Material	Features	Common insertion site (veins)	Recommended indwelling life and common uses
Peripheral cannulae	Teflon Vialon	Winged Non-winged Ported	Cephalic Basilic Dorsal venous network	48–96 hours for short-term access
Midline catheters	Silicone Polyurethane	Single lumen Dual lumen	Basilic Median cubital Cephalic	Used for 1–6 weeks or longer for short- to intermediate-term access
Peripherally inserted central catheters (PICC)	Polyurethane Silicone	Dual lumen Valved	Antecubital fossa	Used primarily for patients requiring several weeks or months of intravenous access
Short-term percutaneous central venous catheters (non-tunnelled)	Polyurethane Silicone	Multiple lumen Antimicrobial collagen cuff Heparin, antibiotic and antiseptic coatings	Jugular Subclavian Femoral	Intended for days to weeks of intravenous access
Skin-tunnelled catheters	Polyurethane Silicone	Valved Antimicrobial collagen cuff Multiple lumen	Cephalic Axillary Subclavian Femoral	Indefinite. Used for long-term intermittent, continuous or daily intravenous access. May be appropriate for short-term use if reliable access needed
Implantable ports	*Catheter* Silicone *Port* Titanium Stainless steel Plastic	Dual ports Peripheral ports Valved	Antecubital fossa Subclavian Femoral	Indefinite. Used for long-term intermittent, continuous or daily intravenous access

Cleaning solutions

Most transient flora can be removed from the skin with soap and water using mechanical friction (Carlson 2001). Chlorhexidine 2% (although difficult to obtain and most hospitals use 0.5%) in 70% alcohol has been shown to be the most effective agent for skin cleaning around the VAD insertion site prior to insertion and between dressing changes (Maki *et al.* 1991; Ryder 2001; DoH 2001; RCN 2003). 70% alcohol acts by denaturing protein and so has excellent properties for destruction of Gram-positive and -negative bacteria, as well as being active against fungi and viral organisms. Alcohol concentration between 70 and 92% provides the most rapid and greatest reduction in microbial counts on skin but does not have any residual activity (Larson 1988). This is where chlorhexidine has an advantage over alcohol used alone, as it has excellent residual activity for 4–6 hours after application (Carlson 2001; DoH 2001). Solutions should be applied with friction for up to 1 minute and allowed to air dry for 30–60 minutes

(INS 2000; Springhouse 2002). It has been found that 1 minute of application with alcohol is as effective as 12 minutes of scrubbing and reduces bacterial counts by 75%. A quick wipe fails to reduce bacterial counts prior to peripheral cannulation (Weinstein 2000; INS 2000). Allowing any cleaning solution to dry is vital in order for disinfection to be completed, and in the case of alcohol, which is a plasticizer, it ensures that plastic equipment will not 'glue together'.

Inspection of insertion site and cleaning of equipment

Cleaning solutions should be used not only on insertion sites, but also to clean junctions and connections, etc. It is recommended that injection caps should be cleaned vigorously with appropriate cleaning agents (Brown *et al.* 1997; DoH 2001). The frequency of cleaning the insertion site is debatable; peripheral sites are rarely cleaned once the device is sited because of their short duration in situ. However, central venous access sites, e.g. peripherally inserted central catheters (PICCs), may be cleaned weekly (at dressing change) and short-term central venous catheters (CVCs) may be cleaned daily or more frequently (being associated with the highest infection risk). The insertion site should be checked regularly for signs of phlebitis (erythema, pain and/or swelling) or for signs of infection (for further actions see Ch. 9, Drug administration). Complaints of soreness, unexpected pyrexia and damaged, wet or soiled dressing are reasons for immediate inspection and renewal of the dressing.

Securement of device and dressings

Securement of devices can be used to prevent movement, which reduces the risk of phlebitis, infiltration, infection and migration (Hanchett 1999; INS 2000; Taylor 2000; Gabriel 2001; Perucca 2001). This can be achieved by suturing, taping or use of securing devices. These would all require a dressing over them. Choice of dressing is usually based upon which is most suitable for a particular VAD site or type of skin. An intravenous dressing is applied to minimize the contamination of the insertion site and provide stability of the device. Therefore the ideal intravenous dressing should provide an effective barrier to bacteria; allow the catheter to be securely fixed; be sterile and easy to apply and remove; be waterproof and adhere well; and finally be comfortable for the patient (Perucca 2001). There are two main types of dressing – dry, sterile low-linting gauze and transparent dressings. A dry, sterile, low-linting dressing secured with the minimum of hypoallergenic tape is most suitable for patients with skin that is prone to allergy or is thin and tears easily, as transparent dressings can damage the skin if not removed correctly.

The benefits of transparent dressings (Springhouse 2002) are that they allow inspection of the insertion site while the dressing is in situ and therefore do not require removal; they are waterproof and many are also moisture permeable. This means that the dressing allows moisture vapour transmission, an important factor related to infection as collection of moisture enhances the proliferation of micro-organisms.

When transparent dressings have been compared with sterile gauze it has been shown that there is no significant difference and that infection rates may have been reduced (Maki & Ringer 1987; DoH 2001; RCN 2003). All central venous catheter dressings must be removed and replaced within 24 hours following insertion of the catheter (Ryder 2001). This is due to the bacterial colonization, 'biofilm', which occurs 6–18 hours following insertion (Ryder 2002). If gauze is used it must be replaced when the dressing becomes damp, loosened, soiled or when inspection of the site is necessary (DoH 2001; RCN 2003). Transparent dressings should be changed every 7 days unless manufacturers recommend otherwise or when the integrity is compromised, i.e. when damp, loose or soiled (INS 2000; Hadaway 2000; Carlson 2001; DoH 2001; Perucca 2001; RCN 2003). When the dressing is changed the insertion site should be inspected for inflammation and/or discharge and the condition of the skin noted.

Maintaining a closed intravenous system

If equipment becomes accidentally disconnected, air embolism or profuse blood loss may occur, depending on the condition and position of the patient (Perucca 2001). Accidental disconnection poses a greater risk in patients with central venous access devices (CVADs) than in those with peripheral devices. This is because of the amount of air that could be introduced via a CVAD and the speed with which it could enter the pulmonary vessels. Luer locks provide a more secure connection and all equipment should have these fittings, i.e. administration sets, extension sets, injection caps. Needle-free systems provide a closed environment, which further reduces the risk of air entry (Perucca 2001). Care should be taken to clamp the catheter firmly when changing equipment. Connections must be double checked and precautions taken to prevent the introduction of air into the system when making additions to, or taking blood from, a central venous catheter.

Maintaining patency

It is important at all times for the patency of the device to be maintained. Blockage predisposes to device damage, infection, inconvenience to patients and disruption to drug delivery. Occlusion of the device is usually the result of:

- clot formation due to: (a) an administration set or electronic infusion device being turned off accidentally and left for a prolonged period or (b) insufficient or incorrect flushing of the device when not in use
- precipitate formation due to inadequate flushing between incompatible medications (Goodman 2000; Weinstein 2000; Perdue 2001).

Kinking or pinch-off syndrome may also impair patency of the device. Meticulous intravenous technique will prevent the majority of these problems.

Two main types of solutions are used to maintain patency in VADs; heparin is used to prevent the build-up of fibrin, and sodium chloride is used to clean the internal diameter of the device of blood and drugs (ONS 1996). All devices should be flushed with 10–20 ml 0.9% sodium chloride after blood withdrawal (Gabriel 1999; Goodman 2000; INS 2000; LSC 2002).

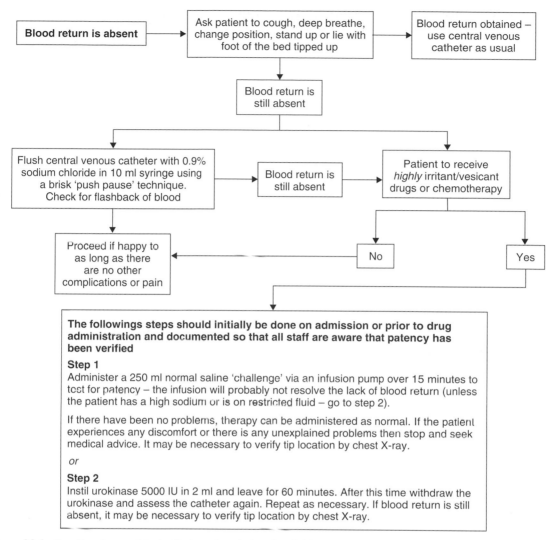

Figure 44.1 Algorithm for persistent withdrawal occlusion, i.e. fluids can be infused freely by gravity but blood cannot be withdrawn from the catheter. (Adapted from UCL Hospital Central Venous Catheter Policy.)

Maintaining patency can be achieved by (a) a continuous infusion to keep the vein open (KVO), either by the patient being attached to an infusion of 0.9% sodium chloride via a volumetric pump, which reduces comfort and mobility, or by use of an elastomeric device, which is less restrictive and has been able to reduce loss of patency by 50% (Heath & Jones 2001), or (b) intermittent flushing (previously known as a 'heparin lock'). The advantages of intermittent flushing compared with a continuous infusion are:

- It reduces the risk of circulatory overload.
- It reduces the risk of vascular irritation.

- It decreases the risk of bacterial contamination as it eliminates a continuous intravenous pathway.
- It increases patient comfort and mobility.
- It may reduce the cost of intravenous equipment.

One of the disadvantages is the necessity for constant vigilance and regular flushing (Weinstein 2000).

When used for intermittent therapy, the device should be flushed after each use with the appropriate flushing solution. (Guidelines for volumes, concentrations and frequency of flushing are commonly established within individual institutions.) It is now well established that flushing with 0.9% sodium chloride can also adequately maintain the patency of the cannula

(Goode *et al.* 1991). This avoids side-effects such as local tissue damage, drug incompatibilities and iatrogenic haemorrhage, which can occur with heparin (Goode *et al.* 1991). As well as being cost effective, it appears that daily or twice daily flushing with a volume of 2–5 ml 0.9% sodium chloride is acceptable (Goode *et al.* 1991).

There has been a lack of general consensus about best practice for maintaining patency in CVCs. This has been resolved within London by the introduction of London Standing Conference Standards on care of external central venous catheters in adults (LSC 2002). It supports the recommendation that heparinized saline is the accepted solution for maintaining the patency of central venous catheters for intermittent use (Randolph 1998; DoH 2001; LSC 2002; NICE 2003; RCN 2003). Use of 0.9% sodium chloride alone is not yet widespread (except with certain types of catheters such as the Groshong valve; INS 2000; LSC 2002) and remains controversial (Mayo 1996). Flushing regimens ranging from once daily to once weekly have been found to be effective. Implanted drug delivery systems such as implanted ports are flushed using a stronger solution of heparin, usually 500 IU heparin in 5 ml 0.9% sodium chloride (Perucca 2001). Recommendations range from monthly (Springhouse 2002) to every 3–4 months when not in use (Goodman 2000).

Using the correct techniques to flush the VAD has been highlighted as one of the key issues in maintaining patency (Baranowski 1993; Goodwin & Carlson 1993). There are two stages in flushing.

1 Using a pulsated (push pause) flush to create turbulent flow when administering the solution, regardless of type and volume. This removes debris from the internal catheter wall (Goodwin & Carlson 1993; Todd 1998; LSC 2002).
2 The procedure is completed using the positive pressure technique. This is accomplished by maintaining pressure on the plunger of the syringe while disconnecting the syringe from the injection cap, which prevents reflux of blood into the tip, reducing the risk of occlusion (INS 2000; Goodman 2000; LSC 2002).

Manufacturers have now produced needleless injection caps which enable a positive 'displacement' flush and achieve positive pressure without practitioners being required to actively achieve the positive pressure (Weinstein 2000). They have been shown to significantly reduce the incidence of catheter occlusions (Berger 2000; Lenhart 2000; Mayo 2001a; Rummel 2001).

Excessive force should never be used when flushing devices. However, when the catheter lumen is totally patent, internal pressure will not increase during flushing (Hadaway 1998a). If resistance is felt (due to partial occlusion), and a force is applied to the plunger, this could result in a high pressure within the catheter, which may then rupture (Conn 1993; Hadaway 1998a; Macklin 1999). It is, therefore, recommended that the device is checked first with a 10 ml or larger syringe containing 0.9% sodium chloride, and if there is no pressure or occlusion smaller syringes may be used to administer drugs where it is not possible to further dilute drugs and administer in a large syringe (Hadaway 1998a; Macklin 1999; LSC 2002). It is then safe to use a small-size syringe (Hadaway 1998a; Macklin 1999). The composition of the individual device determines the maximum pressure that can be exerted. If a catheter becomes occluded the nurse should establish the cause of the clot – occlusion or precipitation (INS 2000). If precipitation, then instillation of hydrochloric acid or ethyl chloride may be required (Holcombe 1992; LSC 2002). There are two types of thrombotic occlusion.

- Partial withdrawal occlusion (PWO) (see Fig. 44.1): this is usually caused by fibrin sheath formation and identified by the absent or sluggish blood return whilst fluids can be infused. Fibrin sheaths can result in seeding of bacteria and drug extravasation (Mayo 2000, 2001b) and can be resolved by the instillation of a thrombolytic agent such as urokinase or alteplase (Haire & Herbst 2000; Weinstein 2000; Rinn 2001).
- Total occlusion: when there is an inability to withdraw blood or infuse fluids or medications. This can be resolved by instillation of a thrombolytic agent (Ponec *et al.* 2001; Deitcher *et al.* 2002; Timoney *et al.* 2002) or by use of an endoluminal brush (Archis *et al.* 2000; Weinstein 2000).

If the occlusion is caused by a clot, gentle pressure and aspiration may be sufficient to dislodge the clot. Silicone catheters expand on pressure and allow fluid to flow around the clot, facilitating its dislodgement. This should only be attempted using a 10 ml or larger syringe. Smaller syringes should never be used as they create a greater pressure (ONS 1996; Perdue 2001; Springhouse 2002) of mmHg or pounds per square inch (psi). This can result in rupture of the catheter, resulting in loss of catheter integrity, or dislodge the clot (Perucca 2001), so manufacturers' instructions should be checked and adhered to (INS 2000). Instillation of thrombolytic agents should be performed using a three-way tap and negative pressure (Gabriel 1999; Simcock 2001a; LSC 2002).

Preventing damage of the VAD and performing a repair

If damage occurs to peripheral devices, they are usually removed and replaced. Most central venous catheters are made of silicone which is prone to cracking or splitting if handled incorrectly (Tingey 2000) but both temporary and permanent repairs can be performed. However, prevention of this occurrence is preferred.

Artery forceps, scissors or sharp-edged clamps should not be used on the catheter. A smooth clamp should be placed on the reinforced section of the catheter provided for clamping. If a reinforced section is not present, placing a tape tab over part of the catheter can create one. A second alternative is to move the clamp up or down the catheter at regular intervals to reduce the risk of wear and tear at one point.

Use of the correct syringe size in accordance with manufacturer's guidelines will reduce the risk of catheter rupture (INS 2000). However, syringe size alone will not be sufficient to prevent catheter rupture. If resistance is felt and more pressure is applied to overcome it, catheter fracture could result regardless of syringe size (Hadaway 1998a; Macklin 1999). The nurse must be familiar with the action to be taken to minimize any risk to patient safety in this event. Immediate clamping of the catheter proximal to the fracture or split is essential to prevent blood loss or air embolism. The split area should be covered with an alcohol swab and emergency repair equipment collected, together with sterile gloves to ensure that all manipulations are aseptic. A permanent repair should be performed as soon as possible using the specific equipment provided by the manufacturer. A member of the medical staff or other designated personnel should do this.

Peripheral cannulae

Definition

A cannula is a flexible tube containing a needle (stylet) which may be inserted into a blood vessel (Anderson & Anderson 1995). Cannulae are usually placed in the peripheral veins in the lower arm but may also be placed in the veins of the foot (an area used particularly in paediatric care) (Weinstein 2000). However, veins of the lower extremities should not be routinely used in adults due to the risk of embolism and thrombophlebitis (INS 2000).

Indications

- Short-term therapy of 3–5 days
- Bolus injections or short infusions in the outpatient/ day unit setting (Perucca 2001).

Reference material

The advantages of using a peripheral cannula are that they are usually easy to insert and have few associated

Table 44.2 Gauge sizes and average flow rates (using water)

Gauge (G)	Flow rate (ml/min)	General uses
14	350	Used in theatres or emergency for rapid transfusion of blood or viscous fluids
16	215	As 14 G
18	104	Blood transfusions, parenteral nutrition, stem cell harvesting and cell separation, large volumes of fluids
20	62	Blood transfusions, large volumes of fluids
22	35	Blood transfusions, most medications and fluids
24	24	Medications, short-term infusions, fragile veins, children

complications; however, they are associated with phlebitis (either mechanical or chemical) and require constant resiting (Dougherty 1999; Hadaway 2000; Taylor 2000; INS 2000; Perucca 2001).

Device information

A number of different types of peripheral cannula are available. It has been shown that the incidence of vascular complications increases as the ratio of cannula external diameter to vessel lumen increases. Therefore most of the literature recommends the smallest, shortest gauge cannula in any given situation (RCN 2003) (Table 44.2). The measurement used for needle and cannulae is standard wire gauge (swg), which measures the internal diameter; the smaller the gauge size, the larger the diameter. Standard wire gauge measurement is determined by how many cannulae fit into a tube with an inner diameter of 1 inch (25.4 mm) and uses consecutive numbers from 13 to 24. The diameter, e.g. 1.2 mm, may be expressed as a gauge, e.g. 18 G (BSI 1997; Nauth Misir 1998). Needles are odd numbers, e.g. 19 G, 21 G, while cannulae are even numbers, e.g. 18 G, 20 G, (Weinstein 2000).

The walls of the device should, therefore, be thin to provide the largest internal diameter without increasing the external diameter. This is to ensure that maximum flow rates may be achieved while reducing complications such as mechanical irritation. Flow rates vary with equipment from different manufacturers. Flow rate through a cannula is related to its internal diameter and is inversely proportional to its length. However, as the length of the cannula increases, so does the likelihood of vascular complications, for example a large-gauge device of longer length (1.6–2 cm) will fill the vessel, preventing blood flow around it, which could result in mechanical trauma to the vessel and encourage the development of phlebitis (Dougherty 1999; Taylor 2001).

The most suitable material is one that is non-irritant and does not predispose to thrombus formation (Payne-James *et al.* 1991). The material should also be radiopaque or contain a stripe of radiopaque material for radiographic visualization in the event of catheter embolus (Fuller & Winn 1999; Perucca 2001). Types of material include polyvinylchloride, Teflon, Vialon, and various polyurethane and elastomeric hydrogel materials. Studies have compared the different types of material available such as Teflon and Vialon, to ascertain which is most likely to be associated with the lowest potential risk of phlebitis (Keradag 2000). When considering the results of these studies, however, it must be noted that investigators often use different phlebitis scales and calculations for creating a total score for each device. Other inconsistencies relate to the differences in catheter size, skin preparation, the use of dressings and the type of solution being infused. This makes comparison between catheter materials difficult.

The 'over the needle' type of cannula is the most commonly used device for peripheral venous access and is available in various gauge sizes, lengths, composition and design features. The cannula is mounted on the needle (known as the stylet) and once the device is pushed off of the needle into the vein, the stylet is removed. A sharp-tipped stylet facilitates penetration into the vein and the type of graduation from the cannula to the needle can affect the degree of trauma to the vessel and the cannula tip (Perucca 2001). A thin smooth-walled cannula tapering to a scalloped end causes less damage than one that is abruptly cut off (Dougherty 1999).

Other features of peripheral cannulae include winged cannulae (which help with the securing of the device to the skin in order to prevent a piston-like movement within the vein and accidental removal) (Perucca 2001) and devices with small ports on the top of the device – which are favoured more in Europe than in the USA. The advantage of a ported device is the ability to administer drugs without interfering with continuous infusion. However, the caps are often not replaced correctly, which leaves the system exposed to contamination and the possible risk of air entering. It has also been found that the ports cannot be adequately sterilized with a swab, as there is no flat surface. The use of ports may encourage the practitioner not to remove the dressing and inspect the site but merely to administer the drug via the port (RCN 1999).

Choice of vein

The main factors to consider prior to inserting a peripheral cannula are the location for siting, condition of the vein, purpose of the infusion (that is the rate of flow required and the solution to be infused) and the duration of therapy.

The suitable vein should always be selected prior to selection of the device. The veins should feel bouncy and refill when depressed and should be straight and free of valves to ensure easy advancement of the cannula. Valves can be felt as small lumps in the vein or may be visualized at bifurcations or more commonly seen in certain vessels (see below). It is best to avoid siting a cannula over a joint as this will lead to an increased risk of mechanical phlebitis and an infusion that will infuse intermittently due to the patient's movement (Dougherty 1999; INS 2000; Perucca 2001; Weinstein 2000; RCN 2003). It can also be very awkward for the patient and may restrict his or her ability to carry out activities.

The veins of choice are either the cephalic or basilic veins, followed by the dorsal venous network (see Fig. 45.1 in Ch. 45, Venepuncture). The practitioner should start distally and cannulate at proximal points (INS 2000; Perucca 2001). However, the best vein should always be selected (Weinstein 2000).

The cephalic vein

The size and position of the cephalic vein make it an excellent vessel for administration of transfusions. It readily accommodates a large-gauge cannula and, by virtue of its position on the forearm, provides a natural splint (Weinstein 2000). However, its position at a joint may increase complications such as mechanical phlebitis and even general discomfort. The tendons controlling the thumb obscure the vein during insertion (Hadaway 2001), and care must be taken not to touch the radial nerve.

The basilic vein

The basilic vein is a large vessel, which is often overlooked due to its inconspicuous position on the ulnar border of the hand and forearm. It is found on palpation when the patient's arm is placed across the chest, with the practitioner opposite the patient (Hadaway 2001). Cannulation can be awkward because of its position, mobility and tendency to have many valves (Hadaway 2001; Springhouse 2002).

The dorsal venous network

Using the veins of the dorsal venous network of the hand will allow for cannulation proximally along the veins when resiting the device (Weinstein 2000). They can usually be visualized and palpated easily.

- The digital veins are small and may be prominent enough to accommodate a small-gauge needle as a last resort for fluid administration. With adequate taping the fingers can be immobilized; thus preventing the cannula from piercing the posterior wall of the vein, leading to bruising or infiltration; and making it more comfortable (Springhouse 2002).
- The metacarpal veins are accessible, and easily visualized and palpated. They are well suited for cannulation as the cannula lies flat and the metacarpal veins provide a natural splint (Weinstein 2000; Springhouse 2002). The veins tend to be smaller than the forearm and therefore may prove difficult in infants due to higher amounts of subcutaneous fat compared to older children and adults. The use of these veins is contraindicated in the elderly as there is diminished skin turgor and loss of subcutaneous tissue, making the vein difficult to stabilize. They are also more fragile and venous distension is slower (Powers 1999; Hadaway 2000; Walther 2001; Springhouse 2002). Metacarpal veins are a better option for short-term or outpatient intravenous therapy.

Insertion

As the most common cause of VAD infection is the patient's own skin flora, it is important to adequately clean the skin prior to cannulation. The patient's skin should be washed with soap and water if visibly dirty which will remove most transient flora (Carlson 2001; Perucca 2001). Then an antiseptic solution such as chlorhexidine solution or 70% alcohol should be applied in an area of 4–5 cm in diameter with friction for 30–60 seconds. A quick wipe fails to reduce bacterial count (Weinstein 2000). It should be allowed to air dry for up to 1 minute to ensure coagulation of the organism and to prevent stinging as the needle pierces the skin (INS 2000; Weinstein 2000; Springhouse 2002). Once the skin has been cleaned it must not be touched or repalpated. If it is necessary to repalpate, then the cleaning regimen should be repeated.

Shaving the skin prior to cannulation is not recommended (INS 2000; Weinstein 2000; Perucca 2001) as the need to remove hair has not been substantiated by scientific evidence (Weinstein 2000). Shaving with a razor should not be performed because of the potential for causing microabrasions, which increase the risk of infection (INS 2000; Carlson 2001). Depilatories should not be used because of the potential for allergic reaction or irritation (INS 2000; Perucca 2001). If hair removal is necessary then this can be accomplished by clipping with scissors or clippers (Carlson 2001; INS 2000). These should be cleaned

between patients or only used once to prevent cross-infection (INS 2000).

Skin stabilization is one of the most important elements for successful venepuncture or cannulation (Perucca 2001; Springhouse 2002). Superficial veins tend to roll and to prevent this the vein must be stabilized by applying traction to the side of the insertion site or below it, using the practitioner's non-dominant hand. This also facilitates a smoother needle entry. Various methods are used:

- The thumb can be used to stretch the skin downwards.
- The hand of the practitioner can be placed under the patient's arm and traction applied with the thumb and forefinger on either side, creating an even traction.
- The vein can be stretched between forefinger and thumb (Springhouse 2002).

Stabilization of the vein must be maintained throughout the procedure until the needle or cannula is successfully sited. If the tension is released half way through the procedure, it can result in the needle penetrating the opposite wall of the vein, resulting in a haematoma formation.

It is important that the needle enters the skin with the bevel up, as this results in a smooth venepuncture as the sharpest part of the needle will penetrate the skin first, and this also reduces the risk of piercing the posterior wall of the vein (Weinstein 2000). The angle the needle enters the skin varies with the type of device used and the depth of the vein in the subcutaneous tissue, and ranges from 10 to 45° (Weinstein 2000; Perucca 2001; Springhouse 2002). Once the device is in the vein, the angle will always be reduced in order to prevent puncturing the posterior wall of the vein (Perucca 2001).

There are two main methods for approaching the vein:

- The direct method is when the device enters through the skin and immediately enters the vein. However, with smaller veins this method may result in puncture of the posterior wall.
- The indirect method is when the device is inserted through the skin and then the vein is relocated and the device advanced into the vessel. This method enables a more gentle entry and may be useful in veins which are palpable and visible for only a short section (Hadaway 2000; Weinstein 2000; Perucca 2001).

When blood appears in the chamber of a cannula, known as 'flashback', this indicates that the initial entry into the vein has been successful. This may be accompanied by a 'giving way' sensation felt by the practitioner, which occurs due to resistance from the vein wall as the device enters the lumen of the vein. This usually occurs with thicker walled cannulae (Weinstein 2000; Springhouse 2002). If the device punctures the posterior wall, the flashback will stop. However, the flashback may be slow with small-gauge cannulae or hypotensive patients.

The cannula should be advanced gently and smoothly into the vein and a number of techniques are used by practitioners. One method which provides the least risk of through puncture but which is more difficult to learn initially is the one-handed technique (Hadaway 2000; Perucca 2001). If one hand is not used to apply traction then on cannula advancement there may be unnecessary damage to the endothelium, resulting in phlebitis (Hadaway 2001). The same hand that performs cannulation also withdraws the stylet and advances the cannula into the vein. This allows skin traction to be maintained while the device is advanced and if the patient is unable to co-operate allows the practitioner to hold onto the patient's arm (Dougherty 1999; Hadaway 2000).

The one-step technique is when the cannula has entered the vein and the practitioner can slide the cannula off the stylet in one movement. The disadvantage with this method is that the stylet must remain completely still in order to prevent damage to the vein. It is best accomplished on a straight vein and when the cannula has a small fingerguard which can be used to 'push' the cannula off. If the cannulation is unsuccessful the stylet should not be reintroduced as this could result in catheter fragmentation and embolism (Perucca 2001). A practitioner should not have more than two attempts before passing the patient onto a more experienced colleague (Dougherty 1999; INS 2000; Perucca 2001).

The two-handed technique is where the practitioner performs the cannulation with one hand but releases the skin traction in order to advance the cannula off the stylet. This method prevents blood spill, but as it necessitates the release of skin traction, it can often lead to the puncturing of the vein wall (Millam 1992).

Local anaesthesia

The use of local anaesthetic prior to insertion of peripheral cannulae has been advocated to reduce pain and anxiety in children and selected adults and is recommended if the cannula is larger than 18 G, dependent on site and at the patient's request (Dougherty 1999; Moureau & Zonderman 2000). Local anaesthetic may be applied in a cream/gel, given as an intradermal injection or administered by iontophoresis – a painless dry electrode pushing the local anaesthetic into the skin within 7–10 minutes to a depth of 10 mm (Moureau & Zonderman 2000; Perucca 2001; Springhouse 2002).

The most commonly used local anaesthetic creams are EMLA (eutectic mixture of local anaesthetics – lidocaine and prilocaine) and Ametop (topical amethocaine). These are applied to the skin 30–60 minutes prior to cannulation and covered with an occlusive dressing. A recent meta-analysis showed that EMLA cream significantly decreased the pain of intravenous cannulation in 85% of adults and children (Fetzer 2002). However, it causes vasoconstriction, making cannulation more difficult. Ametop has been shown to be more effective than EMLA and to cause significantly less vasoconstriction (Brown et al. 1999). However, it can result in an erythematous rash if left in situ longer than the recommended time (BMA & RPS 2003).

Intradermal lidocaine 1% can be slowly injected around the vein to be cannulated after skin sterilization to minimize the discomfort of the procedure. Intradermal injection of lidocaine has been shown to reduce the pain of intravenous cannulation and be less painful than placement of the cannula itself (Brown & Larson 1999). However, it should be used with caution because of the potential to cause an allergic reaction, tissue damage and inadvertent injection of the drug into the vascular system, and it can even obliterate the vein (INS 2000; Perucca 2001). It is not recommended for routine use (Perucca 2001).

Iontophoresis uses a painless electrical current to facilitate the movement of solute ions across the skin. It has been used to administer lidocaine prior to intravenous cannulation without the need for intradermal injection and has been shown to be as effective as EMLA (Galinkin et al. 2002).

Although local anaesthetic reduces the pain of intravenous cannulation, it is not without complications. Irrespective of the method of anaesthesia there is a risk that the symptoms of extravasation may be obscured or may even influence the risk of injury occurring (Stanley 2002). Other methods to help reduce pain and anxiety prior to and during cannulation include distraction and anxiolytics (Moureau & Zonderman 2000).

Care and management in situ

Once sited the peripheral cannula should be flushed using a pulsatile flush, ending with positive pressure (Kamimoto 1996; Weinstein 2000; RCN 2003). The cannula should be secured using clean tape. Non-sterile tape should not cover the insertion site and taping should enable the site to remain visible and the cannula stable. The procedure shown in Figure 44.2 is recommended (Dougherty 1999; Hadaway 2000; Perucca 2001; Springhouse 2002). A dressing should be applied – this can be either a transparent dressing or low-linting

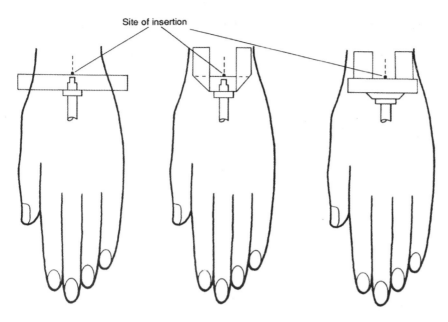

Site of insertion

Figure 44.2 Method of taping a peripheral cannula.

gauze (Madeo *et al.* 1997). Once the gauze is in place a bandage may be applied. However, transparent dressings, particularly moisture-permeable dressings, should not be bandaged as the visibility and moisture permeability are obscured.

Removal

It has been recommended that peripheral devices should be resited every 48–72 hours (INS 2000; Carlson 2001; Frey 2001) but devices may remain in for up to 96 hours with no significant complications providing that non-irritants are administered (Homer & Holmes 1998). Other studies have found that drug irritation is the most significant predictor of phlebitis and infiltration, rather than dwell time, and that extending the dwell time up to 144 hours could be considered under certain circumstances (Bregenzer *et al.* 1998; Catney 2001). Removal of the intravenous device or cannula should be an aseptic procedure. The device should be removed carefully using a slow, steady movement and pressure should be applied until haemostasis is achieved. This pressure should be firm and not involve any rubbing movement. A haematoma will occur if the needle is carelessly removed, causing discomfort and a focus for infection (Perdue 2001). The site should be inspected to ensure bleeding has stopped and the site should then be covered with a sterile dressing (INS 2001). The cannula integrity should be checked to ensure the complete device has been removed (INS 2001; RCN 2003).

Midline catheters

Definition

A midline catheter can be defined as one that is between 7.5 cm and 20 cm in length (Carlson 1999; INS 2000; Hadaway 2000; Perucca 2001). It provides vascular access in a larger peripheral vein without entering the central venous circulation. It is inserted into an antecubital vein and the tip is extended into the vein of the upper arm up to 20 cm, but is not extended past the axilla (Hadaway 2000; Perucca 2001; Frey 2001; Springhouse 2002; RCN 2003).

Indications

Midline catheters are indicated in the following circumstances:

- When patients do not have accessible peripheral veins in the lower arm
- When patients will be undergoing therapy for 1–4 weeks (Carlson 1999), in order to preserve the integrity of the veins and increase patient comfort by removing the need for resites, e.g. antibiotics
- Patient preference.

Reference material

The midline catheter offers an alternative to peripheral and central venous access. Where patients present with poor peripheral venous access and when use of a central venous catheter is contraindicated, the midline catheter provides venous accessibility along with easy, less hazardous insertion at the antecubital fossa (Goetz *et al.* 1998; Weinstein 2000). Because the tip of the catheter does not extend beyond the extremities in which it is placed, radiographic confirmation of tip placement is optional and recommended only when there is difficulty in insertion or flushing (Carlson 1999; Weinstein 2000). The insertion is performed using either an over-the-needle or Seldinger technique: venous access is established with a needle, a guidewire is threaded though the needle, the needle is removed and the catheter is threaded over the guidewire (Weinstein 2000). Benefits to the patient include less frequent resiting of the catheter and a subsequent reduction in associated venous trauma (Weinstein 2000). However, mechanical phlebitis is a common side-effect and close observation and appropriate management are indicated. Once in situ, the catheter should be managed exactly as a central venous catheter. The following therapies are not appropriate for administration via a midline catheter: vesicant medications, especially by continuous infusion; parenteral nutrition, solutions and/or medications with pH less than 5 or greater than 9 and those with osmolarity (Banton & Leahy 1998; INS 2000; Hadaway 2000; Frey 2001).

Device information

Silicone and polyurethane are the most frequently used materials in the manufacture of midline catheters (Kupensky 1998; Hadaway 2000) and they are available as single and double lumen catheters in lengths of up to 20 cm, which can be cut to the desired length following measurement of the arm from the selected vein towards the axilla. They are available in various gauges (16–24) (Perucca 2001; Frey 2001).

Choice of vein

The basilic vein is the vein of choice due to its larger size, straighter course for catheter advancement and improved haemodilution capability (Weinstein 2000; Perucca 2001). The cephalic and median cubital veins would be the second and third choices (INS 2000).

Insertion

The procedure should only be performed by experienced nurses with excellent insertion skills (Weinstein 2000). Adequate assessment of the patient's veins is vital and given the choice the non-dominant arm should be used. The procedure requires a sterile approach and it is recommended that sterile gloves are worn. These should be powder-free, as powder on the catheter can result in mechanical phlebitis (Goodman 2000).

Care and management in situ

It is not usually appropriate to suture these devices in situ, as they can be adequately secured with Steristrips or catheter securement devices such as a Statlock (Perucca 2001). The insertion site can then be covered with a moisture-permeable transparent dressing and changed according to the manufacturer's recommendations, e.g. once a week. The device should be flushed with 0.9% sodium chloride after each use and then with a heparinized solution according to the manufacturer's recommendations, e.g. weekly. Midline catheters can be left in situ for extended periods of time; the optimal time interval for removal of a midline catheter is unknown. Therefore it is recommended that maximum dwell times should be limited to 2–4 weeks (INS 2000). Longer dwell times should be evaluated on site assessment, length of maintaining therapy and patient condition (Kupensky 1998; INS 2000).

Removal

Removal requires gentle firm traction and the catheter will slide out from the insertion site. Pressure should be applied for at least 3–4 minutes and the site inspected prior to applying a dressing to ensure bleeding has stopped. The catheter integrity should be checked and its length measured to ensure that a complete device has been removed.

Central venous access devices (CVAD)

Definition

A central venous access device is one where the catheter is threaded into the central vasculature. If inserted by direct skin puncture into a vein it is percutaneous, e.g. non-tunnelled or PICC; it can also be tunnelled under the skin (INS 2000). A central venous catheter tip will always be in the superior vena cava (SVC) or right atrium.

Indications

- To monitor central venous pressure in seriously ill patients
- For the administration of large amounts of intravenous fluid or blood, e.g. in cases of shock or major surgery
- To provide long-term access for:
  (a) Hydration or electrolyte maintenance
  (b) Repeated administration of drugs, such as cytotoxic and antibiotic therapy
  (c) Repeated transfusion of blood or blood products

Table 44.3 Hazards of central venous catheter insertion (INS 2000; Weinstein 2000; Springhouse 2002)

Sepsis	Air embolism	Pneumothorax
Hydrothorax	Haemorrhage	Haemothorax
Brachial plexus injury	Thoracic duct trauma	Misdirection or kinking
Catheter embolism	Thrombosis	Cardiac tamponade
Arterial puncture and malposition		Cardiac arrhythmias

(d) Repeated specimen collection

(e) Parenteral nutrition (Weinstein 2000; Springhouse 2002).

Hazards of insertion

See Table 44.3.

Complications associated with indwelling central venous catheters

Dislodgement or twiddler's syndrome, catheter migration or occlusion, pinch-off syndrome; catheter-related thrombosis; SVC syndrome; damaged catheters; site infection or site erosion (INS 2000).

Peripherally inserted central catheters

Definition

A peripherally inserted central catheter (PICC) is a catheter that is inserted via the antecubital veins in the arm and is advanced into the central veins, with the tip located in the SVC (usually the lower third) (Todd 1998; INS 2000; Springhouse 2002; RCN 2003). It is not to be confused with a midclavicular catheter ('long line') where the tip is located in a central vein leading to the SVC such as the subclavian or proximal axillary vein (Carlson 1999). Because of the increasing evidence that midclavicular catheters are associated with a high incidence of thrombotic complications (up to 60%), midclavicular placement should only be considered if there are anatomical or pathophysiological reasons, e.g. SVC syndrome (Carlson 1999).

Indications

- Lack of peripheral access
- Infusions of vesicant, irritant, parenteral nutrition or hyperosmolar solutions
- Long-term venous access
- Patient preference

- Patients with needle phobia, to prevent repeated cannulation
- Clinician preference if patients are at risk of haemorrhage or pneumothorax (Goodman 2000; Weinstein 2000).

PICCs should not be considered as a last resort, but introduced early in treatment (Springhouse 2002).

Reference material

The PICC has many advantages over the other central venous access devices: firstly, it eliminates the risks associated with CVC placement, particularly pneumothorax (Carlson 1999; Weinstein 2000; Perucca 2001). Secondly, PICCs have been shown to be associated with a reduction in catheter sepsis when using these devices. This may be related to the temperature of the skin and it has been reported that peripheral sites rarely have more than 50–100 colony-forming units (cfu) of bacteria per $10\,cm^2$ of skin compared with 1000–10 000 cfu per cm^2 on the neck and chest (Carlson 1999, 2001). Thirdly, it is easy to use for both staff and patients and helps to preserve peripheral veins (Goodman 2000; Gabriel 2000; Oakley *et al.* 2000; Weinstein 2000). It has been shown to reduce patient discomfort and provide a reliable form of access (Crawford 2000; Gabriel 2000; Oakley *et al.* 2000; Weinstein 2000; Springhouse 2002). It has also been shown to be cost effective when compared with other long-term and short-term catheters and can be inserted at the bedside (Goodman 2000; Snelling 2001; Springhouse 2002). Disadvantages include an increase in self-care; blood withdrawal is not always easy with the smaller gauges and they may occlude. Over time multiple insertions can cause venous scarring and decrease the ability to reuse the site (Goodman 2000). It has also been found that compared with skin-tunnelled catheters in patients with gastrointestinal cancers, the advantages of a PICC decrease significantly if treatment lasts more than 120 days (Snelling 2001).

Contraindications for using a PICC include the inability to locate suitable antecubital veins; anatomical distortions from surgery, injury or trauma, e.g. scarring from mastectomy, lymphoedema or burns, which may prevent advancement of the catheter to the desired tip location; if a patient is unable to carry out catheter care or is confused; if the patient is unable to lie supine for the insertion period (Macrae 1998).

Device information

PICCs are available as single- and double-lumen catheters, open-ended or valved, and may be made of silicone or polyurethane (Springhouse 2002). Catheters measure 50–65 cm long, with a diameter of 2–7 Fr. PICCs can be cut to the required length, except for valved catheters. The catheter may be inserted through a breakaway needle or peel-away introducer with or without a guidewire (Perucca 2001). With the breakaway needle design the catheter is passed through a splittable needle (Weinstein 2000) and the peel-away introducer is plastic, peeling away once the catheter is inserted. A guidewire within the catheter adds firmness to a silicone catheter, enhancing its advancement. Guidewires are not usually required with a polyurethane catheter (Perucca 2001).

A microintroducer technique can be used to facilitate placement in a smaller difficult vein (Perucca 2001) and improves success (Sansivero 2000). A cannula is inserted and once the needle has been removed, a guidewire is advanced, the cannula is removed and the catheter is threaded over the guidewire (Sansivero 2000; Weinstein 2000; Perucca 2001).

Choice of vein

Careful evaluation and adequate assessment of the patient prior to attempting catheter placement go a long way to ensuring success. Examine both arms with a tourniquet in place, palpate for the healthiest, largest vein, and preferably use the non-dominant arm. Problems associated with vein location have been overcome with the use of a hand-held Doppler, which can identify forearm veins larger than 2 mm in diameter (Whitely et al. 1995). In patients with limited venous access, PICCs may be introduced using ultrasound technology. It has been shown that ultrasonography can increase the chance of successful cannulation of the vein on the first attempt (La Rue 2000) compared with using the traditional landmark method. This method is described as using surface anatomical landmarks and knowing the expected anatomical relationship of the vein to its palpable companion artery (NICE 2002). However, by using ultrasound, the nurse may identify arterial vessels and ultrasound can facilitate visualization of solid material, such as a thrombus, in the lumen of the vessel (Weinstein 2001).

The basilic vein

The median basilic vein is the vein of choice for PICC insertions owing to its larger size, straighter course for catheter advancement and improved haemodilution capability (Perucca 2001; Springhouse 2002) (see Fig. 44.3).

The basilic vein begins in the ulnar (inner aspect) part of the forearm, runs along the posterior, medial surface (back of the arm) and then curves towards the

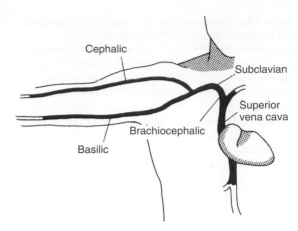

Figure 44.3 Veins of the thorax. (From BD First PICC Clinical Education Class Manual D11 952B 5/98.)

antecubital region, where it is joined by the median cubital vein. It then progresses straight up the upper arm for approximately 5–8 cm and enters the deep tissues. It ascends medially to form the axillary vein (Hadaway 2001).

The median cubital vein

The median cubital vein ascends from just below the middle of the antecubital region and commonly divides into two vessels, one of which joins the basilic and the other the cephalic vein. The median cubital vein is commonly used for blood sampling owing to its size and ease of needle entry. If a practitioner is having difficulty locating and/or cannulating the basilic vein, then the median cubital vein may be used as an alternative insertion route (Sansivero 1998). The catheter will then advance into the basilic (or cephalic) vein.

The cephalic vein

The cephalic vein begins in the radial side (thumb side) of the hand and ascends laterally (along the outer region of the forearm) into the antecubital region, where it forms a junction with the axillary vein. This vein is usually more accessible than the basilic but its size and the sharp angle where it anastomoses with the subclavian make it more difficult to advance the catheter (Perucca 2001; Springhouse 2002) and therefore present a greater potential for catheter tip malposition (Weinstein 2000).

Insertion

Venous assessment and selection play key roles in the successful insertion of a PICC, along with the correct positioning of the patient and careful measurement of the patient and the device. To obtain the correct measurement of the length of catheter to be inserted, using a tape measure, measure diagonally from the selected point for venepuncture with the arm at 45°, to the middle of the clavicle, and then add the length of the clavicle – this gives the measurement for right-sided placement. For left-sided placement add the width of the manubrium (about 2–4 cm) (Lum 1999) (see Fig. 44.10).

The use of local anaesthetic either topically or by injection should be considered to reduce the pain associated with the initial venepuncture with the introducer. It has been found that lidocaine intradermally is superior to EMLA prior to insertion of PICCs (Fry & Aholt 2001). The position of the tip of the PICC should be verified immediately after insertion before any infusion. This is done by chest X-ray (CXR). Ascertaining correct placement is the major reason for ordering CXR but also to rule out malposition and pneumothorax and confirm acceptable tip location for the type of medication being administered (Weinstein 2000; Perucca 2001; Wise 2001; Royer 2001; Springhouse 2002; RCN 2003).

Care and management in situ

Most PICCs are designed with suture wings and these can be used to suture the PICC to the patient's skin. A disadvantage is that patients have reported long-term suturing to be uncomfortable and scarring when the device is removed (Gabriel 2000, 2001). PICCs can be adequately secured using Steristrips or securement devices (self-adhesive anchoring devices applied to the skin such as Statlocks; Gabriel 2000, 2001). These have been shown to result in significantly longer catheter dwell times and fewer total complications (Sheppard *et al.* 1999). The insertion site is then covered with a moisture-permeable transparent dressing and changed according to manufacturer's recommendations, e.g. once a week, to minimize the potential for infection and catheter migration (Gabriel 2000; RCN 2003).

Flushing solution and frequency are usually dependent on the type of catheter and so manufacturer's recommendations should be followed, e.g. valved catheters are usually flushed once a week with 0.9% sodium chloride, while open-ended catheters are flushed with a heparinized solution. Care should be taken when using devices such as power injectors for administering intravenous contrast agents via a PICC as the pressure created may lead to catheter rupture. However, this will depend on the gauge and manufacturer of the catheter (Williamson & McKinney 2001).

Removal

Removal requires gentle firm traction and the catheter will slide out from the insertion site. A PICC may resist removal because of venous spasm, vasoconstriction, phlebitis, valve inflammation, thrombophlebitis or when a fibrin sheath is present (Perucca 2001). Gentle traction and a warm moist compress can be applied to alleviate venous spasm, resulting in easier removal of the catheter (Marx 1995; Perucca 2001). If there is difficulty with removal then wait 20–30 minutes and try again or leave for 12–24 hours. Other interventions include smooth muscle relaxants or relaxation techniques (Marx 1995).

Following removal of the PICC, pressure should be applied for at least 3–4 minutes and the site inspected prior to applying a sterile transparent dressing to ensure bleeding has stopped. The catheter integrity should be checked and its length measured to ensure an intact device has been removed (Springhouse 2002).

Short-term percutaneous central venous catheters (non-tunnelled)

Definition

A short-term non-tunnelled percutaneous central venous catheter is a device that enters through the skin directly into a central vein (Perucca 2001).

Indications

- Short-term therapy of a few days up to several weeks
- Central venous pressure readings
- Emergency use, e.g. fluid replacement
- Absence of peripheral veins (Perucca 2001; Simcock 2001).

Reference material

Percutaneous non-tunnelled CVCs are commonly used for patients in acute settings and insertion may be in response to an emergency or planned event (Simcock 2001b; Springhouse 2002). This catheter is stiff and this aids in CVP monitoring. In addition, its configuration as a multilumen catheter allows administration of several solutions at once and it is easy to remove. However, these catheters are associated with an increased risk of complications such as pneumothorax and infection (Perucca 2001) and catheter material results in irritation of the inner lumen of the vessel and is more thrombogenic (Springhouse 2002).

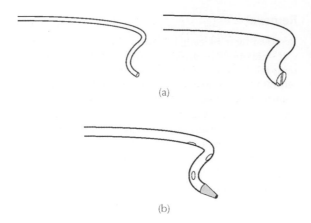

Figure 44.4 Types of catheter tips. (a) Open-ended catheter (single and double lumen). (b) Staggered exit open-ended catheter.

Device information

Most catheters are made of polyurethane and range from single- to multi- (up to five) lumen devices. There are a variety of lumen gauges and the catheters vary in length. The catheters are usually open ended, but lumens can exit at staggered points along the catheter (see Fig. 44.4). Multilumen catheters carry a high risk of infection, which has resulted in the manufacture of coated and impregnated catheters. These can have antimicrobial agents such as chlorhexidine or silver sulphadiazine bonded onto the surface. It has been shown that this can reduce the incidence of catheter-related bloodstream infections and their use is strongly recommended by the DoH (2001) (Collin 1999; Darouiche *et al.* 1999; Xu *et al.* 2000; Veenstra *et al.* 2001; Sampath 2001; Bassetti *et al.* 2001; RCN 2003).

Choice of vein

These catheters are usually placed in the jugular, subclavian (or femoral) veins. The preferred vein for most CVCs is the subclavian (Weinstein 2000; Perucca 2001; Springhouse 2002). It requires the shortest catheters and the most direct route, thus creating a rapid blood flow around the catheter, which reduces irritation and obstructions, the risk of complications and increased dwell time of the catheter (Weinstein 2000; Springhouse 2002). This route also has the lowest risk of infection (Mermel *et al.* 2000) and allows greatest patient mobility after insertion (Springhouse 2002). Disadvantages are an increased risk of pneumothorax and a difficulty controlling bleeding (Springhouse 2002). Its use is contraindicated in patients with radiation burns to the insertion site, fractured clavicle, malignant lesion at base of neck or apex of lungs (Weinstein 2000; Perucca 2001), SVC syndrome or history of central placement problems. The jugular vein approach can be via the internal or external jugular vein. The anatomical location of the internal jugular vein makes it easier to catheterize than the subclavian vein and there is less risk of pneumothorax (Springhouse 2002). The external jugular vein is observable and easily entered and insertion complications are rare (Weinstein 2000; Springhouse 2002). Disadvantages include catheter occlusion and venous irritation as a result of head movement, and difficulty in maintaining an intact dressing, and the position of the catheters may be disturbing for patient and family (Weinstein 2000; Perucca 2001; Springhouse 2002). The femoral veins are primarily used for short-term access when other sites are not suitable (Springhouse 2002). Insertion may be difficult and is associated with an increased risk of infection, inhibiting the patient's mobility and difficulty in maintaining an intact dressing (Perucca 2001; Springhouse 2002).

Insertion

CVC insertion is a sterile procedure and the insertion requires use of a mask, sterile gloves, a gown and sterile drapes (INS 2000; Weinstein 2000; Perucca 2001; RCN 2003). These catheters may be inserted at the patient's bedside but it recommended that the procedure is performed in a controlled environment to reduce the risk of contamination (Perucca 2001). This procedure is usually performed by doctors and so the nurse's responsibilities include the following:

- To ensure, where possible, that the patient understands and has been given a full explanation of the procedure and had the opportunity to discuss any aspects
- To teach the patient techniques that may be required during insertion, the Valsalva manoeuvre and being placed in the Trendelenburg position (where the patient lies flat with their head lowered; knees may be bent) (Weinstein 2000; Perucca 2001; Springhouse 2002) (see Fig. 44.5)
- To explain any specific pre- and post-procedure instructions and the appearance and function of the catheter or device
- To assemble the equipment requested
- To prepare local anaesthesia and dressing materials
- To ensure the correct positioning of the patient during insertion, that is, in the supine or Trendelenburg position

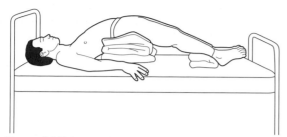

Figure 44.5 Ways of achieving the Trendelenburg position.

- To attend to the physical and psychological comfort of the patient during and immediately following the procedure
- To ensure that no fluid or medication is infused before the correct position of the catheter is confirmed on X-ray by medical staff and documented.

The Valsalva manoeuvre and Trendelenburg position

Placing the patient in the Trendelenburg position facilitates entry to the vein by distending the vein, increasing central venous pressure and venous blood supply, making veins more usable and accessible. It also reduces the chance of air embolism because the venous pressure is higher than atmospheric pressure. This is especially important when the catheter is placed using the subclavian approach. A rolled towel may be placed under the back along the spinal cord and between the shoulders to hyperextend the neck and clavicle (Weinstein 2000) (see Fig. 44.5). The Valsalva manoeuvre can be performed by conscious patients to aid insertion of the catheter and also to prevent air embolism (Weinstein 2000; Springhouse 2002; Verghese 2002). The patient is asked to breathe in and then try to force the air out with the mouth and nose closed (i.e. against a closed glottis). This increases the intrathoracic pressure so that the return of blood to the heart is reduced momentarily and the veins in the neck region become engorged.

Insertion can be aided by the use of two-dimensional imagery. Ultrasound guidance should be used routinely when a CVC is being inserted whether in an elective or emergency situation (NICE 2002). Ultrasound has been shown to increase success, decreasing failure by 83% and reducing complications by 57% (NICE 2002).

It is recommended that these types of catheter remain in for 10–14 days. They can then be removed or the site rotated (Timsit 2000) or they can be replaced over a guidewire (Cook *et al.* 1997). The catheter is easily removed by either nursing or medical staff, using aseptic technique. The site should be cleaned prior to catheter removal to prevent a false-positive result if the catheter tip needs to be sent for microbiological examination (Perucca 2001). CVC removal is associated with air embolism. Precautions are required to prevent this: position the patient in the Trendelenburg position and ask the patient to perform the Valsalva manoeuvre while the catheter is being withdrawn (Perucca 2001; Springhouse 2002). Patients should remain flat for a short time after catheter removal to maintain positive intrathoracic pressure and allow the tissue tract time to seal (Perucca 2001).

Care and management in situ

Flushing is recommended after each use of the catheter. Since these devices are usually in constant use, 0.9% sodium chloride is the flushing solution of choice to reduce the risk of occlusion. It may be appropriate to use continuous infusions to keep the vein open. The types of dressings used at the insertion site may vary according to the type of patient and unit. Staff in some critical care units do not dress the site but clean the insertion site every 4 hours whilst other units may use a moisture-permeable dressing which is changed as necessary. This enables the staff to observe the site regularly for any signs of infection.

Removal

Major vessels usually heal quickly, but direct pressure must be applied to the site until cessation of bleeding confirms this (INS 2000; Springhouse 2002). A sterile transparent occlusive dressing should be applied (INS 2000; Springhouse 2002; RCN 2003), and the site assessed daily until the site has epithelialized (INS 2000; Perucca 2001), usually within 72 hours (Springhouse 2002). The integrity of the catheter should be ascertained and documented (INS 2000; RCN 2003).

Skin-tunnelled catheters

Definition

A skin-tunnelled catheter is a long-term catheter that lies in a subcutaneous tunnel before entering a central vein (usually subclavian). The tunnel commonly exits between the sternum and the nipple. The tip lies at the junction of the SVC and RA or within the lower portion of the SVC or the upper RA (Perucca 2001).

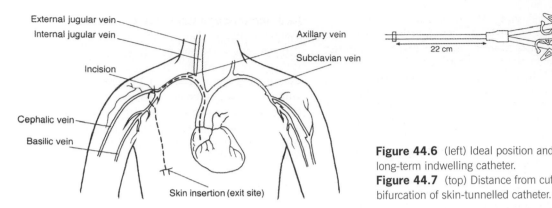

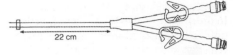

Figure 44.6 (left) Ideal position and site for a long-term indwelling catheter.

Figure 44.7 (top) Distance from cuff to bifurcation of skin-tunnelled catheter.

Indications

A skin-tunnelled catheter is used when long-term venous access is required or if peripheral vascular access is problematic.

Reference material

Tunnelled silicone catheters were first described by Broviac in Seattle in 1973 and were modified by Hickman and his colleagues, creating a larger lumen of 1.6 mm internal diameter (Bjeletich & Hickman 1980). Their special features included an inert anti-thrombogenic flexible material and a subcutaneous Dacron cuff attached to the catheter. The cuff has two functions. First, the cuff is used to secure the catheter as fibrous tissue grows around it and obliterates part of the subcutaneous tunnel within 1–2 weeks of insertion. Second, the cuff impedes the migration of micro-organisms, creating a 'barrier' along the subcutaneous tract and therefore reducing the incidence of catheter-related infection (Wilson 2000; Weinstein 2000; Perucca 2001; Springhouse 2002). The cuff is about 1 cm wide (Perucca 2001) and is usually located about 3–5 cm from the exit site (Stacey 1991; Weinstein 2000).

The Quinton catheter currently used at The Royal Marsden Hospital has a cuff that is situated 22 cm from the top of the bifurcation (Fig. 44.7). This measurement may assist the practitioner in locating the cuff during removal of the catheter. However, the distance of the cuff from the bifurcation may vary according to the type of catheter.

Device information

Polyurethane or silicone skin-tunnelled catheters present as single-, double- or triple-lumen catheters and the tip may be open ended or closed with a slit valve. The disadvantage of an open-ended catheter is the problem

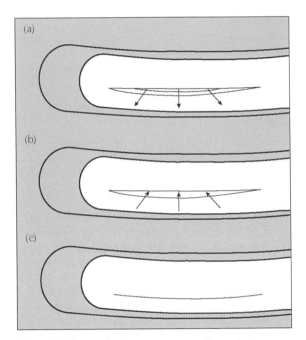

Figure 44.8 The Groshong two-way valve catheter. (a) Infusion (positive pressure). (b) Aspiration (negative pressure). (c) Closed (neutral pressure). (Groshong is a registered trademark of C.R. Bard, Inc. or an affiliate.)

of blood reflux, resulting in occlusion. Catheters such as the Groshong catheter have a round blunt tip which incorporates a two-way valve which remains closed at normal venous caval pressure. Application of a vacuum in order to withdraw blood enables the valve to open inwards; positive pressure into the catheter forces the valve to open outwards (Fig. 44.8). The advantages of valved catheters are the reduced risk of bleeding or air emboli on insertion and during subsequent care; the elimination of catheter clamping; and the elimination of the need for heparin along with a reduction in the frequency of flushing (Weinstein 2000; Perucca 2001). In order for the valved catheter to function properly the tip must be situated in the midsuperior section of the vena cava and not in the right atrium. Thrombus formation around the tip could result, followed by malfunction and loss of valve competence (Weinstein 2000).

Another type of catheter is the pressure-activated safety valve (PASV). The valve opens with minimal positive pressure for infusion but requires four times as much negative pressure for aspiration. This feature reduces the risk of air embolism or bleeding resulting from accidental disconnection. The valve is incorporated within the hub and not the tip and reduces the risk of reflux even during periods of raised central venous pressure (Weinstein 2000).

Choice of vein

The aim of the insertion is to place the catheter tip in the right atrium via the subclavian vein and SVC (Stacey 1991). When there is an SVC obstruction from thrombosis or compression, the femoral vein can be used to access the inferior vena cava. Selection of vessels is as for non-tunnelled central venous catheter.

Insertion

The insertion of a skin-tunnelled catheter is a surgical procedure usually carried out in an operating theatre under aseptic conditions, under fluoroscopic control with monitoring of the patient by pulse oximetry and ECG to detect arrhythmias (Stacey 1991; Weinstein 2000). However, this procedure is now also performed by nurse specialists at the bedside and within radiology departments (Hamilton et al. 1995; Fitzsimmons et al. 1997; Benton and Marsden 2002). The procedure is usually performed under sedation along with the use of local anaesthesia. In some patients, e.g. children, this procedure would be carried out under general anaesthesia.

Access may be gained percutaneously using a needle and a guidewire or via an open surgical cutdown procedure. The percutaneous insertion involves the subclavian vein being accessed using a guidewire and Seldinger technique. After the catheter has been tunnelled subcutaneously, a vein dilator is passed over the guidewire and the catheter is cut to length and introduced using a 'peel-away' sheath (Davidson & Al Mufti 1997). Position is confirmed by the easy aspiration of blood from each lumen and these are then flushed with heparin or a slow infusion of 0.9% sodium chloride (10–20 ml/hour) until correct tip placement has been confirmed. A chest X-ray should be performed 2 hours after insertion to check for correct placement and pneumothorax (Stacey et al. 1991; Davidson & Al Mufti 1997).

Care and management in situ

Following healing of the skin tunnel, which takes approximately 7 days, sutures at the entry site may be removed. The exit sutures should be retained until the fibroblastic response to the Dacron cuff is adequate to secure the catheter, usually in 2–3 weeks (Stacey et al. 1991; Weinstein 2000; Perucca 2001). A transparent dressing should cover the site and be changed weekly until removal of sutures. Thereafter no dressing is usually required unless the patient requests one.

Removal

Removal techniques for skin-tunnelled catheters vary. Removal should only be performed by specially trained nurses or doctors. It is recommended that the patient is placed supine and that aseptic technique is used throughout. There are two methods for removal.

Surgical excision

This method involves locating the cuff and performing a minor surgical excision under local anaesthetic. A small incision is made over the site of the cuff and blunt dissection, i.e. using forceps, is carried out to prise apart tissues (Goodman 2000; Perucca 2001); this causes less damage to the tissues than using a scalpel. The cuff and the catheter are freed from the surrounding fibrous tissue. The catheter is then cut in order to remove the distal end via the exit site and the proximal end through the incision. Once the catheter has been removed, the wound is sutured using interrupted sutures, which can be removed after 7 days.

Traction method

With the traction method there is a greater risk of the catheter breaking, which could result in a catheter embolism. The catheter is gripped firmly and constant traction applied until the cuff is loosened in the tunnel (Goodman 2000). It may take a few minutes for the catheter and cuff to become loose before sliding free. Constant steady pressure will remove the complete catheter; however, the catheter should be checked on removal to ensure it is complete as breakage and splitting can occur (Goodman 2000; INS 2000). The catheter and cuff may be pulled through, but the cuff may remain attached to tissue. This is thought to be of no significance and may be left in place, although some suggest that if the cuff is not removed it could become infected later (Goodman 2000). Difficulty with removal or a break in the catheter will require surgical intervention.

Since the vein closes following removal of the catheter there is usually no bleeding. However, there may be slight bleeding at the exit site immediately after removal because of the passage of the cuff.

Following either removal method, pressure should be applied to the site until the bleeding stops, and a dressing may be required for up to 24 hours. The patient should be encouraged to rest flat for 30–60 minutes to allow the tissue tract time to seal (Perucca 2001).

If the tip is required for microbiological examination, care should be taken to clean the exit site with chlorhexidine in 70% alcohol, prior to removal, to prevent a false positive tip culture. The tip should be placed into a sterile container immediately upon removal and sent to the laboratory (Perucca 2001).

Implantable ports

Definition

An implanted port is a totally implanted vascular access device made of two components: a reservoir with a self-sealing septum is attached to a silicone catheter (see Fig. 44.9). The port is inserted on either the chest or the arm and is accessed using a special non-coring needle (Goodman 2000; Weinstein 2000; Perucca 2001).

Indications

An implanted port can be used for long-term venous access for all types of therapies, both continuous and intermittent, and if patients have problematic venous access (Springhouse 2002).

Reference material

Ports are implanted subcutaneously to provide repeated long-term access (Weinstein 2000) to the vascular system (other ports include arterial, epidural and peritoneal ports). Implanted ports require little care of the site because of the intact skin layer over the accessible port, except when accessed, and when not in use, the only care required is a monthly flush (Weinstein 2000). Other benefits include a reduced risk of infection (Mirro 1989; Bow *et al.* 1999; Moureau 1999) and less interference with daily activities such as bathing or swimming (Goodman 2000), and body image is less threatened than by the presence of an external catheter (Mirro 1989; Bow *et al.* 1999). Patients with ports are often very satisfied with their access devices (Chernecky 2001).

Disadvantages of the port include discomfort when accessing is performed (particularly if placed deeply or in a difficult area to access). This can be overcome with the use of topical local anaesthetic. However, the tissue over the septum becomes calloused or scarred and over time there is loss of sensitivity (Moureau 1999; Perucca 2001). Needle dislodgement with resulting extravasation or needlestick injury are well-documented problems

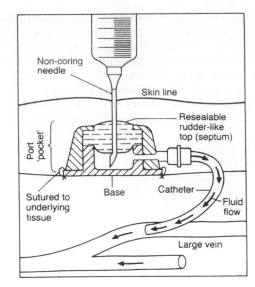

Figure 44.9 Cross-section of an implantable port, accessed with non-coring needle.

associated with ports (Schulmeister 1998; Schulmeister & Camp Sorrel 2000; Nesti & Kovac 2000; Goodman 2000). There are also issues related to occlusion and 'sludge' build-up and newer designs are attempting to reduce this (Stevenis *et al.* 2000). Finally there are often problems with obtaining blood return (Moureau 1999).

Device information

A variety of ports are available and the one chosen is dependent on a number of factors; for example, whether the patient is a child or an adult, the amount of access required and where it is located (Perucca 2001). Ports are usually single lumen, although double-lumen ports are available. However, double-lumen ports have two septums and therefore require needle access into each septum (Goodman 2000). Port reservoirs are about 2.5 cm in height and 0.625 in diameter and can weigh from 21 to 28 g; low-profile ports are smaller and often placed in the arm (Perucca 2001). Entry can be gained via the side or top but most are accessed by top entry (Goodman 2000; Weinstein 2000; Springhouse 2002). Catheters are made of silicone and may be open ended or have a Groshong valve (Biffi *et al.* 2001; Perucca 2001). The portal body may be made of stainless steel, plastic or titanium, although steel is not often used any more as it interferes with electromagnetic imaging procedures and is quite heavy in comparison with other material (Perucca 2001). The self-sealing silicone septum can be accessed 1000–3600 times, often dependent upon the size of the needle used (Goodman

2000; Perucca 2001). Non-coring needles have the penetration of a knife so when the needle is removed the septum closes behind it. The bevel opens on the side of the needle instead of the end (Weinstein 2000; Perucca 2001). They are available in straight or 90° angle configuration with or without extension sets. The needle is available with a metal or plastic hub in gauges 19–24 and lengths from 0.65 to 2.5 cm. Needle gauge is selected dependent on type and rate of infusate as well as the location of the port (Weinstein 2000).

Choice of vein

The most common veins used are subclavian, internal or external jugular veins, cephalic or femoral vein. Ports can also be inserted in the antecubital area of the arm (Goodman 2000; Weinstein 2000; Perucca 2001).

Insertion

Implantation is a surgical procedure usually carried out under general anaesthetic. Some catheters are preattached to the reservoir whilst others require attachment on insertion (Goodman 2000). The catheter is introduced into the SVC via the subclavian, jugular or cephalic vein and fluoroscopy verifies the placement of the tip and the catheter is tunnelled to the pocket (Perucca 2001; Springhouse 2002). The pocket is made just under the skin, usually on a bony area prominence for stabilization (Springhouse 2002). The port is then sutured into place to the underlying fascia. The suture line should be lateral, medial, superior or inferior to the port septum because repeated access could cause stress to the suture line (Weinstein 2000). The area is tender and oedematous for up to a week following implantation and any manipulation/accessing may be painful. When immediate use is indicated the port should be accessed and dressed in theatre (Goodman 2000).

Care and management in situ

When the port is accessed the needle can remain in situ for 7 days (Goodman 2000; Springhouse 2002). Accessing should always be performed by specifically trained nurses owing to the risk of extravasation if the needle is incorrectly placed (Goodman 2000). Patients can also be taught to access their own ports. The needle should be supported with gauze and covered with a transparent dressing to minimize the risk of needle dislodgement. Regular assessment of the port when accessed is essential to check for signs of erthyema, swelling or discomfort, which could indicate infection, infiltration or extravasation (INS 2000; Springhouse 2002). Most manufacturers recommend that only syringes 10 ml or larger should be used for drug administration or when flushing to prevent excessive pressure which could result in separation of the catheter from the reservoir or rupture if the catheter is occluded (Conn 1993). When not in use the port only requires flushing once a month with a concentrated solution of heparin (100 IU in 1 ml), usually a total of 5–6 ml (Weinstein 2000; Perucca 2001; Springhouse 2002).

Removal

Implanted ports may be surgically removed and after removal the site must be assessed for any signs of inflammation (Perucca 2001).

Discharging patients home with a VAD in situ

Patients may be discharged home with a VAD in situ which will allow them to receive treatment at home (e.g. continuous chemotherapy or intermittent antibiotics) or allow for easier access on each admission (e.g. via implantable ports). An early referral to the district nurse is crucial to ensure adequate support for the patient once at home.

Patients may now receive daily treatment over a 3–5 day period with an indwelling peripheral cannula (Shotkin & Lombardo 1996). The degree of care is minimal compared with a central venous catheter, but patients should receive adequate information about the early signs of phlebitis, i.e. pain, redness and swelling, and what to do in the case of accidental dislodgement or removal of the cannula.

Patients with long-term CVADs in situ such as PICCs or skin-tunnelled catheters will require instruction and supervision to ensure adequate understanding of the care and maintenance of their devices. This must start early within the discharge planning process along with an assessment of the home environment, the patient's manual dexterity, physical and medical condition (Cole 1999; Kayley 1999; Weinstein 2000). Patient education is one of the most important aspects of care, but to make teaching effective it is essential to recognize each patient's needs and limitations. It is also vital to acknowledge each patient's past experiences and readiness to learn (Cole 1999; Lonsway 2001). Education of the patient should encompass care and maintenance of the device as well as signs and symptoms of complications (Dougherty et al. 1998; Cole 1999). Educational packages should be prepared in the form of practical demonstrations and clear, succinct handouts (McDermott 1995; Redman 1997; Cole 1999; Kayley 1999). It is also important to recognize the need to prepare patients carefully to participate in their own self-care and therapy treatment. The patient, relative and/or friends should understand the following:

- The frequency of changing the dressing and how to care for the site
- How to maintain patency
- How to inspect for signs of infection or other complications
- How to problem solve and where to seek help.

Care of the site/dressing changes

The dressing of choice for PICC and skin-tunnelled insertion sites is one which is moisture permeable and transparent (DoH 2001; LSC 2002; NICE 2003) which usually requires changing, following the initial change within first 24 hours, once a week (Todd 1998; Ryder 2001). This type of dressing may make it difficult for the patient to change the dressing themselves and so a carer or district nurse will need to be involved. At the dressing change the site should be inspected and any signs of erythema or inflammation should be reported to the hospital at once in order for appropriate treatment to be prescribed. The area should be cleaned using an aseptic technique with a chlorhexidine-based solution (DoH 2001; NICE 2003).

Maintaining patency and handling of equipment

If a patient wishes to be self-caring, the nurse should observe them carrying out the flushing procedure, either in hospital or in the home setting, until competent to do so without supervision of a nurse (INS 2000). However, some patients prefer the district nurse to take responsibility for maintaining patency. Sufficient equipment must be supplied to enable the patient or nurse to care for the CVAD from the time of discharge until the patient's next admission. A kit should be assembled containing the following when a patient has a skin-tunnelled catheter or PICC in situ:

- Needleless injection caps
- Ampoules of heparinized saline (50 IU heparin in 5 ml 0.9% sodium chloride)
- Chlorhexidine 0.5% in 70% alcohol or 70% isopropyl alcohol swabs
- Sterile 10 ml syringes
- 21 G needles
- Instruction leaflet to provide both the community nurse and patient with a point of reference, e.g. Patient Information Series Care of the Skin Tunnelled Catheter
- Sharps container.

Early recognition of complications

Patients should be taught what early signs and symptoms to look out for and who and when to contact. The most common complications associated with CVADs are infection and thrombosis. The patients should be told to report signs of redness and tracking at the exit site, along the skin tunnel or up the arm, any oozing at the exit site and fevers or rigors. Many patients are now prescribed prophylactic warfarin (either 1 mg daily or according to regular international normalized ratio screening) to prevent thrombosis (Bagnell Reeb 1998; Hadaway 1998; Perdue 2001). However, it should be stressed to the patient that any of the following signs or symptoms should be reported immediately: pain and/or swelling over the shoulder, across the chest and into the neck and arm. Early reporting may enable effective treatment and avoid removal of the device.

Problem solving and who and when to ask for help

Patients must be informed what to do if the catheter becomes occluded or damaged and given a contact name and number in order to be able to seek professional advice. This will help to alleviate any anxiety (Dougherty *et al.* 1998). Most problems can be managed at home with the involvement of the community nurses and GP.

Quality of life issues: living with a VAD

Body image and a patient's lifestyle can be issues when living with a CVAD. This is particularly true with an external catheter which can be distressing and embarrassing for some patients (Goodman 2000). It can result in restrictions to normal daily activities, e.g. bathing or involvement in sporting activities such as swimming (Gabriel 2000; Goodman 2000; Robbins 2000); some of these can be resolved by the use of an implantable device (Chernecky 2001).

The following have been listed as ways in which a CVAD can affect body image:

- Physical presence and alteration of body appearance and invasion of body integrity
- It influences the type of clothes that can be worn
- It may interfere with bodily expressions of closeness and sexuality (Daniels 1995).

The presence of a CVAD could also have implications on how others view the role function of the individual, particularly if the patient is attached to an infusion pump (Thompson *et al.* 1989). The psychological impact of an indwelling catheter on body image should not be overlooked, especially when patients are sexually active.

Patients may be well informed about access devices from the media or via the Internet. They may also have gained knowledge from friends or family experiences. Therefore, involving the patient in the decision-making process is vital. Patient choice about the device or even the site of insertion, e.g. use of the non-dominant arm, results in better compliance with care of the device and monitoring of problems (Hudek 1986; Gabriel 1999). It also enables patients to cope better with the changes to their normal activities (Daniels 1995) and the impact on body image can be reduced by involving the individual in the choice and management of the device (Daniels 1995).

Procedure guidelines: **Inserting a peripheral cannula**

Equipment

1 Sterile dressing pack.
2 Various gauge sizes of cannula.
3 Alcohol-based hand scrub.
4 Alcohol-based skin cleaning preparation, e.g. chlorhexidine in 70% alcohol.

5 Extension set.
6 Needleless injection cap.
7 Hypoallergenic tape.
8 Bandage.

Procedure

Action	Rationale
1 Explain and discuss the procedure with the patient.	To ensure that the patient understands the procedure and gives his/her valid consent.
2 If he/she requires topical local anaesthetic, then apply it to chosen venepuncture sites for 30–60 minutes prior to cannulation.	In order to give adequate time for local anaesthetic to be effective.
3 Assemble all the equipment necessary for cannulation.	To ensure that time is not wasted and that the procedure goes smoothly without unnecessary interruptions.
4 Check all packaging before opening and preparing the equipment to be used.	To maintain asepsis throughout and check that no equipment is damaged or out of date.
5 Carefully wash hands using bactericidal soap and water or bactericidal alcohol handrub before commencement, and dry.	To minimize the risk of infection.
6 Check hands for any visibly broken skin, and cover with a waterproof dressing.	To minimize the risk of contamination of the nurse by the patient's blood.
7 In both an inpatient and outpatient situation, the correct lighting, ventilation, privacy and position of the patient must be ascertained.	To ensure that the operator and patient are comfortable and that adequate light is available to illuminate the procedure.
8 Support the chosen limb on a pillow.	To ensure the patient's comfort and ease of access.
9 Apply the tourniquet to the chosen limb.	To dilate the veins by obstructing the venous return. If necessary, use other methods to encourage venous access.
10 Assess and select the vein.	
11 Release the tourniquet.	To ensure that the patient does not feel discomfort while the device is selected and equipment prepared.
12 Select the device based on the vein size.	To reduce damage or trauma to the vein. To reduce the risk of phlebitis and restricted movement.
13 Wash hands using bactericidal soap and water or bactericidal alcohol handrub.	To minimize risk of infection.
14 Open a pack, empty all equipment onto the pack and place a sterile dressing towel under the patient's arm.	To create a sterile working area.
15 Reapply the tourniquet.	To promote venous filling.

Procedure guidelines: Inserting a peripheral cannula (cont'd)

Action	Rationale
16 Clean the patient's skin and the selected vein for at least 30 seconds using an appropriate preparation and allow to dry. Do not repalpate the vein or touch the skin.	To maintain asepsis and remove skin flora.
17 Put on gloves.	To prevent contamination of the nurse from any blood spill.
18 Remove needle guard and inspect the device for any faults.	To detect faulty equipment, e.g. bent or barbed needles. If these are present, do not use and report to company as faulty equipment.
19 Anchor the vein by applying manual traction on the skin a few centimetres below the proposed site of insertion.	To immobilize the vein. To provide countertension, which will facilitate a smooth needle entry.
20 Ensure the cannula is in the bevel-up position and place the device directly over the vein; insert the cannula through the skin at the selected angle according to the depth of the vein.	To ensure a successful, pain-free cannulation.
21 Wait for the first flashback of blood in the flashback chamber of the stylet.	To indicate that the needle has entered the vein.
22 Level the device by decreasing the angle between the cannula and the skin and advance the cannula slightly to ensure entry into the lumen of the vein.	To avoid advancing too far through the vein wall and causing damage to the vein wall. To stabilize the device.
23 Withdraw the stylet slightly and a second flashback of blood will be seen along the shaft of the cannula.	To ensure that the cannula is still in a patent vein. This is called the hooded technique.
24 Maintaining skin traction with the non-dominant hand, and using the dominant hand, slowly advance the cannula off the stylet and into the vein.	To ensure the vein remains immobilized and thus reducing the risk of a 'through puncture'.
25 Release the tourniquet.	To decrease the pressure within the vein.
26 Apply digital pressure to the vein above the cannula tip and remove the stylet.	To prevent blood spillage.
27 Immediately dispose of the stylet into an appropriate sharps container.	To reduce the risk of accidental needlestick injury.
28 Attach an extension set, needleless injection cap or an administration set and flush the cannula with 0.9% sodium chloride.	To ascertain and maintain patency.
29 Observe the site for signs of swelling or leakage, and ask the patient if any discomfort or pain is felt.	To check that the device is positioned correctly.
30 Tape the cannula using the method illustrated in Figure 44.1.	To ensure the device will remain stable and secure.
31 Cover with low-linting swabs and bandage firmly.	To ensure patient comfort and security of device.
32 Discard waste, making sure it is placed in appropriate containers.	To ensure safe disposal in the correct containers and avoid laceration or injury of other staff. To prevent reuse of equipment.

Procedure guidelines: **Inserting a midline catheter**

Equipment

1 Sterile minor operation pack.
2 Sterile powder-free gloves.
3 Alcohol-based hand scrub.
4 Alcohol-based skin cleaning preparation, e.g. chlorhexidine in 70% alcohol.
5 Extension set and needleless injection cap.
6 Sterile low-linting dressing.

7 Hypoallergenic tape.
8 Midline catheter.
9 Introducer.
10 Transparent dressing, securing device and sterile tapes.
11 10 ml syringes.
12 0.9% sodium chloride.
13 Tape measure.

*Procedure guidelines: **Inserting a midline catheter** (cont'd)*

Procedure

Action	Rationale
1 Explain and discuss the procedure with the patient.	To ensure that the patient understands the procedure and gives his/her valid consent.
2 Apply tourniquet to the arm. Assess venous access in both arms and locate veins by sight and palpation.	To ensure the patient has adequate venous access and to select the vein for catheterization.
3 Apply local anaesthetic cream/gel to chosen venepuncture site and leave for allotted time.	To minimize the pain of insertion.
4 Draw screens and position patient in a comfortable position.	To ensure privacy. To aid insertion and correct placement.
5 Measure using the tape measure from the selected venepuncture site up the arm, to just below the axilla.	To enable selection of the most suitable catheter length and to know how far to advance the catheter in order for its tip to be located in the correct position.
6 Take equipment required to patient's bedside. Open outer pack.	
7 Wash hands using a bactericidal handrub.	To minimize the risk of infection.
8 Put on powder-free sterile gloves; open sterile pack, arranging the contents as required. Prefill the syringe with 0.9% sodium chloride.	To prevent contamination. Powder on gloves can increase the risk of mechanical phlebitis.
9 Remove the cap from the extension set and attach 0.9% sodium chloride; gently flush with 2 ml and leave syringe attached.	To check that the catheter is patent and to enable easy removal of guidewire.
10 If the catheter tip can be trimmed, using the graduated markings along the catheter, select the marking required and pull back guidewire 1 cm from desired new tip, and using sterile scissors trim the catheter. *Never trim the guidewire!*	To ensure the catheter will be the correct length for placement and to prevent damage to the vein if the guidewire is damaged.
11 Place sterile towel under patient's arm.	To provide a sterile field to work on.
12 Clean the skin at the selected site with an appropriate disinfectant, e.g. chlorhexidine in 70% alcohol, using concentric circles with friction and prepare an area of 15–25 cm.	To ensure skin flora is destroyed and to minimize the risk of infection.
13 Allow the solution to dry thoroughly.	To ensure coagulation of bacteria and completion of disinfection process.
14 Drape the patient with a fenestrated towel.	To provide a sterile field.
15 Inject local anaesthetic if required using a 25 G needle to area intradermally and wait for a few minutes for it to take effect.	To enable adequate anaesthesia.
16 Reapply tourniquet.	To aid venous distension.
17 Perform venepuncture with introducer by entering the skin, 1 cm from desired point of entry, at a 15–30° angle. Advance 0.5–1 cm once flashback is seen.	To gain venous access.
18 Release tourniquet.	To prevent blood loss and 'through puncture' and enable advancement of catheter.
19 Position fingers in a V, with index finger on wings and middle finger above sheath tip, and gently remove stylet. Apply pressure.	To contain flashback, prevent contamination of the area with blood and minimize the amount of blood loss from patient.
20 Grip catheter 1 cm from the tip and thread through the introducer sheath.	To ensure tip is not contaminated.
21 Continue slow advancement of the catheter to the desired length.	To minimize damage to intima of vein.

Procedure guidelines: Inserting a midline catheter (cont'd)

Action	Rationale
22 Apply pressure above introducer and carefully withdraw the introducer and peel apart.	To ensure there is no movement of the catheter. To remove peel-away introducer.
23 Aspirate for blood return and flush catheter with 0.9% sodium chloride.	To check patency of device and ensure continued patency.
24 Apply gentle pressure on catheter and slowly withdraw the guidewire.	To ensure there is no withdrawal of catheter.
25 Attach needleless injection cap and flush as per midline guidelines.	To ensure patency of the device.
26 Secure the catheter with sterile tape or other securing device. Apply a transparent dressing. Apply gauze and a bandage.	To ensure stability of device and protection of the site.
27 Dispose of equipment appropriately. Dispose of sharps and clinical waste.	
28 Document the procedure in the patient's notes: type, length and gauge of cannula, where it was inserted, any problem, how it was secured.	To ensure adequate records and enable continued care of device and patient.

Procedure guidelines: **Insertion and removal of a peripherally inserted central catheter (PICC)**

Equipment

1 Sterile minor operations pack.
2 Two pairs of sterile powder-free gloves.
3 Alcohol-based hand scrub.
4 Alcohol-based skin cleaning preparation, e.g. chlorhexidine in 70% alcohol.
5 Extension set and needleless injection cap.
6 Sterile low-linting gauze.
7 Hypoallergenic tape.
8 Peripherally inserted central catheter.
9 Introducer.
10 Transparent dressing, securing device and sterile tapes.
11 10 ml syringes.
12 0.9% sodium chloride.
13 Tape measure.

Procedure

Action	Rationale
1 Gain consent from doctor and assess patient's medical and intravenous device history.	To ensure the patient has no underlying medical problems and is suitable to undergo the procedure.
2 Explain and discuss the procedure with the patient.	To ensure that the patient understands the procedure and gives his/her valid written consent.
3 Apply tourniquet and assess venous access, assessing both extremities, and locate veins by sight and palpation.	To ensure the patient has adequate venous access and to select the vein for catheterization.
4 Apply local anaesthetic cream/gel to chosen venepuncture site and leave for allotted time.	To minimize the pain of insertion.
5 Draw screens and position patient in a supine position, with patient's arm at a 45° angle, with ability to move arm to a 90° angle.	To ensure privacy. To aid insertion of introducer and then advancement of catheter.
6 Measure using the tape measure from the selected venepuncture site diagonally across to the middle of the clavicle, then measure total distance of clavicle. Added together, these will give catheter measurement (Fig. 44.10).	To enable selection of the most suitable catheter length and to establish how far to advance the catheter in order for its tip to be located in the correct position, i.e. the SVC.
7 Take equipment required to patient's bedside. Open outer pack.	To ensure appropriate equipment is available for procedure.

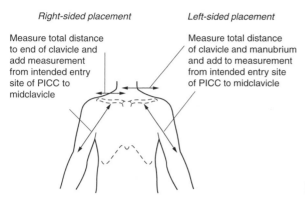

Right-sided placement

Measure total distance
to end of clavicle and
add measurement
from intended entry
site of PICC to
midclavicle

Left-sided placement

Measure total distance
of clavicle and manubrium
and add to measurement
from intended entry site
of PICC to midclavicle

Figure 44.10 Preinsertion measurement of PICC.

Procedure guidelines: **Insertion and removal of a peripherally inserted central catheter (PICC)** *(cont'd)*

Action	Rationale
8 Wash hands using a bactericidal handrub.	To minimize the risk of infection.
9 Put on sterile gown and powder-free sterile gloves; open sterile tray, arranging the contents as required. Prefill the syringe with 0.9% sodium chloride.	To prevent contamination. Powder on gloves can increase the risk of mechanical phlebitis.
10 Remove the cap from the extension set and attach 0.9% sodium chloride; gently flush with 2 ml and leave syringe attached.	To check that the catheter is patent and to enable easy removal of guidewire.
11 If the catheter tip can be trimmed, using the graduated markings along the catheter, select the marking required and pull back guidewire 1 cm from desired new tip, and using sterile scissors trim the catheter. *Never trim the guidewire!*	To ensure the catheter will be the correct length for SVC tip placement and to prevent damage to the vein if the guidewire is damaged.
12 Place sterile towel under patient's arm.	To provide a sterile field to work on.
13 Clean the skin at the selected site with an appropriate disinfectant, e.g. chlorhexidine in 70% alcohol, using concentric circles with friction and prepare an area of 15–25 cm.	To ensure the removal of skin flora and to minimize the risk of infection.
14 Allow the solution to dry thoroughly.	To ensure coagulation of bacteria and disinfection.
15 Drape the patient with a fenestrated towel.	To provide a sterile field.
16 Inject local anaesthetic if required using a 25 G needle to area intradermally and wait a few minutes for it to take effect.	To enable adequate anaesthesia.
17 Reapply tourniquet.	To aid venous distension.
18 Remove gloves and discard. Put on a new pair of sterile gloves.	To minimize risk of contamination of venepuncture site or catheter.
19 Perform venepuncture with introducer by entering the skin, 1 cm from desired point of entry, at a 15–30° angle. Advance 0.5–1 cm once flashback is seen.	To gain venous access.
20 Release tourniquet.	To prevent blood loss and 'through puncture' and enable advancement of catheter.
21 Position fingers in a V, with index finger on wings and middle finger above sheath tip, and gently remove stylet. Apply pressure.	To contain flashback, prevent contamination of the area with blood and minimize the amount of blood loss from the patient.
22 Grip catheter 1 cm from the tip and thread through introducer sheath.	
23 Advance the catheter 10–15 cm.	To ensure the catheter is securely within the vein before moving the patient's arm.

*Procedure guidelines: **Insertion and removal of a peripherally inserted central catheter (PICC)** (cont'd)*

Action	Rationale
24 Ask the patient (assisted) to move the arm to a 90° angle.	To enable further advancement of catheter.
25 Turn patient's head towards the arm of insertion and place the chin on the clavicle if possible.	To prevent the catheter entering the jugular vein and to ensure correct advancement of catheter downwards to the SVC.
26 Continue slow advancement of the catheter to the desired length.	To minimize damage to intima of vein.
27 Apply pressure above introducer and carefully withdraw the introducer and peel apart.	To ensure there is no movement of the catheter. To remove peel-away introducer.
28 Aspirate for blood return and flush catheter with 0.9% sodium chloride.	To check patency of device and ensure continued patency.
29 Apply gentle pressure on catheter and slowly withdraw the guidewire.	To ensure there is no withdrawal of catheter.
30 Attach a needleless injection cap and flush as per PICC guidelines.	To ensure patency of the device.
31 Secure the catheter with a securing device such as Statlock. Apply a small pad of low-linting gauze directly over the insertion site and secure with sterile tape.	To ensure stability of device and to minimize blood leakage at the site which occurs following insertion.
32 Apply a transparent dressing. Apply low-linting gauze under the extension set and cap, then bandage.	To ensure protection of the site. To prevent the tubing pressing into the patient's skin.
33 Dispose of equipment appropriately. Dispose of sharps and clinical waste.	
34 Send patient for chest X-ray. Position of catheter to be assessed by the doctor.	To allow position of tip to be assessed. To ensure correct tip location.
35 Document the procedure in the patient's notes: type, length and gauge of cannula, where it was inserted, tip confirmation, any problem, how it was secured and patient education.	To ensure adequate records and enable continued care of device and patient.

Removal

Action	Rationale
1 Wash hands using a bactericidal handrub and gather equipment required (dressing pack, dressing, tape).	To minimize the risk of infection.
2 Remove transparent dressing and gently remove securing devices and/or sterile tapes.	To prepare for catheter removal.
3 Apply a pair of gloves and, using a steady and constant motion, gently pull catheter until completely removed from exit site.	To remove the catheter and prevent vein damage.
4 Apply digital pressure over exit site for about 2–3 minutes or until bleeding stops, and apply dressing.	To minimize blood loss and bruising. To provide protection of the entry site.
5 Check marking of length removed and check it is same as the length inserted. Document.	To ensure that complete catheter has been removed.

Procedure guidelines: **Changing the dressing on a central venous catheter insertion site**

Equipment

1 Sterile dressing pack.
2 Alcohol-based handrub.
3 Alcohol-based skin cleaning preparation, e.g. chlorhexidine in 70% alcohol.
4 Semi-permeable transparent dressing or other appropriate dressing.
5 Hypoallergenic tape.
6 Bacteriological swab.

Procedure guidelines: Changing the dressing on a central venous catheter insertion site (cont'd)

Procedure

Action	Rationale
1 Explain and discuss the procedure with the patient.	To ensure that the patient understands the procedure and gives his/her valid consent.
2 Perform the dressing using an aseptic technique.	To prevent infection. (For further information on asepsis, see Ch. 4, Aseptic technique.)
3 Screen the bed. Assist the patient into a supine position, if possible.	To allow dust and airborne organisms to settle before the insertion site and the sterile field are exposed.
4 Wash hands with bactericidal soap and water or bactericidal alcohol handrub. Place all equipment required for the dressing on the bottom shelf of a clean dressing trolley.	To reduce the risk of cross-infection.
5 Take the trolley to the patient's bedside, disturbing the screens as little as possible.	To minimize airborne contamination.
6 Open the sterile dressing pack.	
7 Attach a yellow clinical waste bag to the side of the trolley below the level of the top shelf.	So that contaminated material is below the level of the sterile field.
8 Open the other sterile packs, tipping their contents gently onto the centre of the sterile field. Pour lotions into gallipots or an indented plastic tray.	To reduce risk of contamination of contents.
9 Wash hands with bactericidal alcohol handrub.	Hands may have become contaminated by handling the outer packs, etc.
10 Loosen the old dressing gently.	So that the dressing can be lifted off easily.
11 Put on clean gloves.	To protect the nurse from any contact with the patient's blood.
12 Using gloved hands, remove the old dressing and discard it.	
13 If the site is red or discharging, take a swab for bacteriological investigation.	For identification of pathogens. To predict colonization of the site.
14 Remove gloves and put on sterile gloves from pack.	To minimize the risk of introducing infection.
15 Clean the wound with chlorhexidine in 70% alcohol, working from the inside to the outside of the area and dealing with the cleanest parts of the wound first. Allow area to dry prior to applying the dressing.	To minimize the risk of infection spread from a 'dirty' to a 'clean' area. To enable disinfection process to be completed. To prevent skin reaction in response to the application of a transparent dressing to moist skin.
16 Apply appropriate dressing, moulding it into place so that there are no folds or creases.	To minimize skin irritation and reduce risk of dressing peeling or becoming damaged.
17 Remove gloves.	
18 Fold up the sterile field, place it in the yellow clinical waste bag and seal it before moving the trolley. Draw back the curtains. Dispose of waste in appropriate containers.	To prevent environmental contamination.

Procedure guidelines: **Maintaining patency of a central venous access device**

This is a simple procedure which may be performed after each use or once weekly when no therapy is necessary. For implantable ports the procedure requires the port to be accessed and flushed once a month (see Procedure guidelines, p. 756).

Equipment

1 Flushing solution ready prepared in a 10 ml syringe in a clinically clean container.

2 Chlorhexidine in 70% alcohol/swab saturated with 70% isopropyl alcohol.

Procedure guidelines: Maintaining patency of a central venous access device (cont'd)

Procedure

Action	Rationale
1 Explain and discuss the procedure with the patient.	To ensure that the patient understands the procedure and gives his/her valid consent.
2 Wash hands thoroughly or use an alcohol-based handrub.	To reduce the risk of contamination.
3 Clean the needleless injection cap using chlorhexidine in 70% alcohol/swab saturated with 70% isopropyl alcohol and apply with friction, rubbing the cap in a clockwise and anticlockwise manner at least 5 times.	To minimize the risk of contamination at the connections.
4 Attach the syringe to the needleless injection cap.	To establish connection between cap and syringe.
5 Using a push–pause method (inject 1 ml at a time), inject the contents of the syringe.	To create turbulence in order to flush the catheter thoroughly.
6 Maintain pressure on the plunger as the syringe is disconnected from the cap then clamp catheter if necessary.	To maintain positive pressure and prevent back-flow of blood into the catheter, and possible clot formation.
7 Dispose of equipment safely.	To prevent contamination of others.
8 Demonstrate the procedure clearly and methodically. Ensure patient receives written instructions.	To ensure the patient is aware of each step, and the need for good hand washing/drying techniques, etc., as he/she may be performing this procedure on discharge.

Procedure guidelines: **Taking blood samples from a central venous access device**

Obtaining blood samples from a central venous access device can lead to inaccurate results, especially coagulation values, if the correct method is not followed to ensure removal of any drug/solution prior to sampling (Frey 2002). A number of methods may be used to withdraw samples:

1 The discard method – this is the standard accepted method (recommended by The Royal Marsden Hospital) where the first 6–10 ml of blood is withdrawn and discarded (Holmes 1998; Cosca 1998). This ensures removal of any heparin or saline solution but may result in excessive blood removal in small children or those requiring multiple samples, e.g. for pharmacokinetic tests (Cosca 1998).

2 Push–pull/mixing method – a syringe is attached to the catheter, the catheter is flushed with 0.9% sodium chloride, then 6 ml is withdrawn and pushed back without removing the syringe; this is repeated three times. This removes any residual solution and reduces exposure to blood and there is no blood wastage (Holmes 1998).

This method supposes that mixing of blood eliminates intravenous fluids and heparin from the catheter lumen (Cosca 1998). However, it may be difficult to obtain enough blood for 3–4 times push/pull and there is a chance for haemolysis with agitation of blood (Frey 2002).

3 Reinfusion method – this method is performed by taking the first 6 ml of blood, capping off the syringe, taking the samples and then reinfusing the blood first taken (Keller 1994). It does not result in depleted blood volume but there is a risk of blood exposure, the discard syringe could be confused with the specimen sample and there could be contamination or clots in the sample for reinfusion (Frey 2002).

Whichever method is used, once the samples have been taken it is vital that the catheter is adequately flushed with sodium chloride to reduce the risk of clot formation and subsequent infection and/or occlusion.

It is preferable to use the proximal lumen of a multilumen catheter when obtaining a sample and where these catheters have different-sized lumens, the largest should be reserved for blood sampling.

Equipment

1 Sterile dressing pack.
2 Clamp for catheter, if necessary.
3 Alcohol-based hand wash solution.

4 Extra 10 ml blood bottle without heparin or sterile 10 ml syringe.

*Procedure guidelines: **Taking blood samples from a central venous access device** (cont'd)*

5 Vacuum system container holder (shell).
6 Vacuum system adaptor.
7 Appropriate vacuumed blood bottles (*or*)
8 Sterile syringe of appropriate size for sample required.

9 Needleless injection cap (as necessary).
10 10 ml syringe of 0.9% sodium chloride.
11 Flushing solution, as per policy.

Procedure

Action	Rationale
1 Explain and discuss the procedure with the patient. Check forms to ascertain sample bottles required and check patient's identity.	To ensure that the patient understands the procedure and gives his/her valid consent. To ensure correct bottles are used and blood is taken from correct patient.
2 Perform procedure using an aseptic technique.	To reduce the risk of infection. (For further information on asepsis see Ch. 4, Aseptic technique.)
3 Wash hands with bactericidal soap and water or bactericidal alcohol handrub.	To reduce the risk of cross-infection.
4 Prepare a tray or trolley and take it to the bedside. Clean hands as above. Open sterile pack and prepare equipment.	To reduce the risk of contamination of contents.
5 If intravenous fluid infusion is in progress, switch it off and clamp.	
6 Clean hands with a bactericidal alcohol handrub. Put on non-sterile gloves. Clean hub thoroughly with chlorhexidine. Allow to dry.	To minimize the risk of introducing infection into the catheter, and prevent contamination of practitioner's hands with blood. To enable disinfection process to be completed.
7 Where required, disconnect the administration set from the catheter and cover the end of the set with sterile cap.	To reduce the risk of contaminating the end of the administration set.
8 For vacuum sampling this is the method of choice and should always be attempted first:	
(a) Attach vacuum container holder and adaptor via the needleless injection cap and release clamp.	To maintain a closed system and prevent contamination of practitioner or air entry.
(b) Attach extra sample bottle: fill and discard.	To remove blood, heparin and intravenous fluids from the 'dead space' of the catheter. Samples from this 'dead space' are likely to cause inaccuracies in blood tests, because of the risk of contamination of the sample with heparin, sodium or dextrose, etc.
(c) Attach required sample bottles for requested specimens.	To obtain sample. It is not necessary to clamp the catheter when changing collection bottles, as the system is not open.
(d) Re-clamp catheter and detach vacuum container holder.	To prevent blood loss or air embolism.
9 For syringe sampling:	
(a) Attach a 10 ml syringe to the needleless injection cap. Release the clamp and withdraw 5–10 ml of blood.	To remove blood, heparin and intravenous fluids from the 'dead space' of the catheter. Samples from this 'dead space' are likely to cause inaccuracies in blood tests.
(b) Discard the sample and syringe.	
(c) Attach a new syringe of appropriate size. Withdraw the required amount of blood.	To obtain the sample.
(d) Detach the syringe.	
(e) Decant blood into sample bottles.	
10 Flush with 10 ml 0.9% sodium chloride, using the push–pause method (i.e. 1 ml at a time).	To create turbulence, ensure removal of all blood in the catheter and prevent occlusion.
11 Reconnect the administration set, unclamp the catheter and recommence infusion or attach new needleless	To prevent the catheter clotting between uses.

Procedure guidelines: Taking blood samples from a central venous access device (cont'd)

Action	Rationale
injection cap. Release clamp and flush catheter through injection cap using the push–pause method and finishing with the positive pressure technique.	
12 Ensure that blood samples have been placed in the correct containers and agitated as necessary to prevent clotting. Label them with patient's name, number, date of birth, etc., and send them to the laboratory with the appropriate forms.	To make certain that the specimens, correctly presented and identified, are delivered to the laboratory, enabling the requested tests to be performed and the results returned to the correct patient's records.

Difficulty may be encountered when taking blood samples. This is more common when the central venous catheter is made of silicone and has been in place for a long period of time. One of the causes is that the tip of the soft catheter lies against the wall of the vessel and the suction required to draw blood brings this into close contact, leading to temporary occlusion. There could also be a collapse of the catheter walls when using the vacuum system which may necessitate the use of syringes to obtain the blood.

Measures to try to dislodge the tip include asking the patient to:
1 Cough and breathe deeply
2 Roll from side to side
3 Raise his/her arms
4 Perform the Valsalva manoeuvre, if possible
5 Increase general activity, e.g. walk up and down stairs.

Pinch-off syndrome occurs when a central venous catheter inserted via the percutaneous subclavian site is compressed by the clavicle and first rib and aspirating blood becomes difficult (Andris & Krzywda 1997). The tip of the catheter may be covered in a fibrin sheath. This may be resolved with rapid flushing of the catheter with 0.9% sodium chloride or a dilute solution of heparin. Occasionally this results in persistent withdrawal occlusion (PWO) and may require a fibrinolytic agent (Ponec *et al.* 2001; Dietcher *et al.* 2002) to remove the fibrin (Mayo 1998). However, it may be necessary to take blood from a peripheral vein (see Ch. 45, Venepuncture).

Procedure guidelines: **Unblocking an occluded catheter**

Catheters may become occluded for a number of reasons, e.g. not being flushed adequately or using the incorrect flushing technique, infusion being switched off or running too slowly or precipitation formation due to inadequate flushing between solutions/drugs. Clearance of a catheter occlusion is best performed using a negative pressure approach. The establishment of negative pressure within a catheter means creating a vacuum by aspiration of the air or dead space within a catheter (Moureau *et al.* 1999). Unblocking a catheter is not a quick procedure and can take up to 30 minutes to achieve success.

Equipment

1 Sterile dressing pack.
2 Bactericidal handrub.
3 Alcohol-based skin cleaning preparation, e.g. chlorhexidine in 70% alcohol.
4 Extension set or needleless injection cap.

5 10 ml syringes.
6 0.9% sodium chloride.
7 Three-way tap.
8 Heparin 50 IU in a saline solution.

Procedure

Action	Rationale
1 Explain and discuss the procedure with the patient.	To ensure that the patient understands the procedure and gives his/her valid consent.
2 Perform the procedure using an aseptic technique.	To minimize the risk of infection. (For further information on asepsis see Ch. 4, Aseptic technique.)
3 Wash hands with bactericidal soap and water or bactericidal alcohol handrub. Place all equipment required on bottom shelf.	To minimize the risk of cross-infection.
4 Open a sterile pack and empty other equipment onto it.	To create a clean working area.

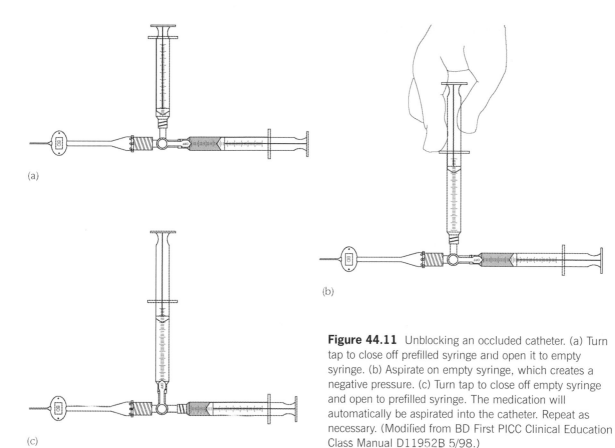

(a)

(b)

(c)

Figure 44.11 Unblocking an occluded catheter. (a) Turn tap to close off prefilled syringe and open it to empty syringe. (b) Aspirate on empty syringe, which creates a negative pressure. (c) Turn tap to close off empty syringe and open to prefilled syringe. The medication will automatically be aspirated into the catheter. Repeat as necessary. (Modified from BD First PICC Clinical Education Class Manual D11952B 5/98.)

*Procedure guidelines: **Unblocking an occluded catheter** (cont'd)*

Action	Rationale
5 Wash hands with bactericidal alcohol handrub.	Hands may have become contaminated by handling the outer packs, etc.
6 Clean connections thoroughly with chlorhexidine in 70% alcohol before disconnection.	To minimize infection risk at connection site.
7 Remove any extension sets or injection caps.	Occlusion may be in extension set/cap and not in catheter.
8 Attempt to flush with 0.9% sodium chloride using a 10 ml syringe.	Smaller syringes create excessive pressure which could result in catheter rupture.
9 If there is pressure within the catheter lumen, attempt to gently instil the 0.9% sodium chloride using a 'to and fro' motion (push–pull) over a few minutes.	To attempt to clear the catheter.
10 If nothing can be aspirated, attach a three-way tap and to this add an empty 10 ml syringe and a 10 ml syringe containing heparin 50 IU in 5 ml saline.	To commence the negative pressure technique (see Fig. 44.11a).
11 Attempt to unblock catheter using the negative pressure technique (see Fig. 44.11b,c).	This enables the solution to be drawn into catheter without creating any pressure which could result in catheter rupture.
12 If still unable to aspirate, then determine the cause of the occlusion:	
(a) Blood – discuss with doctors who may prescribe a fibrinolytic agent, e.g. urokinase, alteplase.	To break down fibrin.

Procedure guidelines: Unblocking an occluded catheter (cont'd)

Action	Rationale
(b) Precipitation – discuss with pharmacy for best antidote, e.g. ethyl alcohol or hydrochloric acid.	To break down drug precipitate or fat emulsion.
13 Draw up prescribed solution in a 10 ml syringe.	To prepare appropriate treatment.
14 Clean gloved hands with bactericidal alcohol handrub.	To minimize the risk of introducing infection.
15 Instil via a three-way tap using negative pressure technique (see above).	To prevent catheter rupture.
16 Cap off catheter and leave for allotted time, e.g. 2–4 hours or overnight.	To allow the drug to destroy fibrin.
17 Attach an empty syringe to catheter and attempt to aspirate any clots and solution.	To unblock catheter and ensure no clots are administered into the patient.
18 If blood returns, withdraw at least 10 ml and discard.	To ensure no fibrinolytic agent or clots are flushed into the patient.
19 Flush catheter with 10 ml 0.9% sodium chloride using a pulsatile flush and then flush with heparinized saline.	To ensure the catheter is flushed and patent.
20 Dispose of waste.	To prevent contamination of others.
21 If still unable to aspirate, discuss the use of a second instillation of fibrinolytic agent. It may be necessary to remove the catheter if a single lumen or if multilumen, to refrain from using the occluded lumen.	To maintain some venous access for the patient. If occlusion cannot be removed the catheter is no longer patent. In multilumen catheters there may be another patent lumen for use.

Procedure guidelines: **Insertion and removal of non-coring needles in implantable ports**

Placement of a non-coring 'Huber' point needle into the implantable port should be performed by a doctor or by nurses who have been specifically assessed as being competent to access ports. The needle may be connected to an extension set and a Luer–Lok injection cap placed at the end of this. The needle and extension set can remain in position for 7 days but will then need to be changed.

Equipment

1 Plastic apron.
2 Sterile gloves.
3 Dressing pack.
4 10 ml Luer–Lok syringes containing 0.9% sodium chloride ×2.

5 Non-coring (Huber point) needle with extension set.
6 Chlorhexidine in 70% alcohol.
7 Heparinized saline in 10 ml syringe.
8 Plaster.

Procedure

Action	Rationale
1 Explain and discuss the procedure with the patient.	To ensure the patient understands the procedure and gives his/her valid consent.
2 If required, apply topical local anaesthetic cream for 30–60 minutes.	To reduce the feeling of pain on insertion of the needle.
3 Place the patient in a comfortable position.	
4 Locate the port and identify the septum; assess the depth of the port and thickness of the skin.	In order to select correct length of needle.
5 Check length and type of therapy.	In order to select correct gauge and configuration of needle.
6 Wash hands using a bactericidal hand soap or rub.	To minimize the risk of contamination.
7 Put on sterile gloves.	To minimize the risk of contamination.
8 Flush port needle and extension set with 0.9% sodium chloride.	To check patency of needle and set.

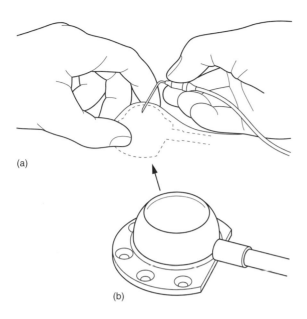

(a)

(b)

Figure 44.12 Flushing a port.

Procedure guidelines: **Insertion and removal of non-coring needles in implantable ports** *(cont'd)*

Action	Rationale
9 Clean the skin over the port with chlorhexidine 70% alcohol in a circular pattern. Allow to dry.	To minimize the risk of contamination and destroy skin flora. To ensure disinfection.
10 Holding the needle in the dominant hand, stabilize the port between the forefinger and index finger of the non-dominant hand (see Fig. 44.12).	To ensure the port is stabilized and will not move on insertion of the needle.
11 Inform the patient you are about to insert the needle.	To prepare the patient for a pushing sensation.
12 Using a perpendicular angle, push the needle through the skin until the needle hits the back plate.	To ensure the needle is well inserted into the portal septum.
13 Draw back on the syringe and check for blood return.	To check the needle is correctly placed and the port is patent.
14 Flush with 0.9% sodium chloride and observe the site for any swelling or pain.	To check for patency and correct positioning.
15 Administer the drug as required.	To carry out instructions as per prescription.
16 Flush with 10 ml 0.9% sodium chloride.	To ensure all of the drug is administered.
17 If the needle is to remain in situ, attach an injection cap and flush with heparinized saline using a pulsatile flush and ending with positive pressure.	To maintain patency.
18 Secure the needle by placing gauze under the needle if necessary and cover with transparent dressing.	To ensure the needle is well supported and will not become dislodged.
19 If needle is to be removed, then heparinize using 500 IU heparin in 5 ml 0.9% sodium chloride.	To maintain patency over a longer period of time, e.g. 1 month.
20 Maintain pressure on the plunger as syringe is disconnected from injection cap.	To prevent back-flow of blood and possible clot formation.
21 Press down on either side of the portal of the implantable port with two fingers.	To support the port while removing the needle.
22 Withdraw the needle using steady traction Discard needle in appropriate sharps container.	To prevent trauma to the skin and the risk of needlestick injury.
23 No dressing is usually required, but a small plaster may be applied.	To prevent oozing at the site.

Procedure guidelines: **Removal of a non-skin-tunnelled central venous catheter**

Equipment

As for Procedure guidelines: Changing the dressing on a central venous catheter insertion site (items 1–6; see p. 750) plus:

7 Sterile scissors.
8 Small sterile specimen container.
9 Stitch cutter.

10 Additional sterile low-linting gauze swab and sterile transparent dressing.

Procedure

Place patient flat in the Trendelenburg position, i.e. head slightly lower than feet (to prevent air entering vein on catheter removal) and then proceed as for a dressing procedure, steps 1–13 (p. 751); then continue as follows:

Action	Rationale
14 Clean the insertion site.	To prevent contamination of the catheter on removal, and a false-positive culture result.
15 Discontinue the infusion, if in progress. Clamp the catheter.	To prevent entry of air or leakage of blood when the catheter is disconnected.
16 Clean gloved hands with a bactericidal alcohol handrub.	To minimize the risk of infection after handling unsterile parts of the system.
17 Cut and remove any skin suture securing the catheter and disconnect the infusion system from the catheter.	To facilitate removal and to ease handling and removal.
18 Ask the patient to perform the Valsalva manoeuvre.	To reduce the risk of air embolus.
19 Cover the insertion site with low-linting gauze.	Swabs are used to discourage the entry of organisms into the insertion site and to absorb any leakage of blood.
20 Hold the catheter with one hand near the point of insertion and pull firmly and gently. As the catheter begins to move, press firmly down on the site with the swabs. Maintain pressure on the swabs for about 5 minutes after the catheter has been removed.	Pressure is applied to prevent haemorrhage and to encourage resealing of the vein wall. It also prevents the entry of air into the vein. Continued pressure is necessary to allow time for the puncture in the vein to close.
21 If the catheter is removed because of infection, carefully cut off the tip (approximately 5 cm) of the catheter using sterile scissors and place it in a sterile container for microbiological investigation.	To detect any infection related to the catheter, and thus provide necessary treatment.
22 When bleeding has stopped (approximately 5 minutes), cover site with transparent dressing.	To detect any infection at exit site. To prevent air entering the vein via the site.
23 Fold up the sterile field, place it in the yellow clinical waste bag and seal it before moving the trolley. Dispose of the equipment in the appropriate containers.	To reduce the risk of environmental contamination.
24 Make the patient comfortable.	

Procedure guidelines: **Surgical removal of a skin-tunnelled central venous catheter**

Equipment

1 Plastic apron.
2 Sterile gloves.
3 Minor operations set.

4 10 ml Luer–Lok syringe.
5 25 G needle.
6 21 G needle.

*Procedure guidelines: **Surgical removal of a skin-tunnelled central venous catheter** (cont'd)*

7 10 ml plain lidocaine 1%.
8 10 × 10 cm low-linting gauze swabs ×5.
9 3/0 Mersilk suture on a curved needle.

10 2 cm hypoallergenic tape.
11 Chlorhexidine in 70% alcohol.
12 Steristrips (to be used if necessary).

Procedure

Action	Rationale
1 Check the patient's full blood count and clotting profile for that day.	To ensure that the patient is not at risk of bleeding or infection from this invasive procedure. The platelets should be above 100×10^9/litre, the white blood count >2 and the international normalized ratio (INR) <1.3.
2 Explain and discuss the procedure with the patient.	To ensure that the patient understands the procedure and gives his/her valid consent.
3 Screen the bed and ask patient to remove clothing down to the waist.	To ensure ease of access to the patient's chest.
4 Ask patient to lie as flat as possible with his or her arms by his/her sides.	To minimize the risk of bleeding from gravitational pressure and to dissuade the patient from touching the sterile field.
5 Palpate and identify the position of the cuff in the patient.	To locate the area for the incision.
6 If the cuff cannot easily be felt, measure 22 cm up from the bifurcation at the end of the catheter distal to the patient dependent on the type of catheter in situ (see Fig. 44.7), then palpate again. If it still cannot be felt ask for assistance from a more experienced colleague.	To locate the probable site of the cuff. To guard against malplaced incisions.
7 Open the outer bag of the minor operation pack. Put on plastic apron and wash hands, then dry hands on sterile towel provided in the pack.	To reduce risk of infection.
8 Accept and put on sterile gloves from assistant and assemble all necessary equipment on the sterile pack.	To maintain asepsis and to prepare for the procedure and maximize efficiency.
9 Advise the patient that you will explain each step of the procedure as you go along if the patient wishes.	This should take into account the patient's individual wish for information.
10 Clean the area directly over the cuff with swabs soaked in chlorhexidine in 70% alcohol. Use a circular motion working out from the centre directly over the cuff. Allow the area to dry.	To reduce the risk of infection. To enable disinfection process to be completed. To prevent stinging on insertion of the needle.
11 Position the two sterile towels – one horizontally across the waist and the other longitudinally down the side of the patient between you and the patient.	To create a sterile field to operate within and therefore reduce the risk of infection.
12 Inform the patient that you are about to administer the local anaesthetic and that this will cause a stinging sensation.	To prepare the patient. The first injection can be painful and causes a stinging sensation.
13 With a 25 G needle, administer the first millilitre of local anaesthetic intradermally directly over the cuff site causing a raised bleb.	To commence the numbing of the area to be incised. To provide a raised area for the next injection and identification of the site.
14 Give a further 1–2 ml of local anaesthetic subcutaneously using the bleb as the area for the insertion of the needle, but directing the needle out and around the area of the cuff site area.	To reduce pain for the patient with repeated injections. To ensure all the incision area is numb.
15 Attach the 21 G needle and with the last remaining 4 ml of local anaesthetic give two deeper injections to either side of the cuff area.	To ensure anaesthesia at a deeper level during the blunt dissection around the cuff.

Problem solving (cont'd)

Problem	Cause	Suggested action
Oedema of the arm on the side of the catheter insertion, may be associated with pain or limb discoloration.	Thoracic duct injury at insertion, resulting in alterations in lymph flow.	Inform a doctor. Removal of the catheter is usually necessary.
Oedema/pain and tenderness of arm, neck and/or chest. Engorged peripheral veins or feelings of tightness.	Thrombosis in major vessel due to irritation/damage by foreign body (catheter).	Report to doctor. Ultrasound and/or venogram may be performed and anticoagulant therapy commenced. May be prevented by use of low-dose warfarin during dwell time. May necessitate removal of catheter.
Pyrexia, tachycardia, rigors indicating systemic infection.	Infection due to poor aseptic technique.	Culture of the blood is required from the catheter and patient's peripheral blood. Take a swab of the insertion site, employing strict asepsis and minimum handling of the equipment. Administer antimicrobials as prescribed. Observe the patient closely. Removal of the catheter is sometimes indicated.
Leakage of fluid onto the dressing.	Loose connection in the system. Cracking of catheter or hub.	Check and tighten connections. Report to the relevant nursing staff and/or doctors. Repair may be possible.
Catheter required for many functions, e.g. blood sampling and extra drug administration.	Limited routes of access available to satisfy the patient's requirements.	Consider multilumen catheter before insertion. Use simple regimens and methods of administration. Use extension sets and administration sets available for this purpose. May require additional peripheral access.
Fluid overload resulting in dyspnoea, oedema, raised pulse rate and blood pressure.	Infusion is too fast. Inaccurate fluid monitoring.	Revise the patient's fluid intake regimen. Use flow control devices. Keep accurate records of the patient's fluid balance and weight. Inform a doctor. Patient may require diuretics.
Potential pulmonary embolus due to catheter tip embolus. Symptoms include chest pain, cool clammy skin, haemoptysis, tachycardia, hypotension.	Occasionally occurs after the removal of the catheter especially when using traction method for removal of skin-tunnelled catheter.	Check catheter length where possible and check integrity of catheter on removal. Avoid using the traction method. Notify a doctor immediately if the patient develops any of the related symptoms.
Bleeding at the insertion site following removal of the catheter.	Opening in the vein wall. Low platelets, anticoagulant therapy.	Apply pressure over the site with sterile low-linting swabs, until bleeding has stopped. Patients prescribed warfarin or heparin will require a longer period of pressure to compensate for the prolonged clotting time. Apply sterile transparent dressing. If bleeding persists, the doctor must be informed.
Pyrexia of unknown origin.	Could be related to CVAD.	Do not remove catheter until site of infection confirmed (unless clinical condition dictates otherwise). Inform doctors. Carry out investigations such as 'blood cultures' (from catheter and peripheral vein), swab of entry site, full blood count, midstream urine, chest X-ray, swabs of areas that could be the source of infection, e.g. throat or wound swabs. If catheter removed, tip should be sent for bacteriological examination.

In addition, the problem solving list associated with intravenous management (Ch. 9, Drug administration) may contain useful and relevant information.

Arterial cannulae

Definition

An arterial cannula is a cannula generally inserted into a peripheral artery, most commonly the radial and dorsalis pedis. The femoral artery can be cannulated if it is not possible to cannulate a peripheral artery, particularly if the patient is haemodynamically compromised, i.e. hypotensive. This is because the femoral artery is accessible and there is 'relative' ease in palpating a weak pulse (Adams & Osbourne 1997).

Reasons for arterial cannulation

- To gain continuous and accurate direct measurement of interarterial blood pressure. Arterial pressures do vary depending upon cannulation location. The blood pressure measured from the dorsalis pedis and radial artery will be higher than that in the femoral artery due to the greater distance from the heart to the smaller vessel lumen, and may not necessarily reflect the perfusion pressure in other regions (Adams & Osbourne 1997). Oh (1997) suggests that the tubing should be non-compliant and <1 m in length.
- For ease of access to blood, thereby avoiding the discomfort of frequent punctures, e.g. regular testing for blood gases, full blood counts, coagulation and urea and electrolytes, and the subsequent risk of infection (Hicks Keen 1997).

Indications

- During and following major surgery involving prolonged anaesthesia, e.g. major intracavity surgery for longer than 1 hour
- Monitoring of acid–base balance and respiratory status in:
  - (a) Acute respiratory failure
  - (b) Mechanical ventilation, especially in response to alteration of support and oxygenation
  - (c) The period during and after cardiorespiratory arrest
  - (d) Severe sepsis
  - (e) Shock conditions
  - (f) Major trauma
  - (g) Acute poisoning
  - (h) Acute renal failure
  - (i) Severe diabetic ketoacidosis
- Patients who require continuous arterial monitoring, e.g. those who are critically ill, or after cardiac surgery. Such patients typically receive intravenous nitrates and numerous inotropic drugs, glyceryl trinitrate and

specifically adrenaline (epinephrine). These drugs have to be titrated as they have a direct impact on mean arterial pressures (MAP), making direct, accurate and continuous measurement of MAP essential for safe practice (Hicks Keen 1997). It should be noted that wave artefacts will affect haemodynamic measurements.

Reference material

Direct haemodynamic monitoring is performed more frequently because there is more awareness of the need for patient safety, and one of these methods, intra-arterial pressure monitoring, is used in operating theatres, recovery rooms, critical care facilities and very rarely on specialized wards and during interhospital transfer of acutely ill patients (Allan 1984; Royal College of Anaesthetists 1990). The monitoring systems necessary and the hazard of disconnection and severe haemorrhage limit its use to specialized areas where personnel are skilled in its care and management. In the event of disconnection the flow from an 18 G cannula can result in blood loss of 500 ml/minute (Oh 1997).

The most convenient site for arterial cannulation is either radial artery (Weinstein 2000). The arterial cannula should not be positioned close to an adjoining intravenous cannula as this may compromise blood flow to the adjoining structures. The radial artery passes along the lateral aspect of the forearm and then through the wrist and hand, supplying these structures with blood. At the wrist the radial artery contacts the distal end of the radius, where it is covered only by fascia and skin. Because of its superficial location at this point it is the most common site for palpating the radial pulse (Tortora 2002).

Before the insertion of a radial artery cannula, circulation to the hand should be evaluated by assessing the circulation of the palmar arch using the Allen test. More than 97% patients have adequate flow through collaterals to prevent ischaemia should either the radial or ulnar artery be interrupted (Durbin 2001). The Allen test should therefore be completed prior to arterial cannulation in order to establish whether there is adequate blood supply to the wrist (see Fig. 44.13). The Allen test consists of simultaneously compressing both the ulnar and radial arteries for approximately 1 minute. During this time, the patient rapidly opens and closes the hand to promote exsanguination (Fig. 44.13a). Approximately 5 seconds after release of the artery (usually the ulnar), the extended hand should blush owing to capillary refilling (Fig. 44.13b). This reactive hyperaemia indicates adequate circulation in the hand. If blanching occurs, palmar arch circulation is inadequate and a

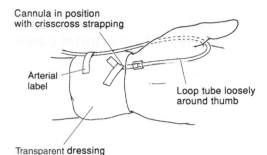

Figure 44.14 Positioning, securing and labelling of cannula.

Procedure guidelines: **Setting up the monitoring set and preparation for insertion of an arterial cannula** *(cont'd)*

Action	Rationale
19 Apply transparent dressing and tape tubing securely. Clearly label 'arterial' (Fig. 44.14).	Leaving the site visible allows the observer to recognize immediately any dislodgement or disconnection. Clear labelling prevents accidental injection of drugs.
20 When the patient is awake, loop the tube around the thumb, ensuring that it is not too tight.	To minimize movement of cannula and damage to vessel. To avoid a pressure ulcer forming.
21 Inform patient of amount of movement permitted, e.g. fingers and arm may be moved gently. Discourage any stress on arm and connections.	To prevent dislodgement.

Procedure guidelines: **Taking a blood sample from an arterial cannula**

Care must be taken not to introduce air or infection and to ensure that three-way tap is left in closed position. The following volumes of blood should be taken and discarded depending on type and use of arterial cannula:

- Peripheral artery cannula – take 3 ml and discard
- Femoral artery cannula – take 5 ml and discard
- Heparinized flush system – take at least 5 ml regardless of site and discard
- Arterial blood gases only – take 3–5 ml and discard
- Other samples, e.g. full blood count, biochemistry – use vacuum system and take one bottle and discard.

Equipment

1 Intravenous sterile dressing pack.
2 Gloves.
3 Appropriate syringes and blood sample bottles, dependent on samples required.

4 Chlorhexidine in 70% alcohol.
5 Bactericidal alcohol handrub.

Procedure

Action	Rationale
1 Explain and discuss the procedure with the patient.	To ensure that the patient understands the procedure and gives his/her valid consent.
2 Prepare the trolley.	To ensure all equipment is ready.
3 Wash hands with bactericidal soap and water or bactericidal alcohol handrub before leaving clinical room.	To minimize the risk of cross-infection.
4 Check that the three-way tap (Fig. 44.15a) is closed.	To prevent back-flow of blood and blood spillage.
5 Clean hands with bactericidal alcohol handrub.	Hands have been contaminated by touching three-way tap.

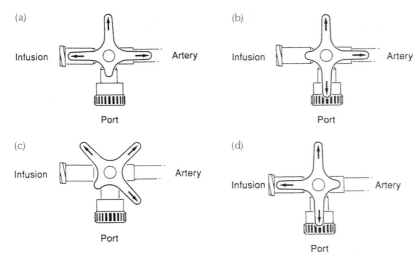

Figure 44.15 Three-way tap: (a) closed to port; (b) turned to artery and port; (c) turned diagonally to close off infusion, artery and port; (d) turned to infusion and port.

Procedure guidelines: **Taking a blood sample from an arterial cannula** *(cont'd)*

Action	Rationale
6 Prepare trolley as described in Ch. 4, Procedure guidelines: Aseptic technique.	
7 Apply gloves. (See Ch. 4 for safe technique and procedure guidelines.)	To prevent contamination of hands with blood.
8 Press silence button on arterial monitor for duration of sampling. Remove cap from three-way tap (Fig. 44.15a) and clean open port with a swab soaked in chlorhexidine in 70% alcohol.	The continual alarm disturbs both patient and others in the unit. To minimize the risk of infection.
9 Connect 5 ml syringe to open port.	
10 Turn three-way tap to artery and port (Fig. 44.15b).	To prevent contamination of blood sample with heparinized saline.
11 Slowly withdraw appropriate volume (see above) of blood until the cannula is clear of infusion fluid.	To prevent contamination of blood with infusion fluid.
12 Turn three-way tap diagonally to close off infusion, artery and port (Fig. 44.15c).	To prevent back-flow of blood from artery, contamination with infusion fluid and blood spillage.
13 Remove syringe and discard.	
14 Connect blood gas syringe.	In order to take the required amount of blood.
15 Turn three-way tap to artery and port (Fig. 44.15b).	To prevent contamination with infusion fluid.
16 Slowly remove the amount of blood.	To prevent any spasm in vessel. To ensure adequate mix with the heparin.
17 Turn three-way tap diagonally to close off infusion, artery and port (Fig. 44.15c).	To prevent back-flow of blood and blood spillage.
18 Remove syringe.	
19 Turn three-way tap to infusion and port (Fig. 44.15d). Flush by squeezing actuator (see instructions with set)	To prevent blood clotting in port.
20 Turn three-way tap to infusion and artery (Fig. 44.15a). Flush cannula gently by squeezing actuator. As cannula is flushed observe digits for signs of blanching, discoloration or complaints of pain from the patient.	To clear blood from cannula. To ensure early recognition of proximal or distal embolization.
21 Clean port with chlorhexidine in 70% alcohol swab.	To minimize the risk of infection.
22 Apply sterile Luer–Lok cap and check it is secure.	To prevent haemorrhage or blood spillage.
23 Check pressure infuser cuff is inflated to 300 mmHg.	To prevent back-flow of blood into circuit.
24 Analyse or send to nearest blood gas analyser.	To ensure identity of sample is correct.

Procedure guidelines: **Removal of an arterial cannula**

Equipment

1 Intravenous sterile dressing pack.
2 Gloves.

3 Hypoallergenic tape.
4 Chlorhexidine in 70% alcohol.

Procedure

Action	Rationale
1 Explain and discuss the procedure with the patient.	To ensure that the patient understands the procedure and gives his/her valid consent.
2 Check for PT, INR levels.	Removal may be delayed until coagulation is corrected.
3 Prepare trolley as described in Ch. 4, Procedure guidelines: Aseptic technique.	
4 Wash hands with bactericidal soap and water or bactericidal alcohol handrub before leaving clinical room.	To reduce the risk of cross-infection.
5 Prepare trolley by patient as described in Ch. 4, Procedure guidelines: Aseptic technique.	
6 Turn three-way tap diagonally (Fig. 44.15c).	To prevent back-flow of blood into cannula.
7 Turn off intravenous set.	To prevent spillage when removing cannula.
8 Deflate pressure cuff.	Pressure no longer required.
9 Loosen transparent dressing and tape from cannula site.	To enable easy removal of cannula.
10 Clean hands with a bactericidal skin cleaning solution.	
11 Apply gloves. (See Ch. 4 for safe technique and procedure guidelines.)	To prevent contamination of hands with blood.
12 Remove dressing and tape. Clean cannula site area with chlorhexidine in 70% alcohol.	To reduce the risk of infection.
13 Place sterile piece of gauze over area and gently remove cannula.	To minimize bleeding.
14 Apply pressure to site for a minimum of 5 minutes or until bleeding stops.	To prevent a haematoma and blood loss.
15 Apply a clean, sterile, low-linting gauze dressing using a non-touch technique.	To maintain asepsis.
16 Apply Elastoplast.	To ensure pressure and prevent haematoma or blood loss.

Following this procedure, check the patient's hand hourly or as frequently as required for warmth, colour, swelling and signs of bleeding. Ask the patient to inform staff if feeling faint or if there is oozing from the dressing. Avoid blood pressure measurement being taken manually on that arm for 12–24 hours to minimize further bleeding or haematoma development. The medical staff must be informed immediately if the hand or forearm becomes discoloured or swollen, or if the patient complains of pain in the limb. Then information must also be carefully documented in the patient's care plan and medical notes. Request for photograph to be taken.

Problem solving

Problem	Cause	Suggested preventive care
Haemorrhage. Severe haemorrhage (hypovolaemia).	Luer–Lok connections are loose or cracked. Blood will be lost from open connection.	Check that Luer locks are fitted securely. Do not force because the locks may crack.
	Blood may ooze around the cannula site.	Place a transparent dressing over the cannula site and observe hourly or more frequently as the situation requires.
	Accidental disconnection.	

Problem solving (cont'd)

Problem	Cause	Suggested preventive care
	Cannula may have become dislodged.	Inform the patient about the danger of dislodging the cannula and amount of movement that is preferred. Take care when moving the patient. Avoid putting stress on the arm and connections. Secure the cannula (Fig. 44.14).
Back-flow of blood into the cannula.	The pressure infusor cuff may not be inflated to the optimal pressure.	Ensure that the pressure infusor cuff is inflated to 300 mmHg. This pressure is higher than arterial blood pressure and an automatic flush mode is activated in the system which delivers 3 ml/hour. This maintains patency of circuit, cannula and artery (Allan 1984).
Ischaemia.	A thrombosis may have formed in the circuit cannula or artery.	Ensure that heparin is added to the saline infusion (Clifton *et al.* 1991). Assess limb pulse, colour and temperature hourly, or more frequently as required. Absent pulses, pallor, cyanosis and coldness denote occlusion. If this occurs, medical advice must be sought and the cannula removed promptly (Hinds 1987).
Erythema or inflammation around the insertion site.	Phlebitis due to sepsis, chemical irritation or mechanical irritation.	Refer to the Problem-solving tips in Ch. 9, Drug administration.
Hypotension, tachycardia, cyanosis, unconsciousness.	Embolism: air particle	Refer to the procedure in Ch. 9, Drug administration.
Arterial spasm.	Forceful flushing or forceful aspiration when withdrawing blood.	Avoid forceful flushing or aspiration and maintain a slow even pressure when withdrawing blood.
Necrosis.	Accidental injection of a drug into the artery, causing local necrosis to vessel wall.	Label the arterial cannula and circuit clearly (Fig. 44.14). In the event of accidental injection of any drug, report the error immediately to medical staff and the senior nurse and perform the following: (a) Gently withdraw blood from the three-way tap to try to withdraw the drug. (b) Stop administering the drug. (c) Assess limb pulse, colour and temperature hourly, or more frequently if required. (d) Complete an accident form and/or other relevant documentation.

References and further reading

Adams, S. & Osbourne, S. (1997) Monitoring the critically ill patient. In: *Critical Care Nursing: Science & Practice*. Oxford University Press, Oxford, pp. 101–4.

Allan, D. (1984) Care of the patient with an arterial catheter. *Nurs Times*, **80**(46), 40–1.

Anderson, K.N. & Anderson, L.E. (eds) (1995) *Mosby's Pocket Dictionary of Nursing, Medicine and Professions Allied to Medicine*. Mosby, London.

Andris, D.A. & Krzywda, E.A. (1997) Catheter pinch off syndrome: recognition and management. *J Intravenous Nurs*, **20**(5), 233–7.

Archis, C.A., Black, J. & Brown, M.A. (2000) Does an endoluminal catheter brush improve flows or unblock haemodialysis catheters? *Nephrology*, **5**, 55–8.

Bagnell, H. & Reeb (1998) Diagnosis of central venous access device occlusions: implications for nursing practice. *J Intravenous Nurs*, 21(Suppl 5), S115–21.

Bahruth, A.J. (1996) PICC insertion problems associated with topical anesthesia. *J Intravenous Nurs*, 19(1), 32–4.

Baranowski, L. (1993) Central venous access devices – current technologies, uses and management strategies. *J Intravenous Nurs*, 16(3), 167–94.

Bassetti, S. et al. (2001) Prolonged antimicrobial activity of a catheter containing chlorhexidine silver sulfadiazine extends protection against catheter infection in vivo. *Antimicrob Agents Chemother*, 45, 1535–8.

Benton, S. & Marsden, C. (2002) Training nurses to place tunnelled central venous catheters. *Prof Nurse*, 17(9), 531–5.

Berger, L. (2000) The effects of positive pressure devices on catheter occlusions. *J Vasc Access Devices*, 5(4), 31–3.

Biffi, R. et al. (2001) A randomised prospective trial of central venous ports connected to standard open ended or groshong catheters in adult oncology patients. *Cancer*, 92(5), 1204–12.

BMA (1991) *A Code of Practice for the Safe Use and Disposal of Sharps*. British Medical Association, London, pp. 20–1.

BMA & RPS (2003) *British National Formulary*. British Medical Association and Royal Pharmaceutical Society, London.

Bow, E.J., Kirkpatrick, M.G. & Clinch, J.J. (1999) Totally implantable venous access ports systems for patients receiving chemotherapy for solid tissue malignancies. *J Clin Oncol*, 17(4), 1267.

Bregenzer, T. (1998) Is routine replacement necessary? *Arch Intern Med*, 158, 151–6.

Brown, J. & Larson, M. (1999) Pain during insertion of peripheral intravenous catheters with or without intradermal lidocaine. *Clin Nurse Specialist*, 13, 283–5.

Brown, J.D. et al. (1997) The potential for catheter microbial contamination from a needleless connector. *J Hosp Infect*, 36, 181–9.

Browne, J. et al. (1999) Topical ametocaine (Ametop) is superior to EMLA for intravenous cannulation. *Can J Anesth*, 46, 1014–18.

BSI (1997) *Sterile Single Use Intravascular Catheters, Part 1: General Requirements*, BSEN ISO 10555–1 1997. British Standards Institution, London.

Carlson, K., Perdue, M.B. & Hankins, J. (2001) Infection control. In: *Infusion Therapy in Clinical Practice*, 2nd edn (eds J. Hankin et al.). W.B. Saunders, Philadelphia, pp. 126–40.

Carlson, K.R. (1999) Correct utilisation and management of PICCs and midline catheters in the alternate care setting. *J Intravenous Nurs*, 22(Suppl 6), S46–50.

Catney, M.R. et al. (2001) Relationship between peripheral IV catheter dwell time and the development of phlebitis and infiltration. *J Intravenous Nurs*, 24(5), 332–41.

Chernecky, L. (2001) Satisfaction versus dissatisfaction with venous access devices in outpatient oncology: a pilot study. *Oncol Nurs Forum*, 28(10), 1613–16.

Ciano, B.A. (2001) Hemodynamic monitoring. In: *Infusion Therapy in Clinical Practice*, 2nd edn (eds J. Hankin et al.). W.B. Saunders, Philadelphia.

Clifton, G.D. et al. (1991) Comparison of 0.9% sodium chloride and heparin solutions for maintenance of arterial catheter patency. *Heart Lung*, 20(2), 115–18.

Cole, D. (1999) Selection and management of central venous access devices in the home setting. *J Intravenous Nurs*, 22(6), 315–19.

Collin, G.R. (1999) Decreasing catheter colonisation through the use of an antiseptic impregnated catheter: a continuous quality improvement project. *Chest*, 115, 1632–40.

Conn, C. (1993) The importance of syringe size when using an implanted vascular access device. *J Vasc Access Networks*, 3(1), 11–18.

Cook, D. et al. (1997) Central venous catheter replacement strategies: a systemic review of the literature. *Crit Care Med*, 25(8), 1417–24.

Cosca, P.A., Smith, S., Chatfield, S. et al. (1998) Reinfusion of discard blood from venous access devices. *Oncol Nurs Forum*, 25(6), 73–6.

Crawford, M. et al. (2000) Peripherally inserted central catheter program. *Nurs Clin North Am*, 35(2), 349–59.

Daniels, L.E. (1995) The physical and psychosocial implications of central venous access devices in cancer patients: a review of the literature. *J Cancer Care*, 4, 141–5.

Darouiche, R.O. (1999) A comparison of two antimicrobial impregnated central venous catheters. *N Engl J Med*, 340, 1–8.

Davidson, T. & Al Mufti, R. (1997) Hickman central venous catheters in cancer patients. *Cancer Topics*, 10(8), 10–14.

Dennis, A.R., Leeson-Payne, C.G., Langham, B.T. & Aikenhead, A.R. (1995) Local anaesthesia for cannulation – has practice changed? *Anaesthesia*, 50, 400–2.

Dick, M.J., Maree, S.M. & Gray, J. (1992) How to boost the odds of a painless IV start. *Am J Nurs*, 6, 49–50.

Dietcher, S.R. et al. (2002) Safety and efficacy of alteplase for restoring function in occluded central venous catheters: results of the Cardiovascular Thrombolytic to Open Occluded Lines trial. *J Clin Oncol*, 20(1), 317–24.

DoH (2001) Guidelines for preventing infections associated with the insertion and maintenance of central venous catheters. *J Hosp Infect*, 47(Suppl), S47–67.

Dougherty, L. (1994) *A study to discover how cancer patients perceive the intravenous cannulation experience*. Unpublished MSc thesis, University of Surrey, Guildford.

Dougherty, L. (1996) Intravenous cannulation. *Nurs Stand*, 11(2), 47–51.

Dougherty, L. (1999) Obtaining peripheral vascular access. In: *Intravenous Therapy in Nursing Practice* (eds L. Dougherty & J. Lamb). Churchill Livingstone, Edinburgh.

Dougherty, L., Viner, C. & Young, J. (1998) Establishing ambulatory chemotherapy at home. *Prof Nurse*, 13(6), 356–60.

Durbin, C.G. (2001) Radial arterial lines and sticks: what are the risks? *Repair Care*, 46(3), 229–31.

Fetzer, S.J. (2002) Reducing venipuncture and intravenous insertion pain with eutectic mixture of local anesthetic: a meta analysis. *Nurs Res*, 51, 119–24.

Fitzsimmons, C.L., Gilleece, M.H., Ranson, M.R. et al. (1997) Central venous catheter placement: extending the role of the nurse. *J R Coll Phys London*, 31(5), 533–5.

Fletcher, S.J. & Bodenham, A.R. (1999) Catheter related sepsis: an overview – part 1. *Br J Intensive Care*, 9(2), 46–53.

Frey, A.M. (2001) IV therapy in children. In: *Infusion Therapy in Clinical Practice*, 2nd edn (eds J. Hankin *et al.*). W.B. Saunders, Philadelphia.

Frey, A.M. (2002) Drawing labs from venous access devices. *Presentation at NAVAN 15th Annual Conference, Virginia*, January.

Frezza, E.E. & Mezghebe, H. (1998) Indications and complications of arterial catheter use in surgical or medical intensive care units. Analysis of 4932 patients. *Am Surg*, **64**(2), 127–31.

Fry, C. & Aholt, D. (2001) Local anaesthetic prior to insertion of a PICC. *J Intravenous Nurs*, **24**(6), 404–8.

Gabriel, J. (1999) Long term central venous access. In: *Intravenous Therapy in Nursing Practice* (eds L. Dougherty & J. Lamb). Churchill Livingstone, Edinburgh.

Gabriel, J. (2000) What patients think of a PICC. *J Vasc Access Devices*, **5**(4), 26–9.

Gabriel, J. (2001) PICC securement: minimising potential complications. *Nurs Stand*, **15**(43), 42–4.

Galinkin, J.L. *et al.* (2002) Lidocaine iontophoresis versus eutectic mixture of local anaesthetics (EMLA) for IV placement in children. *Anesth Analg*, **94**(6), 1484–8.

Gamby, A. & Bennett, J. (1995) A feasibility study of the use of non-heparinised 0.9% sodium chloride for transduced arterial and venous lines. *Intensive Crit Care Nurs*, **11**(3), 148–50.

Goetz, A.M., Miller, J., Wagener, M.M. & Muder, R.R. (1998) Complications related to intravenous midline catheter usage. *J Intravenous Nurs*, **21**(2), 76–80.

Goode, C.J. *et al.* (1991) A meta analysis of effects of heparin flush and saline flush – quality and cost implications. *Nurs Res*, **40**(6), 324–30.

Goodman, M. (2000) Chemotherapy: principles of administration. In: *Cancer Nursing* (eds C. Henke Yarbro *et al.*). Jones & Bartlett, Boston.

Goodwin, M. & Carlson, I. (1993) The peripherally inserted catheter: a retrospective look at 3 years of insertions. *J Intravenous Nurs*, **16**(2), 92–103.

Hadaway, L. (1998a) Catheter connection. *J Vasc Access Devices*, **3**(3), 40.

Hadaway, L. (1998b) Major thrombotic and non thrombotic complications: loss of patency. *J Intravenous Nurs*, **21**(Suppl 5), S143.

Hadaway, L. (2000) Peripheral IV therapy in adults. In: *Self Study Workbook*. Hadaway Associates, Georgia.

Hadaway, L. (2001) Anatomy and physiology related to intravenous therapy. In: *Infusion Therapy in Clinical Practice*, 2nd edn (eds J. Hankin *et al.*). W.B. Saunders, Philadelphia.

Haire, W.D. & Herbst, S.F. (2000) Use of alteplase. *J Vasc Access Devices*, **5**(2), 28–36.

Hamilton, H., O'Byrne, M. & Nicholai, L. (1995) Central lines inserted by clinical nurse specialists. *Nurs Times*, **91**(17), 38–9.

Hanchett, M. (1999) Science of IV securement. *J Vasc Access Devices*, **4**(3), 9–15.

Heath, J. & Jones, S. (2001) Utilisation of an elastomeric continuous infusion device to maintain catheter patency. *J Intravenous Nurs*, **24**(2), 102–6.

Hicks Keen, J. (1997) *Critical Care Nursing Consultant*. Mosby, St Louis.

Hinds, C.J. (1987) *Intensive Care*. Ballière Tindall, Gillingham.

Holcombe, B.J. *et al.* (1992) Restoring patency of long term central venous access devices. *J Intravenous Nurs*, **15**, 36–41.

Holmes, K. (1998) Comparison of push–pull versus discard method from central venous catheters for blood testing. *J Intravenous Nurs*, **21**(5), 282–5.

Homer, L.D. & Holmes, K.R. (1998) Risks associated with 72 and 96 hour peripheral IV catheter dwell times. *J Intravenous Nurs*, **21**(5), 301–5.

Hudek, K. (1986) Compliance in intravenous therapy. *J Can Intravenous Assoc*, **2**(3), 3–8.

ICNA (2003) Reducing sharps injury – prevention and risk management. Infection Control Nurses Association, February.

INS (2000) *Standards for Infusion Therapy*. Infusion Nurses Society, Massachusetts.

Jackson, D. (2001) Infection control principles and practices in the care and management of VADs: alternate care settings. *J Intravenous Nurs*, **24**(Suppl 3), S28–34.

Kamimoto, V. & Olson, K. (1996) Using normal saline to lock peripheral intravenous catheters in ambulatory cancer patients. *J Intravenous Nurs*, **19**(2), 75–8.

Kayley, J. (1999) IV therapy in the community. In: *IV Therapy in Nursing Practice* (eds L. Dougherty & J. Lamb). Churchill Livingstone, Edinburgh.

Keenleyside, D. (1993) Avoiding an unnecessary outcome. A comparative trial between IV 3000 and a conventional film dressing to assess rates of catheter related sepsis. *Prof Nurse*, February, 288–91.

Keller, C.A. (1994) Method of drawing blood samples through central venous catheters in paediatric patients undergoing bone marrow transplants – results of a national survey. *Oncol Nurs Forum*, **21**(5), 879–84.

Keradag, A. & Gorgulu, S. (2000) Vialon better than Teflon. *J Intravenous Nurs*, **23**(3), 158–66.

Kerrison, T. & Woodhull, J. (1994) Reducing the risk of thrombophlebitis – comparison of Teflon and Vialon cannulae. *Prof Nurse*, **9**(10), 662–6.

Kulkarni, M. (1994) Heparinised saline vs normal saline in maintaining patency of the radial artery catheter. *Can J Surg*, **37**(1), 37–42.

Kupensky, D.T. (1998) Applying current research to influence clinical practice – utilization of midline catheters. *J Intravenous Nurs*, **21**(5), 271–4.

La Rue, G.D. (2000) Efficacy of ultrasonography in peripheral venous cannulation. *J Intravenous Nurs*, **23**(1), 29–34.

Lenhart, C. (2000) Prevention vs treatment of vascular access devices occlusions. *J Vasc Access Devices*, **5**(4), 34–5.

Lonsway, R.A. (2001) IV therapy in the home. In: *Infusion Therapy in Clinical Practice*, 2nd edn (eds J. Hankin *et al.*). W.B. Saunders, Philadelphia.

LSC (2002) *Standards of Care of External Central Venous Catheters in Adult Cancer Patients*. London Standing Committee, London.

Lum, P. (1999) Techniques for optimising catheter tip position. *Presentation at NAVAN 13th Annual Conference, Orlando*, September.

Macklin, D. (1999) A review of the physical principles of fluid administration. *J Vasc Access Devices*, **4**(2), 7–11.

Macrae, K. (1998) Hand held Dopplers in central catheter insertion. *Prof Nurse*, **14**(2), 99–102.

Madeo, M. *et al.* (1997) A randomised study comparing IV 3000 (transparent polyurethane dressing) to a dry gauze dressing for peripheral intravenous catheter sites. *J Intravenous Nurs*, **20**(5), 253–6.

Maki, D.G. & Ringer, M. (1987) Evaluation of dressing regimes for prevention of infection with peripheral IV catheters. *JAMA*, **258**(17), 2396–403.

Maki, D.G. *et al.* (1991) Prospective randomized trial of povidone iodine, alcohol and chlorhexidine for prevention of infection associated with CVC and arterial catheters. *Lancet*, **338**, 339–43.

Maki, D.G., Stolz, S.M., Wheeler, S. & Mermel, L.A. (1997) Prevention of central venous catheter related bloodstream infection by the use of an antiseptic impregnated catheter. *Ann Intern Med*, **127**(4), 257–66f.

Marieb, E. (2001) *Human Anatomy and Physiology*, 5th edn. Benjamin Cummings, California.

Marx, M. (1995) The management of the difficult peripherally inserted central venous catheter line removal. *J Intravenous Nurs*, **18**(5), 246–9.

Mayo, D.J. (1996) The effects of heparin flush on patency of Groshong catheter: a pilot study. *Oncol Nurs Forum*, **23**(9), 1401–5.

Mayo, D.J. (1998) Fibrin sheath formation and chemotherapy extravasation: a case report. *Supportive Care in Cancer*, **6**, 51–6.

Mayo, D.J. (2000a) Catheter related thrombosis. *J Intravenous Nurs*, **24**(Suppl 3), S13–22.

Mayo, D.J. (2000b) Catheter-related thrombosis. *J Vasc Access Devices*, **5**(2), 10–20.

Mayo, D.J. (2001) Reflux in vascular access devices – a manageable problem. *J Vasc Access Devices*, **6**(4), 39–40.

McDermott, M.K. (1995) Patient education and compliance issues associated with access devices. *Semin Oncol Nurs*, **11**(3), 221–6.

Mermel, L.A. *et al.* (2001) Guidelines for management of intravascular catheter related infections. *J Intravenous Nurs*, **24**(3), 180–205.

Millam, D. (1992) Starting IVs – how to develop your venepuncture skills. *Nursing*, **92**, 33–46.

Millam, D. (1993) How to teach good venepuncture technique. *Am J Nurs*, **93**(7), 38–41.

Mirro, J. *et al.* (1998) A prospective study of Hickman/Broviac catheters and implanted ports in paediatric oncology patients. *J Clin Oncol*, **7**, 214–22.

Morven, H. (1995) The first years of continuing arterial pressure measurement. *Br J Anaesth*, **67**, 353–9.

Moureau, N. (1999) Practicing prevention with implanted ports. *J Vasc Access Devices*, **4**(3), 30–5.

Moureau, N. & Zonderman, A. (2000) Does it always have to hurt? *J Intravenous Nurs*, **23**(4), 213–19.

Moureau, N. *et al.* (1999) Multidisciplinary management of thrombotic catheter occlusions in VADs. *J Vasc Access Devices*, **4**(2), 22–9.

Nauth Misir, N. (1998) Intravascular catheters. *Prof Nurse*, **13**(7), 463–71.

Nesti, S.P. & Kovac, R. (2000) 5Fu extravasation following port failure. *J Intravenous Nurs*, **23**(3), 176–80.

NICE (2002) *Ultrasound Imaging for Central Venous Catheter Placement*. DoH, London.

NICE (2003) *Infection Control – Prevention of Healthcare Associated Infection in Primary and Community Care*. Clinical Guideline 2. National Institute for Clinical Excellence, London.

Oakley, C., Wright, E. & Ream, E. (2000) The experiences of patients and nurses with a nurse led peripherally inserted central venous catheter line service. *Eur J Oncol Nurs*, **4**(4), 207–18.

Oh, T. (1997) *Intensive Care Manual*, 4th edn. Butterworth Heinemann, Oxford.

Oh, T.E. (1995) *Intensive Care Manual*. Butterworths, Sydney.

ONS (1996) *Cancer Chemotherapy Guidelines and Recommendations for Nursing Education and Practice*. Oncology Nursing Society, Pittsburgh.

Parker, L. (2002) Management of IV devices to prevent infection. *Br J Nurs*, **11**(4), 240–5.

Payne-James, J.J., Rogers, J., Bray, M.J., Rana, S.K., McSwiggon, D. & Silk, D.B. (1991) Development of thrombophlebitis in peripheral veins with Vialon and PTFE-Teflon cannulas: a double blind randomised controlled trial. *Ann R Coll Surg Engl*, **73**, 322–5.

Perdue, M.B. (2001) Intravenous complications. In: *Infusion Therapy in Clinical Practice*, 2nd edn (eds J. Hankin *et al.*). W.B. Saunders, Philadelphia.

Perucca, R. (2001) Obtaining vascular access. In: *Infusion Therapy in Clinical Practice*, 2nd edn (eds J. Hankin *et al.*). W.B. Saunders, Philadelphia.

Pierce, L.R. (1998) Non invasive respiratory monitoring and invasive monitoring of direct and derived tissue oxygenation variables. In: *Guide to Mechanical Ventilation and Intensive Respiratory Care*. W.B. Saunders, Philadelphia, p. 259.

Ponec, D. *et al.* (2001) Recombinant tissue plasminogen activator (alteplase) for restoration of flow in occluded central venous access devices: a double blind placebo controlled trial – the Cardiovascular Thrombolytic to Open Occluded Lines (COOL) efficacy trial. *J Vasc Interv Radiol*, **12**, 951–5.

Powers, F.A. (1999) Can you keep her safe? *Nursing*, **99**, 54–5.

Randolph, A.G. *et al.* (1998) Benefit of heparin use in central venous catheters and pulmonary artery catheters – a meta analysis of randomised controlled trials. *Chest*, **113**, 165–71.

RCN (2003) *Standards for Infusion Therapy*. Royal College of Nursing, London.

RCN and Infection Control Nurses' Association (1992) *Intravenous Line Dressings – Principles of Infection Control*. Smith & Nephew Medical Ltd, Hull.

Rickard, N.A.S. (2001) Central venous catheter – infection and patient susceptibility. *Br J Nurs*, **10**(16), 1044–53.

Rinn, T.L. (2001) Fibrinolytic therapy in CVC occlusion. *J Intravenous Nurs*, **24**(Suppl 3), S9–12.

Robbins, J., Cromwell, P. & Korones, D.N. (2000) Swimming and central venous catheter related infections in children with cancer. In: *Measuring Patient Outcomes* (eds M. Nolan & V. Mock). Sage Publications, California.

Rowley, S. (2001) Theory to practice: aseptic non touch technique. *Nurs Times*, **97**(7), 6–8.

Royal College of Anaesthetists (1990) *The Working Party of the Commission on the Provision of Surgical Services*. Royal College of Surgeons and College of Anaesthetists, London.

Royer, T. (2001) A case for post, anterior and lateral CXR being performed following each PICC placement. *J Vasc Access Devices*, **6**(4), 9–11.

Rummel, M.A., Donnelly, P.J. & Fortenbaugh, C.C. (2001) Clinical evaluation of a positive pressure device to prevent central venous catheter occlusion: results of a pilot study. *Clin J Oncol Nurs*, **5**(6), 261–5.

Ryder, M. (2001) The role of biofilm in vascular catheter related infections. *New Dev Vasc Dis*, **2**(2), 15–25.

Ryder, M. (2002) Biofilm – unlocking the mystery of catheter-related infections. *Presentation at NAVAN 15th Annual Conference, Virginia*, January.

Sampath, L.A. *et al.* (2001) Safety and efficacy of an improved antiseptic catheter impregnated intraluminally with chlorhexidine. *J Intravenous Nurs*, **24**(6), 395–403.

Sansivero, G.E. (1998) Venous anatomy and physiology. *J Intravenous Nurs*, **21**(Suppl 5), S107–14.

Sansivero, G.E. (2000) Microintroducer techniques for PICC placement. *J Intravenous Nurs*, **23**(6), 345–51.

Santolla, A. & Weckel, C. (1983) A new closed system for arterial lines. *Reg Nurse*, **46**(6), 49–52.

Sculmeister, L. & Camp Sorrell, D. (2000) Chemotherapy extravasation from implanted ports. *Oncol Nurs Forum*, **27**(3), 531–60.

Sheppard, K. *et al.* (1999) A prospective study of two intravenous catheter securement techniques in a skilled nursing facility. *J Intravenous Nurs*, **22**(3), 151–6.

Shotkin, J.D. & Lombardo, F. (1996) Use of an indwelling peripheral catheter for 3–5 day chemotherapy administration in the outpatient setting. *J Intravenous Nurs*, **19**(6), 315–20.

Simcock, L. (2001a) Managing occlusion in central venous catheters. *Nurs Times*, **97**(21), 36–8.

Simcock, L. (2001b) The use of central venous catheters for IV therapy. *Nurs Times*, **97**(18), 34–5.

Snelling, R. *et al.* (2001) CVC for infusion therapy in GI cancer. *J Intravenous Nurs*, **24**(1), 38–47.

Springhouse Corporation (2002) *Intravenous Therapy Made Incredibly Easy*. Springhouse, Lippincott, Williams & Wilkins, Philadelphia.

Stacey, R.G.W. *et al.* (1991) Percutaneous insertion of Hickman type catheters. *Br J Hosp Med*, **46**, 396–8.

Stanley, A. (2002) Managing complications of chemotherapy administration. In: *The Cytotoxic Handbook* (eds M. Allwood *et al.*). Radcliffe Medical Press, Oxford.

Stevenis, B., Barton, S.E., Brechbill, M. *et al.* (2000) A randomised prospective trial of conventional vascular ports vs the vortex 'clear-flow' reservoir ports in adult oncology patients. *J Vasc Access Devices*, **5**(2), 37–40.

Taylor, M.J. (2000) A fascination with phlebitis. *J Vasc Access Devices*, **5**(3), 24–8.

Teplitz, L. (1990) Arterial line disconnection: first aid procedure. *Nursing*, **20**(5), 33.

Thompson, A. *et al.* (1989) Long-term central venous access: the patient's view. *Intensive Ther Clin Monit*, **10**(5), 142–5.

Timoney, J.P. *et al.* (2002) Safe and effective use of alteplase for the clearance of occluded central venous access devices. *J Clin Oncol*, **20**(7), 1918–22.

Timsit, J.F. (2000) Rotation of central venous catheter sites. *Infect Control Hosp Epidemiol*, **21**(6), 371–4.

Tingey, K.G. (2000) Desirable properties for vascular catheter materials. *J Vasc Access Devices*, **5**(3), 14–16.

Tinker, J. & Zapol, W. (1991) *Care of the Critically Ill Patient*. Springer, London.

Todd, J. (1998) Peripherally inserted central catheters. *Prof Nurse*, **13**(5), 297–302.

Tortora, G. & Grabowski, S.R. (2002) The cardiovascular system, blood vessels and haemodynamics. In: *The Principles of Anatomy and Physiology*, 10th edn. John Wiley, New York, p. 723.

Veenstra, D.L. *et al.* (1999) Efficacy of antiseptic impregnated central venous catheters in preventing catheter related blood stream infection: a meta analysis. *JAMA*, **281**(3), 261–7.

Verghese, S.T. *et al.* (2002) The effects of the simulated Valsalva maneuver liver compression and/or Trendelenburg position on the cross sectional area of the internal jugular vein in infants and young children. *Anesthes Analg*, **94**(2), 250–4.

Walther, K. (2001) Intravenous therapy in the older adult. In: *Infusion Therapy in Clinical Practice*, 2nd edn (eds J. Hankin *et al.*). W.B. Saunders, Philadelphia.

Weinstein, S. (2000) *Plumer's Principles and Practices of Intravenous Therapy*. Lippincott, Philadelphia.

Whitely, M.S., Change, B.Y.P. & Marsh, H.P. (1995) Use of hand held Doppler to identify 'difficult' forearm veins for cannulation. *Ann R Coll Surg Engl*, **77**, 224–6.

Whitson, M. (1996) Intravenous therapy in the older adult: special needs and considerations. *J Intravenous Nurs*, **19**(5), 251–5.

Williamson, E.E. & McKinney, J.M. (2001) Assessing the adequacy of PICCs for power injection of intravenous contrast agents for CT. *J Comput Assist Tomogr*, **25**(6), 932–7.

Wilson, J. (2001) Preventing infection associated with intravenous therapy. In: *Infection Control in Clinical Practice*, 2nd edn. Baillière Tindall, London.

Wilson, K.J. & Waugh, A. (1998) *Ross and Wilson's Anatomy and Physiology and Illness*, 8th edn. Churchill Livingstone, Edinburgh.

Wise, M. *et al.* (2001) Catheter tip position. *J Vasc Access Devices*, **6**(2), 18–27.

Xu, Q.A. *et al.* (2000) Adequacy of a new chlorhexidine bearing polyurethane central venous catheter for administration of 82 selected parenteral drugs. *Ann Pharmacother*, **34**, 1109–16.

Zideman, D.A. & Morgan, M. (1981) Inadvertent intra-arterial injection of flucloxacillin. *Anaesthesia*, **36**(6), 296–8.

Venepuncture

Chapter contents

Definition

Venepuncture is the procedure of entering a vein with a needle.

Indications

Venepuncture is carried out for two reasons:

- To obtain a blood sample for diagnostic purposes.
- To monitor levels of blood components.

Reference material

Venepuncture is one of the most commonly performed invasive procedures (Castledine 1996) and is now routinely being undertaken by nurses (Ernst & Ernst 2001). In order to perform venepuncture safely the nurse must have basic knowledge of the following:

- The relevant anatomy and physiology.
- The criteria for choosing both the vein and device to use
- The potential problems which may be encountered, how to prevent them and necessary interventions
- The health and safety/risk management of the procedure, as well as the correct disposal of equipment (Intravenous Nursing Society 2000).

Certain principles, such as adherence to an aseptic technique, must be applied throughout (see Ch. 4, Aseptic technique). The circulation is a closed sterile system and a venepuncture, however quickly completed, is a breach of this system providing a means of entry for bacteria.

The nurse must be aware of the physical and psychological comfort of the patient (Weinstein 2000). He/she must appreciate the value of adequate explanation and simple measures to prevent the complications of venepuncture, such as haematoma formation, when it is neither a natural nor acceptable consequence of the procedure (Ernst & Ernst 2001).

Anatomy and physiology

The superficial veins of the upper limb are most commonly chosen for venepuncture. These veins are numerous and accessible, ensuring that the procedure can be performed safely and with minimum discomfort (Marieb 1998; Ernst & Ernst 2001). In adults veins located on the dorsal portion of the foot may be selected but there is an increased risk of deep vein thrombosis (Springhouse 2002) or tissue necrosis in diabetics (Ernst & Ernst 2001). Therefore, veins in the lower limbs should be avoided where possible.

The veins commonly used for venepuncture are those found in the antecubital fossa because they are sizeable veins capable of providing copious and repeated blood specimens (Weinstein 2000). However, the venous anatomy of each individual may differ. The main veins of choice are (see Fig. 45.1a):

- The median cubital veins
- The cephalic vein
- The basilic vein
- The metacarpal veins (used only when the others are not accessible) (Fig. 45.1b).

The median cubital vein may not always be visible, but its size and location make it easy to palpate. It is also well supported by subcutaneous tissue, which prevents it from rolling under the needle.

On the lateral aspect of the wrist, the cephalic vein rises from the dorsal veins and flows upwards along the radial border of the forearm as the median cephalic, crossing the antecubital fossa as the median cubital vein. Care must be taken to avoid accidental arterial puncture, as this vein crosses the brachial artery. It is also in close proximity to the radial nerve (Thrush & Belsole 1995; Masoorli 2002).

The basilic vein is often overlooked as a site for venepuncture and has its origins in the ulnar border of the hand and forearm (Waugh & Grant 2001). It may well be prominent but is not well supported by subcutaneous tissue, making it roll easily, which can result in difficult venepuncture (Dougherty 1999). Owing to its position, a haematoma may occur if the patient flexes the arm on removal of the needle, as this squeezes blood from the vein into the surrounding tissues (Weinstein 2000; McCall & Tankersley 2002). Care must also be taken to avoid accidental puncture of the median nerve and brachial artery (Ernst & Ernst 2001).

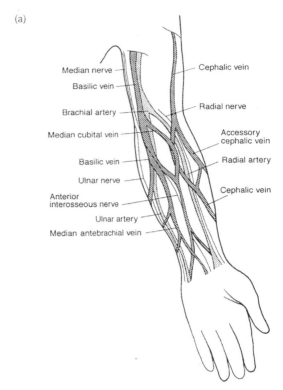

(a)

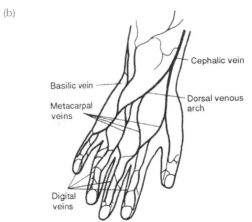

(b)

Figure 45.1 (a) Superficial veins of the forearm. (b) Superficial veins of dorsal aspect of the hand. (Reproduced by permission from Becton Dickinson and Company.)

The metacarpal veins are easily visualized and palpated. However, the use of these veins is contraindicated in the elderly where skin turgor and subcutaneous tissue are diminished (Weinstein 2000).

Veins consist of three layers: the tunica intima is a smooth endothelial lining, which allows the passage of blood cells. If it becomes damaged, the lining may become roughened and there is an increased risk of thrombus formation (Weinstein 2000). Within this layer are folds of endothelium called valves, which keep blood moving towards the heart by preventing back flow of blood. Valves are present in larger vessels and at points of branching and are present as noticeable bulges in the veins (Dougherty 1999; Weinstein 2000). However, when a needle touches a valve, the valve can compress and close the lumen of the vein, thus preventing the withdrawal of blood (Weinstein 2000). Therefore, if detected, venepuncture should be performed above the valve in order to facilitate collection of the sample (Weinstein 2000).

The tunica media, the middle layer of the vein wall, is composed of muscular tissue and nerve fibres, both vasoconstrictors and vasodilators, which can stimulate the vein to contract or relax. This layer is not as strong or stiff as an artery and therefore veins can distend or collapse as the pressure rises or falls (Weinstein 2000; Waugh & Grant 2001). Stimulation of this layer by a change in temperature, mechanical or chemical stimulation can produce venous spasm, which can make a venepuncture more difficult.

The tunica adventitia is the outer layer and consists of connective tissue, which surrounds and supports the vessel.

Arteries tend to be placed more deeply than veins and can be distinguished by the thicker walls, which do not collapse, the presence of a pulse and the blood is bright red. It should be noted that aberrant arteries may be present. These are arteries that are located superficially in an unusual place (Weinstein 2000).

Choosing a vein

The choice of vein must be that which is best for the individual patient. The most prominent vein is not necessarily the most suitable vein for venepuncture (Weinstein 2000). There are two stages to locating a vein:

1 Visual inspection
2 Palpation.

Visual inspection is the scrutiny of the veins in both arms and is essential prior to choosing a vein. Veins adjacent to foci of infection, bruising and phlebitis should not be considered, owing to the risk of causing more local tissue damage or systemic infection. An oedematous limb should be avoided as there is danger of stasis of lymph, predisposing to such complications

as phlebitis and cellulitis (Smith 1998). Areas of previous venepuncture should be avoided as a build-up of scar tissue can cause difficulty in accessing the vein and can result in pain due to repeated trauma (McCall & Tankersley 2002).

Palpation is an important assessment technique, as it determines the location and condition of the vein, distinguishes veins from arteries and tendons, identifies the presence of valves and detects deeper veins (Dougherty 1999). The nurse should use the same fingers for palpation as this will increase the sensitivity and ability of the nurse to know what she or he is feeling. The thumb should not be used as it is not as sensitive and has a pulse, which may lead to confusion in distinguishing veins from arteries in the patient (Weinstein 2000).

Thrombosed veins feel hard and cord-like, and should be avoided along with tortuous, sclerosed, fibrosed, inflamed or fragile veins, which may be unable to accommodate the device to be used and will result in pain and repeated venepunctures. Use of veins which cross over joints or bony prominences and those with little skin or subcutaneous cover, e.g. the inner aspect of the wrist, will also subject the patient to more discomfort. Therefore preference should be given to a vessel that is unused, easily detected by inspection and palpation, patent and healthy. These veins feel soft and bouncy and will refill when depressed (Weinstein 2000).

Influencing factors

• Injury, disease or treatment may prevent the use of a limb for venepuncture thereby reducing the venous access, e.g. amputation, fracture and cerebrovascular accident. Use of a limb may be contraindicated because of an operation on one side of the body, for example mastectomy and axillary node dissection, as this can lead to impairment of lymphatic drainage, which can influence venous flow regardless of whether there is obvious lymphoedema (Smith 1998; Weinstein 2000).

• The age and weight of the patient will also influence choice. Young children have short fine veins, and the elderly have prominent but fragile veins. Care must be taken with fragile veins and the largest vein should be chosen along with the smallest gauge device to reduce the amount of trauma to the vessel. Malnourished patients will often present with friable veins.

• If the patient is in shock or dehydrated there will be poor superficial peripheral access. It may be necessary to take blood after the patient is rehydrated as this will promote venous filling and blood will be obtained more easily.

- Medications can influence the choice of vein in that patients on anticoagulants or steroids or those who are thrombocytopenic tend to have more fragile veins and will be at greater risk of bruising both during venepuncture and on removal of the needle. Therefore choice may be limited by areas of bruising present or the inability to access the vessel without causing bruising to occur.
- The temperature of the environment will influence venous dilatation. If the patient is cold, no veins may be evident on first inspection. Application of heat, e.g. in the form of a warm compress or soaking the arm in warm water, will increase the size and visibility of the veins, thus increasing the likelihood of a successful first attempt (Weinstein 2000; Springhouse 2002).
- Venepuncture itself may cause the vein to collapse or go into a spasm. This will produce discomfort and a reduction in blood flow. Careful preparation and choice of vein will reduce the likelihood of this and stroking the vein or applying heat will help resolve it.
- Patient anxiety about the procedure may result in vasoconstriction. The nurse's manner and approach will also have a direct bearing on the patient's experience (Weinstein 2000). Approaching the patient with a confident manner and giving an adequate explanation of the procedure may reduce anxiety. Careful preparation and an unhurried approach will help to relax the patient and this in turn will increase vasodilatation (Dougherty 1999; Weinstein 2000). It is important to remember that patients may dread venepuncture (Garza & Becan McBride 2002) and if a patient is particularly anxious, or for venepuncture in children, the use of a topical local anaesthetic cream may be appropriate (Weinstein 2000; Garza & Becan McBride 2002; Springhouse 2002). Involving patients in the choice of vein, even if it is simply to choose the non-dominant arm, can increase a feeling of control which in turn helps to relieve anxiety (Hudek 1986).

Improving venous access

There are a number of methods of improving venous access:

- Application of a tourniquet – this promotes venous distension. The tourniquet should be tight enough to impede venous return but not restrict arterial flow. The tourniquet should be placed about 7–8 cm above the venepuncture site. It may be more comfortable for the patient to position it over a sleeve or paper towel to prevent pinching the skin. The tourniquet should not be left on for longer than 1 minute as it may result in haemoconcentration or pooling of the blood, leading to inaccurate blood results (Ernst & Ernst 2001).

There are several types of tourniquet available. A good-quality, buckle closure, single hand release type is most effective but the choice will depend on availability and operator. Consideration should be given to the type of material and the ability to decontaminate the tourniquet (Golder 2000; RCN 2003).

- Opening and closing of the fist ensures the muscles will force blood into the veins and encourages distension. This action may affect certain blood results, e.g. potassium (Ernst & Ernst 2001; Garza & Becan McBride 2002).
- Lowering the arm below heart level also increases blood supply to the veins.
- Light tapping of the vein may be useful but can be painful and may result in the formation of a haematoma in patients with fragile veins, e.g. thrombocytopenic patients (Dougherty 1999).
- The use of heat in the form of a warm pack or by immersing the arm in a bowl of warm water for 10 minutes helps to encourage venodilatation and venous filling.
- Ointment or patches containing small amounts of glyceryl trinitrate have been used to improve local vasodilatation to aid venepuncture (Weinstein 2000).

Choice of device

The intravenous devices commonly used to perform a venepuncture for blood sampling are a straight steel needle and a steel winged infusion device. The optimum gauge to use is 21 swg (standard wire gauge, which measures internal diameter – the smaller the gauge size, the larger the diameter. Standard wire gauge measurement is determined by how many cannulae fit into a tube with an inner diameter of 1 inch (2.5 cm), and uses consecutive numbers from 13 to 24). This enables blood to be withdrawn at a reasonable speed without undue discomfort to the patient or possible damage to the blood cells.

Equipment available will depend on local policy (Table 45.1) but with increasing concern about the possibility of contamination to the practitioner, blood collection systems with integrated safety devices are now readily available and should be used wherever possible (ICNA 2003). However, the nurse must always select the device after assessing the condition and accessibility of the vein.

Skin preparation

Asepsis is vital when performing a venepuncture as the skin is breached and a foreign device is introduced into a sterile circulatory system. The two major sources of

Table 45.1 Choice of intravenous device

Device	swg	Advantages	Disadvantages	Use
Needle	21	Cheaper than winged infusion devices. Easy to use with large veins	Rigid. Difficult to manipulate with smaller veins in less conventional sites. May cause more discomfort Venous access only confirmed when sample tube attached.	Large, accessible veins in the antecubital fossa. When small quantities of blood are to be drawn
Winged infusion device with or without safety shield	21	Flexible due to small needle shaft. Easy to manipulate and insert at any site. Causes less discomfort Usually shows a 'flashback' of blood to indicate a successful venepuncture	More expensive than steel needles The 12–30 cm length of tubing on the device may be caught and dislodge the needle.	Veins in sites other than the antecubital fossa. When quantities of blood greater than 20 ml are required from any site
	23	Flexible due to small needle shaft. Easy to manipulate and insert at any site. Causes less discomfort. Smaller swg and therefore useful with fragile veins	More expensive than steel needles, plus there can be damage to cells which can cause inaccurate measurements in certain blood samples, e.g. potassium	Small veins in more painful sites, e.g. inner aspect of the wrist, especially if measurements are related to plasma and not cellular components

microbial contamination are:

- Cross-infection from practitioner to patient
- Skin flora of the patient.

Good hand washing and drying techniques are essential on the part of the nurse; gloves should be changed between patients (see Ch. 4, Aseptic technique).

To remove the risk presented by the patient's skin flora, firm and prolonged rubbing with an alcohol-based solution, such as chlorhexidine 0.5% in 70% alcohol, is advised (Walther *et al.* 2001). This cleaning should continue for about 30 seconds, although some authors state a minimum of 1 minute or longer (Weinstein 2000). The area that has been cleaned should then be allowed to dry to (1) facilitate coagulation of the organisms, thus ensuring disinfection and (2) prevent a stinging pain on insertion of the needle due to the alcohol on the end of the needle. The skin must not be touched or the vein repalpated prior to venepuncture.

Skin cleaning is a controversial subject and it is acknowledged that a cursory wipe with an alcohol swab does more harm than no cleaning at all as it disturbs the skin flora.

Safety of the practitioner

It is recommended that well-fitting gloves are worn during any procedure that involves handling blood and body fluids, particularly venepuncture and cannulation (RCN 1995; ICNA 2003; RCN 2003). This is to prevent contamination of the practitioner from potential blood spills. Whilst it is recognized that gloves will not prevent a needlestick injury, the wiping effect of a glove on a needle may reduce the volume of blood to which the hand is exposed, thereby reducing the volume inoculated and the risk of infection (Mitchell Higgs 2002; NAO 2003; ICNA 2003). However, there is no substitute for good technique and practitioners must always work carefully when performing venepuncture.

A range of safety devices are now available for venepuncture which can reduce the risk of occupational percutaneous injuries among health care workers, in particular vacuum blood collection systems (Centers for Disease Control 1997). A vacuum system consists of a plastic holder which contains or is attached to a double-ended needle or adaptor. It is important to use the correct Luer adaptor to ensure a good connection and avoid blood leakage (Garza & Becan McBride 2002). The blood tube is vacuumed in order that the exact amount of blood required is withdrawn, when the tube is pushed into the holder. Filling ceases once the tube is full which removes the need for decanting blood and also reduces blood wastage. The system can also be attached to winged infusion devices (Dougherty 1999). It has been shown that the use of vacuum blood collection systems, particularly with winged infusion devices, is associated with a significant reduction in percutaneous injuries (Centers for Disease Control 1997).

Used needles should always be discarded directly into an approved sharps container, without being resheathed (ICNA 2003; RCN 2003). Specimens from patients with known or suspected infections such as hepatitis or HIV should be double-bagged in clear polythene bags with a biohazard label attached. The accompanying request forms should be kept separately from the specimen to avoid contamination. (Health Service Advisory Committee 1991). All other non-sharp disposables should be placed in a universal clinical waste bag.

Removal of the device

It is important to ensure that the needle is removed correctly on completion of blood sampling and that the risk of haematoma formation is minimized. Pressure should be applied as the needle is removed from the skin. If pressure is applied too early, it causes the tip of the needle to drag along the intima of the vein, resulting in sharp pain and damage to the lining of the vessel.

Digital pressure should be applied by the practitioner, as it has been shown that this results in less bruising than if the patient is left to apply the pressure (Godwin *et al.* 1992). The patient should also be instructed to keep his or her arm straight and not bend it as this also results in an increased risk of bruising (McCall & Tankersley 2002). A longer period of pressure may be necessary where the patient's blood may take longer to clot, for example, if the patient is receiving anticoagulants or is thrombocytopenic. The practitioner may choose to apply the tourniquet over the venepuncture site to ensure even and constant pressure on the area (Perdue 1995). Alternatively they can elevate the arm for approximately 5 minutes to decrease venous pressure (Springhouse 2002).

The practitioner should inspect the site carefully for bleeding or bruising before applying a dressing to the site, and the patient leaving the department. If bruising has occurred the patient should be informed of why this has happened and given instructions for what to do to reduce the bruising and any associated pain. Initially the application of an ice pack may help to soothe and decrease bruising. The application of Hirudoid cream, which is used for the treatment of thrombophlebitis, may be helpful (BMA & RPS 2003).

Summary

In order to perform a safe and successful venepuncture, it is important that the practitioner

- Considers carefully the choice of vein and device
- Applies the principles of asepsis
- Adheres to and understands safe technique and practices.

Recently there has been an increase in the number of cases of litigation involving injuries, which have occurred as a result of venepuncture (McConnell & MacKay 1996; Price & Moss 1998). It is therefore vital that nurses receive accredited and appropriate training, supervision and assessment by an experienced member of staff (Dougherty 1996; RCN 1999). The nurse is then accountable and responsible for ensuring that his or her skills and competence are maintained and his or her knowledge is kept up to date, in order to fulfil the criteria set out in the *Code of Professional Conduct* (NMC 2002; Lamb 1999).

Procedure guidelines: **Venepuncture**

Equipment

1 Clean tray or receiver.
2 Tourniquet or sphygmomanometer and cuff.
3 21 swg multiple sample needle or 21 swg winged infusion device and multiple sample Luer adaptor.
4 Plastic tube holder, standard or for blood cultures.
5 Appropriate vacuumed specimen tubes.
6 Swab saturated with chlorhexidine in 70% alcohol, or or isopropyl alcohol 70%.

7 Low-linting swabs.
8 Sterile adhesive plaster or hypoallergenic tape.
9 Specimen request forms.
10 Gloves.
11 Plastic apron (optional).

A number of vacuum systems are available that can be used for taking blood samples. These are simple to use and cost effective. The manufacturer's instructions should be followed if one of these systems is used. Vacuum systems reduce the risk of health care workers being contaminated, because they offer a completely closed system during the process of blood withdrawal and there is no necessity to decant blood into bottles (Dougherty 1999). This makes

Procedure guidelines: Venepuncture (cont'd)

them the safest method for collecting blood samples using venepuncture. If not available, the following items replace the vacuum system:

1 21 swg needle or 21 swg winged infusion device.
2 Syringe(s) of appropriate size.
3 Appropriate blood specimen bottle(s).

Procedure

	Action	Rationale
1	Approach the patient in a confident manner and explain and discuss the procedure with the patient.	To ensure that the patient understands the procedure and gives his/her valid consent.
2	Allow the patient to ask questions and discuss any problems which have arisen previously.	Anxiety results in vasoconstriction; therefore a patient who is relaxed will have dilated veins, making access easier.
3	Consult the patient as to any preferences and problems that may have been experienced at previous venepunctures.	To involve the patient in the treatment. To acquaint the nurse fully with the patient's previous venous history and identify any changes in clinical status, e.g. mastectomy, as both may influence vein choice.
4	Check the identity of the patient matches the details on the request form by asking for their full name and date of birth and checking their identification bracelet.	To ensure the sample is taken from the correct patient.
5	Assemble the equipment necessary for venepuncture.	To ensure that time is not wasted and that the procedure goes smoothly without unnecessary interruptions.
6	Carefully wash hands using bactericidal soap and water or bactericidal alcohol handrub, and dry before commencement.	To minimize risk of infection.
7	Check hands for any visibly broken skin, and cover with a waterproof dressing.	To minimize the risk of contamination to the practitioner.
8	Check all packaging before opening and preparing the equipment on the chosen clean receptacle.	To maintain asepsis throughout and check that no equipment is damaged.
9	Take all the equipment to the patient, exhibiting a competent manner.	To help the patient feel more at ease with the procedure.
10	In both an inpatient and an outpatient situation, lighting, ventilation, privacy and positioning must be checked.	To ensure that both patient and operator are comfortable and that adequate light is available to illuminate this procedure.
11	Support the chosen limb on a pillow.	To ensure the patient's comfort and facilitate venous access.
12 (a)	Apply a tourniquet to the upper arm on the chosen side, making sure it does not obstruct arterial flow. If the radial pulse cannot be palpated then the tourniquet is too tight (Weinstein 2000). The position of the tourniquet may be varied, e.g. if a vein in the hand is to be used it may be placed on the forearm. A sphygmomanometer cuff may be used as an alternative.	To dilate the veins by obstructing the venous return.
(b)	The arm may be placed in a dependent position. The patient may assist by clenching and unclenching the fist.	To increase the prominence of the veins.
(c)	The veins may be tapped gently or stroked.	
(d)	If all these measures are unsuccessful, remove the tourniquet and apply moist heat, e.g. a warm compress, soak limb in warm water or, with medical prescription, apply glyceryl trinitrate ointment/patch.	To promote blood flow and therefore distend the veins.
13	Select the vein using the aforementioned criteria.	

*Procedure guidelines: **Venepuncture** (cont'd)*

	Action	Rationale
14	Select the device, based on vein size, site, etc.	To reduce damage or trauma to the vein.
15	Wash hands with bactericidal soap and water or bactericidal alcohol handrub.	To maintain asepsis, and minimize the risk of infection.
16	Put on gloves.	To prevent possible contamination of the practitioner.
17	Clean the patient's skin carefully for 30 seconds using an appropriate preparation, e.g. chlorhexidine in 70% alcohol, and allow to dry.	To maintain asepsis and minimize the risk of infection. To prevent pain on insertion.
	Do not repalpate the vein or touch the skin.	To minimize the risk of infection.
18	Remove the cover from the needle and inspect the device carefully.	To detect faulty equipment, e.g. bent or barbed needles. If these are present place them in a safe container, record batch details and return to manufacturer.
19	Anchor the vein by applying manual traction on the skin a few centimetres below the proposed insertion site.	To immobilize the vein. To provide countertension to the vein which will facilitate a smoother needle entry.
20	Insert the needle smoothly at an angle of approximately 30°. However, this will depend on size and depth of the vein.	To facilitate a successful, pain-free venepuncture.
21	Reduce the angle of descent of the needle as soon as a flashback of blood is seen in the tubing of a winged infusion device or when puncture of the vein wall is felt. If you are using a needle and syringe, pull the plunger back slightly prior to venepuncture and a flashback of blood will be seen in the barrel on vein entry.	To prevent advancing too far through vein wall and causing damage to the vessel.
22	Slightly advance the needle into the vein, if possible.	To stabilize the device within the vein and prevent it becoming dislodged during withdrawal of blood.
23	Do not exert any pressure on the needle.	To prevent a puncture occurring through the vein wall.

24	Withdraw the required amount of blood using a vacuumed blood collection system or syringes. Collect blood samples in the following order:
	• Blood culture
	• Plain or serum (no additives)
	• Coagulation
	• Additive tubes such as – gel separator tubes (may contain clot activator or heparin)
	  – heparin tubes
	  – EDTA
	• All other tubes (National Committee for Clinical Laboratory Standards 1991, cited in Ernst & Ernst 2001).
		To minimize the risk of transferring additives from one tube to another and bacterial contamination of blood cultures (Ernst & Ernst 2001).

25	Release the tourniquet. In some instances this may be necessary at the beginning of sampling as inaccurate measurements may be caused by haemostasis, e.g. when taking blood to assess calcium levels.	To decrease the pressure within the vein.
	Remove tube from plastic tube holder.	To prevent blood spillage caused by vacuum in the tube (Campbell *et al.* 1999).
26	If using a needle and syringe withdraw a small amount of blood into the syringe.	To reduce the amount of static blood in the vein and therefore the likelihood of leakage at the venepuncture site on removal of the needle.
27	Pick up a low-linting swab and place it over the puncture point.	

*Procedure guidelines: **Venepuncture** (cont'd)*

	Action	Rationale
28	Remove the needle, but do not apply pressure until the needle has been fully removed.	To prevent pain on removal and damage to the intima of the vein.
29	Activate safety device, if applicable, and then discard the needle immediately in sharps bin.	To reduce the risk of accidental needlestick injury.
30	Apply digital pressure directly over the puncture site. Pressure should be applied until bleeding has ceased; approximately 1 minute or longer may be required if current disease or treatment interferes with clotting mechanisms.	To stop leakage and haematoma formation. To preserve vein by preventing bruising or haematoma formation.
31	The patient may apply pressure with the finger but should be discouraged from bending the arm if a vein in the antecubital fossa is used (McCall & Tankersley 2002).	To prevent leakage and haematoma formation.
32	Where a syringe has been used, transfer the blood to appropriate specimen bottles as soon as possible, making sure that the correct quantity is placed in each container.	To prevent clotting in the syringe. To ensure that an adequate amount is available for each test.
33	Gently invert tube at least six times.	To prevent damage to blood cells and to mix with additives.
34	Label the bottles with the relevant details.	To ensure that the specimens from the right patient are delivered to the laboratory, the requested tests are performed and the results returned to the correct patient's records.
35	Inspect the puncture point before applying a dressing.	To check that the puncture point has sealed.
36	Ascertain whether the patient is allergic to adhesive plaster.	To prevent an allergic skin reaction.
37	Apply an adhesive plaster or alternative dressing.	To cover the puncture and prevent leakage or contamination.
38	Ensure that the patient is comfortable.	To ascertain whether patient wishes to rest before leaving (if an outpatient) or whether any other measures need to be taken.
39	Discard waste, making sure it is placed in the correct containers, e.g. sharps into a designated receptacle.	To ensure safe disposal and avoid laceration or other injury of staff. To prevent reuse of equipment.
40	Follow hospital procedure for collection and transportation of specimens to the laboratory.	To make sure that specimens reach their intended destination.
41	Remove gloves and discard in appropriate clinical waste bag.	

Problem solving

Problem	Cause	Prevention	Suggested action
Pain.	Puncturing an artery.	Knowledge of location of an artery. Palpate vessel for pulse.	Remove device immediately and apply pressure until bleeding stops. Explain to patient what has happened. Inform patient to contact doctor if pain continues or there is increasing swelling or bruising. Document in the patient's notes. Provide information leaflet.
	Touching a nerve (sharp, shooting pain along arm and fingers).	Knowledge of location of nerves. Avoid excessive or blind probing after needle has been inserted.	Remove the needle immediately and apply pressure. Explain to the patient what has happened and that the pain or numbness may last a few hours. Document in the patient's notes.

Problem solving (cont'd)

Problem	Cause	Prevention	Suggested action
			Inform patient to contact doctor if pain continues or becomes worse. Provide information leaflet.
	Anxiety.	(See below.)	See below.
	Use of vein in sensitive area (e.g. wrist).	Avoid using veins in sensitive areas wherever possible. Use local anaesthetic cream.	Complete procedure as quickly as possible.
Anxiety.	Previous trauma.	Minimize the risk of a traumatic venepuncture. Use all methods available to ensure successful venepuncture.	Approach patient in a calm and confident manner. Listen to the patient's fears and explain what the procedure involves. Offer patient opportunity to lie down. Suggest use of local anaesthetic cream.
	Fear of needles.		All above and perhaps referral to a psychologist if fear is of phobic proportions.
Limited venous access.	Repeated use of same veins.	Use alternative sites if possible.	Do not attempt the procedure unless experienced.
	Peripheral shutdown.	Ensure the room is not cold.	Put patient's arm in warm water. Apply glycerol trinitrate patch.
	Dehydration.		May be necessary to rehydrate patient prior to venepuncture.
	Hardened veins (due to scarring and thrombosis).		Do not use these veins as venepuncture will be unsuccessful.
Bruising and/or haematoma.	Needle has punctured the posterior wall of the vein.	Lower angle of insertion.	Remove the needle and apply pressure at the venepuncture site until bleeding stops. The following actions apply regardless of cause: (a) Elevate the limb. (b) Apply ice pack if necessary. (c) Apply Hirudoid cream or arnica cream (as per instructions) with pressure dressing.
	Inadequate pressure on removal of needle.	The practitioner should apply pressure.	
	Forgetting to remove the tourniquet before removing the needle.		Explain to patient what has happened. Inform patient to contact doctor if area becomes more painful as haematoma may be pressing on a nerve. Do not reapply tourniquet to affected limb. Provide information leaflet. Document.
	Poor technique/choice of vein or device.	Ensure correct device and technique are used.	
Infection at the venepuncture site.	Poor aseptic technique.	Ensure good hand washing and adequate skin cleaning.	Report to doctor as patient may require systemic or local antibiotics.
Vasovagal reaction.	Fear of needles. Pain.	Spend time listening to patient's fears. Calm, confident manner.	Place patient's head between his or her legs if patient is feeling faint. Encourage patient to lie down. Call for assistance. It may be appropriate to secure the device (short term) in case it is required for the administration of medication.

Problem solving (cont'd)

Problem	Cause	Prevention	Suggested action
	Warm environment.	Ensure environment is comfortable temperature.	Open a window or door.
Needle inoculation of or contamination to practitioner.	Unsafe practice.	Maintain safe practice. Activate safety device if applicable.	Follow accident procedure for sharps injury, e.g. make site bleed and apply a waterproof dressing. Report and document. An injection of hepatitis B immunoglobulin or triple therapy may be required.
	Incorrect disposal of sharps.	Ensure sharps are disposed of immediately and safely.	
Accidental blood spillage.	Damaged/faulty equipment.	Check equipment prior to use	
	Reverse vacuum.	Use vacuumed plastic blood collection system. Remove blood tube from plastic tube holder before removing needle.	Ensure blood is handled and transported correctly.
Missed vein.	Inadequate anchoring. Poor vein selection. Wrong positioning. Lack of concentration.	Ensure that only properly trained staff perform venepuncture or that those who are training are supervised.	Withdraw the needle slightly and realign it, providing the patient is not feeling any discomfort. Ensure all learners are supervised. If the patient is feeling pain, then the needle should be removed immediately.
	Poor lighting.	Ensure the environment is well lit.	
	Difficult venous access.		Ask experienced colleague to perform the procedure.
Spurt of blood on entry.	Bevel tip of needle enters the vein before entire bevel is under the skin; usually occurs when the vein is very superficial.		Reassure the patient. Wipe blood away on removal of needle.
Blood stops flowing.	Through puncture: needle inserted too far.	Correct angle.	Draw back the needle, but if bruising is evident, then remove the needle immediately and apply pressure.
	Contact with valves.	Palpate to locate.	Withdraw needle slightly to move tip away from valve.
	Venous spasm.	Results from mechanical irritation and cannot be prevented.	Gently massage above the vein or apply heat.
	Vein collapse.	Use veins with large lumen. Use a smaller device.	Release tourniquet, allow veins to refill and retighten tourniquet.
	Small vein.	Avoid use of small veins wherever possible.	May require another venepuncture.
	Poor blood flow.	Use veins with large lumens.	Apply heat above vein.

References and further reading

BMA & RPS (2003) *British National Formulary*. British Medical Association and Royal Pharmaceutical Society of Great Britain, London.

Campbell, H., Carrington, M. & Limber, C. (1999) A practice guide to venepuncture and management of complications. *Br J Nurs*, **8**(7), 426–31.

Castledine, G. (1996) Nurses' role in peripheral venous cannulation. *Br J Nurs*, **5**(20), 1274.

Centers for Disease Control (1997) Evaluation of safety devices for preventing percutaneous injuries among health care workers during phlebotomy procedures. *JAMA*, **277**(6), 449–50.

Dougherty, L. (1996) Intravenous cannulation. *Nurs Stand*, **11**(2), 47–51.

Dougherty, L. (1999) Obtaining vascular access. In: *IV Therapy in Practice* (eds L. Dougherty & J. Lamb). Churchill Livingstone, Edinburgh, Chap. 9.

Ernst, D. & Ernst, C. (2001) *Phlebotomy for Nurses and Nursing Personnel*. Health Star Press, Indiana.

Garza, D. & Becan McBride, K. (2002) *Phlebotomy Handbook: Blood Collection Essentials*. Prentice Hall, New Jersey.

Godwin, P.G.R., Cuthbert, A.C. & Choyce, A. (1992) Reducing bruising after venepuncture. *Quality Health Care*, **1**, 245–6.

Golder, M. (2000) Potential risk of cross infection during peripheral venous access by contamination of tourniquets. *Lancet*, **355**, 44.

Health Service Advisory Committee (1991) *Safety in Health Service Laboratories: Safe Working and the Prevention of Infection in Clinical Laboratories Model Rules for Staff and Visitors*. HMSO, London.

Hudek, K. (1986) Compliance in IV therapy. *J Can Intraven Nurs Assoc*, **2**(3), 3–8.

ICNA (2003) *Reducing Sharps Injury – Prevention and Risk Management*. Infection Control Nurses Association.

INS (Intravenous Nursing Society) (2000) *Standards for Infusion Therapy*. INS & Becton Dickinson, New York.

Lamb, J. (1999) Legal and professional aspects of IV therapy. In: *IV Therapy in Practice* (eds L. Dougherty & J. Lamb). Churchill Livingstone, Edinburgh, Chap. 1.

Marieb, E.N. (1998) *Essentials of Human Anatomy and Physiology*, 5th edn. Benjamin/Cummings, California.

Masoorli, S. (2002) Catheter related nerve injury: inherent risk or avoidable outcome? *J Vasc Access Devices*, **7**(4), 49.

McCall, R.E. & Tankersley, C.M. (2002) Blood collection variables and procedural errors. In: *Phlebotomy Essentials*, 3rd edn. Lippincott, Williams & Wilkins, Philadelphia.

McConnell, A.A. & MacKay, G.M. (1996) Venepuncture: the medicolegal hazards. *Postgrad Med J*, **72**, 23–4.

Mitchell Higgs, N. (2002) *Personal protective equipment – improving compliance*. All Points Conference, Safer Needles Network, London, May.

NAO (2003) *A Safer Place to Work – Management of Health and Safety Risks in Trusts*. National Audit Office, London.

NMC (2002) *Code of Professional Conduct*. Nursing and Midwifery Council, London.

Perdue, M. (1995) Intravenous complications. In: *Intravenous Therapy: Clinical Principles and Practices* (eds J. Terry, L. Baranowski, R.A. Lonsway & C. Hedrick). W.B. Saunders, Philadelphia, Chap. 24.

Price, J. & Moss, J. (1998) The pitfalls of practice nursing. *Nurs Times*, **94**(30), 64–6.

RCN (1995) *Universal Precautions*. Royal College of Nursing, London.

RCN (1999) *Guidance for Nurses Giving Intravenous Therapy*. Royal College of Nursing, London.

RCN (2003) *Standards for Infusion Therapy*. Royal College of Nursing, London.

Smith, J. (1998) The practice of venepuncture in lymphoedema. *Eur J Cancer Care*, **7**, 97–8.

Springhouse (2002) *Intravenous Therapy Made Incredibly Easy*. Springhouse Corporation, Philadelphia.

Thrush, D. & Belsole, R. (1995) Radical nerve injury after routine peripheral cannulation. *J Clin Anaesth*, **7**(2), 160–2.

Walther, K. *et al.* (2001) IV therapy in the older adult. In: *Infusion Therapy in Clinical Practice* (eds J. Hankin *et al.*). W.B. Saunders, Philadelphia.

Waugh, A. & Grant, A. (2001) The cardiovascular system. In: *Anatomy and Physiology in Health and Illness*, 9th edn. Churchill Livingstone, Edinburgh, pp. 79–80.

Weinstein, S.M. (2000) *Plumer's Principles and Practice of Intravenous Therapy*, 7th edn. J.B. Lippincott, Philadelphia.

Violence: prevention and management

Chapter contents

Definition

Violence is endemic in our health care system and is, for many staff working in certain areas, an almost daily occurrence (NMC 2002a). Violence at work can be defined as 'any incident in which a health care employee is verbally abused, threatened or assaulted by a patient or member of the public in the circumstances of their employment' (Health Services Advisory Committee 1997). This is a physically and non-physically related definition. Robinson (1983) defines aggression as 'an assertive force which may be expressed through attitude or behaviour and is usually directed to external objects, though it may be turned inward, as reflected in self-destructive behaviour'. She states that 'aggression is a healthy force which sometimes needs to be channelled'. Thus, it can be expressed either physically or non-physically.

The Royal College of Nursing recommends the following definition of violence orientated towards staff members, which can be adapted at local level as necessary:

> 'Any incident in which a health professional experiences abuse, threat, fear or the application of force arising out of the course of their work, whether or not they are on duty.'
> (RCN 1998)

However, as violence is often directed towards other individuals and objects, the local policy should encompass these aspects.

It can therefore be concluded from the above definitions that violence is an act or type of behaviour that may take the form of aggression, abuse, threat or attack.

Indications

Management of violence is necessary:

- When the person shows a predisposition to violence
- When a person makes a physical attack on another person or object

- When a person becomes disturbed to the extent that his/her behaviour is considered a threat to his/her own safety or the safety of others.

Reference material

In the latter part of 1999, ministers developed the NHS Zero Tolerance Campaign in England with the aim of tackling the issue of violence and intimidation against NHS staff. However, violent crime in the UK is steadily increasing and nearly 650 000 workers had experienced at least one violent incident during 1997 (Mahar 2002). In 1999 there were 65 000 reported violent incidents in British hospitals. By 2001 the number had increased by 30% to 85 000 (DoH 2001). Moreover, there is evidence to suggest that acts of violence against NHS staff, for a variety of reasons, are still underreported (Arnetz & Arnetz 2000; Rippon 2000; Beech 2001; Paterson *et al.* 2001). Nonetheless, assaults in the UK are now the third most common type of reported accident after slips, falls and needle accidents. Nurses, ambulance and A&E staff, and those caring for psychologically disturbed patients, are particularly vulnerable (Dobson 1999). Incidents range from threats and abuse to permanently disabling injuries and, rarely, loss of life. This chapter is confined to the prevention and management of violence in the hospital setting.

Principles

The following principles underlie the management of violent persons:

- Prevention of violent incidents is the foremost principle.
- Restraint is always therapeutic, never punitive. As far as possible, the therapeutic regimen should be maintained.
- The risk of physical injury should be minimized. Any restraint applied must be of a degree appropriate to the actual danger or resistance shown by the person. This is particularly important with children and the elderly. Staff must receive training in the use of restraint as training can help prevent injury to staff and patients.
- The locally agreed procedure for the nursing care of violent patients should be adhered to.

Theories of violence

Mechanisms that may combine to explain or produce a violent act are reviewed by Harrington (1972) and Gunn (1973). Generally, theories of violence may be classified as biological (Lorenz 1966; Gray 1971; Montague 1979), psychological (Freud 1955; Dollard & Miller 1961) or sociocultural (Bandura & Walters 1963; Wertham 1968; Gelles 1972). Although the latter of these cannot be completely divorced from organic or biological predisposition, certain factors may increase the risk of violent or aggressive behaviour. For example, aggressive parents often have aggressive children but people who conclude that aggression is learnt from parents in a 'cycle of violence' never consider the possibility that violent tendencies could be inherited as well as learnt (Pinker 2002). Glasser (1998) also discusses the psychoanalytical perspective of violent acts which may be characterized as one of two types: self-preservation violence or sado-masochistic violence. Self-preservation violence is given as an instinctive, primitive response to danger or threat, whereas sado-masochistic violence is premeditated, usually sustained and pleasure is derived from the suffering of the object (Glasser 1998). Studies have shown associations between combat experience, post-traumatic stress disorder, anger and hostility, and involvement in violence (Reilly *et al.* 1994). In the hospital setting where reactions to stress, illness and treatment are prevalent, staff-related factors are also important in predisposing to violence by patients or visitors. Common antecedents include patients' boredom, inadequate staffing levels, lack of opportunity for patients to participate in therapy and social groups, and staff attitudes, including physical abuse, racism, ridicule of service users and matters of confidentiality (NMC 2002a).

Incidents of verbal or physical abuse are more likely to happen in long-term care and emergency areas and may be directed towards nurses and nursing assistants rather than doctors. In the UK, of all health care professions and grades, student nurses were at the greatest risk of being the victim of a work-related violent incident (Beech 1999). Furthermore, male staff were more involved in actual recorded incidents than expected in the given population (Vanderslott 1998). Violence may be viewed as a behaviour influenced by various factors including personality, environment and social culture. Each perspective may add to the development of a body of knowledge about the problem of violence in the hospital setting.

Physiological considerations

Under certain circumstances patients may have little or no ability to exercise control over their aggression. In these instances aggression may be related to pathological physiology. Internal stressors may include endocrine imbalance such as hyperthyroidism, hyperglycaemia, convulsive disorders, HIV encephalopathy, dementia and brain tumours. Krakowski and Czobor (1994) confirmed an association between persistent violence and neurological impairment. The effects of alcohol and substance abuse should also be considered. One study showed that rates for people with schizophrenia perpetrating violent acts were four times those of populations without mental disorders. For the so-called dual diagnosis populations (with co-existing mental illness and drug/alcohol misuse), rates were four times higher than for people with schizophrenia, i.e. 16 times higher than the general population (NMC 2002a). Among the physiological causes given by Kerr and Taylor (1997) are pain, side-effects of medication (including neuroleptic-induced akathisia), childhood disorders such as autism and mental retardation. Worthington (2000) reports that physical assault is associated with post-traumatic stress disorder, impaired immune and endocrine function and increased substance abuse, all of which compromise long-term health and increase demands on the health care system. Preventive measures to reduce the risk of violence may not be possible and the policy for the management of violence should be adhered to.

Legislation

The law on health and safety at work applies to risks from violence, just as it does to other risks at work. Key points are summarized as follows.

1 *Health and Safety at Work etc. Act 1974*
   Employers must:
   (a) Protect the health and safety at work of their employees
   (b) Protect the health and safety of others who might be affected, such as visitors, contractors, students and patients.
2 *Management of Health and Safety at Work Regulations 1999*
   Employers must:
   (a) Assess the risks to the health and safety of their employees
   (b) Identify the precautions needed to reduce the risks of violence
   (c) Make arrangements for the effective management of risks
   (d) Appoint competent people to advise them on health and safety
   (e) Provide information and training to employees.
3 *The Reporting of Injuries, Diseases and Dangerous Occurrences Regulations 1995*
   These Regulations state that employers must report cases in which employees have been off work for 3 days or more following an assault which has resulted in physical injury. This should be in conjunction with the local incident policy in which any psychological injury is also documented.
4 *The Safety Representatives and Safety Committees Regulations 1977* and *The Health and Safety (Consultation with Employees) Regulations 1996*
   Employers must consult with safety representatives and employees on health and safety matters (Health Services Advisory Committee 1997).

Policy formation

NHS trusts must establish targets for reducing violence against their staff and targets will be expected to be met. In addition, NHS trusts will be expected to have systems in place to monitor and record violence against staff and have published strategies in place to achieve a reduction in such incidents (Dobson 1999).

In forming a policy for managing aggression or violence, the following aspects need to be considered:

- Environmental and organizational factors
- Anticipation and prevention of violence
- Action following an incident.

Environmental and organizational factors

Hospital environments can be stressful places and so certain design features can help to maximize a tranquil ambience. Calming features include creating a perception of space, ensuring there is natural daylight and fresh air and noise levels are controlled, providing smoking and non-smoking areas and ensuring privacy in toilet and bathroom areas. In creating a secure environment (in psychiatric settings) there must be a safe room for severely disturbed people, movable objects should be of a safe weight, size and construction, and doors should be easily accessible. This list is not exhaustive and many other features are possible when considering environmental factors (Royal College of Psychiatrists 1998).

The way in which staff are deployed influences the likelihood and outcome of any violent incident. Teaching sessions on the management of violence should be held on a regular basis so that staff benefit from controlled practice of the required techniques for avoiding or containing violence. Topics may include assessment and prediction of risk factors, the dos and don'ts of verbal and non-verbal interaction and breakaway skills training (Beech 1999). After one such 3-day course, students commented on their increased awareness of risky situations, feeling more confident in dealing with patients' aggression and demonstrating a beneficial change in attitude towards aggression and violence at work.

Perhaps the most significant advance in the management of violence in recent years is the documentation on physical restraint. This has been comprehensively reviewed by Wright (1999) and is recognized as being a controversial and emotive topic. Since the mid-1980s, staff in health care and local authority settings have received training in methods for physically managing violence and aggression, termed 'control and restraint' (C&R). The use of this procedure has expanded to such an extent that in a survey of inpatient care in inner London (Gournay *et al.* 1998, cited in Wright 1999), only one of 11 inner London trusts surveyed did not routinely train acute nursing staff in C&R. However, there are many safety, ethical and legal implications to be considered before embarking on these methods. There have been instances of accidental death of patients resulting from restraint procedures being inappropriately or incorrectly applied (Wright 1999). This is particularly relevant when working with patients who are elderly, infirm or sedated. It is also worth noting that while physical restraint may be seen as potentially damaging to a patient's physical or mental well-being, the consequences of not restraining a patient who is attempting to harm themselves or others may be even more damaging to the patient's self-esteem and may preserve life and/ or minimize harm in the short term (Wright 1999). Whatever physical restraint method is employed, it is vital to apply it uniformly and it should only be conducted by appropriately trained and accredited staff. If there is an incident team in the hospital that is expected to respond to urgent situations where there is violence or the threat of violence, then each member of that team should have received training commensurate with their role and contact with patients (NMC 2002a).

'Breakaway' techniques, such as escaping holds and blocking kicks and punches, may be relevant to any member of staff in a hospital environment, whilst training in restraint is more appropriate for staff working in clinical care. Serious consideration should also be given to C&R training for staff other than nurses because if restraint is only applied by nurses, it is easier for nurses to be seen as agents of control (Wright 1999; NMC 2002a).

Anticipation and prevention of violence

The purpose of the assessment of risk of violence is to identify how and why conflict can occur and consider what measures can be taken to reduce the risks of such events within the workplace. The risk assessment process for the identification and control of violence can be separated into the following steps:

Identify hazards

It is helpful if there is an assessment form for the risks that are being assessed which can be completed in discussion with staff within the department. A review of past incidents will provide an opportunity to identify potential sources of conflict, potential aggressors and likely risk factors. For example, the assessment should consider whether any particular areas present a higher risk of violence such as:

- Front line reception areas
- Inpatient clinical areas
- Outpatient clinical areas
- Communal areas
- Community
- Lone working, e.g. interview rooms, isolated offices.

Identify potential aggressors

The complexities of human nature can make people unpredictable in how they will react in different situations. Illness can exacerbate the response in both patients and their relatives, and health care workers need to be particularly sensitive to this. Staff will also have their own issues that may affect how they respond at different times. For example:

Patients

Patients who are at high risk of being violent should be identified. This includes those with physiological conditions as previously discussed or patients with a previous history of violent behaviour. There should be a multi-professional approach in establishing this. Pinker (2002) states that psychologists find that individuals prone to violence have a distinctive personality profile. They tend to be impulsive, low in intelligence, hyperactive and attention deficient. They are described as having an 'oppositional temperament': they are vindictive, easily angered, resistant to control, deliberately annoying and likely to blame everything on other people. Patients may become violent or aggressive for a number of reasons, often these are not directly related to the environment but are as a result of a changed mental state due to treatment, e.g. drug therapy, anxiety or frustration. There may also be language or cultural differences, which can lead to confusion and aggression. Failure to recognize these issues can give the impression of indifference and further exacerbate the situation (The Royal Marsden Hospital 2002). Violent incidents may be spontaneous, without apparent provocation. For example, a patient suffering from a psychotic illness or cerebral lesion may demonstrate these symptoms. However, there may be warning signs, such as increased agitation, which would alert staff to a potentially violent situation and therefore give nurses the opportunity to reduce the risk of violence.

Physical signs may include:

- Increased restlessness
- Bodily tension
- Pacing
- Tense and angry facial expressions

- Increased volume of speech
- Verbal threats or gestures
- Refusal to communicate or withdrawal (Royal College of Psychiatrists 1998; RCN 1998).

Signs of high arousal (boisterousness), irritability, confusion and anger (threats or attacks on inanimate objects) are reliable predictors of imminent assaults on staff (Whittington 1997). Responding to these cues to violence with an appropriate verbal interaction and non-verbal behaviour can prevent the escalation of an incident (NMC 2002a).

Sheffield University has developed a model for de-escalation called 'CASE', the acronym standing for Calming, Accessing and Self Enabling, which takes into account the internal (thoughts and feelings) and external (behaviour) communication factors for both the nurse and the patient (Walker 2002). The nurse uses verbal and non-verbal skills to calm the situation down and access his or her own thoughts and feelings whilst encouraging the patient to do the same. For example, the nurse asks the angry patient if he would like to sit down and talk about what is upsetting him. This is the test and compliance method of interaction. It enables the nurse to assess not only the patient's level of emotion but also his cognitive ability to help resolve the conflict. When the patient sits down as offered and is ready to engage in conversation, the enabling phase comes into effect. There may be more negotiating language in the communication which gives an indication that the anger is subsiding to a level where he is more able to think and behave rationally (Walker 2002).

Knowledge of the propensities of individual patients will enable a nurse to recognize many of the signs of impending violence, thus allowing steps to be taken to help patients find alternative outlets for their aggressive feelings.

Visitors and relatives

It is important to realize that each visitor, contractor, outpatient or relative visiting the hospital will have individual needs, anxieties and expectations. Tension may be released in terms of anger, and on occasions violence, towards other members of their family or staff that they encounter. Factors such as poor sign-posting, failure to find a parking space, long waiting times for an appointment, inadequate welfare facilities, perceived queue-jumping and inadequate information can all increase the risk of conflict and aggression (The Royal Marsden Hospital 2002).

Staff

The response of staff to aggressive situations may be influenced by factors such as workload, stress, illness, confidence and experience. When long hours are worked, or a heavy workload is undertaken, staff may feel under increased stress. Misunderstandings, failure to clarify task requirements or requests can lead to verbal abuse or aggression. It should not be seen as a weakness of staff if they try to avoid violence. It is the responsibility of individual members of staff to state whether they have a physical condition, such as a back injury or pregnancy, which would render them incapable of performing C&R techniques. If so, then help should be summoned from other staff members at the earliest opportunity. It is important also to consider the needs of new or agency staff who may not be aware of the activities of the department. Inappropriate expectations can also lead to conflict or bullying behaviour. The level of training provided for staff (in terms of undertaking the work required, customer care skills, dealing with aggression, how to diffuse awkward situations, etc.) can also influence the degree of risk (The Royal Marsden Hospital 2002).

Agreement within the policy should be considered concerning what criteria are used before calling the police to attend an incident. This will depend on the severity of the situation and persons or property at risk (RCN 1998). The involvement of the police and the criminal justice system is discussed at greater length in the NMC (2002a) document. To summarize:

- Summoning police assistance generally means that the police will assume responsibility for the control of the violent incident, rather than seeing themselves as assisting nursing staff. The police will then deal with the situation as they see fit.
- The police are obliged to take action after any crime, which may take the form of a warning, a caution or a charge.
- The victim may be asked if they wish to take part in proceedings but does not have the responsibility, as is often thought, of 'pressing charges'.

Taking police action is often thought of as a last resort because of staff feeling that they have failed to manage the incident effectively or that the patient's medical or mental health needs will be overlooked, or fearing that a police presence will inflame the situation. However, there may be several benefits: it would increase the likelihood of the incident being recorded in the medical notes; it may lead to more appropriate future treatment; it may also communicate and enforce a firm message that violence will not be tolerated and that the patient is to be held responsible for his or her behaviour (NMC 2002a). *Ex gratia* payments to victims of crime made by the Criminal Injuries Compensation Board are conditional upon police involvement (Cembrowicz 1989).

Implementing additional control measures to reduce risk

Once the hazards and risks have been identified, the next step required is a review of the procedures already in place to reduce the risks. Any additional precautions, procedures or control measures required can then be implemented. These may include providing the features previously discussed in the section on environmental and organizational factors, plus:

- Providing comfortable seating
- Providing access to refreshment
- Providing appropriate facilities for the disabled
- Improving communication systems and multilingual notices and signposts
- Reducing waiting times
- Providing staff training
- Increasing personal security systems, such as closed-circuit television
- Providing staff support
- Introducing an incident reporting system.

Action following an incident

Once violence has occurred, the following may be regarded as among the important management decisions that need to be implemented:

- Medical personnel should be informed immediately because medication may be required as part of the management of the situation.
- Some nurses must be delegated to attend to the needs of the remaining patients, to telephone for help and to prepare any required medication.
- If immobilization is needed, the agreed local policy for restraining a patient must be implemented.

The law regarding assault and self-defence is complicated and often inconsistent. There is further complication in that, while certain responses to violence may be permissible under the law, the actions of health care staff are also regulated by codes of professional practice (Wright 1999). At all times the *Code of Professional Conduct* must be adhered to (NMC 2002b). This is discussed in further detail in *Dealing with Violence Against Nursing Staff* (RCN 1998) but Point 5.3 on confidentiality and information disclosure and Point 8 on identifying and minimizing risk are particularly pertinent. If legal advice needs to be obtained in a particular case, such as financial compensation or prosecution following personal injury or damage to property, this should be obtained from a solicitor, barrister, health and safety representative and/or trade union representative.

Following the incident, staff should be given an opportunity to discuss their feelings about the aggressor(s), other members of staff involved and the way the incident was managed. This should happen as soon as possible after the incident has resolved and with as many of the staff concerned as possible. There should be discussion on:

- What happened
- Any trigger factors
- People's roles in the incident
- How they feel now
- How they might feel in the next few days
- What can be done about it
- Any measures that can be taken to avoid a repeat of the situation (RCN 1998).

Emotional debriefing aims to recognize potential stress, acknowledge it as a normal response and provide a supportive and structured setting to allow people to cope more effectively. Discussion should not be focused on any person's performance but address the effects on them as individuals (Health Services Advisory Committee 1997). In addition to the debriefing procedure, the physical and psychological well-being of the staff involved and the team as a whole need to be addressed. Staff injured as a result of their involvement in the incident may be entitled to industrial injuries benefit or a payment under the criminal injuries compensation scheme and will need to be informed of their rights by the appropriate body (RCN 1998). Consideration must be given to the risk of infection in cases where injury has occurred; for example, bites or needlestick injuries. Staff must receive continued support when returning to work after a violent incident (RCN 1998). Debriefing can be supplemented by making confidential counselling available through in-house counsellors, occupational health departments or independent external bodies (Health Services Advisory Committee 1997).

Some staff view reporting of incidents as admission of failure, especially if violence is rare in the area in which they work, therefore debriefing becomes particularly relevant in order to promote reporting of incidents (Rippon 2000; Paterson *et al.* 2001; NMC 2002a).

All documentation required by law (such as the reporting of staff off work for 3 days or more following an assault) or hospital policy (such as completing an incident form) should be completed and forwarded to the appropriate departments. If restraints have been used, how and by whom they were applied should be documented. Specific and accurate written records will aid recall if it is required, perhaps years later (RCN 1998).

*Procedure guidelines: **Prevention and management of violence** (cont'd)*

Action	Rationale
8 Each person should know which part of the patient's body is to be held and from where to approach the patient. (The policy for immobilization may vary from area to area.)	To achieve full and safe immobilization of the patient.
9 Allocate one member of staff, preferably someone the patient knows, to talk to the patient throughout the procedure.	To inform the patient about what is happening and why.
10 Try to minimize discomfort. Restraint must be of a degree appropriate to the actual resistance given by the patient.	The procedure is not a punitive one but for safety reasons.
11 As the patient calms down, the leader should indicate when restraint can be reduced. This should be done gradually, e.g. release one wrist at a time.	The patient may still be likely to strike.
12 The leader should withdraw staff from the patient gradually. Some staff should stay with the patient.	Gradual withdrawal is safer in case of further outbursts. To observe mood and behaviour and provide reassurance to the patient.

Follow-up

Action	Rationale
1 Attend to any patients and staff injured during the incident. Such people should be informed of their legal rights.	To provide care and to comply with legal obligations and hospital policy.
2 Record details of any violent incidents in the appropriate documents.	To comply with legal obligations and hospital policy.
3 The entire team should discuss the incident.	To vent feelings and evaluate care provided. Violent incidents are to be regarded as learning experiences and an opportunity for reflective practice.

References and further reading

Arnetz, J. E. & Arnetz, B.B. (2000) Implementation and evaluation of a practical intervention programme for dealing with violence towards health care workers. *J Adv Nurs*, **31**(3), 668–80.

Bandura, A. & Walters, R. (1963) *Social Learning and Personality Development*. Holt, Rinehart & Winston, New York.

Beech, B. (1999) Sign of the times or the shape of things to come? A 3-day unit of instruction on 'aggression and violence in health settings for all students during pre-registration nurse training'. *Nurse Educ Today*, **19**(8), 610–16.

Beech, B. (2001) Zero tolerance of violence against health care staff. *Nurs Stand* **15**(16), 39–41.

Cembrowicz, S. (1989) Dealing with difficult patients: what goes wrong? *Practitioner* **233**(5), 486–9.

Dobson, F. (1999) *Dobson steps up major drive to protect NHS staff from assaults: violence and security*. Memorandum from NHS Executive. Press Release, 15 April. Stationery Office, London.

DoH (2001) *Withholding Treatment from Violent and Abusive Patients in NHS Trusts: NHS Zero Tolerance Zone*. HSC 2001/18. Stationery Office, London.

Dollard, J. & Miller, N.E. (1961) *Frustration and Aggression*. Yale University Press, New Haven.

Freud, S. (1955) *The Complete Psychological Works of Sigmund Freud*, Vol. 18. Hogarth Press, London.

Gelles, R.J. (1972) *The Violent Home*. Sage, Beverly Hills.

Glasser, M. (1998) On violence: a preliminary communication. *Int J Psycho-Analysis*, **79**(5), 887–902.

Gray, J.A. (1971) Sex differences in emotional behaviour in mammals including man: endocrine basis. *Acta Psychol*, **35**, 29–44.

Gunn, J. (1973) *Violence*. David & Charles, Newton Abbot.

Harrington, J.A. (1972) *Violence: a clinical viewpoint. Br Med J*, **i**, 228–31.

Health Services Advisory Committee (1997) *Violence and Aggression to Staff in Health Services: Guidance on Assessment and Management*, 2nd edn. HSE Books, Suffolk.

HSE (1996a) *A Guide to the Reporting of Injuries, Diseases and Dangerous Occurrences Regulations 1995 (RIDDOR)*. L73. Stationery Office, London.

HSE (1996b) *A Guide to the Health and Safety (Consultation with Employees) Regulations 1996*. Guidance on Regulations L95. Stationery Office, London.

HSE (1996c) *Safety Representatives and Safety Committees* L87. Stationery Office. London.

HSE (1999) *Management of Health and Safety at Work Regulations 1999*. Approved Code of Practice L21. Stationery Office, London.

Kerr, I.B. & Taylor, D. (1997) Acute disturbed or violent behaviour: principles of treatment. *J Psychopharmacol*, **11**(3), 271–7.

Krakowski, M. & Czobor, P. (1994) Clinical symptoms, neurological impairment, and prediction of violence in psychiatric inpatients. *Hosp Commun Psychiatry*, **45**(7), 711–13.

Lorenz, K. (1966) *On Aggression*. Harcourt, Brace & World, New York.

Mahar, S. (2002) *Influences on Health at Work*. HL 3038. Home Office, London (accessed June 2002).

Montague, M.C. (1979) Physiology of aggressive behaviour. *J Neurosurg Nurs*, **11**, 10–15.

NMC (2002a) *The Recognition, Prevention and Therapeutic Management of Violence in Mental Health Care*. Nursing and Midwifery Council, London. www.nmc-uk.org (accessed 8 October 2003).

NMC (2002b) *Code of Professional Conduct*. Nursing and Midwifery Council, London.

Paterson, B., Leadbetter, D. & Bowie, V. (2001) Zero in on violence. *Nurs Manage*, **8**(1), 16–22.

Pinker, S. (2002) The killer instinct. *The Times,* T2, 3 September; Suppl, 2–3.

RCN (1998) *Dealing with Violence Against Nursing Staff: An RCN Guide for Nurses and Managers*. Royal College of Nursing, London.

Reilly, P. *et al.* (1994) Anger management and temper control: critical components of post traumatic stress disorder and substance abuse treatment. *J Psychoactive Drugs*, **26**(4), 401–407.

Rippon, T.J. (2000) Aggression and violence in health care professions. *J Adv Nurs*, **31**(2), 452–60.

Robinson, L. (1983) *Psychiatric Nursing as a Human Experience*. W.B. Saunders, Philadelphia.

Royal College of Psychiatrists (1998) *Management of Imminent Violence – Clinical Practice Guidelines: Quick Reference Guide*. Royal College of Psychiatrists, London.

Royal Marsden Hospital (2002) *The Violence at Work Policy*. Royal Marsden Hospital, London.

Vanderslott, J. (1998) A study of incidents of violence towards staff by patients in an NHS trust hospital. *J Psychiatr Mental Health Nurs*, **5**, 291–8.

Walker, J. (2002) Safety first. *Nurs Times* **98**(9), 20–1.

Wertham, D.J. (1968) *A Sign For Cain*. Hale, New York.

Whittington, R. (1997) Violence to nurses: prevalence and risk factors. *Nurs Stand* **12**(5), 49–56.

Worthington, K. (2000) Violence in the health care workplace. *Am J Nurs*, **100**(11), 69–70.

Wright, S. (1999) Physical restraint in the management of violence and aggression in in-patient settings: a review of issues. *J Mental Health*, **8**(5), 459–72.

Table 47.1 Factors that may delay wound healing

Disease, disorders and syndromes	Addison's disease; anaemia; arteriosclerosis; autoimmune disorders; Buerger's disease; diabetes; cardiopulmonary disease; Crohn's disease; Cushing's syndrome; hepatic failure; hypovolaemia; hypoxia; immune disorders; infection; inflammatory bowel disease; jaundice; leucopenia; malignancy; protein losing enteropathy; Raynaud's disease; renal failure; respiratory conditions; rheumatoid arthritis; thyroid deficiency; uraemia; vascular diseases; venous stasis
Drugs	Alcohol; antimicrobials; cytotoxics; immunosuppressives; nicotine; non-steroidal anti-inflammatories; penicillamine and penicillin; steroids
Poor nutritional state	Anaemia; malnutrition; mineral deficiency (particularly zinc); protein deficiency; vitamin deficiency (particularly A and C)
Microenvironment of wound	Blood supply; gas composition; humidity; infection; inflammation; high pH; low temperature; oxygen tension
Other	Aetiology of wound; age; fibrous ring round open wound; foreign body in wound; obesity; radiation; stress; suture materials; suture technique; trauma/mechanical stress; treatment (including use of antiseptics and/or linting materials); inadequate sleep

Note: some conditions may affect the healing process via several mechanisms.
From: Sitton 1992a; Cutting 1994; Wells 1994; Benbow 1995; Kiecolt-Glaser *et al*. 1995; Collier 1996; Bale & Jones 1997; Olde Damink & Soeters 1997; Armstrong 1998; Bowler 1998; Donovan 1998; Grey 1998; Lotti *et al*. 1998; Moore & Foster 1998b; Sussman 1998; Thomson 1998; Williams & Young 1998; Gilchrist 1999; Mahony 1999.

of histamine, vasodilatation begins (Flanagan 1996). The liberation of histamine also increases the permeability of the capillary walls, and plasma proteins, leucocytes, antibodies and electrolytes exude into the surrounding tissues. The wound becomes red, swollen and hot.

Polymorphonuclear leucocytes (neutrophils) and macrophages are chemotactically attracted to the wound to defend against infection and begin the process of repair (Hart 2002). The macrophage is also known as the 'director cell' of wound healing (Silver 1994). If the number and function of macrophages is reduced, as may occur in disease, e.g. diabetes (Tooke *et al*. 1988), or due to treatment, e.g. chemotherapy in cancer patients (Souhami & Tobias 1998), healing is seriously affected.

Neutrophils and macrophages combine to destroy and ingest bacteria, debris and devitalized tissue. This involves a great deal of cellular activity which requires up to 20 times the normal resting rate of oxygen of phagocytic cells. Patients with hypoxic wounds are, therefore, more susceptible to wound infection.

The degradation of unwanted material causes an increased osmolarity within the area, resulting in further swelling by osmosis. This may increase pressure in restricted parts of the body, thus precipitating ischaemia.

Proliferative phase (3–24 days)

Macrophages produce factors that are chemotactic to fibroblasts and angioblasts. The macrophage secretes a fibroblast-stimulating factor which in the presence of a growth factor released by the dead platelets causes the fibroplast to migrate into the wound soon after damage has occurred (Silver 1994; Calvin 1998).

The fibroblasts are activated to divide and produce collagen by processes initiated by the macrophages. This develops a network of poorly organized collagen which increases the strength of the wound. Newly synthesized collagen creates a 'healing ridge' below an intact suture line, thus giving an indication of how wound healing is progressing. This mechanism is dependent on the presence of iron, vitamin C and oxygen. Therefore, appropriate levels of nutrition and oxygenation during this phase of wound healing are particularly necessary.

Angioblasts are required to form new blood vessels which grow into the wound under conditions of a hypoxic tissue gradient (Knighton *et al*. 1981; Flanagan 1996). The vessels branch and join other vessels forming loops. The fragile capillary loops are held within a framework of collagen. This complex is known as granulation tissue. Granulation tissue can grow into wound dressings such as gauze. On removal of the dressing any adhered delicate granulation tissue is destroyed.

The process of wound contraction can significantly reduce the size of the wound and the area that new tissue must cover. It is extremely important, and only observable, in open wounds healing by secondary intention. There is debate about the exact method by which wound contraction occurs but two theories prevail: the cell contraction theory and the cell traction theory (Tejero-Trujeque 2001). The cell contraction theory proposes that an altered fibroblast, called a myofibroblast (which has similar properties to a smooth muscle cell), has the ability to contract and pull collagen fibrils towards itself, thereby reducing the size

Table 47.2 Growth factors involved in wound healing

Growth factor	Actions
Epidermal growth factor (EGF)	Induces keratinocyte proliferation, migration, adhesion and differentiation, and fibroplasia
Fibroblast growth factor 2 (FGF-2)	Promotes angiogenesis, stimulates proliferation of epithelial cells and fibroblasts
Transforming growth factor β (TGF-β)	Attracts macrophages, induces production of procollagen and fibronectin (matrix synthesis), inhibits metalloproteases
Insulin-like growth factor 1 (IGF-1)	Stimulates fibroblast proliferation, increases dermal and epidermal synthesis when administered with PDGF-BB
Platelet-derived growth factor (PDGF)	Stimulates fibroblast proliferation and angiogenesis, attracts neutrophils and macrophages

From: Garrett & Garrett 1997; Hart 1999; Krishnamoorthy *et al.* 2001b; Collier 2002.

of the wound (Flanagan 1996; Calvin 1998). In contrast, the cell traction theory states that wound contraction occurs as a result of the movement of fibroblasts. During their migration into the wound they pull tissue along, causing a 'crinkling' effect (Harris *et al.* 1981). It has also been suggested that collagen fibres are involved in wound contraction (Fletcher 2000).

Re-epithelialization usually begins within 24 hours of injury (Garrett 1997; Calvin 1998). Epithelial cells (keratinocytes) may migrate from hair follicles and sweat glands within the wound or from the perimeter of the wound (Moore & Foster 1998b). The migration of epithelial cells across the wound surface may occur via single cell migration or 'leap-frogging' where a cell moves forward and stops while other cells move over the top of it (Calvin 1998). It has been proposed that individual cells move forward by extending a pseudopod, which attaches to a new position, and then the remainder of the cell is pulled to the new position (amoeboid locomotion) (Garrett 1997). Epithelial cells will burrow under contaminated debris and unwanted material (Waldorf & Fewkes 1995) while also secreting an enzyme that separates the scab from underlying tissue. Dissolving dry eschar requires nearly 50% of the cell's metabolic energy (Messer 1989; Johnson 1998a). Through a mechanism called contact inhibition epithelial cells will cease migrating when they come into contact with other epithelial cells (Garrett 1997).

The ability of the epithelium to cover the wound surface is limited to approximately 2 cm^2. This means that the process of contraction is of vital importance to healing wounds (Messer 1989). Epithelialization (migration, mitosis and differentiation) occurs at an increased rate in a moist wound environment, as do the synthesis of collagen and formation of new capillaries (Winter 1972; Eaglstein 1985; Dyson *et al.* 1988; Miller 1998a; Flanagan 1999). A hypoxic (low oxygen) environment has also been shown to increase the motility of epidermal cells (O'Toole *et al.* 1997).

Maturation phase (21 days onward)

This stage begins at around 21 days following the initial injury. Maturation or remodelling of the healed wound may last for more than a year. Collagen is reorganized, the fibres becoming enlarged and orientated along the lines of tension in the wound (at right angles to the wound margin) (Silver 1994). This occurs via a process of lysis and resynthesis. Intermolecular cross-linking aids the tensile strength of the wound. The reorganization of collagen may result in further contraction of the wound, which may potentiate contraction deformities (Silver 1994; Moore & Foster 1998b). During this phase the number of blood vessels within the scar is reduced. Maximum strength is reached in approximately 3 months, although the scar will only achieve about 70–80% of normal skin strength (Calvin 1998; Ehrlich 1999). At the end of the maturation phase the delicate granulation tissue of the wound will have been replaced by stronger avascular scar tissue.

Growth factors

Recent research has indicated that essential cellular activity that occurs during wound healing can be attributed to specific proteins known as growth factors (Cox 1993; Garrett 1997; Krishnamoorthy *et al.* 2001a). They are naturally occurring proteins secreted by cells in response to an injury and 'mediate, co-ordinate and control cellular interactions that occur during skin maintenance and wound healing' (Cox 1993). Table 47.2 lists the most common growth factors involved with the process of wound repair. The discovery of these growth factors has led to advances in wound therapeutics (Devel 1987; Brown *et al.* 1991; Robson 1996; Robson *et al.* 1993, 2001; Wieman 1998; Smiell *et al.* 1999). For example, a small study found that a group of patients with non-healing venous ulcers showed a significantly faster healing rate following treatment with TGF-β2 growth factors (Robson *et al.* 1993).

necrotic tissue by neutrophils and macrophages. This effect is enhanced in a moist wound environment, which can be achieved through the use of hydrogel dressings or semi-occlusive dressings that maintain moisture at the wound surface (Hofman 1996; Bale 1997; Freedline 1999). If autolytic debridement is considered too slow or is not working and the patient is unfit for surgical or sharp debridement then treatment with enzymic debriding agents could be considered (Freedline 1999; Werner 1999). These products actively breakdown dead tissue and blood clots, accelerating removal of devitalized tissue from the wound.

A novel approach to debridement that has recently returned to favour is the use of sterile fly larvae (maggots). The sterile larvae (usually *Lucilia sericata*, the greenbottle blowfly, or *Phormia regina*, the blackbottle blowfly) are applied to and retained at the wound bed (Hinshaw 2000). The larvae move over the surface of the wound, secreting a powerful mixture of proteolytic enzymes which break down necrotic tissue, which they then ingest. They remove devitalized tissue by this method (the enzymes are neutralized by live tissue) while at the same time ingesting and destroying bacteria. This action may cause a significant increase in exudate production due to the rapid debridement of necrotic tissue. It has been proposed that the larval secretions may also change the wound pH and may stimulate healing (Hinshaw 2000).

Controlling oedema

Oedema develops when fluid accumulates in the extracellular space as a result of impaired lymphatic drainage or increased capillary permeability. This may occur in immobile individuals whose dependent limbs develop oedema due to the effect of gravity and inactivation of the calf muscle pump, which assists in return of blood from the lower limbs (Carcary 2001). Poor lymphatic circulation may contribute to the problem. This is commonly seen in patients with venous stasis of the lower limbs, who may also have impaired venous return due to incompetent or damaged valves in the veins (Bennett 1999). Lymphoedema on the other hand occurs as a result of damage to the lymphatic system, commonly through surgery or radiotherapy (Badger 1992). The reversal and control of oedema and lymphoedema need careful assessment and planning. Oedema can usually be controlled with the use of compression bandaging or hosiery, intermittent pneumatic compression, limb evaluation and exercise (Carcary 2001; Vowden & Vowden 2002). In the case of lymphoedema manual lymphatic drainage may also be appropriate (see Ch. 17, External compression).

Achieving a well-vascularized wound bed

Improving the blood flow to the wound bed will increase the availability of nutrients, oxygen, active cells and growth factors within the wound environment (Collier 2002). This may be achieved through the use of compression therapy, topical negative pressure therapy (vacuum-assisted closure or VAC therapy) or wound management products that exert an osmotic pull on the wound bed, increasing capillary growth, e.g. Vacutex (Collier 2002). Surgery may be indicated to correct vascular insufficiency in patients with peripheral vascular disease or to debride the wound down to healthy bleeding tissue.

Decreasing the bacterial burden

It is generally agreed that all chronic wounds harbour a variety of bacteria to some degree and this can range from contamination through colonization to infection. There is also a stage between colonization and infection called 'critical colonization' where the bacterial load has reached a level just below clinical infection (Collier 2002). When a wound becomes infected it will display the characteristic signs of heat, redness, swelling, pain, heavy exudate and malodour. The patient may also develop generalized pyrexia. However, immunosuppressed patients or those on systemic steroid therapy may not present with the classic signs of infection. Instead they may experience delayed healing, breakdown of the wound, presence of friable granulation tissue that bleeds easily, formation of an epithelial tissue bridge over the wound, increased production of exudate and malodour, and increased pain (Miller & Dyson 1996; Miller 1998b; Cutting 1998; Gilchrist 1999). Careful wound assessment is essential to identify potential sites for infection, although routine swabbing of the area is not considered to be beneficial (Donovan 1998). Methods available for the management of wound infection or to decrease the bacterial burden in the wound include debridement, antimicrobial dressings, e.g. those containing iodine or silver, topical negative pressure therapy and antibiotic therapy. Appropriate antibiotic treatment of the infection should be determined from a positive wound swab(s).

Minimizing/eliminating wound exudate

Wound exudate usually performs a useful function of cleaning the wound and providing nutrients to the healing wound bed. However, in the presence of excess exudate the process of wound healing can be adversely affected. This is especially so in chronic wounds where wound fluid may actually prevent the proliferation of cells vital to wound healing, such as fibroblasts, keratinocytes and endothelial cells (Phillips *et al.* 1998; White 2001a; Vowden & Vowden 2002).

Table 47.3 Wound assessment parameters

Factor	Variables
General	Aetiology or cause of wound, location, size, depth and shape, open/closed, presence of haematoma, seroma or oedema
Exudate	Amount, colour, consistency, nature/type (e.g. serous, haemoserous, blood, pus), increase or decrease in amount
Odour	Level, increase or decrease in odour
Type of tissue present	Black (necrotic), yellow (sloughy), red (granulating), pink (epithelializing), green (infected)
Signs of infection	Swelling, heat and redness at the wound site, generalized pyrexia, increases in pain, exudate and odour, friable granulation tissue, bridging of epithelium, swab culture result
Pain	Nature, severity (patient self-assessment), site, frequency, impact on daily living and effectiveness of treatments, pain related to dressing changes and wound cleaning
Condition of surrounding skin	Colour, fragile, dry, scaly, erythema, maceration, oedema, skin nodules, skin stripping, dressing allergy, tape allergy, pre-existing skin conditions (e.g. eczema, psoriasis)
Episodes of bleeding	Amount, frequency, aggravating factors

The control of oedema or lymphoedema and lessening the bacterial burden on the wound will undoubtedly help in the reduction of wound exudate. However, if the methods for achieving these goals are unsuccessful or contraindicated then exudate must be managed through the use of wound management products. These include such products as absorbent wound dressings (e.g. alginates, hydrofibre, foams), non-adherent wound contact layers with a secondary absorbent pad, wound manager bags and topical negative pressure therapy (White 2001b). Immunosuppressive drugs or steroids may be indicated in the treatment of inflammatory exudate produced by wounds such as pyoderma gangrenosum or rheumatoid ulcers (Vowden & Vowden 2002). It is also vital to protect the skin surrounding the wound from maceration by excess exudate and excoriation from corrosive exudate. Useful products for skin protection include ointments/pastes (e.g. zinc oxide BP), alcohol-free skin barrier films and thin hydrocolloid sheets used to 'frame' the wound.

Wound assessment

The wound should be evaluated each time a dressing is applied or if it gives rise for concern. The aim of evaluating the wound is to assess healing and to establish which treatment will best provide the ideal environment for healing. In wounds that are not expected to heal, regular assessment will provide information on the efficacy of symptom management interventions and will highlight aspects of the wound that require further attention. The different classifications of wounds that relate to tissue loss, tissue type and absence or presence of infection may be of assistance in this process.

Factors that should be appraised include the underlying pathology of the wound. For example, if an ulcer is present on the leg, is it venous, arterial, lymphatic, malignant, etc? The surface area or volume of the wound should be measured. This can be carried out using a number of methods, for example manual measurements using a ruler, tracing the wound onto grid paper or using a computer mapping program, and is necessary to ascertain the rate of healing. Photography also provides a useful record of wound progression (Vowden 1995). The amount and type of drainage are also important, in both traumatic and surgical wounds.

A list of variables that require regular assessment is shown in Table 47.3. Figure 47.1 is an example of a wound assessment chart. The use of this type of documentation to assist in the assessment process is recommended to:

- Facilitate continuity of care by providing a central reference point for wound progression
- Facilitate appropriate evaluation of all relevant parameters
- Fulfil legal and professional requirements.

Principles of wound cleaning

The aim of wound cleaning is to help create the optimum local conditions for wound healing by removal of excess debris, exudate, foreign and necrotic material, toxic components, bacteria and other micro-organisms.

If the wound is clean and little exudate is present, repeated cleaning is contraindicated since it may damage new tissue, decrease the temperature of the wound unnecessarily and remove exudate (Morison 1989). A fall in the temperature of the wound of 12°C is possible if the procedure is prolonged or the lotions are cold.

THE ROYAL MARSDEN WOUND ASSESSMENT CHART Complete one chart for each wound					
Patient name: **Hospital number:** **Date of assessment (weekly)**					
Wound dimensions					
Max length (cm)					
Max width (cm)					
Max depth (cm)					
Wound bed – approximate % cover (enter %)					
Necrotic (BLACK)					
Slough (YELLOW)					
Granulating (RED)					
Epithelialising (PINK)					
Skin around wound					
Intact					
Healthy					
Fragile					
Dry					
Scaly					
Erythema					
Maceration					
Oedema					
Eczema					
Skin nodules					
Skin stripping					
Dressing allergy					
Tape allergy					
Other (please state)					
Exudate level					
None					
Low					
Moderate					
High					
Amount increasing					
Amount decreasing					
Odour (see over for rating scale)					
None					
Slight					
Moderate					
Strong					
Bleeding					
None					
Slight					
Moderate					
Heavy					
At dressing change					
Pain from wound (see over for rating scale)					
Level (0–10)					
Continuous					
At specific times (specify)					
Wound infection suspected					
Swab taken (Y/N)					
Swab result					
Treatment					
Assessment review date					
Initials of Assessor					

Figure 47.1 Wound assessment chart (The Royal Marsden Hospital).

Location (mark diagram):	Visual Analogue Scale (VAS) for Patient's Rating of Pain.

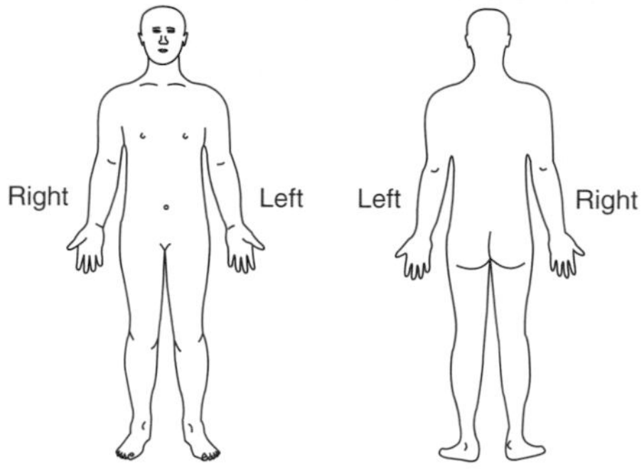

Right   Left   Left   Right

	0	1	2	3	4	5	6	7	8	9	10

No pain

Worst pain imaginable

Rating Scale for Odour

Score	Assessment
None	No odour evident, even when at the patient's bedside with the dressing removed.
Slight	Wound odour is evident at close proximity to the patient when the dressing is removed.
Moderate	Wound odour is evident upon entering the room (1.5 to 3 metres from patient) with the dressing removed.
Strong	Wound odour is evident upon entering the room (1.5 to 3 metres from patient) with the dressing intact.

Diagram of wound if appropriate (or attach tracing/photograph):

Date: _____	Date: _____
Date: _____	Date: _____
Date: _____	Date: _____

Notes on use

Use one chart per wound.

Complete a wound assessment at least once a week.

Measure the wound at its widest points using a clean ruler, use a sterile wound swab or blunt probe to measure wound depth.

For the 'skin around wound' assessment more than one box may be ticked.

Odour and pain should be assessed using the scales at the top of page 2.

Following the assessment a wound management care plan should be written and updated if necessary after each reassessment.

Figure 47.1 Wound assessment chart (The Royal Marsden Hospital) (*continued*).

It can take 3 hours or longer for the wound to return to normal temperature, during which time the cellular activity is reduced and therefore the healing process slowed (Collier 1996).

Sodium chloride (0.9%) is a physiologically balanced solution that has a similar osmotic pressure to that already present in living cells and is therefore compatible with human tissue (Lawrence 1997). Used at body temperature, it is the safest and best cleaning solution for non-contaminated wounds (Miller & Dyson 1996; Fletcher 1997). Although sodium chloride has no antiseptic properties it dilutes bacteria and is non-toxic to tissue (Morgan 2000). Tap water is also advocated for cleaning chronic wounds (Riyat & Quinton 1997). A study demonstrated that, in comparison to sterile 0.9% sodium chloride, lower rates of infection were found in the group where tap water was used (Angeras *et al.* 1992). However, caution should be exercised when using tap water because it can cause pain if applied to raw tissue and lead to further tissue damage if the force of flow is too strong (Clide 1992).

A number of other solutions have been used traditionally to clean wounds, some of which need to be used with caution (Table 47.4).

Principles of dressing the wound

With the exception of wounds where the main aim is to ameliorate symptoms such as malignant wounds, an ideal wound dressing may be described in general terms as follows:

'A material which, when applied to the surface of a wound, provides and maintains an environment in which healing can take place at the maximum rate.'

(Turner *et al.* 1986)

More specifically, to provide such an environment the dressing must be capable of fulfilling the following functions. It must:

- Remove excess exudate and toxic components
- Maintain a high humidity at the wound-dressing interface
- Allow gaseous exchange
- Provide thermal insulation
- Be impermeable to bacteria
- Be free from particulate or toxic components
- Allow change without trauma
- Be acceptable to the patient
- Be highly absorbent (for heavily exuding wounds)

Table 47.4 Suitability of products used on wounds

Suitable	Sodium chloride (0.9%) (safe, non-irritant and non-toxic)
	Tap water (used more frequently, especially on areas already colonized. Some patients prefer to shower prior to dressing changes)
Not ideal, use with caution	Chlorhexidine – antiseptic (can cause sensitization and irritation; do not use alcoholic solutions)
	Fusidic acid (Fucidin) – narrow-spectrum antibiotic for use with penicillin-resistant staphylococci (risk of skin sensitization; not recommended for use on open wounds)
	Hydrogen peroxide – antiseptic (use on superficial, heavily contaminated traumatic wounds only, e.g. from a road traffic accident; do not use on large or deep wounds as may cause air embolism; may be caustic to skin and wound)
	Metronidazole – antibacterial (anaerobes only) (can cause nausea, neuropathy if used systemically)
	Mupirocin (Bactroban) – topical antibiotic (stinging, burning or itching may occur on application; used for bacterial skin infections; may be used in wounds infected with MRSA after advice from a consultant microbiologist)
	Potassium permanganate (0.01%) – mild antiseptic properties (causes staining of skin)
	Povidone-iodine – antiseptic (do not use alcoholic solution; rarely causes skin reactions; some sources suggest that it should not be used on severe or extensive burns, if non-toxic goitre is present, in pregnancy or on lactating women)
	Proflavine – Slow-acting antiseptic (may cause skin hypersensitivity reactions, may stain clothing; used for minor cuts and burns)
Not suitable	Cetrimide – antibacterial and antifungal (toxic to wound tissue and causes skin hypersensitivity)
	Gentian violet – astringent, antiseptic (carcinogenic; is sometimes still used on moist desquamation skin reactions for radiotherapy but this is not recommended; not recommended for use on any open wound)
	Mercurochrome – weak bacteriostatic agent (toxic to tissue)
	Sodium hypochlorite – antiseptic (powerful oxidizing agent which is toxic to tissue)

From: Bloomfield & Sizer 1985; Brennan & Leaper 1985; Sleigh & Linter 1985; Deas *et al.* 1986; Thorp *et al.* 1987; Aidoo *et al.* 1990; Farrow & Toth 1991; Murphy 1995; Miller & Dyson 1996; Trevelyn 1996; Lawrence 1997; Hampton 1999a; Morgan 2000; BNF 2002.

- Be cost-effective
- Provide mechanical protection
- Be conformable and mouldable
- Be able to be sterilized (Field & Kerstein 1994; Hampton 1999a; Morgan 2000).

In addition, the dressing should minimize pain, odour and bleeding and be comfortable when in place.

Occlusive dressings achieve many of these criteria. They affect the wound and healing in several ways. Occlusive dressings have the ability to maintain hydration and prevent the formation of an eschar.

A moist wound environment has been shown to affect a wound in the following ways. It:

- Increases rate of epithelial migration
- Reduces the lag phase between epithelial cell proliferation and differentiation
- Encourages synthesis of collagen and ground substance
- Promotes formation of capillary loops
- Decreases length of inflammatory phase
- Reduces pain and trauma due to dressing adherence
- Promotes breakdown of necrotic tissue
- Speeds wound contraction (Eaglestein 1985; Dyson et al. 1988; Pickworth & De Sousa 1988; Dyson et al. 1992; Miller & Dyson 1996; Garrett 1997; Flanagan 1998; Williams & Young 1998).

Dry dressings do not afford most of the criteria for an ideal dressing and should not be used as a primary contact layer (Dealey 1999). Care should be taken with wounds that are difficult shapes to treat. These include long, narrow cavities which require a dressing that can be comfortably inserted into the space but removed easily without leaving any fibres behind (Bale 1991) and without trauma. (See Table 47.5 for details of groups of dressings.)

Other treatments

Other treatments for wounds include the use of hyperbaric oxygen therapy, topical negative pressure therapy, bio-engineered skin substitutes, topical wound treatments and complementary therapies.

Hyperbaric oxygen therapy

Wound hypoxia is common in patients with chronic wounds and may be exacerbated by diabetes, venous stasis, vascular insufficiency, cardiopulmonary disease or smoking (Messer 1989). Hyperbaric oxygen therapy has been used successfully in healing these wounds (Barr et al. 1990). Treatment involves the patient breathing 100% oxygen while in a chamber where the pressure is elevated above atmospheric pressure, thus increasing the amount of oxygen in solution and therefore the quantity of oxygen reaching the wound bed (Simmons 1999).

Topical negative pressure therapy

Also called vacuum-assisted closure (VAC), topical negative pressure therapy is the application of a uniform negative pressure across the wound bed. This effect is achieved using a mechanical system that includes a sterile open pore foam dressing, which is sealed into the wound, and connected via tubing and a collection chamber to a mechanical pump. An example of such a device is the Vacuum-Assisted Closure Advanced Therapy System – KCI Medical. The main actions of this therapy are to increase blood flow to the wound, remove excess tissue fluid thereby reducing oedema, decrease bacterial load on the wound and debride the wound of moist necrotic tissue (Morykwas et al. 1997; Hampton 1999b). Topical negative pressure therapy encourages the formation of granulation tissue and hastens wound closure (Argenta & Morykwas 1997). See Procedure guidelines on p. 833 for VAC dressing change procedure.

Bio-engineered skin substitutes

Bio-engineered skin substitutes have arisen from a need to find an alternative to skin grafts (autograft, allograft or xenograft) and dressings in the management of extensive burns (Boyce et al. 2002; Harding et al. 2002; Pouliot et al. 2002). Original cultures of human epidermis have been replaced by new skin-equivalent products that contain living cells, predominantly keratinocytes and fibroblasts, within a natural or synthetic scaffolding. Examples of these products are:

- Apligraf (Graftskin) – a cultured human skin equivalent containing viable dermal and epidermal cells (Morgan 2000; Harding et al. 2002)
- Dermagraft – a bio-absorbable mesh containing living neonatal fibroblasts, which produce normal dermal proteins and cytokines (Gentskow et al. 1996)
- Oasis – a sterile, acellular 'biomaterial' composed of a natural collagen matrix derived from porcine (pig) small intestinal submucosa (Benbow 2001; Morgan 2002).

Topical wound treatment dressings

Currently there are two dressing products, Hyalofill and Promogran, which are classified as 'topical treatments' although they are not classed as medicines. Hyalofill is a soft conformable fleece composed entirely of HYAFF, an ester of hyaluronic acid (Edmonds & Foster 2000; Ballard & Baxter 2001). It has been shown to increase angiogenesis and the phagocytic response of macrophages; when used as a wound dressing, it promotes granulation and contraction (Chen & Abatangelo 1999; Hollander et al. 2000).

Promogran is a matrix of freeze-dried collagen (55%) and oxidized regenerated cellulose (45%) (Morgan 2002; Thomas 2002). It forms a gel on contact with wound

Table 47.5 Dressing groups

Dressings	Description	Advantages	Disadvantages
Activated charcoal	Contain a layer of activated charcoal that traps odour-causing molecules thereby reducing/removing wound odour	Easy to apply as either primary or secondary dressing; work immediately to reduce odour	Need to obtain a good seal to prevent leakage of odour; some dressings lose effectiveness when wet
Adhesive island	Consist of a low adherent absorbent pad located centrally on an adhesive backing	Quick and easy to apply; one-piece design negates need for multiple product use; protect the suture line from contamination and absorb exudate/blood	Only suitable for light exudate; some can cause skin damage (excoriation, blistering) if applied incorrectly
Alginates	A textile fibre dressing made from the calcium salt of an alginic acid polymer derived from brown seaweed; contain mannuronic and guluronic acids in varying amounts; available as a sheet, ribbon or packing	Provide a moist wound environment; suitable for moderate to heavy exudate; can be used on infected wounds; useful for sinus and fistula drainage; have haemostatic properties; can be irrigated out of wound with sodium chloride (0.9%)	Cannot be used on dry wounds or wound with hard necrotic tissue (eschar); sometimes a mild burning or 'drawing' sensation is reported on application
Capillary action	Composed of 100% polyester filament outer layers and a 65% polyester and 35% cotton woven inner layer; outer layer draws exudate, interstitial fluid and necrotic tissue into the inner layer via a capillary action	Suitable for light to heavy exudate; debride necrotic tissue; protect and insulate the wound; maintain a moist environment and prevent maceration; encourage development of granulation tissue; can be cut to any shape and are available in large rolls; can be used as a wick to drain sinus and cavity wounds	Can be hard to cut and are quite stiff to fit into wounds; cannot be used on malignant wounds or where there is the risk of bleeding due to the 'drawing' action and resultant increase in blood flow to the wound bed
Debriding enzymes	Consist of natural or synthetic enzymes that break down necrotic tissue	Can be used to remove hard necrotic tissue (eschar) and dry or adherent slough that is resistant to Hydrogel	Cannot be used on wounds actively at risk of bleeding or patients at risk of coronary artery disease due to antigen formation (Varidase); may cause skin maceration
Dextranomers	Consist of highly absorbent beads in powder or paste form, which swell and form a gel on contact with exudate; available as an ointment or paste dressing; may contain iodine	Useful in the treatment of infected wounds	Require retaining dressing; may be difficult to apply, caution in using products containing iodine
Foams	Produced in a variety of forms, most being constructed of polyurethane foam and may have one or more layers; foam cavity dressings are also available	Suitable for use with open, exuding wounds; highly absorbent, non-adherent and provide a moist, thermally insulated wound environment	May be difficult to use in wounds with deep tracts
Honey	Available as impregnated dressing pads or tubes of liquid honey; most widely used is Manuka honey	Suitable for acute and chronic infected, necrotic or sloughy wounds; provide a moist wound environment; non-adherent; antibacterial; assist with wound debridement; eliminate wound malodour; have an anti-inflammatory effect	Can be messy to use and cause leakage if excess exudate is present; caution in diabetes due to absorption of glucose and fructose
Hydrocolloids	Usually consist of a base material containing gelatin, pectin and carboxymethylcellulose combined with adhesives and polymers; base material may be bonded to either a	Suitable for acute and chronic wounds with low to no exudate; provide a moist wound environment; promote wound debridement; provide thermal insulation; waterproof and barrier to	May release degradation products into the wound; strong odour produced as dressing interacts with exudate; some hydrocolloids

(continued)

Table 47.5 Dressing groups (*continued*)

Dressings	Description	Advantages	Disadvantages
	semi-permeable film or a film plus polyurethane foam; some have an adhesive border	micro-organisms; easy to use	cannot be used on infected wounds
Hydrogels	Contain 17.5–90% water depending on the product, plus various other components to form a gel or solid sheet	Suitable for light exudate wounds; absorb small amounts of exudate; donate fluid to dry necrotic tissue; reduce pain and are cooling; low trauma at dressing changes; can be used as carrier for drugs	Cool the wound surface; use with caution in infected wounds; can cause skin maceration due to leakage if too much gel is applied or the wound has moderate to heavy exudate
Hydrofibre	A soft, non-woven dressing composed of 100% hydrocolloid fibres (sodium carboxymethylcellulose); available as sheet or ribbon	Suitable for highly exuding wounds (able to absorb up to 30 times its weight in fluid); holds exudate within its structure and keeps it away from surrounding skin; very easy to remove	Requires a secondary dressing
Paraffin gauze	A fabric mesh of cotton or cotton and viscose/rayon impregnated with soft white or yellow paraffin	Low-adherent; suitable for superficial burns and ulcers, as well as split skin grafts	Can stick to the wound bed if it dries out; may leave residue on the skin
Semi-permeable films	Polyurethane film with a hypoallergenic acrylic adhesive; have a variety of application methods often consisting of a plastic or cardboard carrier	Only suitable for shallow superficial wounds; prophylactic use against friction damage; useful as retention dressing; allow passage of water vapour; allow monitoring of the wound	Possibility of adhesive trauma if removed incorrectly; cool surface of the wound
Skin barrier films	Alcohol-free liquid polymer that forms a protective film on the skin	Non-cytotoxic; do not sting if applied to raw areas of skin; high wash-off resistance; protect the skin from body fluids (including urine, diarrhoea, saliva and wound exudate), friction and shear and the effects of adhesive products	Require good manual dexterity to apply; may cause skin warming on application
Sugar paste	Made from a mixture of icing sugar, caster sugar, propylene glycol and hydrogen peroxide; combined to form either a thin or thick paste	Easy and economical to produce; thin paste suitable for cavity or sinus wounds; thick paste can be moulded and used in open cavities or superficial wounds; antibacterial; assist in wound debridement; may assist in reducing wound malodour	Can be messy to use and cause leakage if excess exudate is present; require a secondary dressing; use with caution in diabetic patients due to sugar absorption
Wound contact layers	Consist of a net (polyamide, knitted viscose) coated with a non-adherent substance, e.g. silicone or hydrocolloid	Specifically designed to be non-adherent and provide 'pain-free' removal; allow exudate to pass through the net; can be cut to size	Require an absorbent secondary dressing

From: Mertz *et al.* 1985; Middleton 1990; Bale & Harding 1991; Thomas & Loveless 1992; Benbow 1994; Rolstad *et al.* 1994; Bennett & Moody 1995; Hampton 1998; Thomas *et al.* 1998a; Williams 1998, 1999a,b; Young 1998; Dealey 1999; Molan 1999a,b; Jones & Milton 2000a,b,c; Morgan 2000; Rutter *et al.* 2000; Thomas 2000; Deeth & Pain 2001; Naylor *et al* 2001; Pudner 2001.
Please refer to manufacturer's recommendations with regard to individual products.

exudate and interacts with products found in wound exudate that impair healing, specifically binding to and inactivating metalloproteases that degrade growth factors. Promogran also binds to and protects growth factors, which are released back into the wound as the dressing is absorbed (Morgan 2002).

Complementary therapies

The use of complementary therapies in wound management is based very much on anecdotal evidence. However, there have been trials using essential oils in wound care, in particular for the relief of pain and wound odour (Price & Price 1995; Baker 1998). Complementary therapies such as relaxation, massage, visualization, imagery and distraction may be very useful in the reduction of wound pain, especially that associated with procedures such as dressing changes (Naylor 2001). Other complementary therapies that may be useful in the management of wound pain include acupuncture, acupressure, autogenic therapy, biofeedback and hypnosis (Rankin-Box 2001).

Complementary therapies should only be administered by health care professionals with the relevant training and qualifications (Stone 2001). When used alongside conventional management treatments, these therapies can be extremely beneficial in reducing pain or the response to pain. Unfortunately, complementary therapies are often underutilized or inappropriately administered and many have poor scientific evidence to back up claims of their effectiveness. These are areas that require further research before they can gain widespread acceptance and nurses should therefore exercise caution when considering the use of these therapies.

Conclusions

With any wound, be it acute or chronic, as a result of surgery, trauma or disease process, assessment is the key to good wound management. It is essential to build a picture of the patient and their wound in order to implement appropriate treatment strategies. This is particularly important in today's era of cost and clinical effectiveness where the use of expensive advanced wound care products must be justifiable and have positive outcomes.

It may be useful for nurses to collect and collate statistics and build up an accurate profile of patients and the nature of their problems, together with the effectiveness of treatment interventions. This would provide valuable information on the effectiveness of care given, potential areas of concern, and aspects of wound care requiring further nursing research. While adding to the knowledge base of nursing and wound care, there would also be benefits in increased efficacy and cost-effectiveness of wound management within both hospital and community settings.

Leg ulceration
Reference material

'Ulceration of the skin of the lower limb has been an affliction of the human race since the time of Hippocrates. It is almost certainly the price we pay for having emerged from the ocean and learnt to stand erect.'

(Burnand 1990)

Prevalence and cost

The prevalence of chronic leg ulceration has been evaluated in a number of studies, most of which are focused on ulcers of venous aetiology. It is estimated that between 0.18% and 1.9% of the population will be suffering from some form of lower leg ulceration (Callam *et al.* 1985; Cornwall *et al.* 1986; Barker *et al.* 1991; Lees & Lambert 1992; Nelzén *et al.* 1996). Prevalence increases with age and the majority of leg ulcers occur in people over 60 (Barker *et al.* 1991; Nelzén *et al.* 1996). Ulceration is often recurrent and persistent and affects more women than men (Franks *et al.* 1995). The annual cost of leg ulcer treatment to the NHS is estimated at between £300 million and £600 million (Thomas 1990a; West & Priestly 1994). Not only do leg ulcers carry financial burdens, they can also significantly affect the patient's quality of life, with pain, odour, sleep interruption and impairments to social activities being common problems (Chase *et al.* 1997; Loftus 2001).

Aetiology

The most common predisposing factors for leg ulceration are chronic venous hypertension and arterial disease (Morison & Moffatt 1999). These factors may be present alone or in combination and lead to tissue hypoxia (Casey 1998a). Other less common causes of lower leg ulceration include:

- Neuropathy – e.g. related to diabetes
- Vasculitis – e.g. related to rheumatoid arthritis
- Malignancy – e.g. squamous/basal cell carcinoma, melanoma, Kaposi's sarcoma
- Blood disorders – e.g. haemolytic anaemia, sickle cell anaemia, polycythaemia
- Infection – e.g. osteomyelitis, leprosy, syphilis
- Metabolic disorders – e.g. necrobiosis lipoidica diabeticorum, pyoderma gangrenosum
- Lymphoedema – e.g. related to poor lymphatic drainage postsurgery/radiotherapy, limb dependency
- Trauma/iatrogenic – e.g. pretibial laceration, incorrect pressure bandaging
- Self-inflicted (Bennett & Moody 1995; Dealey 1999; Morison & Moffatt 1999; Hofman 2000).

Venous disease

Venous disease is the most common cause of leg ulceration, accounting for around 70% of cases (Callam *et al.* 1985; Baker *et al.* 1991; Donayre 1998; Thomas 1998a). Venous hypertension develops as a result of an inefficient calf pump (in which the calf muscle pumps blood back up the leg during movement) and incompetent valves causing back-flow of blood in the venous system. This leads to an increase in capillary permeability which allows fluid and blood components to leak into the surrounding tissues. The end result is varicose veins, oedema, stasis eczema and fibrosis or lipodermatosclerosis (Dealey 1999; Morison & Moffatt 1999).

More women than men suffer from leg ulceration presumably due to the presence of varicose veins and episodes of deep vein thrombosis associated with pregnancy, which can lead to venous damage. In one study, only 12% of women with varicose veins had never been pregnant, compared with 57% who had had four or more pregnancies (Henry & Corless 1989).

Venous ulcers most commonly develop in the medial malleolus/gaiter area and present as shallow, red ulceration that may be quite extensive (i.e. circumferential) with associated changes in the surrounding skin (Bennett & Moody 1995; Thomas 1998a; Collier 1999; Morison & Moffatt 1999). Venous ulcers develop gradually and produce intermittent pain, which may be alleviated by elevating the leg. In patients with venous insufficiency any minor trauma to the leg may precipitate ulcer development (Dealey 1999).

Arterial disease

Between 4 and 30% of patients with leg ulceration have been reported to have arterial insufficiency. This proportion increases with age to 50% in the very elderly (Matthews 1986; Callam *et al.* 1987a,b; Williamson 1988; Perkins 1989). Arterial ulceration is caused by decreased arterial blood supply to the affected limb resulting in tissue ischaemia, usually as a result of arteriosclerosis, which may be compounded by hypertension, diabetes and smoking (Scully 1999). Women are also more prone to arterial ulceration than men (Knight 1990), although some research contradicts this (Callam *et al.* 1987a).

Arterial ulcers tend to be deep and 'punched out' in appearance (Dale & Gibson 1986b; Mani *et al.* 1988; Williamson 1988; Perkins 1989), and found on the feet or the anterior or lateral aspect of the ankle (Thomas 1988a). These ulcers develop rapidly and give continuous or persistent pain, especially at night (Dale & Gibson 1986b; Thomas 1988a; Perkins 1989; RCN 1998).

Other predisposing and aggravating factors

Rheumatoid arthritis causes vasculitis which can lead to small, painful, 'punched out' ulcers (Williamson 1988; Baker *et al.* 1991). In addition, treatment with steroids leads to thinning of the skin and susceptibility to trauma. Patients with rheumatoid arthritis also appear to be at a greater risk of developing the common arterial and venous risk factors associated with leg ulceration (McRorie 2000).

Diabetes is also associated with vasculitis and neuropathy, and has been found to be five times more common in patients with leg ulceration (Callam *et al.* 1987b; Rosenberg 1990).

Vowden (1998) showed that venous ulceration was more common in Caucasians than ethnic minorities. However, this may be due to fewer ethnic patients presenting for treatment.

Diastolic hypertension can lead to (usually) painful bilateral ischaemic ulceration, known as 'Martorell's ulcer' (Alberdi 1988).

Obesity, immobilization and dependency of the lower limb, limitation of ankle joint and poor gait due to ulceration or rheumatoid arthritis (the last two both leading to an inadequately functioning calf muscle pump) can aggravate ulceration and contribute to its persistence (Callam *et al.* 1987b; Autar 1998; Hofman 2000).

Poor nutrition, especially relating to older patients with multiple pathologies, may hinder healing (Casey 1998a).

Treatment

Correct diagnosis of ulcer aetiology is imperative to distinguish between ulcer types, as the management and treatment are very different. Assessment must be carried out to elicit which of the three circulatory systems (arterial, venous and/or lymphatic) is diseased and to identify other contributing factors in order to provide the most appropriate care (Ryan 1988a; Vowden 1998). Commonly this includes the patient's medical history/ risk factors, a vascular assessment, weight/nutritional status, urinalysis and blood tests (e.g. for diabetes, anaemia, renal/liver failure, rheumatoid factor) and an assessment of the ulcer and surrounding skin (RCN 1998; Scully 1999).

Calculation of the ankle brachial pressure index (ABPI) using a sphygmomanometer and Doppler ultrasound probe (in place of a stethoscope) is considered an essential part of any leg ulcer assessment and should be carried out as part of routine patient assessment (Vowden & Vowden 2001). The ABPI is used as an aid to decision making when considering the use of compression therapy in leg ulcer treatment, as an ABPI of less than 0.8 is considered an indication of significant arterial disease and therefore a contraindication to compression (Thomas 1998a). The ABPI can be calculated using a simple equation (Vowden & Vowden 2001):

$$\text{ABPI} = \frac{\text{Highest pressure recorded at the ankle for that leg}}{\text{Highest brachial pressure obtained for both arms}}$$

Systemic management of the underlying disease, as well as topical wound care, are necessary for a successful therapeutic approach.

Venous disease can be treated by improving the function of the calf muscle pump through the application of graduated compression (Callam *et al.* 1987b; Dale & Gibson 1987, 1990; Fletcher *et al.* 1997; McCulloch 1998; Thomas 1998a; Brown & Marshall 2001; Moore 2002). Physiotherapy can also play a major role in improving the calf muscle pump function (McCulloch 1998). While dressing choice will be based on the characteristics of the ulcer, compression has been found to be more important than certain types of dressing in the healing of venous ulcers (Blair *et al.* 1988a). There are various methods available for the application of graduated compression:

- Unna's boot (paste bandage)
- High compression bandage (multilayer or single layer)
- Low compression bandage
- Compression hosiery
- Intermittent pneumatic compression.

High compression, e.g. multiple-layer bandaging, and the use of elastic layered compression have been shown to be cost effective in the treatment of venous ulceration and more effective than no compression or bandages giving low compression (Fletcher *et al.* 1997; Dale 1998; Nelson 1998). Practical problems with patient self-application of compression hosiery have been shown to adversely affect compliance with this treatment (Moffatt & Dorman 1995). Therefore careful consideration must be given to the selection of hosiery, with input from the patient, so that an informed decision can be made regarding treatment (Jones & Nelson 1998). The management of oedema has also been established as an important treatment goal. The presence of oedema inhibits the microcirculation, preventing adequate perfusion and exchange of nutrients (Hofman 1998). Dressings used can be simple low/non-adherent and low cost rather than expensive interactive dressings, as compression is the most important factor in the healing of venous ulcers (RCN 1998).

The treatment of arterial ulcers is based on improving limb perfusion through surgery or angioplasty, although this may be inappropriate in elderly patients and it should be noted that arterial surgery can also lead to a decrease in the venous return time (Struckmann 1988; Morison & Moffatt 1999). Pentoxifylline (oxpentifylline) may be helpful for the treatment of both arterial and venous ulcers (Morison & Moffatt 1999; Jull *et al.* 2000). Careful attention to the maintenance of skin integrity and the control of underlying disease conditions are vital to the success of leg ulcer treatment, especially when complicating factors such as diabetes or rheumatoid arthritis are present. Additionally good supportive care

and appropriate pain control are vital aspects of patient care to improve the patient's quality of life.

It is important to note that often these wounds can be of a chronic nature. In this situation, emphasis should be placed on symptom management and quality of life issues (Armstrong *et al.* 1998; Nelson 1998).

Many additional therapies have been successfully evaluated in the management of leg ulcers. Advanced technology applied to the theory of ulceration means that techniques such as laser, hyperbaric oxygen, growth factors and gene therapies are receiving additional attention (Gilchrist 1997).

Pressure ulcers or decubitus ulcers

Definition

The terms 'decubitus ulcer' or 'pressure ulcer or sore' are used to describe any area of damage to the skin or underlying tissues caused by direct pressure or shearing forces. The extent of this damage can range from persistent erythema to necrotic ulceration involving muscle, tendon and bone (Reid & Morison 1994).

Reference material

Cost

The cost of prevention and management of pressure sores has been a key issue in some reports (e.g. DoH 1993). It is estimated that the cost to the NHS may vary widely from £400 million per year (Bader 1990) up to £1 billion (DoH 1993), although no recent estimates are available. In the early 1990s the cost to the NHS was estimated at between £60 and £321 million per annum for the treatment of pressure ulcers (DoH 1991, 1993). Individual patient costs have been estimated as ranging from £2500 for a stage 1 ulcer to £40 000 for a stage 4 ulcer (Collier 1999b). The risk of developing a pressure ulcer when hospitalized is around 4–10%, rising to about 20% in the elderly, and 4.7–66% in surgical and spinal cord injury patients (Cullum *et al.* 1995; Simpson *et al.* 1996; Bale & Jones 1997; Clay 2000; Ash 2002; Schoonhoven *et al.* 2002).

There is a need to monitor and treat pressure ulcers effectively because they are generally avoidable and lead to unnecessary pain and suffering for the patient (Grewal *et al.* 1999). Clark (2002) discusses the significant reduction in quality of life for patients with pressure ulcers. He comments on the paucity of literature to support this important aspect of patient care and notes that factors such as social isolation, pain and limitations on activity can have detrimental effects on patients and their families. Nurses need to be increasingly aware of the potential for litigation, which may present a considerable drain on limited health service budgets (Tingle 1997).

Prevalence

The prevalance of pressure ulcers in hospital across different countries has been shown to range from 5% to 15% (Haalboom *et al.* 1997). Incident rates in specific areas such as the community, palliative care and nursing homes have been particularly difficult to quantify (Shiels *et al.* 1999; Chaplin 2000). These areas already have limited resources, which are being stretched through lack of money and shortage of experienced staff (Inman & Firth 1998). The National Service Framework for Older People (DoH 2001a) has identified the need to reduce the risk of pressure damage in older persons in both community and inpatient settings, and highlighted the importance of specialist care for this vulnerable group of people. Preventing and managing pressure ulcers has also been highlighted in the Essence of Care benchmarking project and has been the subject of recent guidelines produced by the RCN and the National Institute for Clinical Excellence (NICE) (DoH 2001b; Rycroft-Malone 2001; NICE 2001; Scanlon & Whitfield 2002).

Aetiology

Three major factors have been identified as being significant contributory factors in the development of pressure ulcers:

- *Pressure.* The blood pressure at the arterial end of the capillaries is approximately 35 mmHg, while at the venous end this drops to around 16 mmHg (the average mean capillary pressure equals about 17 mmHg) (Guyton & Hall 2000; Tortora & Grabowski 2002). Any external pressures exceeding this will cause capillary obstruction. Tissues that are dependent on these capillaries are deprived of their blood supply. Eventually, the ischaemic tissues will die (Bridel-Nixon 1999; Tong 1999). Kosiak (1958) identified an inverse relationship between the intensity and duration of pressure in the development of skin damage. Further research has demonstrated that with constant pressure, even in denigrated tissues, a critical period of 1–2 hours exists before pathological changes occur (Kosiak 1958, 1976).
- *Shearing.* This may occur when the patient slips down the bed or is dragged up the bed. As the skeleton moves over the underlying tissue the microcirculation is destroyed and the tissue dies of anoxia. In more serious cases, lymphatic vessels and muscle fibres may also become torn, resulting in a deep pressure ulcer (Simpson *et al.* 1996; Collier 1999b; Clay 2000).

- *Friction.* This is a component of shearing, which causes stripping of the stratum corneum, leading to superficial ulceration (Waterlow 1988; Johnson 1989). Poor lifting and moving techniques may be a major contributory factor (NICE 2001).

The most likely sites for pressure ulcer development are shown in Figure 47.2, with the most common sites being the:

- Sacral area
- Coccygeal area
- Ischial tuberosities
- Greater trochanters

Identification of at-risk patients

Many predisposing factors are involved in the development of pressure ulcers:

- Immunosuppression
- Reduced mobility or immobility
- Moisture
- Inactivity
- Faecal and urinary incontinence
- Decreased level of consciousness
- Infection
- Circulatory diseases, for example, peripheral vascular disease, cardiac disease
- Personal hygiene
- Neurological diseases, for example, multiple sclerosis
- Weight distribution
- Treatment regimens
- Poor nutritional status/malnutrition and dehydration
- Drugs that affect mobility, for example, sedatives
- Anaemia
- Malignancy
- Patient handling methods
- Design of beds, mattresses, chairs and wheelchairs
- Advanced age
- Fracture
- Chronic systemic illness or terminal care
- Sensory impairment
- Acute illness
- Previous history of tissue damage (Barton 1988; Waterlow 1988; EPUAP 1998; Clark 1998; Rycroft-Malone 2001; NICE 2001).

A patient's risk of developing a pressure ulcer should be assessed either on admission to hospital or in the community when the patient first comes into contact with health services. The NMC *Code of Professional Conduct* states that nurses must act to identify and minimize the risk to patients and clients (NMC 2002). Norton,

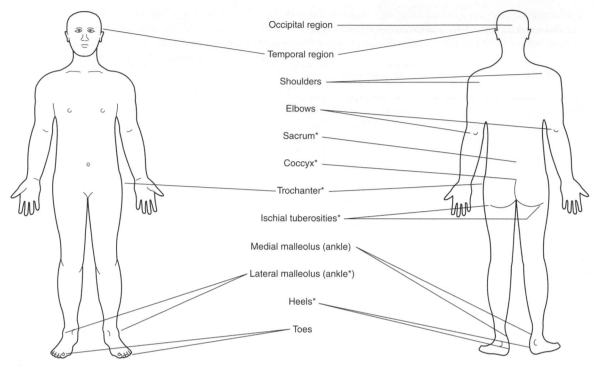

Figure 47.2 Common areas for pressure ulcer formation (* 95% of pressure ulcers develop in these locations).

Physical condition	Score	Mental condition	Score	Activity	Score	Mobility	Score	Incontinent	Score
Good	4	Alert	4	Ambulant	4	Full	4	Not	4
Fair	3	Apathetic	3	Walk/help	3	Slightly limited	3	Occasionally	3
Poor	2	Confused	2	Chairbound	2	Very limited	2	Usually/urine	2
Very bad	1	Stuporous	1	Bedfast	1	Immobile	1	Doubly	1

Figure 47.3 The Norton scale (Norton *et al.* 1985).

Waterlow and Braden have developed risk assessment scales for pressure ulcer development (Norton *et al.* 1985; Braden & Bergstrom 1987; Waterlow 1991, 1998). With the Norton scale (Fig. 47.3) patients with a score of 14 or below are considered to be at greatest risk of pressure ulcer development. A score of 14–18 is not considered at risk but will require reassessment and a score of 18–20 indicates minimal risk. The Waterlow scale (Fig. 47.4) defines a score of 11–15 as being 'at risk', 16–20 as 'high risk' and over 20 as 'very high risk'. In a study of the Norton and Waterlow scales 75.7% of patients identified as 'at risk' by the Waterlow scale developed a pressure ulcer, whereas 62% of those with a score of 16 or less on the Norton scale developed ulcers (Smith 1989). This suggests that the Waterlow scale may give a more accurate prediction of patient risk. The Braden scale (Fig. 47.5) consists of six subscores (sensory perception, activity,

moisture, nutrition, mobility, and friction and shearing) which are scored from 1 to 4 depending on the severity of the condition (with the exception of friction and shearing which is scored 1–3). The total score is then added up with a range possible from 6 to 23. The lower the score, the higher the risk of developing a pressure ulcer. Hospital patients are considered to be at risk if their score is 16 or below. It has been tested in a variety of settings and validated by expert opinion (Bergstrom *et al.* 1987; Bergstrom & Braden 1992).

Deeks (1996) identified 17 different risk assessment tools, which indicates that no one tool is considered reliable and valid for universal use. It has become common for particular areas of care to construct their own hybrid assessment tool as a result of professional discussion and tailoring to specific patient needs (Birtwistle 1994; Chaplin 2000; Lindgren *et al.* 2002).

Name: _____ Hospital No: _____

Instructions for use:
1. Score on admission and update weekly or if significant change in patient's condition
2. Add scores together and insert total score
3. Document actions taken in the evaluation section
4. If total score is 10+ initiate core care plan At Risk of Pressure Damage/Pressure Ulcer Formation

10+ AT RISK   15+ HIGH RISK   20+ VERY HIGH RISK

	Date (Day/Month/Year)									
	Time									
GENDER	Male	1								
	Female	2								
AGE	14–49	1								
	50–64	2								
	65–74	3								
	75–80	4								
	81+	5								
BUILD	Average	0								
	Above average	1								
	Obese	2								
	Below average	3								
APPETITE (select one option ONLY)	Average	0								
	Poor	1								
	NG Tube/fluids only	2								
	NBM/anorexic	3								
VISUAL ASSESSMENT OF AT RISK SKIN AREA (may select one or more options)	Healthy	0								
	Thin and fragile	1								
	Dry	1								
	Oedematous	1								
	Clammy (Temp ↑)	1								
	Previous pressure sore or scarring	2								
	Discoloured	2								
	Broken	3								
MOBILITY (select one option ONLY)	Fully	0								
	Restless/fidgety	1								
	Apathetic	2								
	Restricted	3								
	Inert (due to ↓ consciousness/traction)	4								
	Chairbound	5								
CONTINENCE (select one option ONLY)	Continent/catheterised	0								
	Occasional incontinence	1								
	Incontinent of urine	2								
	Incontinent of faeces	2								
	Doubly incontinent	3								
TISSUE MALNUTRITION (may select one or more options)	Smoking	2								
	Anaemia	2								
	Peripheral vascular disease	5								
	Cardiac failure	5								
	Cachexia	8								
NEUROLOGICAL DEFICIT (score depends on severity)	Diabetes, CVA, MS, motor/sensory paraplegia, epidural	4–6								
MAJOR SURGERY TRAUMA (up to 48 hours post surgery)	Above waist	2								
	Orthopaedic, below waist, spinal > 2 hours on theatre table	5								
MEDICATION	Cytotoxics, high dose steroids, anti-inflammatory	4								
TOTAL SCORE										
NURSE SIGNATURE										

Figure 47.4 Waterlow pressure ulcer risk assessment. (Adapted from the Waterlow Pressure Sore/Ulcer Risk Assessment Scoring System (available from www.judywaterlow.fsnet.co.uk) with permission and acknowledgement of the copyright holder, J. Waterlow 1991, revised 1995 and 1998.)

HIGH RISK: Total score <12   MODERATE RISK: Total score 13–14   LOW RISK: Total score 15–16 if under 75 years old OR 15–18 if over 75 years old   DATE OF ASSESSMENT

	1	2	3	4
SENSORY PERCEPTION Ability to respond meaningfully to pressure related discomfort.	**COMPLETELY LIMITED:** Unresponsive (does not moan, flinch or grasp) to painful stimuli, due to diminished level of consciousness or sedation OR limited ability to feel pain over most of body surface	**VERY LIMITED:** Responds only to painful stimuli. Cannot communicate discomfort except by moaning or restlessness OR has a sensory impairment that limits the ability to feel pain or discomfort over half of the body.	**SLIGHTLY LIMITED:** Responds to verbal commands, but cannot always communicate discomfort or need to be turned OR has some sensory impairment that limits ability to feel pain or discomfort in 1 or 2 extremities.	**NO IMPAIRMENT:** Responds to verbal commands. Has no sensory deficit that would limit ability to feel or voice pain or discomfort
MOISTURE Degree to which skin is exposed to moisture.	**CONSTANTLY MOIST:** Skin is kept moist almost constantly by perspiration, urine etc. Dampness is detected every time patient is moved or turned.	**VERY MOIST:** Skin is often, but not always moist. Linen must be changed at least once a shift.	**OCCASIONALLY MOIST:** Skin is occasionally moist, requiring an extra linen change approximately once a day.	**RARELY MOIST:** Skin is usually dry, linen only requires changing at routine intervals.
ACTIVITY Degree of physical activity.	**BEDFAST:** Confined to bed.	**CHAIRFAST:** Ability to walk severely limited or non-existent. Cannot bear own weight and/or must be assisted into chair or wheelchair.	**WALKS OCCASIONALLY:** Walks occasionally during day, but for very short distances, with or without assistance. Spends majority of each shift in bed or chair.	**WALKS FREQUENTLY:** Walks outside the room at least twice a day and inside room at least once every 2 hours during waking hours.
MOBILITY Ability to change and control body position.	**COMPLETELY IMMOBILE:** Does not make even slight changes in body or extremity position without assistance.	**VERY LIMITED:** Makes occasional slight changes in body or extremity position but unable to make frequent or significant changes independently.	**SLIGHTLY LIMITED:** Makes frequent though slight changes in body or extremity position independently.	**NO LIMITATIONS:** Makes major and frequent changes in position without assistance.
NUTRITION Usual food intake pattern. 1 NBM: Nothing by mouth 2 IV: Intravenously 3 TPN: Total Parenteral Nutrition	**VERY POOR:** Never eats a complete meal. Rarely eats more than1/3 of any food offered. Eats 2 servings or less of protein (meat or dairy products) per day. Takes fluids poorly. Does not take a liquid dietary supplement. OR is NBM 1 and/or maintained on clear fluids or IV 2 for more than 5 days.	**PROBABLY INADEQUATE:** Rarely eats a complete meal and generally eats only about 1/2 of any food offered. Protein intake includes only 3 servings of meat or dairy products per day. Occasionally will take a dietary supplement. OR receives less than the optimum amount of liquid diet or tube feeding.	**ADEQUATE:** Eats over half of most meals. Eats a total of 4 servings of protein (meats, dairy products) each day. Occasionally will refuse a meal, but will usually take a supplement if offered OR is on a tube feeding or TPN 3 regimen that probably meets most of nutritional needs.	**EXCELLENT:** Eats most of every meal. Never refuses a meal. Usually eats a total of 4 or more servings of meat and dairy products. Occasionally eats between meals. Does not require supplementation.
FRICTION AND SHEAR	**PROBLEM:** Requires moderate to maximum assistance in moving. Complete lifting without sliding against sheets is impossible. Frequently slides down in bed or chair, requiring frequent repositioning with maximum assistance. Spasticity, contractures or agitation lead to almost constant friction.	**POTENTIAL PROBLEM:** Moves feebly or requires minimum assistance. During a move skin probably slides to some extent against sheets, chair, restraints, or other devices. Maintains relatively good position in chair or bed most of the time but occasionally slides down.	**NO APPARENT PROBLEM:** Moves in bed and in chair independently and has sufficient muscle strength to lift up completely during move. Maintains good position in bed or chair at all times.	

TOTAL SCORE		Total score of 12 or less represents HIGH RISK		
ASSES	DATE	EVALUATOR/SIGNATURE/TITLE	ASSES	DATE	EVALUATOR/SIGNATURE/TITLE
1	/ /		3	/ /	
2	/ /		4	/ /	

NAME – Last, First, Middle   Attending Physician   ID Number

Figure 47.5 Braden scale for predicting pressure sore risk. (copyright B. Braden and N. Bergstrom 1988. All rights reserved (available from http://www.bradenscale.com).)

Risk assessment strategies are an important factor in clinical governance to ensure quality of care. However, it is often difficult to test the reliability and validity of assessment tools (Butcher 1999). One aspect that is imperative is the inter-rater reliability, which demonstrates the ability of the tool to be used effectively and consistently by nurses in similar areas (Chaplin 2000). NICE (2001) cautions professionals to use risk assessment tools as an *aide mémoire* and recommends their use in conjunction with clinical judgement (Chaplin 2000) and protocols/guidelines in order to influence practice (Deeks 1996).

Grades of pressure ulcers

If a pressure ulcer develops then classification of the wound will assist in determining the most appropriate treatment (see 'Reference material', above). However, grading systems have been produced specifically for use with pressure ulcers (David *et al.* 1983; Reid & Morison 1994; European Pressure Ulcer Advisory Panel 2001). These are valuable in describing the state of the ulcer and the most pertinent care required by the patient.

The Stirling Pressure Sore Severity Scale (SPSSS) is a five-stage classification scale. The scoring is dependent on observation alone and consists of five stages which relate to discoloration of skin, degree of tissue involvement, nature of the wound bed and infective complications. The user can choose the level of detail required, but it is recommended that at least two of the categories are used. The scale can be adapted for local conditions (Reid & Morison 1994) (Fig. 47.6).

Treatment

Treatment of pressure ulcers is the same as for any other wound. The aetiology and underlying or related pathology, as well as the wound itself, must be assessed in order to provide the most appropriate treatment. Care should be aimed at relief of pressure, the minimization of symptoms from predisposing factors and the provision of the ideal microenvironment for wound healing.

Positioning and repositioning of the patient is a prime nursing consideration (Barbenel 1990). Repositioning at least every 2 hours is recommended by the NICE (2001) although this should be determined by the condition of

Stage	0	No clinical evidence of a pressure sore
	0.1	Healed with scarring
	0.2	Tissue damage not assessed as a pressure sore
Stage	1	Discoloration of intact skin
	1.1	Non-blanching hyperaemia (light finger pressure applied to the skin does not alter the discoloration)
	1.2	Blue/purple/black discoloration
Stage	2	Partial-thickness skin loss or damage involving epidermis and/or dermis
	2.1	Blister
	2.2	Abrasion
	2.3	Shallow ulcer, no undermining of adjacent tissue
	2.4	Any of these with underlying blue/purple/black discoloration or induration
Stage	3	Full-thickness skin loss involving damage or necrosis of subcutaneous tissue but not extending to underlying bone, tendon or joint capsule
	3.1	Crater, without undermining of adjacent tissue
	3.2	Crater, with undermining of adjacent tissue
	3.3	Sinus, the full extent of which is uncertain
	3.4	Necrotic tissue masking the full extent of damage
Stage	4	Full-thickness skin loss with extensive destruction and tissue necrosis extending to underlying bone, tendon or joint capsule
	4.1	Visible exposure of bone, tendon or joint capsule
	4.2	Sinus assessed as extending to bone, tendon or joint capsule

Figure 47.6 The Stirling Pressure Sore Severity Scale (Reid & Morison 1994).

the skin and individual needs. An awareness of interface pressures, e.g. creased bed linen and night clothing, is also important to avoid increased friction and further skin breakdown.

Repositioning should take into consideration the overall medical condition of the patient and their comfort. If patients are able, they should be taught the underlying principles of pressure relief and enabled to manage repositioning themselves (NICE 2001) (see Ch. 23, Moving and handling).

The affected area should not be rubbed as this causes maceration and degeneration of the subcutaneous tissues, especially in elderly patients (Dyson 1978). Nurses should possess a basic level of knowledge relating to the underlying principles of pressure ulcer prevention, healing and treatment in order to reduce unnecessary occurrence and discomfort (Mockridge & Anthony 1999).

Devices used for relief of pressure

The most effective way of preventing pressure ulcers or facilitating healing is to minimize the pressure in the affected area(s). Usually it is sufficient for the patient to be nursed on alternating aspects of the body surface, provided the patient is repositioned regularly. Sometimes this is inappropriate or impossible due to individual patients' circumstances, for example, surgical intervention or body deformities.

A wide variety of devices are available to help relieve pressure over susceptible areas, e.g. cushions, overlays, static/dynamic mattresses and replacement beds. These devices differ in function and complexity, and choice must be based on meeting the patient's individual need, sound criteria for decision-making, and effective use of available resources (Table 47.6). Research on the effectiveness of pressure-relieving devices is largely insufficient and inconclusive and does not provide clear guidelines on which equipment is cost effective (Cullum et al. 1995). NICE is currently commissioning the Nursing and Supportive Care Collaboration Centre to update this aspect of the guidelines. A systematic review of beds, mattresses and cushions has been conducted which showed 29 randomized controlled trials supporting the use of high-performance foam mattresses and the effectiveness of using both low air loss beds and air fluidized beds in the management of pressure ulcers (Cullum et al. 1999).

Fungating wounds

Definition

A fungating wound is the result of a cancerous mass that infiltrates the epithelium and surrounding lymph and blood vessels. It can present as an ulcerating crater with a distinct margin or a raised fungating nodule (Moody & Grocott 1993).

Reference material

Aetiology

Fungating wounds can occur almost anywhere on the body. They arise most commonly from cancer of the breast or head and neck, melanoma, soft tissue sarcoma and some cancers of the genito-urinary system (Thomas 1992; Wilks et al. 2001). No two fungating wounds are completely alike. Each patient responds individually to having such a wound, the consequences of which impinge on physical, psychological, social, sexual as well as spiritual well-being. The highest level of nursing expertise is required.

It has been estimated that around 5–10% of people with metastatic cancer will develop such a wound (Haisfield-Wolfe & Rund 1997). Fungating wounds tend to occur in older patients (60–70 years old) with advanced cancer, and usually develop during the last 6 months of life (Haisfield-Wolfe & Rund 1997; Ivetic & Lyne 1990).

Assessment

Assessment and evaluation of a wound are discussed earlier in the chapter, but it is important to emphasize that an accurate history of a malignant lesion should be taken, and that the management of the wound should be documented clearly from the beginning. Assessment is based on the control of symptoms as opposed to the ability and progress of the wound to heal. A wound assessment tool to record the amount and type of odour/exudate/pain, and the dressings used, is a helpful means of evaluating care strategies (see Fig. 47.1).

Grocott (2000a) evaluated a tool that measured patient-centred outcomes using the TELER system (Le Roux 1995) for the key variables of symptom management, dressing performance and the impact that the wound had on the patient's life. This showed that further work was required to develop wound management products in order to meet patients' needs.

Problems associated with fungating wounds

Physical
• Pain/discomfort
• Pruritus/itching in skin around wound
• Heavy exudate
• Malodour/infection
• Bleeding (superficial or large vessel)

Table 47.6 A selection of mechanical methods for relieving pressure

Aid	Use	Advantages	Disadvantages
Sheepskin	Low-risk patients, Waterlow <10. Good for under heels	Warm and comfortable. Decreases friction	Does *not* relieve pressure. Hardens and mats with washing. Needs to be changed frequently. *Not recommended* for use as a pressure-relieving device
Heel and elbow pads: sheepskin, foam, silicone	Waterlow 10+ or patients on prolonged bedrest	Reduce friction and shearing over the elbow and heel	Often have inadequate methods of keeping them in place. Become hardened by washing. Not recommended for use
Silicone-filled mattress pad/cushion (e.g. Transoft)	Waterlow 10+ or patients on prolonged bedrest, able to move spontaneously	Relieves pressure by distributing it over a greater area. Comfortable. Machine (industrial) washable. Acceptable in community settings as well as in hospital. Can be used for incontinent patients. Relatively cheap purchase price. Plastic protective covers available	If the patient is very incontinent of urine, even if the plastic side is uppermost, there is seepage into the core material. Stitching comes undone after several launderings. Not recommended for routine use in pressure ulcer prevention
Roho air-filled mattress/cushions	High–medium-risk patients, Waterlow 10–15	Interlinked air cells transfer air with movement. Patient can be nursed sitting or recumbent. Non-mechanical. Washable	Can be punctured and is expensive to repair. Often incorrectly inflated due to lack of understanding and education. Can be mechanically cleaned in sterile supply department
Alternating pressure beds	High–medium-risk patients, Waterlow 15+	Mechanical alteration of pressure. Reduce the frequency of (but not need for) repositioning. Available on hire at short notice	Must be checked and maintained. May increase pressures in very thin patients. Punctures possible. Patients may complain of nausea due to movement of cells
Mechanaid netbed	Moderate-risk patients, Waterlow 15	Fits any bed. Easy to assemble and dismantle. Easy to store. No servicing, maintenance or laundry difficulties. Patients can be repositioned by one nurse. Appears to encourage relaxation and sleep. Can be lowered onto the bed surface when a firm base is required	Patients do not always like it. Wedge of pillows needed to sit patient up. Patients may lose heat. Not always easy for patients to communicate with people sitting by bed
Water bed	Moderate-risk patients, Waterlow 15+	Spreads pressure. Is warm and comfortable. Available on hire at short notice	Patient is supported on the skin of the water sac thus reducing the pressure-relieving properties. Difficult to get the patient in and out
Water flotation bed	Moderate–high-risk patients, Waterlow 15+	Equalizes pressure and weight. Heated	Expensive to buy, run and maintain. Makes some patients feel 'sea-sick'. Reduces self-motivated movement. Heavy to move. If not filled correctly can create more pressure than conventional bed. Not to be confused with water bed, above
Air fluidized bed	High-risk patients, Waterlow 20+, or indicated because of medical condition	As near to levitation as possible. Warm, sterile air produces a beneficial environment for healing wounds. One nurse can manage even a very heavy or debilitated patient on his/her own. Can be used for incontinent patients or those with heavy wound exudate. May help to alleviate severe pain	Expensive to hire. Need to reinforce floors before it can be installed. Minimizes self-motivation. Can be difficult for the patient to get in and out of bed even with help. Available on hire basis only
Low air loss bed	High-risk patients, Waterlow 20+. Orientated and immobile patients	Pressure-equalizing properties equal to the fluidized air bed. Patient can be nursed in any position including prone. (Patient can control position.) Mobilization easy	Expensive to buy but can be hired. Nurses need education in the use of the equipment. Noise can be disturbing

It is important to remember the risk of cross-infection with the use of special beds. Most companies provide adequate cleaning/sterilizing of their equipment.

- Presence of necrotic tissue
- Wound infection
- Damage to surrounding skin by exudate
- Tunnelling, undermining, fistula and sinus
- The location of wound
- Pain related to dressing changes
- The size and shape of the lesion being dressed
- Side-effects of treatment, e.g. radiotherapy.

Psychosocial
- Body image concerns; cosmetic effect of dressing
- Embarrassment and shame
- Denial
- Depression
- Fear
- Guilt
- Revulsion and disgust
- Self-esteem problems
- Sexual problems
- Communication difficulties
- Impact on family
- Information needs
- Restrictions due to dressing changes
- Social isolation
- Problems with social support and resources.

Aims of treatment

Malignant fungating lesions are an immense challenge. The aim of treatment is rarely to heal: care is focused on reducing the impact of symptoms and maximizing comfort (Saunders & Regnard 1989; Fairbairn 1994; Laverty *et al.* 1997; Naylor *et al.* 2001). Quality of life is the guiding principle of care planning, which should be undertaken in partnership with the patient.

Nurses must ensure that patients are aware that comfort, not cure, is the aim, and respond to patients' needs sensitively. The chronic nature of malignant wounds means that patients are involved in an ongoing process of adjustment. Wounds are also a constant reminder to patients of advanced disease and possible impending death (Laverty *et al.* 1997; Naylor *et al.* 2001).

Management of symptoms

1 *Pain.* Localized pain is sometimes experienced with wounds in addition to generalized pain which is addressed separately (see Ch. 27, Pain assessment and pain management). Assessment provides a means to determine the underlying cause of the pain, e.g. infection, pressure on structures, heightened anxiety, invasion of nerves (Naylor 2001). A short-acting analgesic

such as dextromoramide (e.g. Palfium) or nitrous oxide (e.g. Entonox) may be required to supplement the regular analgesic, for instance when dressings are changed (Hollinworth 1997). Similarly, a breakthrough dose of the patient's regular analgesia may be administered 20–30 minutes before the dressing change (Naylor *et al.* 2001). The use of morphine or diamorphine mixed with a hydrogel (to form a 0.08–0.1% mixture) and applied topically to the wound has been found to be an effective method of pain relief in ulcerating wounds, including fungating wounds (Stein 1995; Back & Finlay 1995; Krajnik & Zylicz 1997; Twillman *et al.* 1999; Grocott 2000b). This is based on the fact that peripheral opioid receptors are present. The results (although on a small group of patients) suggest that the use of topically based analgesia may have a clinically useful analgesic effect.

2 *Itching.* Irritation may occur around the margin of the wound (Fairbairn 1993). A gentle moisturizing cream (e.g. Diprobase) or aqueous cream with menthol may provide relief. The use of a hydrogel sheet can also reduce itching and promote comfort. Advice to the patient regarding the use of light, cool clothing and bathing may be of some benefit. Irritation caused by radiotherapy may respond to topical hydrocortisone.

3 *Exudate.* Exudate from a fungating lesion can act as a reservoir for infection (especially bacterial infection) (Collinson 1992; White 2000). Surgical debridement of necrotic and sloughy areas can control the production of exudate, but may be too extensive a procedure for some patients with advanced disease (Collinson 1992; Fairbairn 1993). Plastic surgical procedures are often not feasible because of local invasion by the tumour (Moss 1989). Less invasive measures (e.g. radiotherapy) may be beneficial in the short term (Thomas 1992; Fairbairn 1993). Wound dressings should be absorbent and non-adhesive (Fairbairn 1994), but can be bulky. The social and psychological effects of large, conspicuous dressings must be taken into account when selecting a suitable dressing (Thomas 1992; White 2000). A high absorbency dressing (e.g. Aquacel) may provide adequate management for a heavily exuding wound (Williams 1999b; Robinson 2000). Care needs to be taken to monitor the condition of the surrounding skin. Medium to high exudate levels can lead to excoriation and maceration of the periwound area. A protective skin barrier film (e.g. Cavilon or SuperSkin) may help to reduce deterioration and prevent pain (Hampton 1998).

4 *Malodour/infection.* Malodour is often an indication that a wound is infected (Dealey 1999). Swabs should be taken to identify the causative organism before systemic measures are adopted. Malodour is commonly

caused by anaerobic organisms that flourish in the necrotic tissue. They release volatile fatty acids as an end product, which are thought to be responsible for the characteristic smell. Metronidazole as a gel has proved an effective agent for deodorization of fungating lesions (Newman *et al.* 1989; Thomas & Hay 1991; Bower *et al.* 1992; Finlay *et al.* 1996; Kelly 2002). Systemic metronidazole can also be beneficial if the odour is extreme. It inhibits anaerobic colonization and decreases associated odours. This should be used with caution in order to avoid any side-effects. Sparrow *et al.* (1980) conducted a small-scale study that showed systemic metronidazole could be given in the lower dose of 200 mg three times daily (as opposed to 400 mg) with equal effectiveness and fewer side-effects. Charcoal dressings are also effective at controlling odour. They attract and bind the molecules which cause odour and prevent their escape from the local area (Thomas 1992; Kelly 2002). Small studies have been conducted on some other topical applications, but there is little substantial research evidence available:

(a) *Natural live yoghurt.* The wound is cleaned with 0.9% sodium chloride and the yoghurt applied for 10 minutes. The yoghurt is then rinsed away thoroughly, again with 0.9% sodium chloride. The wound is dressed according to the plan of care. The process may be repeated three to four times daily (Welch 1981; Schulte 1993).

(b) *Sugar paste.* Useful for debridement and to aid regranulation of tissue. Twice daily application has been recommended for 'optimum antibacterial effect' (Middleton 1990; Topham 2000).

(c) *Icing sugar.* May be effective for deodorizing lesions. The powder is sprinkled over the affected area, washed off and then reapplied as a viscid liquid (Thomlinson 1980).

(d) *Honey.* This has antibacterial properties related to its sugar content and the presence of hydrogen peroxide and plant-derived antibacterial agents. These properties inhibit anaerobe activity, but the antibacterial effect can be destroyed by heat. Frequent dressing changes may be required if there is an increase in the amount of exudate produced, as this makes the honey too dilute and, therefore, affects its activity. The honey is applied directly to the wound and left on with a secondary dressing. It is important to use gamma-irradiated honey in wound care, as this is correctly sterilized. Care should be taken of the surrounding skin, which may be friable and break down easily (Dunford 2000).

(e) *Larval therapy* (see p. 802). This has regained popularity over the last 3–4 years. Patient compliance

is an important consideration and a detailed explanation is required (Jones & Thomas 2000; Thomas *et al.* 2001).

(f) *Tea tree oil.* Early research has shown that tea tree oil demonstrates promising antibacterial properties but there is little evidence to support its long-term use in wound management or the potential systemic uptake when it is applied directly to a wound (Carson *et al.* 1998). Complementary therapies should be used with caution and relevant literature perused to support their use in wound management.

(g) *Deodorizers and environmental air fresheners.* These may help to reduce the odour around the patient but are not particularly effective at masking the odour. Similarly, good ventilation, essential oils and scented candles may be of limited benefit.

5 *Bleeding/haemorrhage.* As the lesion increases in depth and extends at the margins, capillary bleeding may occur (Fairbairn 1994). Dressings should be loosened off by showering or soaking to prevent trauma. The use of non-adherent dressings may prevent the problem of bleeding. Alginate dressings may be useful for controlling capillary bleeding (Thomas *et al.* 1998b). If bleeding is profuse, measures with an immediate effect may be taken:

(a) *Adrenaline 1:1000.* Acts as a vasoconstrictor when applied topically, but must be applied with caution because it is absorbed systemically (Dealey 1999; BNF 2002).

(b) *Tranexamic acid.* Given orally or applied topically to the wound, it stems bleeding and reduces re-bleeding by inhibiting fibrinolysis (breakdown of blood clots) (Dean & Tuffin 1997; Pudner 1998).

(c) *Haemostatic swabs.* Stimulate rapid capillary coagulation. They can be left in place and covered with a secondary dressing. They are most commonly applied in surgical procedures, but are also useful in controlling bleeding in chronic wounds and may be used in primary care as they are easy to apply to the wound and can be left in place under the usual dressing (Naylor 2002).

(d) *Sucralfate.* There have been a few case reports of the effectiveness of adding a suspension or paste of sucralfate directly to a bleeding wound and then covering the area with a non-adherent dressing (Regnard & Mannix 1990; McElligot *et al.* 1992; Lentz *et al.* 1993; Emflorgo 1998).

(e) *Traumacel P.* Tentative reports have suggested that this topical dressing may be beneficial in managing bleeding wounds. It was designed to control capillary bleeding and has been shown to aid healing in chronic wounds. There have been no specific studies to look at this product in relation to fungating wounds (Hofman *et al.* 2000; Hughes *et al.* 2002).

6 *Radiotherapy*. This can reduce the amount of exudate and control bleeding in malignant wounds. It is given either as a single fraction to avoid frequent hospital visits, or in divided doses over 2–3 weeks, in which case patients are admitted for the full course of treatment (Ashby 1991; Young 1997). Occasionally, radiotherapy is used prophylactically to prevent fungation if the skin is intact. If fungation has already occurred, radiotherapy may still be of value in reducing tumour bulk and enabling a degree of healing. Palliative radiotherapy of this kind is designed to spare healthy skin cells surrounding the wound and to avoid damage to the bed and margins of the wound (Horwich 1992).

7 *Hormone therapy*. Hormone therapy can reduce the rate at which a fungating wound progresses and deteriorates (Fairbairn 1993). Chemotherapy is occasionally used for this purpose, but hormone therapy has fewer side-effects and can enhance the patient's sense of well-being.

8 *Psychological/sexual/social issues*. A fungating wound is a constant physical reminder of progressive cancer and impending death. For this reason alone the patient and their family may experience feelings of isolation and fear. The symptoms resulting from the wound (e.g. malodour, exudate) may mean that the patient is unable or reluctant to continue to live their normal life. They may feel immense embarrassment, especially with regard to their relationship with their partner (Bird 2000). Leakage of exudate and strong odour may lead them to live separate lives, and may make the continuation of a sexual relationship extremely difficult, if not impossible (Hallett 1995).

The nurse needs to be aware of these psychosocial issues and allow the patient to express their fears and concerns. Excellent communication skills coupled with empathy and sensitivity can be of great benefit to the patient when having to cope, adapt and readjust to their changing situation (Naylor *et al.* 2001). It is impossible to completely understand the impact that a fungating wound has on a patient and their family but it is possible to offer a realistic and holistic approach to their care that affords them the opportunity to live as full a life as possible within the limitations of their wound and their disease.

Dressings

Numerous dressings are available to help overcome the problems associated with malignant wounds. Table 47.7 lists types of wound and recommended dressings. The FP10 index is the drug tariff that general practitioners use to prescribe wound dressings for patients in the community. There are a few limitations to this guide and it is important that hospital nurses are aware of dressing availability before they do their selection process (Dale 1995).

District nurses and health visitors are now able to prescribe a limited number of drugs and wound management products. Some centres are also using protocolized prescribing or patient group directions (Laverty *et al.* 1997; Naylor *et al.* 2001) to ensure that those professionals with appropriate experience can supply dressings and wound care products without a prescription.

Securing dressings

Tapes should only be applied to healthy skin in order to avoid further tissue damage. Care should be taken to leave a large margin around the wound including any existing cutaneous nodules. If the skin is potentially friable, a skin barrier film, e.g. Cavilon or SuperSkin, can be applied before the dressing to protect the skin.

Plain bandaging or the use of Netelast/Tubifast is helpful where a wound is positioned in a difficult area. Tapeless retention dressings are ideal to use in difficult-to-dress areas and for delicate skin. They are also reusable and can be adapted to suit the individual patient (McGregor 1998; McGregor & Baxter 1999). However, care should be taken when reusing these products owing to potential infection control issues.

Conclusions

Fungating wounds pose a challenge in primary care, where district and Macmillan nurses are an invaluable resource in the important work of assessing wounds and liaising with hospitals and hospices about individual care plans. Clear, rational decision-making is vital to establishing trust with the patient and achieving maximum levels of comfort and quality of life.

Radiotherapy skin damage

Definition

Skin damage from radiotherapy can be defined as skin irritation, erythema and/or loss of skin integrity within the field of radiotherapy treatment. In contrast to a burn, radiotherapy skin reactions develop over a period of weeks and are the result of suppressed cellular replication and a local inflammatory reaction (De Conno *et al.* 1991).

Reference material

Up to 95% of patients treated with external beam radio-therapy will develop an acute skin reaction, sometimes referred to as radiodermatitis or, incorrectly, a radiation burn (De Conno *et al.* 1991). This is due to damage to the rapidly dividing cells in the basal layer of the epidermis (Stratum Basale). There are four main types of skin reaction, which are classified according to the appearance of the skin (Table 47.8).

The degree of skin reaction depends on a number of factors:

- High total dose of radiation
- Low-energy radiation or electrons
- Treatment of the head and neck, breast or pelvic area (increased moisture and friction in skin folds, groin, natal cleft, axilla)

- Large volume of normal tissue included in the area of treatment
- Tangential treatment fields
- Use of 'bolus' materials (e.g. a wax blanket to increase the dose of radiotherapy to the skin)
- Older age
- Immunosuppression
- Concurrent chemotherapy or steroid therapy
- Poor nutritional status
- Tobacco smoking
- Chronic sun exposure (Rigter *et al.* 1994; Blackmar 1997; Porock *et al.* 1998; Maher 2000; Naylor *et al.* 2001).

Assessment

Assessment of the treatment area is imperative and should be ongoing. Measures to promote comfort and

Table 47.7 Dressings for management of fungating wounds

Wound type	Aim	Suggested intervention
Necrotic	Debridement of eschar	Enzymes
		Hydrogel
		(Surgical intervention if appropriate)
Sloughy	Debride slough. Prevent infection	Hydrogel
		Alginate/hydrofibre (if high exudate is present)
		Enzymes (rarely)
		Larval therapy
Infected	Treat infection. Prevent associated symptoms (odour, exudate)	Metronidazole gel (topical) (can be mixed with hydrogel or hydrocolloid gel to manage associated symptoms)
Malodorous	Remove odour	Metronidazole gel (topical)
		Activated charcoal dressings
		Sugar paste prepared under sterile conditions
		Icing sugar
		Honey
		Larval therapy
Highly exuding (cavity)	Contain exudate	Alginate (sheet/ribbon)
		Hydrofibre (sheet/ribbon)
		Foam sheet
		Foam cavity dressings
Lightly exuding	Contain exudate. Prevent increase	Hydrocolloid
		Hydrogel/hydrocolloid gel
		Semi-permeable film
Bleeding	Control bleeding	Alginate
		Surgical haemostatic sponges
		Sucralfate paste
		Trauexamic acid
Itching	Control itching	Hydrogel sheets
		Aqueous cream with menthol

A mixture of these products can be used, depending on the current status of the wound and the number of presenting problems (Mallett *et al.* 1999; Naylor *et al.* 2001; Naylor 2002).

ease any 'burning' sensation should be initiated early on in the treatment plan. It may be useful to use an assessment tool that has been designed specifically for radiotherapy skin reactions to record skin changes during treatment along with treatments and advice given (Noble-Adams 1999). Along with the risk factors listed above, a baseline skin assessment should include:

- Current condition of the skin
- Any previous or current skin disorders
- Surgical changes (e.g. scars)
- Educational needs of the patient and their family or carers
- Information on treatment details and potential side-effects (Maher 2000).

Table 47.8 Categories of acute radiotherapy skin reactions

Category	Description
Erythema	Reddened skin, which may be oedematous and feel hot and irritable
Dry desquamation	Dry, flaky or peeling skin that may be itchy
Moist desquamation	Peeling skin with exposure of the dermis and exudate production, often painful and may become infected
Necrosis	Death of tissue; skin may darken and turn black

Symptom management

In order to minimize the effects of acute skin reactions, a number of management strategies have been suggested, the majority of which rely on topical skin treatments with either pharmaceutical preparations or dressings. A vital aspect of radiotherapy skin reaction management is the use of preventive measures to maintain skin integrity. These measures should be instituted as soon as treatment is started and include washing the skin using warm water and non-perfumed mild soap, avoiding friction on the skin, moisturizing the skin and avoiding extreme cold and sunlight. (For further information see Naylor et al. (2001) and The Royal Marsden Hospital Patient Information Series booklet 'Radiotherapy'.)

Three separate UK-wide surveys have previously been conducted in an attempt to identify skin care practices for radiotherapy skin reactions (Thomas 1992; Barkham 1993; Lavery 1995). All three surveys concluded that there were a wide variety of products and practices in use and that many of these treatments were based not on sound principles but rather on historical practice and personal preference. Similarly, reviews of published literature have found a diverse range of products being recommended for the management of acute radiotherapy skin reactions, many of which have no research evidence to justify their use (Naylor & Mallett 2001; Glean et al. 2001). Recommended skin care products are listed in Table 47.9.

Table 47.9 Recommended treatments for acute radiotherapy skin reactions

Category of skin reaction	Suggested treatment
Erythema and dry desquamation (may be managed in the same way)	• Hydrophilic and moisturizing creams – provide symptomatic relief • Hyaluronic acid 0.2% cream applied twice a day • Natural Care Gel® applied in a thin layer three times a day • Sucralfate cream applied twice a day • 1% hydrocortisone – for itchy, irritable or burning feelings of the skin within the treatment field; should be applied sparingly, 2–3 times a day, but *not to areas of broken or infected skin*
Moist desquamation	• Hydrogel sheets – reduce discomfort and promote healing (soothing and cooling) • Amorphous hydrogels – useful in skin-folds or the perineum • Semi-permeable film dressings – may be applied to areas of low or no exudate and left in place during treatment; reduce pain and are easy to remove • Modern absorbent dressings, e.g. alginate, hydrofibre, foam • Hydrocolloid sheet dressings – may be applied to areas of moist desquamation *once radiotherapy treatment has finished*; provide an aesthetically acceptable dressing that promotes comfort and healing
Necrosis	Debride eschar/slough; use appropriate dressings to promote healing (see Table 47.4)

(From: Shell et al. 1986; Margolin et al. 1990; Pickering & Warland 1992; Crane 1993; Strunk & Maher 1993; Campbell & Lane 1996; Maiche et al. 1994; Blackmar 1997; Korinko & Yurick 1997; Ligouri et al. 1997; Rice 1997; Jones 1998; Boots-Vickers & Eaton 1999; Mak et al. 2000; Glean et al. 2001; Kitchen & Ireland 2001; Naylor & Mallett 2001.)

It is important to remember that the skin reactions will not heal during, or for up to 4 weeks after, treatment and that any dressings used must be removed during the actual treatment session to prevent a 'bolus' effect causing an increased dose of radiation to the skin (Lochhead 1983). Some dressings can be left in place during treatment if they are very thin or if treatment was planned with the dressing in situ.

Products not recommended

There are a number of products that are unsuitable for the management of skin reactions; many of these are traditional treatments that should be replaced with more modern, research-based products.

- Petroleum jelly
- Topical antibiotics
- Topical steroids on moist desquamation
- Gentian violet
- Talcum powder
- Cornstarch
- Silver sulphadiazine cream (Flamazine) (Farley 1991; Sitton 1992b; Rigter *et al.* 1994; Campbell & Lane 1996; Blackmar 1997; Rice 1997; Korinko & Yurick 1997; Jones 1998; Mak *et al.* 2000).

Conclusions

Acute radiotherapy-induced skin reactions, while resembling a burn, should not be classed or treated as such. They are caused by the effect of radiation on the rapidly dividing cells in the skin. Treatment is aimed at maintaining skin integrity and patient comfort and preventing infection. There are many products being used in radiotherapy skin care but the majority have no firm evidence of their efficacy. However, there are a number of products that can be used based on research evidence and expert opinion.

Plastic surgery wounds

Definition

Plastic surgery is the collective term that refers to surgical procedures that are performed to restore function and cosmesis. This is achieved by using flaps and skin grafts for reconstruction purposes, in addition to using the natural elasticity and mobility of the skin. A surgical flap is a strip of tissue, usually consisting of skin, underlying fat, fascia, muscle and/or bone, which is transferred from one part of the body (known as the donor site) to another (known as the recipient site) (Edwards 1994; Brown *et al.* 1998).

A skin graft is living, but devascularized, tissue consisting of all or some of the layers of the skin, which is removed from one area of the body and applied to a wound on another area of the body. The two types of skin graft are full-thickness skin graft (FTSG), in which the entire epidermis and dermis is removed, and split-thickness or split skin graft (SSG), which consists of the epidermis and the upper part of the dermis only (Francis 1998; Young & Fowler 1998).

Reference material

Aetiology

Reconstructive plastic surgery is usually performed following trauma, e.g. burn, surgery, e.g. wide excision of a skin lesion, or to repair congenital defects, e.g. cleft palate. Surgical reconstruction is often required following extensive surgery for cancers of the breast, head and neck, skin (melanoma), soft tissue (sarcomas) and genitourinary system. The aim is to perform the simplest procedure that will provide the best aesthetic and functional outcome (Clamon & Netscher 1994). Each patient will require individually planned, and therefore unique, surgery. Reconstructive surgery of this type often results in altered anatomy, in both appearance and function, which may impact upon the psychological and physical well-being of the patient.

Assessment

Preoperative patient assessment must be as detailed as possible; this should include information on past and present medical conditions that may delay wound healing (see above, Wound assessment and Factors affecting wound healing). For certain patient groups, e.g. those with recurrence of head and neck cancer, anatomy may already have been altered, through previous surgery, thereby narrowing down the possible options for reconstruction.

Postoperative observation of the wound sites, dressings and drains is crucial as deterioration of a wound can occur suddenly, e.g. fluid-filled seromas, necessitating the need for prompt nursing action (see below).

Associated problems

Split skin graft donor site

The two most common problems associated with a split skin graft donor site are slipping of dressing and infection.

Slipping of dressing, resulting in pain and discomfort
The donor sites chosen for SSG harvesting are usually the upper thigh, upper arm or upper buttock. Less conspicuous areas of the body are chosen wherever possible.

As a result of gravity, the dressing has a tendency to slip, resulting in the exposure of raw skin. The excision of the thin layer of skin leaves nerve endings exposed, resulting in pain at the donor site (Wilkinson 1997). Analgesia should therefore be given prior to performing or renewing a dressing. Exposed areas of raw skin should be dressed with an alginate and covered with low-linting gauze. The combination of these two dressings will assist in absorbing exudate. A crêpe bandage and tape are then used to secure the dressings. A tapeless dressing can be used instead of a bandage and tape. This is a hypoallergenic, stretchy bandage that does not require tape to secure it to the primary dressing or to the patient (McGregor & Baxter 1999).

Infection

A high amount of exudate on the dressing, evident by new and excessive strikethrough, can indicate the presence of infection. The entire dressing should be soaked off in order to assess the wound site, and the site should be swabbed for microbial culture and sensitivity. While infected, the wound site should be dressed daily. *Pseudomonas aeruginosa* is a common infecting organism of donor sites and is often evidenced by a strong musty smell and bright blue–green exudate. Flamazine (silver sulphadiazine) is usually an effective treatment for *Pseudomonas* when applied topically to the donor site and covered with a non-adherent dressing (Hamilton-Miller *et al.* 1993). If the patient experiences a raised temperature, increased pain or appears unwell, this may indicate the presence of a systemic infection and they will require a course of antibiotics (Wilkinson 1997).

Split skin recipient site (flap donor site)

When a flap is transferred from its original site or a tumour is widely excised, it leaves a deficit of tissue. Split skin is applied to this site, as primary closure is not usually possible. The most common problem with SSG recipient sites is fluid-filled seromas.

Fluid-filled seromas

On removing the dressing after 5 days, the SSG should be smooth and pink or red in colour. Any seromas, characterized by blisters containing air and haemoserous fluid, must be expelled. Without performing this the graft will not 'take'. A sterile needle is used to evacuate the fluid, enabling the graft to be carefully rolled from the centre outwards (Coull 1991). This can be performed by using a cotton bud and enables the graft to adhere to the underlying tissue. A tulle dressing, low-linting gauze and a bandage, or a tapeless dressing are then applied. The pressure from the dressing assists in expelling the blisters (Coull 1991).

Scarring

Definition

A scar is defined as the mark left after a wound has healed with the formation of connective tissue, giving rise to an altered appearance of the skin (Davis 1993; Eisenbeiss *et al.* 1998). Initially the scar is red and raised; then over a period of 6–12 months this matures to produce a hypopigmented, flat scar (Davies 1985).

Hypertrophic and keloid scars

Occasionally the scar continues to become increasingly red, raised and itchy, defined as hypertrophic. If these symptoms continue, with the scar tissue invading surrounding unaffected tissue as well as increasing in height, a keloid scar is formed (Williams 1996; Eisenbeiss *et al.* 1998). The areas that are most susceptible are the upper back, shoulders, anterior chest, presternal area and the upper arms (Munro 1995a; Beldon 2000). Dark-skinned people have a greater susceptibility to developing keloid scars than those who are lighter skinned (Eisenbeiss *et al.* 1998).

Reference material

Aetiology

There are a number of possible predisposing factors, as stated by Munro (1995a):

- Increased skin tension can contribute to the formation of keloid and hypertrophic scars; however, earlobes, which are free of tension, can also develop keloid scars.
- These scars appear to have a genetic basis. In addition to this, keloid formation is more common in females (3:1 female:male ratio).
- There is thought to be a relationship between endocrine changes and keloid formation, e.g. keloids have been known to occur after a thyroidectomy and with increased hypothalamic activity.
- The production of hypertrophic and keloid scars may have an immunological basis.
- Biochemical differences between healthy scars, keloid and hypertrophic scars have been found, indicating that collagen synthesis is altered.
- Hypoxia may contribute to the formation of abnormal scars. Kischer *et al.* (1982) found that microvessels in these scars are partially or completely occluded, causing excessive fibroblast activity in the scar.
- Growth factors may have a role in keloid formation. Russell *et al.* (1988) found that cultured keloid fibroblasts grew more readily in a medium with reduced growth factors than normal fibroblasts.

Management

Education and support are crucial in assisting the patient to reintegrate into society. Advice may be required regarding specific problems; for example, patients with a history of keloid scar formation should avoid elective surgery or trauma, such as ear piercing (Munro 1995b). Disfigurement should be approached as a total problem, skin deep, mind deep and societal, as stated by Doreen Trust, founder and director of the Disfigurement Guidance Centre (cited in Trevelyan 1996). Patients may be offered a number of treatments to help prevent or improve an abnormal scar.

- *Finger massage* can improve the condition of the scar. A non-perfumed moisturizing cream should be used to prevent friction between the finger and scar. Finger massage can begin when the wound has completely healed and all bruising has subsided. Massage should be performed for 10 minutes, six times each day using firm pressure in a tight circular motion over the scar.
- *Pressure treatment* with individually tailored elastic garments, e.g. a Jobst garment, may be used for both keloid and hypertrophic scars. This treatment is used to prevent secondary contractures and to restore flatness and smoothness to scars. Pressure must be applied continuously for at least 12 months and any break in pressure should not exceed 30 minutes per day (Munro 1995b; Puzey 2001).

- *Intralesional corticosteroid injections* may help reduce scar tissue deposition and to soften and flatten keloid scars (Munro 1995b). There is a risk of scar recurrence with this treatment and it is only suitable for small scars (Eisenbeiss *et al.* 1998).
- *Silicone gel sheeting* will soften, flatten and blanch keloid and hypertrophic scars (Carney *et al.* 1994; Williams 1996).
- *Glycerine-based hydrogel sheet* (Novogel) may be effective in the prevention and treatment of hypertrophic and keloid scars. It can soften, flatten and relieve itching, redness and burning of scars (Baum & Busuito 1997).
- *Surgical excision* may be considered to release scar contractures; for example, a 'W' or 'Z' plasty to release a scar contracture by cutting it in the line of relaxed skin tension (Allsworth 1985; Beldon 2000). In the case of larger scars, surgical excision with or without skin grafting may be performed but there is a high rate of scar recurrence especially with keloid scars. Postoperative radiotherapy may reduce the recurrence rate (Eisenbeiss *et al.* 1998).
- *Cosmetic camouflage*, utilizing specialist cosmetic products, can be used to hide scarring; this is most successful in patients with atrophic (indented) and hypertrophic scars. This service is provided by appropriately trained professionals who also provide advice and education to enable patients to perform their own camouflage make-up.

Procedure guidelines: **Changing wound dressings**

Equipment

1 As for Procedure guidelines: Aseptic technique (Ch. 4, p. 57).

2 Cleaning fluid for irrigation (see Table 47.4).
3 Appropriate dressing (see Table 47.5).

Procedure

See procedure for Aseptic technique (Ch. 4, p. 57) up to and including step 11, then loosen the dressing.

Action	Rationale
12 Where appropriate, loosen the old dressing.	The dressing can then be lifted off without causing trauma.
13 Clean hands with a bactericidal alcohol handrub.	Hands may become contaminated by handling outer packets, dressing, etc.
14 Using the plastic bag in the pack, arrange the sterile field. Pour cleaning solution into gallipots or an indented plastic tray.	The time the wound is exposed should be kept to a minimum to reduce the risk of contamination. To prevent contamination of the environment. To minimize risk of contamination of cleaning solution.
15 Remove dressing by placing a hand in the plastic bag, lifting the dressing off and inverting the plastic bag so that the dressing is now inside the bag. Thereafter use this as the 'dirty' bag.	To reduce the risk of cross-infection. To prevent contamination of the environment.

Procedure guidelines: Changing wound dressings (cont'd)

Action	Rationale
16 Attach the bag with the dressing to the side of the trolley below the top shelf.	Contaminated material should be below the level of the sterile field.
17 Assess wound healing with reference to volume, amount of granulation tissue and epithelialization, signs of infection, underlying pathology, etc. (Table 47.3/Fig. 47.1). (Record assessment in relevant documentation at the end of the procedure.)	To evaluate wound care.
18 Put on gloves, touching only the inside wrist end.	To reduce the risk of infection to the wound and contamination of the nurse. Gloves provide greater sensitivity than forceps and are less likely to traumatize the wound or the patient's skin.
19 If necessary, gently clean the wound with a gloved hand using 0.9% sodium chloride, unless another solution is indicated (Table 47.3). If appropriate, irrigate by flushing with water or 0.9% sodium chloride.	To reduce the possibility of physical and chemical trauma to granulation and epithelial tissue.
20 Apply the dressing that is most suitable for the wound using the criteria for dressings (Table 47.5).	To promote healing and/or reduce symptoms.
21 Remove gloves; fasten dressing as appropriate with hypoallergenic tape/Netelast/bandage/tapeless retention dressing.	To prevent irritation of skin and to avoid trauma to wound.
22 Make sure the patient is comfortable and the dressing is secure.	A dressing may slip or feel uncomfortable as the patient changes position.
Continue with steps 18–21 from the procedure for Aseptic technique, p. 58.	

Procedure guidelines: **Removal of sutures, clips or staples**

Equipment

1 As for Procedure guidelines: Aseptic technique (Ch. 4, p. 57).

2 Sterile scissors, stitch cutter, staple remover.
3 Sterile adhesive sutures.

Procedure

Action	Rationale
1 Explain and discuss the procedure with the patient.	To ensure that the patient understands the procedure and gives his/her valid consent.
2 Perform procedure using aseptic technique.	To prevent infection (for further information see procedure on aseptic technique, Ch. 4).
3 Clean the wound with an appropriate sterile solution such as 0.9% sodium chloride (Table 47.4).	To prevent infection.

For removal of sutures

4 Lift knot of suture with metal forceps. Snip stitch close to the skin. Pull suture out gently.	Plastic forceps tend to slip against nylon sutures. To prevent infection by drawing exposed suture through the tissue.
5 Use tips of scissors slightly open or the side of the stitch cutter to gently press the skin when the suture is being drawn out.	To minimize pain by counteracting the adhesion between the suture and surrounding tissue.

For removal of clips

6 Squeeze wings of clips together with forceps to release from skin.	To release clips atraumatically from the wound.

*Procedure guidelines: **Removal of sutures, clips or staples** (cont'd)*

Action	Rationale
7 If the wound gapes use adhesive sutures to oppose the wound edges.	To improve the cosmetic effect.
8 When necessary, cover the wound with an appropriate dressing (Table 47.5).	To provide the best possible environment for wound healing to take place. To reduce the risk of infection. To prevent the suture line from rubbing against clothing.

For removal of staples

Action	Rationale
9 Slide the lower bar of the staple remover with the V-shaped groove under the staple at an angle of 90°. Squeeze the handles of the staple removers together to open the staple.	To release the staple atraumatically from the wound. If the angle of the staple remover is not correct, the staple will not come out freely.
If the suture line is under tension, use free hand to gently squeeze the skin either side of the suture line.	To reduce tension of skin around suture line and lessen pain on removal of staple.
10 If the wound gapes use adhesive sutures to oppose the wound edges.	To improve the cosmetic effect.

For all suture lines

Action	Rationale
11 Record condition of suture line and surrounding skin (amount of exudate, pus, inflammation, pain, etc.; see Table 47.3).	To document care and enable evaluation of the wound.

Procedure guidelines: **Drain dressing (Redivac – closed drainage systems)**

Equipment

1 As for Procedure guidelines: Aseptic technique (Ch. 4, p. 57).

2 Non-adherent, absorbent dressing.

Procedure

Action	Rationale
1 Explain and discuss the procedure with the patient.	To ensure that the patient understands the procedure and gives his/her valid consent.
2 Perform procedure using aseptic technique.	To prevent infection (for further information on asepsis, see procedure on aseptic technique, Ch. 4).
3 Clean the surrounding skin with an appropriate sterile solution such as 0.9% sodium chloride (Table 47.4).	To prevent infection and remove excess debris.
4 Check condition of surrounding skin.	To assess for any excoriation of the skin.
5 Ensure that the skin suture holding the drain site in position is intact.	To prevent the drain from leaving the wound.
6 Cover the drain site with a non-adherent, absorbent dressing.	To protect the drain site, prevent infection entering the wound and absorb exudate.
7 Tape securely.	To prevent drain coming loose.
8 Ensure that the drain is primed or that the suction pump is in working order.	To ensure continuity of drainage.

Procedure guidelines: **Change of vacuum drainage system**

(See Ch. 20, Intrapleural drainage.)

Equipment

1 Sterile topical swab.

2 Dressing pack.

Procedure guidelines: Change of vacuum drainage system (cont'd)

Procedure

Action	Rationale
1 Explain and discuss the procedure with the patient.	To ensure that the patient understands the procedure and gives his/her valid consent.
2 Perform procedure using aseptic technique.	To prevent infection (see procedure on aseptic technique, Ch. 4).
3 Wash hands using bactericidal soap and water or bactericidal alcohol handrub.	To minimize the risk of infection.
4 Ensure sterile drainage system is readily available.	To ensure sterility during change of system.
5 Measure the contents of the bottle to be changed and record this in the appropriate documents.	To maintain an accurate record of drainage from the wound and enable evaluation of state of wound.
6 Clamp the tube with the tubing clamps on the drainage tube and bottle connector and remove the bottle.	To prevent air and contamination entering the wound via the drain.
7 Clean the end of the tube and attach it to the sterile bottle.	To maintain sterility.
8 Unclamp the tubing clamps.	To re-establish the drainage system.
9 Place used vacuum drainage system into the clinical waste bag.	To safely dispose of used system.

Procedure guidelines: **Removal of drain (Yeates vacuum drainage system)**

Equipment

1 As for Procedure guidelines: Aseptic technique (Ch. 4, p. 57).

2 Sterile scissors or suture cutter.

Procedure

Action	Rationale
1 Check the patient's operation notes.	To establish the number and site(s) of internal and external sutures.
2 Explain and discuss the procedure with the patient.	To ensure that the patient understands the procedure and gives his/her valid consent.
3 If appropriate (in closed drainage systems) release vacuum.	To prevent pulling at wound tissue, causing pain and tissue damage.
4 Perform the procedure using aseptic technique.	To minimize the risk of infection. (For further information on asepsis, see Ch. 4.)
5 Where the wound is covered with an occlusive dressing (e.g. following lumpectomy in the breast), lift and snip the dressing from around the drain. Do not remove it from the entire wound.	To prevent disturbing the incision or contaminating the wound.
6 Only clean the wound if necessary, using an appropriate sterile solution, such as 0.9% sodium chloride (Table 47.4).	To reduce risk of infection.
7 Hold the knot of the suture with metal forceps and gently lift upwards.	Plastic forceps tend to slip against nylon sutures. To allow space for the scissors or stitch cutter to be placed underneath.
8 Cut the shortest end of the suture as close to the skin as possible.	To prevent infection by allowing the suture to be liberated from the drain without drawing the exposed part through tissue.
9 Remove drain gently. If there is resistance, place free gloved hand against the tissue to oppose the tugging of the drain being removed. If the resistance is felt to be excessive, nitrous oxide (e.g. Entonox) may be required.	To minimize pain and reduce trauma.

*Procedure guidelines: **Removal of drain (Yeates vacuum drainage system)** (cont'd)*

Action	Rationale
10 Cover the drain site with a sterile dressing and tape securely.	To prevent infection entering the drain site.
11 Measure and record the contents of the drainage bottle in the appropriate documents.	To maintain an accurate record of drainage from the wound and enable evaluation of state of wound.
12 Dispose of used drainage system in clinical waste bag.	To ensure safe disposal.

Procedure guidelines: **Shortening of drain (Penrose, etc., open drainage systems)**

Procedure

Action	Rationale
1 Follow steps 1–8 above (removal of drain), i.e. to the stage where the suture has been cut.	
2 Using gloved hand, gently ease the drain out of wound to the length requested by surgeons (usually 3–5 cm).	To allow healing to take place from base of wound.
3 Using gloved hand, place a sterile safety pin through the drain as close to the skin as possible, taking great care not to stab either the nurse or patient.	To prevent retraction into the wound and minimize the risk of cross-infection and sharps injury.
4 Cut same amount of tubing from distal end of drain as withdrawn from wound.	So there is a convenient length of tubing to drain into the bag. To ensure patient comfort.
5 Place a sterile, suitably sized drainage bag over the drain site.	To allow effluent to drain into the bag. To prevent excoriation of the skin. To contain any odour.
6 Check bag is secure and comfortable for the patient.	For patient comfort.
7 Record by how much the drainage tube was shortened.	To ensure the length remaining in the wound is known.

Procedure guidelines: **Prevention of pressure ulcers**

Procedure

Action	Rationale
1 Assess every patient on admission using a recognized scale, such as the Norton (Fig. 47.3), Waterlow (Fig. 47.4) or Braden Scale (Fig. 47.5).	To identify the patient at risk of developing pressure ulcers.
2 Reassess every patient on a regular basis and/or if there has been any deterioration or change in condition.	To provide appropriate data on which to base treatment.
3 Do not rub any area at risk.	Rubbing causes maceration and degeneration of subcutaneous tissues, especially in the elderly.
4 Wash areas at risk only if the patient is incontinent or sweating profusely. Use mild soap or a liquid detergent. Ensure that all detergent or soap is rinsed off and that the area is patted dry. Use moisturizer if the skin is very dry. Ask the patient what suits his/her skin.	To maintain skin integrity and prevent the formation of sores. Excessive use of soap can be harmful to the skin. Thorough gentle drying of the skin promotes comfort and discourages the growth of micro-organisms. Dry skin cracks allow entry of micro-organisms.
5 Use barrier creams only when indicated.	Barrier creams prevent damage to the epidermis. They are, however, occlusive and prevent moisture exchange from the skin.
6 Educate the patient to shift position, to pull or push up regularly and to examine the vulnerable areas.	After discharge the patient may be self-caring and possibly still vulnerable to pressure ulcers/tissue damage. To encourage the patient to participate in their own care.
7 Initiate a mobility programme for the patient. Call on the physiotherapist, occupational therapist or dietitian as appropriate.	To reduce further tissue damage and improve the circulation.

*Procedure guidelines: **Prevention of pressure ulcers** (cont'd)*

Action	Rationale
8 Where possible, relieve the pressure over areas vulnerable to tissue breakdown. Use appropriate pressure relief devices (Table 47.6). If necessary, turn the patient at least 2-hourly and record the position on the relevant charts (Clark 1998).	To reduce pressure where possible. Use of inappropriate aids may increase pressure to vulnerable areas.
9 Have the patient recumbent whenever possible. Support with bead bags or pillows in bed. Reduce period spent sitting in chair if pelvic sores develop.	Avoid the use of bedrests as these increase shearing by allowing the patient to slide down the bed.

Procedure guidelines: **Sharp debridement**

Equipment

1 Sterile (disposable) scalpel with size 10 or 15 blade.
2 Sterile scissors (preferable curved or straight iris scissors).
3 Sterile toothed forceps capable of grasping and holding necrotic tissue.
4 Sterile probe for assessing tracking and depth of wound.
5 Sterile low-linting gauze.
6 Haemostatic dressing (alginate or oxidized cellulose).
7 Plastic apron.
8 Dressing procedure pack.
9 Sterile gloves.
10 Appropriate cleaning solution and post-procedure dressing.
11 Camera (optional).
12 Suitable light source.

Note: extra precautions, such as wearing a sterile gown, should be used for immunosuppressed patients.

Procedure

Action	Rationale
1 Explain and discuss the procedure with the patient. Agree a time limit for the procedure.	To ensure the patient understands the procedure and other options available, and gives his/her valid consent.
2 Provide routine analgesia prior to debridement procedure.	To prevent unnecessary procedural pain. Debridement of only necrotic tissue should not increase pain. However, viable tissue pulled or cut may necessitate additional analgesia.
3 Ensure there is adequate lighting and the patient is comfortable and in a position where the wound can be accessed and viewed easily.	To allow access to area for debridement. The patient needs to be discouraged from making unexpected movements and so should be in the most comfortable position possible at the start of the procedure.
4 Perform steps 2–15 of the Aseptic technique guideline (Ch. 4, p. 57).	To reduce the risk of cross-infection and reduce the amount of time the wound is exposed.
5 Take photograph of the wound if appropriate.	To provide a baseline assessment of wound appearance.
6 Put on sterile gloves, touching only the inside wrist.	To reduce the risk of cross-infection and protect the nurse from exposure to blood and wound exudate.
7 Lift the necrotic tissue with forceps and cut it carefully with a scalpel or scissors, taking it down in layers. Debridement should be stopped if the nurse feels uncertain at any time during the procedure.	To reduce the possibility of damaging healthy tissue.
8 If bleeding occurs apply constant local pressure initially. Use haemostatic dressing if necessary. If bleeding persists seek medical advice.	To ensure blood loss is minimal.
9 Take photograph of the wound post debridement if appropriate.	To evaluate and document extent of debridement.
10 Reassess wound bed and re-dress according to local guidelines.	To provide the ideal healing environment for the wound.
11 Dispose of used dressings and disposable equipment in a clinical waste bag/sharps container as appropriate.	To prevent environmental contamination, sharps injury and reuse of disposable equipment.

*Procedure guidelines: **Sharp debridement** (cont'd)*

Action	Rationale
12 Check that the trolley remains dry and physically clean.	To reduce the risk of cross-infection.
13 Wash hands with soap and water or alcohol hand gel.	To reduce the risk of cross-infection.
14 Complete the patient's care plan and other hospital and/or legally required documents.	To ensure all of those involved in this patient's care are aware that debridement of the wound has been undertaken.

Adapted from a generic template document 'Nursing Procedure – Sharp Debridement of Wounds' (Ballard *et al.* 2002; Fairbairn *et al.* 2002).

Procedure guidelines: **VAC ATS dressing**

Equipment

1 1 VAC ATS therapy unit.
2 1 VAC (TRAC) dressing pack.
3 1 VAC canister and tubing.
4 Sterile scissors.
5 Sterile gloves.
6 Apron.
7 Dressing procedure pack.
8 Sterile 0.9% sodium chloride for irrigation (warmed to approx. 37°C in a jug of warm water).

Additional materials as required

- Extra semi-permeable film dressings to seal any leaks.
- Non-adherent wound contact layer to prevent foam adhering to wound bed.
- VAC gel strips (for sensitive or difficult to seal areas).
- Alcohol-free skin barrier film to protect any fragile or macerated skin around the wound
- *or* thin hydrocolloid sheet to 'frame' the wound.

Procedure

Action	Rationale
1 Explain and discuss the procedure with the patient. Agree a time limit for the procedure.	To ensure the patient understands the procedure and other options available, and gives his/her valid consent.
2 Provide routine analgesia prior to dressing procedure.	To prevent unnecessary procedural pain.
3 Ensure there is adequate lighting and the patient is comfortable and in a position where the wound can be accessed and viewed easily.	To allow access to area for dressing change. Dressing application can be complicated and take a long time so the patient should be in a comfortable position for the procedure.
4 Perform steps 2–15 of the Aseptic technique guideline (Ch. 4, p. 57).	To reduce the risk of cross-infection and reduce the amount of time the wound is exposed.

Dressing removal

5 Put on a pair of non-sterile gloves.	To reduce the risk of cross-infection.
6 Clamp the dressing tubing and disconnect it from the canister tubing. Allow any fluid in the canister tubing to be sucked into the canister. Switch off the pump and clamp the canister tubing.	To prevent spillage of body fluid waste from the tubing or canister.
7 Remove and discard the canister (if full or at least weekly).	To prevent pump alarming and for infection control.
8 Carefully remove the occlusive film drape by gently lifting one edge and then stretching the drape horizontally and slowly pulling up from the skin.	To prevent damage to the peri-wound skin.
9 Carefully remove the foam dressing from the wound bed.	To prevent damage to newly formed tissue within the wound bed and prevent pain.
10 Clean the wound with an appropriate sterile solution such as 0.9% sodium chloride (see Table 47.4).	To prevent infection and remove surface debris/necrotic tissue.
11 Debride the wound if applicable.	To remove loose necrotic tissue that may be a focus for infection.

Procedure guidelines: VAC ATS dressing (cont'd)

Dressing application

12 Clean, dry and prepare the peri-wound skin (e.g. with VAC gel strip, barrier film or thin hydrocolloid). — To prevent skin damage and ensure a good seal.

13 Cut the VAC foam to fit the size and shape of the wound, including tunnelling and undermined areas. — The foam should fit the wound exactly to ensure full benefit of the negative pressure therapy.

14 Avoid cutting the foam over the wound bed. — To prevent loose particles of foam falling into the wound.

15 Place the foam into the wound cavity (Note: if the wound is bigger than the largest foam dressing, more than one piece of foam may be used as long as the edges of the foam are in contact with each other). — The whole wound bed must be covered with foam. If the foam is touching it will transfer the negative pressure to the next piece.

16 Avoid foam contact with intact skin. — To prevent skin maceration by wound exudate.

17 Cut the occlusive film drape to size and apply over the top of the foam, ensuring a 3–5 cm border onto intact skin, VAC gel strip or hydrocolloid (Note: do not compress the foam into the wound). — To obtain a good seal around the wound edges.

18 Choose a location on the sealed occlusive film drape to apply the tubing where the tubing will not rub or cause pressure. Cut a hole through the film, approximately 2 cm in diameter, leaving the foam intact. — To reduce the risk of pressure injury to skin.

19 Place the TRAC pad on the film with the hole in the centre of the elbow joint directly over the hole in the film drape. Gently press around the TRAC pad. — To ensure correct position and seal of the pad.

Commencing therapy

20 Insert the canister into the pump until it clicks into place — Indicates the canister is positioned correctly and is secure.

21 Connect the dressing tubing to the canister tubing and open clamps. — The pump will alarm if the tubing is clamped or not connected.

22 Press POWER button and follow the on-screen instructions to set the level and type of pressure required according to instructions from the patient's medical/surgical team (see Table 47.10). — To ensure the therapy is set to the individual requirements of the patient.

23 Start the pump by pressing THERAPY ON/OFF – the foam should collapse into the wound. If it does not, assess the film drape for air leaks and seal with leftover drape or a semi-permeable film dressing. — Any small air leak will prevent the foam dressing from collapsing.

Table 47.10 Suggested VAC therapy protocols (KCI International 2000)

	Pressure ulcers or acute wounds	Flaps	Split skin grafts	Chronic ulcers
Therapy type	Continuous for 48 hours, then intermittent (5 minutes on, 2 minutes off)	Continuous therapy	Continuous therapy	Continuous therapy
Length of therapy	24 hours/day	24 hours/day	24 hours/day for 5 days	24 hours/day
Pressure	125 mmHg	125–150 mmHg	50 mmHg	50–75 mmHg
Dressing change	Every 48 hours (more often if infected)	Every 48 hours (more often if infected)	No dressing change until day 5	Every 48 hours (more often if infected)

(mmHg = millimetres of mercury)

References and further reading

Ågren, M.S., Karlsmark, T., Hansen, J.B. & Rygaard, J. (2001) Occlusion versus air exposure on full-thickness biopsy wounds. *J Wound Care*, **10**(8), 301–4.

Aidoo, A., Gao, N., Neft, R.E., *et al.* (1990) Evaluation of the genotoxicity of gentian violet in bacterial and mammalian cell systems. *Teratogenesis, Carcinogenesis, Mutagenesis*, **10**(6), 449–62.

Alberdi, J.M.Z. (1988) Hypertensive ulcer: Martorell's ulcer. *Phlebology*, **3**, 139–42.

Allsworth, J. (1985) *Skin Camouflage. A Guide To Remedial Techniques*. Arnould–Taylor, Cheltenham.

Angeras, M.H., Brandberg, A., Falk, A. & Seeman, T. (1992) Comparison between sterile saline and tap water for the cleaning of acute traumatic soft tissue wounds. *Eur J Surg*, **58**, 347–50.

Argenta, L.C. & Morykwas, M.J. (1997) Vacuum-assisted closure: a new method for wound control and treatment: clinical experience. *Ann Plast Surg*, **38**(6), 563–76.

Armstrong, S., Duncan, V. & Gibson B. (1998) Venous leg ulcers, Part 4. Wound care. *Prof Nurse*, **13**(11), 798–802.

Ash, D. (2002) An exploration of the occurrence of pressure ulcers in a British spinal injuries unit. *J Clin Nurs*, **11**(4), 470–8.

Ashby, M. (1991) The role of radiotherapy in palliative care. *J Pain Symptom Manage*, **6**(6), 380–8.

Autar, R. (1998) Calculating patients' risk of deep vein thrombosis. *Br J Nurs*, **7**(1), 7–12.

Back, I.N. & Finlay, I. (1995) Analgesic effect of topical opioids on painful skin ulcers. *J Pain Symptom Manage*, **10**(7), 493.

Bader, D.L. (1990) *Clinical Practice and Scientific Approach*. Macmillan, London.

Badger, C. (1992) *Lymphoedema: Assessment and Management* (Educational Leaflet No. 13). Wound Care Society, Huntingdon.

Baker, J. (1998) Essential oils: a complementary therapy in wound management. *J Wound Care*, **7**(7), 355–7.

Baker, S.R., Stacey, M.C., Jopp-McKay, A.G. *et al.* (1991) Epidemiology of chronic venous ulcers. *Br J Surg*, **78**, 864–7.

Bale, S. (1991) A holistic approach and the ideal dressing. *Prof Nurse*, **6**(6), 316–23.

Bale, S. (1997) A guide to wound debridement. *J Wound Care*, **6**(4), 179–82.

Bale, S. & Harding, K.G. (1991) Foams still find favour: wound management using foam dressings. *Prof Nurse*, **6**(9), 510, 512–14, 516.

Bale, S. & Jones, V. (1997) *Wound Care Nursing: A Patient Centred Approach*. Baillière Tindall, London.

Ballard, K. & Baxter, H. (2001) Promoting healing in static wounds. *Nurs Times*, **97**(14), 52.

Ballard, K., Fairbairn, K., Grier, J., Hunter, C., O'Brien, M. & Preece, J. (2002) *Nursing Procedure – Sharp Debridement of Wounds*. Available from Kate Ballard, Clinical Nurse Specialist (Tissue Viability), Tissue Viability Unit, Guys & St Thomas NHS Trust, London.

Banwell, P.E. (1999) Topical negative pressure therapy in wound care. *J Wound Care*, **8**(2), 79–84.

Barbenel, J.C. (1990) Movement studies during sleep. In: *Pressure Sores – Clinical Practice and Scientific Approach* (ed. D. L. Bader). Macmillan, London, pp. 249–60.

Barkham, A.M. (1993) Radiotherapy skin reactions and treatments. *Prof Nurse*, **8**(11), 732, 734, 736.

Barr, P.O. *et al.* (1990) Hyperbaric oxygen and problem wounds. *Care Sci Pract*, **8**(1), 3–6.

Barton, A.A. (1988) Prevention of pressure sores. *Nurs Times*, **73**, 1593–5.

Baum, T.M. & Busuito, M.J. (1998) Use of a glycerin-based gel sheeting in scar management. *Adv Wound Care*, **11**(1), 40–3.

Baxandall, T. (1997) Healing cavity wounds with negative pressure. *Elderly Care*, **9**(1), 20–2.

Beldon, P. (2000) Abnormal scar formation in wound healing. *Nurs Times*, **96**(10), 44–5.

Benbow, M. (1994) The benefits of hydrogel dressings. *Commun Outlook*, October, 29–34.

Benbow, M. (1995) Parameters of wound assessment. *Br J Nurs*, **4**(11), 647–51.

Benbow, M. (2001) Oasis®: an innovative alternative dressing for chronic wounds. *Br J Nurs*, **10**(22), 1489–92.

Bennett, G. & Moody, M. (1995) *Wound Care for Health Professionals*. Chapman & Hall, London.

Bennett, G. (1999) *Graduated Compression Hosiery* (Educational Leaflet No. 6(1)). Wound Care Society, Huntingdon.

Bergstrom, N. & Braden, B. (1992) A prospective study of pressure sore risk among institutionalized elderly. *J Am Geriatr Soc*, **40**(8), 747–58.

Bergstrom, N., Braden, B.J., Laguzza, A. & Holman, V. (1987) The Braden Scale for Predicting Pressure Sore Risk. *Nurs Res*, **36**(4), 205–10.

Bird, C. (2000) Supporting patients with fungating breast wounds. *Prof Nurse*, **15**(10), 649–52.

Birtwistle, J. (1994) Pressure sore formation and risk assessment in intensive care. *Care Crit Ill*, **10**(4), 154–5, 157–9.

Blackmar, A. (1997) Focus on wound care: radiation-induced skin alterations. *Medsurg Nurs*, **6**(3), 172–5.

Blair, S.D. *et al.* (1988) Do dressings influence the healing of chronic venous ulcers? *Phlebology*, **3**, 129–34.

Bloomfield, S.F. & Sizer, T.J. (1985) Eusol BPC and other hypochlorite formulations used in hospitals. *Pharm J*, 3 August, 153–7.

Boots-Vickers, M. & Eaton, K. (1999) Skin care for patients receiving radiotherapy. *Prof Nurse*, **14**(10), 706–8.

Bower, M., Stein, R., Evans, T., Hedley, A., Pert, P. & Coombes, R. (1992) A double-blind study of the efficacy of metronidazole gel in the treatment of malodorous fungating tumours. *Eur J Cancer*, **28**(4/5), 888–9.

Bowler, P. (1998) The anaerobic and aerobic microbiology of wounds: a review. *Wounds*, **10**(6), 170–8.

Boyce, S.T., Kagan, R.J., Yakuboff, K.P. *et al.* (2002) Cultured skin substitutes reduce donor skin harvesting for closure of excised, full-thickness burns. *Ann Surg*, **235**(2), 269–79.

Braden, B.J. & Bergstrom, N. (1987) A conceptual schema for the study of aetiology of pressure sores. *Rehabil Nurs*, **12**(1), 8–12.

Brennan, S.S. & Leaper, D.J. (1985) The effect of antiseptics on the healing wound: a study using the rabbit ear chamber. *Br J Surg*, **72**, 780–2.

Bridel-Nixon, J. (1999) Pressure sores. In: *Nursing Management of Chronic Wounds*, 2nd edn (eds M. Morison, C. Moffatt, J. Bridel-Nixon & S. Bale). Mosby, London.

Brown, A.S., Glickman, L.T., Matthews, M.S. & Slezak, S. (1998) *Essentials for Students – Plastic and Reconstructive Surgery*, 5th edn. Plastic Surgery Information Service. Online: www.plasticsurgery.org/profinfo/essen/essentia.htm (accessed 17 December 2001).

Brown, G.I., et al. (1991) Stimulation of healing of chronic wounds by epidermal growth factor. *Plastic Reconstr Surg*, **88**, 189–94.

Brown, V. & Marshall, D. (2001) Compression therapy in leg ulcer management. *Nurs Stand*, **14**(15), 64–70.

Burnand, K.G. (1990) Aetiology of venous ulceration. *Br J Surg*, **77**, 483–4.

Butcher, M. (1999) Identifying and combating the risk of pressure. *Nurs Stand*, **14**(3), 58–63.

Callam, M.J. et al. (1985) Chronic ulceration of the leg: extent of the problem and provision of care. *Br Med J*, **290**, 1855–6.

Callam, M.J. et al. (1987) Arterial disease in chronic leg ulceration: an underestimated hazard? Lothian and Forth Valley Leg Ulcer Study. *Br Med J*, **294**, 929–31.

Calvin, M. (1998) Cutaneous wound repair. *Wounds*, **10**(1), 12–32.

Campbell, J. & Lane, C. (1996) Developing a skin-care protocol in radiotherapy. *Prof Nurse*, **12**(2), 105–8.

Carcary, M. (2001) Intermittent sequential compression therapy. *Nurs Times*, **97**(48), 48–50.

Carney, S.A., Cason, C.G., Gowar J.P. et al. (1994) Cica-care gel sheeting in the management of hypertrophic scarring. *Burns*, **20**(2), 163–7.

Carson, C.F., Riley, T.V. & Cookson, B.D. (1998) Efficacy and safety of tea tree oil as a topical antimicrobial agent. *J Hosp Infect*, **40**(3), 175–8.

Casey, G. (1998) The importance of nutrition in wound healing. *Nurs Stand*, **13**(3), 51–6.

Chaplin, J. (2000) Pressure sore risk assessment in palliative care. *J Tissue Viability*, **10**(1), 27–31.

Chase, S.K., Melloni, M. & Savage, A. (1997) A forever healing: the lived experience of venous ulcer disease. *J Vasc Nurs*, **15**(2), 73–8.

Chen, W.Y.J. & Abatangelo, G. (1999) Functions of hyaluronan in wound repair. *Wound Repair Regen*, **7**(2), 79–89.

Clamon, J. & Netscher, D.T. (1994) General principles of flap reconstruction: goals for aesthetic and functional outcome. *Plastic Surg Nurs*, **14**(1), 9–14.

Clark, M. (1998) Repositioning to prevent pressure sores – what is the evidence? *Nurs Stand*, **13**(3), 58–64.

Clark, M. (2002) Pressure ulcers and quality of life. *Nurs Stand*, **13**(16), 74–80.

Clay, M. (2000) Pressure sore prevention in nursing homes. *Nurs Stand*, **14**(44), 45–50.

Clide, S. (1992) Cleaning choices. *Nurs Times*, **88**(19), 74–8.

Collier, M. (1996) The principles of optimum wound management. *Nurs Stand*, **10**(43), 47–52.

Collier, M. (1999a) Venous leg ulceration. In: *Wound Management: Theory and Practice* (eds M. Miller & D. Glover). Nursing Times Books, London.

Collier, M. (1999b) Pressure ulcer development and principles for prevention. In: *Wound Management: Theory and Practice* (eds M. Miller & D. Glover). Nursing Times Books, London.

Collier, M. (2001) 'Universal' concepts. *J Wound Care*, **10**(7), 249.

Collier, M. (2002) Wound care. Wound-bed preparation. *Nurs Times*, **98**(2), 55–7.

Collinson, G. (1992) Improving quality of life in patients with malignant fungating wounds. *Proc 2nd Eur Conf on Wound Management*. Macmillan, London.

Cornwall, J.V., Dore, C.J. & Lewis, J.D. (1986) Leg ulcers: epidemiology and aetiology. *Br J Surg*, **73**(9), 693–6.

Coull, A. (1991) Making sense of split skin grafts. *Nurs Times*, **87**(27), 54–5.

Cox, D.A. (1993) Growth factors in wound healing. *J Wound Care*, **12**(6), 339–42.

Crane, J. (1993) Extending the role of a new hydrogel. *J Tissue Viability*, **3**(3), 98–9.

Cullum, N., Deeks, J., Fletcher, A. et al. (1995) *Effective Health Care Bulletin 2(1)*. The prevention and treatment of pressure sores: how useful are the measurements for scoring people's risk of developing a pressure sore? NHS Centre for Reviews and Dissemination and Nuffield Institute for Health/Churchill Livingstone, York. Online: www.york.ac.uk/inst/crd/ehc21.pdf

Cullum, N., Deeks, J., Sheldon, T.A., Song, F. & Fletcher, A. (1999) *Beds, Mattresses and Cushions for Pressure Sore Prevention and Treatment (Cochrane Review)*. Cochrane Library, Oxford.

Cunliffe, W.J. (1990) Eusol – to use or not to use? *Dermatol Pract*, **8**(2), 5–7.

Cutting, K. (1994) Factors influencing wound healing. *Nurs Stand*, **8**(50), 33–7.

Cutting, K.F. (1998) *Wounds and Infection* (Educational Leaflet No. 5(2)). Wound Care Society, Huntingdon.

Dale, J. (1995) Wound dressings on the Drug Tariff. *Prof Nurse*, **10**(7), 461–5.

Dale, J. (1998) Venous leg ulcers. Part 3: compression. *Prof Nurse*, **13**(10), 715–19.

Dale, J.J. & Gibson, B. (1986a) Leg ulcers: the nursing assessment. *Prof Nurse*, **1**(9), 236–8.

Dale, J.J. & Gibson, B. (1986b) The treatment of leg ulcers. *Prof Nurse*, **1**(12), 321–4.

Dale, J.J. & Gibson, B. (1987) Compression bandaging for venous ulcers. *Prof Nurse*, **2**(7), 211–14.

Dale, J.J. & Gibson, B. (1990) Back-up for the venous pump. *Prof Nurse*, **5**(9), 481–6.

David, J.A. et al. (1983) *An Investigation of the Current Methods Used in Nursing for the Care of Patients with Established Pressure Sores*. Nursing Practice Research Unit, University of Surrey.

Davies, D.M. (1985) Plastic and reconstructive surgery. *Br Med J*, **290**, 1056–8.

Davis, M.H., Dunkley, P., Harden, R. et al. (1993) *The Wound Handbook*. Centre for Medical Education, Dundee, and Perspective, London.

De Conno, F., Ventafridda, V. & Saita, L. (1991) Skin problems in advanced and terminal cancer patients. *J Pain Symptom Manage*, **6**(4), 247–56.

Dealey, C. (1999) *The Care of Wounds: A Guide for Nurses*, 2nd edn. Blackwell Science, Oxford.

Dean, A. (1997) Fibrinolytic inhibitors for cancer-associated bleeding problems. *J Pain Symptom Manage*, **13**(1), 20–4.

Deas, J. et al. (1986) The toxicity of commonly used antiseptics on fibroblasts in tissue culture. *Phlebology*, **1**, 205–9.

Deeks, J.J. (1996) Pressure sore prevention: using and evaluating risk assessment tools. *Br J Nurs*, **5**(5), 313–20.

Deeth, M. & Pain, L. (2001) Vacutex®: a dressing designed for patients, tailored by nurses. *Br J Nurs*, **10**(4), 268–71.

Devel, T.F. (1987) Polypeptide growth factors: roles in normal and abnormal cell growth. *Annu Rev Cell Biol*, **3**, 443–64.

DoH (1991) *The Health of the Nation*. HMSO, London.

DoH (1993) *The Health of the Nation: Pressure Sores – A Key Quality Indicator*. Stationery Office, London.

DoH (2001a) *National Service Framework for Older People*. Department of Health, London.

DoH (2001b) *The Essence of Care: Patient-Focussed Benchmarking for Health Care Practitioners*. Department of Health, London.

Donayre, C.E. (1998) Diagnosis and management of vascular ulcers. In: *Wound Care: A Collaborative Practice Manual for Physical Therapists and Nurses* (eds C. Sussman & B.M. Bate-Jensen). Aspen Publishers, Maryland.

Donovan, S. (1998) Wound infection and wound swabbing. *Prof Nurse*, **13**(11), 757–9.

Dunford, C. (2000) The use of honey in wound management. *Nurs Stand*, **15**(11), 63–8.

Dyson, M., Young, S., Pendle, C.L., Webster, D.F. & Lang, S.M. (1988) Comparison of the effects of moist and dry conditions on dermal repair. *J Invest Dermatol*, **91**(5), 434–9.

Dyson, M., Young, S.R., Hart, J., Lynch, J.A. & Lang, S. (1992) Comparison of the effects of moist and dry conditions on the process of angiogenesis during dermal repair. *J Invest Dermatol*, **99**(6), 729–33.

Dyson, R. (1978) Bed sores – the injuries hospital staff inflict on patients. *Nurs Mirror*, **146**(24), 30–2.

Eaglstein, W.H. (1985) The effect of occlusive dressings on collagen synthesis and re-epithelialisation in superficial wounds. In: *An Environment for Healing: The Role of Occlusion*. Royal Society of Medicine International Congress and Symposium Series No. 88 (ed. T.J. Ryan). Royal Society of Medicine, London.

Edmonds, M. & Foster, A. (2000) Hyalofill: a new product for chronic wound management. *Diabetic Foot*, **3**(1), 29–30.

Edwards, M. (1994) *The reliability and validity of the Waterlow pressure sore risk scale when used within district nursing to assess elders nursed in a domiciliary setting*. MSc dissertation, University of London.

Ehrlich, H.P. (1999) The physiology of wound healing: a summary of normal and abnormal wound healing processes. *Adv Wound Care*, **11**(7), 326–8.

Ehrlich, H.P. & Hunt, T.K. (1968) Effects of cortisone and vitamin A on wound healing. *Ann Surg*, **167**(3), 324–8.

Eisenbeiss, W., Peter, F.W., Bakhtiari, C. & Frenz, C. (1998) Hypertrophic scars and keloids. *J Wound Care*, **7**(5), 255–7.

Emflorgo, C. (1998) Controlling bleeding in fungating wounds (Letter). *J Wound Care*, **7**(5), 235.

EPUAP (1998) A policy statement on the prevention of pressure ulcers. *Br J Nurs*, **7**(15), 888–90.

EPUAP (2001) *Pressure Ulcer Prevention Guidelines*. European Pressure Ulcer Advisory Panel, Oxford. Online: www.epuap.com

Fairbairn, K. (1993) Towards better care for women. *Prof Nurse*, **9**(3), 204–12.

Fairbairn, K. (1994) A challenge that requires further research. *Prof Nurse*, **9**(4), 272–7.

Fairbairn, K., Grier, J., Hunter, C. & Preece, J. (2002) A sharp debridement procedure devised by specialist nurses. *J Wound Care*, **11**(10), 371–5.

Falanga, V. (2000) Classifications for wound bed preparation and stimulation of chronic wounds. *Wound Repair Regen*, **8**(5), 347–52.

Farley, K.M. (1991) Cornstarch as a treatment for dry desquamation. *Oncol Nurs Forum*, **18**(1), 134.

Farrow, S. & Toth, B. (1991) The place of Eusol in wound management. *Nurs Stand*, **5**(22), 25–7.

Ferguson, M., Rimmasch, H., Voss, A., Cook, A. & Bender, S. (2000) Pressure ulcer management: the importance of nutrition. *Medsurg Nurs*, **9**(4), 163–75.

Field, C.K. & Kerstein, M.D. (1994) Overview of wound healing in a moist environment. *Am J Surg*, **167**, Suppl 1a, 2–6s.

Finlay, I., Bowszyc, J. & Ramlav, C. (1996) The effect of topical 0.75% metronidazole gel on malodorous cutaneous ulcers. *J Pain Symptom Manage*, **11**(3), 158–62.

Flanagan, M. (1994) Wound care: assessment criteria. *Nurs Times*, **90**(35), 76–88.

Flanagan, M. (1996) A practical framework for wound assessment 1: physiology. *Br J Nurs*, **5**(22), 1391–7.

Flanagan, M. (1997) A practical framework for wound assessment 2: methods. *Br J Nurs*, **6**(1), 6–11.

Flanagan, M. (1998) The characteristics and formation of granulation tissue. *J Wound Care*, **7**(10), 508–10.

Flanagan, M. (1999) The physiology of wound healing. In: *Wound Management: Theory and Practice* (eds M. Miller & D. Glover). Nursing Times Books, London.

Flanagan, M. (2000) The physiology of wound healing. *J Wound Care*, **9**(6), 299–300.

Fletcher, A., Cullum, N. & Sheldon, T.A. (1997) A systematic review of compression treatment for venous leg ulcers. *Br Med J*, **315**(7108), 576–80.

Fletcher, J. (1997) Update: wound cleansing. *Prof Nurse*, **12**(11), 793–6.

Fletcher, J. (2000) The role of collagen in wound healing. *Prof Nurse*, **15**(8), 527–30.

Francis, A. (1998) Nursing management of skin graft sites. *Nurs Stand*, **12**(33), 41–4.

Franks, P., Oldroyd, M. & Dickson, D. (1995) Risk factors for leg ulceration recurrence: a randomised trial of two types of compression stocking. *Age Ageing*, **24**, 490–4.

Freedline, A. (1999) *Types of Wound Debridement*. Wound Care Information Network. Online: www.medicaledu.com/debridhp.htm (accessed 8 October 1999).

Garrett, B. (1997) The proliferation and movement of cells during re-epithelialisation. *J Wound Care*, **6**(4), 174–7.

Garrett, B. & Garrett, S. (1997) Healing messengers. *Nurs Times*, **93**(46), 78, 80, 82.

Gentzkow, G.D., Iwasaki, S.D., Hershon, K.S. *et al.* (1996) Use of Dermagraft, a cultured human dermis, to treat diabetic foot ulcers. *Diabetes Care*, **19**(4), 350–4.

Gilchrist, B. (1997) Should iodine be considered in wound management? *J Wound Care*, **6**(3), 148–50.

Gilchrist, B. (1999) Wound infection. In: *Wound Management: Theory and Practice* (eds M. Miller & D. Glover). Nursing Times Books, London.

Glean, E., Faithfull, S., Meredith, S., Richards, C., Smith, C. & Colyer, M.H. (2001) Intervention for acute radiotherapy induced skin reactions in cancer patients: the development of clinical practice guidelines recommended for use by the College of Radiographers. *J Radiother Pract*, 2(2), 75–84.

Grewal, P.S., Sawant, N.H., Deaney, C.N. *et al.* (1999) Pressure sore prevention in hospital patients: a clinical audit. *J Wound Care*, 8(3), 129–31.

Grocott, P. (2000a) Palliative management of fungating malignant wounds. *J Wound Care*, 9(1), 4–9.

Grocott, P. (2000b) Palliative management of fungating malignant wounds. *J Commun Nurs*, 14(3), 31–2, 35–6, 38.

Guyton, A.C. & Hall, J.E. (2000) *Textbook of Medical Physiology*, 10th edn. W.B. Saunders, Philadelphia.

Haalboom, J.R.E., Van Everdingen, J.J.E. & Cullum, N. (1997) Incidence, prevalence and classification. In: *The Decubitus Ulcer in Clinical Practice* (eds L.C. Parish, J.A. Witkowski & J.T. Crissey). Springer, Berlin.

Haisfield-Wolfe, M.E. & Rund, C. (1997) Malignant cutaneous wounds: a management protocol. *Ostomy Wound Manage*, 43(1), 56–66.

Hallett, A. (1995) Fungating wounds. *Nurs Times*, 91(47), 81–83.

Hamilton, K. (1995) Wound healing and nutrition – a review. *J Aust Coll Nutr Environ Med*, 14(2), 15.

Hamilton-Miller, J.M.T., Shah, S. & Smith, C. (1993) Silver sulphadiazine: a comprehensive in vitro reassessment. *Chemotherapy*, 39, 405–9.

Hampton, S. (1998) Film subjects win the day. *Nurs Times*, 94(24), 80–2.

Hampton, S. (1999a) Choosing the right dressing. In: *Wound Management: Theory and Practice* (eds M. Miller & D. Glover). Nursing Times Books, London.

Hampton, S. (1999b) Wound care: vacuum wrapped. *Nurs Times*, 95(3), 77–8.

Harding, K.G., Morris, H.L. & Patel, G.K. (2002) Healing chronic wounds. *Br Med J*, 324(7330), 160–3.

Harris, A.K., Stopak, D. & Wild, P. (1981) Fibroblast traction as a mechanism for collagen morphogenesis. *Nature*, 290(5803), 249–51.

Hart, J. (1999) Growth factors. In: *Wound Management: Theory and Practice* (eds M. Miller & D. Glover). Nursing Times Books, London.

Hart, J. (2002) Inflammation 1: its role in the healing of acute wounds. *J Wound Care*, 11(6), 205–9.

Henry, M. & Corless, C. (1989) The incidence of varicose veins in Ireland. *Phlebology*, 41, 133–7.

Hilderly, L.J. (2000) Principles of radiotherapy. In: *Cancer Nursing: Principles and Practice*, 5th edn (eds C. Henke Yarbro, M. Hansen Frogge, M. Goodman & S.L. Groenwald). Jones and Bartlett, Boston.

Hinshaw, J. (2000) Larval therapy: a review of clinical human and veterinary studies. *World Wide Wounds*, Online: www.worldwidewounds.com/2000/oct/Janet-Hinshaw/Larval-Therapy-Human-and-Veterinary.html (accessed 20 December 2002).

Hofman, D. (1996) Know how: a guide to wound debridement. *Nurs Times*, 92(32), 22–3.

Hofman, D. (1998) Oedema and the management of leg ulcers. *J Wound Care*, 7(7), 345–8.

Hofman, D. (2000) Quick reference guide 15: management of leg ulcers. *Nurs Stand*, 14(29) (Suppl).

Hofman, D., Wilson, J., Poore, S., Cherry, G. & Ryan, T. (2000) Can Traumacel be used in the treatment of chronic wounds? *J Wound Care*, 9(8), 393–6.

Hollander, D., Schmandra, T. & Windolf, J. (2000) Using an esterified hyaluronan fleece to promote healing in difficult-to-treat wounds. *J Wound Care*, 9(10), 463–6.

Hollinworth, H. (1997) Less pain, more gain. *Nurs Times*, 93(46), 89–91.

Horwich, A. (1992) Radiotherapy update. *Br Med J*, 304, 1554–7.

Hughes, M.A., Yang, Y. & Cherry, G.W. (2002) Effect of Traumacel p on the growth of human dermal fibroblasts *in vitro*. *J Wound Care*, 11(4), 149–54.

Inman, C. & Firth, J. (1998) Pressure sore prevention in the community. *Prof Nurse*, 13(7), 515–20.

Ivetic, O. & Lyne, P.A. (1990) Fungating and ulcerating malignant lesions: a review of the literature. *J Adv Nurs*, 15, 83–8.

James, H. (1998) Classification and grading of pressure sores. *Prof Nurse*, 13(10), 669–72.

Johnson, A. (1988) Natural healing processes: an essential update. *Prof Nurse*, 3, 149–52.

Johnson, A. (1989) Granuflex wafers as a prophylactic pressure sore dressing. *Care Sci Pract*, 7(2), 55–8.

Jones, J. (1998) How to manage skin reactions to radiation therapy. *Nursing (Nurs Aust)*, **December**, Suppl 1–2.

Jones, J.E. & Nelson, E.A. (1998) Compression hosiery in the management of venous leg ulcers. *J Wound Care*, 7(6), 293–6.

Jones, M. (ed.) (1999) Can nurses manage it? In: *Nurse Prescribing: Politics to Practice*. Baillière Tindall, London.

Jones, M. & Thomas, S. (2000) Larval therapy. *Nurs Stand*, 14(20), 47–51.

Jones, V. & Milton, T. (2000a) When and how to use adhesive film dressings. *Nurs Times*, 96(14), NTPlus 3–4.

Jones, V. & Milton, T. (2000b) When and how to use hydrocolloid dressings. *Nurs Times*, 96(4), NTPlus 5–7.

Jones, V. & Milton, T. (2000c) When and how to use hydrogels. *Nurs Times*, 96(23), NTPlus 3–4.

Jull, A.B., Waters, J. & Arroll, B. (2000) Oral pentoxifylline for treatment of venous leg ulcers. *J Tissue Viability*, 10(4), 161.

KCI International (2000) *V.A.C. Recommended Guidelines for Use: Physician and Caregiver Reference Manual*. KCI International, Oxon.

Kelly, N. (2002) Malodorous fungating wounds: a review of current literature. *Prof Nurse*, 17(5), 323–6.

Kiecolt-Glaser, J.K., Marucha, P.T., Malarkey, W.B., Mercado, A.M. & Glaser, R. (1995) Slowing of wound healing by psychological stress. *Lancet*, 346(4), 1194–6.

Kischer, C.W., Shetlar, M.R. & Chvapil, M. (1982) Hypertrophic scars and keloids: a review and new concept concerning their origin. *Scan Microsc*, 4, 1699–713.

Kitchen, A. & Ireland, J. (2001) *Care of the Patient who has Radiotherapy Skin Damage*. London Standing Conference. Online: www.london.nhs.uk/lscn/cancer/index.html (accessed 2 February 2003).

Knight, A. (1990) The skin clinic. *Mod Med*, 35(8), 608.

Knighton, D.R. *et al.* (1981) Regulation of wound healing angiogenesis. Effect of oxygen gradients and inspired oxygen concentration. *Surgery*, 90(2), 262–70.

Korinko, A. & Yurick, A. (1997) Maintaining skin integrity. *Am J Nurs*, **97**(2), 40–4.

Kosiak, M. (1958) Evaluation of pressure as a factor in the production of ischial ulcers. *Arch Phys Med Rehabil*, **40**, 62–9.

Kosiak, M. (1976) A mechanical resting surface: its effect on pressure distribution. *Arch Phys Med Rehabil*, **57**, 481–3.

Krajnik, M. & Zylicz, Z. (1997) Topical morphine for cutaneous cancer pain. *Palliat Med*, **11**(4), 326.

Krishnamoorthy, L., Morris, H.L. & Harding, K.G. (2001a) A dynamic regulator: the role of growth factors in tissue repair. *J Wound Care*, **10**(4), 99–101.

Krishnamoorthy, L., Morris, H.L. & Harding, K.G. (2001b) Specific growth factors and the healing of chronic wounds. *J Wound Care*, **10**(5), 173–8.

Laverty, D., Mallett, J. & Mulholland, J. (1997) Protocols and guidelines for managing wounds. *Prof Nurse*, **13**(2), 79–81.

Lavery, B.A. (1995) Skin care during radiotherapy: a survey of UK practice. *Clin Oncol*, **7**(3), 184–7.

Lawrence, J.C. (1997) Wound irrigation. *J Wound Care*, **6**(1), 23–6.

Le Roux, A.A. (1995) TELER: the concept. *Physiotherapy*, **79**(11), 755–8.

Lees, T.A. & Lambert, D. (1992) Prevalence of lower limb ulceration in an urban health district. *Br J Surg*, **79**, 1032–4.

Lentz, S.S., Barrett, R.J. & Homesley, H.D. (1993) Topical sucralfate in the treatment of vaginal ulceration. *Obstet Gynaecol*, **81**(5), 869–71.

Lewis, B. (1996) Zinc and vitamin C in the aetiology of pressure sores. *J Wound Care*, **5**(10), 483–4.

Liguori, V., Guillemin, C., Pesce, G.F., Mirimanoff, R.O. & Bernier, J. (1997) Double-blind, randomized clinical study comparing hyaluronic acid cream to placebo in patients treated with radiotherapy. *Radiother Oncol*, **42**(2), 155–61.

Lindgren, M., Unosson, M., Krantz, A.-M. & Ek, A. (2002) A risk assessment scale for the prediction of pressure sore development: reliability and validity. *J Adv Nurs*, **38**(2), 190–9.

Lochhead, J.N. (1983) *Care of the Patient in Radiotherapy*. Blackwell Science, Oxford, p. 113.

Loftus, S. (2001) A longitudinal, quality of life study comparing four layer bandaging and superficial venous surgery for the treatment of venous leg ulcers. *J Tissue Viability*, **11**(1), 14–9.

Lotti, T., Rodofili, C., Benci, M. & Menchin, G. (1998) Wound-healing problems associated with cancers. *J Wound Care*, **7**(2), 81–4.

Maher, K.E. (2000) Radiation therapy: toxicities and management. In: *Cancer Nursing: Principles and Practice*, 5th edn (eds C. Henke Yarbro, M. Hansen Frogge, M. Goodman & S.L. Groenwald). Jones and Barlett, Boston.

Mahony, C. (1999) Aids to help district nurses boost patient nutrition and wound care. *Nurs Times*, **95**(32), 49–51.

Maiche, A., Isokangas, O. & Grohn, P. (1994) Skin protection by sucralfate cream during electron beam therapy. *Acta Oncol*, **33**(2), 201–3.

Mak, S.S.S., Molassiotis, A., Wan, W., Lee, I.Y.M. & Chan, E.S.J. (2000) The effects of hydrocolloid dressing and gentian violet on radiation-induced moist desquamation wound healing. *Cancer Nurs*, **23**(3), 220–9.

Mallett, J., Mulholland, J., Laverty, D. *et al.* (1999) An integrated approach to wound management. *Int J Palliat Nurs*, **5**(3), 124–32.

Mani, R. *et al.* (1988) Non-invasive oxygen measurements: have they a role in ulcer investigations? In: *Beyond Occlusion: Wound Care Proceedings. Royal Society of Medicine International Congress and Symposium Series* (ed. T.J. Ryan). Royal Society of Medicine, London.

Margolin, S.G., Breneman, J.C., Denman, D.L., LaChapelle, P., Weckbach, L. & Aron, B.S. (1990) Management of radiation-induced moist skin desquamation using hydrocolloid dressing. *Cancer Nurs*, **13**(2), 71–80.

Martin, E.A. (2002) *Concise Colour Medical Dictionary*. Oxford University Press, Oxford.

Matthews, R.N. (1986) Leg ulcers. *Surgery*, **1**(33), 790–5.

McCulloch, J.M. (1998) The role of physiotherapy in managing patients with wounds. *J Wound Care*, **7**(5), 241–4.

McElligot, E., Quigley, C. & Hanks, G.W. (1992) Tranexamic acid and rectal bleeding. *Lancet*, **337**(8738), 431.

McGregor, F. (1998) *Reusable Non-Adhesive Secondary Dressing System for Difficult to Dress Areas and Delicate Skin*. Guy's and St Thomas' Hospital Trust, London.

McGregor, F. & Baxter, H. (1999) Staying power. *Nurs Times*, **95**(19), 66, 68, 71.

McRorie, E.R. (2000) The assessment and management of leg ulcers in rheumatoid arthritis. *J Wound Care*, **9**(6), 289–92.

Mendez-Eastman, S. (1990) When wounds won't heal. *RN*, **61**(6), 20–3.

Mertz, P.M. *et al.* (1985) Occlusive wound dressings to prevent bacterial invasion and wound infection. *J Am Acad Dermatol*, **12**(4), 662–8.

Messer, M.S. (1989) Wound care. *Crit Care Nurs Q*, **11**(4), 17–27.

Middleton, K. (1990) Sugar pastes in wound management. *Dressings Times*, **3**(2), Online: www.smtl.co.uk/WMPRC/DressingsTimes/vol3.2.txt (accessed 27 June 2000).

Miller, M. (1998a) Moist wound healing: the evidence. *Nurs Times*, **94**(45), 74–6.

Miller, M. (1998b) How do I diagnose and treat wound infection? *Br J Nurs*, **7**(6), 335–8.

Miller, M. & Dyson, M. (1996) *Principles of Wound Care*. Macmillan, London.

Milward, P.A. (1995) Common problems associated with necrotic and sloughy wounds. *Br J Nurs*, **4**(15), 896–900.

Mockridge, J. & Anthony, D. (1999) Nurses' knowledge about pressure sore treatment and healing. *Nurs Stand*, **13**(29), 66–72.

Moffat, C.J. & Dorman, M.C.R. (1995) Recurrence of leg ulcers within a community ulcer service. *J Wound Care*, **4**(2), 57–61.

Molan, P.C. (1999a) The role of honey in the management of wounds. *J Wound Care*, **8**(8), 415–8.

Molan, P.C. (1999b) *The Role of Honey in Wound Care*. Honey New Zealand. Online: www.honeynz.co.nz/publicat.htm (accessed 23 June 2000).

Moody, M. & Grocott, P. (1993) Let us extend our knowledge base. *Prof Nurse*, **8**(9), 586–90.

Moore, P. & Foster, L. (1998a) Acute surgical wound care 1: an overview of treatment. *Br J Nurs*, **7**(18), 1101–6.

Moore, P. & Foster, L. (1998b) Acute surgical wound care 2: the wound healing process. *Br J Nurs*, **7**(19), 1183–7.

Moore, Z. (2002) Compression bandaging: are practitioners achieving the ideal sub-bandage pressures? *J Wound Care*, **11**(7), 265–8.

Morgan, D.A. (2000) *Formulary of Wound Management Products: A Guide for Healthcare Staff*, 8th edn. Euromed Communications, Haslemere.

Morgan, D.A. (2002) *Formulary of Wound Management Products: A Guide for Healthcare Staff*, 8th edn (Internet Update). Euromed Communications. Online: www.euromed.uk.com/formulary6update.htm (accessed 20 December 2002).

Morison, M. & Moffatt, C. (1999) Leg ulcers. In: *A Colour Guide to the Nursing Management of Chronic Wounds* (eds M. Morison, C. Moffatt, J. Bridel-Nixon & S. Bale). Mosby, London.

Morison, M.J. (1989) Wound cleansing – which solution? *Prof Nurse*, 4, 220–5.

Morykwas, M.J., Argenta, L.C., Shelton-Brown, E.I. & McGuirt, W. (1997) Vacuum-assisted closure: a new method for wound control and treatment: animal studies and basic foundation. *Ann Plast Surg*, 38(6), 553–62.

Moss, A. (1989) Treatment of terminal breast cancer. *Br Med J*, 298, 10.

Munro, K.J.G. (1995a) Hypertrophic and keloid scars. *J Wound Care*, 4(3), 143–8.

Munro, K.J.G. (1995b) Treatment of hypertrophic and keloid scars. *J Wound Care*, 4(5), 243–5.

Murphy, A. (1995) Cleansing solution. *Nurs Times*, 91(30), 79.

Naylor, W. (2001) Assessment and management of pain in fungating wounds. *Br J Nurs*, 10(22) (Suppl), S33–56.

Naylor, W. (2002) Malignant wounds: aetiology and principles of management. *Nurs Stand*, 16(52), 45–53.

Naylor, W. & Mallett, J. (2001) Management of acute radiotherapy induced skin reactions: a literature review. *Eur J Oncol Nurs*, 5(4), 221–33.

Naylor, W., Laverty, D. & Mallett, J. (2001) *The Royal Marsden Hospital Handbook of Wound Management in Cancer Care*. Blackwell Science, Oxford.

Nelson, E.A. (1998) The evidence in support of compression bandaging. *J Wound Care*, 7(3), 148–50.

Nelzen, O., Bergqvist, D. & Lindhagen, A. (1996) The prevalence of chronic lower-limb ulceration has been underestimated: results of a validated population questionnaire. *Br J Surg*, 83(2), 255–8.

Newman, V. *et al.* (1989) The use of metronidazole gel to control the smell of malodorous lesions. *Palliat Med*, 3, 303–5.

NICE (2001) *Pressure Ulcer Risk: Assessment and Prevention*. National Institute for Clinical Excellence, London. Online: www.nice.org.uk/Docref.asp?d=16477

NMC (2002) *Code of Professional Conduct*. Nursing and Midwifery Council, London.

Noble-Adams, R. (1999) Radiation-induced skin reactions 2: development of a measurement tool. *Br J Nurs*, 8(18), 1208–11.

Norton, D. *et al.* (1985) *An Investigation of Geriatric Nursing Problems in Hospital*. Churchill Livingstone, Edinburgh.

Olde Damink, S.W.M. & Soeters, P.B. (1997) Nutrition and wound healing. *Nurs Times*, 93(30), (insert 1–6).

O'Toole, E.A., Marinkovich, M.P., Peavey, C.L. *et al.* (1997) Hypoxia increases human keratinocyte motility on connective tissue. *J Clin Invest*, 100(11), 2881–91.

Perkins, P. (1989) A clinic to cope with leg ulcers. *Mims Mag*, April, 73–4.

Phillips, T.J., Al-Amoudi, H.O., Leverkus, M. & Park, H.Y. (1998) Effect of chronic wound fluid on fibroblasts. *J Wound Care*, 7(10), 527–32.

Pickering, D. & Warland, S. (1992) The management of desquamative radiation skin reactions. *Dressing Times*, 5(1), Online: www.smtl.co.uk/WMPRC/DressingsTimes/vol5.1.txt (accessed 7 March 2000).

Pickworth, J.J. & De Sousa, N. (1988) Differential wound angiogenesis: quantitation by immunohistological staining for factor Vlll-related antigen. In: *Beyond Occlusion: Wound Care Proceedings*. Royal Society of Medicine International Congress and Symposium Series No. 136 (ed. T.J. Ryan). Royal Society of Medicine, London.

Porock, D., Kristjanson, L., Nikoletti, S., Cameron, F. & Pedler, P. (1998) Predicting the severity of radiation skin reactions in women with breast cancer. *Oncol Nurs Forum*, 25(6), 1019–29.

Poston, J. (1996) Sharp debridement of devitalised tissue: the nurse's role. *Br J Nurs*, 5(11), 655–62.

Pouliot, R., Larouche, D., Auger, F.A. *et al.* (2002) Reconstructed human skin produced in vitro and grafted on athymic mice. *Transplantation*, 73(11), 1751–7.

Price, S. & Price, L. (1995) *Aromatherapy for Health Professionals*. Churchill Livingstone, New York.

Pudner, R. (1998) The management of patients with a fungating or malignant wound. *J Commun Nurs*, 12(9), 30–4.

Pudner, R. (2001) Low/non-adherent dressings in wound management. *J Commun Nurs*, 15(8), 12, 15–17.

Pudner, R. (2002) Wound bed preparation. *J Commun Nurs*, 16(5), 35.

Puzey, G. (2001) The use of pressure garments on hypertrophic scars. *J Tissue Viability*, 12(1), 11–15.

Rankin-Box, D. (2001) *The Nurse's Handbook of Complementary Therapies*, 2nd edn. Baillière Tindall, London.

RCN (1998) *Clinical Practice Guidelines: The Management of Patients with Venous Leg Ulcers*. Royal College of Nursing, London.

Regnard, C.F.B. & Mannix, K. (1990) Palliation of gastric carcinoma haemorrhage with sucralfate. *Palliat Med*, 4, 329–30.

Reid, J. & Morison, M. (1994) Towards a consensus classification of pressure sores. *J Wound Care*, 3(3), 157–9.

Reynolds, T.M. (2000) The future of nutrition and wound healing. *J Tissue Viability*, 11(1), 5–13.

Rice, A.M. (1997) An introduction to radiotherapy. *Nurs Stand*, 12(3), 49–54.

Rigter, B., Clendon, H. & Kettle, S. (1994) Dermatology. Skin reactions due to radiotherapy. *New Zealand Pract Nurse*, September, 17–19, 21–2.

Riyat, M.S. & Quinton, D.N. (1997) Tap water as a wound cleansing agent in accident and emergency. *J Accid Emerg*, 14, 165–6.

Robinson, B.J. (2000) The use of a hydrofibre dressing in wound management. *J Wound Care*, 9(1), 32–4.

Robson, M.C. (1996) Exogenous growth factor application effect on human wound healing. *Prog Dermatol*, 30, 1–7.

Robson, M.C. *et al.* (1993) Transforming growth factor beta-2 accelerates healing of venous stasis ulcers in an open-label, placebo-controlled clinical study. *Wound Repair Regen*, 1, 91.

Robson, M.C., Phillips, T.J., Falanga V. *et al.* (2001) Randomised trial of topically applied repifermin (recombinant human keratinocytes growth factor-2) to accelerate wound healing in venous ulcers. *Wound Repair Regen*, 9(5), 347–52.

Rollins, H. (1997) Special focus: tissue viability – nutrition and wound healing. *Nurs Stand*, 11(51), 49–52.

Rolstad, B.S., Borchert, K., Magnan, S. & Scheel, N. (1994) A comparison of an alcohol-based and siloxane-based peri-wound skin protectant. *J Wound Care*, **3**(8), 367–8.

Rosenberg, C.S. (1990) Wound healing in the patient with diabetes mellitus. *Nurs Clin North Am*, **25**(1), 247–61.

Royal Marsden Hospital (1999) *Radiotherapy: Your Questions Answered* (Patient Information Series). Royal Marsden Hospital, London.

Russell, L. (2001) The importance of patients' nutritional status in wound healing. *Br J Nurs* **10**(6), Suppl S44–9.

Russell, S.B., Trupin, K.M., Rodriguez-Eaton, S., Russell, J.D. & Trupin, J.S. (1988) Reduced growth-factor requirement of keloid-derived fibroblasts may account for tumor growth. *Proc Natl Acad Sci USA*, **85**, 587–91.

Rutter, P.M., Carpenter, B., Hill, S.S. & Locke, I.C. (2000) Varidase: the science behind the medicament. *J Wound Care*, **9**(5), 223–6.

Ryan, T.J. (1988) Management of leg ulcers. *Practitioner*, **232**, 1014–21.

Rycroft-Malone, J. (2001) *Clinical Practice Guidelines: Pressure Ulcer Risk Assessment and Prevention*. Royal College of Nursing, London.

Saunders, Y. & Regnard, C. (1989) Management of malignant ulcers: a flow diagram. *Palliat Med*, **3**, 153–5.

Scanlon, E. & Whitfield, N. (2002) Benchmarking pressure ulcers. *Nurs Stand*, **16**(2), 50–60.

Schneider, A.M., Morykwas, M.J. & Argenta, L.C. (1998) A new and reliable method of securing skin grafts to difficult recipient bed. *J Plast Reconstruct Surg*, **102**(4), 1195–8.

Scholl, D. & Langkamp-Henken, B. (2001) Nutrient recommendations for wound healing. *J Intravenous Nurs*, **24**(2), 124–32.

Schoonhoven, L., Defloor, T. & Grypdonck, M.H.F. (2002) Incidence of pressure ulcers due to surgery. *J Clin Nurs*, **11**(4), 479–87.

Schulte, M. (1993) Yoghurt helps to control wound odour. *Oncol Nurs Forum*, **20**(8), 1262.

Scully, C. (1999) In on a limb. *Nurs Times*, **95**(27), 59–60, 62, 65.

Shell, J.A., Stanutz, F. & Grimm, J. (1986) Comparison of moisture vapour permeable (MVP) dressings to conventional dressings for management of radiation skin reactions. *Oncol Nurs Forum*, **13**(1), 11–16.

Shiels, C., Moores, J. & Roe, B. (1999) Pressure sore care. *Nurs Stand*, **14**(6), 41–4.

Silver, I.A. (1994) The physiology of wound healing. *J Wound Care*, **3**(2), 106–9.

Simmons, S. (1999) Hyperbaric therapy. In: *Wound Management: Theory and Practice* (eds M. Miller & D. Glover). Nursing Times Books, London.

Simpson, A., Bowers, K. & Weir-Hughes, D. (1996) *Clinical Care: Pressure Sore Prevention*. Whurr, London.

Sitton, E. (1992a) Early and late radiation-induced skin alterations part I: mechanisms of skin changes. *Oncol Nurs Forum*, **19**(5), 801–7.

Sitton, E. (1992b) Early and late radiation-induced skin alterations part II: nursing care of irradiated skin. *Oncol Nurs Forum*, **19**(6), 907–12.

Sleigh, J.W. & Linter, S.P.K. (1985) Hazards of hydrogen peroxide. *Br Med J (Clin Res)*, **291**(6510), 1706.

Smiell, J.M., Wieman, T.J., Steed, D.L., Perry, B.H., Sampson, A.R. & Schwab, B.H. (1999) Efficacy and safety of becaplermin (recombinant human platelet-derived growth factor-BB) in patients with nonhealing, lower extremity diabetic ulcers: a combined analysis of four randomised studies. *Wound Repair Regen*, **7**(5), 335–46.

Smith, I. (1989) Waterlow/Norton scoring system – a ward view. *Care Sci Pract*, **7**(4), 93–5.

Smith, K.P., Zardiackas, L.D. & Didlake, R.H. (1986) Cortisone, vitamin A, and wound healing: the importance of measuring wound surface area. *J Surg Res*, **40**(2), 120–5.

Souhami, R. & Tobias, J. (1998) *Cancer and Its Management*. Blackwell Science, Oxford.

Sparrow, G., Minton, M., Rubens, R.D., Simmons, N.A. & Aubrey, C. (1980) Metronidazole in smelly tumours. *Lancet*, **i**(8179), 1185.

Stein, C. (1993) Peripheral mechanisms of opioid analgesia. *Anaesth Analg*, **76**, 182–91.

Stein, C. (1995) The control of pain in peripheral tissue by opioids. *N Engl J Med*, **332**(25), 1685–90.

Stone, J. (2001) Ethical and legal issues. In: *The Nurse's Handbook of Complementary Therapies*, 2nd edn (ed. D. Rankin-Box). Baillière Tindall, London.

Struckmann, J.R. (1988) Venous muscle pump function following reconstructive arterial surgery. *Phlebology*, **3**, 169–73.

Strunk, B. & Maher, K. (1993) Collaborative nurse management of multifactorial moist desquamation in a patient undergoing radiotherapy. *J ET Nurs*, **20**(4), 152–7.

Sussman, C. (1998) Wound healing biology and chronic wound healing. In: *Wound Care: A Collaborative Practice Manual for Physical Therapists and Nurses* (eds C. Sussman & B.M. Bate-Jensen). Aspen Publishers, Maryland.

Tejero-Trujeque, R. (2001) How do fibroblasts interact with the extracellular matrix in wound contraction? *J Wound Care*, **10**(6), 237–42.

Thomas, C. & Hess (1998) *Nurse's Clinical Guide: Wound Care*, 2nd edn. Springhouse Corporation, Pennsylvania.

Thomas, L. (1988) Treating leg ulcers. *Nurs Stand*, **2**(18), 22–3.

Thomas, S. (1990) Cost-effective management of leg ulcers. *Commun Outlook, Nurs Times*, **86**(11), 21–2.

Thomas, S. (1992) *Current Practices in the Management of Fungating Lesions and Radiation Damaged Skin*. Surgical Materials Testing Laboratory, Bridgend.

Thomas, S. (1998) Compression bandaging in the treatment of venous leg ulcers *World Wide Wounds*. Online: www.worldwidewounds.com/1997/september/Thomas-Bandaging/bandage-paper.html (accessed 23 July 2002).

Thomas, S. (2000) Alginate dressings in surgery and wound management – part 1. *J Wound Care*, **9**(2), 56–60.

Thomas, S. (2002) *SMTL Dressings Datacard: Promogran*. Surgical Materials Testing Laboratory, Bridgend. Online: dressings.org/Dressings/promogran.html (accessed 25 July 2002).

Thomas, S. & Hay, N. (1991) The antimicrobial properties of 2 metronidazole-mediated dressings used to treat malodorous wounds. *Pharm J*, 2 March, 264–6.

Thomas, S. & Loveless, P. (1992) Observations on the fluid handling properties of alginate dressings. *Pharm J*, **248**, 850–1.

Thomas, S., Fisher, B., Fram, P. & Waring, M. (1998a) Odour absorbing dressings: a comparative laboratory study. *World Wide Wounds*. Online: www.smtl.co.uk/World-Wide-Wounds/1998/march/Odour-Absorbing-Dressings/odour-absorbing-dressings.html (accessed 28 June 2000).

Thomas, S., Vowden, K. & Newton, H. (1998b) Controlling bleeding in fragile fungating wounds. *J Wound Care*, **7**(3), 154.

Thomas, T., Jones, M., Wynn, K. & Fowler, T. (2001) The current status of maggot therapy in wound healing. *Br J Nurs*, **10**(22), (Suppl S5–12).

Thomlinson, R. (1980) Kitchen remedy for necrotic malignant breast ulcers (Letter). *Lancet*, 27 September, 707.

Thomson, P. (1998) The microbiology of wounds. *J Wound Care*, **7**(9), 477–8.

Thorp, J.M. *et al.* (1987) Gross hypernatraemia associated with the use of antiseptic surgical packs. *Anaesthesia*, **42**, 750–3.

Tingle, J. (1997) Pressure sores: counting the legal cost of nursing neglect. *Br J Nurs*, **6**(13), 757–61.

Tong, A. (1999) Back to basics wound care. *Nurs Times Nurs Homes*, **1**(1), 20–3.

Tooke, J.E. *et al.* (1988) Diabetes and wound healing: the skin response to injury, and white cell behaviour in vivo in diabetic patients. In: *Beyond Occlusion: Wound Care Proceedings. Royal Society of Medicine International Congress and Symposium Series* (ed. T.J. Ryan). Royal Society Medicine, London, pp. 71–4.

Topham, J. (2000) Sugar for wounds. *J Tissue Viability*, **10**(3), 86–9.

Torrance, C. (1985) Wound care in accident and emergency. *Nursing*, **2**(42), Suppl, 1–3.

Tortora, G.J. & Grabowski, S.R. (2002) *Principles of Anatomy and Physiology*, 10th edn. John Wiley, New York.

Trevelyan, J. (1996) Looking good. Wigs and camouflage. *Nurs Times*, **92**(39), 44–5.

Trevelyan, J. (1996) Wound cleansing: principles and practice. *Nurs Times*, **92**(16), 46–8.

Turner, T.D. (1983) A practical guide to absorbent dressings. *Nursing*, **12**, Suppl.

Turner, T.D. *et al.* (1986) Advances in wound management symposium proceedings. John Wiley, Cardiff. In: *Blueprint for the Treatment of Leg Ulcers and the Prevention of Recurrence* (1987) (eds G.W. Cherry & T.J. Ryan). Squibb Surgicare, Hounslow.

Twillman, R.K., Long, T.D., Cathers, T.A. & Mueller, D.W. (1999) Treatment of painful skin ulcers with topical opioids. *J Pain Symptom Manage*, **17**(4), 288–92.

Vowden, K. (1995) Common problems in wound care: wound and ulcer measurement. *Br J Nurs*, **4**(13), 775–9.

Vowden, K. (1998) Venous leg ulcers, Part 2: assessment. *Prof Nurse*, **13**(9), 633–8.

Vowden, K.R. & Vowden, P. (1999) Wound debridement, part 2: sharp techniques. *J Wound Care*, **8**(6), 291–4.

Vowden, K. & Vowden, P. (2001) Doppler and the ABPI: how good is our understanding? *J Wound Care*, **10**(6), 197–202.

Vowden, K. & Vowden, P. (2002) Wound bed preparation. *World Wide Wounds*. Online: www.worldwidewounds.com/2002/april/Vowden/Wound-Bed-Preparation.html (accessed 20 December 2002).

Waldorf, H. & Fewkes, J. (1995) Advances in dermatology. *J Wound Heal*, **10**, 77–97.

Wandl, U.B. (1997) GM-CSF in the treatment of skin ulceration in breast cancer. *J Wound Care*, **6**(4), 165–6.

Waterlow, J. (1988) Prevention is cheaper than cure. *Nurs Times*, **84**(25), 69–70.

Waterlow, J. (1991) A policy that protects. *Prof Nurse*, **6**(5), 258–64.

Waterlow, J. (1998) The treatment and use of the Waterlow card. *Nurs Times*, **94**(7), 63–7.

Weinberg, R.A. (1996) How cancer arises. *Sci Am*, **275**(3), 62–70.

Welch, L. (1981) Simple new remedy for the odour of open lesion. *Reg Nurse*, February, 42–3.

Wells, L. (1994) At the front line of care, the importance of nutrition in wound management. *Prof Nurse*, **9**(8), 525–30.

Werner, K.G. (1999) *Guideline for the Outpatient Treatment of Pressure Ulcer*. Compliance Network Physicians/Health Force Initiative, Online: www.cnhfi.org/pressure-ulcer.html (accessed 8 October 1999).

West, P. & Priestly, J. (1994) Money under the mattress. *Health Serv J*, **104**(5398), 20–2.

Westaby, S. (1985) *Wound Care*. Heinemann, London.

White, R. (2001a) Managing exudate. *Nurs Times*, **97**(9), XI–XIII.

White, R. (2001b) Managing exudate. *Nurs Times*, **97**(14), 59–60.

White, R.J. (2000) *The Management of Exuding Wounds*. (Educational Leaflet No. 7(3)). Wound Care Society, Huntingdon.

Wieman, T.J. (1998) Clinical efficacy of becaplermin (rhPDGF-BB) gel. *Am J Surg*, **176**(2A) (Suppl), 74–9S.

Wilkinson, B. (1997) Hard graft. *Nurs Times*, **93**(16), 63–4, 66 & 68.

Wilks, L., White, K., Smeal, T. & Beale, B. (2001) Malignant wound management: what dressings do nurses use? *J Wound Care*, **10**(3), 65–70.

Williams, C. (1996) Product focus. Cica-care: adhesive gel sheet. *Br J Nurs*, **5**(14), 875–6.

Williams, C. (1998) 3M Cavilon no sting barrier film in the protection of vulnerable skin. *Br J Nurs*, **7**(10), 613–15.

Williams, C. (1999a) Superskin: a polymer adhesive skin sealant. *Nurs Residential Care*, **1**(1), 56–7.

Williams, C. (1999b) Product focus: an investigation of the benefits of Aquacel Hydrofibre wound dressing. *Br J Nurs*, **8**(10), 676–80.

Williams, C. & Young, T. (1998) *Myth and Reality in Wound Care*. Mark Allen, Dinton.

Williams, L. (2002) Assessing patients' nutritional needs in the wound-healing process. *J Wound Care*, **11**(6), 225–8.

Williamson, D. (1988) Leg ulcers. Taking your time with leg ulcers. *Mims Mag*, 1 May, 105–8.

Winter, G.D. (1972) Epidermal regeneration studied in the domestic pig. In: *Epidermal Wound Healing* (eds H.I. Maibach & D.T. Rovee). Year Book Medical Publishers, Chicago, pp. 71–112.

Young, T. (1997) Wound care: the challenge of managing fungating wounds. *Commun Nurse (Nurse Prescriber)*, **3**(9), 41–4.

Young, T. (1998) Reaping the benefits of foam dressings. *Commun Nurse*, **4**(5), 47–8.

Young, T. & Fowler, A. (1998) Nursing management of skin grafts and donor sites. *Br J Nurs*, **7**(6), 324, 326, 328, 330, 332–4.

Appendix 1: Contributors to previous editions

First Edition edited by
A. Phylip Pritchard
Research Assistant, Department of Nursing Research

Valerie-Anne Walker
Research Assistant, Department of Nursing Research

Second Edition edited by
A. Phylip Pritchard
Assistant to the Director of In-Patient Services/Chief
Nursing Officer

Jill A. David
Director of Nursing Research

Third Edition edited by
A. Phylip Pritchard
Formerly Co-ordinator of European Educational
Initiatives, The Royal Marsden Hospital
and
Executive Secretary, European Oncology Nursing Society

Jane Mallett
Research and Practice Development Co-ordinator

Fourth Edition edited by
Jane Mallett
Research and Practice Development Manager

Christopher Bailey
Macmillan Research Practitioner, Macmillan Practice
Development Unit, Centre for Cancer and Palliative Care
Studies, Institute of Cancer Research

Fifth Edition edited by
Jane Mallett
Research and Practice Development Manager, The Royal
Marsden Hospital

Lisa Dougherty
Clinical Nurse Specialist Intravenous Services, The Royal
Marsden Hospital

Contributors
Caroline Badger, formerly Senior Nurse (Lymphoedema)

Christopher Bailey, Macmillan Research Practitioner,
Institute of Cancer Research

Sophie Baty, Sister (Recovery Theatre)

Chris Berry, formerly Back Care Advisor

Peter Blake, Consultant Clinical Oncologist

Judith Bibbings, formerly Sister (Gastro-intestinal/
Genito-urinary)

Yannette Booth, formerly Lecturer in Cancer Nursing

Derryn Borley, formerly Assistant Director of Nursing
Services

Monica Burchall, formerly Sister (High Dependency)

Nancy Burnett, Senior Nurse Manager

Antoinette Byrne, formerly Dietitian

Jill Carter, formerly Clinical Nurse Specialist
(Palliative Care)

Patrick Casey, formerly Clinical Nurse Specialist/Unit
Manager (Gastro-intestinal/Genito-urinary)

Gay Curling, Clinical Nurse Specialist (Breast Diagnostic
Unit)

Lisa Curtis, formerly Macmillan Lecturer, Institute of
Cancer Research

Tonia Dawson, Clinical Nurse Specialist (Pelvic Cancer)

Barbara Dicks, Director of Patient Services/Chief Nursing
Officer

Emma Dilnutt, formerly Clinical Nurse Specialist
(Palliative Care)

Anne Doherty, formerly Staff Nurse
(Operating Theatres)

Nuala Durkin, formerly Clinical Nurse Specialist/Unit
Manager (High Dependency)

Jean Edwards, Senior Nurse Manager/Private Patient
Co-ordinator

Sarah Faithfull, CRC Nursing Fellow, Institute of Cancer
Research

Deborah Fenlon, formerly Group Clinical Nurse Specialist (Breast Care Services)

Jacqueline Green, Senior Dietitian

Rachel Hair, formerly Senior Nurse (Neuro-oncology)

Cathryn Havard, formerly Senior Nurse (Gastro-intestinal/Genito-urinary)

Pauline Hill, Clinical Nurse Specialist (Community Liaison)

Sian Horn, formerly Sister (High Dependency)

Elizabeth Houlton, formerly Senior Nurse (Community Liaison/Self-Care Unit)

Nest Howells, formerly Information Officer, CancerLink

Jennifer Hunt, Director, Nursing Research Initiative for Scotland

Maureen Hunter, Rehabilitation Services Manager

Elizabeth Janes, formerly Dietitian

Penelope A. Jones, formerly Clinical Nurse Specialist (Community Liaison/Palliative Care)

Margareta Johnstone, formerly Clinical Nurse Specialist (High Dependency Unit)

Danny Kelly, formerly Lecturer in Cancer Nursing, Institute of Cancer Research

Annie Leggett, formerly Clinical Nurse Specialist (Intravenous Therapy)

Anne Lister, formerly Clinical Nurse Specialist/Unit Manager (Palliative Care)

Nicholas Lodge, Clinical Group Research Nurse (Gynaecology)

E. Lopez-Verdugo, Senior Technician/Theatre Manager

Jane Mallett, Research and Practice Development Manager

Glynis Markham, formerly Director of Nursing Services

Catherine Miller, formerly Senior Nurse (Continuing Care)

Marion Morgan, formerly Research Sister (Gynaecology)

Katrina Neal, formerly Clinical Nurse Specialist/Unit Manager (Palliative Care)

Helen Jayne Porter, formerly Clinical Nurse Specialist (High Dose Chemotherapy)

Judith Pretty, formerly Clinical Nurse Specialist (Head and Neck)

Frances Rhys-Evans, formerly Clinical Nurse Specialist/Ward Manager (Head & Neck and Thyroid Cancer)

Helen Roberts, formerly Senior Nurse (Head and Neck)

Tim Root, Chief Pharmacist

Ray Rowden, formerly Director of Nursing Services

Miriam Rushton, formerly Senior Nurse (Gynaecology)

Lena Salter, formerly Patient Services Manager

James Smith, formerly Chaplain

Val Speechley, Patient Information Officer

Mavis Stork, formerly Theatre Services Manager

June Toovey, formerly Sister (Intravenous Therapy Team)

Anne Topping, formerly Senior Nurse (Gastro-intestinal/Genito-urinary)

Jennie Treleaven, Consultant Haematologist

Robert Tunmore, formerly Clinical Nurse Specialist (Psychological Support)

Beverley van der Molen, formerly Clinical Nurse Specialist/Unit Manager (General Oncology)

Richard Wells, formerly Rehabilitation Services Manager

Isabel White, Head of Undergraduate Cancer Care Studies

Jane Wilson, formerly Group Theatre Manager

Karen Wright, formerly Research Assistant, Nursing Research Unit

Karen Young, formerly Physiological Measurement Technician

Appendix 2: Patient information booklets

The Royal Marsden publishes a number of booklets and leaflets about cancer and its treatments in the *Patient Information Series* (see below).

After treatment
Breast care – A guide for women
Breast reconstruction
Cancer of the bladder
Cancer of the breast
Cancer of the cervix
Cancer of the large bowel
Cancer of the lung
Cancer of the ovary
Cancer of the prostate
Care of a skin tunnelled catheter (leaflet)
Chemotherapy
Clinical trials
Colostomy – A guide for cancer patients
Coping with nausea and vomiting – A guide for cancer patients
CT scan (leaflet)
Eating well when you have cancer

Feminine care (during and after radiotherapy to the pelvis) – A guide for women with cancer
Going home after a bone marrow or peripheral blood stem cell transplant
Hair care and hair loss – A guide for cancer patients
Hormone replacement therapy – A guide for women with cancer
Laryngectomy
Lymphoedema – A guide for cancer patients
Lymphoedema (a leaflet)
Lymphomas
MR scan (leaflet)
Radioiodine therapy
Radiotherapy
Tamoxifen (leaflet)
Testicular cancer
Testicular self examination (leaflet)
Ultrasound scan (leaflet)
Your operation and anaesthetic

You may also like to visit our website at www.royalmarsden.org.

Index

Notes: Page numbers in italic denote illustrations and tables (where not already given in text references. Pages with "guidelines" *(procedural guidelines)* are given separately only where there are several subheadings.